RADIATION ONCOLOGY

Management Decisions

RADIATION ONCOLOGY

Management Decisions

Fourth Edition

Editors

K. S. Clifford Chao, MD

Professor and Vice President
China Medical University
Taichung, Taiwan

Carlos A. Perez, MD

Professor Emeritus
Department of Radiation Oncology
Siteman Cancer Center
Mallinckrodt Institute of Radiology
Washington University
St. Louis, Missouri

Tony J. C. Wang, MD

Associate Professor of Radiation Oncology (in Neurological Surgery)
Department of Radiation Oncology
Columbia University College of Physicians and Surgeons
New York, New York

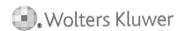

Philadelphia • Baltimore • New York • London
Buenos Aires • Hong Kong • Sydney • Tokyo

Senior Acquisitions Editor: Ryan Shaw
Editorial Coordinator: Kerry McShane
Editorial Assistant: Amy Masgay
Art Director: Jennifer Clements
Marketing Manager: Julie Sikora
Production Project Manager: Linda Van Pelt
Design Coordinator: Elaine Kasmer
Manufacturing Coordinator: Beth Welsh
Prepress Vendor: SPi Global

Fourth Edition

Library of Congress Cataloging-in-Publication Data
Names: Chao, K. S. Clifford, editor. | Perez, Carlos A., 1934- editor. | Wang, Tony J. C., editor.
Title: Radiation oncology : management decisions / editors, K.S. Clifford Chao, Carlos A. Perez, Tony J.C. Wang.
Other titles: Radiation oncology management decisions.
Description: Fourth edition. | Philadelphia : Wolters Kluwer, [2019] | Preceded by Radiation oncology management decisions / [edited by] K.S. Clifford Chao, Carlos A. Perez, Luther W. Brady ; Tim Marinetti, assistant editor. 3rd ed. 2011. | Includes bibliographical references and index.
Identifiers: LCCN 2018022262 | ISBN 9781496391094 (pbk)
Subjects: | MESH: Neoplasms—radiotherapy | Case Management | Neoplasms—diagnosis | Handbooks
Classification: LCC RC271.R3 | NLM QZ 39 | DDC 616.99/40642—dc23 LC record available at https://lccn.loc.gov/2018022262

Sally A. Amundson, ScD
Department of Radiation Oncology
Center for Radiological Research
Columbia University College of Physicians
and Surgeons
New York, New York

Leslie Ballas, MD
Department of Radiation Oncology
Division of Radiation Oncology
The University of Texas
MD Anderson Cancer Center
Houston, Texas

Luther W. Brady, MD
Hylda Cohn/American Cancer Society
Drexel University College of Medicine
Philadelphia, Pennsylvania

Ryan J. Burri, MD
Department of Radiation Oncology
Columbia University College of Physicians
and Surgeons
New York, New York

K.S. Clifford Chao, MD
China Medical University
Taichung, Taiwan

Israel Deutsch, MD
Department of Radiation Oncology
Columbia University College of Physicians
and Surgeons
New York, New York

Mary Katherine Hayes, MD
Department of Radiation Oncology
Weill Cornell Medical College
Department of Radiation Oncology
New York Presbyterian–(Weill Cornell campus)
New York, New York

Leena Mathew, MD
Department of Anesthesiology, Division of
Pain Medicine
Columbia University College of Physicians
and Surgeons
New York, New York

Tim Marinetti, PhD
Department of Radiation Oncology
Columbia University College of Physicians
and Surgeons
New York, New York

Joshua Meyer, MD
Radiation Oncology
Fox Chase Cancer Center
Philadelphia, Pennsylvania

Bhupesh Parashar, MD
Division of Radiation Oncology
Weill Cornell Medical College
New York, New York

Priti Patel, MD
Division of Radiation Oncology
NewYork-Presbyterian Hospital
(Cornell campus)
New York, New York

Carlos A. Perez, MD
Department of Radiation Oncology
Siteman Cancer Center
Mallinckrodt Institute of Radiology
Washington University
St. Louis, Missouri

Amish A. Shah, MD
Department of Radiation Oncology
NewYork-Presbyterian Hospital (Columbia
campus)
New York, New York

Waseet Z. Vance, MD
Department of Radiation Oncology
Joe Arrington Cancer Center
Lubbock, Texas

A. Gabriella Wernicke, MD
Division of Radiation Oncology
Weill Cornell Medical College
New York, New York

Cheng-Shie Wuu, PhD
Department of Radiation Oncology
Columbia University College of Physicians
    and Surgeons
New York, New York

Vishesh Agrawal, MD
Weill Cornell Medicine
New York, New York

Musaddiq Awan, MD
Medical College of Wisconsin
Milwaukee, Wisconsin

Craig D. Blinderman, MD, MA, FAAHPM
NewYork-Presbyterian/Columbia University
    Medical Center
New York, New York

Jonathan J. Chen, MD, PhD
Weill Cornell Medical College
New York City, New York

Christine Chin, MD
NewYork-Presbyterian/Columbia University
    Medical Center
New York, New York

Eileen P. Connolly, MD, PhD
NewYork-Presbyterian/Columbia University
    Medical Center
New York, New York

Neil B. Desai, MD, MHS
University of Texas Southwestern Medical
    Center
Dallas, Texas

Eric D. Donnelly, MD
Northwestern Memorial Hospital
Northwestern University Feinberg School
    of Medicine
Chicago, Illinois

Israel Deutsch, MD
NewYork-Presbyterian/Columbia University
    Medical Center
New York, New York

Michael R. Folkert, MD, PhD
University of Texas Southwestern Medical Center
Dallas, Texas

Naamit Gerber, MD
NYU Langone Health
Department of Radiation
    Oncology
New York, New York

Zahra Ghiassi-Nejad, MD, PhD
Mount Sinai Hospital
New York, New York

Chelain R. Goodman, MD, PhD
Northwestern University Feinberg
    School of Medicine
Chicago, Illinois

Vishal Gupta, MD
Mount Sinai Health System
New York, New York

Tom K. Hei, PhD
NewYork-Presbyterian/Columbia University
    Medical Center
New York, New York

David P. Horowitz, MD
NewYork-Presbyterian/Columbia University
    Medical Center
New York, New York

Mark E. Hwang, MD, PhD
NewYork-Presbyterian/Columbia University
    Medical Center
New York, New York

Anshu K. Jain, MD
Yale School of Medicine
New Haven, Connecticut

Ashish Jani, MD
NewYork-Presbyterian/Columbia University
    Medical Center
New York, New York

Benjamin H. Kann, MD
Yale School of Medicine
New Haven, Connecticut

Jacqueline Kelly, MD, MSc
Yale School of Medicine
New Haven, Connecticut

Atif Jalees Khan, MD
Memorial Sloan Kettering Cancer Center
New York, New York

Percy Lee, MD
University of California, Los Angeles
Los Angeles, California

Baoqing Li, PhD, MD
NewYork-Presbyterian Hospital
New York, New York

Chi Lin, MD, PhD
University of Nebraska Medical Center
Omaha, Nebraska

Lilie Lin, MD
University of Texas MD Anderson Cancer
    Center
Houston, Texas

Joseph A. Miccio, MD
Yale School of Medicine
New Haven, Connecticut

Osama Mohamad, MD, PhD
University of Texas Southwestern Medical
    Center
Simmons Radiation Oncology Center
Dallas, Texas

John Ng, MD
Weill Cornell Medicine
New York, New York

Anurag Saraf, MD
Columbia University
New York, New York

Caitlin A. Schonewolf, MD, MS
University of Pennsylvania
Philadelphia, Pennsylvania

Joshua S. Silverman, MD, PhD
NYU Langone Health
Department of Radiation Oncology
New York, New York

Deborah Smith, BS
NewYork-Presbyterian/Columbia University
    Medical Center
New York, New York

Catherine S. Spina, MD, PhD
NewYork-Presbyterian/Columbia University
    Medical Center
New York, New York

John M. Stahl, MD
Yale School of Medicine
New Haven, Connecticut

Lakshya U. Trivedi, BS
University of Texas Southwestern Medical
    Center
Dallas, Texas

Sriram Venigalla, MD
University of Pennsylvania
Philadelphia, Pennsylvania

Vivek Verma, MD
Allegheny General Hospital
Pittsburgh, Pennsylvania

Jennifer Vogel, MD
Vanderbilt University
Nashville, Tennessee

Horia Vulpe, MD, CM
Department of Radiation Oncology
Columbia University College of Physicians
    and Surgeons
New York, New York

Chenyang Wang, MD, PhD
University of California, Los Angeles
Los Angeles, California

Cheng-Chia (Fred) Wu, MD, PhD
NewYork-Presbyterian/Columbia University
    Medical Center
New York, New York

Shengyang (Peter) Wu, MD
NYU Langone Health
Department of Radiation Oncology
New York, New York

Cheng-Shie Wuu, PhD
Department of Radiation Oncology
Columbia University College of Physicians
    and Surgeons
New York, New York

Eric Xanthopoulos, MD, JD
NewYork-Presbyterian/Columbia University
    Medical Center
New York, New York

Ted K. Yanagihara, MD, PhD
Weill Cornell Medical College
NewYork-Presbyterian Brooklyn
    Methodist Hospital
Brooklyn, New York

Min Yao, MD, PhD
University Hospitals Cleveland
    Medical Center
Case Western Reserve University
Cleveland, Ohio

Elizabeth C. Yoo, MD
Mount Sinai Hospital
New York, New York

Chi Zhang, MD, PhD
Buffett Cancer Center
University of Nebraska Medical Center
Omaha, Nebraska

Andrew Zhang, MD
Rutgers Cancer Institute of New Jersey
New Brunswick, New Jersey

S ince the third edition of *Radiation Oncology Management Decisions (ROMD)*, there have been major advances in the delivery of radiation treatment as well as novel systemic therapy agents including immunotherapy. Image-guided radiotherapy and hypofractionation have been increasingly utilized to achieve tumor control while minimizing burden on patients and their families. Four-dimensional planning taking into account organ motion have been incorporated as well.

This fourth edition is updated to be a bridge for students and radiation oncologists to connect questions arising in the clinic to the comprehensive texts and research journals. We summarize new updates with the AJCC *Cancer Staging Manual*, eighth edition, TNM staging classification for each organ or disease sites. We highlight new treatment paradigms for the management of multiple disease sites with updates on new trials and paradigms shifts. We present updates on dose constraints for stereotactic radiosurgery and hypofractionated radiation doses.

We have updated new figures to highlight treatment planning and advances in our field. We understand that resources may not allow the acquisition of the latest and most expensive technology and have kept classic treatment techniques in place. We welcome your comments and suggestions.

March 23, 2018

Editors
K. S. Clifford Chao
Carlos A. Perez
Tony J. C. Wang

ACKNOWLEDGMENTS

We are grateful to the following contributors to the third edition of *Principles and Practice of Radiation Oncology* for the excellent chapters that formed the basis for the preparation of the original manual:

Sally Amundson, PhD, K. Kian Ang, MD, James J. Augsburger, MD, Hassan I. Aziz, MD, Glenn S. Bauman, MD, Leslie K. Ballas, MD, Steven A. Binnick, MD, Ralph A. Brasacchio, MD, John C. Breneman, MD, Ryan J. Burri, MD, Nicholas J. Cassisi, DDS, MD, J. Donald Chapman, BSc, MSc, PhD, Yuhchyau Chen, MD, PhD, C. Norman Coleman, MD, Louis S. Constine, MD, Jay S. Cooper, MD, Bernard J. Cummings, MB., ChB, Patrick V. De Potter, MD, Venkata Rao Devineni, MD, Sarah S. Donaldson, MD, Robert E. Drzymala, PhD, Michael F. Dzeda, MD, Bahman Emami, MD, Gary A. Ezzell, PhD, Luis F. Fajardo L-G, MD, Scot A. Fisher, DO, Peter J. Fitzpatrick, MB, BS, Jorge E. Freire, MD, Delia M. Garcia, MD, Melahat Garipagaoglu, MD, John R. Glassburn, MD, Mary K. Gospodarowicz, MD, Mary V. Graham, MD, Thomas W. Griffin, MD, Perry W. Grigsby, MD, MBA, Patrizia Guerrieri, MD, Leonard L. Gunderson, MD, Mary Katherine Hayes, MD, Becki Sue Hill, MD, MPA, Richard T. Hoppe, MD, Stephen Horowitz, MD, Nora A. Janjan, MD, A. Robert Kagan, MD, Ulf L. Karlsson, MD, Eric E. Klein, MS, Morton M. Kligerman, MD, Larry E. Kun, MD, John E. Lahaniatis, MD, David A. Larson, MD, PhD, Theodore S. Lawrence, MD, PhD, Henry K. Lee, MD, Seymour H. Levitt, MD, Hsiu-san Lin, MD, PhD, Kenneth H. Luk, MD, Tim Marinetti, PhD, Alvaro A. Martinez, MD Leena Mathew, MBBS, MD, William H. McBride, DSc, PhD, Ann E. MDnald, MN, Cornelius J. McGinn, MD, William M. Mendenhall, MD, Joshua E. Meyer, MD, Bizhan Micaily, MD, Jeff M. Michalski, MD, Rodney R. Million, MD, Curtis T. Miyamoto, MD, Paolo Montemaggi, MD, Eduardo Moros, PhD, Robert J. Myerson, MD, PhD, Colin G. Orton, PhD, Diana M. Ostapovicz, MD, Thomas F. Pajak, PhD, Bhupesh Parashar, MD, James T. Parsons, MD, Priti Patel, MD, Lester J. Peters, MD, Mark H. Phillips, PhD, William E. Powers, MD, James A. Purdy, PhD, Vaneerat Ratanatharathorn, MD, Keith M. Rich, MD, Tyvin A. Rich, MD, Joseph L. Roti Roti, PhD, Marvin Rotman, MD, Philip Rubin, MD, William Serber, MD, Amish A. Shah, MD, Carol L. Shields, MD, Jerry A. Shields, MD, Joseph R. Simpson, MD, PhD, Stephen R. Smalley, MD, Penny K. Sneed, MD, Merrill J. Solan, MD, J. Glershon Spector, MD, Burton L. Speiser, MD, Judith Anne Stitt, MD, Scott P. Stringer, MD, Marie E. Taylor, MD, Joel E. Tepper, MD, Howard D. Thames, PhD, Gillian M. Thomas, MD, Patrick R. M. Thomas, MB, BS, Waseet Z. Vance, MD, Eric C. Vonderheid, MD, William M. Wara, MD, Todd H. Wasserman, MD, A. Gabriella Wernicke, MD, Christopher G. Willett, MD,

Jacqueline P. Williams, PhD, Stephen D. Williams, MD, Jeffrey F. Williamson, PhD, H. Rodney Withers, MD, DSc, Robert A. Zlotecki, MD, PhD

K. S. Clifford Chao, MD
Carlos A. Perez, MD
Tony J. C. Wang, MD

CONTENTS

CHAPTER 1

FUNDAMENTALS OF PATIENT MANAGEMENT

MANAGEMENT OF THE PATIENT WITH CANCER

- The optimal care of patients with malignant tumors is a multidisciplinary effort that combines the classic modalities of surgery, radiation therapy, and chemotherapy.
- The role of the radiation oncologist is to assess all conditions relative to the patient and tumor, systematically review the need for diagnostic and staging procedures, and, in consultation with a multidisciplinary team, determine the best therapeutic strategy.
- Radiation oncology is the clinical and scientific discipline devoted to the use of ionizing radiation in the management of patients with cancer (and other diseases), the investigation of the biologic and physical basis of radiation therapy, and the training of professionals in the field.
- The aim of radiation therapy is to deliver a precisely measured dose of radiation to a defined tumor volume with minimal damage to surrounding healthy tissue.

PROCESS OF RADIATION THERAPY

The goal of therapy should be defined at the onset of therapeutic intervention:
- *Curative*: There is a probability of long-term survival after adequate therapy; some side effects of therapy, although undesirable, may be acceptable.
- *Palliative*: There is little hope of survival for extended periods. Symptoms producing discomfort or an impending condition that may impair comfort or self-sufficiency require treatment. Relatively high doses of irradiation (sometimes 75% to 80% of curative dose) are required to control the tumor for the survival period of the patient.

BASIS FOR PRESCRIPTION OF IRRADIATION

- Evaluation of tumor extent (staging), including diagnostic studies.
- Knowledge of pathologic characteristics of the disease.

- Definition of the goal of therapy (cure or palliation).
- Selection of appropriate treatment modalities (irradiation alone or combined with surgery, chemotherapy, or both).
- Determination of optimal dose of irradiation and volume to be treated, according to anatomic location, histologic type, stage, potential regional nodal involvement (and other tumor characteristics), and normal structures in the region.
- Evaluation of patient's general condition, plus periodic assessment of tolerance to treatment, tumor response, and status of normal tissues treated.
- The radiation oncologist must work closely with physics, treatment planning, and dosimetry staffs to ensure greatest accuracy, practicality, and cost-benefit in the design of treatment plans.
- The ultimate responsibility for treatment decisions, technical execution of therapy, and consequences of therapy always rests with the radiation oncologist.

RADIATION TREATMENT PLANNING

- Different radiation doses are required for given probabilities of tumor control, depending on the tumor type, the initial number of clonogenic cells present, the extent of disease to be treated (1), and the inclusion or exclusion of additional therapeutic modalities (e.g., surgery and/or chemotherapy) in the overall treatment plan.
- International Commission on Radiation Units and Measurements Report Nos. 50 and 62 define the following treatment planning volumes (2,3):
  - *Gross tumor volume (GTV)*: All known gross disease, including abnormally enlarged regional lymph nodes. To determine GTV, appropriate computed tomography (CT) window and level settings that give the maximum dimension of what is considered potential gross disease should be used.
  - *Clinical target volume (CTV)*: Encompasses GTV plus regions potentially harboring microscopic disease.
  - *Planning target volume (PTV)*: Provides margin around CTV to allow for internal target motion, other anatomic motion during treatment (e.g., respiration), and variations in treatment setup. This does not account for treatment machine beam characteristics.
- Treatment portals must adequately cover all treatment volumes plus a margin to account for beam physical characteristics, such as penumbra (Fig. 1-1).
- Simulation is used to accurately identify target volumes and sensitive structures and to document configuration of portals and target volume to be irradiated.
- Treatment aids (e.g., shielding blocks, molds, masks, immobilization devices, compensators) are extremely important in treatment planning and delivery for optimal dose distribution. Repositioning and immobilization devices are critical because effective irradiation is that which accurately hits the clonogenic tumor cells.
- Simpler treatment techniques that yield an acceptable dose distribution are sometimes preferred over more costly and complex ones, which may have a greater margin of error in day-to-day treatment.

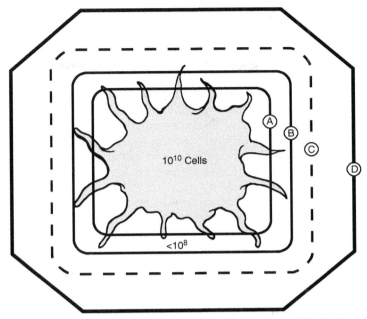

FIGURE 1-1. Schematic representation of "volumes" in radiation therapy. The treatment portal volume includes tumor volume, potential areas of local and regional microscopic disease around tumor, and a margin of surrounding normal tissue. *A* shows gross tumor volume, *B* shows CTV, *C* shows planning treatment volume, and *D* shows treatment portal volume. (Adapted with permission from Halperin EC, Wazer DE, Perez CA. The discipline of radiation oncology. In: Halperin EC, Perez CA, Brady LW, eds. *Principles and practice of radiation oncology*, 6th ed. Philadelphia, PA: Lippincott Williams & Wilkins, 2013:2–60. © Wolters Kluwer.)

- Accuracy is periodically assessed with portal (localization) films or on-line (electronic portal) imaging verification devices, which may be two-dimensional (2-D) (e.g., port films) or three-dimensional (3D) (e.g., on-board kV or MV cone-beam CT imaging) based systems. Portal localization errors may be systematic or may occur at random.

Three-Dimensional Treatment Planning

- CT simulation allows more accurate definition of target volume and anatomy of critical normal structures, 3D treatment planning to optimize dose distribution, and radiographic verification of volume treated (4,5).
- Advances in computer technology have augmented accurate and timely computation, display of 3D radiation dose distributions, and dose-volume histograms that yield relevant information for evaluation of tumor extent, definition of target volume, delineation of normal tissues, virtual simulation of therapy, generation of digitally reconstructed radiographs, design of treatment portals and aids, calculation of 3D dose distributions and dose optimization, and critical evaluation of the treatment plan (6).

- Dose-volume histograms are useful in assessing several treatment plan dose distributions and provide a complete summary of the entire 3D dose matrix, showing the amount of target volume or critical structure receiving more than the specified dose. They do not provide spatial dose information and cannot replace other methods of dose display.
- 3D treatment planning systems play an important role in treatment verification. Digitally reconstructed radiographs based on sequential CT slice data generate a simulation film that can be used in portal localization and for comparison with the treatment portal film for verifying treatment geometry.
- Increased sophistication in treatment planning requires parallel precision in patient positioning and immobilization, as well as in portal verification techniques (7). Several real-time, on-line verification systems allow monitoring of the area to be treated during radiation exposure.
- Computer-aided integration of data generated by 3D radiation treatment planning with parameters used on the treatment machine, including gantry and couch position, may decrease localization errors and enhance the precision and efficiency of irradiation.

Intensity-Modulated Radiation Therapy

- Intensity-modulated radiation therapy (IMRT), a relatively newer approach to 3D treatment planning and conformal therapy, optimizes delivery of irradiation to irregularly shaped volumes through complex forward or inverse treatment planning and results in modulated fluence of multiple photon beam profiles.
- Inverse planning starts with an ideal dose distribution and results in, through trial and error or multiple iterations (simulated annealing), the desired beam characteristics (fluence profiles). It produces the best approximation to the ideal dose defined in a 3D array of dose voxels organized in a stack of 2-D arrays.
- Approaches to IMRT include the following:
  - The step-and-shoot method, which employs a linear accelerator and multileaf collimator, that breaks each treatment field into a set of smaller subfields. Each subfield is delivered one at a time in a predefined sequence. After a subfield is treated, the beam is shut off, the multileaf collimator (MLC) leaves are repositioned for the next subfield, and the beam is turned on again.
  - Dynamic computer-controlled IMRT is delivered when the configuration of the portals with the MLC changes at the same time that the gantry or accelerator changes positions around the patient.
  - In helical tomotherapy, a photon fan beam continually rotates around the patient, as the couch transports the patient longitudinally through a ring gantry (8). The ring gantry enables verification processes for helical tomotherapy; the geometry of a CT scanner allows tomographic processes to be reliably performed. Dose reconstruction is a key process of tomography; the treatment detector sinogram computes the actual dose deposited in the patient. The lengths of the MLC in helical tomotherapy are temporally modulated or binary because they are rapidly driven either in or out by air system actuators rather than by beams slowly pushed by motors driving lead screws, as in the conventional MLC.

- The robotic arm of the IMRT system CyberKnife (Accuray, Sunnyvale, CA) consists of a miniaturized 6-MV photon linear accelerator mounted on a highly mobile arm and a set of ceiling-mounted x-ray cameras to provide near real-time information on patient position and target exposure during treatment.
- The majority of IMRT systems use 6-MV x-rays, but energies of 8 to 18 MV may be more desirable in some anatomic sites to decrease skin and superficial subcutaneous tissue dose.

PROBABILITY OF TUMOR CONTROL

- Various levels of irradiation yield different probabilities of tumor control, depending on the histology and number of clonogenic cells present. Numerous dose-response curves for a variety of tumors have been published with higher doses of irradiation, producing better tumor control.
- For every increment of irradiation dose, a certain fraction of cells will be killed; the total number of surviving cells is proportional to the initial number present and the fraction killed with each dose (9).
- For subclinical disease (deposit of tumor cells too small to be detected clinically or even microscopically), doses of 45 to 50 Gy will result in disease control in more than 90% of patients (10).
- Microscopic tumor, such as at the surgical margin, is not subclinical disease; cell aggregates 10^6 per cm^3 or greater are required for the pathologist to detect them. These volumes must receive higher doses of irradiation (e.g., 60 to 65 Gy in 6 to 7 weeks) (10).
- For clinically palpable tumors, doses of 65 (for T1 tumors) to 75 to 80 Gy or even higher (for T4 tumors) are required (1.8 to 2.0 Gy per day, five fractions weekly) (10).
- A boost is an additional dose administered through small portals to residual disease; it is given to obtain a similar probability of control as for subclinical aggregates.
- Portals can be progressively reduced in size (i.e., the "shrinking-field" technique) to administer higher doses to the central portion of the tumor, where more clonogenic cells (presumably hypoxic) are present, in contrast to the smaller doses required to eradicate disease in the periphery, where a lower number of better oxygenated tumor cells are assumed to be present.

NORMAL TISSUE EFFECTS

- Ionizing radiation induces various changes in normal tissues, depending on the closely interrelated factors of total dose, fractionation schedule (daily dose and total radiation course time), and volume treated. For many normal tissues, the necessary dose to produce a particular sequela increases as the irradiated volume of the organ decreases.
- Higher tolerance doses (TDs) than initially reported have been observed in some organs, stressing the importance of updating information in light of more precise treatment planning and radiation delivery systems and more accurate evaluation of treatment sequelae (11). Tolerance curves for multiple organs have been developed (12).

- The $TD_{5/5}$ is the dose of radiation that could cause no more than a 5% severe complication rate in a particular organ or organ system within 5 years of treatment.
- An acceptable complication rate for moderate to severe injury is 5% to 15% in most curative clinical situations.
- Less clinically significant sequelae occur in 20% to 25% of patients, depending on irradiation dose and the proximity of organs at risk to the target volume.
- The effects of irradiation are described based on the time in which they are observed: *acute* (first 6 months), *subacute* (second 6 months), or *late*. The gross manifestations depend on the kinetic properties of the cells (e.g., slow or rapid renewal) and the dose given.
- Depending on their cellular architecture, organs are classified by functional subunits in either series (e.g., the spinal cord), in which injury of a segment results in a functional deficit of the distal organ, or parallel (e.g., lung, kidney), in which injury of a segment is compensated by function of unaffected adjacent segments.
- Combining irradiation with surgery or various systemic agents frequently modifies the tolerance of normal tissues to a given dose of irradiation, possibly requiring adjustments in treatment planning and dose prescription.
- Radioprotectors, such as amifostine, improve the tolerance of certain normal tissues to a given dose of irradiation, thereby decreasing the likelihood of potential treatment-related morbidities (e.g., xerostomia in patients irradiated for head and neck cancers or pneumonitis in patients with lung or esophageal cancer).

THERAPEUTIC RATIO (GAIN)

- An optimal irradiation dose will produce maximal probability of tumor control with minimal frequency of complications (sequelae of therapy).
- The more the curves of tumor control probability and complication probability diverge, the more favorable the therapeutic ratio.

DOSE-TIME FACTORS

- Fractionation of irradiation with prolongation of radiation course spares acute reactions because of compensatory proliferation of the acute responding tissues.
- A prolonged course of therapy decreases early acute reactions but does not protect against serious late damage to normal tissue. In addition, it may allow the growth of rapidly proliferating tumors and may be inconvenient for the patient.
- For tumors with short potential doubling times, overall treatment course times of less than 6 weeks are optimal. More slowly proliferating tumors can be treated with longer overall courses.
- Late damage is dictated predominantly by radiation fraction size (rather than overall radiation course treatment time).

Prolongation of Overall Treatment Time, Tumor Control, and Morbidity

- The total irradiation dose required to produce a given probability of tumor control must be increased when fractionation is prolonged beyond 4 weeks because of repopulation of surviving cells. Withers et al. (13) estimated that the dose of irradiation is to be increased by 0.6 Gy for every day of interruption of treatment. Taylor et al. (14) estimated the increment, in isoeffect dose per day, to be larger than 1 Gy in squamous cell carcinoma of the head and neck.
- The Radiation Therapy Oncology Group reported no therapeutic advantage in studies of split-course radiation in head and neck, uterine cervix, lung, or urinary bladder tumors; tumor control and survival were comparable with those with conventional fractionation. Late effects were slightly greater in the split-course groups. Single institution reports suggest that tumor control may be compromised by split-course regimens (15,16).

Linear-Quadratic Equation (α/β Ratio)

- Formulations of dose-survival models have been proposed to evaluate the biologic equivalence of various doses and fractionation schedules, based on a linear-quadratic survival curve:

$$\text{Log}_e\ S = \alpha D + \beta D^2$$

  in which α represents the linear (first-order dose-dependent) component of cell killing, and β represents the quadratic (second-order dose-dependent) component of cell killing. β represents the more reparable (over a few hours) component of cell damage. The dose at which the two components of cell killing are equal is the α/β ratio.
- The shape of the dose-survival curve with photons differs for acutely and slowly responding normal tissues.
- Acutely reacting tissues have a high α/β ratio (between 8 and 15 Gy), whereas tissues involved in late effects have a low α/β ratio (1 to 5 Gy). Values obtained in animal experiments and clinical studies have been summarized (17) (see Table 5-2).
- A biologically equivalent dose (BED) can be obtained using this formula:

$$\text{BED} = nd[1 + d/(\alpha/\beta)]$$

  in which n = number of fractions and d = dose per fraction (fractionation).
- If one wishes to compare the two treatment regimens (with some reservations), the following formula can be used:

$$n_1 d_1 [1 + d_1/(\alpha/\beta)] :: n_2 d_2 [1 + d_2/(\alpha/\beta)]$$

  in which $n_1 d_1$ = known total dose (reference dose), $n_2 d_2$ = new total dose (with different fractionation schedule), d_1 = known fractionation (reference), and d_2 = new fractionation schedule.

COMBINATION OF THERAPEUTIC MODALITIES

Preoperative Radiation Therapy

- *Rationale*: Preoperative radiation therapy potentially eradicates subclinical or microscopic disease beyond the margins of surgical resection, diminishes tumor implantation by decreasing the number of viable cells within the operative field, sterilizes lymph node metastases outside the operative field, decreases potential for dissemination of clonogenic tumor cells that might produce distant metastases, and increases the possibility of resectability.
- *Disadvantage*: Preoperative radiation therapy may interfere with normal healing of tissues affected by radiation.

Postoperative Irradiation

- *Rationale*: Postoperative irradiation may eliminate residual tumor in the operative field by destroying subclinical foci of tumor cells after surgery. This is achieved through the eradication of adjacent subclinical foci of cancer (including lymph node metastases) and the delivery of higher doses than with preoperative irradiation; a greater dose is directed to the volume of high-risk or known residual disease.
- *Disadvantages*: Delay in initiation of irradiation until wound healing is completed, and vascular changes produced in tumor bed by surgery may impair radiation effect.

Irradiation and Chemotherapy

- *Enhancement* is any increase in effect on tumor or normal tissues greater than that observed with either modality alone.
- Calculation of the presence of additivity, supra-additivity, or subadditivity is simple when dose-response curves for irradiation and chemotherapy are linear.
- Chemotherapeutic agents should be non–cross-resistant.
- *Primary chemotherapy* is used as part of definitive treatment of the primary lesion (even if followed later by other local therapy).
- *Adjuvant chemotherapy* is used as an adjunct to other local modalities as part of initial curative treatment.
- *Neoadjuvant chemotherapy* is used in initial treatment of patients with localized tumors before surgery or irradiation.
- Use of chemotherapy before irradiation produces some cell killing and reduces the number of cells to be eliminated by the irradiation. Accelerated repopulation of surviving clonogenic tumor cells may decrease therapeutic effectiveness (13).
- Use of chemotherapy during radiation therapy may interact with local treatment (additive or even supra-additive action) and affect distant subclinical disease (18).

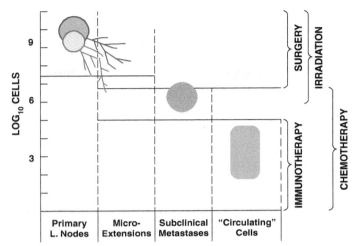

FIGURE 1-2. Use of different treatment modalities to eliminate a given tumor cell burden. Large primary tumors or metastatic lymph nodes must be removed surgically or treated by radiation therapy. Regional microextensions are effectively eliminated by irradiation, and chemotherapy is applied mainly for subclinical disease, although it also has an effect on some larger tumors. (Adapted with permission from Perez CA, Marks JE, Powers WE. Preoperative irradiation in head and neck cancer. *Semin Oncol* 1977; 4:387–397. © Elsevier, 1977.)

Integrated Multimodality Cancer Management

- Combinations of two or even all three modalities are frequently used to improve tumor control and patient survival. Steel (19) postulated the biologic basis of cancer therapy as (a) spatial cooperation, in which an agent is active against tumor cells spatially missed by another agent; (b) antitumor effects by two or more agents; and (c) nonoverlapping toxicity and protection of normal tissues.
- Figure 1-2 illustrates the selective use of a therapeutic modality to achieve tumor control in each compartment: Large primary tumors or metastatic lymph nodes are treated with surgery or definitive radiation therapy; regional microextensions are treated with irradiation, without the anatomic, and at times physiologic deficit produced by equivalent radical surgery; and disseminated subclinical disease is treated with chemotherapy (this modality also has local effect on some macroscopic tumors).
- Organ preservation is vigorously promoted, as it enhances quality of life, improves survival, and provides excellent tumor control, as demonstrated in many tumors.

QUALITY ASSURANCE

- A comprehensive quality assurance (QA) program is critical to ensure the best treatment for each patient and to establish and document all operating policies and procedures.

- QA procedures in radiation therapy vary, depending on whether standard treatment or a clinical trial is carried out, and at single or multiple institutions. In multi-institutional studies, it is important to provide all participants with clear instructions and standardized parameters in dosimetry procedures, treatment techniques, and treatment.
- Reports of the Patterns of Care Study demonstrate a definite correlation between quality of radiation therapy delivered at various types of institutions and outcome of therapy (10).

Quality Assurance Committee

- The director of the department appoints the committee, which meets regularly to review results of the review and audit process, physics QA program report, outcome studies, mortality and morbidity conference, cases of "misadministration" or error in delivery of greater than 10% of intended dose, and any chart in which an incident report is filed.

PSYCHOLOGICAL, EMOTIONAL, AND SOMATIC SUPPORT FOR THE RADIATION THERAPY PATIENT

- Patients who have cancer are often bewildered by the diagnosis, frightened by an unknown environment, concerned with prognosis, and fearful of the procedures they must undergo. It is extremely important for the radiation oncologist and staff (e.g., nurse, social worker, radiation therapist, and receptionist) to be empathetic and to spend time with the patient discussing the nature of the tumor, the prognosis, the procedures to be performed, and possible side effects of therapy.
- The radiation oncologist should discuss details of treatment with relatives (particularly of elderly and pediatric patients) as indicated, provided that this is acceptable to the patient.
- Continued surveillance and support of the patient during therapy are mandatory, with at least one weekly evaluation by the radiation oncologist to assess the effects of treatment and side effects of therapy. Psychological and emotional reinforcement, medications, dietetic counseling, and oral cavity and skin care instructions are integral in the management of these patients.

QUALITY-OF-LIFE STUDIES

- Health-related quality of life is increasingly used as an outcome parameter in clinical trials, effectiveness research, and quality-of-care assessment.
- Radiation oncologists must play a proactive role in improving tumor control and survival, decreasing morbidity, and identifying risk factors that may affect health status and quality of life.

ETHICAL CONSIDERATIONS

- The radiation oncology staff must acknowledge patient's rights and responsibilities that directly influence quality of care and are conducive to establishing the most desirable relationship between patient and staff.
- The patient has the following rights:
  1. *The right to be treated as a human being,* with respect and consideration, regardless of race, sex, creed, or national origin.
  2. *The right to feel secure with the health care program.* The patient must be able to obtain complete, current information concerning individual diagnosis, treatment, and prognosis in understandable terms.
  3. *The right to privacy.* Discussion of the patient's condition is confidential, as are any consultations, examinations, or treatment records. Permission in writing is necessary, except as otherwise provided by law, before any information is released.
  4. *The right to service.* All patients have the right to expect that their requests for services will be fulfilled, within reasonable limits.
  5. *The right to understand the cost of their treatment.* If financial problems arise, suitable arrangements can be made for payment.
  6. *The right to be advised of education or research activities.* Patients should know the identity and professional status of persons directly involved in their care and know which physicians are primarily responsible for their care. In teaching institutions, student, intern, or resident involvement in patient care should be explained to the patient. Patients will be advised if their participation as a subject in research activity is desired, but they have the right to refuse participation. The investigational review board's approval of the protocol and signed investigational consent forms are mandatory.
  7. *The right to counseling on consequences of refusal of treatment.* Patients refusing treatment must clearly have the potential consequences of such refusal of treatment explained to them.

PROFESSIONAL LIABILITY AND RISK MANAGEMENT

- It is important for the radiation oncologist and staff to make every effort to decrease professional liability risks.
- Effective practices include good rapport with patients and relatives, effective communication, QA programs in all activities related to patient management, and clear and accurate records that include documentation of all procedures, discussions, and events that take place before, during, and after treatment.
- The histologic diagnosis must be confirmed at the treating institution, including review of outside pathologic slides.
- All procedures performed should be recorded in the chart, including details of daily treatments, such as the use of special treatment aids (e.g., wedges, immobilization devices) and problems related to equipment operation.

- All treatment parameters and calculations should be accurately recorded and verified by a physicist or dosimetrist, in addition to the radiation oncologist.

Informed Consent

- The need to obtain informed consent for treatment is based on the patient's right to self-determination and the fiduciary relationship between the patient and physician (20).
- The law requires that the treating physician adequately apprise every patient of the nature of the disease, recommended course of therapy and its details, treatment options, benefits of recommended treatment, and all minor and major risks (acute and late effects) associated with the recommended therapy.
- If the plan of therapy is modified, it should be discussed carefully with the patient; if warranted, a second informed consent may be required.
- It is advisable to discuss the informed consent contents in the presence of a witness and have that person sign the informed consent form (or the chart) to verify that the information was discussed with the patient.
- The competent adult patient or a legal representative must agree to the treatment and give approval. For minors or legally incompetent adults, informed consent must be signed by parents, adult brothers or sisters, or a responsible near relative or legal guardian. In some states, spouses may be allowed to provide informed consent for incompetent adults. Emancipated minors may provide their own consent.
- Table 1-1 describes sequelae to be included in the informed consent.

Table 1-1		
Possible Specific Sequelae of Therapy Discussed in Informed Consent		
Anatomic Site	Acute Sequelae	Late Sequelae
Brain	Earache, headache, dizziness, hair loss, erythema	Hearing loss Damage to middle or inner ear Pituitary gland dysfunction Cataract formation Brain necrosis
Head and neck	Odynophagia, dysphagia, hoarseness, xerostomia, dysgeusia, weight loss	Subcutaneous fibrosis, skin ulceration, necrosis Thyroid dysfunction Persistent hoarseness, dysphonia, xerostomia, dysgeusia Cartilage necrosis Osteoradionecrosis of mandible Delayed wound healing, fistulae Dental decay Damage to middle and inner ear Apical pulmonary fibrosis Rare: myelopathy

Table 1-1

Possible Specific Sequelae of Therapy Discussed in Informed Consent *(continued)*

Anatomic Site	Acute Sequelae	Late Sequelae
Lung and mediastinum or esophagus	Odynophagia, dysphagia, hoarseness, cough Pneumonitis Carditis	Progressive fibrosis of lung, dyspnea, chronic cough Esophageal stricture Rare: chronic pericarditis, myelopathy
Breast or chest wall	Odynophagia, dysphagia, hoarseness, cough Pneumonitis (asymptomatic) Carditis Cytopenia	Fibrosis, retraction of breast Lung fibrosis Arm edema Chronic endocarditis, myocardial infarction Rare: osteonecrosis of ribs
Abdomen or pelvis	Nausea, vomiting Abdominal pain, diarrhea Urinary frequency, dysuria, nocturia Cytopenia	Proctitis, sigmoiditis Rectal or sigmoid stricture Colonic perforation or obstruction Contracted bladder, urinary incontinence, hematuria (chronic cystitis) Vesicovaginal fistula Rectovaginal fistula Leg edema Scrotal edema, sexual impotency Vaginal retraction or scarring Sterilization Sexual impotence Damage to liver or kidneys
Extremities	Erythema, dry/moist desquamation	Subcutaneous fibrosis Ankylosis, edema Bone/soft tissue necrosis

Reprinted with permission from Halperin, EC, Wazer DE, Perez CA. The discipline of radiation oncology. In: Halperin EC, Wazer DE, Perez CA, Brady LW, eds. *Principles and practice of radiation oncology*, 6th ed. Philadelphia, PA: Lippincott Williams & Wilkins, 2013:2 -60. © Wolters Kluwer.

References

1. Brahme A. Optimization of stationary and moving beam radiation therapy techniques. *Radiother Oncol* 1988;12(2):129–140.
2. ICRU. International Commission on Radiation Units and Measurements. Prescribing, recording, and reporting photon beam therapy (supplement to ICRU report 50). ICRU report 62. Bethesda, MD: International Commission on Radiation Units and Measurements, 1999.
3. ICRU. International Commission on Radiation Units and Measurements. Prescribing, recording, and reporting photon beam therapy: ICRU report 50. Bethesda, MD: International Commission of Radiation Units and Measurements, 1993.
4. Perez CA, Michalski JM, Purdy JA, et al. Three-dimensional conformal radiation therapy (3-D CRT) in localized carcinoma of prostate. In: Meyer JM, ed. *Frontiers of radiation therapy and oncology*. Basel, Switzerland: Karger, 1996.

5. Purdy JA, Emami B, Graham ML, et al. Three-dimensional treatment planning and conformal therapy. In: Levitt S, Kahn F, Potish R, et al., eds. *Levitt and Tapley's technological basis of radiation therapy: clinical applications*, 3rd ed. Baltimore, MD: Williams & Wilkins, 1999:104–127.

6. Webb S. *The physics of three-dimensional radiation therapy: conformal radiotherapy, radiosurgery and treatment planning*. Bristol, UK: Institute of Physics Publishing, 1993.

7. Suit HD, Becht J, Leong J, et al. Potential for improvement in radiation therapy. *Int J Radiat Oncol Biol Phys* 1988;14(4):777–786.

8. Mackie TR, Balog J, Ruchala K, et al. Tomotherapy. *Semin Radiat Oncol* 1999;9(1):108–117.

9. Fletcher GH. *Textbook of radiotherapy*, 3rd ed. Philadelphia, PA: Lea & Febiger, 1980.

10. Halperin EC, Perez CA, Brady LW. The discipline of radiation oncology. In: Halperin EC, Perez CA, Brady LW, eds. *Principles and practice of radiation oncology*, 5th ed. Philadelphia, PA: Lippincott Williams & Wilkins, 2008:2–75.

11. Emami B, Lyman J, Brown A, et al. Tolerance of normal tissue to therapeutic irradiation. *Int J Radiat Oncol Biol Phys* 1991;21(1):109–122.

12. Burman C, Kutcher GJ, Emami B, et al. Fitting of normal tissue tolerance data to an analytic function. *Int J Radiat Oncol Biol Phys* 1991;21(1):123–135.

13. Withers HR, Taylor JM, Maciejewski B. The hazard of accelerated tumor clonogen repopulation during radiotherapy. *Acta Oncol* 1988;27(2):131–146.

14. Taylor JM, Withers HR, Mendenhall WM. Dose-time considerations of head and neck squamous cell carcinomas treated with irradiation. *Radiother Oncol* 1990;17(2):95–102.

15. Parsons JT, Bova FJ, Million RR. A re-evaluation of split-course technique for squamous cell carcinoma of the head and neck. *Int J Radiat Oncol Biol Phys* 1980;6(12):1645–1652.

16. Parsons JT, Thar TL, Bova FJ, et al. An evaluation of split-course irradiation for pelvic malignancies. *Int J Radiat Oncol Biol Phys* 1980;6(2):175–181.

17. Turesson I, Notter G. The influence of fraction size in radiotherapy on the late normal tissue reaction—I: Comparison of the effects of daily and once-a-week fractionation on human skin. *Int J Radiat Oncol Biol Phys* 1984;10(5):593–598.

18. Phillips TL. Biochemical modifiers: drug-radiation interactions. In: Mauch PM, Loeffler JS, eds. *Radiation oncology: technology and biology*. Philadelphia, PA: WB Saunders, 1994:113–151.

19. Steel GC. The combination of radiotherapy and chemotherapy. In: Steel GC, Adams GE, Peckham MJ, eds. *The biological basis of radiotherapy*. Amsterdam, The Netherlands: Elsevier Science, 1983:239–248.

20. Annas GJ. Informed consent, cancer, and truth in prognosis. *N Engl J Med* 1994;330(3):223–225.

CHAPTER 2

BEAM DOSIMETRY, PHYSICS, AND CLINICAL APPLICATIONS

CLINICAL PHOTON BEAM DOSIMETRY

Single-Field Isodose Distributions

- The central-axis percentage depth dose (PDD) expresses the penetrability of a radiation beam.
- Beam characteristics for x-ray and gamma-ray beams typically used in radiation therapy, the depth at which the dose is maximum (100%), and the PDD value at 10 cm depth are summarized in Table 2-1 and Figure 2-1.
- For a 10- × 10-cm field, 18- and 6-MV x-ray beams and cobalt-60 (^{60}Co) beams (1.25 MV average x-ray energy) lose approximately 2.0%, 3.5%, and 4.5% per cm, respectively, beyond the depth of maximum dose (d_{max}).
- Cobalt units exhibit a large penumbra, and their isodose distributions are rounded toward the source as a result of the relatively large source size (typically 1 to 2 cm in diameter). Linear accelerator (linac) isodose distributions have much smaller penumbras and relatively flat isodose curves at depth.

Buildup Region

- The buildup region is very energy dependent (Fig. 2-1).
- If the x-ray beam is incident normal (at 0 degrees) to the surface, maximum skin sparing is achieved.
- Skin dose increases and d_{max} moves toward the surface as the angle of incidence increases. This is because more secondary electrons are ejected along the oblique path of the beam, a phenomenon called tangential effect (1–4).

Tissue Heterogeneities

- Perturbation of photon transport is more noticeable for lower-energy beams.
- For a modest lung thickness of 10 cm, there will be an approximately 15% increase in the dose to the lung for a ^{60}Co or 6-MV x-ray beam (5) but only an approximately 5% increase for an 18-MV x-ray beam (6) (Fig. 2-2).

Table 2-1

Beam Characteristics for Photon Beam Energies of Interest in Radiation Therapy

200 kV(p) (kilovolt [peak]); 2.0 mm Cu half-value layer (HVL); source to skin distance (SSD) = 50 cm
  Depth of maximum dose = surface
  Rapid falloff with depth because of (a) low energy and (b) short SSD
  Sharp beam edge because of small focal spot
  Significant dose outside beam boundaries because of Compton-scattered radiation at low energies
^{60}Co, SSD = 80 cm
  Depth of maximum dose = 0.5 cm
  Increased penetration (10-cm PDD = 55%)
  Beam edge not as well defined—penumbra because of source size
  Dose outside beam low because most scattering is in forward direction
  Isodose curvature increases as the field size increases
4-MV x-ray; SSD = 80 cm
  Depth of maximum dose = 1.0–1.2 cm
  Penetration slightly greater than cobalt (10 cm PDD = 61%)
  Penumbra smaller
  "Horns" (beam intensity off-axis) because of flattening filter design can be significant (14%)
6-MV x-ray; SSD = 100 cm
  Depth of maximum dose = 1.5 cm
  Slightly more penetration than ^{60}Co and 4 MV (10 cm PDD = 67%)
  Small penumbra
  "Horns" (beam intensity off-axis) because of flattening filter design reduced (9%)
18-MV x-ray; SSD = 100 cm
  Depth of maximum dose = 3.0–3.5 cm
  Much greater penetration (10 cm PDD = 80%)
  Small penumbra
  "Horns" (beam intensity off-axis) because of flattening filter design reduced (5%)
  Exit dose often higher than entrance dose

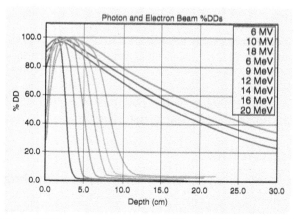

FIGURE 2-1. Central-axis PDD for megavoltage x-rays (^{60}Co to 18 MV—*long-tailed curves to right*) and also electron beams (6 to 20 MeV). (Reprinted with permission from Halperin EC, Perez CA, Brady LW. *Principles and practice of radiation oncology*, 5th ed. Philadelphia, PA: Lippincott Williams & Wilkins, 2008:160. © Wolters Kluwer.)

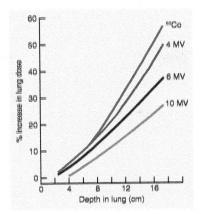

FIGURE 2-2. Percentage increase in lung dose as a function of depth in the lung for selected energies. Field size is 10 × 10 cm. (Reprinted with permission from McDonald SC, Keller BE, Rubin P. Method for calculating dose when lung tissue lies in the treatment field. *Med Phys* 1976;3:210.)

- Measurements performed with a parallel-plate ionization chamber for cobalt showed significant losses of ionization on the central axis following air cavities of varying dimensions. Because of lack of forward-scattered electrons, the losses were approximately 12% for a typical laryngeal air cavity but were recovered within 5 mm in the new buildup region (7).
- Klein et al. (8), using a parallel-plate chamber in both the distal and proximal regions, observed a 10% loss at the interfaces for an air cavity of 2 × 2 × 2 cm for 4- × 4-cm parallel-opposed fields for 4- and 15-MV photons. They also observed losses at the lateral interfaces perpendicular to the beam on the order of 5% for a 4-MV beam.

Prostheses (Steel and Silicon)

- Das et al. (9) measured forward dose perturbation factors following a 10.5-mm-thick stainless steel layer simulating a hip prosthesis geometry. They reported an enhancement of 19% for 24-MV photons but only 3% for 6-MV photons. They also measured backscatter dose perturbation factors for various energies and many high-Z materials, including steel, and observed an enhancement of 30% for steel because of backscattered electrons, independent of the energy, field size, or lateral extent of the steel.
- Klein and Kuske (10) reported on interface perturbations with silicon breast prostheses, which have a density similar to breast tissue but a different atomic number. They observed a 6% enhancement at the proximal interface and a 9% loss at the distal interface.

Wedge Filters

- The term wedge angle refers to the angle through which an isodose curve is tilted at the central ray of a beam at a specified depth.
- For cobalt units, the depth of the 50% isodose line is usually selected for specification of the wedge angle, whereas for higher-energy linacs, higher-percentile isodose curves, such as the 80% curve, or isodose curves at a specific depth (e.g., 10 cm) are used to define the wedge angle. Modern computer-controlled medical linacs have software features that allow the users to create a wedge-shaped dose distribution by moving one collimator jaw across the field with adjustment of the speed and/or dose rate over the course of the daily single-field treatment (11) (i.e., dynamic wedge).
- When a patient's treatment is planned, wedged fields are commonly arranged such that the angle between the beams (the hinge angle, φ) is related to the wedge angle, θ, by the relationship
  $\theta = 90$ degrees $- \varphi/2$.
- As shown in Figure 2-3, 45-degree wedges orthogonal to one another yield a uniform dose distribution.

Parallel-Opposed Fields

- Figure 2-4 shows the normalized relative-axis dose profiles from parallel-opposed photon beams for a 10- × 10-cm field at source to skin distance (SSD) of 100 cm and for patient diameters of 15 to 30 cm in 5-cm increments.
- The maximum patient diameter easily treated with parallel-opposed beams for a mid-plane tumor with low-energy megavoltage beams is approximately 18 cm.
- For thicker patients, higher x-ray energies produce improved dose profiles and reduce hot spots in the entry and exit regions.

FIELD SHAPING

- Cerrobend, probably the most commonly used metal alloy, consists of 13.3% tin, 50.0% bismuth, 26.7% lead, and 10.0% cadmium. The physical density at 20°C is 9.4 g per cm³, compared with 11.3 g per cm³ for lead. The total time required for the block to solidify is typically approximately 45 minutes.
- Doses to critical organs may be limited by using either a full shielding block—usually 5 half-value layer (HVL) (3.125% transmission) or 6 HVL (1.562% transmission)—or a partial transmission block, such as a single HVL (50% transmission) of shielding material.
- The true percentage dose level is generally greater than the percentage stated because of scattered radiation beneath the blocks from adjacent unshielded portions of the field and increases with depth as more radiation scatters into the shielded volume beneath the shield.
- At present, multileaf collimation is increasingly used in lieu of Cerrobend blocking on compatible linacs.

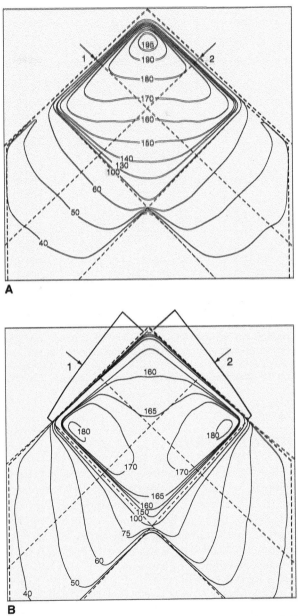

FIGURE 2-3. Isodose distribution for two angle beams. **A:** Without wedges. **B:** With wedges. (4 MV; field size, 10 × 10 cm; SSD, 100 cm; wedge angle, 45 degrees.) (Reprinted with permission from Khan FM. *The physics of radiation therapy*, 4th ed. Baltimore, MD: Williams & Wilkins, 2009:193. © Wolters Kluwer.)

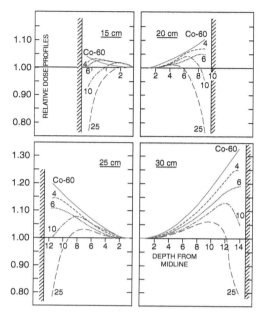

FIGURE 2-4. Relative central-axis dose profiles as a function of x-ray energy (^{60}Co or 4, 6, 10, and 18 MV) and patient thickness (15, 20, 25, and 30 cm). The parallel-opposed beams are equally weighted, and the profiles are normalized to unity at midline. Because of symmetry, only half of each profile is shown. (Reprinted with permission from Purdy JA, Klein EE. Photon external beam dosimetry and treatment planning. In: Halperin, EC, Perez CA, Brady LW, eds. *Principles and practice of radiation oncology*, 5th ed. Philadelphia, PA: Lippincott Williams & Wilkins, 2008:167. © Wolters Kluwer.)

COMPENSATING FILTERS

- A compensating-filter system includes methods for measuring the missing-tissue deficit, demagnifying patient topography, constructing the compensating filter, aligning and holding the filter in the beam, and performing quality control.
- Purdy et al. (12) developed a one-dimensional compensating system designed for individual patient chest curvatures using Lucite plates. The SSD is set to the highest point of the anatomic area (chest) to be irradiated (Fig. 2-5). A sagittal contour of the chest is obtained, and the number of layers of Lucite, each with thickness equivalent to 1 cm of tissue, is obtained as well.
- A practical two-dimensional compensator system is still widely used (13). A rod-box device (a formulator) is used to measure the tissue deficit in a 1-cm grid over the treatment surface. Blocks of aluminum or brass of appropriate thickness are then mounted on a tray above the patient to attenuate the beam by the desired amount. Beam divergence also may be incorporated into this system.

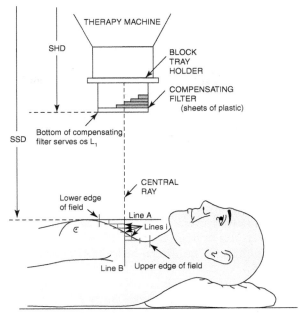

FIGURE 2-5. One-dimensional chest compensating-filter system using sheets of plastic. (Reprinted with permission from Purdy JA, Klein EE. External photon beam dosimetry and treatment planning. In: Perez CA, Brady LW, eds. *Principles and practice of radiation oncology*, 3rd ed. Philadelphia, PA: Lippincott–Raven, 1998:281–320. © Wolters Kluwer.)

BOLUS

- Tissue-equivalent material placed directly on the patient's skin surface to reduce the skin sparing of megavoltage photon beams is referred to as bolus.
- A tissue-equivalent bolus should have electron density, physical density, and atomic number similar to that of tissue or water, and it should be pliable, so that it conforms to the skin surface contour.
- Inexpensive, nearly tissue-equivalent materials used as a bolus in radiation therapy include slabs of paraffin wax, rice bags filled with soda, and gauze coated with petrolatum.

SEPARATION OF ADJACENT X-RAY FIELDS

Field Junctions

- A commonly used method matches adjacent radiation fields at depth.
- The necessary separation between adjacent field edges needed to produce junction doses similar to central-axis doses follows from the similar triangles formed by the

half-field length and SSD in each field. The field edge is defined by the dose at the edge that is 50% of the dose at d_{max}.
- Consider two contiguous fields of lengths L_1 and L_2; the separation, S, of these two fields at the skin surface follows from these expressions:

$$S = \frac{1}{2}L_1\left(\frac{d}{SSD}\right) + \frac{1}{2}L_2\left(\frac{d}{SSD}\right)$$

where d is the depth-dose specification, and L_1 and L_2 are the respective field lengths at the surface. A slight modification of this formula is needed when sloping surfaces are involved (14).

Orthogonal Field Junctions

- Figure 2-6 illustrates the geometry of matching abutting orthogonal photon beams.
- Such techniques are necessary (particularly in the head and neck region, where the spinal cord can be in an area of beam overlap) in the treatment of medulloblastoma with multiple spinal portals (5) and lateral brain portals and in multiple-field treatments of the breast (15).
- A common solution to avoid overlap is to use a half-block, so that abutting anterior and lateral field edges are perpendicular to the gantry axis (16).
- In addition, a notch in the posterior corner of the lateral oral cavity portal is commonly used to ensure overlap avoidance of the spinal cord when midline cord blocks cannot be used on anteroposterior portals irradiating the lower neck and matched to the oral cavity portals.
- Other techniques rotate the couch about a vertical axis to compensate for the divergence of the lateral field (15). With a source-axis distance (SAD), the angle of rotation given by

$$\arctan\theta = \left(\frac{1}{2}\frac{\text{field width}}{\text{SAD}}\right)$$

- or to leave a gap, S, on the anterior neck surface between the posterior field of length L and lateral field edges (17), where d is the depth of the spine beneath the posterior field and where

$$S = \frac{1}{2}(L)\left(\frac{d}{SAD}\right)$$

- Craniospinal irradiation is well established as a standard method of treatment of suprasellar dysgerminoma, pineal tumors, medulloblastomas, and other tumors involving the central nervous system. Uniform treatment of the entire craniospinal target volume is possible using separate parallel-opposed lateral whole-brain portals rotated so their inferior borders match with the superior border of the spinal portal, which is treated with either one or two fields (depending on the length of the spine to be treated).
- Lim (18,19) described the dosimetry of optional methods of treating medulloblastoma with excellent descriptions and diagrams.

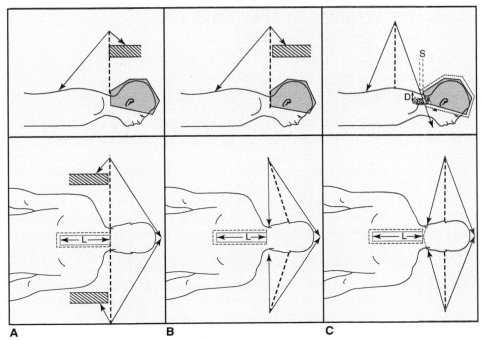

FIGURE 2-6. Some solutions for the problem of overlap for orthogonal fields. **A:** A beam splitter, a shield that blocks half of the field, is used on the lateral and posterior fields and on the spinal cord portal to match the nondivergent edges of the beams. **B:** Divergence in the lateral beams may also be removed by angling the lateral beams, so that their caudal edges match. Because most therapy units cannot be angled like this, the couch is rotated through small angles in opposite directions to achieve the same effect. **C:** A gap technique allows the posterior and lateral field to be matched at depth using a gap, *S*, on the skin surface. The *dashed lines* indicate projected field edges at depth *D*, where the orthogonal fields meet. (Adapted with permission from Williamson TJ. A technique for matching orthogonal megavoltage fields. *Int J Radiat Oncol Biol Phys* 1979;5:111–116.)

- Two junctional moves are made at one third and two thirds of the total dose. The spinal-field central axis is shifted away from the brain by 0.5 cm, and the field-size length is reduced by 0.5 cm, with corresponding increases in the length of the whole-brain field, so that a match exists between the inferior border of the brain portal and the superior border of the spinal portal. The whole-brain portals are rotated by an angle

$$\arctan\theta = \left(\frac{1}{2} \frac{\text{spinal field length}}{\text{SSD}} \right)$$

- to achieve the match. To eliminate the divergence between the brain portal and spinal portal, the table is rotated through a floor angle:

$$\arctan\alpha = \left(\frac{1}{2} \frac{\text{skull field length}}{\text{SAD}} \right)$$

RADIATION THERAPY IN PATIENTS WITH CARDIAC PACEMAKERS

- Modern pacemakers are radiosensitive and have a significant probability of failing catastrophically at radiation doses well below normal tissue tolerance; therefore, they should never be irradiated by the direct beam.
- The devices are well shielded electrically, so that transient malfunction because of stray electromagnetic (EM) (20) fields around a modern linac is unlikely.
- Potential interactions between a functioning pacemaker and the radiation therapy environment fall into two categories:
  1. Transient malfunctions can be caused by strong high- or low-frequency EM fields created by the treatment machine when producing high-energy photon and electron beams. Ambient EM fields arise in linacs from the microwave transport system used to accelerate electrons and from the low-frequency, high-voltage pulses used to energize the electron gun and microwave sources.
  2. Excessive exposure of the pacer to primary or scatter ionizing radiation may cause permanent malfunction of circuit components.

- Following is a widely accepted set of clinical management guidelines based on recommendations by the American Association of Physicists in Medicine (AAPM) (21):
  1. Pacemaker-implanted patients should never be treated with a betatron.
  2. A patient's coronary and pacemaker status must be evaluated by a cardiologist before and soon after completion of therapy.
  3. The pacemaker should always be kept outside the machine-collimated radiation beam during treatment and during the taking of portal films.
  4. Patients must be carefully observed during the first therapy session to verify that no transient malfunctions are occurring and during subsequent treatments if magnetron or klystron misfiring (sparking) occurs.
  5. Before treatment, the dose (from scatter) to be received by the pacemaker must be estimated and recorded. The total accumulated dose should not exceed approximately 2 Gy.
  6. If treatment within these guidelines is not possible, the physician should consider having the pacemaker either temporarily or permanently removed before irradiation.

DOSIMETRY FOR PERIPHERAL RADIATION TO THE FETUS

- Major components of peripheral dose can be divided into the following regions:
  1. Within 10 cm from beam edge, the dose is primarily because of collimator scatter and internal patient scatter.
  2. From 10 to 20 cm from beam edge, the dose is primarily because of internal patient scatter.
  3. From 20 to 30 cm from beam edge, patient scatter and head leakage contribute equally.
  4. Beyond 30 cm, the dose is primarily from head leakage.

- The AAPM suggests that pregnant patients be treated with energies less than 10 MV whenever possible (22).
- Two methods can be used to reduce the dose to the fetus: (a) modification of treatment techniques and (b) use of special shields.
- Modifications include changing field angle (avoiding placement of the gantry close to the fetus, i.e., treatment of a posterior field with the patient lying prone on a false table top), reducing field size, choosing a different radiation energy (avoiding ^{60}Co because of high leakage or energies greater than 10 MV because of neutrons), and using tertiary collimation to define the field edge nearest to the fetus.
- When shields are designed, the shielding device must allow for treatment fields above the diaphragm and on the lower extremities. Safety to the patient and personnel is a primary consideration in shield design.
- Commonly used shielding arrangements include bridge over patient, table over treatment couch, and mobile shield.

Effects by Gestational Age Postconception

- *Preimplantation*: 0 to 8 days postconception: Death of the embryo or early fetus is an acute effect of radiation exposure. Most data come from experiments on mice and rats. The maximum risk to the embryo or fetus of rodents suggests a 1% to 2% chance of early death after doses on the order of 0.1 Gy corresponding to an LD_{50} (i.e., lethal dose in 50% of cases) of 1 Gy.
- *Embryonic period*: 8 to 56 days PC: The principal risk during this period is malformation of specific organs. Small head size (SHS) is common. Atomic bomb survivor data show that the risk of SHS increases with dose above a threshold of a few cGy and is approximately 40% for a uterine-absorbed dose of 0.5 Gy. A risk of growth retardation with a threshold dose of 0.05 to 0.25 Gy has been observed. A possible late cancer risk of 14% per Gy exists for an acute single dose to the fetus at this stage. Fractionation of the dose would probably reduce this risk. Data from pregnant patients receiving large therapeutic radiation doses to the abdomen indicate that abortions are induced with doses of 3.6 to 5.0 Gy.
- *Early fetal*: 56 to 105 days PC: SHS and severe mental retardation (SMR) are the principal risks. Risk of SHS decreases after week 11. Risk of SMR is approximately 40% per Gy, with a threshold of at least 0.12 Gy. Risk of growth retardation is smaller than in the embryonic stage. For doses higher than 1 Gy, there is a risk of sterility and a continuing risk (presumably with no threshold) for a subsequent cancer.
- *Midfetal*: 105 to 175 days PC: Irradiation during this period is not likely to induce gross malformations. SMR has been observed with a threshold of approximately 0.65 Gy among persons irradiated *in utero* during the atom bombing. SHS and growth retardation have also been observed at doses exceeding 0.5 Gy. There is a continuing risk of subsequent cancer development.
- *Late fetal*: more than 175 days PC: Risks of malformation and mental retardation are negligible. The major risk is subsequent cancer development, according to data obtained from diagnostic x-ray exposure of pregnant women in the third trimester. There is a continuing risk of growth retardation for doses exceeding 0.5 Gy.

- The risks of the dominant effects after a dose of 0.1 Gy are SMR, 1:25; malformation, 1:20; and cancer mortality, 1:14. These are conservative estimates because a linear dose-response model has been used for cancer induction and mental retardation.
- The risk of malformation is assumed to have a threshold of 0.5 Gy and a 50% risk at fetal dose of 1 Gy.
- The AAPM report suggests that the fetal dose should be kept below 0.1 Gy, acknowledging an uncertain risk between 0.05 and 0.10 Gy.

PHYSICS AND CLINICAL APPLICATIONS OF ELECTRON BEAM THERAPY

Physical Characteristics of Electron Beams

- Historically, high-energy electron beams have been provided by Van de Graaff, betatron, and linear accelerators for use in radiation oncology. The medical electron linear accelerator design dominates today. Modern designs typically are multienergy and multimodality, using two x-ray energies (e.g., 6 and 18 MV), and five to six electron energies (e.g., between 4 and 20 MeV).
- Electron beams are small (approximately 3 to 4 mm in diameter) and essentially monoenergetic on exit from the waveguide-accelerating component. They are magnetically steered and focused to interact with an energy-dependent selection of electron-scattering metallic foils, which provide the circular, scattered, broad, uniform doses required for radiation treatment. The electron beam then passes through a dual, structured parallel-plate ionization chamber system for dose monitoring. The circular electron beams are collimated to square beams using a set of individual electron collimators, typically ranging in size from 4 × 4 cm to 25 × 25 cm. Low melting point alloys can be used to make irregularly shaped field inserts into the electron collimators for individual patient treatment. The collimators terminate approximately 5 to 8 cm from the patient's skin surface setup at 100-cm SSD.
- The electron beam dose rates are selectable, from 100 to 400 cGy per minute typically. A high-dose rate option is usually available at ≥1,000 cGy per minute for use in the treatment of total skin at extended distances of 4 to 6 m.
- Electron beams, although essentially monoenergetic when they first exit from the waveguide, lose energy continuously as they interact with the air, the metallic scattering foils, the dose monitor chamber system, and the patient's tissues. When this kinetic energy is fully dissipated, the electron is said to be "thermalized," and it enters the atomic milieu of the matter in which it stops. The further it penetrates, the less monoenergetic it becomes. The linear energy transfer (23), or linear stopping power, of the electron beams has the value 2 MeV energy loss per cm travel in water, approximately independent of the energy in the range of 4 to 20 MeV. Thus, we say that a 10-MeV beam has a range of approximately 5 cm in water. This energy loss is predominately because of collisional (elastic) interactions of the electrons with electrons and nuclei in the media.

- Because of these collisional interactions, the electrons scatter away from a straight inline path. This angular spread of the beam increases as the electrons penetrate into the media. The rate of angular spread is greater for lower-energy electrons. This phenomenon, together with the approximate constant linear energy transfer (LET), explains why higher-energy clinical electron beams (unlike high-energy x-ray beams) have a higher surface dose and lower-energy electrons have a lower surface dose.
- Radiative (inelastic) interactions by these clinical electron beams produce a weak field of bremsstrahlung (x-rays). In tissue at the treatment distance, for example, this is approximately 0.1% of the total dose for 6-MeV electron beams and less than 2% for 18-MeV electrons. Bremsstrahlung contamination has the obvious penetration ability of the respective 6- to 18-MV x-ray beams. This is clinically significant only for therapy around the lens of the eye with high-Z blocking and for multifield total skin electron beams used in the treatment of mycosis fungoides.
- Optimum scatterer-collimator design produces electron fields that have uniform dose (flat and symmetric), good surface dose preservation, and minimum bremsstrahlung contamination.

Clinical Characteristics of Electron Beams

- The central-axis depth dose of several electron beams is shown in Figure 2-7. Unlike megavoltage photon beams, electron beams exhibit rapid falloff, especially if the energy is below 15 MeV. This is clinically significant because tissues lying beyond the practical range of the electron beam absorb almost no dose other than that from x-ray contamination.

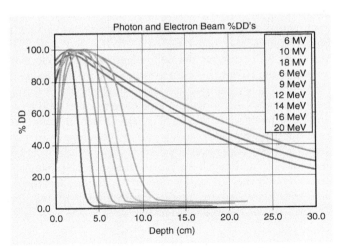

FIGURE 2-7. Central-axis PDD for electron beams (6 to 20 MeV—*sharply attenuated curves to left*) and also megavoltage x-rays (⁶⁰Co to 18 MV). (Reprinted with permission from Halperin EC, Perez CA, Brady LW. *Principles and practice of radiation oncology*, 5th ed. Philadelphia, PA: Lippincott Williams & Wilkins, 2008:160. © Wolters Kluwer.)

Table 2-2					
Electron Beam Surface Dose (% Values)					
	Energy (MeV)				
Applicator Size (cm²)	6	9	12	16	20
6 × 6	82	86	90	94	96
15 × 15	80	86	88	92	94

Reprinted with permission from Perez CA, Lovett RD, Gerber R. Electron beam and x-rays in the treatment of epithelial skin cancer: dosimetric considerations and clinical results. In: Vaeth JM, Meyer JL, eds. *The role of high-energy electrons in the treatment of cancer. Frontiers of radiation therapy and oncology*, vol 25. Basel, Switzerland: Karger, 1991:90–106. © Wolters Kluwer.

- The most commonly used prescription is to the depth of the 90% depth-dose line (therapeutic range). This therapeutic range is approximately given by $E/3.2$ cm. E is the most probable energy of the electron beam at the patient surface. The depth of the 80% depth-dose line is given approximately by $E/2.8$ cm.
- Skin-surface percent depth doses range from approximately 80% for low-energy electrons to 93% for 18-MeV electrons, as shown in Table 2-2.
- The depth at which maximum dose is reached below the skin surface is proportional to E, up to approximately 12 to 16 MeV (ranging from 1.0 to 2.5 cm), and then decreases at greater energies (ranging from 2.5 down to 1.5 as energy goes from 16 MeV up to 20 MeV). The region of uniform maximum dose is narrow for low-energy electrons and broad for high-energy electrons.
- The rate of decrease in percent depth dose versus depth, between the 80% and 20% level, is greater for small field sizes than for large field sizes and greater for low-energy electrons than for high-energy electrons.
- Isodose curves show ballooning at the field edges caused by electron scattering at depth. This results in the 10% to 30% lines ballooning to the outside of the field and the 80% to 95% lines constricting to the inside of the field. To treat uniformly at a depth of the 80% to 90% line, one may thus have to use a field that is as much as 2 cm larger than the tumor at that depth. This phenomenon is more important with higher energy and for smaller fields.
- This summary of clinical and physical characteristics of electron beams does not replace the need for exact and detailed measurements of each parameter for each individual accelerator, even if they are of the same make, model, and upgrade.
- Calibration and treatment planning require measurements of each machine parameter and individual patient treatment parameter, such as SSD, air-gap field size, and blocking (24).

Clinical Applications

- Electron beams may be the primary mode of therapy or may be combined with photon beams.

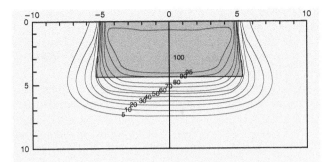

FIGURE 2-8. Isodose curves for a 15-MeV, 10 by 10 cm² electron beam in water (source to surface distance or SSD = 100 cm). Note the shape of the 90% isodose contour with respect to the *shaded area*, which is framed by the diverging field edges and the R_{90} depth. (Reprinted with permission from Halperin EC, Perez CA, Brady LW. *Principles and practice of radiation oncology*, 5th ed. Philadelphia, PA: Lippincott Williams & Wilkins, 2008:201. © Wolters Kluwer.)

- It is mandatory that radiation oncologists be familiar with the idiosyncrasies of their machines, in addition to isodose distributions, energies available for treatment, parameters of the tumor, and volume to be irradiated.
- Output measurements, central-axis depth dose, and off-axis profiles should be measured for all energies and for each standard electron collimator and its insert combinations. Beams are considered to be clinically uniform (flat and symmetric) when dose measurements in the plane perpendicular to the central axis, at the depth of the 95% depth dose on the far side of the depth of dose maximum, do not exceed plus or minus 5% across the area confined within 2 cm of the geometric field edge for fields of 10 × 10 cm or greater. See Figure 2-8.
- Surface air gaps (skin curvature), bolus, and tissue inhomogeneities in the treatment field significantly affect the dose distribution.
- Electron output at the depth of maximum dose (d_{max}) for SSD (different from the nominal SSD 100 cm) will vary as an inverse square factor using an "effective" SSD rather than the nominal SSD of 100 cm. Effective SSD is determined experimentally as a function of electron energy and collimator size and is ≤100 cm. It is smaller for lower energies and smaller collimator sizes.
- Compact bone (e.g., mandible) causes an approximate 4 MeV loss per cm of bone and thus proportionately lessens the electron beam. Failure to consider this may lead to underdose behind the mandible. Spongy bone (e.g., sternum) should have much less effect.
- In lung tissue, the range of the electron is increased by a factor of approximately 3. If one ignores this, then one will underestimate the dose to deeper lung points and the volume of lung irradiated.
- When tissue-equivalent bolus is used on the skin surface to increase surface dose, one must not forget that the entire central-axis depth dose has effectively been shifted toward the surface by an amount equal to the thickness of the bolus. One may have to increase the energy to get proper dose at depth below the skin surface in the presence of the bolus.
- Better dose distribution can be achieved by placing a secondary collimation near the patient's skin surface.

- The penumbra increases dramatically with distance from the applicator; this is particularly significant at low energies and for small fields.
- Small blocks of bolus that do not cover the whole field should be avoided because they behave like large air or tissue inhomogeneities and may generate significant scatter hot spots in tissue at their edges.
- Shielding should be applied carefully because of the hot spots that exist at shield edges. The minimum thickness of lead, in millimeters, needed to block electron beams of energy E in MeV is given by $E/2$ mm lead. Thickness should be increased by approximately 20% if low melting point lead-cadmium alloys are used.
- The choice of an appropriate gap between abutted fields is critical. The gap may vary with field size, distance, and beam characteristics.
- Matching for uniform dose at the surface causes 20% to 50% hot spots at depth, and matching for uniform dose at depth causes 20% to 50% cold spots at the surface. Use of 1- to 2-cm plastic wedges in each penumbra region improves the ability to optimize uniform dose in overlapping regions.
- The current standard of care in computerized treatment planning for clinical use of electron beams—either alone or in conjunction with photon beams—is to choose computer planning systems that use implementations of pencil electron beam algorithms, preferably in a fully three-dimensional (3D) computational and clinical environment, which requires a volume set of CT scans.

Normal Tissue Reactions

- Clinical electron beams are low LET radiations, and expected radiobiologic equivalent and oxygen enhancement ratio characteristics are identical to that of photon beams to within plus or minus 5%.
- The higher the electron beam energy, the greater the surface buildup dose, and the more intense the skin reactions.
- Widely varying accelerator designs for flattening and collimating clinical electron beams lead to differing skin surface dose buildup for the same nominal energy settings.
- Tapley (25) developed skin tolerance tables correlating the factors of dose, time, area, electron energy, and anatomic site, including the lateral face, upper and lower neck, and chest wall.
- The intensity of skin reactions at high energies suggests that electron beams should be used in combination with megavoltage photon beams (Table 2-3).

Table 2-3				
Tolerance Doses for Different Anatomic Locations, Field Sizes, and Electron Energies				
Anatomic Location	Field Size (cm²)	Electron Energy (MeV)	Dose (Gy)	Total Time (weeks)
Lateral face	50	15–18	65	6.0–6.5
Neck and chest wall	50	7–11	50–55	4

- The acute mucous membrane reactions seen with electron beam therapy are similar to those produced by photon beams at the same doses but are advantageously, sharply localized to the ipsilateral side.
- If electron beam therapy is used exclusively to treat lateralized lesions of the head and neck, fibrosis and late radiation sequelae usually become unacceptable; electron beam therapy should be combined with other radiation modalities.

Techniques

Intraoral tumors
- For the treatment of lesions of the oral cavity, intraoral stents containing lead offer protection to adjacent tissues distal to the tumor; they should be covered with dental wax to decrease scattered radiation effects on the adjacent mucosa. Similar protection can be achieved by increasing distance with tissue-equivalent Lucite "spacers."

Skin and lip tumors
- For small, superficial basal cell carcinomas, a 1.0- to 1.5-cm margin surrounding the gross lesion is adequate. In large, infiltrative lesions, 2- to 3-cm margins are required, with wide borders of uninvolved tissue.
- For squamous cell carcinoma, the field usually can be reduced at 50 Gy.
- Most lesions located on the eyelids, external nose, cheeks, and ears are not deeply invasive and can be treated with electron beam energies of 6 to 9 MeV.
- If the lesion approaches 2 cm in thickness, 9- to 12-MeV electron beams should be used.
- Protective devices should be designed to delineate the treatment field and conform to the irregular shape of the lesion.
- Lead shields should be placed beneath the lid in eyelid lesions or in lesions near the eye. Eye shields should be wax-coated to decrease backscatter electron dose to the eyelid. Thicker external blocks may be necessary to protect the eye at higher-energy levels.
- Shielding devices (wrapped in wet gauze or dipped in dental wax) should also be placed within the cavity of the area being treated to protect opposite tissues.
- If there is potential skin involvement, appropriately chosen bolus and energy adjustment should be used.

Upper respiratory and digestive tracts
- Electron beams alone may be used to treat lateralized tumors of the oral cavity, oropharynx, hypopharynx, or supraglottic larynx, frequently combined with external beam high-energy photons or interstitial brachytherapy.
- In the oral cavity, electron beams may be used with intraoral cones, providing coverage of the lesion with a 1-cm margin of normal mucosa on all sides. An intraoral stent may be necessary to position the cone and to reproduce its placement at each treatment.
- Electron energy is chosen at 6, 9, or 12 MeV, depending on the characteristics and depth of the tumor.

Salivary gland tumors

- In treatment for salivary gland tumors, electrons generally are used alone for 75% to 80% of the dose and are combined with photon beams for 20% to 25% of the dose.
- The application of electron beam therapy, either alone or with photon beams, is most effective after the bulk of the tumor has been removed.

Breast cancer

- Electron beam therapy is of particular value for administration of boost dose to the tumor excision volume in breast conservation treatment and for treatment of subclinical, relatively superficial disease in patients who have had surgical removal of the primary breast lesion and axillary lymphatics.
- Radiation therapy may be designed for the chest wall using an electron beam, a combination of electrons and photons, or a combination of electron beams at varying energies.
- Computed tomography and 3D treatment planning offer excellent means to measure the thickness of the chest wall and aid in the choice of appropriate energy level to be used and volume to be treated.

Neoplasms of other sites

- Certain lymphomas that present as subcutaneous masses or dermal lesions can be treated by electron beam therapy.
- In many soft tissue sarcomas, electron beam therapy can be used as total treatment, an adjunct to photon beam treatment, or a boost to photon beam treatment, with the electron beam portion being given at the time of the surgical excision procedure.
- Primary or recurrent carcinomas of the vulva, distal vagina, urethra, suburethral area, or other areas that recur after surgical removal may be treated by electrons incorporating the appropriate bolus.

Intraoperative irradiation

- Intraoperative electron beam used as a boost followed by photon beam treatment is an innovative regimen for pancreatic, gastric, and rectal cancers; retroperitoneal sarcomas; head and neck cancers; and genitourinary and some gynecologic cancers.
- There are two low kV x-ray devices currently on the market. The ASTRO emerging technology committee published a report in 2010 that reviews these technologies (26). Both devices are well suited to spherical targets such as breast cancer.

References

1. Gagnon WF, Horton JL. Physical factors affecting absorbed dose to the skin from cobalt-60 gamma rays and 25-MV x rays. *Med Phys* 1979;6(4):285–290.
2. Gerbi BJ, Meigooni AS, Khan FM. Dose buildup for obliquely incident photon beams. *Med Phys* 1987;14(3):393–399.
3. Jackson W. Surface effects of high-energy X rays at oblique incidence. *Br J Radiol* 1971;44(518):109–115.
4. Svensson GK, Bjarngard BE, Chen GT, et al. Superficial doses in treatment of breast with tangential fields using 4 MV x-rays. *Int J Radiat Oncol Biol Phys* 1977;2(7–8):705–710.

5. Van Dyk J, Jenkin RD, Leung PM, et al. Medulloblastoma: treatment technique and radiation dosimetry. *Int J Radiat Oncol Biol Phys* 1977;2(9–10):993–1005.
6. Mackie TR, el-Khatib E, Battista J, et al. Lung dose corrections for 6- and 15-MV x rays. *Med Phys* 1985;12(3):327–332.
7. Epp ER, Lougheed MN, Mc KJ. Ionization build-up in upper respiratory air passages during teletherapy with cobalt 60 radiation. *Br J Radiol* 1958;31(367):361–367.
8. Klein EE, Chin LM, Rice RK, et al. The influence of air cavities on interface doses for photon beams. *Int J Radiat Oncol Biol Phys* 1993;27(2):419–427.
9. Das IJ, Kase KR, Meigooni AS, et al. Validity of transition-zone dosimetry at high atomic number interfaces in megavoltage photon beams. *Med Phys* 1990;17(1):10–16.
10. Klein EE, Kuske RR. Changes in photon dose distributions due to breast prostheses. *Int J Radiat Oncol Biol Phys* 1993;25(3):541–549.
11. Leavitt DD, Martin M, Moeller JH, et al. Dynamic wedge field techniques through computer-controlled collimator motion and dose delivery. *Med Phys* 1990;17(1):87–91.
12. Purdy JA, Keys DJ, Zivnuska F. A compensation filter for chest portals. *Int J Radiat Oncol Biol Phys* 1977;2(11–12):1213–1215.
13. Ellis F, Hall EJ, Oliver R. A compensator for variations in tissue thickness for high energy beams. *Br J Radiol* 1959;32(378):421–422.
14. Keys R, Grigsby PW. Gapping fields on sloping surfaces. *Int J Radiat Oncol Biol Phys* 1990;18(5):1183–1190.
15. Siddon RL, Tonnesen GL, Svensson GK. Three-field technique for breast treatment using a rotatable half-beam block. *Int J Radiat Oncol Biol Phys* 1981;7(10):1473–1477.
16. Karzmark C, Huisman P, Palos B, et al. Overlap at the cord in abutting orthogonal fields: a perceptual anomaly. *Int J Radiat Oncol Biol Phys* 1980;6:1366.
17. Williamson TJ. A technique for matching orthogonal megavoltage fields. *Int J Radiat Oncol Biol Phys* 1979;5:111–116. (See also Gillon MT, Kline RW. Field separation between lateral and anterior fields on a 6-MV linear accelerator. *Int J Radiat Oncol Biol Phys* 1980;6:233–237.)
18. Lim M. Evolution of medulloblastoma treatment techniques. *Med Dosim* 1986;11:25.
19. Lim M. A study of four methods of junction change in the treatment of medulloblastoma. *Med Dosim* 1985;10:17.
20. Freeman CR, Farmer J, Taylor R. Central nervous system tumors in children. In: Halperin EC, Perez CA, Brady LW, eds. *Principles and practice of radiation oncology*, 5th ed. Philadelphia, PA: Lippincott Williams & Wilkins, 2008:1822–1849.
21. Marbach JR, Sontag MR, Van Dyk J, et al. Management of radiation oncology patients with implanted cardiac pacemakers: report of AAPM Task Group No. 34. American Association of Physicists in Medicine. *Med Phys* 1994;21(1):85–90.
22. Stovall M, Blackwell CR, Cundiff J, et al. Fetal dose from radiotherapy with photon beams: report of AAPM Radiation Therapy Committee Task Group No. 36. *Med Phys* 1995;22(1):63–82.
23. Fletcher GH. *Textbook of radiotherapy*, 3rd ed. Philadelphia, PA: Lea & Febiger, 1980.
24. Cunningham J. Tissue inhomogeneity corrections in photon-beam treatment planning in progress in modern radiation physics. In: Orton C, ed. *Progress in medical radiation physics*. New York, NY: Plenum Publishing, 1982.
25. Tapley N. Skin and lips. In: Tapley N, ed. *Clinical applications of the electron beam*. New York, NY: John Wiley & Sons, 1976:93–122.
26. Park CC, Yom SS, Podgorsak MB, et al. American Society for Therapeutic Radiology and Oncology (ASTRO) Emerging Technology Committee Report on electronic brachytherapy. *Int J Radiat Oncol Biol Phys* 2010;76(4):963–972.

THREE-DIMENSIONAL PHYSICS AND TREATMENT PLANNING

- Technologic and computer developments have allowed three-dimensional conformal radiation therapy (3DCRT) planning.
- Computed tomography (CT) and magnetic resonance imaging (MRI) provide a 3D model of the patient's anatomy and tumor, which allows radiation oncologists to accurately prescribe irradiation to the target volume while sparing neighboring critical normal organs.

THREE-DIMENSIONAL TREATMENT PLANNING SYSTEMS

- Conformational treatment methods were pioneered by Takahashi (1) in Japan; Proimos, Wright, and Trump in the United States (2–4); and Green, Jennings, and Christie in Great Britain (5,6).
- Computer-controlled radiation therapy was initiated by the work of Kijewski et al. (7) at the Harvard Medical School and Davy et al. (8,9) at the Royal Free Hospital in London.
- Sterling et al. (10) demonstrated the first 3D approach to radiation treatment planning (RTP), using a computer-generated film loop technique that gave the illusion of a 3D view of anatomic features and isodose distribution (two-dimensional [2D] color washes) throughout a treatment volume.
- McShan et al. (11,12) implemented a clinically usable 3D RTP system based on beam's eye view (BEV), which provided the treatment planner with a viewing point from the perspective of the source of radiation, looking out along the axis of the radiation beam, similar to that obtained when viewing simulation radiographs.
- Goitein and Abrams (13,14) reported on a system that took advantage of CT scanning and interactive scan displays, increased minicomputer capabilities, produced high-quality color BEV displays, and computed and displayed radiographs from the digital CT data, called digitally reconstructed radiographs (DRRs).
- Other groups developed even more powerful 3D RTP systems, including use of nonaxial (noncoplanar) beams (15–18).

CONFORMAL RADIATION THERAPY

- The goal of 3DCRT is to conform the prescription dose to the configuration of the target volumes while delivering lower doses to surrounding normal tissues.

Preplanning and Localization

- After the proposed treatment position of the patient is determined, immobilization devices are fabricated in a CT simulator suite.
- Radiopaque marks are placed on the patient's skin, and the immobilization device is used for the volumetric 3D planning CT study in the treatment position.
- CT topograms are reviewed, and patient alignment is adjusted.

Computed Tomography Imaging for Three-Dimensional Planning

- A volumetric planning CT scan is performed on the CT simulator with the patient in the treatment position, typically with 50 to 100 slices that are 0.5 to 8 mm thick (19).
- CT images are transferred to a 3D RTP or virtual simulation computer workstation via a computer network.

Critical Structure, Tumor, and Target Volume Delineation

- The task of critical structure, tumor, and target volume delineation is performed by treatment planning staff and the radiation oncologist.
- Most structures are contoured manually using a mouse or digitizer, although some structures with distinct boundaries (e.g., skin) can be contoured automatically (Fig. 3-1).
- Many critical structures require the expertise of the radiation oncologist.
- Consultation with a diagnostic radiologist is often helpful.
- Advances in treatment planning software allow autocontouring of critical structures but still requires review by a radiation oncologist.

Designing Beams and Field Shaping

- 3D RTP systems have the ability to simulate all treatment machine motions, including gantry angle, collimator width, length and angle, multileaf collimator (MLC) leaf settings, couch latitude, longitude, height, and angle, thus providing the capability to generate plans that involve nonaxial beams.
- BEV display is used to select optimal beam directions and design beam apertures. This task is complemented by a room-view display, which is used to graphically set isocenter position and to better appreciate multiple-beam treatment techniques (19).

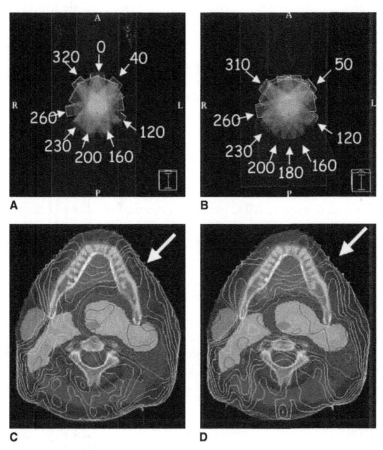

FIGURE 3-1. Patient with carcinoma of the base of the tongue treated with IMRT. Beam angle arrangement (**A** and **B**) and the resulting isodose distributions (**C** and **D**). *Arrow* in **C** indicates a "horn" of high dose to the left oral tongue and buccal mucosa. In **B**, the anterior beam placement was rearranged, leading to the improved dose distribution to the normal mucosa of the left anterior oral cavity **(D)**. (Reprinted with permission from Chao KSC, Mohan R, Lee NA, et al. Intensity-modulated radiation treatment techniques and clinical applications. In: Halperin EC, Perez CA, Brady LW. *Principles and practice of radiation oncology*, 6th ed. Philadelphia, PA: Lippincott Williams & Wilkins, 2013:228. © Wolters Kluwer.)

Dose Calculation

- After the beam geometries are designed, the dose distribution is calculated through-out a defined 3D volume with appropriate algorithms (20).

Plan Optimization and Evaluation

- 3DCRT plans are typically optimized by iteratively changing beam directions and apertures and recalculating the dose distribution until an optimal plan is obtained.

- Plans are evaluated qualitatively using dose-display tools, such as dose-volume histograms (DVHs); 2D axial, sagittal, and coronal isodose sections; and 3D room-view isodose surface displays.
- If warranted, changes are made and the dose distribution recalculated and reevaluated; this process is repeated until the radiation oncologist approves the plan as meeting both target volume goals and normal tissue dose constraints (19).

Treatment Documentation

- Once the treatment plan has been designed, evaluated, and approved, documentation for plan implementation is generated.
- Documentation includes beam parameter settings, hard-copy block templates for block fabrication room or MLC parameters communicated over a network to the computer system that controls the MLC subsystem of the treatment machine (19), DRR generation and printing, and transfer of these documents to the medical record database.

Plan and Treatment Verification

- Independent check of the treatment plan and monitor unit calculation by a physicist, radiographic verification simulation, first-day treatment portal films or electronic portal imaging devices, diode, TLD, or MOSFET *in vivo* dosimetry, and record-and-verify systems are used to confirm the validity and accuracy of the 3D-based plan (19).
- The elements of 3DCRT are summarized in Figure 3-2.

VOLUME AND DOSE SPECIFICATION FOR THREE-DIMENSIONAL CONFORMAL RADIATION THERAPY

- The recommendations for specifying gross tumor volume (GTV), clinical target volume (CTV), and planning target volume (PTV) for 3DCRT follow the International Commission on Radiation Units and Measurements (ICRU) Report Nos. 50 (21) and 62 (22) guidelines.
- Two dose volumes retained from ICRU Report No. 29 (23) are the treated volume, which is the volume enclosed by an isodose surface that is selected and specified by the radiation oncologist as being appropriate to achieve the purpose of treatment (e.g., 95% isodose surface), and the irradiated volume, which is the volume that receives a dose considered significant in relation to normal tissue tolerance (e.g., 50% isodose surface).
- ICRU Report No. 50 (21) recommends that dose to the PTV be reported for the ICRU reference point, along with the minimum, maximum, and mean doses. Information on how the mean dose was computed should be included to ensure consistency among reported mean dose values.

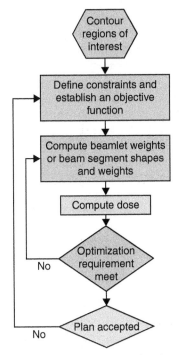

FIGURE 3-2. Elements of IMRT: planning phase. (Reprinted with permission from Chao KSC, et al. Intensity-modulated radiation treatment techniques and clinical applications. In: Halperin EC, Perez CA, Brady LW. *Principles and practice of radiation oncology*, 6th ed. Philadelphia, PA: Lippincott Williams & Wilkins, 2013:225. © Wolters Kluwer.)

- ICRU Report No. 62 (22) further defines the PTV, incorporating interval margins for expected physiologic movements and variations in size, shape, and position of the CTV during therapy in relation to an internal reference point. The volume formed by the CTV and the internal margin is known as the internal target volume.
- A setup margin accounts for inaccuracies and lack of reproducibility in patient positioning and alignment of the therapeutic beams during treatment.
- DVHs for GTVs, CTVs, PTVs, and all organs at risk should be reported to facilitate interpretation of treatment outcome and comparison of the relative merits of different techniques.

Practical Use of Gross Tumor Volume, Clinical Target Volume, and Planning Target Volume

- The radiation oncologist must specify GTV, CTV, and PTV on a volumetric CT scan of the patient, independent of the dose distribution; the GTV in terms of the patient's anatomy; the CTV in terms of the patient's anatomy or of knowledge of natural history and tumor biology data to be added to the GTV; and the PTV in terms of a quantitative margin to be added to the CTV to account for internal organ motion and repositioning uncertainties.

- The imaging study should be performed with the patient in the treatment position, using reliable patient immobilization devices.
- Radiopaque fiducial markers visible on the CT images are needed to coordinate transformation for planning and eventual treatment implementation.
- Large data sets with spiral CT scanning greatly improve the quality of the DRR; however, the contouring effort and the data storage requirements are increased.
- Defining the CTV is even more difficult and must be done by the radiation oncologist based on clinical experience, because current imaging techniques are not capable of directly detecting subclinical tumor involvement.
- Assistance from a diagnostic radiologist and/or surgeon is frequently useful in defining target volumes and normal tissues on axial CT slices.
- Image-based cross-sectional anatomy training is an essential part of radiation oncology training programs in order to improve the radiation oncologist's expertise in image recognition of normal tissue anatomy and gross tumor delineation.
- The PTV margin is specified by the radiation oncologist, taking into account the asymmetric nature of positional uncertainties and/or whether daily nonvolumetric or volumetric image guidance will be used.
- Certain limitations and practical issues must be clearly understood when ICRU Report No. 50 or 62 methodologies are adopted (21,22).
- In our clinic, the radiation oncologist specifies the PTV margin as an estimate based on clinical experience, use of daily image guidance, taking into account published literature, and intramural uncertainty studies; it is not treated as a simple summation.
- When a PTV overlaps a contoured normal structure, a quandary arises as to which volume the overlapping voxels should be assigned for DVH calculations. We assign the overlapping voxels to both volumes, which ensure that the clinician is aware of the potential for this high-dose region to include the normal structure as well as the CTV/GTV when reviewing the DVHs (19).
- CT is the principal source of image data for 3D RTP. However, it is encouraged to use complementary information from MRI (24–27), single photon emission computed tomography (SPECT), and positron emission tomography (PET) into the 3D RTP process. MRI provides excellent soft tissue contrast and allows precise delineation of normal critical structures and treatment volumes; SPECT and PET imaging provides detailed functional information concerning tissue metabolism and radioisotope transport, which results in better therapeutic strategies and more accurate target definition.
- The treated volume encompasses the tissue volume planned to receive a prescribed irradiation dose that will achieve the objectives of the treatment. The treated volume is enclosed by the isodose corresponding to the prescribed dose level.
- The irradiated volume receives a radiation dose that is significant in relation to normal tissue tolerance. A concept described in ICRU Report No. 62 (22) is the planning organ at risk volume (PRV), which should describe the size of the PRV in different directions for each specific organ within the irradiated volume.
- Figure 3-3 gives a schematic representation of the various volumes specified by the ICRU reports.

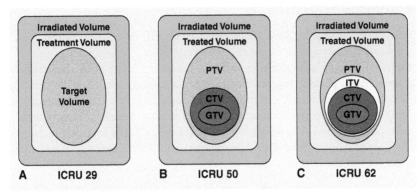

FIGURE 3-3. **A:** Schematic illustration of the boundaries of the volumes defined by ICRU Report No. 29: target volume, treatment volume, and irradiated volume. **B:** Boundaries in ICRU Report No. 50: gross tumor volume, clinical target volume, and planning target volume. **C:** Boundaries in ICRU Report No. 62: GTV, CTV, internal target volume, and PTV. (Adapted with permission from Purdy JA. Three-dimensional conformal radiation therapy: physics, treatment planning, and clinical aspects. In Halperin EC, Perez CA, and Brady LW. *Principles and practices of radiation oncology*, 6th ed. Philadelphia, Lippincott Williams & Wilkins, 2013:204. © Wolters Kluwer.)

DOSE-VOLUME HISTOGRAMS

- Differential and cumulative DVHs are used in 3DCRT.

Differential Dose-Volume Histograms

- First, the volume under consideration is divided into a 3D grid of volume elements (voxels); their size is small enough so that the dose can be assumed to be constant within one voxel.
- The volume's dose distribution is divided into dose bins, and the voxels are grouped according to dose bin without regard to anatomic location.
- A plot of the number of voxels in each bin (x axis) versus the bin dose range (y axis) is a differential DVH.
- The size of the dose bin determines the height of each bin of the differential DVH. For example, if the bin widths increase, the heights of the histogram bins generally increase because more voxels fall into any given bin.

Cumulative Dose-Volume Histograms

- A cumulative DVH is a plot in which each bin represents the volume or percentage of volume (y axis) that receives a dose equal to or greater than an indicated dose (x axis).
- In a cumulative DVH, the value at any dose bin is computed by summing the number of voxels of the corresponding differential DVH to the right of that dose bin. The volume value for the first bin (dose origin) is the full volume of the structure, because the total volume receives at least zero dose, and the volume for the last bin is that which receives the maximum dose bin (19).

Dose-Volume Statistics

- Explicit values of dose-volume parameters, which can be extracted from the DVH data, are called dose-volume statistics or dose statistics.
- Examples of dose-volume statistics include maximum point dose, minimum point dose, mean dose, percent volume receiving equal to or greater than the prescription dose for target volumes and maximum point dose, mean dose, and percent volume receiving equal to or greater than an established tolerance dose for organs at risk.
- There is some question as to whether point doses are clinically meaningful, suggesting that perhaps maximum dose should be reported for the dose averaged over a small but clinically significant volume.

Plan Evaluation Using Dose-Volume Histograms and Dose-Volume Statistics

- The DVH is an essential tool for 3DCRT plan comparison, because the planner can superimpose DVHs from several competing plans on one plot and compare them directly for each organ of interest.
- Sophisticated concepts and software improve our ability to quantitatively evaluate dose optimization in treatment planning (28–31).
- Sometimes, the differences between the DVHs of all the volumes of interest of two compared plans are clear, and one can easily determine which is the better plan. However, this is not the case for DVHs for a normal tissue that crosses over in midrange, with one being higher than the other at low doses and lower at high doses. This difficulty has prompted the development of biologic indices for plan evaluation.

BIOLOGIC MODELS

- Because 3DCRT plans provide both dose and volume information, the traditional practice of determining the "best plan" is extremely difficult (32,33). For example, it is not clear which degree of dose uniformity in the PTV can be tolerated as dose levels are escalated using 3DCRT, or how high of a dose can be tolerated by a small portion of a normal structure.
- Researchers are developing biophysical models that attempt to translate dose-volume information into estimates of biologic impact, such as tumor control probability and normal tissue complication probability models.

DIGITALLY RECONSTRUCTED RADIOGRAPHS

- DRRs are computer-generated projection images produced by mathematically passing divergent rays through a CT data set and acquiring x-ray attenuation information along the rays during 3D RTP; they are essential for implementing 3DCRT (14,34).
- The method for calculating DRRs is described in detail elsewhere (34).

- The DRR serves as a reference image for transferring the 3D treatment plan to the clinical setting; thus, its role is similar to that of a simulation film.
- DRR images can be printed on film using laser cameras and stored in the patient's film jacket just as if they were physical radiographs.

INTENSITY-MODULATED RADIATION THERAPY

- Intensity-modulated radiation therapy (IMRT) is a cutting-edge technology that can precisely deliver radiation to the target area while sparing surrounding normal tissues.
- In IMRT, the beam intensity varies across the treatment field. Rather than being treated with a single, large, uniform beam, the tumor is treated with many very small beams with different intensities. Multiple small beams of variable intensity are achieved by the use of a MIMiC, MLC, or dynamic MLC.
- The modulator of the radiation beam, MIMiC, consists of 40 leaves in two rows of 20, each defining a beam approximately 1 cm². By cross-firing the tumor with these beams, the dose to the tumor is uniform, but surrounding tissues receive a significantly lower radiation dose (35,36).
- A standard MLC is used to deliver the optimized fluence distribution in rather dynamic mode (defined as the leave moving while the radiation is on) or static mode, that is, "step-and-shoot" mode (defined as sequential delivery of radiation subportals that combine to deliver the desired fluence distribution), to deliver a set of intensity-modulated fields incident from fixed gantry angles (37).
- The next development was to use the conventional linac and MLC and to perform the dynamic delivery throughout an arc, which is called volumetric-modulated arc radiotherapy (VMAT). This is sometimes referred to by its original development name of intensity-modulated arc radiotherapy (IMAT) (38).
- By contrast, conventional 3DCRT uses radiation beams of uniform intensity. Its limitation is seen when a tumor is wrapped around an organ. Beams of uniform intensity usually cannot safely separate the tumor from the adjacent normal organ.
- With advances in IMRT technology, more precise separation of the target volume from adjacent tissue, such as in the spinal cord, is now feasible (Fig. 3-4).

QUALITY ASSURANCE FOR THREE-DIMENSIONAL CONFORMAL RADIATION THERAPY AND INTENSITY-MODULATED RADIATION THERAPY

- The precision and accuracy required for the 3D treatment planning process exceed accepted tolerances generally found in 2D treatment planning.
- A 3DCRT quality assurance program must address all of the individual procedures that make up the 3D process, including systematic testing of the hardware and software used in the 3D treatment planning process and careful review of each patient's treatment plan and its physical implementation (39).
- The 3DCRT quality assurance program requires the active involvement of physicists, dosimetrists, physicians, and radiation therapists.

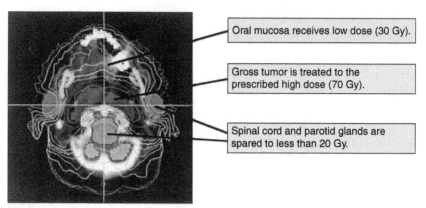

Oral mucosa receives low dose (30 Gy).

Gross tumor is treated to the prescribed high dose (70 Gy).

Spinal cord and parotid glands are spared to less than 20 Gy.

FIGURE 3-4. Coronal dose distribution for treatment with IMRT (6-MV x-rays, Nomos Peacock System; NOMOS, Sewickley, PA) in a patient with stage T3 carcinoma of the nasopharynx with left oropharyngeal extension.

FUTURE DIRECTIONS IN THREE-DIMENSIONAL CONFORMAL RADIATION THERAPY AND INTENSITY-MODULATED RADIATION THERAPY

- Software for contouring normal structures and target volumes and virtual simulation that previously required a significant investment of time and effort by the radiation oncology staff will continue to be improved.
- Use of Monte Carlo calculations to account for the effects of scattered photons and secondary electrons appears promising (19); it is likely that Monte Carlo–based algorithms will be practical for clinical 3D RTP early in this century.
- Computer-controlled 3DCRT delivery systems (e.g., beam intensity modulation) will require that the planning system generates the computer files needed to implement the 3DCRT technique. Integrated on-line electronic portal imaging, dose monitoring, verify-and-record, and computer-controlled feedback systems will play a role in verifying 3DCRT treatments (40).
- The advantage of 3DCRT, with its inverse treatment design, is easily demonstrated in planning exercises; however, we must show that this advantage translates to improved outcome in prospective clinical trials.
- Integrated 3D technology likely will lead to improved efficiency of planning, delivery, and verification procedures, which will result in lower overall costs of radiation therapy (40).

References

1. Takahashi S. Conformation radiotherapy. Rotation techniques as applied to radiography and radiotherapy of cancer. *Acta Radiol Diagn (Stockh)* 1965;242(Suppl):241.
2. Proimos BS. Shaping the dose distribution through a tumor model. *Radiology* 1969;92(1):130–135.
3. Trump JG, Wright KA, Smedal MI, et al. Synchronous field shaping and protection in 2-million-volt rotational therapy. *Radiology* 1961;76:275.

4. Wright K, Proimos B, Trump J, et al. Field shaping and selective protection in megavoltage therapy. *Radiology* 1959;72:101.

5. Green A. Tracking cobalt project. *Nature* 1965;207(5003):1311.

6. Green A, Jennings WA, Bush F. Rotational roentgen therapy in the horizontal plane. *Acta Radiol* 1949;31(4):273–320.

7. Kijewski PK, Chin LM, Bjarngard BE. Wedge-shaped dose distributions by computer-controlled collimator motion. *Med Phys* 1978;5(5):426–429.

8. Davy T, Bruce J. Dynamic 3-D treatment using a computer-controlled cobalt unit. *Br J Radiol* 1979;53:612–616.

9. Davy T, Johnson P, Redford R, et al. Conformation therapy using the tracking cobalt unit. *Br J Radiol* 1975;48:122–130.

10. Sterling TD, Knowlton KC, Weinkam JJ, et al. Dynamic display of radiotherapy plans using computer-produced films. *Radiology* 1973;107(3):689–691.

11. McShan DL, Silverman A, Lanza DM, et al. A computerized three-dimensional treatment planning system utilizing interactive colour graphics. *Br J Radiol* 1979;52(618):478–481.

12. Reinstein LE, McShan D, Webber BM, et al. A computer-assisted three-dimensional treatment planning system. *Radiology* 1978;127(1):259–264.

13. Goitein M, Abrams M. Multi-dimensional treatment planning: I. Delineation of anatomy. *Int J Radiat Oncol Biol Phys* 1983;9(6):777–787.

14. Goitein M, Abrams M, Rowell D, et al. Multi-dimensional treatment planning: II. Beam's eye-view, back projection, and projection through CT sections. *Int J Radiat Oncol Biol Phys* 1983;9(6):789–797.

15. Mohan R, Barest G, Brewster LJ, et al. A comprehensive three-dimensional radiation treatment planning system. *Int J Radiat Oncol Biol Phys* 1988;15(2):481–495.

16. Purdy JA. Defining our goals: volume and dose specification for 3-D conformal radiation therapy. In: Meyer JL, Purdy JA, eds. *Frontiers of radiation therapy oncology*. Basel, Switzerland: Karger, 1996:24–30.

17. Purdy JA, Harms WB, Matthews JW, et al. Advances in 3-dimensional radiation treatment planning systems: room-view display with real time interactivity. *Int J Radiat Oncol Biol Phys* 1993;27(4):933–944.

18. Sherouse GW, Chaney EL. The portable virtual simulator. *Int J Radiat Oncol Biol Phys* 1991;21(2):475–482.

19. Purdy JA. Three-dimensional conformal radiation therapy physics, treatment planning, and clinical aspects. In: Halperin EC, Perez CA, Brady LW, eds. *Principles and practice of radiation oncology*, 5th ed. Philadelphia, PA: Lippincott Williams & Wilkins, 2008:218–238.

20. Purdy JA. Photon dose calculations for three-dimensional radiation treatment planning. *Semin Radiat Oncol* 1992;2(4):235–245.

21. International Commission on Radiation Units and Measurements. *ICRU Report No. 50: prescribing, recording, and reporting photon beam therapy*. Bethesda, MD: ICRU, 1993.

22. International Commission on Radiation Units and Measurements. *ICRU Report No. 62: prescribing, recording, and reporting photon beam therapy (supplement to ICRU Report 50)*. Bethesda, MD: ICRU, 1999.

23. International Commission on Radiation Units and Measurements. *ICRU Report No. 29: dose specification for reporting external beam therapy with photons and electrons*. Washington, DC: ICRU, 1978.

24. Austin-Seymour M, Chen GT, Rosenman J, et al. Tumor and target delineation: current research and future challenges. *Int J Radiat Oncol Biol Phys* 1995;33(5):1041–1052.

25. Chaney EL, Pizer SM. Defining anatomical structures from medical images. *Semin Radiat Oncol* 1992;2(4):215–225.

26. Kessler M. Integration of multimodality image data for three-dimensional treatment planning. In: Purdy JA, Fraass B, eds. *Syllabus: a categorical course in physics*. Oak Brook, IL: Radiological Society of North America, 1994.

27. Kuszyk BS, Ney DR, Fishman EK. The current state of the art in three dimensional oncologic imaging: an overview. *Int J Radiat Oncol Biol Phys* 1995;33(5):1029–1039.

28. Brahme A. Optimization of radiation therapy. *Int J Radiat Oncol Biol Phys* 1994;28:785–787.

29. Brahme A. Optimization of stationary and moving beam radiation therapy techniques. *Radiother Oncol* 1988;12(2):129–140.

30. Drzymala RE, Holman MD, Yan D, et al. Integrated software tools for the evaluation of radiotherapy treatment plans. *Int J Radiat Oncol Biol Phys* 1994;30(4):909–919.

31. Niemierko A, Urie M, Goitein M. Optimization of 3D radiation therapy with both physical and biological end points and constraints. *Int J Radiat Oncol Biol Phys* 1992;23(1):99–108.

32. Goitein M. The comparison of treatment plans. *Semin Radiat Oncol* 1992;2(4):246–256.

33. Kutcher GJ. Quantitative plan evaluation: TCP/NTCP models. 3-D conformal radiotherapy. In: Meyer JL, Purdy JA, eds. *Frontiers of radiation therapy oncology*. Basel, Switzerland: Karger, 1996:67–80.

34. Sherouse GW, Novins K, Chaney EL. Computation of digitally reconstructed radiographs for use in radiotherapy treatment design. *Int J Radiat Oncol Biol Phys* 1990;18(3):651–658.

35. Mackie TR, Holms TW, Swerdloff S, et al. Tomotherapy: a new concept for the delivery of conformal radiotherapy. *Med Phys* 1993;20:1709–1719.

36. Mackie TR, Kapatoes J, Ruchala K, et al. Image guidance for precise conformal radiotherapy. *Int J Radiat Oncol Biol Phys* 2003;56:89–105.

37. Bortfeld T. IMRT: a review and preview. *Phys Med Biol* 2006;51:R363–R379.

38. Yu CX, Amies CJ, Svatos M. Planning and delivery of intensity-modulated radiation therapy. *Med Phys* 2008;35:5233–41.

39. Harms W, Purdy J, Emami B, et al. Quality assurance for three-dimensional treatment planning. In: Purdy J, Fraass B, eds. *Syllabus: a categorical course in physics*. Oak Brook, IL: Radiological Society of North America, 1994.

40. Boyer AL. Present and future developments in radiotherapy treatment units. *Semin Radiat Oncol* 1995;5(2):146–155.

CHAPTER 4

ADVANCED TREATMENT TECHNOLOGY

(IMRT, SRS, SBRT, IGRT, PROTON BEAM THERAPY)

- Intensity-modulated radiation therapy (IMRT) is capable of generating complex three-dimensional (3D) dose distributions to conform closely to the target volume, even in tumors with concave features. With IMRT, the beam intensity (fluence) is optimized, using computer algorithms, as it is oriented around the patient (1).
- This form of computer algorithm considers not only target and normal tissue dimensions but also user-defined constraints such as dose limits. This process is based on the "inverse method" of treatment planning ("inverse planning") and is capable of generating significant dose gradients between the target volume and adjacent tissue structures to accomplish the intended dose-volume prescription (2).
- Because of this specific feature, a precise mechanical system to deliver and validate the intended radiation dose to the desired area is crucial. An inverse prescription guideline that optimizes tumor target coverage and normal tissue sparing is another pertinent component of IMRT treatment.
- A variety of techniques have been developed to deliver optimized IMRT. The major differences among the various approaches are in the mechanisms they use for the delivery of nonuniform fluencies.

BASIC PHYSICAL PRINCIPLES OF INTENSITY-MODULATED RADIATION THERAPY

- For IMRT delivery, the fluence is to be modulated as a function of the entry angle at each point within the target volume. The dose at any point within the patient will be generated by a series of beamlets incident on that point, each with a unique entry angle.
- The radiation fluence can be modulated within the cone beam using a physical modulator, a scanning dynamic multileaf collimator (MLC), a scanning bremsstrahlung photon beam, or a combination of these techniques.
- Alternatively, the accelerator can be operated using dynamic motion of one or more of the angular degrees of freedom (couch, collimator, and gantry).

INVERSE TREATMENT OPTIMIZATION AND CRITERION

- Reported optimization methods include (a) exhaustive search, (b) image reconstruction approaches, (c) quadratic programming, and (d) simulated annealing.
- The optimization criteria in terms of dosimetric and clinical objectives are expressed as a mathematical entity in the form of an objective or cost function. The objective function defines a plan's quality and is to be maximized or minimized, as appropriate, to satisfy a set of mathematical constraints.
- Plan optimization criteria historically have been based on dose parameters. The optimization software iteratively adjusts the beam parameters to obtain the best possible results of the desired dose distribution. Recent efforts are examining the use of biologically based indices (e.g., tumor control probability and normal tissue complication probability) (3,4).

INTENSITY-MODULATED RADIATION THERAPY TREATMENT DELIVERY SYSTEMS

- *Robotic pencil beam*: Robot-mounted linear accelerators producing fairly narrow photon beams that move around the patient.
- *Rotary fan beam with intensity modulation*: A commercial implementation of a fan-beam approach to IMRT, using a mini-MLC system (MIMiC) that is mounted on an unmodified linear accelerator. Treatment is delivered to a narrow slice of the patient using arc rotation (5).
- The beam is collimated to a narrow slit, and beamlets are turned on and off by driving the mini-MLC leaves in and out of the beam path, respectively, as the gantry rotates around the patient. A complete treatment is accomplished by sequential delivery to adjoining slices.
- Helical tomotherapy, proposed by Mackie et al. (6), uses MIMiC to perform rotation IMRT while the patient is translated through the doughnut-shaped aperture in a fashion similar to the helical computed tomography (CT) scanner. In this form of tomotherapy, the problem of interslice matchlines is minimized because of the continuous helical motion of the beam around the longitudinal axis of the patient. The geometry of tomotherapy provides the opportunity to provide CT images of the body in the treatment setup position.
- A system that can generate tomographic images while receiving fan-beam tomotherapy on a megavoltage linac, with the patient in the treatment position, is under development (7).

Fixed Field Multileaf Collimator

- For this type of IMRT, the MLC is operated in either dynamic mode (the leaves moving while the radiation is on) or static mode, that is "step-and-shoot" mode (a sequential delivery of radiation subportals that combine to deliver the desired fluence distribution), in which the gap formed by each opposing leaf sweeps under computer control across the target volume to produce the desired fluence profile.

Intensity-Modulated Arc Therapy

- This technique, developed by Yu (8), uses a combination of dynamic multileaf collimation and arc therapy. The shape of the field formed by the MLC changes continuously during gantry rotation. Multiple superimposing arcs are used, and the field shape for a specific gantry angle changes from one arc to the next so that the cumulative fluence distribution is equal to the desired distribution. In the late 2000s, both Varian and Elekta introduced variable dose rate rotational delivery options into their linear accelerators. The delivery of a rotational cone beam with variable shape and intensity is commonly called volumetric-modulated arc therapy (VMAT).

Fixed Field with Compensating Filter

- Filters can be designed by calculating a thickness along a ray line using an effective attenuation coefficient for the filter material. The filter construction process can be automated using numerically controlled milling machines and generates the desired IMRT fluence profile.
- Comparisons of IMRT dose distributions delivered using physical modulators and MLC-based approaches are under investigation, with indications that the dose distributions provided by these modalities are similar (9).

PATIENT IMMOBILIZATION AND IMAGE ACQUISITION

- A noninvasive immobilization method is used. In the treatment of head and neck cancers, for example, the patient is placed in the supine position on a custom-made head support, and a reinforced thermoplastic immobilization mask is placed around the head. This procedure allows precise repositioning over the course of treatment (10).
- A volumetric CT image is acquired from a dedicated CT simulator with the patient immobilized in the treatment position, and the data are transferred to an inverse planning system.
- The scan slice thickness can range from 0.5 to 2.5 mm depending on the clinical scenario. Intended target volumes representing gross and microscopic tumor and organs at risk are defined on the prescription page of the inverse planning system.
- Double-exposure portal films are obtained weekly and compared with the corresponding digitally reconstructed radiograph from initial simulation.

SPECIFICATION OF PRESCRIPTION DOSE

- The desired minimum dose to target(s) and the maximum allowable dose to non-target structures are defined in the prescription. Unlike conventional beam arrangement, the isocenter of each treatment segment may not be located within the target. Therefore, the dose is specified to each target volume.
- Table 4-1 shows examples of dose prescriptions for head and neck cancer. The prescribed fraction size for the primary target is set to 1.9 Gy to increase the minimal fraction size in the lower-risk region to 1.5 Gy.

Table 4-1

Target Dose Specifications for Head and Neck Cancer

Target Volume	Type of Treatment					
	Definitive			Postoperative		
	IMRT/35	IMRT/33	3DCRT	IMRT/33	IMRT/30	3DCRT
Low risk (CTV3)	56/1.6	54/1.64	50/2.0	54/1.64	54/1.8	50/2.0
Intermediate risk (CTV2)	63/1.8	59.4/1.8	60/2.0	59.4/1.8	60/2.0	60/2.0
High risk (CTV1)	70/2.0	70/2.12	70/2.0	66/2.0	—	66/2.0

Number pairs are total dose/fraction dose (Gy); IMRT, intensity-modulated radiation therapy; 3DCRT, three-dimensional conformal radiation therapy; number following IMRT is the number of fractions; CTV1, CTV2, and CTV3 defined in text.

- To compensate for decrease in daily fraction dose to the secondary or tertiary targets, the biologically equivalent dose (BED) was implemented, using a linear-quadratic model. An α/β ratio of 10 Gy was used to convert tumor target dose.
- Based on institutional treatment guidelines for head and neck cancer, and depending on tumor volume, target doses are divided into four categories. Low-risk regions include primarily a prophylactically treated region. Intermediate-risk regions were those adjacent to the gross tumor but not directly involved by tumor. High-risk regions included the surgical bed with soft tissue invasion by the tumor or extracapsular extension by metastatic lymph nodes (5). Gross residual disease is treated with the highest dose.

TARGET DELINEATION

- Execution of IMRT requires proper knowledge of the volumes to be irradiated, based on clinical, pathologic, and radiologic information and on patterns of disease failure in addition to accurate delineation of these volumes on a 3D basis.

DOSIMETRIC ADVANTAGE OF INTENSITY-MODULATED RADIATION THERAPY

- IMRT has been shown to improve target coverage and normal tissue sparing in head and neck, cervical, prostate, and breast cancers.
- The emergent use of the combined-modality approach (chemotherapy and radiation therapy) for the treatment of patients with cervical cancer is associated with

significant gastrointestinal and genitourinary toxicity. The unique dosimetric advantage of IMRT is the potential to deliver an adequate dose to the target structures while sparing the normal organs. It could also allow for dose escalation to grossly enlarged metastatic lymph nodes in pelvic or paraaortic areas without increasing gastrointestinal/genitourinary complications.

- Portelance et al. reported that the volume of small bowel receiving the prescribed dose (45 Gy) with fixed-field dynamic MLC technique was four fields, $11.01\% \pm 5.67\%$; seven fields, $15.05\% \pm 6.76\%$; and nine fields, $13.56\% \pm 5.30\%$. These were all significantly better than with two-field ($35.58\% \pm 13.84\%$) and four-field ($34.24\% \pm 17.82\%$) conventional techniques ($p < 0.05$) (11).

STEREOTACTIC IRRADIATION

Radiosurgery Techniques

- For intracranial techniques, a stereotactic headframe is temporarily affixed to the patient's skull, providing highly accurate fiducial landmarks that allow for stereotactic localization of intracranial targets after registration (i.e., image fusion) of the treatment planning CT with diagnostic neuroimaging studies, such as magnetic resonance imaging (MRI), CT, or angiography (12).
- The frame provides the basis by which a target can be identified in the image study set with respect to the stereotactic frame and specified in an X-, Y-, and Z-coordinate system after registration. This coordinate system is used during target localization to define the shape and extent of the lesion to be treated (13).
- Stereotactic external beam radiation therapy (EBRT) differs from conventional EBRT in several important respects.
- Small volumes of 1 to 30 cm³ are treated.
- When a single fraction of stereotactically guided conformal irradiation is delivered to a defined target, the term stereotactic radiosurgery (SRS) is used. The term fractionated stereotactic radiosurgery or fractionated stereotactic radiation therapy (fSRS or SRT or FSRT) is used when more than one fraction is delivered over the course of several days or weeks.
- Extra precision with target localization and treatment geometries is required. The best achievable mechanical accuracy is less than 0.5 mm, although a maximum error of ±1.0 mm is commonly accepted in view of the unavoidable uncertainties in target localization.
- High-dose gradients at field edges minimize dose deposition outside the target volume. The volume of tissue beyond the target that receives significant dose is strongly dependent on target size and the conformity of the isodose to the target.
- Beams intersect at a common point within the skull after entering through points distributed over the surface of the skull. Three-dimensional distribution of beams reduces the volume of normal tissue receiving moderate or high doses of radiation.

INDICATIONS FOR STEREOTACTIC RADIOSURGERY

- Indications for SRS include the presence of a suitably sized (generally less than 4 cm), radiographically distinct lesion that has the potential to respond to a single, large dose of radiation.
- SRS can be used for arteriovenous malformations (AVMs), malignant primary brain tumors, metastatic brain tumors, benign brain tumors, and functional disorders including essential tremors and obsessive-compulsive disorder.
- Ideal target volumes for radiosurgery are nearly spherical and small (less than 3 cm in maximum dimension).

RADIOSURGERY SYSTEMS

- A radiosurgery system consists of a stereotactic frame, a radiation delivery system, and computer hardware and treatment planning software.
- Combined with the use of a conventional MRI or CT scanner, the system allows accurate determination of target size and location, treatment planning, and delivery of radiation.
- Different systems that meet these requirements equally should produce equivalent outcomes in similar groups of patients.

Gamma Knife

- The Gamma Knife system (Elekta AB, Stockholm, Sweden) requires a large capital purchase of approximately $3.5 million with construction of new space. The cobalt sources decay and need to be replaced, at a high cost, after 7 years.
- The Gamma Knife performs SRS, and more recent models allow fractionated SRS.
- The unit consists of a permanent 18,000-kg shield surrounding a hemispheric array 5,500 to 6,000 Ci of ^{60}Co, distributed in 192 sources over a portion of a hemisphere in such a way that circular beams from collimators may enter the skull through a large number of points distributed relatively uniformly over the convexity.
- Interchangeable collimators with beam diameters of 4 to 16 mm are used to vary the target volume. Individual collimators may be plugged in to conform the dose distribution to the target shape. It produces a target size of approximately 3 to 16 mm, with a target accuracy of 0.1 mm.
- The Perfexion model introduced in 2006 uses a larger patient aperture and has improved shielding.
- The Icon model is the latest advance in Gamma Knife radiosurgery. Icon provides the flexibility for single dose administration or multiple treatment sessions over time using a frameless approach and CBCT, which enables treatment of larger tumor volumes, targets close to critical brain structures and new or recurring brain metastases.

Linac-Based System

- A linear accelerator (linac) can be modified to perform stereotactic irradiation at a cost of $50,000 to $300,000, depending on whether external treatment planning devices need to be purchased.
- The linac can give a target size of 10 to 50 mm, with a target accuracy of 0.1 to 1.0 mm.
- Linacs have been applied for radiosurgery in various ways: (a) multiple noncoplanar arcs with circular cones; (b) noncoplanar 3DCRT (12 to 18 fields); (c) noncoplanar 3D conformal arc (12 to 18 fields); (d) IMRT and intensity-modulated arc therapy; and (e) CyberKnife (Accuray Inc., Sunnyvale, CA), which combines a miniaturized linac mounted on an industrial robot with a system for target tracking and beam realignment to deliver the desired dose with 6 degrees of freedom.
- Conventionally, a film technique allows verification of all positioning adjustments after the coordinates of the isocenter are determined. The film technique has been gradually replaced by the modern technologies including EPID (electronic portal imaging) and OBI (on-board imaging).

TARGET VOLUME DETERMINATION AND LOCALIZATION

- The technique used to determine target volume to be treated depends on the type of lesion.

Arteriovenous Malformations

- The target volume should include the entire nidus of the vascular lesion, which can be visualized with radiographic angiograms, MRI, or CT.
- It is important to include MRI or CT to accurately conform treatment plans with the 3D shape of the nidus, while avoiding excessive irradiation to surrounding brain.

Neoplasms

- MRI and CT are used to define treatment volumes for neoplastic lesions.
- Potential limitations include errors of localization or lack of knowledge of the actual (rather than apparent) extent of the lesion, especially with infiltrative glial neoplasms.
- Positron emission tomography (PET), or single-photon emission computed tomography (SPECT), is not routinely used as the primary imaging modality for stereotactic localization because of poor spatial resolution and inconsistency in determining tumor margins.

ARTERIOVENOUS MALFORMATIONS

- AVMs may be symptomatic as a result of seizure disorders, vascular steal from surrounding tissue, or intracranial hemorrhage.

- Hemorrhage is the most dangerous complication. AVMs bleed at a rate of 2% to 4% per year (14). The mortality associated with a bleed is generally 10% to 15%.
- The best treatment option is to surgically resect the AVM, if it can be done with acceptable morbidity (15). A second treatment modality is endovascular embolization.
- The radiosurgery principles applicable to AVMs are similar to those established for surgery. The goal is to remove the nidus of the AVM from the circulation while preserving surrounding brain parenchyma.
- AVMs respond to doses of 15 Gy or lower in a certain number of cases. Doses closer to 20 to 25 Gy may provide greater responses but also may be associated with a higher incidence of radiation-induced complications.
- It is reasonable to obtain 6- to 12-month serial CT or MRI scans of the vascular lesion.
- The posttreatment angiogram must show complete obliteration of the nidus of the AVM to predict a "cure."
- Irradiation of AVMs can lead to intimal proliferation and vascular occlusion. Small vessels are occluded more easily than large ones.
- Radiosurgery of AVMs may lead to an intense gliosis around the malformation, possibly producing endarteritis obliterans.
- Doses are selected so that the dose at the 80% isodose surface (which encloses the target volume) lies near the 1% brain necrosis line.
- Most AVMs have been treated with doses of 15 to 25 Gy, depending on size and location. For small lesions treated with a single isocenter, the dose at the periphery (approximately 25 Gy) corresponds to the 80% to 90% isodose surface. For somewhat larger lesions (collimator sizes less than 18 mm), more than one isocenter is used. In this situation, the dose at the periphery (approximately 20 to 25 Gy) corresponds to the 50% to 60% isodose surface. For somewhat larger lesions (collimator sizes less than 18 mm), more than one isocenter is used. In this situation, the dose at the periphery (approximately 20 to 25 Gy) corresponds to the 50% to 60% isodose surface.
- Steiner (16) reported 2-year complete and partial angiographic response rates of 87% and 11%, respectively.
- There has been no consistent statistically significant change in the rate of intracerebral hemorrhage in most reports after radiosurgery for AVMs, as compared with the rate of hemorrhage predicted by the natural history.
- Kjellberg (17) described neurologic complications in 9 of 444 patients (2%), with improvements in complication rates attributed to changes in dose and field size.

GLIOMAS

- Both low- and high-grade gliomas have been treated with SRS.
- The Joint Center for Radiation Therapy reported similar median survival results with either SRS or brachytherapy for recurrent malignant gliomas (10.9 versus 10.2 months) (18).
- The Radiation Therapy Oncology Group (RTOG) conducted a phase III randomized study (RTOG 93-05) for newly diagnosed glioblastoma to evaluate the impact of the

addition of an SRS boost to EBRT and chemotherapy on patient outcome (19). The results suggest that SRS does not significantly improve outcomes over standard EBRT and chemotherapy.
- In focal recurrent gliomas, reirradiation with SRS may be feasible for local control benefit.

BRAIN METASTASES

- RTOG 95-08 was a phase III trial of conventional irradiation (whole-brain radiation therapy [WBRT] 37.5 Gy in 15 fractions) followed by an SRS boost dose versus conventional WBRT alone in patients with up to three brain metastases. SRS improved survival in patients with a single unresectable brain metastasis in the setting of WBRT but did not impact survival in patients with two or three brain metastases (20).
- Cost is less than with surgical treatment.

MENINGIOMAS

- A linac-based radiosurgery report from Rome showed the results of radiosurgical management of 72 middle fossa meningiomas; 50 patients showed shrinkage of tumor from 24% to 91% of the initial tumor volume (21).

ACOUSTIC NEUROMAS

- Acoustic neuroma (a.k.a., vestibular schwannoma) is the most frequent cause of the cerebellopontine angle syndrome (22).
- Tumors involve the vestibular portion of cranial nerve VIII. More than half of the patients have facial weakness, disturbance of taste, and facial sensory loss; deafness and vestibular dysfunction also may occur.
- The surgical goal is complete removal via the suboccipital, translabyrinthine, or, rarely, middle cranial fossa approach.
- SRS has recently been recognized as an acceptable alternative to surgical resection of acoustic neuromas, especially for patients with hearing loss or significant comorbid medical conditions. Long-term control rates are as high as 85%.
- The peripheral tumor dose is usually 18 to 25 Gy, depending on lesion size and patient age.
- The Pittsburgh group reported on 26 patients with a median follow-up of 13 months and a tumor response of 42% (23,24).

IMAGING STUDIES AFTER RADIOSURGERY

- Beginning at approximately 6 months after radiosurgery, MRI is useful for monitoring the possible development of edema or signs of radiation damage.
- AVM patients can be followed with MRI and stereotactic angiography.

- PET recently has emerged as a useful way to differentiate tumor from necrosis in previously irradiated patients. It may also have potential for evaluating recurrent brain tumors for malignant degeneration (25) and predicting prognosis after therapy (26).

TOTAL-BODY AND HEMIBODY IRRADIATION

Total-Body Irradiation

- Total-body irradiation (TBI) has been used as a form of systemic therapy for various malignant diseases since the turn of this century.

Applications

Immunosuppression

- Low-dose TBI (less than 2 Gy given as a single fraction or multiple 0.05- to 0.15-Gy fractions given two to five times per week) has been used for patients with autoimmune diseases (27).
- In allogeneic bone marrow transplantation (BMT), higher doses (greater than 9.5 Gy) are often required to prevent graft rejection (28).
- When patients with aplastic anemia are prepared for BMT, a single dose of 3 Gy has been used in conjunction with cyclophosphamide to reduce the probability of graft rejection (29).

Low-dose systemic therapy for chronic lymphocytic leukemia and non-Hodgkin's lymphoma

- Patients receive 0.05 to 0.15 Gy two to five times per week for leukocytosis.
- It is generally recommended to give 4 to 8 weeks off after each 0.5-Gy TBI to avoid severe thrombocytopenia (30).

High-dose cytoreductive therapy before bone marrow or peripheral blood stem cell transplantation

- Shank et al. (31) used 1.2 Gy given three times per day, as well as partial lung blocks to protect the lungs. Use of this hyperfractionation schedule has reduced the incidence of interstitial pneumonitis to 33%, compared to 70% with single-dose TBI (10 Gy).

Technique

The general dosimetry approach recommended by the American Association of Physicists in Medicine (AAPM) (32) for calibration is a three-step process: (a) an absolute calibration of the radiation beam using the AAPM TG-21 protocol (33) for large-field geometry at TBI distance must be determined; (b) this dose must be corrected so that it represents the dose that would be obtained under full scattering conditions; and (c) corrections should be made for patient dimensions in terms of the area of the patient intersecting the radiation beam and patient thickness.

- Blankets provide an 8-mm tissue-equivalent bolus.

- A 2-cm-thick Plexiglas screen placed approximately 10 cm from the patient as the source of scattered electrons provides near-maximum dose to the skin for both 6- and 18-MV x-rays.
- Dose rate lower than 0.05 Gy per minute is expected to reduce the incidence of interstitial pneumonitis.

Complications

Low-dose total-body irradiation
- The major side effect of low-dose TBI is thrombocytopenia, which usually occurs after doses exceeding 1.0 to 1.5 Gy (34).

High-dose total-body irradiation
- Nausea, vomiting, and diarrhea are the most common early side effects with a single fraction or multiple fractions totaling 8 to 10 Gy (35).
- Dry mouth, reduction in tear formation, and sore throat develop within 10 days.
- A side effect that is unique to TBI is parotitis, which usually occurs after the first day of irradiation and subsides within 24 to 48 hours (36).
- Venoocclusive disease of the liver, characterized by hepatic enlargement, ascites, jaundice, encephalopathy, and weight gain, occurs in 10% to 20% of patients (37).
- Interstitial pneumonitis occurred in approximately 50% of BMT patients who received a single large fraction of TBI; approximately half of these patients died of this complication (38). Use of fractionated or low dose rate TBI has greatly diminished its incidence (39). Approximately 26% of interstitial pneumonitis cases are directly attributed to TBI or chemotherapy; 42% are associated with cytomegalovirus (40). The median time to diagnosis of interstitial pneumonitis is approximately 2 months. A dose-response curve for interstitial pneumonitis based on the experience at Toronto, using high dose rates of 0.5 to 4.0 Gy per minute, is steep and indicates that the onset of radiation pneumonitis occurs at approximately 7.5 Gy (absolute dose, which is 10% to 24% higher than the uncorrected dose), with the 5% actuarial incidence occurring at approximately 8.2 Gy (41). The sigmoidal complication curve rises dramatically, demonstrating a 50% and 95% incidence at 9.3 and 10.6 Gy, respectively.
- Approximately 85% of patients who receive a single, large dose of TBI develop cataract within 11 years; the incidence is 34% when 12 Gy of fractionated TBI is used (42).
- High-dose TBI produces primary gonadal failure in almost all patients. Thyroid dysfunction has been observed in approximately 43% of patients (43). Deterioration of renal function occurs in most patients undergoing BMT (44).
- The risk of developing a second tumor 10 years after intensive chemoradiation and BMT is estimated to be approximately 20% (39).

Hemibody Irradiation

- Hemibody irradiation (HBI) was developed as a method to treat patients with disseminated tumors involving multiple sites (45).
- Prospective randomized trials by RTOG showed that single high-dose HBI is as effective as conventional fractionated irradiation in achieving pain control in patients with

multiple metastases (46). The most effective HBI doses found by the RTOG study were 6 Gy for upper HBI and 8 Gy for lower and middle HBI, with 80% pain improvement at 1 week. Doses beyond these levels do not appear to increase pain relief or duration of relief or give a faster response.

- Poulter et al. (47) reported the results of RTOG 82-06, which compared HBI added to local irradiation with local radiation therapy alone, and showed that adjuvant single-dose, half-body irradiation delayed the progression of the existing disease, reduced the frequency of new disease (68% versus 50%), and delayed (as well as reduced) the need for retreatment (78% versus 60%). When prostate cancer patients in this trial were analyzed separately, there was also a trend toward survival benefit at 1 year (44% versus 33%) in favor of the patients who received HBI (48).
- When treatment of the other half of the body is indicated, it is advisable to wait 6 to 8 weeks to allow for sufficient recovery of blood cells (45).

Technique

- Subtotal body irradiation is usually divided into upper, lower, and middle HBI.
- A line passing across the bottom of L4 is commonly used to separate upper and lower HBI (49).
- When upper HBI is given, appropriate lung blocks should be used to limit the midline lung dose to less than 7 Gy.

Sequelae

- Hematologic toxicity (bone marrow depression) usually disappears in 4 to 6 weeks.
- Potentially fatal interstitial pneumonitis can be avoided if the dose of upper HBI is limited to 6 Gy.

IMAGE-GUIDED RADIOTHERAPY

- All current cancer radiotherapy is image-guided in the sense that some picture of the tumor region (most often CT) is used to plan the course of treatment whether by brachytherapy or external beam irradiation. However, the new image-guided radiotherapy (IGRT) methods coming onstream are using dynamic and/or functional imaging of the tumor. See Mell et al. (50) for a recent review.
- Standard RT is static in that a single treatment plan is developed by the radiation oncologist and medical physicist. Fiducial markers, either external (e.g., molds, tattoos) or internal (gold pins), may be used to register the patient on the couch prior to each treatment session. For sites such as thoracic, where respiratory motion is a significant factor, treatment margins are increased to adequately cover the tumor through the inspiration-exhalation cycle.

Interfraction Adjustments

- These treatment alterations are concerned with changes in the target location and size, which occur on a timescale much longer than breathing motions. Many patients are treated with combined modalities, for example, chemotherapy and RT. Hence, one can expect (and anticipate) significant movements of the tumor due to cell kill, anatomical changes in the body (e.g., weight loss), and long-term shifts in the placement of the parent organ as tumor burden is lowered.

- PET can be used to image the biologically active tumor sites. Advantages are relatively low radiation dose (comparable to a pelvic CT) specificity to metabolically active tumor, especially in soft tissues, which have poor contrast on CT or ultrasound (US). Disadvantages are high cost, short half-life of positron-emitting nuclides, limited spatial resolution, and complications of image registration.

- US. This is a relatively inexpensive, widely available imaging method, which images anatomical features based on differences in the local density. Image registration is still a task, but unlike CT or PET, no ionizing radiation is employed. Given the speed of sound in typical biologic tissues (about 1,500 m per second) and US transducers operating at or above 2 MHz, the spatial resolution should be better than 1 mm. A key advantage is the small size of the transducers, which allows presence in the linac treatment area. Potential pitfalls are improper probes to skin placement, leading to deterioration of image quality and reproducibility and difficulty in resolving structures with similar mass density (e.g., soft tissues).

- MRI. MRI can give high resolution images, and by use of specific rf pulse sequences, the view can contrast-select for certain tissue types (e.g., CNS) and even malignant versus nonmalignant regions because of known variations in the spin-lattice (T1) or spin-spin (T2) relaxation times. No ionizing radiation is used, but MRI is still relatively expensive compared to CT and requires a high-field open bore magnet, typically superconducting with cryogenic cooling. This makes placement in the linac treatment area rather difficult.

- CT. Various methods have been used to get coregistered x-ray pictures while the patient is on the RT treatment couch. Some linac machines simply incorporate kV x-ray tubes and detectors orthogonal to the MV beam line; others place the CT source and detector on a movable rail or on the MV gantry. New machines are using x-rays from the treatment beam itself to generate images, such as the so-called cone beam CT. The latter either uses MV photons generated at lower voltages from treatment, or with an in-line target to generate kV photons. In all cases, the CT scan is used to readjust the treatment, in many cases using dynamic multileaf collimators (DMLC).

Intrafraction Alternations

- The most serious tumor motions on the second timescale are due to the respiratory motions of the patient. Efforts have been made to coach patients to control breathing during irradiation, to restrict it with external restraints (and oxygen masks), but some of these are not options for patients with poor pulmonary function. The goal is to track (or estimate) the tumor movement in real time and interactively modulate the treatment beam accordingly.

- The most common method being used now is called 4D gated imaging: either 4D CT or 4D PET (or both in combination), that is, images formed in three spatial dimensions with the fourth being time. The idea is that for both CT and PET, one can gate data acquisition into separate time windows, depending upon where one is in the respiratory cycle. (Similarly, the treatment beam can be gated in synchrony with breathing motions.) Determination of the actual respiratory cycle can be done externally (infrared reflectors on the patient's chest or abdomen) or internally from the images themselves. In the simplest case, one waits for the extremum of exhalation for high-dose irradiation with tight margins. Irradiation throughout the breathing cycle requires rather sophisticated computer control of the treatment beam using DMLC. These in turn require strict redundant shutoff mechanisms to prevent overdosage or misdosage caused by a software problem.

- As the spatial and temporal demands of imaging increase, so will the need for better algorithms and more powerful computing equipment. Fortunately, this is one area where the speed and data-handling capacity are growing while the size and cost of data storage and price per megaflop are ever decreasing. Not all technical upgrades are equally sensational—side by side with spectacular time-resolved CT images, one has MLC controller cards operating with serial communication protocols as antiquated as an Internet connection with a 14.4-kbps modem.

PARTICLE BEAM RADIOTHERAPY

- When high-energy charged particles, protons or carbon ions, for example, move through the matter, these ionized atoms deposit their energy along their path. At the end of their path immediately before the particles come to rest, they release most of the energy before rapidly dropping to zero. This is called Bragg peak, after William Henry Bragg who discovered it in 1903.
- To vary the width of the peak, a technique named spread-out Bragg peak or SOBP can be used to encompass the location and depth of tumor into the irradiated tissue. Figure 4-1 illustrates the dose penetration for MV photons compared to monoenergetic protons at various beam energies, using water as a target. Notice the sharp spike for each proton beam at the end of its range. By allowing a range of proton energies, one can obtain quite an isotropic beam profile over a targeted depth range (51)
- At the end of 2008, there were a total of 26 proton therapy centers in Canada, China, England, France, Germany, Italy, Japan, Korea, Russia, South Africa, Sweden, Switzerland, and United States; over 60,000 patients had been treated (52).
- Indication for particle therapy can be categorized into two clinical scenarios.
- To escalate tumor dose while maintaining normal tissue exposure at a similar level of photon therapy. These include (but are not limited to) uveal melanoma (ocular tumors), skull base and paraspinal tumors (chondrosarcoma and chordoma), and unresectable sarcomas. In all these cases, proton therapy achieves significant improvements in the probability of local control over conventional radiotherapy (53–55).
- Charged particle therapy for ocular tumor (uveal melanoma) requires only a low-energy (about 70 MeV) proton beam.
- To reduce short- and long-term side effects but limiting the dose to normal tissue. In this case, tumor dose will remain the same so that there is no increase in tumor

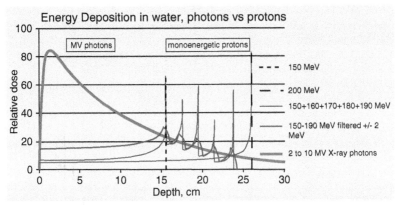

FIGURE 4-1. Dose penetration of MV photons and protons in water. The blue curve is a simple model-based exponential attenuation of the incident x-rays, convoluted with a shorter exponential falloff in energy deposition due to forward scattered electrons. Here, the forward scatter was given a characteristic length (1/e) of 0.5 cm and the attenuation as 10 cm. This curve is similar to the attenuation data in Figure 2 of Ahuja et al. (56). The spiked curves on the right are theoretical spectra for monoenergetic protons based on the model in Bortfeld (57). The curves exhibit the "Bragg peak" caused by the fact that charged particles lose their energy to the surrounding medium mostly at the end of their trajectory. Note that the depth of penetration is dependent on the initial energy of the proton. By the use of attenuating filters, one can create a distribution of incident particle energies and achieve a spread-out Bragg peak with a reasonably isotropic dosage in a range of depth. The figure shows the dosage of the sum of monoenergetic proton beams of 150 to 190 MeV in 10 MeV steps. With even minimal band-pass filtering, the spikes can be smoothed. Clearly, a beam containing all energies within a window could be made essentially flat in the region of the Bragg peaks.

control. These include but are not limited to pediatric neoplasms (such as medulloblastoma) and prostate cancer.

- In the case of pediatric cancers, there are convincing clinical data showing the advantage of sparing developing organs by using protons, and the resulting reduction of long-term damage to the surviving child.
- Currently, there is no prospective phase III study comparing proton therapy with IMRT for prostate cancer.

References

1. Low D, Purdy JA, Perez CA, et al. Intensity modulated radiation therapy. In: Levitt SH, Potish RA, Khan FM, et al., eds. *Levitt and Tapley's technological basis of radiation therapy: clinical applications*, 3rd ed. Baltimore, MD: Lippincott Williams & Wilkins, 1999:128–146.
2. Mackie R, Deasy J, Holmes T, et al. Letter in response to "Optimization of radiation therapy and the development of multileaf collimation" by Anders Brahme. *Int J Radiat Oncol Biol Phys* 1994;28(3):784–787.
3. Brahme A. Treatment optimization using physical and radiobiological objective functions. In: Smith A, ed. *Medical radiology, radiation therapy physics*. Berlin, Germany: Springer-Verlag, 1995:209–246.

4. Graham MV, Jain NL, Kahn MG, et al. Evaluation of an objective plan-evaluation model in the three dimensional treatment of nonsmall cell lung cancer. *Int J Radiat Oncol Biol Phys* 1996;34(2):469–474.

5. Chao KS, Low DA, Perez CA, et al. Intensity-modulated radiation therapy in head and neck cancers: the Mallinckrodt experience. *Int J Cancer* 2000;90(2):92–103.

6. Mackie TR, Holmes T, Swerdloff S, et al. Tomotherapy: a new concept for the delivery of dynamic conformal radiotherapy. *Med Phys* 1993;20(6):1709–1719.

7. Ruchala KJ, Olivera GH, Kapatoes JM, et al. Megavoltage CT image reconstruction during tomotherapy treatments. *Phys Med Biol* 2000;45(12):3545–3562.

8. Yu CX. Intensity-modulated arc therapy with dynamic multileaf collimation: an alternative to tomotherapy. *Phys Med Biol* 1995;40(9):1435–1449.

9. Stein J, Hartwig K, Levegrun S, et al. *Intensity-modulated treatments: compensators vs. multileaf modulation.* In: Leavitt D, Starkschall G, eds. *XII International Conference on the Use of Computers in Radiation Therapy.* Salt Lake City, UT: Medical Physics Publishing, 1997:338–341.

10. Low DA, Chao KS, Mutic S, et al. Quality assurance of serial tomotherapy for head and neck patient treatments. *Int J Radiat Oncol Biol Phys* 1998;42(3):681–692.

11. Portelance L, Chao KS, Grigsby PW, et al. Intensity-modulated radiation therapy (IMRT) reduces small bowel, rectum, and bladder doses in patients with cervical cancer receiving pelvic and para-aortic irradiation. *Int J Radiat Oncol Biol Phys* 2001;51(1):261–266.

12. Wasserman TH, Rich KM, Drzymala RE, et al. Stereotactic irradiation. In: Perez CA, Brady LW, eds. *Principles and practice of radiation oncology*, 3rd ed. Philadelphia, PA: Lippincott–Raven, 1998:387–404.

13. Verhey LJ, Smith VV. The physics of radiosurgery. *Semin Radiat Oncol* 1995;5(3):175–191.

14. Graf CJ, Perret GE, Torner JC. Bleeding from cerebral arteriovenous malformations as part of their natural history. *J Neurosurg* 1983;58(3):331–337.

15. Jane JA, Kassell NF, Torner JC, et al. The natural history of aneurysms and arteriovenous malformations. *J Neurosurg* 1985;62(3):321–323.

16. Steiner L. Stereotactic radiosurgery with the cobalt 60 gamma unit in the surgical treatment of intracranial tumors and arteriovenous malformations. In: Schmidek H, Sweet W, eds. *Operative neurosurgical techniques.* Philadelphia, PA: WB Saunders, 1988:515–529.

17. Kjellberg RN. Stereotactic Bragg peak proton beam radiosurgery for cerebral arteriovenous malformations. *Ann Clin Res* 1986;18(Suppl 47):17–19.

18. Shrieve DC, Alexander E III, Wen PY, et al. Comparison of stereotactic radiosurgery and brachytherapy in the treatment of recurrent glioblastoma multiforme. *Neurosurgery* 1995;36(2):275–282; discussion 282–274.

19. Souhami L, Seiferheld W, Brachman D, et al. Randomized comparison of stereotactic radiosurgery followed by conventional radiotherapy with carmustine to conventional radiotherapy with carmustine for patients with glioblastoma multiforme: report of Radiation Therapy Oncology Group 93-05 protocol. *Int J Radiat Oncol Biol Phys* 2004;60(3):853–860.

20. Andrews DW, Scott CB, Sperduto PW, et al. Whole brain radiation therapy with or without stereotactic radiosurgery boost for patients with one to three brain metastases: phase III results of the RTOG 9508 randomised trial. *Lancet* 2004;363(9422):1665–1672.

21. Valentino V, Schinaia G, Raimondi AJ. The results of radiosurgical management of 72 middle fossa meningiomas. *Acta Neurochir (Wien)* 1993;122(1–2):60–70.

22. Levin V, Gutin P, Leibel S. Neoplasms of the central nervous system. In: DeVita V, Hellman S, Rosenberg S, eds. *Cancer: principles and practice of oncology*, 4th ed. Philadelphia, PA: JB Lippincott Co., 1993.

23. Linskey ME, Lunsford LD, Flickinger JC. Radiosurgery for acoustic neurinomas: early experience. *Neurosurgery* 1990;26(5):736–744; discussion 744–735.

24. Marks L. Complications following radiosurgery: a review. *Radiat Oncol Invest* 1994;2:111.

25. Francavilla TL, Miletich RS, Di Chiro G, et al. Positron emission tomography in the detection of malignant degeneration of low-grade gliomas. *Neurosurgery* 1989;24(1):1–5.

26. Alavi JB, Alavi A, Chawluk J, et al. Positron emission tomography in patients with glioma. A predictor of prognosis. *Cancer* 1988;62(6):1074–1078.

27. Engel WK, Lichter AS, Galdi AP. Polymyositis: remarkable response to total body irradiation. *Lancet* 1981;1(8221):658.

28. Thomas ED, Storb R, Clift RA, et al. Bone-marrow transplantation. *N Engl J Med* 1975;292:832–843.

29. Feig SA, Champlin R, Arenson E, et al. Improved survival following bone marrow transplantation for aplastic anaemia. *Br J Haematol* 1983;54(4):509–517.

30. Del Regato JA. Proceedings: total body irradiation in the treatment of chronic lymphogenous leukemia. *Am J Roentgenol Radium Ther Nucl Med* 1974;120(3):504–520.

31. Shank B, Hopfan S, Kim JH, et al. Hyperfractionated total body irradiation for bone marrow transplantation: I. Early results in leukemia patients. *Int J Radiat Oncol Biol Phys* 1981;7(8):1109–1115.

32. Van Dyk J, Galvin JM, Glasgow GP, et al. The physical aspects of total- and half-body photon irradiation: a report of Task Group 29 Radiation Therapy Committee, AAPM report no. 17. College Park, MD: American Association of Physicists in Medicine, American Institute of Physics, 1986.

33. AAPM protocol for the determination of absorbed dose from high-energy photon and electron beams. *Med Phys* 1983;10(6):741–771.

34. Johnson RE, Ruhl U. Treatment of chronic lymphocytic leukemia with emphasis on total body irradiation. *Int J Radiat Oncol Biol Phys* 1976;1(5–6):387–397.

35. Goolden AW, Goldman JM, Kam KC, et al. Fractionation of whole body irradiation before bone marrow transplantation for patients with leukaemia. *Br J Radiol* 1983;56(664):245–250.

36. Deeg HJ. Delayed complications and long-term effects after bone marrow transplantation. *Hematol Oncol Clin North Am* 1990;4(3):641–657.

37. Ayash LJ, Hunt M, Antman K, et al. Hepatic venoocclusive disease in autologous bone marrow transplantation of solid tumors and lymphomas. *J Clin Oncol* 1990;8(10):1699–1706.

38. Keane TJ, Van Dyk J, Rider WD. Idiopathic interstitial pneumonia following bone marrow transplantation: the relationship with total body irradiation. *Int J Radiat Oncol Biol Phys* 1981;7(10):1365–1370.

39. Barrett AJ. Bone marrow transplantation. *Cancer Treat Rev* 1987;14(3–4):203–213.

40. Pecego R, Hill R, Appelbaum FR, et al. Interstitial pneumonitis following autologous bone marrow transplantation. *Transplantation* 1986;42(5):515–517.

41. Van Dyk J, Keane TJ, Kan S, et al. Radiation pneumonitis following large single dose irradiation: a re-evaluation based on absolute dose to lung. *Int J Radiat Oncol Biol Phys* 1981;7(4):461–467.

42. Benyunes MC, Sullivan KM, Deeg HJ, et al. Cataracts after bone marrow transplantation: long-term follow-up of adults treated with fractionated total body irradiation. *Int J Radiat Oncol Biol Phys* 1995;32(3):661–670.

43. Sklar CA, Kim TH, Ramsay NK. Thyroid dysfunction among long-term survivors of bone marrow transplantation. *Am J Med* 1982;73(5):688–694.

44. Bergstein J, Andreoli SP, Provisor AJ, et al. Radiation nephritis following total-body irradiation and cyclophosphamide in preparation for bone marrow transplantation. *Transplantation* 1986;41(1):63–66.

45. Fitzpatrick PJ, Rider WD. Half body radiotherapy. *Int J Radiat Oncol Biol Phys* 1976;1(3–4):197–207.

46. Salazar OM, Rubin P, Hendrickson FR, et al. Single-dose half-body irradiation for the palliation of multiple bone metastases from solid tumors: a preliminary report. *Int J Radiat Oncol Biol Phys* 1981;7(6):773–781.
47. Poulter CA, Cosmatos D, Rubin P, et al. A report of RTOG 8206: a phase III study of whether the addition of single dose hemibody irradiation to standard fractionated local field irradiation is more effective than local field irradiation alone in the treatment of symptomatic osseous metastases. *Int J Radiat Oncol Biol Phys* 1992;23(1):207–214.
48. Lin H-S, Drzymala RE. Total body and hemibody irradiation. In: Perez CA, Brady LW, eds. *Principles and practice of radiation oncology*, 3rd ed. Philadelphia, PA: Lippincott–Raven, 1998:333–342.
49. Rubin P, Salazar O, Zagars G, et al. Systemic hemibody irradiation for overt and occult metastases. *Cancer* 1985;55(9 Suppl):2210–2221.
50. Nell LK, Pawlicki T, Jiang SB, et al. Image-guided radiation therapy. In Halperin EC, Perez CA, Brady LW. *Principles and practice of radiation oncology*, 5th ed. Philadelphia, PA: Lippincott Williams & Wilkins, 2008:263-298
51. Park I. A new approach to produce spread-out Bragg peak using MINUIT fit. *Curr Appl Phys* 2009;9:852–855.
52. PTCOG. Particle therapy facilities in operation, 2010. http://ptwg.web.psi.ch/ptchentres.html
53. Gragoudas E, Li W, Goitein M, et al. Evidence-based estimates of outcome in patients irradiated for intraocular melanoma. *Arch Ophthalmol* 2002;120(12):1665–1671.
54. Munzenrider JE, Liebsch NJ. Proton therapy for tumors of the skull base. *Strahlenther Onkol* 1999;175(Suppl 2):57–63.
55. St Clair WH, Adams JA, Bues M, et al. Advantage of protons compared to conventional X-ray or IMRT in the treatment of a pediatric patient with medulloblastoma. *Int J Radiat Oncol Biol Phys* 2004;58(3):727–734.
56. Ahuja SD, Stroup SL, Bolin MG. Semi-empirical model for depth dose distributions of megavoltage x-ray beams. *Med Phys* 1980;7(5):537–544.
57. Bortfeld T. An analytical approximation of the Bragg curve for therapeutic proton beams. *Med Phys* 1997;24(12):2024–2033.

CHAPTER 5

ALTERED FRACTIONATION SCHEDULES

IRRADIATION FRACTIONATION REGIMENS (TABLE 5-1)

- *Conventional fractionation* consists of daily fractions of 1.8 to 2.0 Gy, 5 days per week; the total dose is determined by the tumor being treated and the tolerance of critical normal tissues in the target volume (usually 60 to 75 Gy).
- *Hyperfractionation* uses an increased number of fractions with the dose per fraction significantly reduced. Although the overall time is relatively unchanged, the total dose delivered is increased.
- *Quasi-hyperfractionation* is the same as hyperfractionation, except that total dose is not increased.
- In *accelerated fractionation*, overall time is significantly reduced; the number of fractions, total dose, and size of dose per fraction are unchanged or somewhat reduced, depending on the overall time reduction.
- *Quasi-accelerated fractionation* is the same as accelerated fractionation, except that overall time is not reduced because of treatment interruption, which defeats the rationale of accelerated fractionation.
- *Accelerated hyperfractionation* has features of both hyperfractionation and accelerated fractionation.
- *Concomitant boost* is an additional dose delivered one or more times per week to selected target volumes (i.e., gross tumor volume) through smaller field(s), along with the conventional dose to larger irradiated volumes.
- *Hypofractionation* is a dose given over a shorter period of time than standard radiotherapy and typically larger doses.
- To achieve an increase in tolerance of late-responding tissues through dose fractionation, the time interval between the dose fractions must be long enough (6 hours) to allow cellular repair to approach completion.
- Two Radiation Therapy Oncology Group (RTOG) reports showed an increased rate of late complications with hyperfractionated protocols when the mean interfraction interval was less than 4.5 hours (1). Most protocols now stipulate a minimum 6-hour interval between dose fractions. Clinical data suggest that this is adequate for normal tissues other than the spinal cord.

Table 5-1

Comparison of Various Fractionation Schedules

	Conventional	Split Course	Accelerated Fractionation	Hyperfractionation
Indication, in tumors, of growth rate	Average	Average or slow	Rapid	Slow (with large cell loss factors)
Normal tissue effects, acute	Standard	Standard or greater	Greater	Standard or greater
Normal tissue effects, late	Standard	Greater	Standard (if complete repair of sublethal damage occurs) or greater	Lower
Advantages	—	Shorter actual treatment time (fewer fractions)	Destroys more tumor cells; prevents tumor cell repopulation; less overall treatment time	Lower OER (5) with small doses; spares late damage; allows reoxygenation; allows stem cell repopulation
Disadvantages	—	May permit tumor repopulation	—	More fractions

OER, oxygen enhancement ratio.

OVERALL TIME

- The intensity of acute reactions is determined primarily by the rate of dose accumulation.
- The importance of the dose per fraction is a reflection of the biologic fact that acute reactions represent a deficit in the balance between the rate of cell killing by radiation and cell regeneration from surviving stem cells.
- After the stem cell population is depleted to the point at which it is unable to renew the functional layers of the epithelium, the acute reaction peaks, and further depopulation produces no increase in the severity of the reaction.
- The time taken to heal depends on the total dose, provided the weekly dose rate exceeds the regenerative ability of the surviving stem cells. This is because healing is a function of the absolute number of stem cells surviving the course of treatment, and the higher the total dose, the fewer stem cells will survive.
- Curability of many cancers (particularly squamous cell carcinomas) is highly dependent on overall treatment time; this has been interpreted in terms of accelerated regeneration of surviving tumor clonogens.
- Evidence for accelerated regeneration of surviving tumor cells after therapeutic intervention comes from three observations: time-to-recurrence data for tumors not sterilized by radiation therapy, comparison of split-course and continuous-course treatment regimens, and analysis of tumor control doses as a function of time (with correction for fraction size differences) (2).

SPLIT-COURSE VERSUS CONTINUOUS-COURSE TREATMENT

- In earlier studies, inferior results were found with split-course treatment for head and neck cancer, compared to continuous-course treatment, when daily and total doses were not adjusted to compensate for treatment interruptions (3).
- To compensate, approximately 0.6 Gy per day is needed to compensate for treatment interruptions and, therefore, a prolongation in treatment time (4).

LINEAR-QUADRATIC EQUATION

- The linear-quadratic equation is internally consistent for a wide range of tissue types and end points.
- Clinical application of the model for derivation of new fractionation schedules is limited by a lack of precise estimates of α/β.
- The α/β ratios of available human data are consistent with experimentally determined α/β ratios, with wide confidence limits (Table 5-2).

Table 5-2

α/β Ratios for Human Normal Tissues and Tumors

Tissue or Organ	End Point	α/β (Gy)[a]
Early Reactions		
Skin	Erythema	8.8–12.3
	Desquamation	11.2
Oral mucosa	Mucositis	8.8–15[b]
Late Reactions		
Skin/vasculature	Telangiectasia	2.8–3.9[b]
Subcutis	Fibrosis	1.9[b]
Muscle/vasculature/cartilage	Impaired shoulder movement	3.5
Nerve	Brachial plexopathy	<3.5[b]
	Brachial plexopathy	~2
	Optic neuropathy	1.6
Spinal cord	Myelopathy	<3.3
Eye	Corneal injury	2.9
Bowel	Stricture/perforation	2.2–8[b]
Lung	Pneumonitis	<3.8[b]
	Fibrosis (radiologic)	3.1
Head and neck	Various late effects	3.5–3.8
Oral cavity and oropharynx	Various late effects	0.8
Tumors		
Head and neck		
Larynx	—	13–18[b]
Vocal cord	—	>9.9[b]
Oropharynx	—	~16[b]
Buccal mucosa	—	6.6
Tonsil	—	14.7[b]
Nasopharynx	—	16
Skin	—	8.5[b]
Melanoma	—	0.6
Liposarcoma	—	0.4

[a]Studies related to these data may be found in the original publication.
[b]Reanalysis of original published data.
Data compiled by Bentzen and Thames (unpublished) from Thames HD, Bentzen SM, Turesson I, et al. Time-dose factors in radiotherapy: a review of the human data. *Radiother Oncol* 1990;19:219; Joiner MC, van der Kogel AJ. The value of α/β. In: Steel GG, ed. *Basic clinical radiobiology*, 2nd ed. London, UK: Arnold, 1997:111.

HYPERFRACTIONATION

- Small dose fractions allow higher total doses to be administered within the tolerance of late-responding normal tissues, and a higher biologically effective dose can be delivered to the tumor.
- Radiosensitization is achieved through redistribution and lesser dependence on oxygen effect.
- More severe acute reactions occur than with conventional fractionation, but a therapeutic gain should be realized in tumors with large α/β ratios.

ACCELERATED FRACTIONATION

- Reduction in overall treatment time decreases the opportunity for tumor cell regeneration during treatment and increases the probability of tumor control for a given total dose.
- Because overall treatment time has little influence on probability of late, normal tissue injury (provided the size of the dose per fraction is not increased and the interval between dose fractions is sufficient for complete repair to take place), a therapeutic gain should be realized.
- When the overall duration of treatment is markedly reduced, the total dose should be reduced as well, to prevent excessively severe acute reactions. Therapeutic gain is realized only if the dose that inhibits regeneration of tumor cells during the time by which treatment is shortened is below the maximum tolerated dose for acute reactions.
- Type A accelerated fractionation is a short course of treatment; overall duration of treatment is markedly reduced, and total dose is substantially decreased.
- In types B and C, duration of treatment is more modestly reduced, and total dose is kept in the similar range as conventional treatment by using split-course (type B) or concomitant-boost (type C) technique.
- In type D accelerated fractionation, the total dose delivered per week progressively increases during treatment; less-intensive therapy at the outset of treatment stimulates a regenerative response in normal mucosa so that it can better tolerate more intensive treatment as the course progresses. There is a slightly greater reduction in overall time (without decreasing total dose) than with types B and C.
- Techniques are differentiated on the basis of the strategy adopted to circumvent intolerable acute reactions: type A, reduction in dose; type B, break in treatment; type C, reduction in volume of mucosa exposed to accelerated treatment; and type D, stimulation of mucosal regenerative response by starting with a milder fractionation schedule (1) (Fig. 5-1).
- The overall take-home message with dose fractionation scheme is to use an optimal dose per fraction to deliver the total prescribed dose in as short a total treatment time as possible in order to maximize clinical gains.

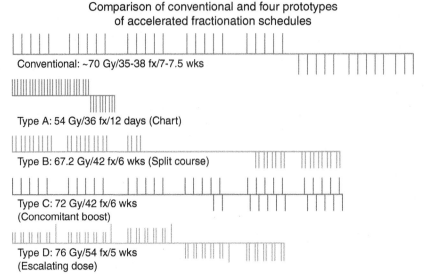

FIGURE 5-1. Conventional and accelerated fractionation schedules. For each regimen, the large-field treatment is depicted by bars above the horizontal line and the boost-field irradiation by the bars below the line. fx, fraction. (Reprinted with permission from Ahamad A. Altered fractionation schedules. In: Halperin EC, Wazer DE, Perez CA, et al., eds. *Principles and practice of radiation oncology*, 6th ed. Philadelphia, PA: Lippincott Williams & Wilkins, 2013:278–296; © Wolters Kluwer.)

CLINICAL STUDIES

Predominantly Hyperfractionation: Phase I and II Studies

- In head and neck studies, 2 daily fractions of 1.1 to 1.2 Gy were used, with interfraction intervals of 3 to 8 hours. Increased mucosal reactions were associated with improved tumor control; there was an increased risk of late complications with total doses over 76.8 Gy (5,6).
- In four brainstem glioma studies (2 daily fractions of 1.00 to 1.26 Gy, minimum 4-hour interfraction interval), there was no increase in brainstem necrosis; median survival time improved in one study (7).
- In the RTOG 83-11 lung cancer study (2 daily fractions of 1.2 Gy, minimum 4-hour interfraction interval, total doses of 60.0 to 79.2 Gy), no dose response for survival was noted; best survival (29% at 2 years) was with a total dose of 69.6 Gy in a subset of patients with favorable presentation. There was a trend toward an increased incidence of severe complications at the highest dose level (8).
- An RTOG bladder dose-escalation protocol (2 daily fractions of 1.2 Gy, minimum 4-hour interfraction interval, total dose of 60.0 to 69.6 Gy) reported a 10% 2-year actuarial incidence of grade 3 and 4 late complications, suggesting that acceptable tolerance of pelvic organs may be significantly increased through hyperfractionation (9).

Predominantly Hyperfractionation: Phase III Studies

- Multiple prospective randomized phase III clinical trials have been performed (four in head and neck carcinomas, one in bladder cancer, two in non–small cell lung cancer, one in brainstem tumors, and more) (10–17).
- In a study of T2-3N0-1 tumors of the oropharynx comparing 2 fractions of 1.15 Gy, 6- to 8-hour interfraction interval, total dose of 80.5 Gy in 7 weeks versus 1 daily fraction of 2 Gy, total dose of 70 Gy in 7 weeks, with hyperfractionation, there was an improved overall 5-year locoregional control rate (59%) ($p = 0.02$) (improvement in T3 but not in T2 primary tumors), improved overall survival ($p = 0.08$), and more severe mucosal reactions; late treatment-related morbidity was the same (10).

Type A: Continuous Short Intensive Courses

- In Burkitt's lymphoma, with 3 daily fractions of 1.00 to 1.25 Gy, there were greatly improved response rates compared with 1 daily fraction to similar total doses (18).
- With continuous hyperfractionated accelerated radiation therapy (CHART) for head and neck cancer, primarily stage III or IV cancers of the oral cavity, oropharynx, hypopharynx, and larynx, a short, intensive irradiation schedule was used (3 daily fractions of 1.5 Gy, 6-hour intervals, for 12 consecutive days, total dose of 54 Gy) (19). Three-year local tumor control was 49% compared to 36% in matched historic controls. Healing of acute reactions was delayed beyond 6 months in approximately 20%; late effects were no worse or were less severe than with conventional fractionation, except for radiation-induced myelitis (four patients with spinal cord doses of 45 to 48 Gy).
- In a phase III trial of CHART (66 Gy in 33 fractions in 6.5 weeks) versus conventional fractionation in 918 patients with head and neck cancer, including all sites and stages except T1N0, there was no significant difference in tumor control or survival, although there was a trend for CHART to be more effective in achieving control of higher-stage tumors (20). Acute mucosal reactions were more severe with CHART, although there was no difference in late reactions; myelopathy did not occur when spinal cord dose was limited to 40 Gy.
- In a phase III postoperative accelerated fractionation study, patients with stage T3-4N0-2 carcinomas of various head and neck sites were randomized, after surgical resection, to receive either 50 Gy in 25 fractions in 5 weeks or 42 Gy in 30 fractions, three times a day with 4-hour intervals in 11 days (21). Accelerated hyperfractionation was associated with higher actuarial disease-free survival and a lower late complication rate at 3 years in 56 patients and with higher survival in patients with fast-proliferating tumors (thymidine labeling index greater than 10.4% or T^{pot} less than 4.5 days). The overall late complication rate was very high (approximately 75%).
- A study of 103 patients with inoperable breast cancer treated with a short, intensive course showed 34.6% tumor control at 5 years; significant late effects occurred when total doses exceeded 45 Gy (22). In 42 patients with inflammatory breast cancer who were treated with accelerated fractionation (51 to 54 Gy in 4 weeks, plus a boost),

the locoregional control rate significantly improved over historic controls treated with protracted Baclesse technique (23).

- Two studies of non–small cell lung cancer treated with accelerated fractionation (66 Gy in 1.8 to 2.0 Gy fractions in 4 weeks (24) or the CHART regimen described earlier (19,20)) reported encouraging tumor responses, but esophagitis was severe.

- In a randomized, phase III trial of non–small cell lung cancer patients with disease apparently confined to chest, CHART was compared with conventional fractionation (60 Gy in 30 fractions in 6 weeks); there was a significant survival advantage with CHART (29% 2-year rate versus 20% with conventional treatment) and a 21% reduction in local progression (25). Intrathoracic tumor control was not significantly different. The incidence of severe dysphagia was 49% with CHART and 19% with conventional therapy.

Type C: Concomitant Boost

- In 79 patients with moderately advanced oropharyngeal primary lesions, overall 2-year locoregional tumor control was 68%, with best results obtained when boost was given during the last 2.0 to 2.5 weeks of basic treatment course (2-year locoregional control of 78%). There was an increase in severe acute reactions but no increase in late treatment complications (23). In an update in 127 patients treated with concomitant boost, delivered during the later part of the basic treatment, 4-year locoregional tumor control was 72%, increasing to 81% with surgical salvage (26).

- In a nonrandomized study of 100 patients, 50 received accelerated fractionation (total doses of 68.4 to 73.4 Gy in 42 to 65 days), and 50 received conventional fractionation (total dose of 70.6 Gy in 52 to 54 days); concomitant boost was given during the first and middle thirds of the basic treatment course. Significantly higher 3-year locoregional control (62% versus 33%) and disease-specific survival (66% versus 38%) occurred with concomitant boost; there was increased acute toxicity in the accelerated fractionation group (27).

Other Randomized Trials

- Although altered fractionation regimens have been the focus of intense study to improve locoregional tumor control for radiation therapy of head and neck cancers, the results of a recently reported RTOG study were below expectations (13). In RTOG 9003, 1,073 patients with locally advanced head and neck cancer were randomly assigned to four different fractionation schemes: standard fractionation (70 Gy, 35 fractions, 7 weeks), hyperfractionation (81.6 Gy, 1.2 Gy per fraction, twice daily for 7 weeks), accelerated fractionation with split course (to 67.2 Gy, 1.6 Gy per fraction, twice daily for 6 weeks including a 2-week rest after 38.4 Gy), and accelerated fractionation with concomitant boost (72 Gy, 1.8 Gy daily fraction, and 1.5 Gy boost as a second daily treatment for the last 12 treatments over 6 weeks). Approximately, 60% of patients analyzed had cancer in the oropharynx. With a median follow-up of 23 months, the results indicated a small but significantly better locoregional control in patients treated with hyperfractionation (54.4%) and accelerated fractionation with concomitant boost (54.5%) than those treated with standard fractionation (46%).

- In patients with locally advanced head and neck cancer, a combination of hyper-fractionated irradiation (75 Gy, 1.25 Gy twice a day) and cisplatin/5-fluorouracil chemotherapy (cisplatin 12 mg/m^2 daily and fluorouracil 600 mg/m^2/d during weeks 1 and 6 of irradiation) was more efficacious than hyperfractionated irradiation alone (28,29). The relapse-free survival rate was higher in the combined-treatment group (61% versus 41%, p = 0.08). The rate of locoregional control of disease at 3 years was 70% in the combined-treatment group and 44% in the hyperfractionation group (p = 0.01).

Hypofractionation

- Hypofractionation has been a common practice in the United Kingdom and Canada, and data are available in breast, prostate, and brain cancer.
- UK Standardisation of Breast Radiotherapy Trial B randomized early breast cancer patients to conventional fractionation of 50 Gy in 25 fractions versus hypofraction-ation of 40 Gy in 15 fractions. At 5 years, locoregional tumor relapse was 2.2% in the hypofractionated group versus 3.3% in the conventional group (30).
- The sister trial, UK Standardisation of Breast Radiotherapy Trial A, tested two differ-ent hypofractionation regimens of 41.6 and 39 Gy, both in 13 fractions. At 5 years, locoregional tumor relapse was 3.6% in the conventional group, 3.5% in the 41.6 Gy group, and 5.2% in the 39 Gy group (31).
- A Canadian trial of conventional radiotherapy versus hypofractionated radiotherapy for early breast cancer patients found no difference in locoregional control (32).
- The American Society for Radiation Oncology has developed a guideline to pro-vide direction for the fractionation of breast cancer (33). In brief, hypofractionation should be reserved for patients 50 years or older, pathologic stage T1-2N0 with breast-conserving surgery, not been treated with systemic chemotherapy, minimum dose no less than 93% and maximum dose no greater than 107%.
- Fox Chase Cancer Center performed a randomized trial of prostate cancer patients to conventional fractionation of 78 Gy in 38 fractions to hypofractionation of 70.2 Gy in 26 fractions using intensity-modulated radiotherapy. They found that GI toxicity was mildly increased during weeks 2, 3, and 4 in the hypofractionation arm (34).
- Multiple ongoing randomized trials of hypofractionation versus conventional radio-therapy for prostate cancers will provide more answer on long-term efficacy and toxicity.
- A Canadian trial randomized glioblastoma patients 60 years of age or older with a KPS greater than 50 to conventional radiotherapy of 60 Gy in 30 fractions versus hypofractionation of 40 Gy in 15 fractions. Of note, temozolomide was not given concurrently. The overall survival between both arms was similar (35).
- Additional randomized trial of hypofractionation for glioblastoma patients has been published (36,37). The American Society for Radiation Oncology has recently pub-lished guidelines for glioblastoma patients for consideration of hypofractionation (38).

CONCLUSIONS

- In some trials for head and neck cancer, altered fractionated schedules have been proven to be more efficacious than standard irradiation.
- In other tumors, altered fractionation schedules should be further investigated in additional clinical trials.
- Hypofractionation is increasingly utilized for breast, prostate, and brain cancer as well other sites and should be considered in the appropriate group of patients.

References

1. Ahamad A. Altered fractionation schedules. In: Halperin EC, Wazer DE, Perez CA, et al., eds. *Principles and practice of radiation oncology*, 6th ed. Philadelphia, PA: Lippincott Williams & Wilkins, 2013:278–296.
2. Withers HR, Taylor JM, Maciejewski B. The hazard of accelerated tumor clonogen repopulation during radiotherapy. *Acta Oncol* 1988;27(2):131–146.
3. Million RR, Zimmermann RC. Evaluation of University of Florida split-course technique for various head and neck squamous cell carcinomas. *Cancer* 1975;35(6):1533–1536.
4. Budihna M, Skrk J, Smid L, et al. Tumor cell repopulation in the rest interval of split-course radiation treatment. *Strahlentherapie* 1980;156(6):402–408
5. Parsons JT, Mendenhall WM, Stringer SP, et al. Twice-a-day radiotherapy for squamous cell carcinoma of the head and neck: the University of Florida experience. *Head Neck* 1993;15(2):87–96.
6. Wendt CD, Peters LJ, Ang KK, et al. Hyperfractionated radiotherapy in the treatment of squamous cell carcinomas of the supraglottic larynx. *Int J Radiat Oncol Biol Phys* 1989;17(5):1057–1062.
7. Linstadt DE, Edwards MS, Prados M, et al. Hyperfractionated irradiation for adults with brain-stem gliomas. *Int J Radiat Oncol Biol Phys* 1991;20(4):757–760.
8. Cox JD, Azarnia N, Byhardt RW, et al. A randomized phase I/II trial of hyperfractionated radiation therapy with total doses of 60.0 Gy to 79.2 Gy: possible survival benefit with greater than or equal to 69.6 Gy in favorable patients with Radiation Therapy Oncology Group stage III non-small-cell lung carcinoma: report of Radiation Therapy Oncology Group 83-11. *J Clin Oncol* 1990;8(9):1543–1555.
9. Cox JD, Guse C, Asbell S, et al. Tolerance of pelvic normal tissues to hyperfractionated radiation therapy: results of Protocol 83-08 of the Radiation Therapy Oncology Group. *Int J Radiat Oncol Biol Phys* 1998;15(6):1331–1336.
10. Horiot J, LeFur RN, Schraub S, et al. Status of the experience of the EORTC Cooperative Group of Radiotherapy with hyperfractionated and accelerated radiotherapy regimes. *Semin Radiat Oncol* 1992;2:34–37.
11. Pinto LH, Canary PC, Araujo CM, et al. Prospective randomized trial comparing hyperfractionated versus conventional radiotherapy in stages III and IV oropharyngeal carcinoma. *Int J Radiat Oncol Biol Phys* 1991;21(3):557–562.
12. Cummings B, O'Sullivan B, Keane T. 5-Year results of a 4 week/twice daily radiation schedule: the Toronto trial. *Radiother Oncol* 2000;56:S8.
13. Fu KK, Pajak TF, Trotti A, et al. A Radiation Therapy Oncology Group (RTOG) phase III randomized study to compare hyperfractionation and two variants of accelerated fractionation to standard fractionation radiotherapy for head and neck squamous cell carcinomas: first report of RTOG 9003. *Int J Radiat Oncol Biol Phys* 2000;48(1):7–16.
14. Naslund I, Nilsson B, Littbrand B. Hyperfractionated radiotherapy of bladder cancer. A ten-year follow-up of a randomized clinical trial. *Acta Oncol* 1994;33(4):397–402.

15. Sause W, Kolesar P, Taylor SI, et al. Final results of phase III trial in regionally advanced unresectable non-small cell lung cancer: Radiation Therapy Oncology Group, Eastern Cooperative Oncology Group, ad Southwest Oncology Group. *Chest* 2000;117(2):358–364.

16. Curran WJ, Paulus R, Langer CJ, et al. Sequential vs. concurrent chemoradiation for stage III non-small cell lung cancer: randomized phase III trial RTOG 9410. *J Natl Cancer Inst* 2011;103(19):1452–1460.

17. Mandell LR, Kadota R, Freeman C, et al. There is no role for hyperfractionated radiotherapy in the management of children with newly diagnosed diffuse intrinsic brainstem tumors: results of a Pediatric Oncology Group phase III trial comparing conventional vs hyperfractionated radiotherapy. *Int J Radiat Oncol Biol Phys* 1999;43(5)959–964.

18. Norin T, Onyango J. Radiotherapy in Burkitt's lymphoma: conventional or superfractionated regime—early results. *Int J Radiat Oncol Biol Phys* 1977;2(5–6):399–406.

19. Dische S, Saunders MI. The CHART regimen and morbidity. *Acta Oncol* 1999;38(2):147–152.

20. Dische S, Saunders M, Barrett A, et al. A randomised multicentre trial of CHART versus conventional radiotherapy in head and neck cancer. *Radiother Oncol* 1997;44(2):123–136.

21. Awwad HK, Khafagy Y, Barsoum M, et al. Accelerated versus conventional fractionation in the postoperative irradiation of locally advanced head and neck cancer: influence of tumour proliferation. *Radiother Oncol* 1992;25(4):261–266.

22. Svoboda VH, Krawczyk J, Krawczyk A. Seventeen years experience with accelerated radiotherapy for carcinoma of the breast. *Int J Radiat Oncol Biol Phys* 1992;24(1):65–71.

23. Ang KK, Peters LJ, Weber RS, et al. Concomitant boost radiotherapy schedules in the treatment of carcinoma of the oropharynx and nasopharynx. *Int J Radiat Oncol Biol Phys* 1990;19(6):1339–1345.

24. von Rottkay P. Remissions and acute toxicity during accelerated fractionated irradiation of non-small-cell bronchial carcinoma. *Strahlenther Onkol* 1986;162(5):300–307.

25. Saunders M, Dische S, Barrett A, et al. Continuous, hyperfractionated, accelerated radiotherapy (CHART) versus conventional radiotherapy in non-small cell lung cancer: mature data from the randomised multicentre trial. CHART Steering Committee. *Radiother Oncol* 1999;52(2):137–148.

26. Ang K, Peters LJ. Concomitant boost radiotherapy in the treatment of head and neck cancers. *Semin Radiat Oncol* 1992;2:31–33.

27. Johnson CR, Schmidt-Ullrich RK, Wazer DE. Concomitant boost technique using accelerated superfractionated radiation therapy for advanced squamous cell carcinoma of the head and neck. *Cancer* 1992;69(11):2749–2754.

28. Brizel DM, Albers ME, Fisher SR, et al. Hyperfractionated irradiation with or without concurrent chemotherapy for locally advanced head and neck cancer. *N Engl J Med* 1998;338(25):1798–1804.

29. Barker JL, Montague ED, Peters LJ. Clinical experience with irradiation of inflammatory carcinoma of the breast with and without elective chemotherapy. *Cancer* 1980;45(4):625–629.

30. Bentzen SM, Agrawal RK, Aird EG, et al. The UK Standardisation of Breast Radiotherapy (START) Trial B of radiotherapy hypofractionation for treatment of early breast cancer: a randomised trial. *Lancet* 2008;371(9618):1098–1107.

31. Bentzen SM, Agrawal RK, Aird EG, et al. The UK Standardisation of Breast Radiotherapy (START) Trial A of radiotherapy hypofractionation for treatment of early breast cancer: a randomised trial. *Lancet Oncol* 2008;9(4):331–341.

32. Whelan TJ, Pignol JP, Levine MN, et al. Long-term results of hypofractionated radiation therapy for breast cancer. *N Engl J Med* 2010;362(6):513–520.

33. Smith BD, Bentzen SM, Correa CR, et al. Fractionation for whole breast irradiation: an American Society for Radiation Oncology (ASTRO) evidence-based guidelines. *Int J Radiat Oncol Biol Phys* 2011;81(1):59–68.

34. Pollack A, Hanlon AL, Horwitz EM, et al. Dosimetry and preliminary acute toxicity in the first 100 men treated for prostate cancer on a randomized hypofractionation dose escalation trial. *Int J Radiat Oncol Biol Phys* 2006;64(2):518–526.
35. Roa W, Brasher PM, Bauman G, et al. Abbreviated course of radiation therapy in older patients with glioblastoma multiforme: a prospective randomized clinical trial. *J Clin Oncol* 2004;22(9):1583–1588.
36. Malmström A, Grønberg BH, Marosi C, et al. Temozolomide versus standard 6-week radiotherapy versus hypofractionated radiotherapy in patients older than 60 years with glioblastoma: the Nordic randomised, phase 3 trial. *Lancet Oncol* 2012;13(9):916–926.
37. Perry JR, Laperriere N, O'Callaghan CJ, et al. Short-course radiation plus temozolomide in elderly patients with glioblastoma. *N Engl J Med* 2017;376(11):1027–1037.
38. Cabrera AR, Kirkpatrick JP, Fiveash JB, et al. Radiation therapy for glioblastoma: executive summary of an American Society for Radiation Oncology Evidence-Based Clinical Practice Guidelines. *Pract Radiat Oncol* 2016;6(4):217-225.

CHAPTER 6

PHYSICS AND DOSIMETRY OF BRACHYTHERAPY

BRACHYTHERAPY TECHNIQUES

- Brachytherapy (*brachy*, from the Greek for "short distance") consists of placing sealed radioactive sources close to, or in contact with, the target tissue.
- Implantation techniques may be broadly characterized in terms of the following: surgical approach to the target volume (interstitial, intracavitary, transluminal, or mold techniques), means of controlling the dose delivered (temporary or permanent implants), source loading technology (preloaded, manually afterloaded, or remotely afterloaded), and dose rate (low, medium, or high).
- Intracavitary insertion consists of positioning applicators containing radioactive sources into a body cavity in close proximity to the target tissue. The most widely used intracavitary treatment technique is insertion of a tandem and colpostats for cervical cancer.
- All intracavitary implants are temporary; they are left in the patient for a specified time (usually 24 to 168 hours after source insertion for low dose rate [LDR] therapy) to deliver the prescribed dose.
- Interstitial brachytherapy consists of surgically implanting small radioactive sources directly into the target tissues.
- A permanent interstitial implant remains in place forever. The initial source strength is chosen so that the prescribed dose is fully delivered when the implanted radioactivity has decayed to a negligible level.
- Surface-dose applications (sometimes called *plesiocurie* or *mold therapy*) consist of an applicator containing an array of radioactive sources, usually designed to deliver a uniform dose distribution to the intraoperative tumor bed, skin, or mucosal surface.
- Transluminal brachytherapy consists of inserting a line source into a body lumen to treat its surface and adjacent tissues (1,2).
- Radiation exposure to nursing staff (and other hospital staff responsible for source loading and the care of implant patients) can be greatly reduced or eliminated by using remote afterloading devices, which consist of a pneumatically or motor-driven source transport system for robotically transferring radioactive material between a shielded safe and each treatment applicator (3).

DOSE RATE

- According to International Commission on Radiation Units and Measurements (ICRU) Report No. 38 (4), LDR implants deliver doses at a rate of 40 to 200 cGy per hour (0.4 to 2.0 Gy per hour), requiring treatment times of 24 to 144 hours.
- High dose rate (HDR) brachytherapy uses dose rates in excess of 0.2 Gy per minute (12 Gy per hour). Modern HDR remote afterloaders contain sources capable of delivering dose rates of 0.12 Gy per second (430 Gy per hour) at 1-cm distance, resulting in treatment times of a few minutes. A heavily shielded vault and remote afterloading device are essential components of an HDR brachytherapy facility.
- Temporary LDR implant patients must be confined to the hospital during treatment to manage the radiation safety hazard posed by the ambient exposure rates around the implant. HDR implants are usually performed as outpatient procedures.
- Although not recognized by ICRU Report No. 38, the ultralow dose rate range (0.01 to 0.30 Gy per hour) is important; it is the dose rate used for permanent iodine-125 (^{125}I) and palladium-103 (^{103}Pd) seed implants.
- The clinical utility of any radionuclide depends on physical properties such as half-life, radiation output per unit activity, specific activity (Ci per g), and photon energy. Detailed properties of radionuclides are listed in Table 6-1.

CLASSIC SYSTEMS FOR INTERSTITIAL IMPLANTS

- The traditional implant systems (Manchester, Quimby, and Paris) were developed before the advent of computer-aided dosimetry for implant therapy.
- For target volumes identified intraoperatively by palpation and direct visualization, classic systems continue to guide the radiation oncologist in arranging and positioning sources relative to the target volume. They also serve as the basis of dose prescription, whether or not computer-assisted treatment planning is used.
- For all types of implants, classic systems are useful for advanced planning of interstitial implants and for manually verifying postinsertion computer plans.
- An interstitial implant system consists of the following elements:
  - *Distribution rules*: Given a target volume, these rules determine how to distribute the radioactive sources and applicators in and around the target volume.
  - *Dose-specification and implant-optimization criteria*: At the heart of each system is a dose-specification criterion (definition of prescribed dose). In the Manchester or Paterson-Parker (P-P) system, for example, the prescribed dose is the modal dose in the volume bounded by the peripheral sources. The distribution rules and dose-specification criterion together constitute a compromise among implant quality indices, such as dose homogeneity within the target volume, normal tissue sparing, number of catheters implanted (amount of trauma inflicted), dosimetric margin around the target, and presence of high-dose regions outside the target.
  - *Dose calculation aids*: These are used to estimate the source strengths required to achieve the prescribed dose rate (as specified by the system) for source arrangements

Table 6-1

Physical Properties and Uses of Brachytherapy Radionuclides

Element	Isotope	Energy (MeV)	Half-Life	HVL-Lead (mm)	Exposure Rate Constant^a ($\Gamma\delta$)	Source Form	Clinical Application
Obsolete Sealed Sources of Historic Significance							
Radium	^{226}Ra	0.83 (average)	1,626 y	16	8.25^b	Tubes and needles	LDR intracavitary and interstitial
Currently Used Sealed Sources							
Cesium	^{137}Cs	0.662	30 y	6.5	3.28	Tubes and needles	LDR intracavitary and interstitial
Iridium	^{192}Ir	0.397 (average)	73.8 d	6	4.69	Seeds	LDR temporary interstitial / HDR interstitial and intracavitary
Cobalt	^{60}Co	1.25	5.26 y	11	13.07	Encapsulated spheres	HDR intracavitary
Iodine	^{125}I	0.028	59.6 d	0.025	1.45	Seeds	Permanent interstitial
Palladium	^{103}Pd	0.020	17 d	0.013	1.48	Seeds	Permanent interstitial
Gold	^{198}Au	0.412	2.7 d	6	2.35	Seeds	Permanent interstitial
Strontium	^{90}Sr-^{90}Y	2.24 β_{max}	28.9 y	—	—	Plaque	Treatment of superficial ocular lesions
Unsealed Radioisotopes Used for Radiopharmaceutical Therapy							
Strontium	^{89}Sr	1.4 β_{max}	51 d	—	—	SrCl$_2$ i.v. solution	Diffuse bone metastases
Iodine	^{131}I	0.61 β_{max} / 0.364 MeV γ	8.06 d	—	—	Capsule / NaI oral solution	Thyroid cancer / —
Phosphorus	^{32}P	1.71 β_{max}	14.3 d	—	—	Chromic phosphate / Na$_2$PO$_3$ solution	Chromic phosphate / PCV, chronic leukemia

^{a}No filtration in units of R cm^2 mCi^{-1} h^{-1}.

^{b}0.5 mm Pt filtration; units of R cm^2 mg^{-1} h^{-1}

HDR, high dose rate; HVL, half-value layer; LDR, low dose rate; PCV, polycythemia vera.

Reprinted with permission from Williamson JF, Li XA, Brenner DJ. Physics and biology of brachytherapy. In: Halperin EC, Perez CA, Brady LW, eds. *Principles and practice of radiation oncology*, 6th ed. Philadelphia, PA: Lippincott Williams & Wilkins, 2013:423. © Wolters Kluwer.

satisfying its distribution rules. Older systems (Manchester and Quimby) use tables that give dose delivered per mgRaEq-h as a function of treatment volume or area. The more recent Paris system makes extensive use of computerized treatment planning to relate absorbed dose to source strength and treatment time.

Manchester System

* The Manchester system, developed by Ralston Paterson and Herbert Parker (5–7), is called the Paterson-Parker (P-P) system.
* The P-P system is the most relevant of the classic systems to the practice patterns of North American radiation oncologists.
* Table 6-2 lists the rules of the Manchester system. Table 6-3 lists the stated dose per mgRaEq-h and integrated reference air kerma as a function of treated area or volume.

Table 6-2
Manchester System Characteristics

Feature	Paterson and Parker (Manchester System) Rules				
Dose and dose rate	6,000–8,000 R in 6–8 d (1,000 R/d, 40 R/h)				
Dose specification criterion	Effective minimum dose is 10% above the absolute minimum dose in treatment plane or volume				
Dose gradient	Dose in treatment volume or plane varies by no more than ±10% from stated dose, except for localized hot spots				
Linear activity	Variable: 0.66 and 0.33 mgRaEq/cm				
Source strength distribution Planar	Area < 25 cm²: 2/3 periphery, 1/3 center 25 < area < 100 cm²: 1/2 periphery, 1/2 center Area > 100 cm²: 1/3 periphery, 2/3 center				
Source strength distribution volume	Cylinder: belt:core:end:end = 4:2:1:1 Sphere: belt:core = 6:2 Cube: 1/8 of the activity in each face 2/8 of the activity in the core				
Spacing	Constant uniform spacing				
Crossing needles	Planar implant: Target area effectively treated is reduced in length by 10% per uncrossed end				
	Volume implant: Target volume effectively treated is reduced by 7.5% per uncrossed end				
Elongation corrections	Long:short dimension:	1.5:1.0	2:1	2.5:1.0	3:1	4:1
Correction factors for mgRaEq-h	Planar:	1.025	1.05	1.07	1.09	1.12
	Volume:	1.03	1.06	1.10	1.15	1.23

Table 6-3

Manchester Implant Tables

Volume Implants			Planar Implants		
Volume (cm³)	mgRaEq·hᵃ / 1,000 P·PR	Minimum Dose/ IRAKᵇ cGy/(µ Gy m²)	Area (cm²)	mgRaEq·hᵃ / 1,000 P·PR	Minimum Dose/ IRAKᵇ cGy/(µGy m²)
1	34	3.49	0	30	4.48
2	54	2.20	2	97	1.38
3	70	1.68	4	141	0.953
4	85	1.38	6	177	0.759
5	99	1.194	8	206	0.652
10	158	0.752	10	235	0.572
15	207	0.574	12	261	0.515
20	251	0.474	14	288	0.466
25	291	0.408	16	315	0.426
30	329	0.361	18	342	0.393
40	398	0.298	20	368	0.365
50	462	0.257	24	417	0.322
60	522	0.228	28	466	0.288
70	579	0.206	32	513	0.262
80	633	0.188	36	558	0.241
90	684	0.174	40	603	0.223
100	734	0.162	44	644	0.209
110	782	0.152	48	685	0.196
120	829	0.143	52	725	0.185
140	919	0.129	56	762	0.176
160	1,005	0.118	60	800	0.168
180	1,087	0.110	64	837	0.160
200	1,166	0.102	68	873	0.154
220	1,242	0.0958	72	908	0.148
240	1,316	0.0904	76	945	0.142
260	1,389	0.0857	80	981	0.137
280	1,459	0.0815	84	1,016	0.132
300	1,528	0.0779	88	1,052	0.128
320	1,595	0.0746	92	1,087	0.124
340	1,661	0.0716	96	1,122	0.120
360	1,725	0.0690	100	1,155	0.116

continued

Table 6-3

Manchester Implant Tables *(continued)*

Volume Implants			Planar Implants		
Volume (cm³)	mgRaEq-h[a] 1,000 P-PR	Minimum Dose/ IRAK[b] cGy/(μ Gy m²)	Area (cm²)	mgRaEq-h[a] 1,000 P-PR	Minimum Dose/ IRAK[b] cGy/(μGy m²)
380	1,788	0.0665	120	1,307	0.103
400	1,851	0.0643	140	1,463	0.0918
—	—	—	160	1,608	0.0835
—	—	—	180	1,746	0.0769
—	—	—	200	1,880	0.0715
—	—	—	220	2,008	0.0669
—	—	—	240	2,132	0.0630
—	—	—	260	2,256	0.0595
—	—	—	280	2,372	0.0566
—	—	—	300	2,495	0.0538

[a]Original Manchester values from Paterson R, Parker HM. A dosage system for interstitial radium therapy. *Br J Radiol* 1938;11:313–339, with permission.
[b]Modified from original values for ¹⁹²Ir, assuming 8.6 Gy minimum peripheral dose per 1,000 P-PR and 7.227 μGy·m²/mgRaEq-h.
1,000 P-PR, 1,000 Manchester system roentgens; IRAK, integrated reference air kerma.
Reprinted with permission from Williamson JF, Li XA, Brenner DJ. Physics and biology of brachytherapy. In: Halperin EC, Perez CA, Brady LW, eds. *Principles and practice of radiation oncology*, 6th ed. Philadelphia, PA: Lippincott Williams & Wilkins, 2013:443. © Wolters Kluwer.

- Figure 6-1 illustrates a classic Manchester implant with crossed ends, using iridium-192 (^{192}Ir) line sources and 1-cm spacing to treat a cylindrical target volume 5 cm in diameter and 5 cm high. The required source strength is calculated as follows:

Target volume height = active needle length = 5 cm

$$\text{Treated volume} = \pi \cdot (2.5)^2 \cdot 5.0 = 98.3 \text{ cm}^3 \Rightarrow \frac{726 \text{ mg-h}}{1,000 \text{ P-PR}} = \frac{726 \text{ mg-h}}{860 \text{ cGy minumum dose}}$$

Assume: minimum peripheral dose rate = 45 cGy per hour and belt:core:end:end = 4:2:1:1

$$\text{mgRaEq/belt wire} = \frac{4}{8} \cdot \frac{45 \text{ cGy/h}}{860 \text{ cGy}} \cdot \frac{726 \text{ mg-h}}{15 \text{ needles}} = 1.27 \text{ mgRaEq/wire}$$

$$\text{mgRaEq/core wire} = \frac{2}{8} \cdot \frac{45 \text{ cGy/h}}{860 \text{ cGy}} \cdot \frac{726 \text{ mg-h}}{12 \text{ needles}} = 0.791 \text{ mgRaEq/wire}$$

$$\text{mgRaEq/AL end wires} = \frac{1}{8} \cdot \frac{45 \text{ cGy/h}}{860 \text{ cGy}} \cdot \frac{726 \text{ mg-h}}{2 \cdot (3 + 4.5)} = 0.317 \text{ mgRaEq/cm}$$

P-P Volume Implant: Crossed Ends, Ir-192 Wires and 1 cm Spacing

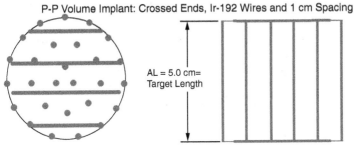

AL = 5.0 cm=
Target Length

A Arrange wires on three concentric cylinders: 15 wires on 5 cm diameter cylinder, 9 wires on 3 cm diameter cylinder, and three wires on 1 cm diameter cylinders. Use 4 wires to cross ends, with AL of 3 and 4.5 cm.

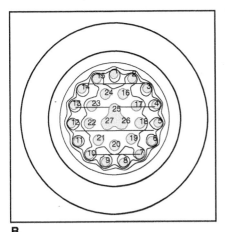

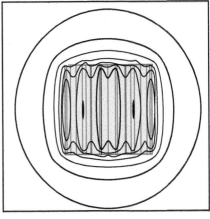

B

FIGURE 6-1. **A:** A 5-cm high by 5-cm diameter cylindrical target volume implanted with 35 differentially loaded wires spaced at 1-cm intervals. **B:** Resultant central transverse and coronal isodose curves plotted as percentages of the computer-calculated mean control dose (MCD) value of 56.3 cGy per hour (100%): 110% (62 cGy per hour), 100% (56 cGy per hour), 90% (51 cGy per hour), 80% (45 cGy per hour), 60% (34 cGy per hour), 40% (23 cGy per hour), and 11% (12 cGy per hour). Note that 80% of MCD, 45 cGy per hour, agrees exactly with the minimum peripheral dose rate of 45 cGy per hour predicted by the P-P tables. (Reprinted with permission from Williamson JF, Brenner DJ. Physics of brachytherapy. In: Halperin EC, Perez CA, Brady LW, eds. *Principles and practice of radiation oncology*, 5th ed. Philadelphia, PA: Lippincott Williams & Wilkins, 2008. © Wolters Kluwer.)

mgRaEq of each 3-cm wire = 3.0. 3.317 = 0.95 mgRaEq

mgRaEq of each 4.5-cm wire = 4.5. 0.317 = 1.42 mgRaEq

- Figure 6-2 demonstrates that by increasing the interneedle spacing to 1.3 cm, the need for differential loading can be eliminated.

  Because ends are uncrossed, required active length = target length/0.85 = 5.9 cm

  Effective volume = $\pi (2.5)^2.5.9.0.85 = 98.5$ cm^3, where

  From the original P–P volume table, $\dfrac{728 \text{ mg-h}}{1,000 \text{ P-PR}} = \dfrac{728 \text{ mg-h}}{840 \text{ cGy minimum dose}}$

Paterson-Parker Implant: CS-137 Needles with uncrossed ends

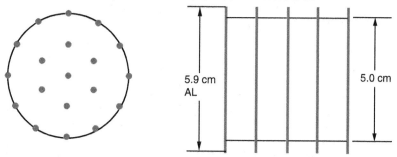

1.3 cm spacing can be approximately achieved by arranging 12 needles on the 5 cm diameter belt, 6 needles on the 2.5 cm diameter inner cylinder and 1 central needle. The resulting belt:core ratio is 12.7 = 0.63:0.37 which is close to the 0.67:0.33 Manchester ration for a cylinder implant with uncrossed ends.

FIGURE 6-2. A 5 × 5-cm cylindrical volume implanted by uniform strength ^{137}Cs needles spaced at 13-cm intervals. (Reprinted with permission from Williamson JF, Brenner DJ. Physics of brachytherapy. In: Halperin EC, Perez CA, Brady LW, eds. *Principles and practice of radiation oncology*, 5th ed. Philadelphia, PA: Lippincott Williams & Wilkins, 2008:448. © Wolters Kluwer.)

Assuming a minimum peripheral dose rate of 45 cGy per hour and belt:core = 4:2,

$$\text{mgRaEq/core needle} = \frac{1}{3} \cdot \frac{45}{840 \cdot 7} \cdot 728 = 1.86 \text{ mgRaEq}$$

$$\text{mgRaEq/belt needle} = \frac{2}{3} \cdot \frac{45}{840 \cdot 12} \cdot 728 = 2.17 \text{ mgRaEq}$$

Assuming uniform strength needles: $\text{mgRaEq/needle} = \dfrac{45}{840 \cdot 19} \cdot 728 = 2.05 \text{ mgRaEq}$

- Figure 6-3 illustrates application of the Manchester system to the same 5 × 5-cm cylindrical target volume, using ^{192}Ir ribbons with seed-to-seed spacing of 1 cm and an intercatheter spacing of 1.3 cm. Note that the distribution rules are satisfied almost exactly by using uniform seed strengths.

  Assuming uncrossed ends, active length = target length/0.85 = 5.9 cm ⇒ 6 seeds/ribbon

  Equivalently, the first and last seeds can be treated as "end" seeds, bisecting the target boundaries.

  Either way, treated volume = $\pi \cdot (2.5)^2 \cdot 5.0 = 98.2 \text{ cm}^3$

  Hence: $\dfrac{726 \text{ mg-h}}{1.000 \text{ P-PR}} = \dfrac{726 \text{ mg-h}}{860 \text{ cGy minimum dose}}$

  By choice of spacing, distribution rules are met by using seeds of equal strength.

  To give 45 cGy/h, $\text{mgRaEq/seed} = \dfrac{45 \text{ cGy/h}}{860 \text{ cGy}} \cdot \dfrac{726 \text{ mg-h}}{19 \text{ ribbons} \times 6 \text{ seeds/ribbon}}$

  $= 0.33 \text{ mgRaEq/seed}$

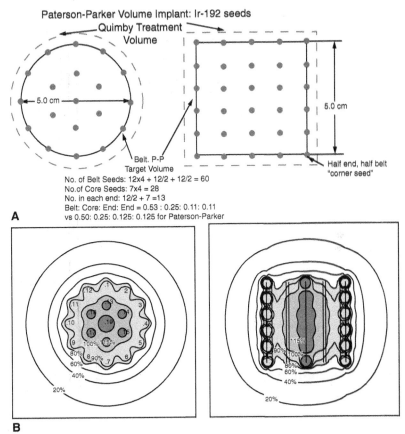

A:

Paterson-Parker Volume Implant: Ir-192 seeds

Quimby Treatment Volume

5.0 cm

5.0 cm

Belt. P-P Target Volume

Half end, half belt "corner seed"

No. of Belt Seeds: 12x4 + 12/2 + 12/2 = 60
No.of Core Seeds: 7x4 = 28
No. in each end: 12/2 + 7 =13
Belt: Core: End: End = 0.53 : 0.25: 0.11: 0.11
vs 0.50: 0.25: 0.125: 0.125 for Paterson-Parker

B

FIGURE 6-3. **A:** A 5 × 5-cm cylindrical target volume implanted with uniform-strength ^{192}Ir ribbons spaced at 1.3-cm intervals. **B:** Resultant central transverse and coronal isodose curves normalized to the mean control dose (MCD) value of 58.9 cGy per hour (100%): 115% (68 cGy per hour), 100% (59 cGy per hour), 90% (53 cGy per hour), 80% (47 cGy per hour), 60% (35 cGy per hour), 40% (24 cGy per hour), and 20% (12 cGy per hour). Note that 80% of MCD, 47 cGy per hour, agrees closely with the minimum peripheral dose rate of 45 cGy per hour predicted by the P-P tables. (Reprinted with permission from Williamson JF, Li XA, Brenner DJ. Physics and biology of brachytherapy. In: Halperin EC, Perez CA, Brady LW, eds. *Principles and practice of radiation oncology*, 6th ed. Philadelphia, PA: Lippincott Williams & Wilkins, 2013:445. © Wolters Kluwer.)

- Figure 6-4 illustrates application of the P-P system to a modern planar implant.

  As both ends are uncrossed, active length is greater than target length/0.92

  = 5/0.81 = 6.2 cm

  The shortest ribbon of active length ≥6.2 cm contains seven seeds

  (AL = 7 cm)

  Lookup area = area treated = 4 × 7 × 0.92 = 22.7 cm²

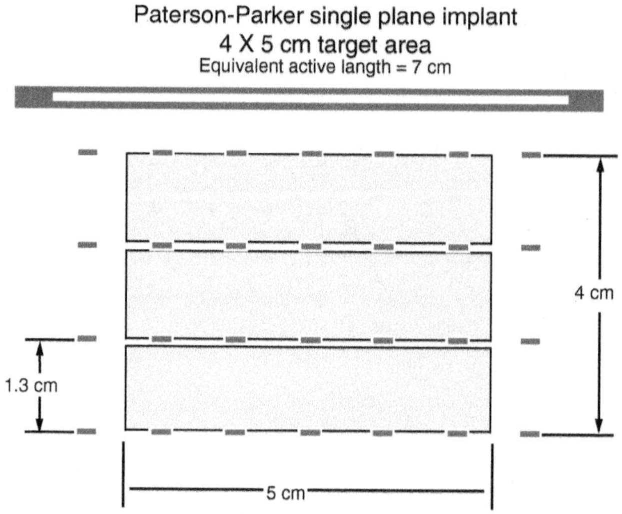

Paterson-Parker single plane implant
4 X 5 cm target area
Equivalent active length = 7 cm

FIGURE 6-4. A 1-cm-thick target with an area of 4 × 5 cm is to be treated with a single-plane Manchester implant using ^{192}Ir ribbons. A minimum dose rate of 45 cGy per hour is desired, and interneedle spacing is 1.3 cm. (Reprinted with permission from Williamson JF, Brenner DJ. Physics of brachytherapy. In: Halperin EC, Perez CA, Brady LW, eds. *Principles and practice of radiation oncology*, 5th ed. Philadelphia, PA: Lippincott Williams & Wilkins, 2008:448. © Wolters Kluwer.)

• Note that there are 10 central seeds and 18 peripheral seeds, a ratio of 0.64:0.36, which closely approximates the recommended 2/3:1/3 ratio. For this spacing, uniform-strength seeds can be used.

$$\text{Area} = 22.7 \text{ cm}^2 \Rightarrow \frac{402 \text{ mg-h}}{1{,}000 \text{ P-PR}} = \frac{402 \text{ mg-h}}{860 \text{ cGy minimum dose}}$$

$$\text{Elongation ratio} = \frac{\text{longest}}{\text{shortest}} \text{ side} = \frac{0.81 \cdot 7}{4} \cong 1.4 \Rightarrow \text{additional correction} = 1.02$$

Assuming a minimum peripheral dose rate of 45 cGy per hour:

$$\text{mgRaEq/peripheral seed} = \frac{2}{3} \cdot \frac{945 \text{ cGy/h}}{860 \text{ cGy}} \cdot \frac{402 \cdot 1.02 \text{ mg-h}}{18 \text{ seeds}} = 0.795 \text{ mgRaEq/seed}$$

$$\text{mgRaEq/central seed} = \frac{1}{3} \cdot \frac{45 \text{ cGy/h}}{860 \text{ cGy}} \cdot \frac{402 \cdot 1.02 \text{ mg-h}}{10 \text{ seeds}} = 0.720 \text{ mgRaEq/seed}$$

Quimby System

• The Quimby system was developed by Quimby and Castro (8) at New York Memorial Hospital between 1920 and 1940 (Table 6-4).
• This system is much less complex than the P-P system and was intended to be used with the limited radium-226 (^{226}Ra) needle inventories (usually 1 mgRaEq per cm) used in clinics in the United States during that period.

Table 6-4

Quimby System Characteristics

Feature	Quimby System Rules
Dose and dose rate	5,000–6,000 R in 3–4 d (60–70 R/h).
Dose specification criterion	Planar implants/molds: the point 5 mm from the needle plane along the perpendicular line passing through the center of the source array Volume implant: Dose appears to be delivered to a point located 3–5 mm outside implanted volume near the peripheral needle tips.
Dose gradient	Large central high-dose regions are characteristic of volume implants, whereas planar implants underdose the edges of the target area relative to the stated dose.
Linear activity	Constant (1.0 mgRaEq/cm used historically; 0.5 mgRaEq/cm commonly used)
Activity distribution: planar and volume	Identical strength needles spaced uniformly throughout target area or volume
Spacing	Preferably 1.5 cm and for seeds not <1 cm
Crossing needles	Planar: not clear Volume: if not used, active ends should extend beyond target volume margin by 7.5%.
Elongation corrections	Planar: not used Volume: Use Manchester system corrections.

Reprinted with permission from Williamson JF. Physics of brachytherapy. In: Perez CA, Brady LW, eds. *Principles and practice of radiation oncology*, 3rd ed. Philadelphia, PA: Lippincott–Raven, 1998:405–468. © Wolters Kluwer.

Paris System

- The Paris system was developed in the early 1960s by Pierquin, Chassange, and Marinello (9,10) and was motivated by the ^{192}Ir afterloading techniques developed by Henschke and coworkers (11).
- Outside the United States, the Paris system is the most widely used approach for definitive brachytherapy of localized lesions in the head and neck, breast, and many other sites.

INTRACAVITARY TREATMENT OF CARCINOMA OF THE UTERINE CERVIX

- The focus is restricted to common systems (Fletcher and Mallinckrodt) derived from the Manchester system.

Manchester Therapy System

- The Manchester system, developed in 1938 by Tod and Meredith (12), was the first to use applicators and loadings designed to satisfy specific dosimetric constraints (13).
- It was the first system to use a radiation field quantity, exposure at point A, rather than mgh, to specify treatment. The reference point A originally was defined as the point "2 cm lateral to the center of the uterine canal and 2 cm cephalad from the mucous membrane of the lateral fornix in the plane of the uterus."
- This seemingly arbitrary definition reflected the system developers' view that "radiation necrosis is not due to direct effects of radiation on the bladder and rectum, but high-dose effects in the area in the medial edge of the broad ligament where the uterine vessels cross the ureter" (12). They believed that the radiation tolerance of this area, termed the paracervical triangle, was the limiting factor in the treatment of cervical cancer and used point A exposure to represent its average dose.
- In current practice, point A dose is used to approximate the average or minimum dose to the tumor.
- Point B, defined as 5 cm from the patient's midline at the same level as point A, was intended to quantify the dose delivered to the obturator lymph nodes.
- Many radiation oncologists use a revised definition of point A that references its location to the cervical os (tandem collar, tip of caudalmost tandem source, or gold seed implanted in the cervix) rather than to the lateral fornix (Fig. 6-5). Doses may be very different, depending on the definition used.

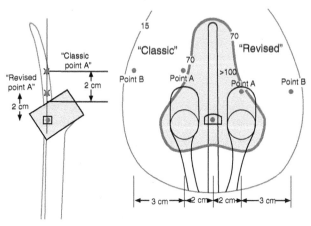

FIGURE 6-5. Radiographic definition of classic point A (2 cm above the cephalic most aspect of the colpostat in the tilted coronal plane) and the revised point A (2 cm above the cervical collar top or center). Because the distance from caudalmost intrauterine source tip to colpostat center (tandem-to-colpostat displacement) varies from one patient to another, the vaginal contribution to revised point A is highly variable. The revised definition was suggested by Tod and Meredith (13) in their 1953 paper. (Reprinted with permission from Williamson JF, Li XA, Brenner DJ. Physics and biology of brachytherapy. In: Halperin EC, Perez CA, Brady LW, eds. *Principles and practice of radiation oncology*, 6th ed. Philadelphia, PA: Lippincott Williams & Wilkins, 2013:455. © Wolters Kluwer.)

Volumetric Specification of Intracavitary Treatment: International Commission on Radiation Units and Measurements Report No. 38

- The ICRU (4) introduced the concept of reference volume enclosed by the reference isodose surface for reporting and comparing intracavitary treatments performed in different centers, regardless of the applicator system, insertion technique, and method of treatment prescription used.
- ICRU Report No. 38 recommended that the reference volume be taken at the 60-Gy isodose surface, resulting from the addition of dose contributions from any external beam whole-pelvis irradiation and all intracavitary insertions.
- Figure 6-6 illustrates the bladder and rectal reference points recommended by the ICRU.
- For nonstandard loadings using miniovoids, large-diameter colpostats, or nonstandard-length tandems, the vaginal and uterine target mgRaEq-h prescriptions are modified according to the following principles:
- The target mgRaEq-h is considered to be divided equally between the vaginal and uterine components. When nonstandard applications are used, these two components are manipulated independently. For the loadings shown in Figure 6-7, this results in different treatment times for the vaginal and intrauterine loadings.
- The vaginal mgRaEq-h deliverable with minicolpostats is constrained by the vaginal surface dose limit. This surface dose, called rad surface dose, is specified at the midpoint of the lateral cylindrical surface of a single colpostat, including its cap. The rad surface dose includes a 6% average applicator shielding correction and any whole-pelvis dose but excludes dose contributions from the tandem and

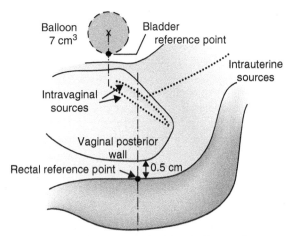

FIGURE 6-6. Reference points for bladder and rectal brachytherapy doses proposed by the ICRU. (Reprinted with permission from Chassagne D, Dutreix A, Almond P, Burgers JMV, Busch M, Joslin CA. Dose and volume specification for reporting intracavitary therapy in gynecology (Report 38). *Journal of the International Commission on Radiation Units and Measurements.* 1985;os20(1). doi:10.1093/jicru/os20.1.201)

Mallinckrodt Intracavitary Loadings

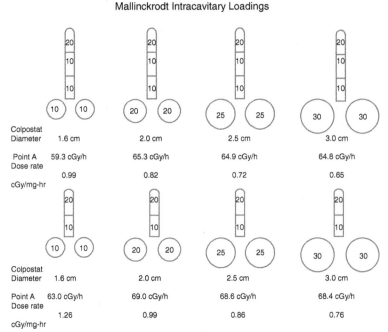

FIGURE 6-7. Applicator loadings used with Fletcher-Suit applicators for treatment of cervical carcinoma. Because the system uses model 6500 3M ^{137}Cs tubes, equivalent mass of radium is used to specify loadings and mgRaEq-h rather than mg-h to prescribe intracavitary therapy. The point A dose rates assume the classic Manchester definition and average colpostat separations and tandem-colpostat alignments. (Reprinted with permission from Williamson JF, Li XA, Brenner DJ. *Physics and biology of brachytherapy.* In: Halperin EC, Perez CA, Brady LW, eds. *Principles and practice of radiation oncology,* 6th ed. Philadelphia, PA: Lippincott Williams & Wilkins, 2013:455. © Wolters Kluwer.)

contralateral colpostat. Current treatment guidelines limit this dose to approximately 150 Gy in the upper vagina and 90 Gy in the distal vagina. For medium and large colpostats, the vaginal mgRaEq-h is increased by specified fractions to compensate for the increased source to surface distance.

- When medium and short tandems are used for the intrauterine tandem, the target mgRaEq-h is reduced in proportion to the fraction of cesium-137 (^{137}Cs) "missing," relative to the standard tandem. Consequently, the treatment time for the tandem component is constant and independent of its loading.

- Table 6-5 shows that as tumor size increases and therapeutic emphasis shifts from intracavitary insertions to external beam therapy, point A doses increase from 70 Gy for small stage IB lesions (less than 1 cm) (schema A) to 94 Gy for stage IV lesions (schema E).

- The mgRaEq-h actually administered within a given treatment group may deviate from the target mgRaEq-h prescriptions by as much as –30% to +40% for very small and large insertions, respectively.

Table 6-5

Prescriptions for Carcinoma of the Cervix

Treatment Scheme	Indication	External Beam Treatment			Intracavitary Treatment		Total: Smallest to Largest Insertion		
		Whole Pelvis (Gy)	Split Field (Gy)	Target mgRaEq-h	Maximum Vaginal Vault Dose (Gy)	Point A Dose (Gy)	Point B Dose (Gy)	mgRaEq-h
A	IB < 2 cm	0	45	7,000	150	70–80	56–60	5,580–7,980
B	IB 2–4 cm	10	40	7,500	150	80–85	61–66	5,580–8,550
C	IB/IIA/IIB/IIIA bulky (>4 cm), limited parametrial extension	20	30	8,000	150	84–90	61–67	5,600–9,100
D	IIB/IIB bulky, extensive parametrial extension	20	40	8,000	150	84–90	71–77	5,600–9,100
E	IIB, IIIB, IV, poor anatomy, poor regression	40	20	6,500	150	92–94	69–74	4,610–7,410

Note: Treatment scheme is selected according to disease stage, lesion location, volume, histology, and extent of vaginal and parametrial invasion.
Reprinted with permission from Williamson JF, Li XA, Brenner DJ. Physics and biology of brachytherapy. In: Halperin EC, Perez CA, Brady LW, eds. *Principles and practice of radiation oncology*, 6th ed. Philadelphia, PA: Lippincott Williams & Wilkins, 2013:459. © Wolters Kluwer.

- Despite reliance on the mgRaEq-h prescription philosophy, treatment times are approximately constant, and total point A doses are nearly independent of applicator size, the defining features of the Manchester system.
- When whole-pelvis doses are limited to 20 to 40 Gy even for locally advanced disease, relatively high bladder (80 Gy) and rectal (75 Gy) doses are acceptable (14).
- Table 6-6 illustrates detailed application of the prescription schema rules, listing total doses for point A, point B, and the vaginal mucosa, along with the volumes of tissue enclosed by point A and ICRU 60-Gy reference isodose surfaces.

Intracavitary Brachytherapy Dose Specification

- For Manchester-type loadings and applicators, point A dose rate is approximately constant and independent of loading, leading to a linear relationship between point A dose and time, not mgRaEq-h.
- Intracavitary implants delivering the same mgRaEq-h are volumetrically equivalent in the clinical dose range, despite significant differences in geometry and loading. Delivery of a specified mgRaEq-h prescription is equivalent to treating the patient until a reference isodose expands to occupy a specified volume.
- Practical mgRaEq-h systems use other parameters as constraints and guides and are more Manchester-like than the "strict" mg-h philosophy would suggest. These parameters have the following roles: (a) mgRaEq-h or mg-h: limit the volume of tissue treated to a high dose; (b) point A: ensure that tumor periphery receives adequate dose; (c) vaginal surface dose: ensure that dose to mucosal surfaces in contact with applicator system remains within tolerance; and (d) treatment time: indirect control of point A dose.
- In current practice, implant placement is guided by direct visualization and palpation, and treatment prescription is determined by the radiation oncologist's knowledge of treatment outcome, averaged over groups of uniformly treated patients with similar medical condition and tumor size and location.
- The implant system must be applied as a whole; mixing dose-specification methods, insertion techniques, and normal tissue dose-response relationships from different clinical systems is a dangerous practice that can lead to suboptimal or indeterminate clinical outcomes. For example, the use of the maximum rectal tolerance dose (75 to 80 Gy) to guide prescription in a system using higher whole-pelvis doses or less packing will not guarantee an acceptable level of complication (15).
- Because classic dose-specification quantities fail to completely describe the dose distribution, a radiation oncologist must be trained in all details of an intracavitary system to duplicate the results of its developers.
- For the clinical physicist, consistency of current dosimetric practice with past clinical experience is often more important than absolute accuracy of the computed dose distributions or consistency with some practice standard or definition external to the treatment system (16).

Table 6-6

Loading Schema: 8,000 mg-h, 20-Gy Whole Pelvis, and 30-Gy Split Pelvis

Applicator	Loading	Time	mgRaEq-h	Vaginal Surface Dose[a]	Total Point A Dose (Volume)	Total Point B Dose	ICRU Volume (60 Gy)
Miniovoids, small tandem	20	×100 h =	3,000		83.5 Gy (85 cm³)	61.0 Gy	165 cm³
	10			152.3 Gy			
	10–10	×130 h =	2,600				
			5,600				
2-cm colpostats, standard tandem	20	×100 h =	4,000		86.3 Gy	65.2 Gy	281 cm³
	10			150.1 Gy	(131 cm³)		
	10						
	20–20	×100 h =	4,000				
			8,000				
3-cm colpostats, standard tandem	20	×100 h =	4,000		85.6 Gy	66.9 Gy	343 cm³
	10			98.6 Gy	(160 cm³)		
	10						
	30–30	×85 h =	5,100				
			9,100				

[a]On surface of single colpostat, neglecting other source.

Reprinted with permission from Williamson JF, Li XA, Brenner DJ. Physics and biology of brachytherapy. In: Halperin EC, Perez CA, Brady LW, eds. *Principles and practice of radiation oncology*, 6th ed. Philadelphia, PA: Lippincott Williams & Wilkins, 2013:459. © Wolters Kluwer.

HIGH DOSE RATE BRACHYTHERAPY

- Most HDR units use iridium-192 (^{192}Ir) or cobalt-60 (^{60}Co). ^{192}Ir offers smaller source sizes, but sources must be changed more frequently (usually every 3 to 4 months). A similar decay source exchange for ^{60}Co takes 6 to 8 years.
- The smaller ^{192}Ir sources permit access to more body sites via interstitial or intraluminal applications. ^{60}Co and cesium-137 (^{137}Cs) sources are suitable only for intracavitary and some intraluminal treatments, such as for the esophagus.
- Virtually any applicator designed for LDR manual afterloading has been, or could be, adapted for HDR systems.
- The applicator, transfer tube, and afterloader must form a closed system so that there is no possibility of any part of the HDR source becoming dislodged in the patient.
- Users converting from an LDR to HDR system must carefully evaluate the features of the new applicator dosimetry system for any changes that may occur in the dose distribution.
- The shielding of the HDR brachytherapy room must be sufficient to protect workers and the public and must be evaluated by a competent physicist.
- For HDR units using ^{192}Ir, with the wall and ceiling being at least 5 feet from the remote afterloader, typical shielding requirements are 4 to 5 cm of lead or 43 to 50 cm of concrete wall. For larger rooms, the required concrete wall thickness will be lower. Because the radiation is uncollimated, all barriers in direct line of sight must be similarly shielded; it may be necessary to limit the mobility of the unit to prevent direct irradiation of the door.

Dosimetry

- For all sources used in HDR brachytherapy, the basic specification of source strength should be determined by measurement of air kerma rate at a reference distance along the perpendicular bisector of the source. Slightly different terminology and measurement techniques have been recommended, but the basic concept remains the same (4,17–22).
- The magnitude of any error in delivered dose depends on the source speed, source strength, dwell times, and implant geometry (23–26). The error is unlikely to exceed 2% for common afterloaders and implant situations, but should not be assumed always to be negligible, especially when dwell times are short.
- Even if the transit times between dwell positions within a channel are accounted for, the dose delivered, while the source moves to the first dwell position and back from the last one in the channel, can be significant, on the order of 0.10 to 0.15 Gy at the surface of a 2-mm catheter. The clinical importance depends on the number of fractions and proximity to sensitive structures, but clearly the routing of the tubes deserves some consideration.

Dose or Volume Optimization

- To treat a given volume, unoptimized implants need to be larger than optimized implants.
- A radiation oncologist converting from unoptimized LDR techniques to optimized HDR techniques will need to alter implant geometry, as well as dose and fractionation.

- One attractive feature of HDR remote afterloaders, especially the stepping-source type, is the possibility of manipulating the dose distribution by controlling the dwell time used at each dwell position.
- Optimization based on varying dwell times is fundamentally limited in its ability to alter a dose distribution. The dose from a small source varies linearly with time and as the inverse square of the distance.
- Optimization algorithms can be divided into two classes:
  - "Dose point" optimization: The clinical problem can be described as needing to achieve a desired dose at defined points.
  - "Geometric" optimization: The implanted catheters or needles are assumed to permeate a target volume, the idea being to use the source locations themselves to drive the solution without the introduction of separate dose points (27).

RADIOBIOLOGIC DOSIMETRY

- Because of a lack of personal or documented experience, radiation oncologists frequently resort to the use of bioeffect dose models to convert from LDR to HDR.
- The linear-quadratic (LQ) model is most commonly used.

Linear-Quadratic Model for Brachytherapy

- The LQ equation for N equal exposures, each of dose rate R and duration t, with correction for repopulation during the course of irradiation in overall treatment time T (days), is

$$-\ln S = N[\alpha(Rt) + G\beta(Rt)^2] - 0.693\,T/T_{pot}$$

  where T_{pot} is the potential doubling time of cells (in days), and 0.693 is ln 2 (28–31).
- Rearranging this equation and dividing both sides by α leads to the formula for the biologically effective dose (BED), sometimes referred to as the extrapolated response dose:

$$\frac{-\ln S}{\alpha} = \text{BED} = NRt\left[1 + G\frac{Rt}{(\alpha/\beta)}\right] - \frac{0.693T}{\alpha T_{pot}}$$

  where the single parameter α/β represents the "curviness" of the log cell-survival curve (28–30,32,33).
- For HDR treatments, where the time for each treatment is so short that negligible repair takes place during each exposure, but the time between fractions is long enough for complete repair to occur (30):

$$G = 1$$

- For continuous irradiation (LDR brachytherapy) at a constant dose rate, the value of G is:

$$G = \frac{2}{\mu t}\left[1 - \frac{1 - e^{-\mu t}}{\mu t}\right]$$

where μ is the repair-rate constant (i.e., 0.693 per μ is the half-time for repair) (30). Typical values for μ used in the literature for LQ model calculations are

For late-responding normal tissues: $\mu = 0.46$ h^{-1} ($t_{1/2} = 1.5$ h)

For tumor: $\mu = 0.46 - 1.40$ h^{-1} ($t_{1/2} = 1.5$–0.5 h).

Thomadsen and Das (27) note that most tissues have an approximate repair time of 1.5 hours, but the actual behavior is more complex, with a fast component of 20 minutes and a slow one of about 2.2 hours.

- The BED is essentially a "bioeffect dose," which takes into account not only the physical dose but also the dose rate, time for each exposure, dose per fraction, and time between fractions.
- This bioeffect dose can be used to convert LDR regimens to HDR; however, it is neither advisable nor safe to blindly use a mathematical model such as this without first understanding the radiobiologic principles of LDR and HDR equivalence.

Biologically Effective Dose Calculation of Equivalence

- For the determination of the HDR regimen equivalent to the LDR course of 57.6 Gy in 72 hours at 0.8 Gy per hour, all that is needed is to equate the BEDs for LDR and HDR for both tumor and late-reacting normal tissue cells as follows:

$$BED_{LDR} = BED_{HDR}$$

- For tumor: Assume that repopulation can be ignored and $\alpha/\beta = 10$ Gy, $\mu = 1.4$ h^{-1}. Then equations (1), (2), and (3) give

$$57.6\left[1 + \frac{2 \times 0.8}{1.4 \times 10}\left(1 - \frac{1 - e^{-1.4 \times 72}}{1.4 \times 72}\right)\right] = Nd\left(1 + \frac{d}{10}\right) = 64.1$$

where N and d are the number of fractions and tumor dose per fraction required for equivalence, respectively.

- For late-reacting tissues: $\alpha/\beta = 2.5$ Gy, $\mu = 0.46$ h^{-1}, and the effective dose to normal tissues

$$57.6 \times 0.8\left[1 + \frac{2 \times 0.8 \times 0.8}{0.46 \times 2.5}\left(1 - \frac{1 \cdot e^{-0.46 \times 72}}{0.46 \times 72}\right)\right] = 0.8Nd\left(1 + \frac{0.8d}{2.5}\right) = 95.8$$

equals 0.8 times the effective tumor dose.

- Then dividing equation (6) by equation (4) gives

$$\frac{0.8\,(1+032d)}{1+0.1d} = 1.495$$

or $d = 6.53$ Gy

- Substitution of this value of d in equations (4) or (6) gives $N = 5.94$ fractions, but because it is not possible to deliver a nonintegral number of fractions, equations (4) and (6) can be used to calculate the dose per fraction required in exactly six fractions; for this example, this works out to be 6.5 Gy.

HIGH DOSE RATE APPLICATIONS

- In brachytherapy, normal-tissue cells are in close proximity to tumor cells; the dose per fraction of HDR required for equivalence to LDR is very low; and several fractions are needed.
- LQ model calculations show that to replace a 60-Gy LDR implant at 0.5 Gy per hour requires 13 fractions of HDR at 3.5 Gy per fraction. Fortunately, HDR has one potential advantage: the ability to "optimize" dose distributions by varying the dwell times of the stepping source.
- HDR offers the potential of some "extra" geometric sparing. For the implant described above, if $f = 1$ for LDR, even with just a modest extra sparing of 10% ($f = 0.9$ for HDR), the LQ model calculations show that the equivalent number of HDR fractions reduces dramatically from 13 down to only 6 (33).
- This potential optimization advantage of HDR over LDR is lost if the LDR implant also uses stepping-source technology. This is the basis of pulsed dose rate brachytherapy.

DOSE FRACTIONATION IN HIGH DOSE RATE BRACHYTHERAPY

- The relationship between dose and fractionation for HDR and LDR intracavitary irradiation of stage I and II carcinoma of the cervix was examined by Arai et al. (34). They concluded that the optimal dose fractionation schedules for intracavitary irradiation were (a) for HDR, 28 ± 3 Gy in 4 to 5 fractions or 34 ± 4 Gy in 8 to 10 fractions or 40 ± 5 Gy in 12 to 14 fractions at point A and (b) for LDR, 51 ± 5 Gy in 3 or 4 fractions at point A. The dose at point A with LDR technique appears low compared with those used in European and American practice.
- Liu et al. (35) developed isoeffect tables, based on the LQ model, to convert traditional LDR doses and number of fractions to point A to HDR brachytherapy. Depending on dose rate, different exposure values can be calculated for various fractionation schedules. They predicted that, using the therapeutic gain ratio, similar results would be obtained with either brachytherapy modality, using 2 to 4 fractions of LDR and 4 to 7 fractions of HDR.

Table 6-7

Mean Values of the Number of Fractions and Dose/Fraction to Point A for HDR and Treatment Time and Dose Rate for Low Dose Rate (37), with Standard Errors and the Ratio of Total Doses

| | HDR | | LDR | | |
Stage	Fractions	Dose Per Fraction (Gy)	Treatment Time (h)	Dose Rate (Gy/h)	Ratio of Total Doses (HDR/LDR)
I	5.3 ± 0.4	7.6 ± 0.4	75.4 ± 7.3	0.87 ± 0.14	0.60 ± 0.13
II	4.7 ± 0.3	7.4 ± 0.3	80.2 ± 7.0	0.80 ± 0.11	0.54 ± 0.10
III	4.6 ± 0.4	7.4 ± 0.4	77.3 ± 8.9	0.87 ± 0.14	0.50 ± 0.11
IV	4.7 ± 0.7	7.5 ± 0.6	79.6 ± 18.5	0.89 ± 0.27	0.50 ± 0.21
All	4.82 ± 0.21	7.45 ± 0.20	78.1 ± 4.4	0.85 ± 0.07	0.54 ± 0.06

Reprinted with permission from Orton CG, Seyedsadr M, Somnay A. Comparison of high and low dose rate remote afterloading for cervix cancer and the importance of fractionation. *Int J Radiat Oncol Biol Phys* 1991;21: 1425–1434. © Elsevier.

- Orton et al. (36) analyzed more than 17,000 patients treated with HDR remote afterloading at 56 institutions; the approximate mean value used was 5 fractions, with a 7.5-Gy dose per fraction. The ratio of HDR to LDR total dose was 0.5 to 0.6 (Table 6-7). Survival was equivalent with either HDR or LDR. HDR fraction doses greater than 7.5 Gy resulted in a higher incidence of morbidity.
- Petereit and Pearcey (38) published recommendations for dose fractionation with HDR brachytherapy in carcinoma of the cervix (Table 6-8), based on clinical experience. Except for patients with stage III tumors, results of therapy with HDR or LDR were found to be equivalent (39).

Table 6-8

Carcinoma of the Cervix: Dose Per Fraction for 3, 4, and 5 Fractions of HDR Brachytherapy and Whole-Pelvis Irradiation

Whole Pelvis	3 HDR Fractions (LDR Equivalent) (Gy)	4 HDR Fractions (LDR Equivalent) (Gy)	5 HDR Fractions (LDR Equivalent) (Gy)	Point A Gy$_{10}$	LQED
45/25/1.8	8 (35)	6.5 (35)	5.5 (35)	96	80
45/25/1.8	8.8 (40)	7.2 (40)	6.0 (40)	102	85
50.4	—	—	6.0 (40)	109	90

LQED, linear-quadratic effective dose for 2-Gy fraction.
Data from Petereit DG. Refresher Course No. 103. High dose rate brachytherapy for carcinoma of the cervix. Presented at 40th Annual Meeting of the American Society for Therapeutic Radiology and Oncology. Phoenix, AZ, October 1998.

Table 6-9

Dose Fractionation Schedules for HDR Prostate Brachytherapy and Normal Tissues Constraints Used by Experienced HDR Centers

Current Dose Fractionation Schedules

Institution	Dose Fractionation	Bladder	Urethra	Rectum
MSKCC	Boost 7 Gyx3 Mono 9.5 Gyx4 Salvage 8 Gyx4		<120% prescription	D_{2cc} < 70%
UCSF	Boost 15 Gyx1 Mono 10.5 Gyx3 Salvage 8 Gyx4[a]	V75 < 1 cc	V_{125}< 1 cc, V_{150} = 0 cc	V75 < 1 cc
WBH	Boost 10.5 Gyx2 Mono 4 × 9.5 Gy (historical) 12–13.5 Gyx2 (current) Salvage 7 Gyx4 combined with hyperthermia	No constraint (intra-op TRUS- based dosi)	V_{100} < 90% of prescription V_{115} < 1% of prescription	V_{75} < 1% of prescription
TCC	Boost 6 Gyx2 × 2 implants	<80% of Rx	<125% of prescription	<80% of Rx to outer wall
GW	Boost 6.5 Gyx3 Mono two sessions of 6.5 Gyx3	<100% prescription	<110% prescription	Mucosa <60%, outer wall <100%
Toronto	Boost 15 Gyx 1	n/a	D_{10} < 118% Max < 125%	V_{80}< 0.5 cc
UCLA-CET	Boost 6 Gyx4 Mono 7.25 Gyx6	90%–100% wall 80% balloon	120% combo 105% any TUR 110% mono	Rectal wall 80% Rectal wall 80%–85%

[a]Dose tunnel whenever possible.
D_{10}: dose that covers the highest 10% of the organ; GW, Gamma West Brachytherapy; MSKCC, Memorial Sloan-Kettering Cancer Center; Rx, prescription; TCC, Texas Cancer Center; Toronto, University of Toronto; TUR, transurethral resection; UCLA-CET, University of California Los Angeles-California Endocurietherapy Cancer Center; UCSF, University of California San Francisco; V_{80}: fractional volume covered by 80% of the prescription dose; V_{100}, fractional volume covered by 100% of the prescription dose; V_{115}: fractional volume covered by 100% of the prescription dose; V_{125}: fractional volume covered by 125% of the prescription dose; V_{150}: fractional volume covered by 150% of the prescription dose; WBH, William Beaumont Hospital.
Reprinted with permission from Yamada Y, Rogers L, Demanes DJ, et al. American Brachytherapy Society consensus guidelines for high-dose-rate prostate brachytherapy. *Brachytherapy.* 2012;11(1):20-32. doi:10.1016/j.brachy.2011.09.008. © Elsevier.

- The American Brachytherapy Society (ABS) recently published guidelines for the use of HDR brachytherapy in carcinoma of the cervix (40).
- Mate et al. (41) and Martinez et al. (42) have used HDR brachytherapy in combination with 45 Gy to the pelvis (four fields) for the treatment of patients with high-risk localized carcinoma of the prostate.
- The American Brachytherapy Society (ABS) has published consensus guidelines for high-dose-rate prostate brachytherapy. Current dose fractionation schedules are shown in Table 6-9 (43).

- The ABS recommended prostate high-dose-rate prescriptions are summarized as follows:

  Monotherapy

  10.5 Gy x 3

  8.5-9.5 Gy x 4

  6.0-7.5 Gy x 6

  Boost

  15 Gy x 1 (with 36-40 Gy XRT)

  9.5-10.5 Gy x 2 (with 40-50 Gy XRT)

  5.5-7.5 Gy x 3 (with 40-50 Gy XRT)

  4.0-6.0 Gy x 4 (with 36-50 Gy XRT)

IMAGE-GUIDED BRACHYTHERAPY IN CERVICAL CANCER

Introduction

- Advantages include shaping the spatial dose distribution to conform to the target volume and reduce the dose to normal tissues.
- Three-dimensional imaging such as computed tomography (CT), magnetic resonance imaging (MRI), and/or positron emission tomography (PET) scans allows for better soft tissue delineation of gynecological tissues as well as organs at risk (OARs), compared to 2-D imaging.
- OARs include small bowel, sigmoid, rectum, and bladder.
- In 2005, the ABS and GEC-ESTRO agreed to advocate and adopt the GEC-ESTRO guidelines (44,45) for 3-D image-based planning for cervical cancer in the United States (46).

Methods

- Following the completion of applicator insertion, the patient will undergo imaging to aid in treatment planning.
- Imaging includes orthogonal films, a CT scan, and/or an MRI.
- MRI allows for contouring residual cervical tumor.
- CT allows for visualizing the cervix and parametrium as one structure, resulting in potential overcontouring of the lateral aspect of the volume (47). CT still can identify tumor beyond point A, allowing expansion of target volume when necessary.
- Contour guidelines include identifying a high-risk clinical target volume (HR-CTV) and an intermediate-risk clinical target volume (IR-CTV).
- HR-CTV entails contouring the entire cervix (for stage I) and extension of disease (for stage IIA to IVA) to surrounding tissues as seen on CT or MRI including residual disease as determined from clinical examination at brachytherapy.
- IR-CTV entails adding a 1-cm expansion around HR-CTV, modifying for disease extent at diagnosis, and deleting contours extending into the bladder, sigmoid, or rectum.

Dose Specification to Tumor and Organs at Risk

- Prescription options include point A, 3-D–based CTV, or a combination of the two.
- OARs can be reported based on ICRU definitions, dose-volume histogram (DVH) parameters, or both (Fig. 6-8).
- The most frequently reported 3-D–based DVH parameters include D_{2cc}, D_{1cc}, $D_{0.1cc}$, D_{5cc}, D_{90}, D_{100}, D_{150}, D_{200}, V_{100}, V_{150}, and V_{200}.
- CTV plans are modified based on dose to point A reaching 100% of dose, and/or modifying treatment plan based on D_{90}.
- Bladder ICRU points include a dose less than 80 Gy, or a DVH parameter of D_{2cc} less than 90 Gy.
- Rectum ICRU points include a dose less than 75 Gy, or a DVH parameter of D_{2cc} less than 75 Gy. Sigmoid D_{2cc} dose recommended less than 75 Gy.
- 3-D thresholds for small bowel, urethra, and vagina have not been elucidated.

Future Directions

- Correlation between CT-defined doses and toxicities continues to be evaluated.
- Large prospective trials would more clearly define benefit of MRI-, CT-, and PET-based therapy.

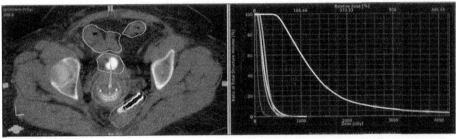

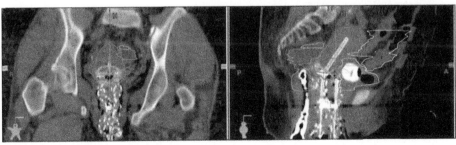

FIGURE 6-8. A 65-year-old female with IIB cervical cancer status post chemotherapy and external beam radiation therapy to the pelvis to 45 Gy. This is the first of 5 fractions with HDR cervical brachytherapy with a ring and tandem applicator. Six hundred centigray is prescribed to point A, and DVH was analyzed to determine dose to the target and OARs.

References

1. Bottcher HD, Schopohl B, Liermann D, et al. Endovascular irradiation—a new method to avoid recurrent stenosis after stent implantation in peripheral arteries: technique and preliminary results. *Int J Radiat Oncol Biol Phys* 1994;29(1):183–186.
2. Wiedermann JG, Marboe C, Amols H, et al. Intracoronary irradiation markedly reduces restenosis after balloon angioplasty in a porcine model. *J Am Coll Cardiol* 1994;23(6):1491–1498.
3. American Association of Physicists in Medicine. *Remote afterloading technology: report of the Radiation Therapy Task Group No. 41* (G. Glasgow, Chair). New York, NY: American Institute of Physics, 1993.
4. International Commission on Radiation Units and Measurements. *Dose and volume specification for reporting intracavitary therapy in gynecology*. Report no. 38. Bethesda, MD: ICRU, 1985.
5. Parker HM. A dosage system for interstitial radium therapy. II Physical aspects. *Br J Radiol* 1938;11:252–266.
6. Parker HM. Limitations of physics in radium therapy. *Radiology* 1943;41:330–336.
7. Paterson JR. *The treatment of malignant disease by radium x-rays, being a practice of radiotherapy*. London, UK: Edward Arnold Ltd., 1948.
8. Quimby EH, Castro V. The calculation of dosage in interstitial radium therapy. *Am J Roentgenol Radium Ther* 1953;70:739–749.
9. Pierquin B, Marinello G. *Manuel practique de curietherapie*. Paris, France: Hermann, 1992.
10. Pierquin B, Wilson JF, Chassange D. *Modern brachytherapy*. New York, NY: Masson Publishing USA, 1987.
11. Henschke UK, Hilaris BS, Mahan GD. Afterloading in interstitial and intracavitary radiation therapy. *Am J Roentgenol Radium Ther Nucl Med* 1963;90:386–395.
12. Tod M, Meredith WJ. A dosage system for use in the treatment of cancer of the uterine cervix. *Br J Radiol* 1938;11:809–824.
13. Tod M, Meredith WJ. Treatment of cancer of the cervix uteri, a revised Manchester method. *Br J Radiol* 1953;26(305):252–257.
14. Perez CA, Fox S, Grigsby PW, et al. Impact of dose in outcome of radiation alone in carcinoma of uterine cervix: analysis of two different methods. *Int J Radiat Oncol Biol Phys* 1991;21:885–898.
15. Williamson JF. Physics of brachytherapy. In: Perez CA, Brady LW, eds. *Principles and practice of radiation oncology*, 3rd ed. Philadelphia, PA: Lippincott–Raven, 1998:405–468.
16. Williamson JF, Brenner DJ. Physics and biology of brachytherapy. In: Halperin EC, Perez CA, Brady LW, eds. *Principles and practice of radiation oncology*, 5th ed. Philadelphia, PA: Lippincott Williams & Wilkins, 2008:423–475.
17. American Association of Physicists in Medicine (AAPM) Task Group 32. *Specification of brachytherapy source strength*. New York, NY: American Institute of Physics, 1987.
18. Comite Français Mesure des Rayonnements Ionisants. *Recommendations pour la determination des doses absorbees en curietherapie*. CFMRI Report No. 1. Paris, France: Bureau National de Metrologie, 1983.
19. Specification of brachytherapy sources. Memorandum from the British Committee on Radiation Units and Measurements. *Br J Radiol* 1984;57(682):941–942.
20. DeWerd LA, Thomadsen BR. Source strength standards and calibration of HDR/PDR sources. In: Williamson J, Thomadsen B, Nath R, eds. *Brachytherapy physics*. Madison, WI: Medical Physics Publishing, 1995:541–556.
21. Williamson JF, Anderson LL, Grigsby PW, et al. American Endocurietherapy Society recommendations for specification of brachytherapy source strength. *Endocurie/Hypertherm Oncol* 1993;9:1–7.
22. Williamson JF, Nath R. Clinical implementation of AAPM Task Group 32 recommendations on brachytherapy source strength specifications. *Med Phys* 1991;18:439–448.

23. Bastin KT, Podgorsak MB, Thomadsen BR. The transit dose component of high dose rate brachytherapy: direct measurements and clinical implications. *Int J Radiat Oncol Biol Phys* 1993;26(4):695–702.

24. Houdek PV, Glasgow GP, Schwade J, et al. Design and implementation of a program for high dose rate brachytherapy. In: Nag S, ed. *High dose rate brachytherapy: a textbook.* Armonk, NY: Futura Publishing, 1994:27–40.

25. Houdek PV, Schwade JG, Wu X, et al. Dose determination in high dose-rate brachytherapy. *Int J Radiat Oncol Biol Phys* 1992;24(4):795–801.

26. Thomadsen BR, Houdek PV, van der Laarse R, et al. Treatment planning and optimization. In: Nag S, ed. *High dose rate brachytherapy: a textbook.* Armonk, NY: Futura Publishing, 1994:79–145.

27. Thomadsen B, Das R. The physics and dosimetry of high–dose-rate brachytherapy. In: Halperin E, Perez C, Brady L, eds. *Principles and practice of radiation oncology,* 5th ed. Philadelphia, PA: Lippincott Williams & Wilkins, 2008:540–559.

28. Fowler JF. Brief summary of radiobiological principles of fractionated radiotherapy. *Semin Radiat Oncol* 1992;2:16–21.

29. Fowler JF. The linear-quadratic formula and progress in fractionated radiotherapy. *Br J Radiol* 1989;62(740):679–694.

30. Orton CG, Brenner DJ, Dale RG, et al. Radiobiology. In: Nag S, ed. *High dose rate brachytherapy: a textbook.* Armonk, NY: Futura Publishing, 1994:11–25.

31. Orton CG, Ezzell GA. Physics and dosimetry of high-dose-rate brachytherapy. In: Perez CA, Brady LW, eds. *Principles and practice of radiation oncology,* 3rd ed. Philadelphia, PA: Lippincott–Raven, 1998:469–485.

32. Barendsen GW. Dose fractionation, dose rate and iso-effect relationships for normal tissue responses. *Int J Radiat Oncol Biol Phys* 1982;8(11):1981–1997.

33. Orton CG. The radiobiology of brachytherapy. In: Nag S, ed. *Principles and practice of brachytherapy.* Armonk, NY: Futura Publishing, 1997.

34. Arai T, Morita S, Iinuma T, et al. Radiation treatment of cervix cancer using the high dose rate remote afterloading intracavitary irradiation: an analysis of the correlation between optimal dose range and fractionation. *Jpn J Cancer Clin* 1979;25:605–612.

35. Liu WS, Yen SH, Chang CH, et al. Determination of the appropriate fraction number and size of the HDR brachytherapy for cervical cancer. *Gynecol Oncol* 1996;60(2):295–300.

36. Orton CG, Seyedsadr M, Somnay A. Comparison of high and low dose rate remote afterloading for cervix cancer and the importance of fractionation. *Int J Radiat Oncol Biol Phys* 1991;21(6):1425–1434.

37. Moore SV, Aldrete JS. Primary retroperitoneal sarcomas: the role of surgical treatment. *Am J Surg* 1981;142(3):358–361.

38. Petereit DG, Pearcey R. Literature analysis of high dose rate brachytherapy fractionation schedules in the treatment of cervical cancer: is there an optimal fractionation schedule? *Int J Radiat Oncol Biol Phys* 1999;43(2):359–366.

39. Petereit DG, Sarkaria JN, Potter DM, et al. High-dose-rate versus low-dose-rate brachytherapy in the treatment of cervical cancer: analysis of tumor recurrence—the University of Wisconsin experience. *Int J Radiat Oncol Biol Phys* 1999;45(5):1267–1274.

40. Nag S, Erickson B, Thomadsen B, et al. The American Brachytherapy Society recommendations for high-dose-rate brachytherapy for carcinoma of the cervix. *Int J Radiat Oncol Biol Phys* 2000;48(1):201–211.

41. Mate TP, Gottesman JE, Hatton J, et al. High dose-rate afterloading [192]Iridium prostate brachytherapy: feasibility report. *Int J Radiat Oncol Biol Phys* 1998;41(3):525–533.

42. Martinez AA, Kestin LL, Stromberg JS, et al. Interim report of image-guided conformal high-dose-rate brachytherapy for patients with unfavorable prostate cancer: the William Beaumont phase II dose-escalating trial. *Int J Radiat Oncol Biol Phys* 2000;472:343–352.

43. Yamada Y, Rogers L, Demanes DJ, et al. American Brachytherapy Society consensus guidelines for high-dose-rate prostate brachytherapy. Brachytherapy 2012;11(1):20–32.

44. Haie-Meder C, Potter R, Van Limbergen E, et al. Recommendations from Gynaecological (GYN) GEC-ESTRO Working Group (I): concepts and terms in 3D image based 3D treatment planning in cervix cancer brachytherapy with emphasis on MRI assessment of GTV and CTV. *Radiother Oncol* 2005;74(3):235–245.

45. Potter R, Haie-Meder C, Van Limbergen E, et al. Recommendations from gynaecological (GYN) GEC ESTRO working group (II): concepts and terms in 3D image-based treatment planning in cervix cancer brachytherapy-3D dose volume parameters and aspects of 3D image-based anatomy, radiation physics, radiobiology. *Radiother Oncol* 2006;78(1):67–77.

46. Viswanathan AN, Erickson BA. Three-dimensional imaging in gynecologic brachytherapy: a survey of the American Brachytherapy Society. *Int J Radiat Oncol Biol Phys* 2010;76(1):104–109.

47. Viswanathan AN, Dimopoulos J, Kirisits C, et al. Computed tomography versus magnetic resonance imaging-based contouring in cervical cancer brachytherapy: results of a prospective trial and preliminary guidelines for standardized contours. *Int J Radiat Oncol Biol Phys* 2007;68(2):491–498.

CHAPTER 7

UNSEALED RADIONUCLIDES: PHYSICS AND CLINICAL APPLICATIONS

- Guidelines for therapeutic use of unsealed radionuclide sources have been published by the American College of Radiology (1). Clinically used radionuclides are listed in Table 7-1.
- Primary uses of nonsealed radionuclide therapy include treatment of the following: benign or malignant thyroid disease, hematologic disease, malignant bone disease, and benign or malignant disease within a body cavity (2–4).
- It is mandatory to verify that female patients are not pregnant or breast-feeding at the time of oral or intravenous radionuclide therapy.
- Pregnancy may be ruled out by a negative beta human chorionic gonadotropin test obtained within 48 hours before administration of the radiopharmaceutical, documented hysterectomy or tubal ligation, a postmenopausal state with absence of menstrual bleeding for 2 years, or premenarche.
- Breast-feeding must be discontinued for 1 to 2 weeks before administration of a radiopharmaceutical (5).

IODINE-131 (^{131}I)

- The biologic half-life (T_{bio}) of iodine in normal adults is 20 to 200 days. With a physical half-life (T_{phy}) of 8.06 days, the effective half-life (T_{eff}) may range from 5.74 to 7.74 days, according to the following formula:

$$T_{eff} = \frac{T_{phy} \times T_{bio}}{T_{phy} + T_{bio}}$$

- The T_{eff} of ^{131}I in postoperative patients with thyroid carcinoma, although not extensively investigated, is estimated to be approximately 17 hours (6).
- Three strategies are used to determine the administered activity for patients with hyperthyroidism:
  - *Empiric strategy*: Most patients receive 3 to 5 mCi (110 to 185 MBq); those who are not euthyroid after 6 months receive a second administration.

Table 7-1				
Clinically Used Nonsealed Radionuclides				
Radionuclide	**Emitted Particles** E_{max}		**Physical Half-Life (Days)**	**Decays to**
	Beta (β⁻)	Gamma (γ)		
¹³¹I	606 keV (10%)	364 keV (81%) 337 keV (7.3%) 284 keV (6%)	8.06	¹³¹Xe
³²P	1.70 MeV	—	14.3	³²S
¹⁵³Sm	0.81 MeV	0.29 MeV	1.9	¹⁵³Eu
⁸⁹Sr	1.46 MeV	—	50.6	⁸⁹Y
¹⁸⁶Re	1.07 MeV (19%)	137 keV (9%)	3.8	¹⁸⁶Os
⁹⁰Y	934 keV	—	2.7	⁹⁰Zr

- *Fixed-administered activity strategy*: Calculated by determining a fixed activity per gram of tissue:

$$\text{Administered Activity } (\mu Ci) = \frac{\mu Ci/g \text{ selected} \times \text{gland weight (g)} \times 100}{\% \text{ uptake @ 24 h}}$$

The μCi per g selected, ranging from 55 to 110 μCi per g (1.5 to 3.0 MBq per g), is based on clinical experience.
- *Delivered dose method*: Irradiation dose of 50 to 100 Gy is selected as a target dose for the gland:

$$\text{Administered Activity } (\mu Ci) = \frac{\text{Gy selected} \times \text{gland weight (g)} \times 100}{\% \text{ uptake @ 24 h} \times 90}$$

where 90 is a constant based on tissue-absorbed fraction of the dose and T_{bio} of 24 days.
- Treatment strategies for postoperative patients with thyroid carcinoma are either empiric, with administered activities of 30 to 250 mCi, or are based on the delivered dose method.

Benign Thyroid Conditions

- ¹³¹I for hyperthyroidism is used to treat diffuse toxic goiter (Graves' disease), toxic nodular goiter, and solitary toxic nodule.
- A recent radioiodine thyroid uptake is necessary; the size of the thyroid gland should be estimated by palpation or some other means.
- The patient's system should be free of iodide-containing medications, iodine contrast agents, exogenous thyroid hormone, and antithyroid medications.

- Usual initial absorbed doses are 50 to 200 µCi (1.85 to 7.40 MBq) per g of thyroid (after adjusting for current 24-hour radioiodine uptake).
- For hyperthyroidism, the usual dose is 3 to 5 mCi (110 to 185 MBq).
- For toxic nodular goiter, doses of up to 30 mCi (1,110 MBq) typically are used; however, higher doses may be necessary for large multinodular glands (1).
- Current Nuclear Regulatory Commission (7) regulations require hospital confinement if the patient's body contains 30 or more mCi (1,110 MBq).
- Thionamides (propylthiouracil, methimazole) inhibit organification of iodide; if ^{131}I therapy is administered during the first 2 weeks after discontinuing thionamide, the dose may need to be increased.
- If the patient does not adequately respond to a dose of ^{131}I, subsequent treatments may be given, at least 2 months after, to allow for the full effect of the initial treatment to occur.

Malignant Thyroid Conditions

Ablation of Thyroid Remnant

- Thyroid hormones should be depleted so that the level of serum thyroid-stimulating hormone is elevated; this is done by withholding thyroid hormone replacement (4 to 6 weeks for thyroxin, 2 weeks for triiodothyronine) after surgery.
- All routine blood work should be performed, and laboratory specimens obtained, before treatment.
- If the remnant is large, thyroid scintigraphy with technetium-99m (^{99m}Tc) (pertechnetate) or iodine-123 (^{123}I) may be used to determine the thyroid remnant uptake of radioiodide. For a very small remnant, a whole-body survey with ^{131}I may be useful.
- Usual oral doses of ^{131}I (sodium iodine) are 100 to 150 mCi (3,700 to 5,500 MBq).
- Side effects include radiation gastritis, radiation sialitis, and diarrhea. With larger or multiple doses, xerostomia may rarely occur.
- The patient must be isolated from others and placed on radiation precautions until radioactivity is equivalent to 29.9 mCi (1,100 MBq) or less and the exposure rate at 1 m is lower than 5 mR per hour.
- On May 29, 1997, the NRC promulgated new rules that allow administration of ^{131}I for thyroid diseases on an outpatient basis. The new regulation is contained in Section 10, Code of Federal Regulations, Part 35 (10 CFR 35), and the specific changes are noted in Section 35.75 (5).
- Activity below which the patient can be discharged, depending on fractional thyroid uptake, is shown in Table 7-2.
- Health care providers (licensees) are authorized to release from their control any individual who has received a radiopharmaceutical or permanent implant(s) containing radioactive materials if the total effective dose equivalent (TEDE) to any other individual from exposure to the released individual is not likely to exceed 5 mSv (500 mrem) (8).

Table 7-2	
Postthyroidectomy for Thyroid Cancer	
Fractional Thyroid Uptake of ^{131}I	Administered Activity Below Which Patient Can be Released (mCi)[a]
0.025	257
0.035	241
0.05	220
0.075	193
0.10	171
0.125	154
0.15	140
0.175	128
0.20	119
0.225	110
0.25	103
0.275	96
0.30	91
0.325	86
0.35	81
0.375	77
0.40	73
0.425	70

[a]The maximum releasable activity for thyroid uptakes not listed can be computed from the equation $Q_0 = 500/[1.621 + 12.98 F_2]$, where Q_0 = maximum administered activity in mCi, and F_2 = the measured fractional thyroid uptake.

- There are three additional requirements imposed by the new ruling:
  - It is required by 10 CFR 35.75(b) that the licensee provides the released individual with instructions, including written instructions, on actions recommended to maintain doses to other individuals As Low As Is Reasonably Achievable (ALARA), if the TEDE is likely to exceed 1 mSv (100 mrem). If the dose to a breast-feeding infant or child could exceed 1 mSv (100 mrem), assuming no interruption of breast-feeding, the instructions would also include (a) guidance on the interruption or discontinuation of breast-feeding and (b) information on the consequences of failure to follow the guidance.
  - It is required by 10 CFR 35.75(c) that the licensee maintains a record, for 3 years after the date of release, on the basis for authorizing the release of an individual, if the TEDE is calculated by (a) using the regained activity rather than the activity

administered, (b) using an occupancy factor of less than 0.25 at 1 m, (c) using the biologic or effective half-life, or (d) considering the shielding by tissue.

- In 10 CFR 35.75(d), the licensee is required to maintain a record, for 3 years after the date of release, that instructions were provided to a breast-feeding woman if the radiation dose to the infant or child from continued breast-feeding could result in a TEDE exceeding 5 mSv (500 mrem).
- It is common policy to determine a 48-hour whole-body retention of ^{131}I; this measurement is made with a thyroid uptake detector.
- This whole-body retention percentage is a very conservative assumption of the long-lived thyroidal component. This retention percentage is inserted into the equation for the three-component model, and the dose to infinity to the maximally exposed individual is determined.
- The maximum ^{131}I activity that can be administered to a patient who is to be immediately released can be determined such that the dose to infinity to the maximally exposed individual is less than 5 mSv (500 mrem). This administered activity is easily determined from a lookup table of activity, based on the whole-body retention percentage (8).
- The NRC published the companion Regulatory Guide 8-39 in (1).
- Grigsby et al. (9) monitored radiation exposure to household members and four rooms of 30 patients who received ^{131}I after thyroidectomy for differentiated thyroid carcinoma. All dose measurements were well below the limit (5 mSv) mandated by NRC regulations.
- If exposure levels are higher than 5 mSv and the patient must temporarily remain in the hospital:
  - It is not normally necessary to store body effluents (urine, stool, or vomitus), but the commode should be flushed after use to ensure sufficient dilution of radioactivity.
  - Surfaces that the patient is likely to touch (floor, faucets, light switches, telephone) should be protected with absorbent pads or plastic.
  - Food trays and linens should be stored in the room until monitored and cleared, or until the patient is discharged.
  - All trash and residual nondisposable items must be monitored after the patient's release and stored until radiation levels reach the statutory level defined for safe disposal or reuse.
  - After all contaminated materials are removed, the room must be surveyed to verify that radiation levels are sufficiently low to permit general use (1).

Residual Thyroid Cancer

- A whole-body scan performed with ^{131}I should demonstrate abnormal concentration of tracer.
- Rising thyroglobulin radioimmunoassay titer or absolute levels above 30 ng per dL may be used in lieu of scintigraphic studies to demonstrate functioning tissue as an indication for treatment.
- For residual tumor in thyroid bed, usual doses are 100 to 150 mCi (3,700 to 5,550 MBq).

Thyroid Metastases

- Usual doses are 150 to 200 mCi (5,550 to 7,400 MBq); larger doses have been used, but at the risk of bone marrow depression.
- Pulmonary fibrosis may occur after therapy of widespread lung metastases with doses over 175 mCi (6,475 MBq).
- Appropriate testing (e.g., complete blood count, pulmonary function studies) should be considered before treatment.

PHOSPHORUS-32 (^{32}P)

- In healthy adults, sodium ^{32}P distributes uniformly throughout the body after injection.
- After 72 hours, bone marrow, spleen, and liver concentrate approximately 10 times as much activity per unit weight as other organs.
- Once equilibrium is established (after approximately 72 hours), the body loses approximately 6% of activity daily (T_{eff} of 11 days).
- Administered activity of 4 mCi given to treat polycythemia vera in a 70-kg person is estimated to be 115 cGy to bone and 17 cGy to body soft tissue.
- In an organ in which the concentration of ^{32}P is C μCi per g, the dose rate D is

$$D(\text{cGy/day}) = 2.13C \times \bar{E}_b$$

  where $\bar{E}$ is the average energy (0.69 MeV) per decay of the isotope. The total dose to the organ is

$$D(\text{cGy}) = 73.8C_{max} \times \bar{E}_b\, T_{eff}\, (1 - e^{T_{eff} \times t})$$

  where C_{max} is the maximum concentration in microcuries per gram, and t is the total elapsed time that the radioisotope is present in the organ (10).
- Chromic ^{32}P is a radiocolloid, with biokinetics and dosimetry different from sodium ^{32}P; the colloid particles are 0.05 to 1.00 μm in diameter in a glucose suspension.
- Chromic ^{32}P is not absorbed systemically but tends to collect on intracavitary surfaces; dose calculations are based on the assumption of uniform distribution of colloid particles over the surface of the cavity. When this assumption is used, dose is calculated by

$$D(z) = \frac{dA}{d\sigma}\tau k \sum_i n_i \bar{E}_i \int_z^{R_{max}} 2\pi \times \Phi(x)\, dx$$

  where $D(z)$ = absorbed dose at a distance z from an infinitely extended plane source (cGy), $dA/d\sigma$ = number of disintegrations per second per unit area (dis · s^{-1} · cm^{-2}), and τ = residence time of the activity.

Polycythemia Vera

- Intravenous sodium ^{32}P is indicated for polycythemia vera and thrombocytosis.
- The dose may be standard (3 mCi [111 MBq]) or based on body surface area (2.3 mCi [85 MBq] per m^2), but usually should not exceed 5 mCi (185 MBq).
- Relapse or failure to respond within 12 weeks may require retreatment with doses up to 7 mCi (260 MBq).
- ^{32}P should not be given if platelet count is less than 100,000 per mL or leukocyte count is lower than 3,000 per mL (1).

Malignant Ascites or Pleural Effusion

- The most common use of colloidal chromic ^{32}P is adjuvant therapy of intraperitoneal metastasis from ovarian or endometrial carcinoma.
- Usual intraperitoneal dose is 10 to 20 mCi (370 to 740 MBq); the average is 15 mCi, administered with approximately 1,000 mL of sterile normal saline. Procedures are detailed elsewhere (3). However, the use of intraperitoneal ^{32}P has widely been replaced by taxane and platinum-based chemotherapy because of lower bowel toxicity (11).
- Uniform spread of the radiopharmaceutical throughout the affected cavity should be documented using ^{99m}Tc sulfur colloid or intraperitoneal injection of sterile radiographic contrast, followed by appropriate imaging.
- Chromic ^{32}P is used to treat malignant pleural effusions, pleural mesotheliomas (doses of 6 to 12 mCi [222 to 444 MBq]), and malignant pericardial effusions.
- Other indications include cystic craniopharyngiomas and, in smaller doses, as an agent for radiation synovectomy.

SAMARIUM-153 (^{153}SM) (QUADRAMET)

- Quadramet is a therapeutic agent consisting of radioactive ^{153}Sm and a tetraphosphonate chelator, ethylenediaminetetramethylenephosphonic acid (EDTMP).
- Quadramet is formulated as a sterile, nonpyrogenic, clear, colorless to light-amber isotonic solution for intravenous administration.
- ^{153}Sm-EDTMP has an affinity for bone and concentrates in areas of bone turnover, in association with hydroxyapatite. Quadramet accumulates in osteoblastic lesions at a greater rate than in normal bone, with a lesion to normal bone ratio of approximately 5:1 (12).
- The recommended dose of Quadramet is 1 mCi per kg (37 MBq per kg) administered intravenously over a period of 1 minute through a secure indwelling catheter and followed with a saline flush.
- The total administered activity of ^{153}Sm-EDTMP, predicted on a 2-Gy bone marrow dose, varied from 35% to 63% of the standard recommended dose of 1 mCi per kg (37 MBq per kg). Doses of 38 MBq per kg resulted in bone marrow doses of 3.27 to 5.90 Gy, at which myelotoxicity would have been anticipated. Caution should be exercised when the dose is determined for a very thin or very obese patient.

STRONTIUM-89 (^{89}SR)

- ^{89}Sr is an analog of calcium and concentrates in osteoblastic bone cancer lesions.
- After intravenous injection of ionic ^{89}Sr, it is cleared rapidly from the blood; approximately 50% of injected activity is deposited in bone, where it may remain for as long as 100 days.
- The standard dose is 40 to 60 μCi (1.48 to 2.22 MBq) per kg of body weight, given intravenously; current available formulation is 4 mCi per vial.
- ^{85}Sr scans have been used to calculate absorbed doses (6 to 61 cGy per MBq administered activity) (13). Estimated doses to normal tissue in a normal adult (70 kg) are 59 cGy per mCi to surface of bone, 40 cGy per mCi to red bone marrow, 3 cGy per mCi to whole body, and 0.23 cGy per mCi to urinary bladder wall.

Bony Metastases

- Patients with osseous metastases with increased tracer uptake on bone scintigraphy and competent bone marrow (white cell count greater than 2,400 per mm^3 and platelet count greater than 60,000 per mm^3) are candidates for radiopharmaceutical therapy.
- A "flare" of bone pain, lasting several days, occurs in approximately 10% of patients.
- Extravasation of ^{153}Sm or ^{89}Sr can cause skin necrosis near the injection site; thus, it is imperative to have excellent intravenous access for injection.
- Bone marrow depression occurs transiently (nadir at approximately 4 weeks), with recovery in 3 to 6 additional weeks.
- Complete blood and platelet counts should be performed routinely for 10 to 12 weeks (1).
- External beam irradiation may be used with ^{153}Sm or ^{89}Sr for local treatment of severely painful sites.
- Wide-field hemibody irradiation should not be given within 2 to 3 months of radiopharmaceutical administration because of potential myelotoxicity.
- Patients should not have received long-acting myelosuppressive chemotherapy for 6 to 8 weeks, or other forms of myelosuppressive chemotherapy for at least 4 weeks, before administration of ^{153}Sm or ^{89}Sr, because of potential marrow toxicity.
- Retreatment may be given in the case of initial treatment failure; the dose is 40 to 60 μCi (1.48 to 2.22 MBq) per kg of body weight. Special attention should be paid to recovery of bone marrow and blood counts. Retreatment generally should not be given sooner than 90 days from the last ^{153}Sm or ^{89}Sr administration, unless white blood cell and platelet counts have adequately recovered (5).

RHENIUM-186 (^{186}RE)

- ^{186}Re has been complexed with a bone-seeking phosphorate, hydroxyethylenediphosphonate, to form ^{186}Re-HEDP.

- After intravenous injection, ^{186}Re-HEDP is rapidly cleared from blood; approximately 50% is deposited in bone, with minimal extraosseous uptake.
- Excretion is through the kidneys into the urine.
- Based on 50% absorption rates, administered activities of 33 to 35 mCi will deliver maximum doses of 0.75 Gy to the red marrow (14).
- Evaluation of pharmacokinetics of ^{186}Re-HEDP therapy in 11 patients with breast or prostate metastases showed that the bone marrow absorbed dose can be predicted from a diagnostic pretherapy ^{99m}Tc-MDP (methylene diphosphonate) scintigram (15).
- ^{186}Re remains largely experimental but has been investigated for radiation synovectomy, cystic craniopharyngioma, cystic astrocytoma, medullary thyroid carcinoma, and bone metastasis.
- Intraperitoneal administration has been used for metastatic ovarian carcinoma.

YTTRIUM-90 (^{90}Y)

- ^{90}Y microspheres have recently been utilized in the management of hepatic metastases with a good response rate and acceptable complications (16).

QUALITY ASSURANCE AND NUCLEAR REGULATORY COMMISSION

- Quality assurance (QA) policies and procedures should be developed by each institution performing nonsealed radionuclide therapy to protect the patient, public, and medical personnel from unnecessary radiation exposure.
- Specific QA procedures are beyond the scope of this chapter; however, areas that should be addressed in such a program are outlined below.
- Care should be taken in ordering the specific isotope, formulary, and quantity for each patient; different foundations of the same isotope must be recognized, such as chromic ^{32}P (used for pleural or peritoneal instillation) versus sodium ^{32}P (used intravenously for polycythemia vera).
- Timing and vendor delivery capabilities should be taken into account to ensure that the appropriate activity of the isotope is available on the date of administration.
- Packaging must be surveyed on delivery; appropriate protection should be used in opening it.
- The activity of the radioisotope should be determined with a dose calibrator that has been evaluated for linearity, constancy, and accuracy.
- According to Title 10, Code of Federal Regulations 35 (5), administration of an activity of a radiopharmaceutical that differs from the prescribed activity by more than 20% (smaller or larger) constitutes a "misadministration." If the difference is between 10% and 20%, administration is a "recordable event." The activity of record of ^{131}I, ^{32}P, ^{153}Sm, ^{89}Sr, ^{186}Re, and ^{90}Y shall be administered only if it differs by less than 10% (larger or smaller) from the activity prescribed by the authorized user. Compliance with NRC regulations regarding prescribed activity is mandatory.

- Before administration of the radioisotope, the following items must be confirmed in accordance with our QA program: informed consent signed; written directive signed and dated by authorized user; prescribed activity correct to within 10%; and patient identified by two methods.
- Previous NRC regulations (10 CFR 35.75) have been revised (5). At present, patients are hospitalized until the total body burden of ^{131}I is less than 33 mCi or the exposure rate at 1 m from the patient is less than 7 mrem per hour. Patients receiving 30 mCi or less, and those who will not subject anyone to more than 5 mSv (500 mrem), receive ^{131}I administration as outpatients (7).
- Consistent with their patient care responsibilities, nurses should reduce their exposure to radiation emitted from the patient by reducing their time with the patient, increasing their distance from the patient, and using shielding.
- Institutions should develop standard emergency procedures for radioisotope spill.

References

1. ACR. *Standard for therapy with unsealed radionuclide sources.* Philadelphia, PA: American College of Radiology, 1996.
2. Clarke SE. Radionuclide therapy in oncology. *Cancer Treat Rev* 1994;20(1):51–71.
3. Grigsby PW. Nonsealed radionuclide therapy. In: Perez CA, Brady LW, eds. *Principles and practice of radiation oncology*, 3rd ed. Philadelphia, PA: Lippincott–Raven, 1998:583–592.
4. Serafini AN. Current status of systemic intravenous radiopharmaceuticals for the treatment of painful metastatic bone disease. *Int J Radiat Oncol Biol Phys* 1994;30(5):1187–1194.
5. US-CFR. Title 10, Code of Federal Regulations: August 31, 1990, Part 35, 1990.
6. Kovalic JJ, Grigsby PW, Slessinger E. The relationship of clinical factors and radiation exposure rates from iodine-131 treated thyroid carcinoma patients. *Med Dosim* 1990;15(4):209–215.
7. US-NRC. U.S. Nuclear Regulatory Commission. *Regulatory guide 8.39: release of patients administered radioactive materials.* Washington, DC: NRC, 1997.
8. Grigsby PW, Baker SM, Siegel BA, et al. New NRC patient release guidelines: major quality of life & cost-containment benefits. *Adm Radiol J* 1998;17(4):18–21.
9. Grigsby PW, Siegel BA, Baker S, et al. Radiation exposure from outpatient radioactive iodine (^{131}I) therapy for thyroid carcinoma. *JAMA* 2000;283(17):2272–2274.
10. Bayouth JE, Macey DJ. Dosimetry considerations of bone-seeking radionuclides for marrow ablation. *Med Phys* 1993;20(4):1089–1096.
11. Gehrig PA, Varia M, Apisarnthanarax S, et al. Ovary. In: Halperin EC, Perez CA, Brady LW, eds. *Principles and practice of radiation oncology*, 5th ed. Philadelphia, PA: Lippincott Williams & Wilkins, 2008:1629–1649.
12. Serafini AN, Houston SJ, Resche I, et al. Palliation of pain associated with metastatic bone cancer using samarium-153 lexidronam: a double-blind placebo-controlled clinical trial. *J Clin Oncol* 1998;16(4):1574–1581.
13. Blake GM, Zivanovic MA, McEwan AJ, et al. Sr-89 therapy: strontium kinetics in disseminated carcinoma of the prostate. *Eur J Nucl Med* 1986;12(9):447–454.
14. Maxon HR, Deutsch EA, Thomas SR, et al. Re-186(Sn) HEDP for treatment of multiple metastatic foci in bone: human biodistribution and dosimetric studies. *Radiology* 1988;166(2):501–507.
15. de Klerk JM, van Dijk A, van het Schip AD, et al. Pharmacokinetics of rhenium-186 after administration of rhenium-186-HEDP to patients with bone metastases. *J Nucl Med* 1992;33(5): 646–651.
16. Cianni R, Urigo C, Notarianni E, et al. Selective internal radiation therapy with SIR-spheres for the treatment of unresectable colorectal hepatic metastases. *Cardiovasc Intervent Radiol* 2009;32(6):1179–1186.

CHAPTER 8

LATE EFFECTS OF CANCER TREATMENT AND THE QUANTEC REVIEW

In this chapter, we provide an overview of radiation-induced late organ toxicities, grading of late toxicities, and recommended normal tissue dose constraints for both conventional fractionation and hypofractionated treatment courses based on the Quantitative Analysis of Normal Tissue Effects in the Clinic (QUANTEC) Study and Radiation Therapy Oncology Group (RTOG) protocols. Although recommended dose constraints are listed for consideration, final decisions should remain at the discretion of the treating physician. We also strongly encourage readers to refer to the original papers from the QUANTEC study, relevant RTOG protocols, and later chapters for site-specific information regarding late toxicity.

BACKGROUND

- Modern treatment planning technologies such as three-dimensional conformal radiotherapy (3D-CRT), intensity-modulated radiation therapy (IMRT), stereotactic radiosurgery (SRS), stereotactic body radiation therapy (SBRT), helical tomotherapy, arc-based therapies, and proton beam therapy allow for highly precise and customizable dose delivery to target volumes, resulting in highly nonuniform dose distributions to surrounding normal tissues.
- In the modern era, combined-modality treatments (e.g., radiation therapy combined with chemotherapy, immunotherapies, and biologic-response modifiers) are increasingly common, with important implications toward potential normal tissue toxicity. When combined with additional treatment modalities, radiation doses customarily deemed safe may no longer be so because such doses may produce increasingly severe late effects.
- When evaluating plans, dose-volume histograms (DVHs) allow for effective two-dimensional visualization of cumulative dose distribution to both target volumes and organs at risk (OARs). Risks of injury to OARs are typically evaluated as a function of dose-volume relationships. Despite important limitations discussed in the QUANTEC study (1–5), DVHs allow for rapid comparison of projected dose distributions between potential treatment plans.

- Normal tissue complication probabilities (NTCPs) are estimated using the linear-quadratic equation, α/β ratio and its clinical applicability (6).
- Late toxicities following radiation therapy are commonly graded using the RTOG/European Organization for Research and Treatment of Cancer (EORTC) Late Radiation Morbidity Scoring Schema (Table 8-1), as well as the National Cancer Institute (NCI) Common Terminology Criteria for Adverse Events (CTCAEs) (7).
- Descriptive summaries of late radiation-induced toxicities for selected critical structures are provided below.
- Recommended dose constraints for critical structures are summarized in Tables 8-2 (QUANTEC recommendations for conventional fractionation), 8-3 (RTOG protocol constraints for conventional fractionation), 8-4 (QUANTEC recommendations for SRS/SBRT), and 8-5 (RTOG protocol constraints for SRS/SBRT). We strongly encourage readers to refer to the QUANTEC literature and relevant RTOG protocols. Although provided for consideration, final decisions on dose constraints remain at the discretion of the treating physician.

BRAIN

(See Chapter 10: Management of Adult Central Nervous System Tumors)

- *Clinical Presentation*: Headache, somnolence, intellectual deficits, functional neurologic losses, and memory alterations may occur during, shortly after, or, most commonly, as a delayed effect after completing treatment.
- *Time Course*: Radiation necrosis and gliosis develop approximately 6 to 12 months after radiation therapy. Early-delayed neurocognitive effects occur at approximately 3 to 12 months, whereas long-term neurocognitive effects occur beginning at 1 year. Whole-brain radiation therapy is associated with higher risks of neurocognitive side effects, although partial-brain irradiation may also cause delayed neurocognitive toxicity.
- *Dose/Time/Volume*: Doses of 50 Gy to the whole brain in 1.8 to 2.0 Gy fractions are generally well tolerated in adults with minimal risk of radiation necrosis, whereas pediatric threshold doses are 30 to 35 Gy (8–11). The brain is particularly sensitive to fraction sizes greater than 2 Gy, and total fractionated RT doses greater than 60 Gy are not generally indicated for most tumors (12,13). A 5% risk and a 10 risk of symptomatic radiation necrosis are predicted to occur with BEDs of 120 Gy and 150 Gy, respectively (corresponding to 72 Gy and 90 Gy delivered in 2 Gy fractions, respectively). Toxicity associated with SRS increases rapidly when brain volume exposed to ≥ 12 Gy exceeds 5 to 10 cm³. For the brainstem, cumulative dose using conventional fractionation should not exceed 54 Gy, although small brainstem volumes (1 to 10 mL) can be treated to 59 Gy (14). For single-fraction SRS to the brainstem, maximum point dose (D_{max}) less than 12.5 Gy correlates with low risk for radiation necrosis (12).
- *Chemical/Biologic Modifiers*: Concurrent temozolomide and carmustine (BCNU) are generally well tolerated. Immediate subsequent use of methotrexate (intrathecally or intravenously) is of concern.

Table 8-1

RTOG/EORTC Late Radiation Morbidity Grading Scale

Organ	Grade 1	Grade 2	Grade 3	Grade 4
Brain	Mild headache Slight lethargy	Moderate headache Great lethargy	Severe headache Severe neurologic dysfunction (partial loss of power/dyskinesia)	Seizures Paralysis Coma
Spinal cord	Mild Lhermitte's syndrome	Severe Lhermitte's syndrome	Objective neurologic findings at/below cord level treated	Monoplegia Paraplegia Quadriplegia
Eye	Asymptomatic cataract Minor corneal ulceration or keratitis	Symptomatic cataract Moderate corneal ulceration Minor retinopathy/glaucoma	Severe keratitis Severe retinopathy or detachment	Panophthalmitis Blindness
Salivary glands	Slight dryness of mouth Good response on stimulation	Moderate dry mouth Poor response on stimulation	Complete dryness of mouth No response on stimulation	Fibrosis
Larynx	Hoarseness Slight arytenoid edema	Moderate arytenoid edema Chondritis	Severe edema Severe chondritis	Necrosis
Heart	Asymptomatic or mild symptoms Transient T wave inversion & ST changes Sinus tachycardia > 110 at rest	Moderate exertional angina Mild pericarditis Normal cardiac size Persistent abnormal ST or T-wave changes Low-voltage QRS	Severe angina Pericardial effusion Constrictive pericarditis Moderate heart failure Cardiac enlargement EKG abnormalities	Cardiac tamponade Severe heart failure Severe constrictive pericarditis
Lung	Asymptomatic or mild symptoms (dry cough) Slight radiographic appearances	Moderate symptomatic fibrosis or pneumonitis (severe cough) Low-grade fever Patchy radiographic appearance	Severe symptomatic fibrosis or pneumonitis Dense radiographic changes	Severe respiratory insufficiency Continuous oxygen Assisted ventilation

continued

Table 8-1

RTOG/EORTC Late Radiation Morbidity Grading Scale *(continued)*

Organ	Grade 1	Grade 2	Grade 3	Grade 4
Esophagus	Mild fibrosis Slight dysphagia to solids with- out odynophagia	Unable to take solid food normally Swallowing semisolid food Dilatation may be indicated	Severe fibrosis Able to swallow only liquids May have odynophagia Dilatation required	Necrosis Perforation fistula
Small Intestine/ large intestine	Mild diarrhea Mild cramping Bowel movement five times daily Slight rectal discharge/bleeding	Moderate diarrhea/colic BMs > five times daily Excessive rectal mucus Intermittent rectal bleeding	Obstruction or bleeding requiring surgery	Necrosis Perforation fistula
Liver	Mild lassitude Nausea Dyspepsia Slightly abnormal liver function	Moderate symptoms Some abnormal LFTs, no hypoalbuminemia	Disabling hepatic insufficiency Liver function tests grossly abnormal Hypoalbuminemia Edema or ascites	Necrosis Hepatic encephalopathy/ coma
Kidney	Transient albuminuria Normotensive Mildly impaired renal function (urea 25–35 mg/dL; creatinine 1.5–2.0 mg/dL; CrCl > 75%)	Persistent moderate albuminuria (2+) Mild HTN No related anemia Moderately impaired renal func- tion (urea > 36–60; CrCl 50%–74%)	Severe albuminuria Severe hypertension Persistent anemia (<10) Severe renal failure (urea > 60; creatinine > 4.0; CrCl < 50%)	Malignant hypertension Uremic coma Hyperuricemia > 100
Bladder	Slight epithelial atrophy Minor telangiectasia (microscopic hematuria)	Moderate urinary frequency Intermittent macroscopic hematuria Generalized telangiectasia	Severe frequency and dysuria Severe telangiectasia (often with petechiae) Frequent hematuria Reduction in bladder capacity <150 cc	Necrosis Contracted bladder (capacity < 100 cc) Severe hemorrhagic cystitis

Bone	Asymptomatic; no growth retardation Reduced bone density	Moderate pain or tenderness Growth retardation Irregular sclerosis	Severe pain/tenderness Complete arrest of bone growth Dense bone sclerosis	Necrosis Spontaneous fracture
Joint	Mild joint stiffness Slight limitation of movement	Moderate stiffness Intermittent/moderate joint pain Moderate movement limitation	Severe joint stiffness Pain with severely limited movement	Necrosis Complete fixation
Skin	Slight atrophy Pigmentation change Some hair loss	Patch atrophy Moderate telangiectasia Total hair loss	Marked atrophy Gross telangiectasia	Ulceration
Subcutaneous tissue	Slight induration (fibrosis) and loss of subcutaneous fat	Moderate fibrosis, asymptomatic Slight field contracture <10% linear reduction	Severe induration/loss of subcutaneous tissue Field contracture >10% linear measurement	Necrosis
Mucous membranes	Slight atrophy and dryness	Moderate atrophy, telangiectasia Little mucous	Marked atrophy with complete dryness	Ulceration

Adapted with permission from Cox JD, Stetz J, Pajak TF. Toxicity criteria of the Radiation Therapy Oncology Group (RTOG) and the European Organization for Research and Treatment of Cancer (EORTC). *Int J Radiat Oncol Biol Phys* 1995;31(5):1341–1346. © Elsevier.

Table 8-2

QUANTEC Normal Tissue Dose Constraints for Conventional Fractionation

Organ	Dose or Dose/Volume Parameter	Toxicity Rate	Toxicity End Point
Brain	Dmax < 60 Gy	<3%	Symptomatic necrosis
	Dmax = 72 Gy	5%	
	Dmax = 90 Gy	10%	
Brainstem	Dmax < 54 Gy	<5%	Symptomatic necrosis or permanent cranial neuropathy
	Dmax < 64 Gy	<5%	
	D1–10 cc ≤ 59 Gy	<5%	
Spinal cord	Dmax = 50 Gy	0.2%	Myelopathy
	Dmax = 60 Gy	6%	
	Dmax = 69 Gy	50%	
Optic nerve/optic chiasm	Dmax < 55 Gy	<3%	Optic neuropathy
	Dmax = 55–60 Gy	3%–7%	
	Dmax > 60 Gy	>7%–20%	
Cochlea	Mean dose ≤ 45 Gy	<30%	Sensorineural hearing loss
Parotid gland	Mean dose < 20 Gy (unilateral parotid)	<20%	Long-term reduction of salivary function <25% pre-RT
	Mean dose < 25 Gy (bilateral parotids)	<20%	
	Mean dose < 39 Gy (bilateral parotids)	<50%	
Pharynx	Mean dose ≤ 50 Gy	<20%	Symptomatic dysphagia/aspiration
Larynx	Dmax < 66 Gy	<20%	Vocal dysfunction
	Mean dose < 50 Gy	<30%	Aspiration
	Mean dose < 44 Gy	<20%	Edema
	V50 < 27%	<20%	Edema
Lung	V20 ≤ 30% (bilateral)	<20%	Symptomatic pneumonitis
	Mean dose = 7 Gy	5%	
	Mean dose = 13 Gy	10%	
	Mean dose = 20 Gy	20%	
	Mean dose = 24 Gy	30%	
	Mean dose = 27 Gy	40%	

Table 8-2

QUANTEC Normal Tissue Dose Constraints for Conventional Fractionation *(continued)*

Organ	Dose or Dose/Volume Parameter	Toxicity Rate	Toxicity End Point
Heart	Mean dose < 26 Gy	<15%	Pericarditis
	V30 < 46%	<15%	Pericarditis
	V25 < 10%	<15%	Long-term cardiac mortality
Esophagus	Mean dose < 34 Gy	5%–20%	Grade ≥3 esophagitis
	V35 < 50%	<30%	Grade ≥2 esophagitis
	V50 < 40%	<30%	Grade ≥2 esophagitis
	V70 < 20%	<30%	Grade ≥2 esophagitis
Stomach	D100 < 45 Gy	<7%	Ulceration
Small intestine	V15 < 120 cc (individual bowel loops)	<10%	Grade ≥3 enteritis
	V45 < 195 cc (bowel bag)	<10%	
Liver	Mean dose < 30–32 Gy	<5%	RILD (normal liver)
	Mean dose < 42 Gy	<50%	RILD (normal liver)
	Mean dose < 28 Gy	<5%	RILD (Child-Pugh A or HCC)
	Mean dose < 36 Gy	<50%	RILD (Child-Pugh A or HCC)
Kidney (Bilateral)	Mean dose < 15–18 Gy	<5%	Clinical renal dysfunction
	Mean dose < 28 Gy	<50%	Clinical renal dysfunction
	V12 < 55%	<5%	Clinical renal dysfunction
	V20 < 32%	<5%	Clinical renal dysfunction
	V23 < 30%	<5%	Clinical renal dysfunction
	V28 < 20%	<5%	Clinical renal dysfunction
Bladder (bladder cancer)	Dmax < 65 Gy	<6%	Grade ≥3 late toxicity
Bladder (prostate cancer)	V65 ≤ 50% V70 ≤ 35% V75 ≤ 25% V80 ≤ 15%		
Rectum	V50 < 50%	<15%	Grade ≥2 late toxicity
		<10%	Grade ≥3 late toxicity
	V60 < 35%	<15%	Grade ≥2 late toxicity
		<10%	Grade ≥3 late toxicity

continued

Table 8-2

QUANTEC Normal Tissue Dose Constraints for Conventional Fractionation *(continued)*

Organ	Dose or Dose/Volume Parameter	Toxicity Rate	Toxicity End Point
	V65 < 25%	<15%	Grade ≥2 late toxicity
		<10%	Grade ≥3 late toxicity
	V70 < 20%	<15%	Grade ≥2 late toxicity
		<10%	Grade ≥3 late toxicity
	V75 < 15%	<15%	Grade ≥2 late toxicity
		<10%	Grade ≥3 late toxicity
Penile bulb	Mean dose to 95% <50 Gy	<35%	Severe erectile dysfunction
	D90 < 50 Gy	<35%	
	D60–70 < 70 Gy	<55%	

Adapted with permission from Marks LB, Yorke ED, Jackson A, et al. Tolerance. Use of Normal Tissue Complication Probability Models in the Clinic. *Int J Radiat Oncol Biol Phys* 2010;76(3):S10–S19. © Elsevier.

Table 8-3

RTOG Normal Tissue Constraints for Conventional Fractionation

Organ/Tissue	RTOG Protocol	Treated Site	Dose or Dose/Volume Constraint	Dose Per Fraction
Brainstem	0539	Intermediate-risk meningioma	Dmax to 0.03 cc < 55 Gy	1.8–2 Gy
	0615	Nasopharynx	54 Gy	33 fxs
	0539, 0825	High-risk meningioma, GBM	Dmax to 0.03 cc < 60 Gy	1.8–2 Gy
Brainstem PRV	1016	Oropharynx	Dmax to 0.03 cc < 52 Gy	2 Gy
Spinal cord	0623, 0615	Lung, nasopharynx	Dmax = 45 Gy	1.8 Gy
	0619, 0522	Postop/definitive H&N	Dmax to 0.03 cc < 48 Gy	2 Gy
	0617	Lung	Dmax = 50.5	2 Gy
	0436	Esophagus	Dose to 10 cm < 50 Gy	1.8 Gy
	0436	Esophagus	Dose to 20 cm < 47 Gy	1.8 Gy
	0937	Lung	Dmax = 36 Gy	3 Gy
	0937	Lung	Dmax = 30 Gy	4 Gy
Spinal cord PRV	1016	Oropharynx	Dose to 0.03 < 48 Gy	2 Gy
Optic chiasm	0615	Nasopharynx	Dmax < 50 Gy	33 fxs

Table 8-3

RTOG Normal Tissue Constraints for Conventional Fractionation *(continued)*

Organ/Tissue	RTOG Protocol	Treated Site	Dose or Dose/Volume Constraint	Dose Per Fraction
	0539	Intermediate-risk meningioma	Dmax to 0.03 cc < 54 Gy	1.8–2 Gy
	0539	High-risk meningioma, GBM	Dmax to 0.03 cc < 56 Gy	1.8–2 Gy
Optic nerve	0539	Intermediate-risk meningioma, nasopharynx	Dmax to 0.03 cc < 50 Gy	1.8–2 Gy
	0539	High-risk meningioma, GBM	Dmax to 0.03 cc < 55 Gy	1.8–2 Gy
Retina	0539	Intermediate-risk meningioma	Dmax 0.3 cc < 45 Gy	1.8–2 Gy
	0539, 0825, 0615	High-risk meningioma, GBM, nasopharynx	Dmax to 0.3 cc < 50 Gy	1.8–2 Gy
Lens	0539	Intermediate-risk meningioma	Dmax to 0.03 cc < 5 Gy	1.8–2 Gy
	0825	High-risk meningioma, GBM	Dmax to 0.03 cc < 7 Gy	1.8–2 Gy
	0615	Nasopharynx	Dmax = 25 Gy	33 fxs
Cochlea	0615	Nasopharynx	V55 < 5%	33 fxs
Parotid gland (unilateral)	0619, 0522, 1016	Postop H&N, definitive H&N, oropharynx	Mean < 26 Gy	2 Gy
	0619, 0522	Postop H&N, definitive H&N	D50 < 30 Gy	2 Gy
Parotid gland (bilateral)	0619, 0522	Postop H&N, definitive H&N	Dose to 20 cc < 20 Gy	2 Gy
Oral cavity	0615	Nasopharynx	Mean dose < 40 Gy	33 fxs
	1016	Oropharynx	Mean dose < 30 Gy Dmax = 60 Gy	2 Gy
Mandible	1016	Oropharynx	Dmax = 66 Gy	2 Gy
	0615	Nasopharynx	Dose to 1 cc < 75 Gy, Dmax = 70 Gy	33 fxs
Submandibular gland	1016	Oropharynx	Mean dose < 39 Gy	2 Gy
Pharynx (postcricoid)	0615	Nasopharynx	Dmax < 45 Gy	33 fxs

continued

Table 8-3

RTOG Normal Tissue Constraints for Conventional Fractionation *(continued)*

Organ/Tissue	RTOG Protocol	Treated Site	Dose or Dose/Volume Constraint	Dose Per Fraction
Pharynx (posterior wall)	1016	Oropharynx	V50 < 33%	2 Gy
	1016	Oropharynx	V60 < 15%	2 Gy
	1016	Oropharynx	Mean dose < 45Gy	2 Gy
Larynx	1016	Oropharynx	Mean dose < 20 Gy	
	0619, 0615, 0522	Postop/definitive H&N, nasopharynx	Dmax = 45 Gy	2 Gy
Lung (total)	0630	Sarcoma	V20 < 20%	2 Gy
	0617, 0623	Lung	V20 < 37%	2 Gy
	0617	Lung	Mean dose = 20 Gy	2 Gy
	0937	Lung	Mean dose = 20 Gy	3 Gy
	0937	Lung	V20 ≤ 30%	3 Gy
Heart	0623, 0617	Lung	V60 < 33%	1.8 Gy
	0436	Esophagus	V50 < 33%	1.8 Gy
	0623, 0617, 0436	Lung, esophagus	V45 < 67%	1.8 Gy
	0623, 0617, 0436	Lung, esophagus	V40 < 100%	1.8 Gy
	0937	Lung	Dmax = 47	3 Gy
	0937	Lung	V45 < 30%	3 Gy
Brachial plexus	0619	Postop H&N	V60 < 5%	2 Gy
	0522	Definitive H&N	Dmax = 60 Gy	2 Gy
	0619, 0617, 0615	Postop H&N, lung, nasopharynx	Dmax = 66 Gy	2 Gy
	0937	Lung	Dmax = 36 Gy	3 Gy
	0937	Lung	Dmax = 30 Gy	4 Gy
Esophagus	0623, 0617	Lung	Mean dose = 34 Gy	1.8 Gy
	0623	Lung	Dose to 10 cm < 60 Gy	1.8 Gy
	0937	Lung	Dmax = 47 Gy	3 Gy
Esophagus (cervical)	1016	Oropharynx	Mean dose = 30 Gy	2 Gy
Small intestine	0529	Anus	Dose to 200 cc < 30 Gy	1.8 Gy
	0529	Anus	Dose to 150 cc < 35 Gy	1.8 Gy
	0822	Rectum	Dose to 180 cc < 35 Gy	1.8 Gy
	0822	Rectum	Dose to 100 cc < 40 Gy	1.8 Gy

Table 8-3

RTOG Normal Tissue Constraints for Conventional Fractionation *(continued)*

Organ/Tissue	RTOG Protocol	Treated Site	Dose or Dose/Volume Constraint	Dose Per Fraction
	0529	Anus	Dose to 20 cc < 45 Gy	1.8 Gy
	0822	Rectum	Dose to 65 cc < 45 Gy	1.8 Gy
	0822, 0529	Rectum/anus	Dmax < 50 Gy	1.8 Gy
	0418	Endometrial	V40 < 30%	1.8 Gy
	0937	Lung	Dose to 150 cc < 30 Gy	3 Gy
	0937	Lung	Dose to 100 cc < 35 Gy	3 Gy
	0937	Lung	Dose to 50 cc < 40 Gy	3 Gy
	0937	Lung	Dose to 1 cc < 45 Gy	3 Gy
	0937	Lung	Dose to 100 cc < 30 Gy	4 Gy
	0937	Lung	Dose to 50 cc < 35 Gy	4 Gy
	0937	Lung	Dose to 1 cc < 40 Gy	4 Gy
Liver	0436	Esophagus	V35 < 50%	1.8 Gy
	0937	Lung	Dose to >700 cc <18 Gy	3 Gy
Large intestine	0529	Anus	V35 < 50%	1.8 Gy
	0529	Anus	V40 < 35%	1.8 Gy
	0529	Anus	V50 < 5%	1.8 Gy
Kidney	0436	Esophagus	V23 < 100%	1.8 Gy
	0436	Esophagus	V30 < 67%	1.8 Gy
	0436	Esophagus	V50 < 33%	1.8 Gy
	0630	Sarcoma	V14 < 50%	2 Gy
	0937	Lung	V18 < 25%	3 Gy
Bladder	0621	Prostate	V50 < 60%	1.8 Gy
	0534	Postop prostate	V40 < 70%	1.8 Gy
	RTOG Prostate Consensus 2009		V50 < 55%	1.8 Gy
	0529	Anus	V35 < 50%	1.8 Gy
	0415	Prostate	V65 < 50%	1.8 Gy
	0822	Rectum	V40 < 40%	1.8 Gy
	0534	Postop prostate	V65 < 50%	1.8 Gy
	0621	Prostate	V66.6 < 40%	1.8 Gy
	0529	Anus	V40 < 35%	1.8 Gy
	0418	Endometrial	V45 < 35%	1.8 Gy
	0415	Prostate	V70 < 35%	1.8 Gy
	RTOG Prostate Consensus 2009		V70 < 30%	1.8 Gy

continued

Table 8-3

RTOG Normal Tissue Constraints for Conventional Fractionation *(continued)*

Organ/Tissue	RTOG Protocol	Treated Site	Dose or Dose/Volume Constraint	Dose Per Fraction
	0415	Prostate	V75 < 25%	1.8 Gy
	0822	Rectum	V45 < 15%	1.8 Gy
	0415	Prostate	V80 < 15%	1.8 Gy
	0529	Anus	V50 < 5%	1.8 Gy
	0822	Rectum	Dmax = 50 Gy	1.8 Gy
Femoral head	0529	Anus	V30 < 50%	1.8 Gy
	0418	Endometrial	V30 < 15%	1.8 Gy
	0822	Rectum	V40 < 40%	1.8 Gy
	0529	Anus	V40 < 35%	1.8 Gy
	0822	Rectum	V45 < 25%	1.8 Gy
	0534	Postop prostate	V50 < 10%	1.8 Gy
	0529	Anus	V44 < 5%	1.8 Gy
	RTOG Prostate Consensus 2009		V50 < 5%	1.8 Gy
	0630	Sarcoma	V60 < 5%	2 Gy
	0822	Rectum	Dmax = 50 Gy	1.8 Gy
	0712	Bladder	Dmax = 45 Gy	1.8 Gy
Rectum	0418	Endometrial	V30 < 60%	1.8 Gy
	0712	Bladder	V55 < 50%	1.8–2 Gy
	0621	Prostate	V50 < 50%	1.8 Gy
	0415	Prostate	V60 < 50%	1.8 Gy
	0415	Prostate	V65 < 35%	1.8 Gy
	0621	Prostate	V66.6 < 25%	1.8 Gy
	0415	Prostate	V70 < 25%	1.8 Gy
	0415	Prostate	V75 < 15%	1.8 Gy
	0534	Postop prostate	V40 < 55%	1.8 Gy
	0534	Postop prostate	V65 < 35%	1.8 Gy
	RTOG Prostate Consensus 2009		V70 < 20%	1.8 Gy
Anus	0630	Sarcoma	V30 < 50%	2 Gy
Penile bulb	0415	Prostate	Mean dose < 51 Gy	1.8 Gy
Testis	0630	Sarcoma	V3 < 50%	2 Gy
Vulva	0630	Sarcoma	V30 < 50%	2 Gy

Source: Radiation Therapy Oncology Group (RTOG) Clinical Trial Protocols (15–38).

- *Radiologic Imaging*: Four stages of radiation necrosis have been described on magnetic resonance imaging (MRI), from early whitening in the periventricular region to a diffuse coalescence of white and gray matter into an intense signal region along with structural loss (9).
- *Differential Diagnosis*: Hypometabolic and hypermetabolic zones on positron emission tomography/computed tomography (PET/CT), respectively, may suggest necrosis versus recurrent tumor. Although distinguishing recurrence from radiation necrosis is often challenging, MR spectroscopy may also be helpful.
- *Pathologic Diagnosis*: Only indicated for suspected tumor recurrence or progression. Hallmarks include alterations in vasculature and loss of myelination due to oligodendrocytic cell death.
- *Management*: Use analgesics, anticonvulsants, and high-dose corticosteroids as needed for worsening headaches and neurologic deficits.
- *Prevention*: For primary brain tumors, IMRT may confer lower risks of neurotoxicity (39) and is especially appropriate for tumors adjacent to critical structures including the brainstem, optic nerves, optic chiasm, lens, and retina. For brain metastases, SRS alone (40), hippocampal avoidance (HA)-WBRT (41), or 6-month courses of systemic therapy using memantine combined with WBRT (42) may be used for appropriate patients.

SPINAL CORD

- *Clinical Presentation*: May include paresthesias (including tingling, pain, and Lhermitte's syndrome), numbness, weakness, or loss of sphincter control that can progress to total paraparesis and paraplegia.
- *Time Course*: Lhermitte's syndrome occurs 2 to 4 months after irradiation and persists (or returns) at 6 to 9 months. Classically, radiation-induced spinal cord transection presents with paresis, numbness, and altered sphincter control approximately 6 to 12 months following treatment (43).
- *Dose/Time/Volume*: Using conventional fractionation, total dose of 45 Gy correlates with less than 0.2% incidence of myelopathy (44). Full spinal cord cross-sectional irradiation to cumulative doses of 50, 60, and 69 Gy is associated with myelopathy rates of approximately 0.2%, 6.0%, and 50.0% (45). For reirradiation (2 Gy per fraction) after prior conventionally fractionated treatment, spinal cord tolerance appears to increase by at least 25% after 6 months. For spine SRS, maximum cord dose of 13 Gy delivered in a single fraction or 20 Gy delivered in three fractions appears associated with less than 1% injury risk (45).
- *Chemical/Biologic Modifiers*: Concomitant intrathecal and intravenous (IV) use of concomitant methotrexate, cisplatin (CDDP), and etoposide (VP-16) can enhance neurotoxicity.
- *Radiologic Imaging*: MRI may show spinal cord edema or atrophy, T1-weighted hypointensity, or T2-weighted hyperintensity.
- *Differential Diagnosis*: Epidural metastasis or spinal cord compression secondary to vertebral metastases should be excluded.
- *Pathologic Diagnosis*: Only possible postmortem.
- *Management*: IV corticosteroids with 1,000 mg daily methylprednisolone for 3 to 5 days followed by gradual dose tapering.

LUNG

(See Chapter 19: Lung)

- *Clinical Presentation*: Radiation pneumonitis may present with cough, dyspnea, pleuritis, and pink-colored sputum. Plain films may reveal diffuse opacifications, coarse reticular markings or patchy consolidations most commonly corresponding to irradiated lung, although CT imaging is more sensitive for detecting radiation-induced lung injury. Radiation fibrosis can lead to decreased pulmonary function (with PFTs consistent with restrictive lung disease and reduced DLCO). Patients can develop pulmonary hypertension and right-heart failure in severe cases.
- *Time Course*: Radiation pneumonitis occurs 1 to 4 months after fractionated and single-dose therapy. Radiation fibrosis typically occurs within 6 to 24 months. Radiation-induced lung injury can occur during treatment when given with chemotherapy (e.g., total-body irradiation and bone marrow transplant conditioning regimens).
- *Dose/Time/Volume*: Percent of total lung volume exceeding 20 Gy (V20) is predictive of radiation pneumonitis (46). For treatment of NSCLC using conventional fractionation, mean lung dose (MLD) should be constrained below 20 Gy and V20 below 35% to 40% to limit risk of radiation pneumonitis to less than 20% (47). Limiting central airway dose to ≤80 Gy may reduce risks of bronchial stricture. For adjuvant radiation in mesothelioma, V5 should be constrained less than 60%, V20 less than 4% to 10%, and MLD to less than 8 Gy (47). Current data for locally advanced NSCLC support routine use of IMRT over 3D-CRT for lower associated risk of Grade 3 radiation pneumonitis (48,49). Retrospective data suggest low rates of Grades II and III lung toxicities for lung SBRT (9.1% and 1.8%, respectively) (50).
- *Chemical/Biologic Modifiers*: Actinomycin D, doxorubicin, taxanes, bleomycin, BCNU, cyclophosphamide, interferons (α, β, and γ), and gemcitabine may enhance RP (46,51). Concurrent rather than sequential chemotherapy appears associated with increased risk of radiation pneumonitis (52). Patients with baseline interstitial lung disease are especially high risk for radiation-induced lung injury (53,54).
- *Radiologic Imaging*: CT should be used to confirm pneumonitis or fibrosis, demonstrating ground-glass attenuation, patchy focal consolidation, scarring or volume loss coinciding with irradiated volumes, comparing to high isodose-curve outlines in cross-sectional contours.
- *Differential Diagnosis*: Includes recurrence, pneumonia, metastatic cancers (Hodgkin's disease, lymphomas), and infiltrates such as lymphangitic spread patterns.
- *Pathologic Diagnosis*: Tissue diagnosis can rule out recurrent disease.
- *Management*: Treatment of pneumonitis most often involves high-dose steroids (beginning with 1 mg per kg prednisone). Patients often experience rapid symptomatic improvement within 24 to 48 hours. No standard-of-care treatment exists for radiation fibrosis.
- *Follow-up*: Patients should be maintained on steroids for several months, after which the dose should be tapered and weaned.

HEART

- *Clinical Presentation*: Pericardial disease is the most common cardiac complication, although coronary artery disease (CAD), cardiomyopathies, conduction defects, and valvular disease can also occur as late complications (55–59). Importantly, electrocardiographic (EKG) changes during treatment are generally not attributable to radiation-induced cardiac injury.
- *Time Course*: Pericardial effusion, which may persist as constrictive pericardial disease, usually appears within 6 to 12 months. Notably, although absolute risks remain low, radiation also appears to increase risk for both CAD and cardiac death within the first and second decades after completing therapy, respectively (60).
- *Dose/Time/Volume*: For conventional fractionation, mean heart dose (MHD) < 26 Gy and V30 < 46% are associated with less than 15% risk of pericardial disease (61,62). Heart dose constraint of V25 <10% is associated with less than 1% probability of cardiac mortality 15 years after completing radiation (61).
- *Chemical/Biologic modifiers*: Doxorubicin (associated with cardiomyopathy) should be kept to lowest minimum possible dose when given with radiation.
- *Radiologic Imaging*: Plain films may demonstrate increased cardiac diameter. Echocardiograms and multigated acquisition (MUGA) scans may be helpful for ruling out pericardial effusion and measuring ejection fraction.
- *Differential Diagnosis*: Recurrent lung or esophageal cancers, relapsing mediastinal Hodgkin's disease and non-Hodgkin's lymphoma should be excluded.
- *Pathologic Diagnosis*: Pericardial biopsy can be performed to rule out malignant pericardial effusion when necessary.
- *Management*: Chronic pericardial effusion is often asymptomatic, although symptomatic disease may require partial pericardiotomy or pericardial window. Cardiac tamponade requires urgent pericardiocentesis. Preventive measures and lifestyle modifications can reduce incidence of symptomatic CAD.
- *Follow-up*: Children and young adults should be closely followed given risk for developing cardiac disease.

ESOPHAGUS

(See Chapter 20: Esophagus)
- *Clinical Presentation*: Acute esophagitis may present with chest discomfort, dysphagia, or odynophagia. Late complications may include esophageal strictures, ulcers, or rarely tracheoesophageal (TE) fistula.
- *Time Course:* Acute esophagitis presents within several weeks of starting treatment. Late esophageal complications can occur beginning 3 to 6 months after treatment
- *Dose/Time/Volume:* Acute esophagitis risk correlates with esophageal volume receiving at least 40 to 50 Gy (63). With mean esophageal dose constraint less than 34 Gy, chemoradiation for Stage III NSCLC appears to be associated with toxicity rates of Grade ≥3 dysphagia and esophagitis of 3.2% and 5.0% (for total dose of 60 Gy) and 12.1% and 17.4% (for total dose of 74 Gy), respectively (64).

- *Chemical/Biologic Modifiers:* Concurrent chemotherapy delivered during radiation increases risk of Grade 3+ toxicity.
- *Radiologic Imaging:* Esophageal manometry can be used for evaluation of dysphagia. Barium swallow is helpful for diagnosing esophageal structures. Endoscopy may demonstrate mucosal inflammation, ulceration, or strictures.
- *Differential Diagnosis:* Differential diagnosis for dysphagia secondary to late esophageal toxicity includes recurrent esophageal tumors and mediastinal masses, as well as achalasia and motility disorders.
- *Pathologic Diagnosis:* May demonstrate inflammation, epithelial prominence, and fibrosis of either submucosa or muscularis mucosa.
- *Management:* Symptomatic treatment may include dietary modifications, topical analgesics, proton-pump inhibitors, or histamine H2-receptor blockers. Esophageal strictures typically require endoscopic dilatation.

LIVER

(See Chapter 24: Pancreas and Hepatobiliary Tract)
- *Clinical Presentation*: Radiation-induced liver disease can present with weight gain, ascites, or hepatomegaly. Patients may present with vague-to-intense right upper quadrant pain.
- *Time Course:* With radiation therapy alone, anicteric ascites develops 2 to 4 months after treatment. Chemoradiotherapy-induced liver disease develops within 1 to 4 weeks.
- *Dose/Time/Volume*: Total liver generally tolerates cumulative doses of 20 to 30 Gy without complications. Using conventional fractionation, mean liver dose for palliative whole-liver radiation should not exceed 28 Gy for primary tumors or 30 Gy for liver metastases (65). For partial-liver irradiation using conventional fractionation, mean normal liver dose should not exceed 28 Gy for primary tumors or 32 Gy for metastatic disease (66). Recommended constraints for liver SBRT are detailed in Tables 8-4 and 8-5. For liver SBRT delivered using three-to-five fractions, at least 700 mL of normal liver should be constrained under 15 Gy.
- *Chemical/Biologic Modifiers*: Nitrosoureas (BCNU, lomustine [CCNU]) can lead to cholestasis and necrosis. Platinum-based agents, hydroxyurea, chlorambucil, and busulfan may also cause hepatotoxicity.
- *Radiologic Imaging*: Imaging may reveal hepatic enlargement or well-delineated hyper- or hypoattenuated regions coinciding with radiation fields.
- *Laboratory Tests*: Most commonly presents with elevated alkaline phosphatase but not hyperbilirubinemia.
- *Differential Diagnosis*: Metastatic liver disease and Budd-Chiari syndrome caused by hepatic vein occlusion (often secondary to metastases in the porta hepatic and para-aortic nodes) should also be considered.
- *Pathologic Diagnosis*: Liver biopsy demonstrates venoocclusive disease with occlusion and obliteration of the central veins of hepatic lobules, leading to hepatic congestion and secondary hepatocyte necrosis. Pathologic findings can progress to fibrosis and cirrhosis.
- *Management*: Supportive care. Radiation-induced liver disease is often self-limited, resolving within six months, although patients may develop chronic liver failure.

Table 8-4

QUANTEC Normal Tissue Constraints for Stereotactic Radiosurgery and Stereotactic Body Radiation Therapy

Organ	Dose or Dose/Volume Parameter	Toxicity End Point	Rate
Brain	V12 < 5–10 cc	Symptomatic necrosis	<20%
Brainstem	Dmax < 12.5 Gy	Cranial neuropathy/ necrosis	<5%
Spinal cord (hypofractionation)	Dmax = 20 Gy	Myelopathy	1%
Spinal cord (single-fraction)	Dmax = 13 Gy	Myelopathy	1%
Optic nerve/chiasm	Dmax < 12 Gy	Optic neuropathy	<10%
Cochlea	Prescription dose ≤ 14 Gy	Sensorineural hearing loss	<25%
Liver (3 fractions)	At least 700 cc < 15 Gy	RILD	<5%
Liver (Mets)	Mean dose < 15 Gy	RILD	<5%
Liver (HCC)	Mean dose < 13 Gy	RILD	<5%

Adapted with permission from Marks LB, Yorke ED, Jackson A, et al. Tolerance. Use of normal tissue complication probability models in the clinic. *Int J Radiat Oncol Biol Phys* 2010;76(3): S10–S19. © Elsevier.

KIDNEY

(See Chapter 27: Upper Urinary Tract)

- *Clinical Detection*: Multiple clinical syndromes may overlap including benign hypertension, malignant hypertension, acute radiation nephropathy, chronic radiation nephropathy, and renovascular (hyperreninemic) hypertension.
- *Time Course*: Acute radiation nephropathy develops within 3 to 12 months. Malignant hypertension generally occurs within 12 to 18 months. Chronic radiation nephropathy and renovascular hypertension develop beginning at 18 months.
- *Dose/Time/Volume*: For bilateral kidney radiation, mean dose to bilateral kidneys should be constrained under 18 Gy (67). For partial unilateral renal irradiation, V20 and V30 should be constrained below 28 and 23 Gy, respectively (67). In the pediatric setting, impaired renal function has been reported with cumulative doses of 12 to 14 Gy (68).
- *Chemical/Biologic Modifiers*: Cisplatin, BCNU, and actinomycin D can be nephrotoxic.
- *Radiologic Imaging*: Renal ^{99m}Tc scintigraphy may demonstrate altered blood flow correlating with biochemical and clearance end points (69). Findings on abdominal CT may reveal asymmetric IV contrast uptake or late-stage renal atrophy.
- *Laboratory Tests*: Radiation nephropathy may present with azotemia, increased serum creatinine reflecting reduced glomerular filtration rate (GFR), and normocytic anemia. Urinalysis may demonstrate microscopic hematuria, proteinuria, and urinary casts.

Table 8-5				
RTOG Normal Tissue Constraints for Stereotactic Radiosurgery and Stereotactic Body Radiation Therapy				
Organ/Tissue	RTOG Protocol	Treated Site	Dose or Dose/ Volume Constraint	Dose & Fractionation
Spinal cord	0631	Spine SBRT	1.2 cc < 7 Gy	16 Gy × 1
	0631	Spine SBRT	10% < 10 Gy	16 Gy × 1
	0631	Spine SBRT	0.35 cc < 10 Gy	16 Gy × 1
	0813	Lung SBRT	0.25 cc < 4.5 Gy/fx	10–12 Gy × 5
	0813	Lung SBRT	0.5cc < 2.7 Gy/fx	10–12 Gy × 5
	0813	Lung SBRT	Dmax = 6 Gy/fx	10–12 Gy × 5
	0915	Lung SBRT	0.35 cc < 5.2 Gy/fx	12 Gy × 4
	0915	Lung SBRT	1.2 cc < 3.4 Gy/fx	12 Gy × 4
	0618	Lung SBRT	Dmax = 6 Gy/fx	20 Gy × 3
	0438	Liver SBRT	Dmax < 34 Gy	7–10 Gy × 5
Trachea/ bronchus	0618	Lung SBRT	4 cc < 3.6 Gy/fx Dmax = 105% PTV	10–12 Gy × 5
	0813	Lung SBRT	Dmax = 8 Gy/fx	10–12 Gy × 5
Trachea/larynx	0631	Spine SBRT	Dmax = 20.2 Gy	16 Gy × 1
	0631	Spine SBRT	5 cc < 11.9 Gy	16 Gy × 1
Lungs (total)	0813	Lung SBRT	1,500 cc < 2.5 Gy/fx	10–12 Gy × 5
	0813	Lung SBRT	1,000 cc < 2.7 Gy/fx	10–12 Gy × 5
	0618	Lung SBRT	V20 < 10% Dmax = 8 Gy/fx	20 Gy × 3
	0631	Spine SBRT	1,000 cc < 7.4 Gy	16 Gy × 1
Heart	0813	Lung SBRT	15 cc < 5.5 Gy/fx	10–12 Gy × 5
	0813	Lung SBRT	Dmax < 105% PTV	10–12 Gy × 5
	0618	Lung SBRT	Dmax = 8 Gy/fx	20 Gy × 3
	0631	Spine SBRT	15 cc < 16 Gy	16 Gy × 1
	0631	Spine SBRT	Dmax = 22 Gy	16 Gy × 1
Brachial plexus	0813	Lung SBRT	3 cc < 6 Gy/fx	10–12 Gy × 5
	0813	Lung SBRT	Dmax = 6.4 Gy/fx	10–12 Gy × 5
	0618	Lung SBRT	Dmax = 8 Gy/fx	20 Gy × 3
	0631	Spine SBRT	3 cc < 14 Gy	16 Gy × 1
	0631	Spine SBRT	Dmax = 17.5 Gy	16 Gy × 1

Table 8-5

RTOG Normal Tissue Constraints for Stereotactic Radiosurgery and Stereotactic Body Radiation Therapy *(continued)*

Organ/Tissue	RTOG Protocol	Treated Site	Dose or Dose/ Volume Constraint	Dose & Fractionation
Esophagus (non-adjacent wall)	0813	Lung SBRT	5 cc < 5.5 Gy/fx	10–12 Gy × 5
	0813	Lung SBRT	Dmax = 105% PTV	10–12 Gy × 5
Esophagus	0618	Lung SBRT	Dmax = 9 Gy/fx	20 Gy × 3
	0631	Spine SBRT	5 cc < 11.9 Gy	16 Gy × 1
	0631	Spine SBRT	Dmax = 16 Gy	16 Gy × 1
Stomach	0631	Spine SBRT	10 cc < 11.2 Gy	16 Gy × 1
	0631	Spine SBRT	Dmax = 16 Gy	16 Gy × 1
	0438	Liver SBRT	V37 ≤ 1cc	7–10 Gy × 5
Liver	0438	Liver SBRT	V27 ≤ 30% & V24 ≤ 50%	7–10 Gy × 5
Small intestine	0438	Liver SBRT	V37 ≤ 1cc	7–10 Gy × 5
Duodenum	0631	Spine SBRT	10 cc < 11.2 Gy	16 Gy × 1
		Spine SBRT	Dmax = 16 Gy	16 Gy × 1
Jejunum/ileum	0631	Spine SBRT	5 cc < 11.9 Gy	16 Gy × 1
		Spine SBRT	Dmax = 15.4 Gy	
Colon	0631	Spine SBRT	20 cc < 14.3 Gy	16 Gy × 1
		Spine SBRT	Dmax = 18.4 Gy	16 Gy × 1
Kidney (cortex)	0631	Spine SBRT	200 cc < 8.4 Gy	16 Gy × 1
Kidney (hilum)	0631	Spine SBRT	2/3 of total volume	16 Gy × 1
		Spine SBRT	< 10.6 Gy	
Kidney (combined)	0438	Liver SBRT	V18 < 67% (both kidneys functional)	10 Gy × 5
		Liver SBRT	V10 < 90% (one kidney functional)	
Cauda equina	0631	Spine SBRT	5 cc < 14 Gy	16 Gy × 1
			Dmax = 16 Gy	

Source: Radiation Therapy Oncology Group (RTOG) Clinical Trial Protocols.

- *Differential Diagnosis*: Includes hypertension and renal failure due to benign causes.
- *Pathologic Diagnosis*: Although histopathologic findings demonstrate glomerular scarring with tuft obliteration and tubular degeneration, biopsy is often unnecessary.
- *Management*: Angiotensin-converting enzyme inhibitors (ACEis) or angiotensin receptor blockers (ARBs) may be helpful. Other interventions include reducing renal workload, blood pressure control and treatment of associated anemia, hypocalcemia, and hyperphosphatemia. Patients may ultimately require dialysis or renal transplantation.

SMALL AND LARGE INTESTINES

(See Chapter 25: Colon and Rectum)
- *Clinical Detection*: Acute radiation enteritis presents with abdominal pain, nausea, vomiting, or diarrhea. Radiation proctitis can also present with tenesmus, fecal urgency, or rectal bleeding. Late radiation-induced bowel toxicities may include abdominal pain, weight loss, malabsorption, bowel strictures, bowel obstruction, ulceration, or fistula formation.
- *Time Course:* Although acute radiation enteritis and proctitis generally occur within six weeks, late radiation-induced bowel toxicities (including strictures and ulceration) typically occur 6 to 24 months after treatment.
- *Dose/Time/Volume*: If contouring individual bowel loops, absolute small bowel volume receiving $\geq$15 Gy should be less than 120 mL; using the bowel bag contouring technique, absolute volume receiving >45 Gy should be less than 195 mL (70). For single-fraction SBRT, small bowel volume receiving more than 12.5 Gy should be kept under 30 mL. For three-to-five fraction SBRT, maximum point dose should be kept below 30 Gy. For pelvic irradiation using conventional fractionation, rectal volume receiving at least 60 Gy correlates with risk of Grade 2+ rectal toxicity. Rectal dose constraints of V75 <15%, V70 <20%, V65 <25%, V60 < 5%, and V50 <50% correlate with projected rates of late rectal toxicity less than 15% (Grade 2+) and less than 10% (Grade 3+), respectively (71). Without compromising coverage, clinicians should strive to minimize rectal volumes receiving 70 Gy and 75 Gy below recommended constraints. In the modern era, IMRT achieves better low-to-intermediate dose-volume constraints than does 3D-CRT producing lower rates of rectal toxicity (72–74).
- *Chemical/Biologic Modifiers*: 5-fluorouracil infusions are generally well tolerated, although prolonged high-dose maintenance chemotherapy can lead to radiation enteritis. Additional risk factors include collagen vascular disease, ulcerative colitis, and Crohn's disease.
- *Radiologic Imaging*: Abdominal CT may demonstrate bowel wall thickening or dilated bowel loops. Endoscopy may reveal mucosal surface irregularity on haustral markings, narrowing, or ulceration.
- *Differential Diagnosis*: Includes recurrent abdominal malignancies, IBD, diverticulitis, and colitis.
- *Pathologic Diagnosis*: Histopathologic features include infarction necrosis associated with arterial thromboses, sclerosis, and obliterated microvasculature in the bowel wall.

• *Management*: Conservative acute measures include antiemetic and antidiarrheal agents. Serious bleeding occurs with significant danger of ulceration, and perforation may require surgical resection of affected loops. Cholestyramine can be offered for choleric diarrhea.

SALIVARY GLANDS

(See Chapter 13: Salivary Glands)
• *Clinical Detection*: Xerostomia presents with a wide range of severity, from mild inconvenience in eating/speaking to debilitating dysfunction. Deterioration of oral health and alteration of eating function from reduced salivary flow can dramatically impact patient quality of life.
• *Time Course*: Acute xerostomia occurs as early as 1 to 2 weeks into treatment courses. Salivary output can improve even years after completion of radiotherapy. However, xerostomia is often permanent.
• *Dose/Time/Volume*: For avoidance of severe xerostomia (defined as long-term salivary function reduction to less than 25% baseline), mean unilateral parotid dose should be constrained under 20 Gy or bilateral mean parotid dose under 25 Gy (75). However, mean parotid dose should be kept as low as possible without compromising target coverage to help maintain better salivary function, even for relatively low mean parotid doses (<10 Gy). Similarly, even if unable to meet recommended constraints, mean parotid dose should be kept as low as possible (75). When deemed oncologically safe, submandibular gland sparing can also reduce risk of xerostomia. Although IMRT provides significant advantages over 3D-conformal radiation therapy, proton therapy offers exciting promise toward reducing toxicity rates (76).
• *Chemical/Biologic Modifiers*: Amifostine helps reduce moderate-to-severe salivary gland toxicity. However, in clinical practice, patients often find it difficult to tolerate because of potential side effects including infusion site reactions, hypotension, nausea, and vomiting.
• *Management*: Xerostomia symptoms are usually permanent. Pilocarpine may increase saliva output.
• *Follow-up*: Dental evaluations should be performed every three months.

CORNEA, LACRIMAL GLAND, AND LENS

• *Clinical Detection*: Mild radiation-induced keratitis presents with tearing, discomfort, or foreign body sensation. Lacrimal gland toxicity can lead to keratoconjunctivitis sicca, which in severe cases may lead to corneal ulceration. Irradiation of lenses commonly causes radiation-induced cataracts.
• *Time Course*: Acute keratitis occurs beginning 24 hours after radiation injury. Severe radiation keratopathy typically begins at least four months after completing therapy. Radiation-induced cataracts commonly occur approximately 2 to 8 years later.
• *Dose/Time/Volume*: Fractionated radiation doses exceeding 12 Gy are believed to cause cataracts, although even small doses (2 to 3 Gy) can result in cataract formation.

Retrospective data suggest high incidence of cataracts from both single-dose total body irradiation (approximately 60%) and fractionated total body irradiation (43%) (77). Cumulative doses of 30 Gy delivered using large fractions (10 Gy) may cause keratoconjunctivitis and corneal ulcers. However, cumulative corneal tolerance is higher (approximately 50 Gy) using conventional fractionation. Transient eyelash loss, erythema, and conjunctivitis may occur at 30 to 40 Gy, whereas doses above 50 Gy may cause permanent lash loss. Doses above 60 Gy can cause keratoconjunctivitis sicca and permanent loss of lacrimal gland function.

* *Management*: Management of keratitis and dry eye consists of ocular lubrication and topical antibiotic drops as needed. Cataracts require surgical intervention.

RETINA AND OPTIC TRACT

* *Clinical Detection*: Optic neuropathy and radiation retinopathy are often asymptomatic, but may present with visual distortion or painless visual impairment. Microaneurysms, telangiectasias, macular edema, and retinal hemorrhages may occur.
* *Time Course*: Radiation retinopathy develops months to years after treatment. Optic neuropathy can occur beginning 6 months after treatment but may not become symptomatic for another 5 to 10 years.
* *Dose/Time/Volume*: To minimize risk of radiation retinopathy, cumulative dose should be constrained under 45 Gy (78,79). Radiation-induced optic neuropathy is rare below D_{max} less than 55 Gy (80).
* *Chemical/Biologic Modifiers*: Chemotherapy increases toxic effects to the eye.
* *Management*: No effective treatment. Prevention is critical.

References

1. Bentzen SM, Constine LS, Deasy JO, et al. Quantitative analyses of normal tissue effects in the clinic (QUANTEC): an introduction to the scientific issues. *Int J Radiat Oncol Biol Phys* 2010;76(3 suppl):S3–S9.
2. Deasy JO, Bentzen SM, Jackson A, et al. Improving normal tissue complication probability models: the need to adopt a "data-pooling" culture. *Int J Radiat Oncol Biol Phys* 2010;76 (3 suppl):151–154. doi:10.1016/j.ijrobp.2009.06.094.
3. Emami B, Lyman J, Brown A, et al. Tolerance of normal tissue to therapeutic irradiation. *Int J Radiat Oncol Biol Phys* 1991;21(1):109–122.
4. Jackson A, Marks LB, Bentzen SM, et al. The lessons of QUANTEC: recommendations for reporting and gathering data on dose-volume dependencies of treatment outcome. *Int J Radiat Oncol Biol Phys* 2010;76(3 Suppl.):155-160.
5. Marks LB, Yorke ED, Jackson A, et al. Use of normal tissue complication probability models in the clinic. *Int J Radiat Oncol Biol Phys* 2010;76(3 SUPPL.). doi:10.1016/j.ijrobp.2009.07.1754.
6. Rubin P, Constine LS, Williams JP. Late effects of cancer treatment: radiation and drug toxicity. In: Perez CA, Brady LW, eds. *Principles and practice of radiation oncology*, 3rd ed. Philadelphia, PA: Lippincott–Raven, 1998:155–210.
7. National Cancer Institute, Division of Cancer Treatment and Diagnosis, Cancer Therapy Evaluation Program. Common Terminology Criteria for Adverse Events. https://ctep.cancer.gov/ protocoldevelopment/electronic_applications/ctc.htm#ctc_50. Updated January 16, 2018.

8. Constine LS. Tumors in children: cure with preservation of function and aesthetics. In: Wilson JF, ed. *Syllabus: a categorical course in radiation therapy*. Oak Brook, IL: Radiological Society of North America, 1988:75–91.

9. Constine LS, Konski A, Ekholm S, et al. Adverse effects of brain irradiation correlated with MR and CT imaging. *Int J Radiat Oncol Biol Phys* 1988;15(2):319–330.

10. Leibel SA, Sheline GE. Tolerance of the brain and spinal cord to conventional irradiation. In: Gutin PH, Leibel SA, Sheline GE, eds. *Radiation injury to the nervous system*. New York, NY: Raven Press, 1991:239–256.

11. Marks JE, Baglan RJ, Prassad SC, et al. Cerebral radionecrosis: incidence and risk in relation to dose, time, fractionation and volume. *Int J Radiat Oncol Biol Phys* 1981;7(2):243–252.

12. Lawrence YR, Li XA, el Naqa I, et al. Radiation dose-volume effects in the brain. *Int J Radiat Oncol Biol Phys* 2010;76(3 suppl):S20–S27.

13. Murray KJ, Nelson DF, Scott C, et al. Quality-adjusted survival analysis of malignant glioma. Patients treated with twice-daily radiation (RT) and carmustine: a report of Radiation Therapy Oncology Group (RTOG) 83–02. *Int J Radiat Oncol Biol Phys* 1995;31(3):453–459.

14. Mayo C, Yorke E, Merchant TE. Radiation associated brainstem injury. *Int J Radiat Oncol Biol Phys* 2010;76(3 suppl):S36–S41.

15. Ang K, Axelrod R, Sherman E, et al. A randomized phase III trial of concurrent accelerated radiation and cisplatin versus concurrent accelerated radiation, cisplatin, and cetuximab (C225) [Followed by Surgery for Selected Patients] for stage III and IV head and neck carcinomas: Radiation Therapy Oncology Group (RTOG). https://www.rtog.org/ClinicalTrials/ ProtocolTable/StudyDetails.aspx?action=openFile&FileID=4637. Updated January 26, 2016.

16. Amin MB, Bruner DW, Swanson GP, et al. A phase III randomized study of hypofractionated 3DCRT/IMRT versus conventionally fractionated 3DCRT/IMRT in patients treated for favorable-risk prostate cancer: Radiation Therapy Oncology Group (RTOG). https:// www.rtog.org/ClinicalTrials/ProtocolTable/StudyDetails.aspx?action=openFile&FileID=4624. Updated December 18, 2014.

17. Bezjak A, Bradley J, Gaspar L, et al. Seamless phase I/II study of stereotactic lung radiotherapy (SBRT) for early stage, centrally located, non-small cell lung cancer (NSCLC) in medically inoperable patients: Radiation Therapy Oncology Group (RTOG). https://www.rtog.org/ClinicalTrials/ ProtocolTable/StudyDetails.aspx?action=openFile&FileID=9067. Updated June 8, 2015.

18. Bradley J, Choy H, Komaki R, et al. A randomized phase III comparison of standard-dose (60 Gy) versus highdose (74 Gy) conformal radiotherapy with concurrent and consolidation carboplatin/paclitaxel +/- cetuximab (IND #103444) in patients with stage IIIA/IIIB non-small cell lung cancer: Radiation Therapy Oncology Group (RTOG). https://www.rtog.org/ClinicalTrials/ ProtocolTable/StudyDetails.aspx?action=openFile&FileID=4649. Updated January 19, 2016.

19. Coen JJ, Saylor PJ, Lee CT, et al. A phase II randomized study for patients with muscle-invasive bladder cancer evaluating transurethral surgery and concomitant chemoradiation by either BID irradiation plus 5-fluorouracil and cisplatin or QD irradiation plus gemcitabine followed by selective bladder preservation and gemcitabine/cisplatin adjuvant chemotherapy: Radiation Therapy Oncology Group (RTOG). https://www.rtog.org/ClinicalTrials/ProtocolTable/StudyDetails.asp x?action=openFile&FileID=4659. Updated December 18, 2014.

20. Garofalo MC, Hong M, Bendell J et al. A phase II evaluation of preoperative chemoradiotherapy utilizing intensity modulated radiation therapy (IMRT) in combination with capecitabine and oxaliplatin for patients with locally advanced rectal cancer: Radiation Therapy Oncology Group (RTOG). https://www.rtog.org/ClinicalTrials/ProtocolTable/StudyDetails.aspx?action=openFile &FileID=4663. Updated August 17, 2011.

21. Gilbert MR, Mehta MP, Blumenthal DT, et al. Phase III double-blind placebo-controlled trial of conventional concurrent chemoradiation and adjuvant temozolomide plus bevacizumab versus conventional concurrent chemoradiation and adjuvant temozolomide in patients with newly diagnosed

glioblastoma: Radiation Therapy Oncology Group (RTOG). https://www.rtog.org/ClinicalTrials/ProtocolTable/StudyDetails.aspx?action=openFile&FileID=4664. Updated November 25, 2014.

22. Gore E, Sun A, Ramalingam SS, et al. Randomized phase II study comparing prophylactic cranial irradiation alone to prophylactic cranial irradiation and consolidative extra-cranial irradiation for extensive disease small cell lung cancer (ED-SCLC): Radiation Therapy Oncology Group (RTOG). https://www.rtog.org/ClinicalTrials/ProtocolTable/StudyDetails.aspx?action=openFile&FileID=13697. Updated June 24, 2014.

23. Hurwitz M, Xiao Y, Shayegan B, et al. Adjuvant 3DCRT/IMRT in combination with androgen suppression and docetaxel for high risk prostate cancer patients post-prostatectomy: a phase II trial: Radiation Therapy Oncology Group (RTOG). https://www.rtog.org/ClinicalTrials/ProtocolTable/StudyDetails.aspx?action=openFile&FileID=4652. Updated April 16, 2014.

24. Jhingran A, Miller BE, Portelance L, et al. A phase II study of intensity modulated radiation therapy (IMRT) to the pelvis +/- chemotherapy for postoperative patients with either endometrial or cervical carcinoma: Radiation Therapy Oncology Group (RTOG). https://www.rtog.org/ClinicalTrials/ProtocolTable/StudyDetails.aspx?action=openFile&FileID=13703. Updated August 17, 2011.

25. Kachnic LA, Goodyear M, Myerson R, et al. A phase II evaluation of dose-painted IMRT in combination with 5-fluorouracil and mitomycin-C for reduction of acute morbidity in carcinoma of the anal canal: Radiation Therapy Oncology Group (RTOG). https://www.rtog.org/ClinicalTrials/ProtocolTable/StudyDetails.aspx?action=openFile&FileID=4641. Updated August 17, 2011.

26. Katz AW, Dawson LA, Elsaleh H et al. Phase I trial of highly conformal radiation therapy for patients with liver metastases: Radiation Therapy Oncology Group (RTOG). https://www.rtog.org/ClinicalTrials/ProtocolTable/StudyDetails.aspx?action=openFile&FileID=4630. Updated March 1, 2011.

27. Lee N, Garden A, Kim J, et al. A phase II study of concurrent chemoradiotherapy using three-dimensional conformal radiotherapy (3D-CRT) or intensity-modulated radiation therapy (IMRT) + bevacizumab (BV) for locally or regionally advanced nasopharyngeal cancer: Radiation Therapy Oncology Group (RTOG). https://www.rtog.org/ClinicalTrials/ProtocolTable/StudyDetails.aspx?action=openFile&FileID=4648. Updated November 25, 2014.

28. Lilenbaum R, Komaki R, Martel MK, et al. A phase II trial of combined modality therapy with growth factor support for patients with limited stage small cell lung cancer: Radiation Therapy Oncology Group (RTOG). https://www.rtog.org/ClinicalTrials/ProtocolTable/StudyDetails.aspx?action=openFile&FileID=4654. Updated December 20, 2007.

29. Pollack A, Balogh A, Low D et al. A phase III trial of short term androgen deprivation with pelvic lymph node or prostate bed only radiotherapy (SPPORT) in prostate cancer patients with a rising PSA after radical prostatectomy: Radiation Therapy Oncology Group (RTOG). https://www.rtog.org/ClinicalTrials/ProtocolTable/StudyDetails.aspx?action=openFile&FileID=13044. Updated November 16, 2015.

30. Raben D, Wong S, Galvin J, et al. A randomized phase II trial of chemoradiotherapy versus chemoradiotherapy and vandetanib for high-risk postoperative advanced squamous cell carcinoma of the head and neck: Radiation Therapy Oncology Group (RTOG). https://www.rtog.org/ClinicalTrials/ProtocolTable/StudyDetails.aspx?action=openFile&FileID=4651. Updated February 25, 2010.

31. Radiation Therapy Oncology Group Foundation. Clinical Trials Protocol Table. https://www.rtog.org/ClinicalTrials/ProtocolTable.aspx. Accessed December 15, 2017.

32. Rogers CL, Vogelbaum MA, Perry A, et al. *hase II trial of observation for low-risk meningiomas and of radiotherapy for intermediate- and high-risk meningiomas: Radiation Therapy Oncology Group (RTOG).* https://www.rtog.org/ClinicalTrials/ProtocolTable/StudyDetails.aspx?action=openFile&FileID=4644. Updated September 11, 2014.

33. Ryu S, Gerszten P, Yin FF, et al. *Phase II/III study of image-guided radiosurgery/SBRT for localized spine metastasis—RTOG CCOP study: Radiation Therapy Oncology Group (RTOG).* https://www.rtog.org/ClinicalTrials/ProtocolTable/StudyDetails.aspx?action=openFile&FileID=12804. Updated September 23, 2016.

34. Suntharalingam M, Ilson D, Dicker AP, et al. A phase III trial evaluating the addition of cetuximab to paclitaxel, cisplatin, and radiation for patients with esophageal cancer who are treated without surgery: Radiation Therapy Oncology Group (RTOG). https://www.rtog.org/ClinicalTrials/ProtocolTable/StudyDetails.aspx?action=openFile&FileID=4629. Updated May 3, 2012.

35. Timmerman RD, Galvin J, Gore E, et al. A phase II trial of stereotactic body radiation therapy (SBRT) in the treatment of patients with operable stage I/II non-small cell lung cancer: Radiation Therapy Oncology Group (RTOG). https://www.rtog.org/ClinicalTrials/ProtocolTable/StudyDetails.aspx?action=openFile&FileID=4650. Updated March 6, 2014.

36. Trotti A, Gillison M, Adelstein DJ, et al. Phase III trial of radiotherapy plus cetuximab versus chemoradiotherapy in HPV-associated oropharynx cancer: Radiation Therapy Oncology Group (RTOG). https://www.rtog.org/ClinicalTrials/ProtocolTable/StudyDetails.aspx?action=openFile&FileID=8629. Updated February 23, 2016.

37. Videtic GMM, Singh AK, Chang JY, et al. A randomized phase II study comparing 2 stereotactic body radiation therapy (SBRT) schedules for medically inoperable patients with stage I peripheral non-small cell lung cancer: Radiation Therapy Oncology Group (RTOG). https://www.rtog.org/ClinicalTrials/ProtocolTable/StudyDetails.aspx?action=openFile&FileID=4673. Updated March 6, 2014.

38. Wang D, Kirsch DG, Okuno SH, et al. A phase II trial of image guided preoperative radiotherapy for primary soft tissue sarcomas of the extremity: Radiation Therapy Oncology Group (RTOG). https://www.rtog.org/ClinicalTrials/ProtocolTable/StudyDetails.aspx?action=openFile&FileID=9379. Updated April 3, 2014.

39. Narayana A, Yamada J, Berry S, Shah P, Hunt M, Gutin PH, Leibel SA. Intensity-modulated radiotherapy in high-grade gliomas: clinical and dosimetric results. *Int J Radiat Oncol Biol Phys* 2006;64(3):892.

40. Brown PD, Jaeckle K, Ballman KV, et al. Effect of radiosurgery alone vs radiosurgery with whole brain radiation therapy on cognitive function in patients with 1 to 3 brain metastases: a randomized clinical trial. *JAMA* 316(4):401–409.

41. Gondi V, Pugh SL, Tome WA, et al. Preservation of memory with conformal avoidance of the hippocampal neural stem-cell compartment during whole-brain radiotherapy for brain metastases (RTOG 0933): a phase II multi-institutional trial. *J Clin Oncol* 2014;32(34):3810.

42. Brown PD, Pugh S, Laack NN, et al. Memantine for the prevention of cognitive dysfunction in patients receiving whole-brain radiotherapy: a randomized, double-blind, placebo-controlled trial. *Neuro Oncol* 2013;15(10):1429–1437.

43. Rubin P, Casarett GW. *Clinical radiation pathology.* Philadelphia, PA: WB Saunders, 1968.

44. Marcus RB, Jr, Million RR. The incidence of myelitis after irradiation of the cervical spinal cord. *Int J Radiat Oncol Biol Phys* 1990;19(1):3–8.

45. Kirkpatrick JP, van der Kogel AJ, Schultheiss TE. Radiation dose-volume effects in the spinal cord. *Int J Radiat Oncol Biol Phys* 2010;76(3 suppl):S42–S49.

46. Arrieta O, Gallardo-Rincon D, Villarreal-Garza C, et al. High frequency of radiation pneumonitis in patients with locally advanced non-small cell lung cancer treated with concurrent radiotherapy and gemcitabine after induction with gemcitabine and carboplatin. *J Thorac Oncol* 2009;4(7):845–852.

47. Marks LB, Bentzen SM, Deasy JO, et al. Radiation dose-volume effects in the lung. *Int J Radiat Oncol Biol Phys* 2010;76(3 suppl):S70–S76.

48. Chun SG, Hu C, Komaki RU, et al. Impact of intensity-modulated radiation therapy technique for locally advanced non-small-cell lung cancer: a secondary analysis of the NRG oncology RTOG 0617 randomized clinical trial. *J Clin Oncol* 2017;35(1):56–62.

49. Graham MV, Purdy JA, Emami B, et al. Preliminary results of a prospective trial using three dimensional radiotherapy for lung cancer. *Int J Radiat Oncol Biol Phys* 1995;33(5):993–1000.

50. Zhao J, Yorke ED, Li L, et al. Simple factors associated with radiation-induced lung toxicity after stereotactic body radiation therapy of the thorax: A pooled analysis of 88 studies. *Int J Radiat Oncol Biol Phys* 2016;95(5):1357–1366.

51. Blackstock AW, Ho C, Butler J, et al. Phase Ia/Ib chemo-radiation trial of gemcitabine and dose-escalated thoracic radiation in patients with stage III A/B non-small cell lung cancer. *J Thorac Oncol* 2006;1(5):434–440.

52. Vogelius IR, Bentzen SM. A literature-based metaanalysis of clinical risk factors for development of radiation-induced pneumonitis. *Acta Oncol* 2012;51:975–983.

53. Chen H, Senan S, Nossent EJ, et al. Treatment-related toxicity in patients with early stage non-small cell lung cancer and coexisting interstitial lung disease: a systematic review. *Int J Radiat Oncol Biol Phys* 2017;98(1):245–246.

54. Ueki N, Matsuo UY, Togashi Y, et al. Impact of pretreatment interstitial lung disease on radiation pneumonitis and survival after stereotactic body radiation therapy for lung cancer. *J Thorac Oncol* 2015;10(1):116–125.

55. Boivin JF, Hutchison GB, Lubin JH, et al. Coronary artery disease mortality in patients treated for Hodgkin's disease. *Cancer* 1992;69(5):1241–1247.

56. Cosset JM, Henry-Amar M, Pellae-Cosset B, et al. Pericarditis and myocardial infarctions after Hodgkin's disease therapy. *Int J Radiat Oncol Biol Phys* 1991;21(2):447–449.

57. Hancock SL, Donaldson SS. *Radiation-related cardiac disease: risks after treatment of Hodgkin's disease during childhood and adolescence.* Proceedings of second international conference on the long-term complications of treatment of children and adolescents for cancer. Buffalo, NY, 1992.

58. Rutqvist LE, Lax I, Fornander T, et al. Cardiovascular mortality in a randomized trial of adjuvant radiation therapy versus surgery alone in primary breast cancer. *Int J Radiat Oncol Biol Phys* 1992;22(5):887–896.

59. Truesdell S, Schwartz C, Constine L, et al. Cardiovascular effects of cancer therapy. In: Schwartz C, Hobbie W, Constine LC, eds. *Survivors of childhood cancers: assessment and management.* St. Louis, MO: Mosby–Year Book, 1994:159–176.

60. Cheng YJ, Nie XY, Cheng-Cheng J, et al. Long-term cardiovascular risk after radiotherapy in women with breast cancer. *J Am Heart Assoc* 2017;6(5):1–14.

61. Gagliardi G, Constine LS, Moiseenko V, et al. Radiation dose-volume effects in the heart. *Int J Radiat Oncol Biol Phys* 2010;76(3 suppl):S77–S85.

62. Wei X, Liu HH, Tucker SL, et al. Risk factors for pericardial effusion in inoperable esophageal cancer patients treated with definitive chemoradiation therapy. *Int J Radiat Oncol Biol Phys* 2008;70(3):707–714.

63. Werner-Wasik M, Yorke E, Deasy J, et al. Radiation dose-volume effects in the esophagus. *Int J Radiat Oncol Biol Phys* 2010;76(3 suppl):S86–S93.

64. Bradley JD, Hu C, Komaki RU, et al. Long-term results of RTOG 0617: a randomized phase 3 comparison of standard dose vs. high-dose conformal chemoradiation therapy +/- cetuximab for stage III NSCLC [ASTRO abstract 227]. *Int J Radiat Oncol Biol Phys* 2017;99(2):S105.

65. Pan CC, Kavanagh BD, Dawson LA, et al. Radiation-associated liver injury. *Int J Radiat Oncol Biol Phys* 2010;76(3 suppl):S94–S100.

66. Dawson LA, Ten Haken RK. Partial volume tolerance of the liver to radiation. *Semin Radiat Oncol* 2005;15(4):279–283.

67. Dawson LA, Kavanagh BD, Paulino AC, et al. Radiation-associated kidney injury. *Int J Radiat Oncol Biol Phys* 2010;76(3 suppl):S108–S115.
68. Peschel RE, Chen M, Seashore J. The treatment of massive hepatomegaly in stage IV-S neuroblastoma. *Int J Radiat Oncol Biol Phys* 1981;7(4):549–553.
69. Dewit L, Anninga JK, Hoefnagel CA, et al. Radiation injury in the human kidney: a prospective analysis using specific scintigraphic and biochemical endpoints. *Int J Radiat Oncol Biol Phys* 1990;19(4):977–983.
70. Kavanagh BD, Pan CC, Dawson LA, et al. Radiation dose-volume effects in the stomach and small bowel. *Int J Radiat Oncol Biol Phys* 2010;76(3 suppl):S101–S107.
71. Michalski JM, Gay H, Jackson A, et al. Radiation dose-volume effects in radiation-induced rectal injury. *Int J Radiat Oncol Biol Phys* 2010;76(3 suppl):S123–S129.
72. Michalski JM, Yan Y, Watkins-Bruner D, et al. Preliminary toxicity analysis of 3-dimentional conformal radiation therapy versus intensity modulated radiation therapy on the high-dose arm of the Radiation Therapy Oncology Group 0126 prostate cancer trial. *Int J Radiat Oncol Biol Phys* 2013;87(5):932–938.
73. Zelefsky MJ, Fuks Z and Happersett L. Clinical experience with intensity modulated radiation therapy (IMRT) in prostate cancer. *Radiother Oncol* 2000; 55(3): 241-249.
74. Zelefsky MJ, Levin EJ, Hunt M, et al. Incidence of late rectal and urinary toxicities after three-dimensional conformal radiotherapy and intensity-modulated radiotherapy for localized prostate cancer. *Int J Radiat Oncol Biol Phys* 2008;70(4): 1124–1129.
75. Deasy JO, Moiseenko V, Marks L, et al. Radiotherapy dose-volume effects on salivary gland function. *Int J Radiat Oncol Biol Phys* 2010;76(3 suppl):S58–S63.
76. Blanchard R, Gunn GB, Lin A, et al. Proton therapy for head and neck cancers. *Semin Radiat Oncol* 2018;28(1):53–63.
77. Merriam GR Jr Focht EF. A clinical study of radiation cataracts and the relationship to dose. *Am J Roentgenol Radium Ther Nucl Med* 1957;77(5):759–785.
78. Nakissa N, Rubin P, Strohl R, et al. Ocular and orbital complications following radiation therapy of paranasal sinus malignancies and review of literature. *Cancer* 1983;51(6):980–986.
79. Parsons JT, Bova FJ, Fitzgerald CR, et al. Radiation optic neuropathy after megavoltage external-beam irradiation: analysis of time-dose factors. *Int J Radiat Oncol Biol Phys* 1994;30(4):755–763.
80. Mayo C, Martel MK, Marks LB, et al. Radiation dose-volume effects of optic nerves and chiasm. *Int J Radiat Oncol Biol Phys* 2010;76(3 suppl):S28–S35.

CHAPTER 9

SKIN CANCER, KAPOSI'S SARCOMA, AND CUTANEOUS LYMPHOMA

SKIN

Anatomy

- The integumentary system comprises the skin and the appendageal structures traversing the skin.
- The epidermis is composed of two layers: the outermost layer is the stratum corneum, and the basal layer rests on the basement membrane that separates the epidermis from the dermis. Melanocytes, which are pigment-producing cells, are located between the basal cells of the epidermis.
- The dermis consists of spindle-shaped fibroblasts that produce collagen, giving the skin much of its strength. It contains two vascular plexuses as well as sensory and autonomic nerves.
- The skin contains smooth muscles in the form of the musculi arrectores pilorum, which attach to the hair shaft and are responsive to cold and sweat.
- Appendageal structures of the skin include the sebaceous, eccrine, and apocrine glands. Sebaceous glands are found throughout the skin, except on the palms and soles. The apocrine glands are found mainly in the anal and genital areas.

Epidemiology

- Carcinomas of the skin account for nearly one third of all cancers diagnosed in the United States each year. The incidence is estimated to be over 800,000 new cases per year (1,2).
- Exposure to (ultraviolet) solar radiation, especially ultraviolet B, is the most common cause of skin cancer (3).
- Other etiologic factors include ionizing radiation, genetic predisposition (xeroderma pigmentosa, albinism), immunosuppression, arsenic exposure, preexisting chronic skin ulcers related to syphilis or burns, and human papillomavirus (4–6).

Diagnostic Workup

- The diagnosis of skin cancer requires a detailed clinical history.
- Physical examination should focus on appreciation of changes in the normal appearance of the skin.
- The size, diameter, depth of invasion, and multifocality of the tumor must be precisely defined.
- Regional lymph nodes must be clinically assessed.
- Various tools to assess the skin, including Wood's light and potassium hydroxide preparations, fungal cultures, skin biopsies, Tzanck smears, and patch testing, should be used.

Staging

- Updates to the staging systems for skin cancer are shown below, including the American Joint Committee on Cancer (AJCC) designations for cutaneous carcinoma of the head and neck, melanoma, and Merkel cell carcinoma (MCC).

NEW!   **SUMMARY OF CHANGES TO AJCC STAGING**

CUTANEOUS SQUAMOUS CELL CARCINOMA OF THE HEAD AND NECK

- Staging of nonmelanoma cutaneous cancers of the head and neck is a new chapter in the American Joint Committee on Cancer (AJCC) 8th edition.
- Includes all nonmelanoma and non–Merkel cell carcinomas of the head and neck, including those of the vermilion border.

See: Amin MB, Edge SB, Greene FL, et al., eds. *AJCC cancer staging manual*, 8th ed. New York, NY: Springer Verlag, 2017.

NEW!   **SUMMARY OF CHANGES TO AJCC STAGING**

MERKEL CELL CARCINOMA

- New category of N2 denotes in-transit metastasis without lymph node metastasis.
- New category of N3 denotes in-transit metastasis with lymph node metastasis.
- M classifications are subcategorized as M1a, M1b, and M1c, by location of distant metastases. M1a is metastasis to distant skin, distant subcutaneous tissue, or distant lymph node. M1b is metastasis to lung. M1c is metastasis to all other visceral sites.

See: Amin MB, Edge SB, Greene FL, et al., eds. *AJCC cancer staging manual*, 8th ed. New York, NY: Springer Verlag, 2017.

MELANOMA OF THE SKIN

- T0 designates disease with clinical suspicion of primary cutaneous melanoma, but no evidence of primary site of disease.
- T1 is subcategorized by tumor thickness at 0.8 mm threshold.
- Tumor mitotic rate has been removed as a staging criterion for T1 tumors.
- Lymph node metastases are now defined as clinically occult—found at time of sentinel lymph node biopsy—or clinically detected.
- Gross extranodal extension is no longer an N-category criterion, but presence of matted nodes is retained as an N-category criterion.
- M1 is now defined by site of distant metastatic disease and serum LDH level.
- M1d designation is new, and includes metastases to the CNS.

See: Amin MB, Edge SB, Greene FL, et al., eds. *AJCC cancer staging manual*, 8th ed. New York, NY: Springer Verlag, 2017.

Clinicopathologic Manifestations

- Malignant tumors of the skin include BCC, SCC, melanoma, MCC, adnexal tumors, connective tissue tumors, malignant lymphomas, mycosis fungoides (MFs), Kaposi's sarcoma, keratoacanthoma (acute epithelial cancer), and metastases.
- BCCs occur most often on hair-bearing skin of the head and neck; they rarely metastasize.
- SCCs frequently are preceded by premalignant lesions, most commonly actinic keratosis. They also can arise from old burn scars or areas of chronic inflammation or radiation dermatitis. Lesions that arise from areas of chronic inflammation or develop *de novo* are more aggressive and metastasize in 10% of cases (7).

General Management

- Surgical excision and radiation therapy offer equivalent, excellent cure rates. The treatment modality selected should offer the greatest potential for cure with the most acceptable cosmetic and functional results (8).
- Factors that influence treatment decisions include size and anatomic location of the lesion, involvement of adjacent cartilage or bone, depth of invasion, tumor grade, previous treatment, and the general medical condition of the patient.
- Computed tomography or magnetic resonance imaging (MRI) should be done for lesions around the eye to determine the magnitude of the tumor, depth of invasion, and bony involvement, particularly for recurrent tumors after surgery.

Surgery

- Small BCCs and SCCs may be surgically excised (9,10).
- Curettage and electrodesiccation is used for small nodular BCCs (<1.5 cm) with distinct margins. The cure rate is approximately 90% in properly selected cases. This technique is contraindicated for diffusely infiltrating tumors, recurrent tumors, and lesions in areas where significant tissue trauma may result from the procedure
- Mohs' microsurgery involves fixation of the tumor and adjacent scar with zinc chloride, followed by mapping and surgical excision. Frozen-section samples are taken to locate areas of residual tumor; these are further excised until negative margins are obtained. Treatment is indicated for BCCs and SCCs. It is contraindicated for Merkel cell tumor, because of its noncontiguous growth pattern. The literature reports a 5-year cure rate of 95% or better (11–13).
- Cryotherapy consists of the application of liquid nitrogen to skin neoplasms, which causes necrosis of malignant cells by destruction of the microvasculature. The indications and contraindications are similar to those for curettage and electrodesiccation. It can result in cure rates of 90% or higher. However, margin assessment is not possible for such therapy.

Radiation Therapy

- For small lesions of the lip, eyelid, ear, or nose, irradiation may offer an advantage over surgical techniques with respect to cosmesis and function (14,15).
- Radiation therapy is indicated for lesions larger than 2 cm, lesions with deep fixation, and lesions with involvement of adjacent structures, in which surgery may result in poor cosmetic or functional outcome (8,16,17).
- A meta-analysis showed a 5-year recurrence risk of 6.7% for primary SCC and 10% for recurrent SCC treated with definitive radiation (18).
- Radiation therapy is beneficial for the treatment of multiple lesions or lesions that involve regional lymph nodes (19).
- Postoperative irradiation is indicated for patients with incomplete resection of squamous cell tumors, as well as SCC with extensive perineural or large nerve involvement (20–24).
- Chemoradiotherapy has shown some effectiveness for high-risk patients in the adjuvant setting (25).

Chemotherapy

- Superficial therapies, including fluorouracil cream, imiquimod cream, and photodynamic therapy, are associated with 75% to 80% recurrence-free survival at 1 to 5 years, with good-to-excellent cosmesis for most patients.
- Cisplatin-based therapy has shown some (26) efficacy for metastatic disease.
- EGFR inhibitors additionally show some efficacy in phase II trials, and cetuximab has a low-toxicity profile,
- Neoadjuvant chemotherapy has been used for very large SCCs and may be appropriate on an individualized basis (27).

- Immunotherapy has shown promise for SCC, though data are currently limited.
- Hedgehog pathway inhibitors are approved metastatic BCC.

Radiation Therapy Techniques

- Various radiation sources are available for the treatment of skin cancer.
- Most skin cancers can be treated with superficial or orthovoltage x-rays; however, superficial x-ray units are no longer widely available in the United States. Megavoltage electrons and photons generated by linear accelerators are most commonly employed in nonmelanoma skin cancer (NMSC) management: (28,29)
- The choice of radiation modality depends on tumor size, depth, and anatomic location.
- Most skin cancers are treated with electrons. Optimal use of modality requires knowledge of its specific beam characteristics.
- Electron beams offer the advantages of rapid dose falloff and the sparing of underlying normal tissue.
- For most tumors, the electron beam energy is selected based on delivering the treatment to the 90% isodose line. Bolus is usually required to enhance surface dose.
- Photon beam irradiation (with surface bolus) must be employed in conjunction with electrons for more advanced lesions with deep penetration and involvement of bone or cartilage.
- IMRT is often indicated for locally advanced disease of the head and neck, particularly for disease requiring tracking of nerves to the skull base (extensive perineural invasion, clinical perineural involvement, and involvement of named nerves).
- Choice of field size depends on the size and site of the lesion and the quality of the radiation beam. Photon margins of 0.5 to 1 cm and electron margins of 1 to 1.5 cm are employed for tumors up to 2 cm and photon margins of 1.5 to 2 cm and electron margins of 2 to 2.5 cm for tumors greater than 2 cm.
- If a lesion is treated with low-energy electron beams, a wider margin of normal tissue is required for adequate coverage, in view of the constriction of the isodose lines at depth for low-energy electron beams.
- Radiation doses and fractionation depend on the histologic type, size, and depth of the tumor, as well as the size of the treatment field and overall time of treatment delivery.
- Multiple dose and fractionation regimens have demonstrated effectiveness. For tumors less than 2 cm in diameter, 60 to 64 Gy in 6 to 7 weeks, 50 to 55 Gy in 3 to 4 weeks, 40 Gy in 2 weeks, and 30 Gy in 5 fractions are highly effective. For larger tumors or those with invasion of bone or deep tissue, 60 to 70 Gy over 6 to 7 weeks and 45 to 55 Gy in 3 to 4 weeks are effective.
- In the adjuvant setting, 60 to 64 Gy in 6 to 7 weeks and 50 Gy in 4 weeks are highly effective. Adjuvant radiation is indicated for large nerve involvement or extensive perineural invasion, as well as tumors unable to be fully resected.
- Protracted radiation courses are associated with improved cosmetic results and should be used for poorly vascularized or cartilaginous areas (15).

- Radiation therapy techniques should give special attention to protection of eyes by using external or intraocular eye shields.
- With proper radiation therapy planning, the incidence of treatment failure should be very low. However, patients for whom irradiation fails can often be successfully treated by surgical excision if recurrence is identified early. This necessitates proper follow-up after irradiation.
- For most BCC or SCC lesions, surgical treatments or radiation therapy offer equivalent excellent cure rates of 90% to 95%.

MELANOMA

- Melanoma is a malignant tumor that accounts for 1.5% of all skin cancers.
- Melanomas occur most frequently in white adults and are rare in dark-skinned ethnicities.
- The incidence is equal in men and women, and peaks in the fourth and fifth decades of life. Women have an apparent survival advantage.
- Superficial spreading melanoma accounts for about 70% of all cases and shows a radial growth pattern within the epidermis.
- Nodular melanoma accounts for 30% of all cases and shows a vertical growth pattern. It is the most aggressive form.
- Lentigo maligna melanoma is the least common form of melanoma; it occurs in elderly patients, with a mean age of 70 years. It has the most benign behavior.
- Tumor depth and thickness have prognostic significance.

Staging

- Breslow's staging system classifies the tumor according to the depth of invasion.
- The AJCC 8th edition stages melanoma on thickness and ulceration.
  - Tis is *in situ* disease, without invasion.
  - T1a is less than 0.8 mm without ulceration. T1b is less than 0.8 mm with ulceration or 0.8 to 1 mm with or without ulceration.
  - T2a is greater than 1 to 2 mm without ulceration. T2b is greater than 1 to 2 mm with ulceration.
  - T3a is greater than 2 to 4 mm without ulceration. T3b is greater than 2 to 4 mm with ulceration.
  - T4a is greater than 4 mm without ulceration. T4b is greater than 4 mm with ulceration.
  - N1 disease has one involved node or in-transit, satellite, or microsatellite metastases without lymph nodes. N1a is one lymph nodes detected by SLNB. N1b is one clinically detected node. N1c is in-transit, satellite, or microsatellite metastases without lymph nodes
  - N2 disease has two to three involved nodes or one involved node plus in-transit, satellite, or microsatellite metastases. N2a is two to three lymph nodes detected by

SLNB. N2b is two to three clinically detected nodes. N2c is in-transit, satellite, or microsatellite metastases with one involved lymph node.
- N3 disease is four or more involved node or matted nodes. N3a is 4+ nodes detected by SLNB. N3b is four or more nodes that were clinically detected, as well as matted nodes. N3c is two or more nodes or matted nodes plus in-transit, satellite, or microsatellite metastases.
- Metastatic sites are differentiated by skin/soft tissue and nonregional lymph node metastases (M1a) versus lung (M1b) versus non-CNS visceral sites (M1c) versus CNS (M1d). LDH level is also used.
- Both level of invasion and maximum thickness should be recorded.
- Satellite lesions and cutaneous and subcutaneous metastases more than 2 cm from the primary tumor, but not beyond the site of the primary lymph node drainage, are considered "in-transit" metastases.

General Management of Malignant Melanoma

- Current recommendations for primary melanoma excision margins are 0.5 to 1 cm for *in situ* melanoma, 1 cm for lesions up to 1 cm and less than 1 mm thick, and 2 cm for lesions greater than 1 cm in size or 1 to 4 mm thick (30).
- Early lesions with relatively little or no invasion are curable in over 95% of cases.
- Sentinel lymph node status is the strongest predictor of survival for stages I and II melanoma (31,32). SLNB is recommended for >1 mm thickness, as well as considered for Breslow's depth less than 0.8mm with ulceration or 0.8 to 1 mm with or without ulceration. High mitotic rate and lymphovascular invasion are important risk factors as well.
- Melanomas have a propensity for distant metastasis, and treatment must be tailored to the type and location of the disease.
- Immunotherapy with anti-PD-1 antibodies pembrolizumab or nivolumab, as well as nivolumab combined with the CTLA-4 inhibitor ipilimumab, show high rates or responsiveness for stages III and IV melanoma.
- Metastatic tumors with BRAF V600 activating mutations can see rapid responses to BRAF/MEK dual inhibition.
- Interleukin-2 and cytotoxic chemotherapy are rarely given as first-line systemic therapy.

Radiation Therapy

- Malignant melanoma cells show a wide shoulder under the cell-survival curve, suggesting that higher-than-conventional doses per fraction are required for cell kill.
- Potential enhancement of cell kill using high-dose fractionation must be weighed against potential increases in late normal tissue complications.
- Definitive radiation to primary lesions has a role for inoperable patients or those with grossly positive margins and inability to undergo further surgical resection. Optimal doses are not well established, but include 64 to 70 Gy in 32 to 25 fractions, 50 to 57.5 Gy in 20 to 23 fractions, and 35 Gy in 5 fractions given every other day.

- Definitive radiotherapy technique depends on the site of treatment and extent of disease. For small lesions, electrons or orthovoltage therapy may be appropriate, but photon techniques, including IMRT, are often required for complex lesions of the head and neck region.
- Adjuvant radiation is not routinely recommended to the primary site after resection, except for select cases with unresectable residual disease or desmoplastic melanoma with close margins and/or extensive neurotropism (33,34).
- Adjuvant radiation to lymph node regions decreases regional failure, although it is not associated with improved survival. Doses of 48 Gy in 20 fractions or 30 Gy in five fractions show efficacy. Toxicity, particularly lymphedema, is high for inguinal irradiation compared to other lymph nodes sites (35–38).
- Risk factors for regional recurrence include extranodal extension, ≥1 parotid node, ≥2 cervical or axillary nodes, ≥3 inguinofemoral nodes. Additionally, cervical or axillary nodes ≥3 cm in size and inguinofemoral lymph nodes ≥4 cm in size are risk factors for regional recurrence (35).
- Multiple palliative regimens for unresectable nodal satellite or in-transit disease show efficacy. These include 24 to 27 Gy in three fractions, 32 Gy in four fractions (over 4 weeks), 40 Gy in eight fractions (over 4 weeks), 50 Gy in 20 fractions, and 30 Gy in five to 10 fractions.
- Given the increasing effectiveness of systemic therapy for melanoma, interactions between radiation and systemic therapies need to be considered. BRAF and MEK inhibitors given concurrently with radiation may increase dermatologic, CNS and pulmonary toxicity, and should be held for at least 3 days before and after fractionated radiation, and 1 day before and after stereotactic radiosurgery. Immunotherapies such as CTLA-4 and PD-1/PD-L1 inhibitors are under investigation in combination with radiotherapy to potentially increase the abscopal effect by which nonirradiated sites respond after radiation to an index lesion.

MERKEL CELL CARCINOMA

- MCC is an aggressive, rare, small neuroendocrine cell skin tumor that usually presents in the sixth and seventh decades.
- The Merkel cell polyomavirus (MCV) is found in 43% to 100% of patient samples, and its role in pathogenesis of MCC is currently under investigation.
- MCC is disproportionately found in immunosuppressed patients.
- Merkel cell tumors involve the reticular dermis and subcutaneous tissue, with only occasional extension to the papillary dermis.
- MCCs frequently infiltrate vascular and lymphatic channels and often behave aggressively, presenting with early regional and nodal metastasis.
- Tumors occur most frequently in the head and neck region, and are associated with a high rate of local recurrence (25% to 75%) after surgical excision.
- Merkel cell tumors have three subtypes: trabecular, intermediate, and small cell; prognosis and treatment approach are similar.

- Regardless of histology, the most important prognostic factor is tumor extent at the time of initial diagnosis.

General Management of Merkel Cell Carcinoma

- The initial approach in the treatment of MCC is excision of the primary tumor with 2- to 3-cm margins, which often requires skin grafting and plastic reconstruction.
- Sentinel lymph node biopsy for clinically node-negative disease is recommended, but false-negative rates are higher in the head and neck region because of aberrant lymph node drainage and multiple sentinel lymph node basins. Lymph node dissection is indicated for clinically involved lymph nodes
- Observation after surgery may be used if primary tumor is less than 1 cm, wide excision is possible, and no lymphovascular invasion is present in a patient without immunosuppression.
- Because the most common site of these tumors is the head and neck region, obtaining adequate surgical margins is often difficult.
- PET/CT changes stage and primary treatment in 22% of patients, as well as changing radiation dose or technique in 15% of patients. The sensitivity and specificity of PET/CT are 90% and 98%, respectively.
- Because of the high recurrence rate after excision and the need to obtain wide negative margins, radiation therapy has become an integral part of the treatment program (39).
- Data in the literature strongly support the role of postoperative irradiation to reduce the relapse rate and enhance local tumor control (40,41).
- Patients with stage I disease treated with wide excision were randomized to adjuvant regional radiation versus observation. This trial closed early because of poor accrual, likely because of adoption of sentinel lymph node biopsy. No overall survival benefit was seen with radiation, but patients treated with radiation had a 0% regional recurrence rate versus 16.7% regional recurrence rate for observation (42).
- A SEER analysis showed a significant improvement in survival of patients receiving adjuvant RT, with the largest improvement seen for tumors greater than 2 cm. A subsequent analysis showed overall survival benefit in those who received RT, but no cause-specific survival benefit, raising the possibility of selection bias among those who receive RT (40,43).
- Adjuvant systemic therapy is not indicated for resected local disease. For regional disease, adjuvant chemotherapy with cisplatin or carboplatin and/or etoposide has not demonstrated survival benefit, but is used on an individual basis (44).
- Immunotherapy with PD-1 and PD-L1 antibodies has a role in advanced unresectable or metastatic disease. For patients with contraindications to immunotherapy, platinum-based chemotherapy shows responsiveness.

Radiation Therapy Techniques

- Radiation therapy fields should include the original tumor volume along with adequate margin of normal tissue (3 to 5 cm), as well as the entire surgical scar.

- Patients with unresectable primary disease can receive radiation as primary therapy.
- MCC exhibits a dose-response relationship, with higher doses needed to control gross disease versus microscopically positive disease versus fully resected disease.
- The primary tumor site receives 50 to 56 Gy for subclinical disease with negative margins, 56 to 60 Gy for microscopically positive margins, and 60 to 66 Gy for gross residual disease at conventional fractionation. Nodal doses of 46 to 50 Gy are employed for prophylaxis of subclinical disease and 56 to 60 Gy for resected gross nodal disease.
- Adjuvant nodal irradiation after lymph node dissection is only indicated for multiple involved lymph nodes and/or the presence of extracapsular extension.
- Palliation of metastatic disease can be done with less protracted courses of 30 Gy in 10 fractions.

Sequelae of Skin Irradiation

- Erythema of the skin is the earliest noticeable radiation effect.
- The intensity of radiation dermatitis depends on dose, field size, fractionation, and beam quality. Treatment involves avoidance of trauma to the skin through shaving, scratching, or sun exposure.
- At intermediate dose levels, dry desquamation often occurs.
- At higher dose levels, in the therapeutic range for skin cancers, moist desquamation occurs. Dilute hydrogen peroxide or silver sulfadiazine cream (Silvadene) is recommended.
- If symptoms of burning and itching develop, a mild steroid cream, such as 1% hydrocortisone, can treat skin erythema and pruritus.
- Radiation necrosis may occur at any time after radiation therapy, but is more likely in patients receiving large-fraction doses.

NON–AIDS-ASSOCIATED KAPOSI'S SARCOMA

Natural History

- In the United States, non–AIDS-related Kaposi's sarcoma ("classic" KS, CKS) constitutes only a small fraction of 1% of all cancers.
- The greatest concentration of non–AIDS-associated KS occurs in the rain forests of Central Africa, where KS ("endemic" KS) accounts for more than 5% of all tumors.
- In the United States, most patients are older than 60 years of age; in Africa, peak age is between 25 and 45.
- In the typical American patient, a violaceous macule, generally in the region of the ankle, is the most common site of onset, followed by the arms.
- Progression of disease typically occurs by local extension, growing predominantly laterally.
- Visceral organs are involved in less than 5% of patients, most commonly in the gastrointestinal (GI) tract.

Diagnostic Workup

- CKS has a sufficiently nonspecific appearance to require a biopsy.
- The diagnostic workup for KS is shown in Table 9-1.

TABLE 9-1

Diagnostic Workup of Kaposi's Sarcoma

For All Patients

History including

    Age

    Ancestry

    Behavior (sexual, drug use)

    Receipt of blood products

    Prior opportunistic infections

    Visceral symptoms (GI, central nervous system)

    Constitutional symptoms (fever, weight loss)

Physical examination

    All cutaneous surfaces

    Visible mucosal surfaces

    Lymph nodes

    Body temperature

    Body weight

Biopsy of suspected lesion

Try to Obtain HIV Titer If

Patient < 60 year old or

High-risk factors present

    Homosexual or bisexual behavior

    Intravenous drug use

    Receipt of blood products

Extracutaneous disease present

If HIV Infection Exists, Add

Blood count (including CD4 lymphocyte count)

Serum chemistries

Chest x-ray

Tuberculin test

Screen for anergy

Screen for sexually transmitted diseases

If GI symptoms exist, add endoscopy

Pathology

- KS has both spindle cell and vascular elements within the lesion. The spindle-shaped cells look much like fibroblasts, and generally are considered the neoplastic element.

General Management

- Because CKS tends to be a slowly progressing disease confined to the legs, locoregional therapy can provide long-term disease-free survival.
- Solitary, small lesions can be surgically excised, vaporized by laser, injected with topical chemotherapy, or frozen with liquid nitrogen, but radiation therapy generally is considered the treatment of choice for localized or regionalized disease, with the best cosmetic result.
- Radiation therapy also often represents the optimal local therapy for palliation of pain, bleeding, or edema.
- For rapidly progressing or life-threatening disease, combinations such as vincristine and actinomycin D (with or without dacarbazine [DTIC]) produce response rates of almost 100%.

Radiation Therapy

- Local irradiation of KS includes the lesion plus a normal tissue border of approximately 1.5 to 2.0 cm.
- Thin, cutaneous lesions can be treated effectively either by low-energy electron beams (4 or 6 MeV covering the lesions, with bolus material).
- Thick plaques or nodules are best treated by higher energy electron beams.
- Eyelid lesions are treated most easily by superficial x-rays, with protective shields over the optic lens.
- When substantial edema is present, parallel-opposed portals and megavoltage therapy are needed to treat the deep tissues. Treatment within a water bath provides both bolus and homogeneity of dose. Wrapping the leg with bolus material and dosing to the mid-thickness of the field will suffice.
- A dose of 24 Gy in 12 fractions or 30 Gy in 10 fractions provides 85% local control for small lesions in patients who are in good general condition. About 8 Gy in one fraction can be used to treat large fields, or patients who are in poor general condition.
- The appearance of KS in tissues adjacent to those treated by local irradiation is a sufficiently common problem to prompt the elective use of wide-field, megavoltage electron irradiation with overlying bolus for localized lesions.
- More than 90% of lesions respond to therapy and approximately 70% respond completely (45).

Kaposi's Sarcoma in Immunosuppressed States

- KS and lymphomas preferentially arise in kidney transplant recipients. The disease often regresses in iatrogenically immunosuppressed patients if immunosuppressive therapy is discontinued
- The sensitivity of this disease to radiation therapy is similar to that in nonimmunosuppressed circumstances.

AIDS-ASSOCIATED KAPOSI'S SARCOMA

Natural History

- The 1981 discovery of KS in eight young homosexual men is generally considered the beginning of our awareness of AIDS. KS is the most common malignancy in patients with HIV
- Intense competition occurs between the destruction caused by the human immunodeficiency virus (HIV) and replacement of CD4 T lymphocytes by the body's immune system. Although the body replaces 2 billion CD4 cells per day, the virus (with a half-life of only 2 days and an ability to replace itself with drug-resistant variants in only 2 weeks) slowly but inevitably erodes the CD4 population (28).
- The risk of developing epidemic KS (EKS) as part of AIDS is approximately 20,000 times greater than developing KS otherwise.
- The legs most commonly are involved in EKS, followed by the tip of the nose and around the eyes and ears.
- Visceral lesions occur in most patients, and can involve any organ.

Diagnostic Workup

- In addition to inspection of all visible skin and mucosal surfaces, the likelihood of visceral KS is sufficiently high that endoscopic evaluation of the GI tract is appropriate for any patient with GI symptoms (Table 9-1).

Pathology

- Despite the major differences in behavior between EKS and other forms of KS, the microscopic findings are extremely similar.

Prognostic Factors

- It is now generally accepted that a CD4 lymphocyte count less than 150 per mL, presence of systemic symptoms, and presence of opportunistic infections or thrush are the key poor prognostic features for both AIDS and EKS.

General Management

- The role of HAART is now well established and appears to result in durable clinical response rates of over 60% of patients. Antiretroviral therapy is a mainstay of therapy for KS for HIV-positive patients. If lesions are asymptomatic and cosmetically acceptable, no therapy beyond antiretroviral therapy may be required. If symptomatic, additional therapy is recommended.
- Liposomal doxorubicin is the preferred systemic treatment option, with a 59% response rate.

- Small doses of dilute vinblastine (e.g., 0.2 mg/mL), injected directly into small lesions in three to five injections (spaced 1 to 2 weeks apart), will produce regression of disease.
- Imiquimod 5% cream or alitretinoin 0.1% gel produce high response rates.
- Liquid nitrogen cryotherapy provides a faster means of treating small lesions, with 80% complete response for a minimum of 6 weeks.

Radiation Therapy

- Currently, radiation therapy should be reserved for specific indications: pain, ulceration, bleeding, functional impairment (dyspnea from pulmonary lesions, incapacitating edema from lesions obstructing lymphatic flow, and loss of flexion at a joint space from thick cutaneous lesions), or improvement of the appearance of cosmetically disfiguring lesions.
- It is important to remember that irradiated regions sometimes are left with a purple hemosiderin stain, but with no tumor mass. This fact limits the cosmetic benefit of radiation therapy.
- The general principles of palliative irradiation for EKS are (a) sufficient dose (8 Gy in a single fraction for small lesions, 24 Gy in 12 fractions, or 30 Gy in 10 fractions) should be delivered to accomplish the desired goal and maintain that state for as long as possible; (b) treatment should be delivered as rapidly as possible; and (c) distressing side effects should not be induced by treatment (4). Radiation therapy technique is similar to that for CKS (46).
- Pulmonary KS occurs with cutaneous EKS in 18% to 47% of patients. When symptomatic pulmonary lesions (bleeding, obstruction) do not respond to chemotherapy, irradiation can provide effective palliative treatment.
- A randomized trial of 24 Gy in 12 fractions versus 20 Gy in five fractions showed equivalent response rates and local control (47).

CUTANEOUS T-CELL LYMPHOMA

- Cutaneous T-cell lymphoma (CTCL) has two major subgroups in its clinical spectrum: MFs and Sézary's syndrome.
- They usually display CD4 positivity and show a propensity to infiltrate the epidermis (epidermotropism).
- The etiology of CTCL is unknown, but an association with industrial exposures and genetic factors has been implicated.
- The incidence of MF in the United States has hit a plateau at an annual incidence of six new cases per 1,000,000 population.
- It occurs more frequently in men than in women, by a ratio of approximately 2:1, and blacks are twice as likely to be afflicted as whites.
- As with other lymphomas, the incidence of CTCL increases sharply with age, with peak incidence being between the ages of 55 and 60. The disease can be seen in patients at younger ages, with a similar clinical course.

NATURAL HISTORY

- Lesions of MF can be found anywhere in the body; however, they are most often seen in "sun-shaded" areas.
- Most cases of MF evolve slowly and progressively through three clinical phases: premycotic phase, infiltrated plaque/mycotic phase, and tumor/fungoid phase.
- The premycotic phase of classic MF is the most variable in clinical appearance and duration. These early lesions are frequently mistaken for other dermatoses. Lesions may spontaneously resolve. After many years, they ultimately develop superimposed infiltrative plaques or tumors more typical of MF.
- The plaque and the tumor phases of MF are characterized by clinically palpable lesions, as a result of the accumulation of atypical lymphoid cells within the skin. Individual lesions tend to regress spontaneously or merge with adjacent lesions to form larger lesions of irregular shape. Cutaneous ulcerations and secondary infections frequently are encountered in the tumor stage.
- Additional skin findings of hypopigmentation, generalized erythroderma alopecia, and ichthyosis-like lesions can be noted.
- Clinical variants include folliculotropic MFs, pagetoid reticulosis, granulomatous slack skin, unilesional MFs, and MFs palmaris et plantaris, among others.
- Most investigators consider Sézary's syndrome to be an erythrodermic and leukemic expression of CTCL. Sézary syndrome is differentiated from MF with erythroderma by the presence of malignant T cells in the peripheral blood possessing an atypical cerebriform microscopic appearance (Sézary cells). An absolute count ≥1,000 Sézary cells/cubic mm or ≥1,000/microL CD4+CD26– or CD4+CD7– cells by flow cytometry is a diagnostic criterion for Sézary syndrome.
- Seventeen percent of patients with CTCL present with generalized erythroderma; about 50% of these have clear-cut Sézary's syndrome.
- The median duration from onset of skin lesions to histologic diagnosis of CTCL is 8 to 10 years, with considerable variation from patient to patient.
- The median survival for all patients has historically been less than 5 years. However, earlier diagnosis and improvement in treatment approaches have increased the median survival to approximately 10 years.
- Extracutaneous infiltration is present in greater than 80% of cases at autopsy. It is associated with a significantly worse prognosis than disease confined to the skin.
- Any organ may be infiltrated by malignant lymphocytes; however, the most common sites are lymph nodes (68%), spleen (56%), lungs (50%), liver (49%), and bone marrow (42%).
- The median survival of patients with confirmed lymph node or visceral disease is 2 years and 1 year, respectively.

DIAGNOSTIC WORKUP

- Procedures used in staging and evaluation are outlined in Table 9-2.

Table 9-2
Diagnostic Workup for Cutaneous T-Cell Lymphoma
General
History with attention to pace of disease evolution Total body skin evaluation examination to assess degree of lesion infiltration and surface involvement Routine physical examination, including palpation for lymphadenopathy, hepatosplenomegaly, and other visceral abnormalities
Radiographic Studies
Chest x-ray Computed tomography of abdomen and pelvis Isotope scans of liver and spleen or bone (when clinically indicated)
Laboratory Studies
Complete blood cell count, blood chemistry Lactate dehydrogenase Serum protein electrophoresis Blood smear for presence and quantification of atypical mononuclear (Sézary) cells
Biopsy Studies
Punch biopsy samples from most infiltrated lesions Biopsy of palpable lymph nodes Bone marrow biopsy

- Several punch biopsy specimens should be taken from the most infiltrated lesions to establish the diagnosis and define the character of the malignant infiltrate.
- The status of the lymph nodes in the cervical, axillary, and inguinal regions should be evaluated. If there are any palpable lymph nodes, a biopsy should be obtained. An effort should be made to confirm the presence of extracutaneous involvement, if suspected.

STAGING SYSTEMS

- A unifying staging system based on the tumor-node-metastasis (TNM) system was originally proposed at a Mycosis Fungoides Cooperative Group Workshop on CTCL at the National Cancer Institute. This system was revised in 2007 (30) as suggested by the International Society for Cutaneous Lymphoma (ISCL) and the European Organization of Research and Treatment of Cancer (EORTC) and emphasizes the prognostic importance of cutaneous tumors, lymphadenopathy, and extracutaneous involvement.

PATHOLOGIC CLASSIFICATION

- The cellular infiltrate of CTCL consists of malignant T cells mixed with various numbers of normal white blood cells (a polymorphous cellular infiltrate).
- Characteristically, atypical lymphoid cells in classic MF and Sézary's syndrome invade the epidermis and follicular epithelium to form small groups surrounded by a halolike clear space (Pautrier's microabscess).
- The cytomorphology of atypical lymphoid cells varies from small cells with hyperchromatic convoluted nuclei (cerebriform cells) to large cells with pale-staining vesicular nuclei and prominent nucleoli.
- Malignant T cells frequently can be demonstrated in lymph nodes.
- Immunophenotyping is used to support standard histologic findings. Expression of CD2, CD3, CD5, and CD7 are key factors in determining the immunophenotype, and lack of one or more mature T cell markers helps establish the diagnosis of lymphoma. T-cell receptor (TCR) gene rearrangements are detected through PCR amplification or high-throughput sequencing, and although clonality is not diagnostic of MF, it helps establish the diagnosis.
- Histologic variants, which can have prognostic importance, include folliculotropic MFs (characterized by lack of epidermotropism and an atypical CD4+ lymphocytic population permeating the hair follicles), large cell histology (associated with worse prognosis), and granulomatous reaction.
- The IASCL/EORTC uses a point-based algorithm to diagnose MF, using clinical, histopathologic, molecular, and immunopathologic criteria.

PROGNOSTIC FACTORS

- Both increasing age and TNM stage are associated with decreased survival after diagnosis.
- Patients older than 60 years of age at the time of diagnosis have a significantly shorter survival than younger patients because they often present with more advanced disease
- Five-year survival of stages T1, T2, T3, and T4 disease is 90%, 67%, 35%, and 40%, respectively.
- Defacement of nodal architecture by malignant T cells is associated with a median survival of less than 2 years.
- Three-year survival rates of patients without nodal involvement, with enlarged nodes in one region, and with enlarged nodes in more than one region are 85%, 68%, and 60%, respectively.
- Visceral involvement is associated with a median survival of less than 1 year.
- Malignant T cells (Sézary cells) found in the peripheral blood is associated with an unfavorable prognosis. The median survival ranges from less than 1 year to approximately 3 years, depending on which criteria are used for the definition of blood involvement.
- Markedly aneuploid cells by DNA cytophotometry or cytogenetic studies are correlated with an even shorter survival.

GENERAL MANAGEMENT

- Staging procedures define two general situations, based on the localization of CTCL: (a) patients with disease apparently limited to the skin and (b) patients with pathologic evidence of extracutaneous involvement.
- Patients with limited involvement (stage IA) have the possibility of cure with intensive therapy directed at the skin alone. Long-term remission rates approaching 40% have been observed in these patients after treatment with total-skin electron beam (TSEB) irradiation, topical mechlorethamine chemotherapy, and photochemotherapy with methoxsalen.
- Patients with stage IIB (T3) tumor tend to have aggressive disease with a poor prognosis. Therefore, more active therapy is needed to clear tumors, and it includes TSEB therapy, denileukin diftitox (recombinant fusion toxin protein), and oral bexarotene (a retinoid). These treatments are generally well tolerated and effective; however, systemic treatment may be required in refractory disease
- A randomized trial compared TSEB irradiation to topical mechlorethamine chemotherapy. No difference in overall survival was found between the two treatments.
- Stage III disease or Sézary's syndrome is best treated with extracorporeal photopheresis with the addition of biologic response modifiers as needed. These patients may also be treated with oral low-dose methotrexate, which is also active in erythrodermic CTCL. Alemtuzumab is an anti-CD52 cell surface glycoprotein (a protein normally found on malignant B and T cells) monoclonal antibody. It has been shown to have some potential efficacy; however, it is associated with severe neutropenia and cardiac toxicity.
- Treatment for patients with widespread intracutaneous disease in the presence of cutaneous tumors should include TSEB irradiation with concomitant multiagent systemic chemotherapy, or total lymph node irradiation if the treatment intent is curative.
- If treatment is for palliation alone, patients should be placed on maintenance topical mechlorethamine chemotherapy or well-tolerated systemic drugs after a course of TSEB irradiation.
- Several single-agent chemotherapy regimens have been shown to have some efficacy. These include alkylating agents (mechlorethamine, cyclophosphamide, chlorambucil, and temozolomide), antimetabolites (methotrexate, gemcitabine, and pralatrexate), and antibiotics (bleomycin and doxorubicin). Some preliminary studies using combination drugs have been encouraging; of these regimens, CHOP has been the most frequently used, and it has demonstrated a complete response rate of up to 38%. However, most single or multiple drug cytotoxic chemotherapy regimens have resulted in a complete response in only 20% to 25% of patients with advanced CTCL. Furthermore, there are generally no long-term disease-free survivors among patients who undergo chemotherapy alone, highlighting the need for additional therapy.
- Systemic drugs fail to control advanced CTCL usually as a result of the incomplete response of cutaneous lesions, while a complete response is typically seen in extracutaneous foci. This is likely a result of malignant cells readily circulating between the skin and extracutaneous tissues; hence the rationale for further local therapy for cutaneous lesions (e.g., topical mechlorethamine chemotherapy or TSEB irradiation).

- Excellent response rates (greater than 90%) with the combination of TSEB and cytotoxic chemotherapy, either concurrently or sequentially, have been shown by several groups. However, a NCI trial comparing this aggressive regimen with the traditional conservative regimen of topical treatment and the addition of sequential single-agent systemic drugs as needed failed to show a significant difference in survival between the two groups.
- Autologous bone marrow transplantation with systemic therapy has been tried in the treatment of advanced CTCL. However, it has been unable to achieve a sustained response, as not all malignant T cells are generally eradicated from the marrow.
- Allogeneic transplantation has a higher potential for success in the treatment of CTCL if graft-versus-host disease can be appropriately prevented or treated.

RADIATION THERAPY TECHNIQUES

- Ionizing radiation is one of the most effective treatments for CTCL. Generous portals should be used to cover defined anatomic areas, with margins of ≥2 cm.
- The need for subsequent treatment in adjacent areas may arise; therefore, it is important to document treated areas with photographs, accurate portal drawings, and/or tattooing of the corners of the fields with India ink.
- The International Lymphoma Radiation Oncology Group (ILROG) has established guidelines for treatment of cutaneous lymphoma (48).
- Although extremely radiosensitive, 2 Gy × 2 fractions are associated with a complete response rate of <30%, and doses of >8Gy achieve complete response in over 90% of patients.
- Experience based on more than 1,000 individual lesions indicates excellent local control with modest doses of fractionated radiation (10 to 20 Gy administered over 1 to 2 weeks) (49–51).
- Bulky tumors and lesions in locations where retreatment could compromise functional or cosmetic outcome should be treated to a higher dose (e.g., 30 Gy over 3.0 to 3.5 weeks) for optimal control. Complete clinical response may take up to 6 to 8 weeks.
- Unilesional MF can be cured with radiation alone, and local recurrence is rare with doses of ≥24 Gy (52).
- In the United States, the most common radiotherapeutic approach for extensive CTCL is TSEB irradiation.
- The European Organization for Research and Treatment of Cancer and Cutaneous Lymphoma Project Group reached a consensus on the acceptable methods and clinical indications for TSEB in the treatment of MF, which recommends high dose treatment to 30 to 36 Gy (53). However, even after complete response with high dose treatment, relapse is common. Low-dose radiation TSEBT to 10 to 12 Gy has gained interest as providing excellent response rates, with fewer side effects and the opportunity for retreatment if required (50).
- Presently, the optimal technique with reasonable uniformity of dose is a six-dual-field technique described originally by Karzmark and later refined by Page et al. (32).
- An electron beam with an effective central-axis energy of 3 to 6 MeV is used to treat three anterior and three posterior stationary treatment fields, each of which has a superior and inferior portal with beam angulation 20 degrees above and 20 degrees below the horizontal axis (Fig. 9-1).

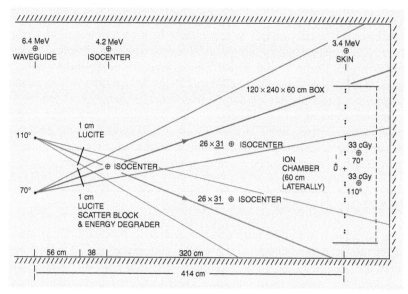

FIGURE 9-1. The portal geometry of total-skin electron beam therapy, as administered at the Columbia University Department of Radiation Oncology, as per the Stanford Technique.

- The patient is placed in front of the beam in six positions during treatment. The straight anterior, right posterior oblique, and left posterior oblique fields are treated on the first day of each treatment cycle, and the straight posterior, right anterior oblique, and left anterior oblique fields are treated on the second day of each cycle.
- The entire wide-field skin surface receives 1.5 to 2 Gy during each 2-day cycle. Most patients can tolerate 2 Gy per cycle; however, those patients with atrophic skin or a previous course of TSEB irradiation may tolerate 1.5 Gy per cycle better.
- The radiation generally is administered on a 4-day per week schedule, with the total dose depending on curative or palliative intent.
- During wide-field skin irradiation, internal or external eye shields are routinely used to protect the cornea and the lens. If internal metallic uncoated eye shields are used, the energy buildup at the surface of the eye shields could result in significant overdosage of the eyelids.
- Shielding of the digits and lateral surfaces of the hands or feet may be necessary because of overlapping treatment fields in these areas.
- Shielding of uninvolved skin is recommended in palliative treatment.
- Areas not directly exposed to the path of the electron beam, such as the soles of the feet, perineum, medial upper thighs, axillae, posterior auricular areas, inframammary regions, vertex of the scalp, and areas under the skin folds are treated with separate electron beam fields with an appropriate energy. *In vivo* dosimetry with optically stimulated luminescent dosimeters or thermoluminescent dosimeters should be used to confirm dose homogeneity and demonstrate areas requiring boost treatments.
- Thick tumors requiring boost should be treated with localized radiation prior to TSEBT, in order to enhance penetration by the TSEBT.

SEQUELAE OF TREATMENT

Short-Term Sequelae

- The skin of patients treated with TSEB irradiation at doses of more than 10 Gy usually develops mild erythema, dry desquamation, and hyperpigmentation.
- At higher doses (greater than 25 Gy), some patients develop transient swelling of the hands, edema of the ankles, and occasionally large blisters, necessitating local shielding or temporary discontinuation of therapy.
- Unless hair and nails are shielded, loss of these skin appendages occurs by the end of treatment. They usually regenerate within 4 to 6 months.
- Gynecomastia may also develop; the mechanism for this is unknown.
- Using current treatment methods patients may develop a mild leukopenia from TSEB, but they are no longer generally susceptible to significant bone marrow suppression from photon contamination.

Long-Term Sequelae

- Chronic cutaneous damage from TSEB irradiation is mild at doses of less than 10 Gy and acceptably mild up to 25 Gy.
- The nature and the severity of acute and chronic radiation effects are a function of technique, fractionation, total dose, concomitant use of topical or systemic cytotoxic drugs, previous treatments, and the condition of the skin before irradiation.
- Superficial atrophy with wrinkling, telangiectasia, xerosis, and uneven pigmentation are the most common changes.
- Higher doses may produce frank poikiloderma, permanent alopecia, skin fragility, and subcutaneous fibrosis; however, these sequelae are relatively rare.

References

1. Rogers HW, et al. Incidence estimate of nonmelanoma skin cancer (keratinocyte carcinomas) in the U.S. population, 2012. *JAMA Dermatol* 2015;151(10):1081–1086.
2. Goon PK, et al. Squamous cell carcinoma of the skin has more than doubled over the last decade in the UK. *Acta Derm Venereol* 2016;96(6):820–821.
3. Wehner MR, et al. Indoor tanning and non-melanoma skin cancer: systematic review and meta-analysis. *BMJ* 2012;345:e5909.
4. Ramsay HM, et al. Factors associated with nonmelanoma skin cancer following renal transplantation in Queensland. *Australia J Am Acad Dermatol* 2003;49(3):397–406.
5. Senet P, et al. Malignancy and chronic leg ulcers: the value of systematic wound biopsies: a prospective, multicenter, cross-sectional study. *Arch Dermatol* 2012;148(6):704–708.
6. Manyam BV, et al. A multi-institutional comparison of outcomes of immunosuppressed and immunocompetent patients treated with surgery and radiation therapy for cutaneous squamous cell carcinoma of the head and neck. *Cancer* 2017;123(11):2054–2060.
7. Karasoy Yesilada A, et al. Marjolin ulcer: clinical experience with 34 patients over 15 years. *J Cutan Med Surg* 2013;17(6):404–409.
8. Avril MF, et al. Basal cell carcinoma of the face: surgery or radiotherapy? Results of a randomized study. *Br J Cancer* 1997;76(1):100–106.

9. Khan AA, et al. Guidelines for the excision of cutaneous squamous cell cancers in the United Kingdom: the best cut is the deepest. *J Plast Reconstr Aesthet Surg* 2013;66(4):467–471.

10. Petit JY, et al. Evaluation of cosmetic results of a randomized trial comparing surgery and radiotherapy in the treatment of basal cell carcinoma of the face. *Plast Reconstr Surg* 2000;105(7):2544–2551.

11. Mosterd K, et al. Surgical excision versus Mohs' micrographic surgery for primary and recurrent basal-cell carcinoma of the face: a prospective randomised controlled trial with 5-years' follow-up. *Lancet Oncol* 2008;9(12):1149–1156.

12. Leibovitch I, et al. Scalp tumors treated with Mohs micrographic surgery: clinical features and surgical outcome. *Dermatol Surg* 2006;32(11):1369–1374.

13. Leibovitch I, et al. Cutaneous squamous cell carcinoma treated with Mohs micrographic surgery in Australia II. Perineural invasion. *J Am Acad Dermatol* 2005;53(2):261–266.

14. Lovett RD, et al. External irradiation of epithelial skin cancer. *Int J Radiat Oncol Biol Phys* 1990;19(2):235–242.

15. Silva JJ, et al. Results of radiotherapy for epithelial skin cancer of the pinna: the Princess Margaret Hospital experience, 1982-1993. *Int J Radiat Oncol Biol Phys* 2000;47(2):451–459.

16. Kwan W, D Wilson, V Moravan. Radiotherapy for locally advanced basal cell and squamous cell carcinomas of the skin. *Int J Radiat Oncol Biol Phys* 2004;60(2):406–411.

17. Wilder RB, et al. Recurrent basal cell carcinoma treated with radiation therapy. *Arch Dermatol* 1991;127(11):1668–1672.

18. Rowe DE, Carroll RJ, Day CL Jr., Prognostic factors for local recurrence, metastasis, and survival rates in squamous cell carcinoma of the skin, ear, and lip. Implications for treatment modality selection. *J Am Acad Dermatol* 1992;26(6):976–990.

19. Samstein RM, et al. Locally advanced and unresectable cutaneous squamous cell carcinoma: outcomes of concurrent cetuximab and radiotherapy. *J Skin Cancer* 2014;2014:284582.

20. Carter JB, et al. Outcomes of primary cutaneous squamous cell carcinoma with perineural invasion: an 11-year cohort study. *JAMA Dermatol* 2013;149(1):35–41.

21. Gluck I, et al. Skin cancer of the head and neck with perineural invasion: defining the clinical target volumes based on the pattern of failure. *Int J Radiat Oncol Biol Phys* 2009;74(1):38–46.

22. Lin C, et al. Perineural infiltration of cutaneous squamous cell carcinoma and basal cell carcinoma without clinical features. *Int J Radiat Oncol Biol Phys* 2012;82(1):334–340.

23. Mendenhall WM, et al. Cutaneous head and neck basal and squamous cell carcinomas with perineural invasion. *Oral Oncol* 2012;48(10):918–922.

24. Warren TA, et al. Outcomes after surgery and postoperative radiotherapy for perineural spread of head and neck cutaneous squamous cell carcinoma. *Head Neck* 2016;38(6):824–831.

25. Tanvetyanon T, et al. Postoperative concurrent chemotherapy and radiotherapy for high-risk cutaneous squamous cell carcinoma of the head and neck. *Head Neck*, 2015;37(6):840–845.

26. Love WE, Bernhard JD, Bordeaux JS. Topical imiquimod or fluorouracil therapy for basal and squamous cell carcinoma: a systematic review. *Arch Dermatol* 2009;145(12):1431–1438.

27. Maubec E, et al. Phase II study of cetuximab as first-line single-drug therapy in patients with unresectable squamous cell carcinoma of the skin. *J Clin Oncol* 2011;29(25):3419–3426.

28. Cognetta AB, et al. Superficial x-ray in the treatment of basal and squamous cell carcinomas: a viable option in select patients. *J Am Acad Dermatol* 2012;67(6):1235–1241.

29. Griep C, et al. Electron beam therapy is not inferior to superficial x-ray therapy in the treatment of skin carcinoma. *Int J Radiat Oncol Biol Phys* 1995;32(5):1347–1350.

30. Thomas JM, et al. Excision margins in high-risk malignant melanoma. *N Engl J Med* 2004;350(8):757–766.

31. Morton DL, et al. Final trial report of sentinel-node biopsy versus nodal observation in melanoma. *N Engl J Med* 2014;370(7):599–609.

32. Leiter U, et al. Complete lymph node dissection versus no dissection in patients with sentinel lymph node biopsy positive melanoma (DeCOG-SLT): a multicentre, randomised, phase 3 trial. *Lancet Oncol* 2016;17(6):757–767.

33. Strom T, et al. Radiotherapy influences local control in patients with desmoplastic melanoma. *Cancer* 2014;120(9):1369–1378.

34. Guadagnolo BA, et al. The role of adjuvant radiotherapy in the local management of desmoplastic melanoma. *Cancer* 2014;120(9):1361–1368.

35. Burmeister BH, et al. Adjuvant radiotherapy versus observation alone for patients at risk of lymph-node field relapse after therapeutic lymphadenectomy for melanoma: a randomised trial. *Lancet Oncol* 2012;13(6):589–597.

36. Henderson MA, et al. Adjuvant lymph-node field radiotherapy versus observation only in patients with melanoma at high risk of further lymph-node field relapse after lymphadenectomy (ANZMTG 01.02/TROG 02.01): 6-year follow-up of a phase 3, randomised controlled trial. *Lancet Oncol* 2015;16(9):1049–1060.

37. Hallemeier CL, et al. Adjuvant hypofractionated intensity modulated radiation therapy after resection of regional lymph node metastases in patients with cutaneous malignant melanoma of the head and neck. *Pract Radiat Oncol* 2013;3(2):e71–e77.

38. Chang DT, et al. Adjuvant radiotherapy for cutaneous melanoma: comparing hypofractionation to conventional fractionation. *Int J Radiat Oncol Biol Phys* 2006;66(4):1051–1055.

39. Lewis KG, et al. Adjuvant local irradiation for Merkel cell carcinoma. *Arch Dermatol* 2006;142(6):693–700.

40. Mojica P, D Smith, JD Ellenhorn. Adjuvant radiation therapy is associated with improved survival in Merkel cell carcinoma of the skin. *J Clin Oncol* 2007;25(9):1043–1047.

41. Garneski KM, P Nghiem. Merkel cell carcinoma adjuvant therapy: current data support radiation but not chemotherapy. *J Am Acad Dermatol* 2007;57(1):166–169.

42. Jouary T, et al. Adjuvant prophylactic regional radiotherapy versus observation in stage I Merkel cell carcinoma: a multicentric prospective randomized study. *Ann Oncol* 2012;23(4): 1074–1080.

43. Kim JA, Choi AH. Effect of radiation therapy on survival in patients with resected Merkel cell carcinoma: a propensity score surveillance, epidemiology, and end results database analysis. *JAMA Dermatol* 2013;149(7):831–838.

44. Poulsen M, et al. High-risk Merkel cell carcinoma of the skin treated with synchronous carboplatin/etoposide and radiation: a Trans-Tasman Radiation Oncology Group Study--TROG 96:07. *J Clin Oncol* 2003;21(23):4371–4376.

45. Hauerstock D, W Gerstein, T Vuong. Results of radiation therapy for treatment of classic Kaposi sarcoma. *J Cutan Med Surg* 2009;13(1):18–21.

46. Kirova YM, et al. Radiotherapy in the management of epidemic Kaposi's sarcoma: a retrospective study of 643 cases. *Radiother Oncol* 1998;46(1):19–22.

47. Singh NB, RH Lakier, B Donde. Hypofractionated radiation therapy in the treatment of epidemic Kaposi sarcoma--a prospective randomized trial. *Radiother Oncol* 2008;88(2): 211–216.

48. Specht L, et al. Modern radiation therapy for primary cutaneous lymphomas: field and dose guidelines from the International Lymphoma Radiation Oncology Group. *Int J Radiat Oncol Biol Phys* 2015;92(1):32–39.

49. Kamstrup MR, et al. Low-dose (10-Gy) total skin electron beam therapy for cutaneous T-cell lymphoma: an open clinical study and pooled data analysis. *Int J Radiat Oncol Biol Phys* 2015;92(1):138–143.

50. Kroeger K, et al. Low-dose total skin electron beam therapy for cutaneous lymphoma : Minimal risk of acute toxicities. *Strahlenther Onkol* 2017;193(12):1024–1030.

51. Morris S, et al. The Results of Low-Dose Total Skin Electron Beam Radiation Therapy (TSEB) in Patients With Mycosis Fungoides From the UK Cutaneous Lymphoma Group. *Int J Radiat Oncol Biol Phys* 2017;99(3):627–633.
52. Micaily B, et al. Radiotherapy for unilesional mycosis fungoides. *Int J Radiat Oncol Biol Phys* 1998;42(2):361–364.
53. Jones GW, et al. Total skin electron radiation in the management of mycosis fungoides: Consensus of the European Organization for Research and Treatment of Cancer (EORTC) Cutaneous Lymphoma Project Group. *J Am Acad Dermatol* 2002;47(3):364–370.

MANAGEMENT OF ADULT CENTRAL NERVOUS SYSTEM TUMORS

BRAIN, BRAINSTEM, AND CEREBELLUM

Anatomy

- The tentorium cerebelli is the dense extension of dura that separates the supratentorial and infratentorial compartments (see anatomical drawings in Figures 10-1 and 10-2).
- The posterior fossa is the cavity between the tentorium cerebelli and foramen magnum within which the brainstem and cerebellum are housed.
- In the supratentorial cerebrum, primary motor and somatosensory areas on opposite sides of the central sulcus (motor in precentral gyrus and somatosensory in postcentral gyrus) control the body from the knees to the feet in the medial cortex, and the trunk, arms, and head in the lateral cortex.
- The motor-speech area of Broca is located posteriorly in the dominant frontal lobe just superior to the lateral sulcus; damage causes expressive aphasia. Damage to the dominant temporal lobe at the posterior end of the superior temporal gyrus immediately inferior to the lateral sulcus (Wernicke's area) results in receptive aphasia. During brain tumor resection adjacent to language areas, intraoperative functional mapping can identify spatial proximity to these important structures and may be aided by preoperative techniques, such as functional imaging or Wada testing.
- Most of the primary visual cortex is represented on the medial and inferior surface at the occipital pole.
- The telencephalon consists of the cerebral cortex, basal ganglia, and olfactory bulb.
- The diencephalon includes the thalamus, hypothalamus, posterior pituitary, and pineal region.
- The mesencephalon rides on the upper part of the clivus at the tentorial notch; its interior is partially occupied by cranial nerve nuclei (for the oculomotor, trochlear, and proprioceptive portion of trigeminal nerves).
- The mesencephalic dorsal plate (tectum) houses the superior and inferior colliculi, which regulate eye movements/visual processing and auditory processing, respectively; the trochlear nerve is the only cranial nerve that exits from this dorsal location.

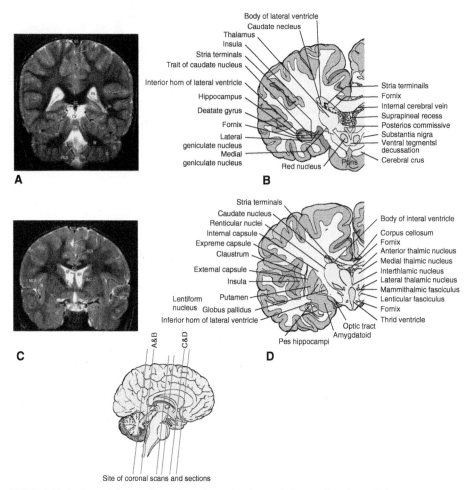

FIGURE 10-1. Frontal (coronal) sections through telencephalon at the plane of the anterior commissure. MRI (T2 weighted) shows same sections (**A** and **B**) as the drawings (**C** and **D**). (Reprinted with permission from Agur AMR, Dalley AF, eds. *Grant's atlas of anatomy*, 14th ed. Philadelphia, PA: Wolters Kluwer, 2017:697.) **Inset** shows side view of brain with lines of intersections of the planes for the MRI-drawing pairs (**A** and **C**) and (**B** and **D**).

- The mesencephalic ventral region (cerebral peduncles) includes the midbrain tegmentum, substantia nigra (extrapyramidal motor function), and crus cerebri (houses longitudinal tracts).
- Pathology may be referenced relative to the brainstem, which is synonymously referred to as "nuclear." For example, supranuclear palsy refers to damage to neural structures above the brainstem (e.g., motor or sensory pathway disruption).
- The pons (part of the metencephalon along with the cerebellum) relays information between the two cerebellar hemispheres, carries the major pathways from the mesencephalon down to the medulla oblongata, and houses the major motor and tactile sensory nuclei for the trigeminal nerve, which emerges from its lateral surface.

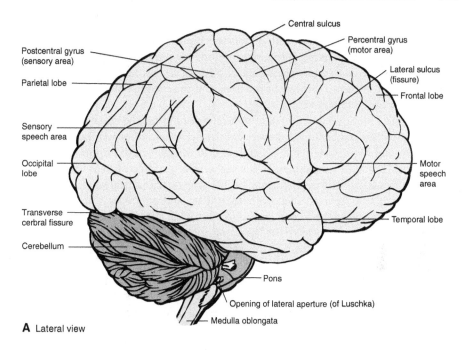

Central sulcus

Percentral gyrus
(motor area)

Postcentral gyrus
(sensory area)

Lateral sulcus
(fissure)

Parietal lobe

Frontal lobe

Sensory
speech area

Occipital
lobe

Motor
speech
area

Transverse
cerbral fissure

Temporal lobe

Cerebellum

Pons

Opening of lateral aperture (of Luschka)

A Lateral view

Medulla oblongata

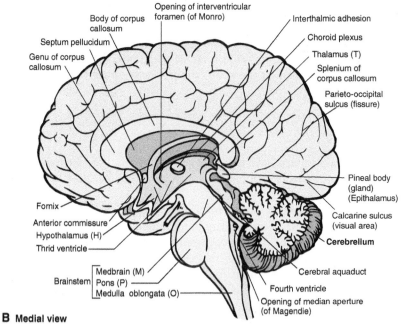

Opening of interventricular
foramen (of Monro)

Body of corpus
callosum

Interthalmic adhesion

Septum pellucidum

Choroid plexus

Genu of corpus
callosum

Thalamus (T)

Splenium of
corpus callosum

Parieto-occipital
sulcus (fissure)

Pineal body
(gland)
(Epithalamus)

Fornix

Calcarine sulcus
(visual area)

Anterior commissure

Hypothalamus (H)

Cerebrellum

Thrid ventricle

Brainstem
Medbrain (M)
Pons (P)
Medulla oblongata (O)

Cerebral aquaduct

Fourth ventricle

Opening of median aperture
(of Magendie)

B Medial view

FIGURE 10-2. Medial section of brain, showing cerebrum, cerebellum and brainstem. **A:** Lateral view; **B:** Medial view. (Reprinted with permission from Agur AMR, Dalley AF, eds. *Grant's atlas of anatomy*, 14th ed. Philadelphia, PA: Wolters Kluwer, 2017:698.)

- The border between the pons and the medulla oblongata is noteworthy for the emergence of the abducens, facial, and vestibulocochlear (acoustic) cranial nerves.
- The cerebellum develops laterally and posteriorly from the pons region and differentiates into the median vermis cerebelli and bilateral hemispheres. Anteriorly, the cerebellum faces the dorsal aspects of the pons and the medulla oblongata (in the form of the floor of the fourth ventricle).
- The medulla oblongata (portion of myelencephalon) forms the link between the pons, spinal cord, and cerebellum; it houses cranial nerve nuclei (glossopharyngeal, vagal, accessory, and hypoglossal) and is implicated in the control of important autonomic functions. Damage to structures in this region is often referred to as "bulbar" palsies and manifest as dysarthria, dysphagia, or difficulty with mastication.
- The ventricular system is lined with ependyma and produces cerebrospinal fluid (CSF) in the roofs of the fourth and third ventricles, the medial walls of the central body, and the inferior horns of the lateral ventricles.
- The foramen of Monro transmit CSF between the third and lateral ventricles at the superolateral corners of the third ventricle.
- The aqueduct of Sylvius in the midbrain (connecting the third and fourth ventricles) is the narrowest canal of the intracranial nervous system and is also the most common location of obstruction of flow by compression, which causes noncommunicating (obstructive) hydrocephalus.
- CSF escapes the ventricular system into the subarachnoid space through the median foramen of Magendie and the two lateral foramen of Luschka (which are located in the roof and lateral corners of the fourth ventricle at the level of the medulla oblongata).
- The subarachnoid space widens into several cisterns; the largest are the cisterna magna (posterior to medulla oblongata just at foramen magnum), the cistern of the lateral sulcus bilaterally at the base of the brain, and the ambient cistern posterior to the midbrain.

Natural History

- Some primary brain tumors have well-defined borders (e.g., meningioma and pilocytic astrocytomas), whereas many, such as high-grade glioma, tend to spread invasively in the brain.
- Intracranial primary neoplasms do not metastasize through the lymphatics.
- Extracranial true metastases from primary brain tumors are rare, but sometimes can occur with high-grade medulloblastoma, germinoma, hemangiopericytoma, sarcoma, and high-grade astrocytoma. These hematogenous metastases often appear in the lung; medulloblastoma has an affinity for bone, bone marrow, and lymph nodes.
- Peritoneal metastases infrequently occur in patients receiving ventriculoperitoneal shunts to relieve obstructive hydrocephalus from tumors.
- Some high-grade neoplasms in the brain and meninges metastasize by "seeding" into the subarachnoid and ventricular spaces and in the spinal canal, particularly in patients with recurrent tumors. Tumors with a propensity for such CSF spread include medulloblastoma, ependymoblastoma, pineoblastoma, and central nervous system (CNS) lymphomas.

Clinical Presentation

- Presenting signs and symptoms depend on tumor location, associated expansion, and surrounding edema.
- Local tumor growth, edema, or both may cause focal neurologic dysfunction, increased intracranial pressure, and/or hydrocephalus. The neurologic effects of an intracranial tumor may be somewhat predicted by its location. With significant cerebral edema or hydrocephalus, signs and symptoms of increased intracranial pressure (e.g., nausea/vomiting, headache, and papilledema), and generalized cerebral dysfunction may predominate.
- Increased intracranial pressure or local pressure on sensitive intracranial structures (dura and vessels) may cause headaches, which may be worse in the morning.
- Long-standing increases in intracranial pressure may lead to optic atrophy and blindness.
- Seizures are common and may be partial (simple, complex, and secondarily generalized) or generalized (tonic-clonic and absence); the highest incidence is with low-grade neoplasms.
- Lumbar back pain or bowel or bladder dysfunction may suggest CSF metastasis in the lumbar cistern.

Diagnostic Workup

- The initial workup of patients with brain tumors must include a complete history and a general physical examination.
- Complete neurologic examination includes assessment of mental condition, cranial nerves, coordination/cerebellar function, sensation, power, and reflexes.
- Ophthalmoscopy checks for papilledema as a sign of increased intracranial pressure.
- The most commonly useful magnetic resonance imaging (MRI) studies are T1-weighted images (with and without gadolinium contrast), T2-weighted images, and fluid attenuated inversion recovery (FLAIR) images. T1 images better demonstrate anatomy and areas of contrast enhancement (CE); T2 and FLAIR images are more sensitive for detecting edema and tumor hyperintensity. Computed tomography (CT) scans with contrast material may be useful when MRI is unavailable or contraindicated. See Table 10-1.
- Staging of the neuraxis is essential for neoplasms at high risk of spread to the CSF (e.g., germ cell tumor, primitive neuroectodermal tumor [PNET], medulloblastoma, and CNS lymphoma). Neuraxis imaging is usually achieved with gadolinium-enhanced MRI of the spine. Ideally, neuraxis imaging should be done preoperatively to avoid surgical artifacts and false-positive scans. Spinal imaging is usually combined with CSF cytology for complete neuraxis staging. CSF sampling preoperatively is typically contraindicated with tumors that may obstruct the ventricular system. Sampling in the immediate postoperative period may lead to false-positive studies and is best done either preoperatively or at least 2 to 3 weeks postoperatively.
- Biopsy of a CNS tumor is generally recommended, but often tissue diagnosis is achieved through frank resection. Selected patients with imaging and symptoms consistent with low-grade glioma may be followed closely without biopsy.

Table 10-1

Differential Diagnosis of Space-Occupying Lesions on CT or MRI

Pathology	Features on CT or MRI
Neoplasm	
Primary	Solitary, no prior cancer, thick nodular CE
Metastatic	Multiple, prior cancer, ++ edema, located at gray/white junction
Infectious	
Abscess	Fever, acutely ill, ±systemic infection, cyst cavity with smooth thin walls and CE
Cerebritis	Fever, acutely ill, ±systemic infection, diffuse T2 change, no CE mass
Meningitis	Diffuse enhancement of meninges on T1-weighted imaging (may simulate leptomeningeal metastases)
Vascular	
Infarct	Gray and white matter involvement, wedge like vascular distribution
Bleeding	Homogenous, clears quickly, residual hemosiderin ring
Treatment-related necrosis	Central hypodensity, ring CE, edema, >3–6 mo after radiation therapy or chemotherapy, metabolic scan shows low activity

CE, contrast enhancement.
Reprinted with permission from Siker ML, Donahue BR, Vogelbaum MA, et al. Primary intracranial neoplasms. In: Halperin EC, Perez CA, Brady LW, eds. *Principles and practice of radiation oncology*, 5th ed. Philadelphia, PA: Lippincott Williams & Wilkins, 2008. © Wolters Kluwer.

Histopathology and Staging

- Primary intracranial tumors arise from the brain, cranial nerves, meninges, pituitary, and vessels and derive from the ectoderm (brain) and mesoderm (vessels, meninges, and blood components).
- The 1979 World Health Organization (WHO) classification of primary CNS tumors lists distinct pathologic subtypes of CNS tumors in broad histologic categories (1).
- The 2016 update to the WHO classification (2) modernized the classification to include laboratory studies that may take precedence over histologic tumor characteristics. Glioblastoma (GBM) remains primarily distinguished by histologic features though more nuanced subclassifications are emerging that include genetic and imaging features. Astrocytoma, oligoastrocytoma, and oligodendroglioma are distinguished based on isocitrate dehydrogenase-1 (IDH-1) status. IDH-1 wild-type gliomas are almost exclusively now graded as GBM. IDH-1 mutant tumors are either classified as oligodendroglioma (i.e., in the presence of 1p/19q codeletion) or diffuse astrocytoma, which are typically associated with alpha-thalassemia/mental retardation syndrome X-linked [ATRX] mutation and TP53 mutation.

- In summary, under the modern classification scheme, brain tumors continue to be characterized by traditional WHO grading (i.e., WHO grade I-IV), but most IDH-wild-type tumors are GBM, oligodendroglial histology requires 1p/19q codeletion with mutation in IDH and a diagnosis of "oligoastrocytoma" is highly discouraged.

Prognostic Factors

- Many prognostic models have been developed. The most common factors that influence outcomes have traditionally been age, tumor type, tumor grade, seizure/other neurologic symptoms, duration of symptoms, performance status, extent of surgery performed, and, in some settings, irradiation dose.
- The strongest prognostic factors for malignant astrocytomas, before irradiation has been given, are age, tumor type, performance status, and extent of surgery (3).
- A recursive partitioning analysis by the Radiation Therapy Oncology Group (RTOG) showed that patients with brain gliomas stratified according to age, Karnofsky performance status, histology, mental status, extent of surgery, time between symptoms and treatment onset, neurologic function, and irradiation dose could be classified into six groups with regard to prognosis and response to treatment (4,5).
- The previous RTOG glioblastoma RPA was updated in 2017 (6) with added cooperative group data. This demonstrated the factors most associated with poor prognosis are high MGMT (O^6-methylguanine DNA methyltransferase) protein expression (as opposed to epigenetic methylation), age greater than 50 years and elevated levels of c-Met. Because these laboratory studies are not readily available at most centers, application outside cooperative group studies may not be routine.

General Management

- Given the poor prognosis of adult CNS malignancies, quality of life, and management of patient's expectations are of the utmost importance.
- Medications, performance and neurologic status, laboratory values, and the patient's social situation must be monitored to optimize the patient's ability to receive the appropriate treatment.
- Glucocorticoids (usually dexamethasone) are used preoperatively, postoperatively, and often during the early phases of irradiation to decrease cerebral edema. They should be tapered to the lowest dose necessary to control symptoms, but most patients do not require steroids through the course of chemoradiation.
- Concomitant medications (such as glucocorticoids) may alter anticonvulsant medication pharmacokinetics (particularly phenytoin); serum anticonvulsant levels should be checked regularly, particularly after medication changes.
- In most tumors, maximal safe surgical resection (MSR) is associated with improved prognosis; in some low-grade tumors, complete surgical resection may be curative.
- Some chemotherapy agents have demonstrated significant radiosensitizing effects in the CNS (7). In particular, temozolomide, an oral alkylating agent with good penetration across the blood-brain barrier, is an effective treatment of gliomas and provides potent radiosensitization (8).

- Tumor-treating fields (TTFields) are a local therapy for supratentorial glioma that involve alternating electric currents (200 kHz). Preclinical data have demonstrated the ability of continuous administration of intermediate frequency alternating fields to disrupt cell division and organelle function, which slows tumor growth. In a randomized study, administration of TTFields provided an overall survival (OS) benefit of a magnitude similar to that of adding temozolomide to radiotherapy (9) and further data have shown efficacy in the recurrent setting (10). Use of TTFields has been limited for several reasons (11), including the unorthodoxy of the treatment device.

Radiation Therapy

- Radiation therapy can be delivered to the CNS by fractionated external-beam radiation therapy, radiosurgery or stereotactic irradiation, or interstitial brachytherapy.
- *External beam irradiation*: Therapy is commonly started 2 to 4 weeks after surgery to allow for wound healing. There does not appear to be a strong relationship between the wait-time to start radiotherapy and survival (12). A range of dose fractionation schemes have been explored for glioma with most modern dose-escalation studies showing no survival benefit and the presence of viable tumor even at doses associated with radionecrosis (13). Current treatment regimens for primary CNS tumors generally include (dependent principally on histology) doses of 45 to 60 Gy (1.8- to 2.0-Gy fractions) with three-dimensional (3-D) conformal irradiation or intensity-modulated radiation therapy (IMRT). Treatment schedules delivering higher doses or using larger fraction sizes (greater than 2 Gy per fraction) may be associated with higher risks of late CNS toxicity, but modest hypofractionation (e.g., 40.05 Gy in 15 fractions of 2.67 Gy) is noninferior to standard fractionation (14). In addition to dose considerations, the volume of brain irradiated to high dose must be minimized; this is best accomplished by multiple treatment beams with careful blocking of the uninvolved brain in 3-D conformal irradiation or by use of IMRT. Interestingly, the duration of each treatment beam-on time may be important to minimize the integral blood volume irradiated. Hyperfractionated and accelerated fractionated schemes have been explored in clinical trials but have not shown a clear benefit (15,16). For tumors at high risk of spread to the CSF space, elective irradiation of the whole craniospinal axis, with a localized boost to the area of gross tumor volume (GTV), may be necessary. Matching of orthogonal, diverging beams of radiation when the brain and spinal cord are treated necessitates careful planning and patient immobilization to avoid overdose in junction areas between treatment fields.
- *Radiosurgery or stereotactic irradiation*: Delivery can be achieved with a linear accelerator (LINAC) or specialized equipment (e.g., Gamma Knife and CyberKnife). Targets typically do not exceed 3 to 4 cm and must be sufficiently distant from critical structures (e.g., optic nerves and brainstem) so that they are not included in the high-dose volume (17). Dose conformality to the target volume is generally an important component of treatment planning. Despite early enthusiasm for dose escalation in the treatment of high-grade glioma, the randomized experience has been disappointing, although the emergence of new systemic agents has renewed interest in high-dose radiation (18).

- *Brachytherapy*: Selection criteria for implant have included the following: tumor confined to one hemisphere; no transcallosal or subependymal spread; size less than 5 to 6 cm; well circumscribed on CT or MRI; and accessible location for implant. Direct infusion of specific radioimmunoglobulins in primary and recurrent brain gliomas has been used (19).
- *Particles*: Proton and charged-particle beam radiation therapy has been used in some intracranial tumors, particularly clivus and base of skull tumors such as chordomas and chondrosarcomas (20–23). There is some interest in combining dose escalation with proton therapy with the radiosensitizing effects of temozolomide for patients with newly diagnosed GBM (i.e., the phase II NRG-BN001, NCT02179086).
- *Radiation modifiers*: Phase I and II studies in malignant glioma have suggested a potential benefit to treatment with halogenated pyrimidines during radiation therapy for anaplastic astrocytoma (AA) (24). Temozolomide is a potent radiosensitizing alkylating agent that is a component of standard management of high-grade glioma patients; others studies on radiosensitizers for gliomas have focused on agents such as motexafin gadolinium, mammalian target of rapamycin inhibitors, and farnesyltransferase inhibitors (8).
- *Follow-up*: The follow-up schedule must be frequent to monitor side effects and properly taper any steroid medications. The physician must ensure that neurologic status is optimized. Tumor recurrence may be detected with periodic MRI (preferred) or CT scans. Assessment of intellectual functioning and quality of life is especially important in patients with benign tumors, as well as in long-term survivors with malignant tumors; patients should also be monitored for neuroendocrine and ophthalmologic side effects.

Radiation Therapy Techniques

Pertinent Anatomic Landmarks

- The external acoustic meatus are bilaterally symmetric; they participate in the definition of anatomic reference planes in the head (Reid's baseline and Frankfort horizontal plane, connecting points in the two external acoustic meatus and one anterior infraorbital edge).
- On a lateral projection radiograph, the sella turcica is centrally located and marks the lower border of the median telencephalon and diencephalon. The hypothalamic structures are located an additional 1 cm superior to the sellar floor, and the optic canal runs, at the most, 1 cm superior and 1 cm anterior to that point.
- The pineal body (tentorial notch) usually sits approximately 1 cm posterior and 3 cm superior to the external acoustic meatus.
- The cribriform plate, the most inferior part of the anterior cranial fossa, is an important reference point for the inferior border of whole-brain irradiation fields; adequate coverage of the cribriform plate is particularly important for conditions with a predilection for recurrences in the frontobasal fossa above the cribriform plate, such as medulloblastoma. In most patients, little distance is found between the lateral projections of the lenses and the most inferior part of the cribriform plate. It may not be possible to both completely block out the lenses and include the cribriform plate in whole-brain irradiation (25).

Treatment Setup

- The head should be positioned so that its major axes are parallel and perpendicular to the central axis incident beam and the treatment table; the most common errors are rotation of the head and longitudinal axis deviation (tilting).
- Reproducibility of head positioning is achieved with a fixation device such as the table-fixed thermoplastic net mask, Flixster stereotactic device (table-fixed reference plate attached to a plastic turban plus mouthpiece), or an individually made mouthpiece attached to a table frame.

Irradiation of Entire Intracranial Contents (Whole-Brain Irradiation)

- Whole-brain irradiation is administered through parallel-opposed lateral portals, which should always be individualized.
- The inferior field border should be 0.5 to 1.0 cm inferior to the cribriform plate, middle cranial fossa, and foramen magnum, which should be distinguishable on simulation radiographs (2-D planning) or digitally reconstructed radiographs (CT-based 3-D planning).
- The anterior border must be about 3 cm posterior to the ipsilateral eyelid for the diverging beam to exclude the contralateral lens; however, this supplies the posterior ocular bulbs with only about 40% of the prescribed dose. A better alternative is to angle the gantry about 5 to 7 degrees anteriorly from true lateral, so that the beam's anterior border traverses the head in a frontal plane about 0.5 cm posterior to the lenses (about 2 cm posterior to eyelid markers). This arrangement provides full dose to the posterior parts of the ocular globe (26).

Treatment Volume in Brain Tumors

- For high-grade gliomas, it was initially recommended that large volumes or even the entire intracranial contents should be irradiated because of their diffuse nature. However, in 35 patients who had a CT scan within 2 months of an autopsy, 78% of recurrences were within 2 cm of the margin of the initial tumor bed, and 56% were within 1 cm or less of the volume outlined by the CT scan (27). No unifocal tumor recurred as a multifocal lesion. These findings were confirmed by others (16).
- In a review of CT scans and pathologic sections of 15 patients with GBM, if radiation treatment portals had been designed to cover the contrast-enhancing volume along with a 3-cm margin around the edema, they would have covered all histologically identified tumors in all cases (28).
- Relatively generous margins (i.e., 2 to 3 cm) and inclusion of all radiographic evidence of tumor and associated edema is generally the rule in designing treatment fields for high-grade gliomas. The classic RTOG method entails irradiating enhancing tumor plus peritumoral edema plus a 2 cm margin to 46 Gy, followed by a boost of 14 Gy to enhancing tumor plus a 2.5 cm margin (24,29). However, some investigators have reported that it is potentially safe (i.e., no change in failure patterns) not to deliberately use the peritumoral edema region to generate the clinical target volume (CTV) but rather simply expand 2 cm from enhancing tumor in high-grade glioma irradiation as in EORTC approach (30).

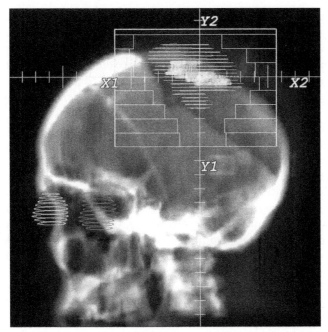

FIGURE 10-3. Initial portal used for the treatment of a multifocal anaplastic astrocytoma (WHO grade III) with some brain edema to deliver 45 Gy, and the reduced portal to deliver an additional 14.4-Gy boost.

- Figure 10-3 illustrates the initial portal used for the treatment of a multifocal AA (WHO grade III) with some brain edema to deliver 45 Gy, and the reduced portal to deliver an additional 14.4 Gy boost.

Two-Dimensional Irradiation Techniques

- Bilateral or medial cerebral hemispheric tumors are often best treated with parallel-opposed portals.
- If the tumor is asymmetric or lateralized, combinations of dual-photon energies (e.g., 6 and 20 MV) may provide better dose distributions, yielding higher tumor doses, and diminishing the dose to the uninvolved normal brain (31).
- Frontal lesions encompassing only the anterior parts of the lobe can be treated with anterior and lateral isocentric perpendicular beams; the dose distribution can be optimized with wedges in either or both beams.
- Midcerebral tumors (posterior frontal or anterior parietal) may best be treated with parallel-opposed anterior and posterior portals and lateral portals, all isocentric and with or without wedges.
- Posterior parietal or occipital lesions can be treated with posterior and lateral isocentric beams, both suitably wedged for dose homogenization.
- Lesions in the temporal lobe tip may be difficult to treat with other than lateral portals unless the patient is flexible enough to tuck the chin against the chest so that a sagittal beam can be added that does not traverse the optic structures/lenses.

- Craniopharyngiomas and pituitary, optic nerve, hypothalamic, and brainstem tumors are deep and centrally located. Depending on the extent, they may be treated—for example—with isocentric three-portal, four-portal, rotation, or arc-rotation treatment techniques. Stationary beams give adequate dose homogeneity in and around the sella turcica. The three-field technique consists of parallel-opposed lateral portals and an anterior vertex portal (i.e., superior anterior oblique). The lateral portals may be wedged to compensate for the declining anteroposterior dose gradient from the anterior portal. The four-field box technique uses both lateral and sagittal parallel-opposed portals. A 360-degree rotation technique can be used if fixation is adequate to avoid geographic misses. Because of the shorter distance from the anterior surface, the cylindrical dose distribution becomes flattened posteriorly. Arc rotation with reversed edges enables an ellipsoid dose distribution.
- Brainstem lesions may be adequately treated with parallel-opposed lateral portals combined with a posterior midline portal that does not irradiate the eyes.
- Unilateral cerebellar lesions also can be covered by appropriately wedged posterior and lateral portals.
- Pineal lesions can often be treated with parallel-opposed lateral portals.
- Superficial lesions (e.g., superior sagittal sinus meningiomas) can be treated with parallel-opposed isocentric tangential fields or half-beam block technique to avoid inferior divergence of beams into the normal brain.

Three-Dimensional Conformal Irradiation and Intensity-Modulated Radiation Therapy

- 3-D conformal therapy (3-DCRT) has supplanted 2-D irradiation techniques in the treatment of primary and metastatic brain tumors.
- Sometimes the CT scan defines abnormalities not always perceptible on MRI studies. Integration of MRI and CT scan data may be necessary for optimal 3-D treatment planning of brain tumors. This can be achieved through computerized CT-MRI registration functions available in many commercial treatment planning software platforms.
- The GTV encompasses the enhancing tumor (and surrounding edema for select histologic types) on CT or MRI scans. The CTV adds 1 to 2 cm, depending on histologic type/grade. The planning target volume (PTV) adds 0.5 cm or smaller if with IGRT.
- Multiple planar and noncoplanar fields encompassing the tumor (and surrounding edema for some tumors) with appropriate margin (PTV) are used—sometimes with static or dynamic wedges and multileaf collimation—to deliver the therapeutic dose. The treated volume should generally be encompassed by at least the 95% isodose volume.
- Marks et al. (32) described some of these techniques; they reported that noncoplanar beams may be preferable to coplanar beams when the target is in the central regions of the head.
- 3-D conformal arc therapy, dynamic arc therapy, and volumetric-modulated arc therapy (VMAT) have also been used for brain tumor treatment planning. Planning study comparing dynamic conformal arc therapy, coplanar VMAT, and non-coplanar

VMAT showed that no-coplanar VMAT is more appropriate than the others for patients with central tumors such as craniopharyngiomas with significantly reduced doses to the bilateral hippocampus without increasing the doses to normal brain tissue and other organ at risk (OAR) (33).

- IMRT appears to offer particular advantages for irradiation of certain brain tumors (e.g., gliomas and pituitary adenomas), including improved target dose homogeneity and improved sparing of critical normal structures (34–38).

- IMRT planning methods to deliver RT are not uniform. IMRT may use beams that remain on as multileaf collimators (MLCs) move around the patient (dynamic MLC) or that are off during movement and turn on once the MLC reaches pre-specified positions ("step and shoot" technique). Tomotherapy can also be used to deliver IMRT using a very narrow single beam that moves spirally around the patient.

- VMAT is one type or a variation of IMRT that delivers radiation from a continuous rotation of the radiation source with greater efficiency in treatment delivery time, reducing radiation exposure, and improving target radiation delivery because of less patient motion.

Craniospinal (Neuraxis) Irradiation

- Brain tumors that generally require craniospinal irradiation of the CNS and the entire subarachnoid space (neuraxis) include medulloblastoma, supratentorial PNETs, disseminated ependymoma, pineoblastoma, disseminated germ cell tumors, and other CNS tumors with dissemination/metastases.

- The patient is typically irradiated with boost, whole-brain ("helmet"), and spine fields. Generally, the entire craniospinal axis is initially irradiated (whole-brain and spine fields), followed by treatment with boost fields to the tumor itself (plus appropriate margin as needed).

- The boost is an individualized portal arrangement that depends on tumor size and location. Multiple portals (with wedges as necessary) or rotational fields may be used; 3-DCRT and more recently IMRT are delivery techniques commonly employed for boost irradiation.

- For craniospinal irradiation, the patient is simulated prone with thermoplastic mask immobilization and with the neck hyperextended to minimize posteroanterior (PA) spinal field exit through the mandible/oral cavity (but not so hyperextended as to cause excessive posterior neck skin creasing and compromise in dose uniformity for the spinal field).

- *Spinal field(s)*: The spine fields are usually simulated first. In adults, the spinal fields are commonly one superior and one inferior field (whereas in children, the entire spinal subarachnoid space can often be covered with one field, especially with the use of an extended source-to-surface distance [SSD] technique such as SSD = 120 to 130 cm) (Fig. 10-4). The superior spinal field has a stationary central ray location, with its initial superior edge typically immediately above the level of the shoulders. This superior border is then usually moved cranially (junction shift) by about 1 cm after each 9 Gy (i.e., five 1.8-Gy fractions) is delivered, with the inferior border of the whole-brain fields appropriately moved cranially by 1 cm as well. Although no gap between the

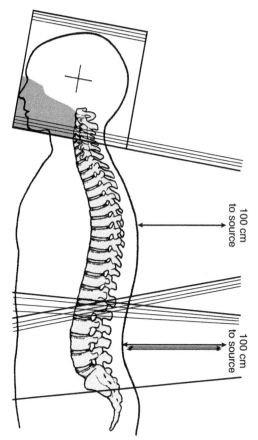

FIGURE 10-4. Lateral whole-brain ("helmet") field with blocking (stripes) and spinal fields. The whole-brain field central ray is stationary. The inferior whole-brain field border traverses the lowest possible cervical vertebra, which allows a moving junction of about 1 cm for each 9 Gy of dose delivered. Abutment adaptation to the superior spinal field border is achieved by collimating (rotating) the whole-brain field about 9 to 11 degrees against the transverse plane through the body. With ideal head fixation, the whole-brain anterior block border is about 0.5 cm inferior to the projection of the cribriform plate, 3 cm posterior to the ipsilateral eyelid surface (1.5 cm between eyelid and posterior lens surface plus 1 cm to protect the contralateral lens from the diverging beam plus 0.5 cm safety margin), and 1 cm inferior to the middle cranial fossa floor. Spinal beams for neuraxis irradiation abut the whole-brain field often with a safety 0.5 cm skin gap. The superior spinal beam has a stationary central ray in a transverse plane of the body, which enables optimal reproducibility of simultaneous movement of superior and inferior junctions after each 9 Gy. If possible, the superior spinal beam should reach caudally to the L1-2 space to avoid junctions over the inferior part of the spinal cord. The inferior spinal beam has a stationary inferior border placed at about S3 (to cover, with margin, the thecal sac, which generally ends at S2). The central ray and superior border must move with step junctions (unless a modern asymmetric jaw technique is used, in which case the central ray is fixed). (Reprinted with permission from Wara WM, Bauman GJ, Sneed PK, et al. Brain, brainstem, and cerebellum. In: Perez CA, Brady LW, eds. *Principles and practice of radiation oncology*, 3rd ed. Philadelphia, PA: Lippincott–Raven, 1998:777–828. © Wolters Kluwer.)

whole-brain and superior spinal light fields is needed if appropriate collimator rotation of the whole-brain fields is performed (see below), many institutions prefer adding an approximately 0.5 cm safety gap between the whole-brain and superior spinal fields. The inferior border of the superior spinal field has a skin gap with the superior border of the inferior spinal field such that these edges of the two fields do not overlap within the spinal cord (i.e., calculation of the gap such that the field edges intersect at anterior spinal cord/posterior vertebral body corpus). After each 9 Gy, this junction between spine fields is either moved superiorly or inferiorly (depending on institutional convention) by about 1 cm; however, if at all possible, this junction between spinal fields should always be below the level of the true cord (in adults, generally cord ends at L1). The inferior border of the inferior spinal field must cover the thecal sac (often at S2) with appropriate margin of about 2 cm; a sagittal MRI view should be used to determine the termination of the thecal sac. The central ray for the inferior spinal field is moved with the moving junction between the two spinal fields because the caudal border of the inferior spinal field is fixed; however, the central ray location for the inferior spinal field is fixed if using a modern asymmetric jaw technique in order to change the length of the inferior spinal field that lies above the central ray axis. The spinal field width(s) should be adjusted so that the lateral field borders are at least 1 cm lateral to the lateral edge of each ipsilateral pedicle; most institutions recommend a widening of the inferior spinal field width at its inferior end by about 1 to 2 cm to cover the more widely spaced sacral nerve roots, although the need to extend out to the sacroiliac joints is controversial ("spade" field design) (39).

- *Whole-brain fields*: Parallel-opposed whole-brain lateral fields are simulated with the central ray approximately in the pineal region. The inferior field border is allowed to reach the most inferior cervical vertebra (usually around C4-5) without traversing the ipsilateral shoulder. When the whole-brain/spinal field junctions are moved, the whole-brain field can be conveniently decreased without a change in the position of the isocenter. The gantry can be angled up from the horizontal position for each whole-brain field (until markers placed on the two lateral orbital canthi align) so that each whole-brain field avoids the contralateral lens. Although this technique allows the ocular bulb behind the lens to reach full-dose levels (26), it risks underdosing the cribriform plate region. Blocks are drawn on the whole-brain fields so that the irradiated volume includes the olfactory groove (cribriform plate), the orbits 3 cm posterior to the eyelid markers (2 cm if gantry is angled anteriorly from true lateral), the middle cranial fossa plus about 1 cm margin, and the included cervical vertebral bodies (Fig. 10-4). As described above, the junction between the whole-brain and superior spinal fields is usually gapped about 0.5 cm, with this junction usually moved cranially by approximately 1 cm after every 9 Gy delivered.
- To match the divergence of the superior spinal field anteriorly, a collimator rotation is applied to whole-brain fields (Fig. 10-4).
- One method to avoid caudal divergence of whole-brain fields into the superior spinal field is to rotate the foot of the couch toward the gantry for each of the whole-brain fields.
- Proton beam should be strongly considered for pediatric patients to reduce the volume of normal tissue irradiated, though proton facilities are not widely available.

Chemotherapy

- Primary chemotherapy is rarely used as the sole treatment for intracerebral malignancies. Exceptions include patients who are poor-functioning and elderly, particularly in those with malignant glioma and a favorable tumor molecular profile.
- Nitrosoureas, vincristine, procarbazine, cisplatin, and carboplatin have been used in conjunction with surgery and irradiation.
- The current standard of care for the treatment of high-grade gliomas (40) after tumor resection or biopsy is concurrent chemoradiation with use of the oral alkylating agent temozolomide, followed by adjuvant temozolomide: 5-year OS in the landmark EORTC/NCIC Phase III trial of 9.8% with concurrent temozolomide plus irradiation followed by up to six cycles of adjuvant temozolomide versus 1.9% with irradiation alone (41). Methylation of the promoter of MGMT, a DNA repair gene, strongly predicts benefit from temozolomide (41,42).
- Alternating low-intensity electrical fields delivered 18 hours per day by an external transducer array attached to the patient's scalp were evaluated in a phase III study of patients with recurrent GBM demonstrated the device was well-tolerated (10). Although failed to show an effect on survival, this chemotherapy-free treatment device showed comparable efficacy to physician's choice chemotherapy and less toxic. The same device was evaluated in a phase III study of patients with GBM as part of primary management of their disease given after completion of chemoradiation (9). This latter trial was positive for a benefit in both progression-free survival (PFS) and OS (median 15.6 months with temozolomide alone versus median 20.5 months in the experimental arm, by per-protocol analysis). Despite these results, utilization has been limited due to criticisms of the trial and skepticism related to the unconventional nature of the device (11).
- Newer agents such as bevacizumab (an antiangiogenic agent) have also been employed; bevacizumab as monotherapy and bevacizumab/irinotecan have yielded some promising results in the recurrent high-grade glioma setting with reduced use of steroids and prolonged PFS but failed to show OS benefit when used for newly diagnosed GBM (43–48).
- The addition of PCV (procarbazine, CCNU, vincristine) to irradiation has demonstrated improved PFS (but not OS) in the treatment of anaplastic oligodendroglioma (49,50). Tumors with chromosome 1p and 19q codeletions appear to be associated with improved survival and greater chemosensitivity to PCV and potentially also to temozolomide (even as monotherapy without irradiation) (51–54). Results from randomized trials comparing PCV and temozolomide are still pending.
- For tumors with leptomeningeal spread or at high risk of CSF involvement, direct intrathecal injection of chemotherapeutic agents into the CSF space has been used. A limited number of agents (thiotepa, methotrexate, and cytosine arabinoside) are suitable for intrathecal injections (55). Some novel agents that have been delivered intrathecally for select cases include liposomal cytarabine, rituximab (for lymphoid malignancies), and trastuzumab (for breast cancer).

Sequelae of Treatment

- Nausea and vomiting independent of changes in intracranial pressure may occur, particularly with posterior fossa or brainstem irradiation.
- Radiation dermatitis is usually mild and may be treated with topical petrolatum, lanolin, or hydrocortisone.
- Alopecia within the irradiated area may be permanent with higher total doses.
- Otitis externa may occur if the ear is included in the irradiation fields; serous otitis media also may occur.
- Inclusion of the inner ear may be associated with high-tone hearing loss and, occasionally, vestibular damage.
- Mucositis, esophagitis, and diarrhea may develop with craniospinal irradiation because of the exit of the spinal fields through the oropharynx, mediastinum, and abdomen.
- Fatigue may occur and blood counts may decrease during treatment, particularly with large-volume cranial or craniospinal irradiation.
- In the 6 to 12 weeks after irradiation, neurologic deterioration may occur as a subacute side effect (somnolence syndrome). This is attributed to changes in capillary permeability and transient demyelination secondary to damage to oligodendroglial cells.
- The most serious late reaction to irradiation is radiation necrosis, which may appear 6 months to many years (peak at 3 years) after treatment; it can mimic recurrent tumor. Management of symptomatic radiation necrosis may include surgical debulking in combination with steroid treatment. Focal necrosis is more often a result of irradiation alone, whereas a more diffuse leukoencephalopathy is more commonly seen after combined treatment with chemotherapy (particularly methotrexate) and irradiation.
- Inclusion of the eye may lead to retinopathy or cataract formation. Optic chiasm and nerve injury may cause a general decrease in visual acuity, visual field changes, or blindness at doses greater than 50 to 54 Gy.
- Onset of hormone insufficiency from irradiation of the hypothalamic-pituitary axis is variable but may be seen with doses as low as 20 Gy (especially growth hormone [GH] deficiency).
- Cranial irradiation can produce neuropsychologic changes such as decreased learning ability, deficits in short-term memory, and difficulties with problem solving, particularly in older adults and after whole-brain irradiation.

Management of Individual Tumors

- A summary of treatment recommendations for selected malignancies is given in Table 10-2.

Anaplastic Astrocytoma and Glioblastoma (High-Grade Gliomas)

- Because malignant gliomas are infiltrative, even gross total resection (GTR) inevitably results in tumor recurrence.

Table 10-2		
General Treatment Recommendations for Selected CNS Malignancies		
Disease	Evidence-Based Treatment (Summary)	RT Dose
Pilocytic astrocytoma	• Maximal surgical resection, although not tested in a prospective trial, is associated with more favorable outcome and is recommended whenever feasible. • RT may be considered postoperatively in patients with incompletely resected tumors or in recurrence. • Chemotherapy does not have an established role in pilocytic astrocytoma in adults.	50.4–54 Gy
Nonpilocytic low-grade glioma	• Maximal surgical resection (as with pilocytic astrocytomas). • Postoperative radiotherapy has not been shown to provide a survival advantage in the only clinical trial testing this question, although progression-free survival and seizure control were superior. • CCNU and PCV do not provide a survival advantage over radiotherapy alone. Temozolomide has not been tested in a phase III trial.	The typical radiotherapy dose is 50.4–54 Gy; randomized trials do not show a survival advantage with higher doses.
Anaplastic astrocytomas, and anaplastic oligodendroglioma	• Maximal surgical resection (as with pilocytic astrocytomas). • Postoperative radiotherapy has been shown to provide a survival advantage in several clinical trials. These trials included patients with WHO grade III and IV tumors; no trial for only grade III tumors has been conducted. • The role of chemotherapy remains undefined. The most widely tested agent, BCNU, and combination, PCV, have no definite survival benefit. Temozolomide is active in recurrent anaplastic astrocytoma and is currently being tested in the up-front setting. • Patients with codeletions of 1p and 19q have a more favorable prognosis and respond better to both chemotherapy and radiotherapy, but even in this subset, chemoradiotherapy does not have proven survival advantage over radiotherapy alone.	The standard of care is as for GBM in terms of radiotherapy target volume and dose, typically 60 Gy in 6 wk.

Table 10-2

General Treatment Recommendations for Selected CNS Malignancies *(continued)*

Disease	Evidence-Based Treatment (Summary)	RT Dose
GBM	• Maximal surgical resection (as with pilocytic astrocytomas). • Postoperative radiotherapy has been shown to provide a survival advantage in several clinical trials. Although there is much interest in incorporating advanced imaging in treatment planning and in using newer treatment modalities, their benefits in GBM remain to be demonstrated. • Temozolomide, given during and after radiotherapy, provides a significant survival advantage that is greatest in patients with methylation of the promoter region of the MGMT gene.	60 Gy in 30–33 fractions; the typical radiotherapy dose is 60 Gy in 6 wk; dose-escalation strategies have generally failed
Adult brainstem glioma	• Surgical resection is indicated for patients with favorable tumor types, but is not an achievable goal in patients with intrinsic pontine gliomas. • For intrinsic pontine tumors, radiotherapy is considered the standard. Dose-escalation strategies have been ineffective.	55.8–60.0 Gy in 1.8–2.0 Gy fractions per day
Oligodendroglioma-ependymoma	• Maximal surgical resection should be performed when feasible. • Postoperative radiotherapy is considered the standard, but no prospective trials have validated its role. Craniospinal irradiation is used only in patients with disseminated disease. • The role of chemotherapy remains to be defined.	Improved tumor control with doses >50 Gy; doses of 54.0–59.4 Gy are typically prescribed
Medulloblastoma (adult and pediatric)	• There are no prospective randomized trials evaluating major therapeutic issues in this disease in adults. • Maximal surgical resection should be performed, where feasible. • Standard treatment consists of postoperative radiotherapy to the craniospinal axis followed by a boost to the posterior fossa or tumor bed with a margin. • The use of chemotherapy generally follows the pediatric indications and guidelines.	CSI (23.4 Gy) with chemo; total dose to the posterior fossa or tumor bed plus a margin should be 54.0–55.8 Gy Fractions are 1.8 Gy

continued

Table 10-2

General Treatment Recommendations for Selected CNS Malignancies *(continued)*

Disease	Evidence-Based Treatment (Summary)	RT Dose
Meningiomas	• Small asymptomatic meningiomas in noncritical locations, especially in the elderly or in patients with other comorbidities can be observed. • The goal of surgery is to completely resect the meningioma, with negative margins as Patients with WHO grades I and II completely resected meningiomas have low rates of relapse and can be observed postoperatively. • For subtotally resected or unresectable progressive meningioma radiotherapy is frequently used but has not been tested in a prospective clinical trial. Local control appears to be improved with postoperative radiotherapy. Both radiosurgery and radiotherapy have been used in this context, but have not been directly compared. • For high-grade and especially malignant meningioma, postoperative radiotherapy is routinely recommended. • Primary radiotherapy or radiosurgery could be used for unresectable, progressive meningiomas. • Systemic therapy does not have a defined role in meningioma.	Per RTOG 0539: Low risk (group I): observe; Intermediate risk (group II): 54 Gy in 1.8–2.0 Gy per fraction; High risk (group III): 60 Gy in 30 fractions. GTV is typically expanded by 1.0–2.0 cm around the contrast-enhancing visible tumor to generate CTV accounting for microscopic invasion of brain parenchyma SRS: 14 Gy (12–18 Gy) to 50% isodose line for GKRS and 50%–90% for LINAC-based SRS
Craniopharyngioma	• Surgical resection is recommended, when feasible. • The use of postoperative radiotherapy has not been tested in prospective trials, but reduces the risk of recurrence and improves survival in incompletely resected tumors. Cyst decompression and biopsy followed by radiotherapy may be an acceptable treatment for patients for whom resection is not considered feasible. • Intracavitary bleomycin or radiocolloids may be useful in cystic tumors.	50–54 Gy in 1.8-Gy fractions

continued

Table 10-2

General Treatment Recommendations for Selected CNS Malignancies (continued)

Disease	Evidence-Based Treatment (Summary)	RT Dose
Vestibular schwannoma and neurofibroma	• Small nonprogressive tumors can be observed • Surgical resection is generally considered the standard of care for symptomatic lesions. • Radiosurgery produces outcomes equivalent to surgery, although these modalities have not been prospectively compared. • Fractionated stereotactic radiotherapy is being increasingly employed, with institutional reports suggesting a lower incidence of cranial neuropathies than radiosurgery, but this has not been prospectively validated	50–55 Gy in 25–30 fractions over 5–6 wk
Hemangioblastoma and hemangiopericytoma	• Surgical resection is recommended, when feasible, for both of these diseases. • Radiotherapy is generally reserved for subtotally resected progressive hemangioblastoma, but there are no prospective data. • Postoperative radiotherapy is recommended for subtotally resected hemangiopericytoma, but there are no prospective data. • Radiotherapy or radiosurgery may be considered for unresectable tumors.	Postoperative radiotherapy to total doses of 50–60 Gy reduces the risk of recurrence rate and improves overall survival; doses >50 Gy are associated with superior outcome
Primary CNS lymphoma	• Surgical resection is not necessary. • For most patients, whole-brain radiotherapy is considered the standard to a volume that includes the posterior orbits. • High-dose methotrexate-based regimens, generally used in preradiotherapy, have become widely accepted in patients fit enough to tolerate them and appear to be associated with improved survival.	Younger patients in complete remission after chemotherapy are usually offered 23.4 Gy in 1.8 Gy per fraction of WBRT. All patients who have not achieved complete response to chemotherapy are generally given WBRT of 30–36 Gy, followed by a boost to 45 Gy to the sites of gross lymphomatous disease.

continued

Table 10-2

General Treatment Recommendations for Selected CNS Malignancies *(continued)*

Disease	Evidence-Based Treatment (Summary)	RT Dose
	• Chemotherapy alone with deferred radiotherapy may be preferred in elderly patients because of substantial risk of neurotoxicity associated with combined chemotherapy-radiotherapy regimens.	For patients who are not chemotherapy candidates, WBRT with doses of 24–36 Gy followed by a boost to the gross disease to a total dose of 45 Gy is recommended. In patients with ocular involvement, the whole eye should be treated to 30–40 Gy, with shielding of the anterior chamber and lacrimal apparatus after this dose; for immunosuppressed patients (e.g., AIDS) modification of dose and schedule may be required
Spinal cord	• Complete surgical resection, consistent with preservation of neurologic function	50.4 Gy in 1.8 Gy daily fractions; GTV consists of the preoperative tumor plus a CTV margin of 0.5–1.0 cm for low-grade astrocytoma or ependymoma; increase margin to 1.5 cm for high grade

Adapted with permission from Siker ML, Donahue BR, Vogelbaum MA, et al. Primary intracranial neoplasms. In: Halperin EC, Perez CA, Brady LW, eds. *Principles and practice of radiation oncology*, 5th ed. Philadelphia, PA: Lippincott Williams & Wilkins, 2008, with permission; spinal cord adapted from Michalski JM. Spinal canal. In: Halperin EC, Perez CA, Brady LW, eds. *Principles and practice of radiation oncology*, 5th ed. Philadelphia, PA: Lippincott Williams & Wilkins, 2008. © Wolters Kluwer.

• Current standard care for GBM call for MSR (or biopsy if no resection possible) followed by adjuvant irradiation with concurrent and adjuvant temozolomide (41). Tumor-treating fields (TTFields) device can be offered concurrently with adjuvant temozolomide with significant improvement in PFS and OS (56).

• Treatment of AA and GBM is similar. MSR followed by adjuvant irradiation with concurrent and adjuvant temozolomide is generally recommended. The CATNON trial demonstrated the significant improvement in both PFS (HR 0.62, 95% CI 0.50 to 0.76) and OS (median 44.1 months versus not yet reached; HR 0.65, 95% CI 0.45 to 0.93) by adding 12 cycles of adjuvant temozolomide (57). The data for whether there is benefit for concurrent temozolomide (during RT) are pending.

- Localized irradiation volumes generally encompass either the peritumoral edema with a 2- to 3-cm margin if tumor is not contrast enhancing, or the contrast-enhanced volume (plus any resection cavity) with an approximately 2- to 3-cm margin, or the RTOG technique of enhancing tumor plus peritumoral edema with a 2-cm margin (CTV) to 46 Gy followed by a boost of 14 Gy to enhancing tumor (plus any resection cavity) with a 2-cm margin (CTV) (58).
- Postoperative irradiation is to a total standard dose of 60 Gy in 2-Gy daily fractions (59–61).
- Attempts at radiation dose escalation, often with use of hyperfractionation or stereotactic boost techniques, have failed to demonstrate consistent survival benefit for high-grade glioma patients (62).
- For patients with poor pretreatment prognostic factors and limited expected survival, palliative treatment (30 Gy in 10 fractions in 2 weeks, 34 Gy in 10 fractions, or 25 Gy in 5 fractions) may provide adequate symptom control without excessively protracted treatment (63–65).
- A regimen of 40 Gy in 15 fractions has been shown to be noninferior to the standard 60 Gy in 30 fractions for GBM patients aged 60 years or older (14).
- Even for elderly patients, radiotherapy has been shown to provide a survival benefit without a reduction in quality of life or cognition when compared with supportive care measures alone (66).
- Methylation of the MGMT promoter is prognostic and strongly predicts benefit from temozolomide in GBM (41,42).
- IDH1 mutation and MGMT methylation status predict survival in patients with AA treated with temozolomide-based chemoradiotherapy (67).
- Following chemoradiation development of "pseudoprogression" (treatment effect–related apparent tumor progression on imaging such as increasing CE and/or necrosis in the immediate postchemoirradiation period usually within 12 weeks, which subsequently stabilizes or wanes with further follow-up) occurs in approximately 20% of patients receiving temozolomide with irradiation, appears to be more common in patients with tumor MGMT methylation with some report occurring in greater than 90% cases, and may be associated with improved survival (68,69).

Low-Grade Astrocytomas and Oligodendrogliomas

- The relative rarity of these lesions, absence of randomized trials, reliance on institutional retrospective reviews, and long natural history make it difficult to make dogmatic treatment recommendations (70).
- Currently, the 2016 CNS WHO grading is predicated on the basis of combined phenotypic and genotypic classification, and on the generation of "integrated" diagnoses.

Pilocytic Astrocytomas

- Pilocytic astrocytomas are more amenable to total resection than other low-grade gliomas. In solid neoplasms, resection of the contrast-enhancing portion is sufficient.
- Fenestration of the cyst and resection of the mural nodule are usually curative.

- In completely resected pilocytic astrocytomas, no adjuvant therapy is needed.
- Postoperative irradiation in subtotally resected pilocytic astrocytoma may be appropriate depending on symptoms, extent of residual disease, availability for follow-up, and feasibility of repeat surgical excision.
- Chemotherapy (e.g., carboplatin/vincristine) is often used as first-line therapy for optic-hypothalamic tumors.
- If radiation therapy is indicated, 50.4 to 54.0 Gy (1.8-Gy fractions) usually is sufficient.

Diffuse Astrocytomas, Supratentorial

- Although observation is reasonable for selected patients, treatment is often instituted for patients with increasing tumor size, progressive/uncontrolled neurologic symptoms (e.g., refractory seizures), or evidence of malignant transformation.
- The treatment regimen is generally maximal safe resection (biopsy if no resection possible), followed by adjuvant radiotherapy in high-risk patients. However, immediate (rather than salvage) postoperative irradiation is associated with a PFS benefit, not OS benefit (71). Postoperative irradiation is often deferred in patients with complete resection who are 40 years of age or younger per RTOG 9802 although a high probability of progression is expected (50% risk of progression at 5 years) (72).
- Postoperative radiation therapy delivers approximately 54 Gy, with no benefit to dose escalation (73,74). Irradiation fields generally cover the FLAIR/T2 tumor volume with a 2-cm margin.
- The addition of PCV chemotherapy to irradiation has demonstrated improved PFS and OS in the treatment of low-grade gliomas (72).

Oligodendrogliomas

- Management of oligodendroglioma and mixed oligoastrocytoma is similar to that for low-grade astrocytoma. However, a reasonable conservative approach for small, asymptomatic, completely resected lesions in young patients is close follow-up with deferred irradiation after resection.
- Adjuvant irradiation (approximately 54 Gy) can be offered for incompletely resected or symptomatic tumors (75).
- Oligodendrogliomas are markedly more sensitive to chemotherapy than astrocytomas, or more specifically, tumors with 1p19q codeletion are more sensitive than non codeleted one (76). However, the optimal chemotherapy regimen, PCV (procarbazine, CCNU, vincristine) or temozolomide, remains uncertain and could potentially vary based on molecular subgroup or other patient characteristics.
- The addition of PCV chemotherapy to irradiation has demonstrated improved PFS and OS in the treatment of low-grade gliomas with 10-year OS being 60% versus 40% with or without six cycles of PCV (72).
- Chemotherapy, particularly with temozolomide, has an evolving role in the primary treatment of low-grade glioma. Temozolomide may be considered as primary treatment for those low-grade gliomas with both 1p/19q codeletion and IDH mutation. In a phase III intergroup study (EORTC 22033-26033), standard radiotherapy versus primary temozolomide chemotherapy were compared in patients with low-grade glioma.

The interim reports showed no significant treatment-dependent differences in PFS for patients with IDH mutant/codeleted tumors, indicating potential role of single modality treatment, either RT alone or temozolomide alone in this particular group of patient. However, patients with tumors with IDH mutation and non-codeletion treated with radiotherapy had a significantly longer PFS than those treated with temozolomide (HR 1.86 [95% CI 1.21 to 2.87], log-rank p = 0.0043), indicating the potential detrimental outcome if RT is not offered upfront (77).

- Anaplastic oligodendroglioma is more aggressive than low-grade oligodendroglioma, although the outlook is still considerably better compared to GBM or AA. MSR is followed by adjuvant irradiation (60 Gy with technique used for high-grade gliomas). Many clinicians now incorporate temozolomide in therapeutic management, often concurrent with irradiation and/or adjuvantly postirradiation.
- The addition of PCV chemotherapy to irradiation has demonstrated improved PFS (but not OS) in the treatment of anaplastic oligodendroglioma (49,50).
- Chromosome 1p and 19q codeletions is prognostic for improved survival and is predictive for greater chemosensitivity to PCV and potentially also to temozolomide (even as monotherapy without irradiation) (51,52).
- Preliminary data from a truncated randomized trial (initial phase of "CODEL" trial) in which temozolomide alone was one of three treatment arms in patients with newly diagnosed anaplastic glioma with 1p/19q codeletion found that patients treated with temozolomide alone did worse than those treated with radiation with or without temozolomide. Thus temozolomide alone for anaplastic oligodendrogliomas is in general not recommended.

Brainstem Gliomas

- Most brainstem neoplasms are high-grade astrocytomas; the remainder are low-grade astrocytomas and ependymomas. The exact distribution of these tumors is difficult to assess, given the low rates of biopsy confirmation in most series because of significant morbidity and mortality.
- Use of CT and MRI has increased the accuracy of diagnosis of brainstem lesions.
- Intrinsic diffuse brainstem lesions that originate in the pons and have rapid onset of symptoms at a younger age are usually high-grade glioma on biopsy. Lesions in the midbrain or thalamus, those with discrete focal lesions, or those with dorsally exophytic tumors often occur at an older age and have a more indolent clinical course; biopsy, when available, usually confirms a low-grade malignancy.
- Intense homogenous enhancement, particularly within a focal lesion, may suggest a juvenile pilocytic astrocytoma rather than a high-grade glioma.
- Other processes confused with primary brainstem tumors include abscess, neurofibromatosis, demyelinating plaque, brainstem arteriovenous malformation, and encephalitis.

Treatment

- Corticosteroids are usually necessary to stabilize neurologic symptoms; patients with severe hydrocephalus may require emergency shunting.

- Surgery has a limited role in brainstem glioma; patients with diffuse pontine lesions (most patients) do not benefit from surgical resection. Dorsally exophytic tumors, cervicomedullary tumors, and focal brainstem tumors may be amenable to resection.
- Radiation therapy is the mainstay of treatment. For diffuse lesions, inclusion of the entire brainstem, from the diencephalon to the C2 vertebral level, may be required; cerebellar extension must also be covered with a 2- to 3-cm margin. More focal lesions may be treated with smaller fields with approximately 2-cm margins. Irradiation dose of approximately 54 Gy (but up to 60 Gy) is recommended. Because most brainstem tumors fail in the irradiated volume, attempts have been made to escalate the dose to improve local control, often with use of hyperfractionation; however, no consistent improvement in outcomes has been demonstrated.
- Temozolomide has recently been incorporated into the treatment regimen, typically concurrent with irradiation, by many clinicians.
- In a historical phase III trial, the Children's Cancer Study Group found no benefit to adjuvant chemotherapy versus irradiation alone. Aggressive high-dose chemotherapy with bone marrow rescue was not of benefit in phase I and II trials. Neoadjuvant chemotherapy has produced clinical and radiographic response, but without clear improvement in survival.

Ependymoma

- Ependymal tumors may arise anywhere within the brain or spinal cord, in close proximity to or distant from the ventricular system.
- Myxopapillary and subependymoma (WHO grade I) variants may behave more indolently than ependymomas in general and can be cured by surgery alone.
- A more malignant variant of ependymoma termed malignant ependymoma or anaplastic ependymoma is recognized.
- Ependymoblastoma, a poorly differentiated embryonal variant with a marked propensity for CSF dissemination, is believed to be a variant of the PNET and is thus treated as such rather than as classical ependymomas are managed.

Treatment

- Emergency management may require corticosteroids or CSF diversion for a symptomatic mass or hydrocephalus.
- Because modern series confirm a survival benefit and a lower risk of CSF dissemination in patients with total excision of the tumor, it should be attempted in all patients before adjuvant radiation therapy. In fact, for patients with initial subtotal resection (STR), an approach that is being explored is chemotherapy after STR in order to facilitate potential complete excision with a second surgery (which is followed by irradiation).
- Surgery alone may be sufficient in selected patients with low-grade (nonanaplastic), noninvasive tumors with complete resections (particularly supratentorial tumors), although a substantial risk of recurrence, even in gross totally resected tumors, may argue for adjuvant therapy in all patients.

- Patients commonly have invasive tumors amenable only to STR, and in these cases postoperative irradiation should be considered mandatory.
- Patients should have spinal MRI and CSF sampling to rule out disseminated disease. If not done prior to surgery, spine MRI should be delayed 2 to 3 weeks after surgery to avoid post-surgical artifacts. CSF sampling/lumbar puncture should be done after spine MRI to avoid false-positive MRI results. Lumbar puncture should be done at least 2 weeks after surgery to avoid a false-positive cytology.
- Patients without evidence of tumor dissemination should be treated with limited field/partial-brain irradiation only, because substantial evidence exists that these tumors are more likely to fail at the primary site than in other areas of the brain (78,79).
- Patients should be treated with local irradiation fields encompassing the tumor bed plus any residual tumor (ensuring coverage of involved areas on preoperative imaging) with approximately a 1 to 2 cm margin to doses of 54.0 to 59.4 Gy.
- For posterior fossa tumors, special attention should be directed to the upper cervical spinal cord, because 10% to 30% extend down through the foramen magnum to the upper cervical spine (78,79).
- The incidence of high-grade and infratentorial tumors relapsing within the CSF led to the historical recommendation to treat with craniospinal irradiation. More recent series document a low overall incidence of isolated spinal relapses, even among the highest risk patients; most spinal failures are associated with local recurrences. Because of the morbidity of craniospinal irradiation, especially in young patients, more selective use of this modality is appropriate and thus craniospinal irradiation is not recommended in the absence of documented disseminated disease.
- Patients with neuraxis spread require craniospinal irradiation (36 Gy), followed by primary tumor bed boost (54.0 to 59.4 Gy), as well as boost to gross spinal disease to 45 Gy (gross metastatic lesions below the conus could receive higher doses of 54 to 60 Gy) (80).
- Anaplastic ependymoma is typically treated in a manner similar to low-grade ependymoma.
- Pathologic review is essential to rule out ependymoblastoma, as this histologic type has a much higher risk of neuraxis spread and thus warrants craniospinal irradiation.
- Chemotherapy is not routinely recommended for patients with ependymoma; previous trials of adjuvant chemotherapy have not demonstrated a survival benefit. However, on protocol, chemotherapy is being used after STR to facilitate potential GTR at second surgery. Recurrent ependymoma is sensitive to agents such as nitrosoureas, platinum compounds, and procarbazine.

Medulloblastoma and Supratentorial Primitive Neuroectodermal Tumor

- Cranial PNET are embryonal neoplasms that can locate infratentorially (medulloblastoma) and supratentorially (cerebral neuroblastoma, pineoblastoma, or esthesioneuroblastoma).

- Medulloblastoma, a posterior fossa tumor, is rare in adults but a common pediatric CNS tumor.
- Extent of disease workup should include CSF sampling and spinal MRI. CSF dissemination may manifest as positive CSF cytology or macroscopic seeding of the subarachnoid space visualized on spinal imaging. The incidence of CSF spread is up to one third of patients at diagnosis, but metastatic disease has been noted in more than 50% of autopsies of patients who died of recurrent disease (81).
- Systemic metastatic incidence is about 5%, especially to lymph nodes and bone.
- Gender and age (males and children younger than 5 years of age have the worst survival) are prognostic factors in medulloblastoma and PNET.
- Locally extensive tumors (invading brainstem or extension beyond fourth ventricle) and those with CSF spread are associated with lower survival.
- Patients with total or near-total resection have survival superior to those with STR or biopsy only.
- Patients with PNET other than medulloblastoma are believed to have a worse prognosis.
- Data regarding medulloblastoma in adults are scarce. A retrospective multivariate analysis of a large series of adults revealed that brainstem or fourth ventricular involvement, classic histologic subtype, and poor pretreatment neurologic status were predictive of worse outcome, as was an irradiation dose of less than 30 Gy to the craniospinal axis.
- A separate staging system for medulloblastoma is available (82), although modern pediatric protocols stratify patients as standard-risk (less than 1.5 cm² residual tumor, age more than 3 years, and no evidence of dissemination) versus high-risk (not meeting standard-risk criteria).

Treatment

- Hydrocephalus and increased intracranial pressure may be managed with corticosteroids or shunting.
- The association of systemic and peritoneal metastases with CSF diversion procedures has led some to recommend against shunting, but currently the benefits are believed to outweigh this risk.
- Complete resection should be attempted in all patients with PNET or medulloblastoma. Gross total or near-total resection is preferred, but extension of the tumor into the brainstem may preclude complete resection without significant morbidity.
- Postoperative irradiation is recommended for patients with medulloblastoma; elective treatment of the whole craniospinal axis (or therapeutic treatment for those patients with evidence of dissemination) with a boost to the posterior fossa is the standard of care.
- The recommended irradiation dose for pediatric patients is 23.4 Gy to the craniospinal axis for standard-risk patients and 36 Gy for high-risk patients, followed by a posterior fossa boost to 54 Gy (with boost also to any gross spinal disease). Chemotherapy is a critical component of the regimen if the craniospinal irradiation dose is limited to 23.4 Gy for standard-risk patients, with a typical regimen of weekly vincristine

concurrent with irradiation followed by adjuvant cisplatin, vincristine, and CCNU (sometimes cyclophosphamide as component of regimen) (83). Indeed, reduced-dose craniospinal irradiation (i.e., 23.4 Gy rather than 36 Gy) without chemotherapy for standard-risk patients is associated with a higher risk of isolated neuraxis failures (84). Chemotherapy is also an integral part of the treatment regimen for high-risk patients.

* Limited tumor bed/residual tumor boost (rather than posterior fossa boost) for standard-risk pediatric patients appears to be a safe approach (85), and is recommended after this strategy being explored formally in a Phase III protocol setting by the Children's Oncology Group (COG ACNS0331). However, lower doses of craniospinal axis irradiation (18 Gy CSI) were associated with higher event rates and worse OS for the youngest patients (ages 3 to 7). Findings from this phase III randomized trial indicate that physicians can adopt smaller boost volumes for posterior fossa RT but should maintain the standard RT dose (23.4 Gy CSI) for craniospinal irradiation.
* Present treatment recommendations for the management of adult medulloblastoma are essentially based on experience in children. The general treatment approach for adult (and older pediatric) medulloblastoma patients is 36 Gy craniospinal irradiation, followed by posterior fossa boost to 54 to 55.8 Gy. The role of chemotherapy is less clear in adults than in pediatric patients.
* Adult patients with large cell or anaplastic medulloblastoma, supratentorial PNET, disease dissemination, unresectable tumors, or residual tumors more than 1.5 cm^2 after surgery are at higher recurrence risk (86,87). These patients should undergo radiation therapy after surgery (36 Gy CSI with boosting primary brain site to 54 to 55.8 Gy) followed by chemotherapy. Alternatively, data from the prospective trial by Brandes et al. suggested that after surgery, up-front chemotherapy using the DEC (cisplatin/etoposide/cyclophosphamide) regimen, followed by radiotherapy (36 Gy CSI followed by boosting posterior fossa to 54.8 Gy) and more adjuvant chemotherapy is feasible, and provides long-term outcomes similar to that obtained with radiotherapy alone in standard-risk patients (88).
* For adult patients with standard-risk profile, 30 to 36 Gy CSI and boosting the primary brain site to 54 to 55.8 Gy after surgery is recommended. Adjuvant chemotherapy is not routinely offered due to lack of evidence. Reduced dose of 23.4 Gy CSI and boosting the primary brain site to 54 to 55.8 Gy can be considered if adjuvant chemotherapy is planned in those standard risk patients.
* It is important to include the cribriform plate in the anterior fossa in the irradiation volume because recurrences appear there, probably as a result of inappropriate concern for blocking the ocular lenses out of the fields. The most common site of failure is in the posterior fossa at the primary tumor site.

Pineal Region

* Pineal tumors are diverse and are grouped together because of their location.
* Germ cell tumors predominate among older patients; pineal parenchymal tumors (pineocytoma, pineal parenchymal tumor of intermediate differentiation (PPTID), and pineoblastoma) are seen occasionally.

- Reluctance to biopsy lesions in this area because of associated morbidity led to empiric treatment of many lesions with irradiation.
- In modern series with routine biopsy, benign lesions account for up to 50% of pineal lesions, highlighting the need for histopathologic confirmation. Elevated CSF and/or serum tumor marker levels, such as alpha-fetoprotein (AFP) or β-human chorionic gonadotropin (β-hCG), may be indicative of the presence of a germ cell tumor.
- Pineal region tumors include pineocytoma, PPTID, pineoblastoma, papillary tumor of pineal region, and germ cell tumors with first three being pineal parenchymal tumors. The first four tumors are rare, and the incidence of germ cell tumors is less than 1% of all intracranial tumors (89).
- When originating in the CNS, germinomas commonly present in the pineal or sellar/suprasellar regions; multifocal presentation is not uncommon.
- Nongerminomatous germ cell tumors (NGGCTs) of the CNS include embryonal carcinoma, Yolk sac tumor (endodermal sinus tumor), choriocarcinoma, teratoma, and mixed tumors.
- Pineocytoma, WHO grade I, is a well-circumscribed, slowly growing lesion composed of well-differentiated, mature-appearing pineal cells.
- Pineoblastoma, WHO grade IV, is generally regarded as pineal PNET; like other PNETs, it has a propensity to spread to the CSF space and thus is treated with craniospinal irradiation.
- PPTID is a rare disease, first classified by the WHO in 2000 as grade III. In WHO 2016 classification, it can be grade II or III.
- The biologic behavior of papillary tumour of the pineal region (PTPR) is variable and may correspond to WHO grades II or III.
- Baseline ophthalmologic assessment is necessary for patients with visual disturbances.
- Serum and CSF β-hCG and AFP markers should be measured in all patients with pineal region masses.
- Neuraxis staging (CSF cytology and spinal imaging) should be performed on all patients except those with biopsy-confirmed benign lesions and low-grade glial tumors.
- Treatment of pineal region tumors is somewhat controversial. Small numbers of patients, incomplete histologic information, nonuniform imaging of the primary tumor, variable staging of CSF, and widely variable treatment using various combinations of surgery, irradiation, and chemotherapy make interpretation of results difficult.
- In the past, many patients with pineal region masses had shunts placed to relieve symptoms of hydrocephalus, followed by irradiation without biopsy; tumors with a good response to irradiation were presumed to be germinoma. Given the known incidence of benign tumors in 10% to 50% of patients, this policy will lead to unnecessary treatment of a substantial proportion of patients.
- Histologic information allows tailoring of the treatment regimen. Response to radiation therapy does not always correlate with histology.

Germinoma

- Aggressive surgical resection is not generally indicated, but adequate sampling is typically essential as nongerminomatous elements are present in 10% to 40% of cases.

- Correlation with serum and tumor markers is essential, as germinoma may be associated with mildly elevated β-hCG but not AFP.
- Although irradiation is the treatment of choice for intracranial germinomas, controversy exists as to the exact volume of the CNS to be irradiated. Most series indicating a benefit to prophylactic irradiation of the neuraxis include nonbiopsied tumors, tumors treated before contemporary CT or MRI was available, and incomplete neuraxis staging. Series with biopsy-proven germinoma and negative neuraxis staging treated to limited fields have a low incidence of isolated spinal canal recurrence (less than 10%).
- Craniospinal irradiation is reserved for neuraxis spread (positive imaging or CSF cytology), subependymal spread, and possibly multiple midline tumors. Craniospinal doses are generally 30.6 to 36.0 Gy (sometimes lower) with a local-field boost to the primary tumor to 50.4 Gy (sometimes lower).
- For patients in whom craniospinal irradiation is not indicated, partial cranial fields are sufficient. Whole-ventricular irradiation of 19.8 to 30.6 Gy, followed by a local-field boost with a 1 to 2 cm margin to a total dose of 45.0 to 50.4 Gy is recommended.
- Response to cisplatin-based chemotherapy in primary intracranial germinoma has been noted; chemotherapy response–adapted irradiation with reduced dose/volume is being explored for pediatric germinoma patients.

Nongerminomatous Germ Cell Tumors

- NGGCTs should be suspected in patients with elevated serum or CSF AFP, as well as those with marked elevation of β-hCG.
- NGGCTs are less radiosensitive than germinomas; maximal safe resection is recommended for most patients as initial therapy.
- For patients with elevated AFP and evidence of neuraxis spread, stereotactic biopsy only may be preferable, as aggressive resection may not improve survival.
- It is not clear if patients with NGGCT and negative neuraxis staging are at higher risk of neuraxis failure than those with germinoma. Poor survival in NGGCT patients has led some to recommend routine craniospinal irradiation after surgery, although it may not be necessary in those with negative neuraxis staging.
- More recently, platinum-based chemotherapy has been used to improve survival. Maximal surgical resection, followed by platinum-based chemotherapy (e.g., bleomycin, etoposide, and cisplatin) is typically used. Consolidative local-field (negative neuraxis) or craniospinal irradiation (positive neuraxis) should be added after chemotherapy. One irradiation approach is 19.8 to 36.0 Gy of whole-ventricular or craniospinal irradiation, followed by local-field boost to 54 Gy.

Pineocytoma, PPTID, and Pineoblastoma

- Pineocytoma is treated in a manner similar to low-grade glioma. Patients with complete surgical resection may be observed. Patients with STR should receive postoperative irradiation. Local-field irradiation (54 Gy) generally encompasses the preoperative tumor volume with a 2-cm margin.
- Pineoblastoma generally is regarded as a variant of PNET and is treated in a manner similar to medulloblastoma. Patients should receive maximal safe resection, followed

by craniospinal irradiation to 36 Gy and local boost to 54 Gy. Adjuvant chemotherapy similar to that for high-risk medulloblastoma is recommended.

- The optimal management for PPTID has not yet been determined. Some clinicians recommend that patients with cerebrospinal dissemination at diagnosis to receive biopsy-only surgery, craniospinal and whole-ventricular irradiation and chemotherapy. Patients with locally limited disease at diagnosis may receive local or whole-ventricular irradiation after surgery. Although PPTID may be aggressive and has CSF seeding potential, PPTID patients may survive long-term (90).

Primary Central Nervous System Lymphomas

- There has been a large increase in the diagnosis of primary CNS lymphomas, particularly in patients with acquired immunodeficiency syndrome (AIDS).
- Most primary CNS lymphomas are B-cell lymphomas. Histologically, most tumors are intermediate- or high-grade lymphomas.
- Immunohistochemical analysis is performed to confirm monoclonality and B versus T cell type.
- Stereotactic biopsy is sufficient for tissue diagnosis, and obviates the morbidity of open craniotomy.
- Staging investigations include MRI of brain, CSF cytology, MRI of spine (especially if is CSF positive or patient is symptomatic), an ophthalmologic assessment (with slit-lamp exam) to rule out ocular involvement, complete blood cell count, and Epstein-Barr virus and human immunodeficiency virus (HIV) serologies.
- Systemic staging (CT of chest/abdomen/pelvis, PET scan, and bone marrow biopsy) is rarely positive in patients with typical findings of CNS lymphoma, but should be performed if signs or symptoms suggestive of systemic involvement are present (e.g., night sweats, fever, or lymphadenopathy).
- The extent of surgical resection does not correlate with survival.
- Treatment with corticosteroids dramatically improves symptoms in most cases, but response is temporary; patients usually relapse within 6 months.
- For nonimmunosuppressed patients, treatment begins with a high-dose methotrexate-based chemotherapy regimen (91). In patients treated with chemotherapy, whole-brain radiation therapy (WBRT) may be withheld in the primary setting. Those who enter complete remission after chemotherapy can most reasonably have whole-brain irradiation deferred, especially if they are older (more than 50 to 60 years old) because of a significant risk of treatment-related severe neurotoxicity (33). If WBRT is used, younger patients in complete remission after chemotherapy are usually offered 23.4 Gy in 1.8 Gy per fraction of WBRT. All patients who have not achieved complete response to chemotherapy are generally given WBRT of 30 to 36 Gy, followed by a boost to 45 Gy to the sites of gross lymphomatous disease.
- For patients who are not chemotherapy candidates, WBRT with doses of 24 to 36 Gy followed by a boost to the gross disease to a total dose of 45 Gy is recommended.
- The posterior orbits are included in the whole-brain fields.
- In patients with ocular involvement, both eyes are generally treated to 36 Gy (delivered concurrent with cranial irradiation to doses described previously if disease is present intracranially as well). The frequent association of ocular lymphoma with

synchronous or metachronous cranial CNS lymphoma has led some clinicians to recommend prophylactic brain irradiation in all patients; however, it is reasonable to treat isolated ocular involvement with irradiation of the eyes only. Craniospinal irradiation is suggested for patients with documented CSF involvement, but intrathecal chemotherapy may be equally efficacious and less toxic.

- For immunosuppressed patients, modification of the irradiation dose and schedule may be necessary. Patients with good prognostic features (non-HIV immunosuppression, HIV-positive patients with no other AIDS-defining diagnoses, and CD4 lymphocyte counts greater than 200) can reasonably receive standard treatment; those with poor prognostic features (low Karnofsky performance status, CD4 count less than 200, and advanced AIDS) may be treated with irradiation alone and even with an abbreviated course of irradiation.

Meningioma

- Meningioma occurs in regions including the cerebral convexities, falx cerebri, tentorium cerebelli, cerebellopontine angle, and sphenoid ridge.
- Meningioma management is typically a problem of local control, with local recurrence being the most troublesome aspect.
- The WHO 2016 classification system recognizes three grades of meningioma: I (benign), II (atypical), III (malignant/anaplastic).
- Malignant/anaplastic varieties (those with obvious malignant cytology such as appearance similar to sarcoma, carcinoma, or melanoma; or those with more than 20 mitoses per 10 high-power microscopic fields) occasionally occur and demonstrate aggressive behavior. Brain invasion is not sufficient to classify a meningioma as malignant/anaplastic histologic subtype; this tumor characteristic (in the absence of features of frank malignant/anaplastic meningioma) merits classification as atypical (WHO grade II) tumor in the WHO 2016 system. Other criteria for diagnosing an atypical meningioma include a mitotic count of four or more, and/or having at least three of the other five histologic features: spontaneous necrosis, sheeting (loss of whirling or fascicular architecture), prominent nucleoli, high cellularity and small cells (high nuclear: cytoplasmic ratio).
- Location of the lesion, extent of surgical resection, and histopathologic features of the tumor (WHO grade) are the most important prognostic factors.
- Treatment of choice for benign meningioma is generally complete surgical resection, if it can be accomplished with low morbidity. Tumor control has been consistently correlated to the extent of resection. The most commonly used system for resection extent is the Simpson grading (92), which is still widely used today.
- No adjuvant irradiation is typically indicated after GTR of a benign meningioma.
- Complete resection may be difficult without significant morbidity in base of skull, cerebellopontine angle, or cavernous sinus meningioma. For these patients, conservative STR followed by postoperative irradiation, rather than complete resection, may give good local control with decreased morbidity (44,93,94).
- Adjuvant radiation therapy plays a role in local control of the meningioma after surgery.

- Target volume for benign meningioma external-beam irradiation is generally restricted to a 1-cm margin beyond the tumor volume defined by CT or MRI scan and modified by the neurosurgeon's description of the location of residual tumor; more generous margins may be necessary for extensive skull base meningiomas (95).
- For atypical meningiomas, postoperative irradiation is generally indicated after STR; immediate postoperative irradiation after GTR is controversial, although many clinicians favor this approach. The external-beam irradiation dose delivered for atypical meningioma is also controversial; a dose between 54 and 60 Gy is reasonable, with many clinicians favoring treatment with a dose at the high end of this range.
- Postoperative irradiation after maximal safe resection is recommended for all malignant meningiomas; recurrence after surgery alone is high (50% to 100%), even with complete surgical resection. The target volume for malignant meningioma external-beam irradiation is more generous (2 to 3 cm margin) than that used for benign lesions; recommended dose is 60 Gy (93).
- Risk stratified treatment options are being tested in a prospective RTOG 0539 trial and are adopted by many physicians as a guideline:
- For low risk (group I) patients with a newly diagnosed WHO grade I meningioma with GTR or STR: observation;
- For intermediate (group II) patients with a newly diagnosed WHO II meningioma with GTR or a recurrent WHO grade I tumor irrespective of the resection extent: radiation therapy with 54 Gy in 30 fractions; CTV will be the GTV plus a margin of 1.0 cm;
- For high risk (group III) patients with a newly diagnosed or recurrent WHO grade III meningioma of any resection extent or a recurrent WHO grade II meningioma of any resection extent or a newly diagnosed WHO grade II meningioma with STR: radiation therapy with 60 Gy in 30 fractions. CTV_{60} from the GTV plus a 1.0 cm margin will receive 60 Gy. CTV54 from GTV plus a 2.0 cm margin will receive 54 Gy. Neither cerebral edema nor the dural tail is to be included in GTV. CTV expansion will be reduced around the natural barriers.
- Current reports from RTOG 0539 showed that the margins proposed for adjuvant RT field may be more than sufficient.
- Patients with intermediate-risk meningioma treated with RT had excellent outcome with the 3-year actuarial local failure rate being 4.1%, and the 3-year OS rate of 96%, as well as a low risk of toxicities (96).
- Alternatives to primary management with surgery for benign meningioma are fractionated external-beam irradiation (typically with modern 3-D conformal or IMRT techniques, sometimes with use of rotational/arc therapy), fractionated stereotactic radiotherapy (fSRT), and stereotactic radiosurgery (SRS); these techniques generally yield 5-year local control rates of 90% or better, comparable to outcomes with primary surgical management (97–99).
- External-beam irradiation doses of 50.4 to 54.0 Gy as definitive treatment are usually recommended for patients with unresectable or recurrent benign meningioma (93). A typical Gamma Knife SRS tumor marginal dose (generally tumor margin at 50% isodose line) is 14 Gy (12 to 16 Gy) (100,101). LINAC-based SRS has also been practiced with 14 Gy prescribed to 50% to 90% isodose line (102).

- For elderly patients with comorbidities, expectant management with deferred irradiation may be appropriate for small asymptomatic lesions or even after STR.
- Chemotherapy is not used as standard therapy, and the efficacy of antiprogesterone agents has not been demonstrated.

Craniopharyngioma

- Craniopharyngioma is a benign neoplasm of the suprasellar region.
- It is more common in children but is occasionally seen in adults, who typically present with craniopharyngioma early and with visual symptoms (e.g., quadrantanopia, bitemporal hemianopsia, or even complete blindness).
- The cystic nature of craniopharyngioma is usually evident on CT and MRI scans; calcifications in the wall are common.
- Complete surgical resection can result in long-term local control and cure; however, some tumors may recur even with presumed complete resection.
- Partial resection or cyst aspiration and biopsy rapidly relieve local compressive symptoms, establish diagnosis and have less operative morbidity, but are associated with eventual tumor progression in most cases. Recurrence is associated with worse prognosis (103).
- Irradiation combined with limited surgical procedures (partial resection or aspiration plus biopsy) minimizes the potential morbidity of aggressive resections (e.g., diabetes insipidus) (103–108).
- Typical doses are 50.4 to 54.0 Gy, delivered to the tumor volume (solid and cystic components) with an approximately 1-cm margin. Techniques used include three fields (opposing lateral and frontal-vertex portals), 3-D conformal irradiation, or IMRT.
- In patients with compressive symptoms, surgical decompression before irradiation is essential, as the tumor typically responds slowly to radiation therapy; in some patients radiation-induced edema or cystic component enlargement can worsen compressive symptoms, thus interim scans during RT are suggested.

Acoustic Neuroma and Neurofibroma

- Neurilemoma, also known as schwannoma and neurinoma, arises from Schwann cells of the myelin sheath of the peripheral nerves.
- Acoustic neuroma (AN) occurs in proximity to the eighth cranial nerve.
- Neurofibroma differs from neurilemoma in cellular composition and growth pattern.
- Neurofibroma arises from peripheral nerves, is most commonly multiple, and is associated with neurofibromatosis type I (von Recklinghausen's disease).
- Initial growth within the internal acoustic canal causes vestibular and hearing abnormalities in up to 95% of patients with AN. Expansion into the cerebellopontine angle may lead to trigeminal symptoms; unilateral corneal reflex depression is an early sign of trigeminal involvement.
- Large ANs may impinge on the cerebellum and brainstem, leading to ataxia, long tract signs, and involvement of lower cranial nerves (IX to XII).

- Pure tone and speech audiometry are the most useful screening tests for suspected AN. Thin-slice, gadolinium-enhanced MRI through the cerebellopontine angle is the imaging modality of choice for suspected AN. Thin-slice, contrast-enhanced, high-resolution CT scans are acceptable alternatives when MRI is not obtainable.
- Patients with suspected neurofibromatosis should have complete imaging of the craniospinal axis to document other neurilemomas, neurofibromas, and meningiomas.
- Treatment of AN should offer a high chance of local control and preservation of cranial nerve function. Preservation of current hearing is a realistic goal in patients with pretreatment "useful hearing."
- The mainstay of treatment of AN has classically been microsurgical resection.
- Primary treatment of AN with external-beam irradiation (often with fractionated stereotactic irradiation) is reported to be successful in many series (5-year local control greater than 90%), and may offer an improved chance of preservation of useful hearing when compared with surgery (109,110). A typical dose is 46.8 to 54 Gy delivered in 1.8-Gy fractions. Andrews et al. reported that, comparing to 54 Gy, a lower total dose at 46.8 Gy with fSRT was associated with a 100% local control tumor rate and a greater hearing preservation rate (111).
- Radiosurgery is also an acceptable alternative to microsurgical resection (12 to 13 Gy to the tumor margin—typically 50% isodose line at tumor margin—is a common prescription dose for Gamma Knife radiosurgical treatment; 12.5 to 13 Gy to 75 to 80% isodose line at tumor margin is commonly prescribed for LINAC-based SRS); at many centers, radiosurgery in fact constitutes first-line therapy for small- and medium-sized lesions (112). AN's well-circumscribed nature and typical intense enhancement on MRI facilitate localization and treatment by stereotactic techniques. SRS also appears to provide potentially an improved chance for preservation of useful hearing when compared with surgery, with dose delivered to the cochlea being one important factor influencing the likelihood of hearing preservation (113,114).
- A retrospective study from Combs et al. showed that the radiation dose for LINAC-based SRS (less than 13 Gy versus greater than 13 Gy) significantly influenced hearing preservation rates. For patients treated with less than 13 Gy, cranial nerve toxicity was comparable to that of the fSRT group.
- SRS doses of less than 12 Gy, for example, 11.5 Gy, have been used in some institutions with high success (115,116).
- Hypofractionated stereotactic radiotherapy using LINAC or CyberKnife in a frameless approach with 21 Gy in three fractions or 25 Gy in five fractions also showed high tumor control probability (98% to 100%) and equivalent rate of hearing preservations as in SRS or fSRT (117–121). Hypofractionation approach might be an alternative for treating tumor with relatively large size or concerns of brainstem/other cranial nerve toxicities.
- Despite of the overall high rate of hearing preservation with SRS, continued hearing deterioration is still very possible contributed by the RT toxicity with useful hearing preserved in only 40% to 60% of all patients. Useful or intact hearing was defined as Gardner-Robertson scale I (specifically speech discrimination scores of ≥70% and/or PTA less than 30 dB) by Kano et al., or as Gardner-Robertson scale I or II by Iwai et al., with the latter specification more commonly cited (115,122).

- Other toxicities with SRS include trigeminal neuropathy or hyperesthesia and motor facial nerve neuropathy, each of which have been reported occurring in less than 5% of patients.
- Adjuvant external irradiation may play a role in subtotally resected AN to decrease local recurrence risk.
- Observation alone may be appropriate in AN patients willing to undergo regular clinical and imaging follow-up, and may allow deferred treatment for some time.
- Treatment for neurofibroma is usually complete resection of compressive lesions with expectant observation of asymptomatic synchronous lesions; local extension may preclude complete resection. Adjuvant irradiation (50.4 to 54.0 Gy) after maximal resection may prevent tumor progression.

Hemangioblastoma and Hemangiopericytoma

- Hemangioblastoma is a benign vascular tumor that presents during the third and fourth decades. Most lesions are found in the cerebellum (and constitute the most common primary cerebellar tumor in adults), but they also may be found in the spinal cord. Treatment is primarily surgical, with complete resection curative. By analogy to arteriovenous malformations, radiosurgical treatment may be useful and offers tumor control rates of 90% or better (123).
- Hemangiopericytoma is a sarcomatous lesion developing from smooth muscle cells in blood vessels. Presentation along intracranial meningeal sites and the base of the skull is common, although isolated intraparenchymal lesions are seen. Treatment is surgical resection followed by postoperative irradiation to a typical dose of 54 to 60 Gy (124). In contrast to other primary CNS tumors, hemangiopericytoma commonly develops systemic metastases (in addition to local recurrences).

PITUITARY

Anatomy

- The pituitary gland is a midline structure situated in the sella turcica in the body of the sphenoid bone (Fig. 10-5).
- In most cases, the optic chiasm overlies the diaphragma sellae and the pituitary.
- The anterior cerebral arteries are superior; the cavernous sinuses, containing the internal carotid arteries and multiple cranial nerves, are lateral to the sella turcica. The sphenoid sinus and nasopharynx are inferior.
- The posterior lobe of the pituitary arises as an evagination from the floor of the third ventricle, with the infundibular recess representing an outpocketing of the anterior floor into the pituitary stalk.
- Nerve fibers of the hypothalamus terminate in the pituitary stalk (infundibulum) or in the posterior lobe (neurohypophysis).
- The anterior (adenohypophysis) and intermediate lobes of the pituitary arise from Rathke's pouch, an evagination of ectodermal tissue from the embryonic buccal cavity.

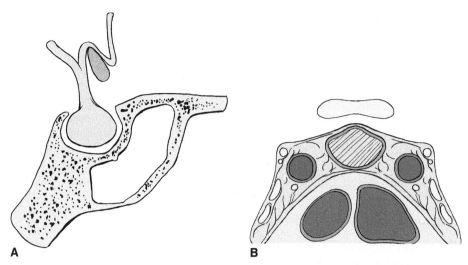

FIGURE 10-5. Frontal (coronal) (**A**) and median (mid-sagittal) (**B**) planes of pituitary fossa region. (Reprinted with permission from Grigsby PW. Pituitary. In: Perez CA, Brady LW, eds. *Principles and practice of radiation oncology*, 3rd ed. Philadelphia, PA: Lippincott–Raven, 1998:829–848. © Wolters Kluwer.)

Natural History

- Pituitary adenomas are benign tumors that vary greatly in size and direction of spread.
- Small tumors tend to be smooth and round; but as size increases, they often become irregular, with nodules extending in various directions.
- Microadenomas (less than 1 cm in diameter) do not generally cause gross enlargement of the sella turcica, but may cause focal anterior bulging, asymmetry, or sloping of the sella floor.
- Pituitary tumors have a long natural history. Onset of symptoms and signs tends to be insidious; symptoms range from a few days to more than 10 years.
- In 121 patients treated with surgery and postoperative irradiation, the risk of developing recurrent disease was less than 0.5% during the first 5 years after treatment, but progressively increased to 4.4% with 25- to 30-year follow-up (125).
- A 22% autopsy incidence of previously undiagnosed adenomas in presumably normal pituitary glands was reported; most were microscopic adenomas, but a few were large enough to displace optic nerves (126).
- If an asymptomatic pituitary tumor (diagnosed from an incidental imaging study) is not treated, it must be evaluated periodically for the duration of the patient's life so that growth can be detected before any potential irreversible damage occurs.
- MRI has detected pituitary abnormalities in approximately 10% of the normal adult population (127).
- Hyperfunctional adenomas progress slowly; mean duration of symptoms is 9.6 years.

Clinical Presentation and Diagnostic Workup

- Pituitary adenomas are the most common cause of pituitary dysfunction in adults. Their presentation may be a consequence of hormonal malfunction or local tumor growth with pressure effects.
- Procedures used for diagnosis are outlined in Table 10-3.
- Decreased visual acuity, papilledema, ophthalmoplegia, and ocular motor abnormalities may occur. Patients may be asymptomatic but have significant visual field defects (128,129). The most common visual field defects are bitemporal hemianopsia and superior temporal defects. Other visual field defects are homonymous hemianopsia, central scotoma, and inferior temporal field cut (130,131).

Table 10-3
Diagnostic Workup for Pituitary Tumors

General
History and physical examination
Neurologic examination with special attention to cranial nerves

Special Tests
Formal testing of visual fields

Imaging Studies
MRI
Skeletal survey (for acromegaly)
CT (if MRI unavailable)

Laboratory Studies
Complete blood count, blood chemistry, urinalysis
Endocrine evaluation of abnormal secretion:
Prolactin hypersecretion: prolactin
GH hypersecretion: basal GH, IGF-I, glucose suppression, insulin tolerance, thyrotropin-releasing hormone stimulation
ACTH hypersecretion: serum ACTH, 24-h urine for 17-hydroxy-corticosteroids and free cortisol, dexamethasone suppressed corticotropin-releasing hormone test
In Cushing's disease with negative neuroimaging studies: selective bilateral simultaneous venous sampling of ACTH from inferior petrosal sinuses

Evaluation of Normal Endocrine Function
Gonadal function: FSH, LH, estradiol, testosterone
Thyroid function: thyroxine, free thyroxine index, TSH
Adrenal function: basal plasma or urinary steroids; cortisol response to insulin-induced hypoglycemia and plasma ACTH response to metyrapone administration

ACTH, adrenocorticotropic hormone; FSH, follicle-stimulating hormone; IGF, insulin growth factor-I; LH, luteinizing hormone; TSH, thyroid-stimulating hormone.
Reprinted with permission from Roberge D, Shenouda G, Souhami L. Pituitary. In: Halperin EC, Perez CA, Brady LW, eds. *Principles and practice of radiation oncology*, 5th ed. Philadelphia, PA: Lippincott Williams & Wilkins, 2008. © Wolters Kluwer.

- Endocrine abnormalities may result from hypersecretion or hyposecretion of one or more of the pituitary hormones.
- Endocrine evaluation (including tests of GH, gonadal, thyroid, and adrenal function) before and after therapy permits assessment of response to treatment and determines necessity for hormonal replacement therapy.

Staging

- Hardy and Vezina (132) developed a staging system that has gained partial acceptance (particularly by neurosurgeons) that classifies pituitary tumors into four grades according to extent of expansion or erosion of the sella:
  - Grade I: normal-sized sella with possible asymmetry of the floor.
  - Grade II: enlarged sella with an intact floor.
  - Grade III: localized erosion or destruction of the sellar floor.
  - Grade IV: diffusely eroded floor.
- It is assumed that grades I and II represent enclosed adenomas and grades III and IV represent invasive adenomas.
- Suprasellar extension requires a secondary designation by type:
  - Type A: tumor bulges into chiasmatic cistern.
  - Type B: tumor reaches floor of third ventricle.
  - Type C: tumor is more voluminous, with extension into third ventricle up to foramen of Monro.
  - Type D: tumor extends into temporal or frontal fossa.
- This system is based primarily on radiologic evidence and tends to emphasize inferior extensions; it assigns a lesser degree of importance to extension or invasion other than through the floor of the sella.

Pathologic Classification

- Modern classification is based on electron microscopy and immunohistochemistry:
  - Prolactin cell adenoma
  - GH cell (somatotropic) adenoma
  - Mixed prolactin-GH cell adenoma
  - Corticotropic cell adenoma
  - Thyrotropic cell adenoma
  - Gonadotropic cell adenoma
  - Nonfunctioning (null cell) adenoma

Prognostic Factors

- Prognosis varies with type of adenoma and depends on a combination of factors: extent of the abnormality present at the time of diagnosis (secondary to either mass or endocrine effect); degree to which injury is reversible; success of therapy in normalizing endocrine activity and/or relieving pressure effects; and permanency of response to treatment (freedom from recurrence) (133).

General Management

Medical Management

- Medical management to suppress pituitary hyperfunction with drugs—such as bromocriptine or cabergoline (dopamine receptor agonists) for prolactinomas; ketoconazole, metyrapone/aminoglutethimide, or mitotane for corticotropic adenomas; octreotide or lanreotide for somatotrophic (and thyrotropic) adenomas—can be used as primary therapy, and may provide temporary control or remission while awaiting the slower but potentially permanent response of irradiation.

Surgical Management

- Transsphenoidal microsurgery, effective in selective removal of microadenomas, is also used for adenomas extending outside the sella.
- Contraindications may include dumbbell-shaped adenomas with constriction at diaphragma sellae, lateral suprasellar extension, massive suprasellar tumor, and incompletely pneumatized sphenoid.
- Delayed surgical complications may occur.
- Anterior pituitary function may be affected with nonfunctioning adenomas.
- Excellent vision improvement can occur with surgery alone.
- Recurrence may be delayed by many years in larger tumors, but the recurrence rate is relatively high with surgery alone.

Radiation Therapy

- Radiation therapy is effective in controlling hypersecretion and destructive/invasive or mass effects of large or recurrent tumors (134–138).
- External irradiation controls hypersecretion in approximately 80% of patients with acromegaly, 50% to 80% of those with Cushing's disease, and one third of those with hyperprolactinemia (139).
- Normalization of circulating hormone levels requires anywhere from a few months to several years for acromegaly and approximately 3 months to 1 year for Cushing's disease.
- Primary radiation therapy can be effective to control mass effects of larger tumors, but it may be preferable to perform surgery to decompress the optic chiasm, and irradiate postoperatively to prevent recurrence for such presentations.
- External irradiation is used to treat tumors that are recurrent after primary surgery (140). It is also commonly employed after STR (especially for patients with persistent hormonal hypersecretion refractory to medical therapy), as well as for medically inoperable patients.
- Reirradiation is sometimes used for recurrences (129).
- In contrast to conventional irradiation, proton and α-particle irradiation and implantation of radioactive sources (^{90}Y or ^{198}Au) deliver very large doses to highly restricted volumes within the pituitary gland; thus, their application is limited to small, essentially intrasellar tumors. Brachytherapy is rarely utilized in the modern management of pituitary tumors.

- SRS has emerged as a viable alternative to surgery and conventional irradiation for pituitary adenoma treatment (especially for small- to medium-sized target volumes) in the primary, adjuvant postoperative, or recurrent setting (141–143). Normalization of hormonal secretion is more common for corticotropic and somatotropic tumors and less common for prolactinomas after radiosurgery (144). Eligibility for SRS includes tumor target being at least 3 to 5 mm away from the chiasm and less than 3 cm in diameter (145). However, if there is insufficient distance between the adenoma/tumor bed and the optic chiasm, conventional fractionated irradiation should be pursued instead of SRS to minimize the likelihood of visual damage.
- Total external-beam irradiation dose is generally 45.0 to 50.4 Gy in 1.8 Gy per fraction for nonfunctioning tumors, and 50.4 to 54 Gy for functioning tumors as recommended by Loeffler and Shih (145). Even higher doses of 54 to 60 Gy were favored by some for functioning tumors with doses at the higher end of this range administered for especially thyroid-stimulating hormone (TSH) and ACTH (adrenocorticotropic hormone)-secreting tumors, although data suggest the optimal doses for secreting tumors being similar to nonfunctioning ones (145).
- SRS may provide a faster biochemical response to treatment than fractionated RT. SRS achieves normalization of ACTH levels in a median time of approximately 7.5 to 33 months.
- Tumor control efficacy appears similar among all forms of SRS: Gamma Knife, LINAC, and proton (146).
- If temporary control of hormonal secretion and/or tumor size is not a concern, withholding pharmacologic treatment during RT is recommended. Concomitant pharmacologic treatment such as somatostatin analogs for acromegaly and dopamine agonists for lactotrophic adenomas at the time of irradiation was associated with lower rates of hormonal control and a higher incidence of hypopituitarism. Size control of the adenoma most likely is not affected (147).

Posttherapy Evaluation

- In acromegaly, posttreatment GH values of less than 10 ng per mL (or even lower at some centers) and normalization of insulin-like growth factor-1 (IGF-1) levels indicate a successful response to therapy. GH and IGF-1 levels should be followed to predict tumor recurrence.
- With prolactin-secreting tumors, the objective is to lower the prolactin level to the normal range.
- Plasma and urine steroids and plasma ACTH levels allow for evaluation of the response to therapy in Cushing's disease.
- For all patients treated for pituitary tumors, periodic assessment of GH, gonadal, thyroid, and adrenal function is necessary because hypopituitarism may occur as a result of irradiation or surgery. Patients treated with irradiation may develop hypopituitarism a number of years after treatment.

Radiation Therapy Techniques

- All diagnostic evidence, including that from imaging studies, as well as clinical and surgical findings, should be combined to define the tumor volume.

- CT simulation helps define the treatment volume, which should be slightly larger (by approximately 0.5 to 1.0 cm of PTV expansion) to include a margin for error in estimation of tumor volume and variation in daily setup.
- For well-defined adenomas, the uncertainty of margin is small; with invasive tumors, there is greater uncertainty. This must be considered in determining the volume to be included and specifically whether the extension is into the sphenoid, cavernous sinus or into intracranial structures.
- Variability of setup should be no more than 2 to 3 mm. To ensure accuracy and reproducibility, the patient's head must be fixed in a thermoplastic mask for external-beam irradiation. Use of three localizing light or laser beams permits easy repositioning.
- Both lateral and sagittal beam-check films or a conebeam CT scan if available are typically obtained at the beginning of therapy and periodically thereafter.
- The irradiation technique should be designed to restrict the high-dose region to the treatment volume.
- Special care must be taken to avoid exposure to the eyes; this requires careful CT-based treatment planning and/or observation of the actual setup on the treatment machine. Radiopaque markers, placed on the contralateral eye when field verification films are taken, can document the location of the eye with respect to the radiation beam. The eye is approximately 2.5 cm in length, and the lens lies in the anterior 1 cm.
- Volume treated includes the pituitary fossa and adjacent tissues, as determined by evaluation of the extent of the adenoma ideally based on MRI.
- In classical external-beam irradiation technique, portals 5 × 5 to 6 × 6 cm or shaped fields 5 to 6 cm in diameter, were used. Although parallel-opposed lateral portals alone were used historically, the isodose distribution of such an arrangement is not ideal and there is a high dose delivered to the temporal lobes. Accordingly, a frontal-vertex (superior anterior oblique) noncoplanar field should generally be incorporated into the field arrangement, yielding a three-field technique (Fig. 10-6). To localize

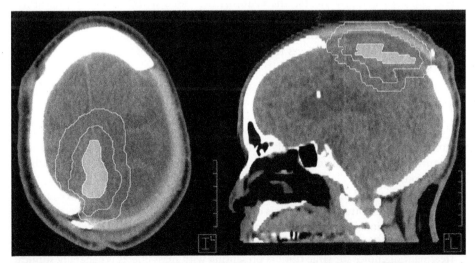

FIGURE 10-6. Targets of treatment planning: GTV (innermost *gray* shaded region), CTV (inner contour), and PTV (outer contour) for patient in Figure 10-3 shown in coronal **(left)** and sagittal **(right)** sections.

the frontal-vertex portal, the patient is placed in the supine position, with head flexed and chin close to the lower neck. A beam entering through the vertex of the head, at approximately the midline of the hairline, is directed posteriorly to pass approximately 1 cm behind the posterior clinoid processes (Fig. 10-6). With modern 3-D CT-based planning, positioning of the frontal-vertex field is greatly simplified through the use of beam's-eye view. Wedges in the lateral fields, with the heel placed anteriorly, assist in obtaining a more homogeneous dose distribution and in decreasing the dose delivered to the optic chiasm and temporal lobes in the three-field technique of parallel-opposed lateral portals plus a frontal-vertex field (92).

- Modern techniques using 3-D conformal radiotherapy, often in noncoplanar beam arrangement, is now the standard of care, A five-field irradiation technique (parallel-opposed laterals, midline superior anterior oblique, right superior anterior oblique, and left superior anterior oblique) may provide improved temporal lobe dose-sparing compared with the standard three-field technique (parallel-opposed laterals and midline superior anterior oblique). IMRT techniques have also been used frequently for the treatment of pituitary adenomas (37). fSRT with tight margins (1.5 mm to 3 mm PTV expansion from GTV) also showed excellent results in the treatment of pituitary adenomas (148–150).

Stereotactic Radiosurgery

- SRS with Gamma Knife delivers focused radiation from ^{60}Co sources to a pituitary tumor (or tumor bed) in a single session, with minimal radiation to the adjacent normal brain tissue. A tumor marginal dose of approximately 14 to 16 Gy for nonfunctioning adenomas and higher—at least 20 Gy, preferably 20 to 25 Gy but up to 30 Gy—for functioning adenomas, should be delivered; generally, the therapeutic dose that can be delivered is restricted by the dose received by the optic chiasm, which should be limited to less than 8 to 10 Gy. Tumor growth control with such an SRS approach is nearly 100%. The neuronal and vascular structures running in the cavernous sinus are much less radiosensitive than the chiasm, thus allowing an ablative dose to be administered to tumors showing lateral invasion to cavernous sinus and impinging on cranial nerves III, IV, V, and VI if the borders of the adenomas are clearly defined (151,152).

Adenomas with Mass Effect

- This section deals with mass effects from pituitary tumors, with the exception of tumors associated with acromegaly or Nelson's syndrome (rapid pituitary adenoma expansion after bilateral adrenalectomy because of loss of cortisol-mediated feedback inhibition).
- In addition to visual field deficits or decreased visual acuity, hypopituitarism caused by pressure-induced pituitary atrophy is common. Previously, such tumors were thought to be nonfunctioning chromophobe adenomas, but in light of present information, it is probable that most such pituitary tumors secrete prolactin.
- Treatment of choice for large tumors presenting with mass effects is generally surgical resection for decompression, followed by irradiation.

- Large, invasive tumors should be treated with irradiation because complete resection is usually not possible; attempted radical removal is associated with high morbidity and even potential mortality.

Sequelae of Treatment

- Epilation, scalp swelling, and otitis are typical side effects during or immediately after irradiation.
- Irradiation-induced pituitary hormonal hypofunction commonly occurs; repeated courses of therapy, occasionally necessary for tumor recurrence, carry an increased risk. Endocrine replacement therapy should be instituted as needed.
- Growth failure with delayed bone age frequently occurs in children or young adults.
- Injuries to optic nerves or chiasm are rare but have been reported in patients treated for pituitary tumors. Most cases reported have had either doses higher than 50 Gy or daily fractions greater than 2 Gy, or both.

SPINAL CANAL

- Primary spinal canal tumors are classified as either intramedullary, arising from the intrinsic substance of the spinal cord and including astrocytoma, ependymoma, and oligodendroglioma; or intradural-extramedullary, arising from connective tissues, blood vessels, or coverings adjacent to the cord or cauda equina. Common primary histologies of the latter include ependymoma, nerve sheath tumors, meningioma, and vascular tumors. Primary spinal GBM is a rare entity with a particularly poor prognosis (153,154).
- Extradural tumors are commonly metastatic, although primary tumors may arise from the vertebral bodies.
- Nonmetastatic extradural tumors include chordoma, chondrosarcoma, osteogenic sarcoma, epidural hemangioma, lipoma, extradural meningioma, nerve sheath tumors, and lymphoma.

Anatomy

Spinal Cord

- The spinal cord is a slender cylinder organized into somatotopically distinct regions and composed of functional segments corresponding to 31 pairs of spinal nerves: 8 cervical, 12 thoracic, 5 lumbar, 5 sacral, and 1 coccygeal.
- The white matter is located in the periphery and surrounds the central gray matter.
- The spinal nerves that enter and exit the spinal cord are sheathed by Schwann cells and frequently possess a myelin sheath.
- The spinal cord is nearly 25 cm shorter than the vertebral column; by adulthood it ends near the level of the L1 vertebral body. Because of this differential growth, the exit level of each pair of spinal nerves within the spinal cord is generally higher than the corresponding vertebral body level.

- The lower lumbar, sacral, and coccygeal nerves form the cauda equina, the collection of nerves that fill the thecal sac below L1.
- At its most caudal extent, the cord tapers to a thin segment, the conus medullaris.

Spinal Canal

- The spinal canal is formed by the posterior body surfaces and arches of the stacked vertebrae, and is triangular in the lumbar and cervical regions.
- It is surrounded by the meninges; the innermost is the pia mater, which covers the spinal cord and its blood vessels. Meningiomas are commonly attached to the dentate ligaments.
- The dura mater forms a dense, fibrous barrier between the bony spinal canal and the spinal cord. The dura ends inferiorly at the level of the S2 vertebra but continues with the filum terminale down to the coccyx.
- Between the dura mater and the pia mater is the arachnoid mater, which encloses the subarachnoid space filled with CSF. The subarachnoid space follows the arachnoid down to the end of the dural (thecal) sac.

Natural History

- Most primary tumors of the spinal canal are histologically benign but often cause significant disability because they compress or invade the spinal cord and interfere with neurologic function.
- Intramedullary tumors produce local invasion or cystic compression of the cord; extramedullary lesions compress, stretch, or distort the cord or the spinal nerves.
- Complications of paraplegia or quadriplegia, such as infection or respiratory compromise, are the major causes of death in patients with spinal canal tumors.
- CSF seeding is possible but uncommon (155).
- Because the CNS has no lymphatics, spread to lymph nodes is not seen; hematogenous spread is extremely rare.
- Primary spinal cord tumors may be focal, relatively localized, or may involve nearly the entire length of the cord.

Clinical Presentation

- Pain, often localized to the involved region, is the presenting symptom in nearly 75% of patients with primary spinal canal neoplasms; radicular pain reflects the distribution of the involved root.
- Numbness replacing pain is a more advanced sign, indicating compromise of spinal nerve or nerve tract conduction.
- Other CNS symptoms include weakness (75% of patients), sensory changes (65%), and sphincter dysfunction (15%) (156,157).
- Low-grade tumors generally have a longer duration of symptoms than high-grade tumors.

- Initial bladder and bowel dysfunction are relatively uncommon except in tumors of the conus medullaris and filum terminale.
- In a cauda equina tumor, saddle anesthesia and absent ankle reflexes (S1) or plantar responses (S2) may occur. Impotence and loss of anal or bulbar cavernous reflexes may also be present.

Diagnostic Workup

- A meticulous and accurate patient history and physical and neurologic examination are necessary.
- The differential diagnosis for spinal cord tumors includes syringomyelia, multiple sclerosis, amyotrophic lateral sclerosis, diabetic neuropathy, viral myelitis, or paraneoplastic syndromes.
- A patient with a suspected spinal canal neoplasm should not be subjected to lumbar puncture before MRI. Symptoms may be exacerbated after a spinal tap because of shifting of the spinal cord and incarceration before the tumor can be adequately localized. The CSF usually has increased protein levels and may exhibit xanthochromia, especially with extradural compression conditions; lower values are found with intramedullary disease and compression in the cervical region (43).
- Plain X-ray films of the spine show abnormalities in approximately 50% of patients with primary spinal canal neoplasms; changes are more likely to be detected in children than in adults (158). Abnormalities caused by increased intracanal pressure include erosion of vertebral pedicles, enlargement of the anteroposterior diameter of the bony canal, and scalloping of the posterior wall of the vertebral bodies. Spinal canal tumors also may be associated with scoliosis or kyphoscoliosis, especially in children. Calcification may be seen in extramedullary tumors, especially meningiomas; and, less frequently, in nerve sheath tumor.
- Myelography has essentially been replaced by high-quality MRI of the spine; however, it is still useful in patients unable to undergo MRI scanning because of implanted ferromagnetic materials.
- CT scanning is frequently combined with myelography to evaluate the presence of intradural pathology, but it is probably most helpful in evaluating the spine for extradural pathology. Bone tumors or paraspinal soft tissue masses that secondarily involve the spinal cord (dumbbell tumors) can be imaged with contrast-enhanced CT scans (159).
- MRI has replaced myelography and CT as the study of choice for evaluating spinal canal tumors. Some cystic tumors, vascular lesions, or lipomas can be diagnosed based on characteristic signals on T1- and T2-weighted images, without contrast. Intravenous gadolinium-diethylenetriamine pentaacetic acid (Gd-DTPA) administration improves the sensitivity of MRI by enhancing the solid component of intramedullary tumors, differentiating them from surrounding edema or syrinx cavities. Nearly all spinal cord gliomas, regardless of grade, enhance with Gd-DTPA (160). Sagittal T1-weighted images usually localize intramedullary masses along with adjacent cysts. Intradural-extramedullary lesions show considerable enhancement on T1-weighted images after administration of Gd-DTPA.

- Intraoperative ultrasonography is an indispensable adjunct in the surgical management of intramedullary spinal cord neoplasms after the posterior spinal bony elements have been removed.

Pathologic Classification

- Suspected primary tumors of the spinal cord and spinal canal should be pathologically confirmed.
- Strong consideration should be given to biopsy of any presumed metastatic tumors if they are the first sites of disease recurrence.
- Primary tumors of the spinal cord are histopathologically similar to those found intracranially, but distribution of the various tumor types depends on the relationship of the neoplasm to the spinal cord and dura (Table 10-4).

Table 10-4

Primary Spinal Canal Tumors: Locations, Types, and Frequencies

Location	Frequency (%)	Type	Comments
Extradural	Few	Meningioma	~10% of spinal meningiomas
Intradural-extramedullary	70	Nerve sheath tumor	45% of primary tumors in this location, thoracic preference
		Meningioma	<40% of primary tumors at this location, thoracic preference
		Ependymoma in cauda	60% of all spinal ependymomas
		Vascular malformations	<10% of primary tumors at this location
		Teratoma, dermoid, squamous cell neoplasia	10% of primary tumors at this location, sacrococcygeal preference
		Lipoma	Few, subpial
Intradural-intramedullary	30	Ependymoma in cord	<40% of all spinal canal ependymomas
		Astrocytoma	<45% of primary tumors at this location
		Vascular malformations	Rare
		Oligodendroglioma	~15% of primary tumors at this location
		Teratoma	Rare
		Hemangioma	Rare

Reprinted with permission from Michalski JM. Spinal canal. In: Halperin EC, Perez CA, Brady LW, eds. *Principles and practice of radiation oncology*, 5th ed. Philadelphia, PA: Lippincott Williams & Wilkins, 2008. © Wolters Kluwer.

Prognostic Factors

- Major clinical prognostic factors include tumor type, grade, extent, and location, in addition to patient age and presenting neurologic function.
- Treatment-related factors that influence outcome in selected patients include tumor resectability and use of radiation therapy.
- Neurologic function at diagnosis is an important clinical prognostic factor (161).
- Young age at time of diagnosis is associated with a good 5-year recurrence-free survival in patients with astrocytoma (162), but it is unclear if age is important in patients with ependymoma (163–166).
- Some series suggest surgical resection may be favored over biopsy alone, particularly for certain low-grade malignancies (167).

General Management

- The treatment of choice for most tumors is complete surgical excision; gross total excision with preservation of neurologic function is the goal.
- Piecemeal resection can often be accomplished with little neurologic disability; however, the risk of recurrence is significant, and adjuvant irradiation is warranted (165,168,169).
- For completely excised tumors, the prognosis is excellent, and no additional therapy is generally indicated; however, high-grade tumors such as malignant gliomas generally merit postoperative irradiation.
- For incompletely excised tumors, adjuvant radiation therapy should be strongly considered to provide durable local tumor control and potentially to improve survival.
- Radiation therapy has been used for postoperative treatment of intramedullary astrocytomas and ependymomas. Observation is a reasonable option for subtotally resected meningiomas.
- Although irradiation is advocated after STR, there are some clinical circumstances—such as when young children are diagnosed before pubertal growth—in which careful follow-up after surgery should be considered, with radiation therapy deferred until after a second operation for clinical recurrence. Most spinal cord tumors in young children are low-grade astrocytomas or well-differentiated ependymomas with a very slow growth rate; delaying radiation therapy until recurrence or early tumor progression may allow the child to grow at a normal rate for several years before receiving irradiation.
- Postoperative irradiation is used in patients with ependymoma after incomplete or piecemeal excision. In some series, increasing doses of irradiation are associated with better tumor control in patients with ependymoma (165).
- Data supporting routine use of adjuvant irradiation in subtotally resected astrocytic tumors of the spinal cord are less conclusive; the slow growth of these neoplasms makes it difficult to prove that radiation therapy is beneficial. However, for high-grade gliomas postoperative irradiation should be delivered.
- Use of chemotherapy for gliomas of the spinal cord remains experimental; however, data are emerging for possible use of temozolomide for spinal cord gliomas (analogous to the intracranial setting) (170–173).

Radiation Therapy Techniques

- Primary tumors of the spinal canal can often simply be treated with a direct posterior field, but conformal techniques may be preferred when treating to higher doses, larger fields, and younger patients. In some settings, particle therapy can be considered, such as in spinal sarcomas and in the pediatric setting (174–176).
- Some lumbar region tumors, including those of the cauda equina, may require opposed anteroposterior and PA portals because of lumbar lordosis and the location of the vertebral bodies near the midline of the trunk.
- Other techniques should be considered when exit dose to the anterior midline structures of the thorax/abdomen/pelvis would be excessive.
- Tumors exclusively involving the cervical spine can be treated with opposed lateral fields to avoid incidental irradiation of the hypopharynx and oral cavity.
- Tumors involving the thoracic and lumbar spinal canal can be treated with a paired set of oblique-wedged fields to get a superior dose distribution, compared with a single posterior field. The oblique-paired field plan, although more complex, treats the midline structures anterior to the spinal column to a lower cumulative irradiation dose; it also avoids the high dose to the subcutaneous tissues that is delivered with a single PA field. In some parts of the trunk, the exit dose delivered to the lungs or kidneys with paired oblique fields may require use of a PA treatment technique either exclusively or in combination with the oblique fields.
- In females requiring treatment to the lumbosacral spine for cauda equina tumors, a lateral technique can be used to avoid exit irradiation to the pelvis and ovaries. This technique may treat more of the back musculature and even some of the retroperitoneum, yet spares the more radiosensitive ovaries and uterus. Wedges may be required on these lateral lumbosacral fields to provide a homogeneous dose distribution. Care should be taken to avoid irradiating the kidneys at the L1 through L3 levels with this technique. The arm should be positioned appropriately to avoid entrance or exit irradiation from these lateral beams.
- The width of PA fields is typically 7 to 8 cm, although fields as small as 5 cm may be considered for young children. Classically, the superior and inferior borders encompass one to two vertebral bodies above and below the tumors, which are defined by MRI or CT (myelogram); this is generally adequate to avoid marginal miss. A more accurate definition of gross tumor on the MRI scan may allow the tumor boost to encompass the lesion plus 2 cm.
- The field width should encompass the anterior vertebral foramina, if tumor extension is suspected.
- In young children, the anterior vertebral bodies and developing epiphyseal plates may be partially spared by using posterior oblique-wedged fields or opposed lateral fields.
- For small-treated segments of the spinal cord, the depth of the cord beneath the skin surface can be determined from CT or MRI scans; classically, it can also be determined by obtaining a lateral radiograph of the spine on a fluoroscopic simulator, using a wire on the skin surface and calculating the spinal cord depth by employing the magnification factor used for the film.

- If large segments of the spinal cord are irradiated, the spinal cord dose should be computed at multiple points because of variation in curvature and depth of the spinal cord, as well as different source-to-skin distances above and below the central axis of the beam. A transverse and sagittal treatment plan using CT and MRI scans should be performed. A sagittal treatment plan can be discerned from a sagittal CT reconstruction or MRI scan, or from a lateral spine radiograph with the midline skin wired and documentation of the magnification factor for the film.
- The most accurate delineation of the spinal cord and thecal sac is with CT myelography, which can be performed at the time of simulation to allow radiation planning in the treatment position. However, T2 MRI is typically adequate for anatomic delineation, thus a high-quality MRI has largely replaced the role of CT myelography in treatment planning.
- For small cervical spinal cord lesions in which lateral fields will be used, radiation beam energies of 4- to 6-MV photons achieve a homogeneous dose distribution. Lesions involving the thoracic and lumbar spine often require combinations of low-energy (4 to 6 MV) and high-energy (10 to 25 MV) photons to achieve a homogeneous dose distribution when posterior fields are used. Parallel-opposed posterior and anterior fields, or paired oblique-wedged fields, can give homogeneous dose distributions with x-ray energies as low as 4 to 6 MV.
- Craniospinal or spinal-axis irradiation generally is not indicated for spinal cord tumors. Local failure is a predominant site of tumor recurrence (155,162,165). Patients with high-grade ependymoma (166) or malignant glioma (177) have a high rate of neuraxis dissemination; consideration can be given to treating the spinal axis or the entire craniospinal axis, although this is generally not standard practice.

RADIATION THERAPY DOSES

Intramedullary Ependymomas and Astrocytomas

- Total dose is 50.4 Gy, given in 1.8-Gy daily fractions.
- If more than half of the spinal cord is irradiated, the total tumor dose should not exceed 45 Gy; however, small segments may tolerate 55 Gy.
- High-grade (malignant) gliomas should receive 54 Gy.

Ependymomas of the Cauda Equina

- Total dose is 45.0 to 50.4 Gy in 1.8-Gy fractions.
- The treatment field should encompass the entire thecal sac, with the field widened inferiorly to approximately the sacroiliac joints to ensure adequate coverage of the meningeal sleeves within the intervertebral foramina.
- In children, an attempt should be made to limit the dose to the spinal cord to approximately 40 to 45 Gy.

- Hyperfractionation has been suggested to treat spinal cord tumors to a higher cumulative irradiation dose while minimizing the risks of spinal cord injury (155), but the merits of hyperfractionation are not proven.

Meningiomas

- Total dose is typically 50.4 to 54.0 Gy for subtotally resected meningiomas, although observation is also a reasonable management strategy for low-grade tumors. Like the case for low-grade gliomas, completely excised benign meningiomas should not generally receive adjuvant irradiation.
- In general, any recurrent meningioma or those with atypical or malignant histology are considered for radiation.
- Treatment with single fraction radiosurgery and hypofractionated radiation have become accepted alternatives, but prospective data are lacking.

Sequelae of Radiation Therapy

- Transient, reversible myelopathy can manifest itself within 2 to 6 months after irradiation. Lhermitte's sign, characterized by shocklike sensations radiating to the hands and feet when the neck is flexed, is a classic finding in patients with transient myelopathy. Although the volume of spinal canal irradiated has been thought to impact the risk of Lhermitte's, this is not well established (178).
- Chronic, progressive, or delayed myelopathy can occur months to years after radiation therapy.
- Progressive myelopathy is dependent on total dose, fraction size, volume, and region irradiated (179,180). A conservative estimate of spinal cord tolerance historically is 45 to 50 Gy in conventional 1.8- to 2.0-Gy fractions or 30 Gy in 3-Gy fractions; the actual incidence of myelopathy is less than 0.2% to 0.5% after 50 Gy, 1% to 5% after 60 Gy, and 50% after 68 to 73 Gy (181). The cervical spinal cord and cauda equina may tolerate slightly higher doses of irradiation than the thoracic or lumbar spinal cord.
- Irradiation of the spine in a child may produce spinal deformity (scoliosis or kyphosis) because of retardation of bone growth. Other organs that may receive a significant dose include thyroid, heart, bowel, and ovaries. Children should receive long-term follow-up for development of functional sequelae.

NORMAL TISSUE COMPLICATIONS—QUANTEC RESULTS

- Numerous retrospective series have evaluated the risk to nervous structures following irradiation and there is particular interest in understanding dose tolerances in the era of hypofractionation and stereotactic techniques. The linear-quadratic model remains a valuable tool to estimate the risk of late effects along with QUANTEC guidelines (182).

Brain

Recommendations of Lawrence et al. (183) are summarized below:

- For standard fractionation, a 5% and 10% risk of symptomatic radiation necrosis is predicted to occur at a BED of 120 Gy (range, 100 to 140) and 150 Gy (range, 140 to 170), respectively (corresponding to 72 Gy [range, 60 to 84] and 90 Gy [range, 84 to 102] in 2-Gy fractions). The brain is especially sensitive to fraction sizes greater than 2 Gy and, surprisingly, twice-daily RT.
- Cognitive changes occur in children after ≥18 Gy to the entire brain. The effect of irradiation on the cognitive performance of adults is less well-defined. We have concluded that the 5% risk at 5 years of the partial brain for normally fractionated RT is 72 Gy (range, 60 to 84).
- For most cancers, there is no clinical indication for giving fractionated RT greater than 60 Gy and that, in some scenarios, an incidence of 1% to 5% radiation necrosis at 5 years would be unacceptably high.
- For radiosurgery, toxicity increases rapidly once the volume of the brain exposed to greater than 12 Gy is greater than 5 to 10 cm³. Eloquent areas of the brain (brain stem and corpus callosum) require more stringent limits.
- The data for fractionated irradiation at or below 2.5 Gy are shown graphically in Figure 10-7. The data points are taken from Table 2 of (178); a few were omitted because they were at variance with all the other low-dose reports. The theoretical curves were calculated using the phenomenologic binomial model of Zaider and Amols (184).

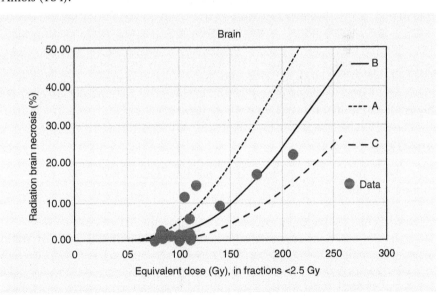

FIGURE 10-7. Modeling of brain necrosis QUANTEC data. The low-dose (less than 2.5 Gy) data from Lawrence et al. (178) are plotted with superimposed curves calculated from the binomial model (equation 10) of Zaider and Amols (179). The first adjustable parameter ($a1$) affects the steepness of the probability curve. The second adjustable parameter, here called $a2$, can be thought of as the inverse of the characteristic dosage where damage will become apparent. The data are reasonably well covered by a characteristic dose of approximately 80 to 120 Gy. $1/a2$ values are 80, 100, and 125 Gy for curves A, B, and C.

Optic Nerve and Chiasm

Recommendations of Mayo et al. (185) are summarized below:
- The incidence of RION (radiation-induced optic neuropathy) was unusual for a D_{max} less than 55 Gy, particularly for fraction sizes less than 2 Gy. The risk increases (3% to 7%) in the region of 55 to 60 Gy and becomes more substantial (greater than 7% to 20%) for doses greater than 60 Gy when fractionations of 1.8 to 2.0 Gy are used. The patients with RION treated in the 55 to 60 Gy range were typically treated to doses in the very high end of that range (i.e., 59 Gy).
- For particles, most investigators found that the incidence of RION was low for a D_{max} less than 54 CGE. One exception to this range was for pituitary tumors, in which investigators used a constrained D_{max} of less than 46 Gy for 1.8 Gy per fraction.
- For single fraction SRS, the studies have indicated the incidence of RION is rare for a D_{max} less than 8 Gy, increases in the range of 8 to 12 Gy, and becomes greater than 10% in the range of 12 to 15 Gy. Consistent agreement has been reached on the low risk of RION for a D_{max} of ≤10 Gy, and one major study indicated a low risk with a D_{max} of ≤12 Gy.

Brainstem

Recommendations of Mayo et al. (186) are summarized below:
- The entire brainstem may be treated to 54 Gy using conventional fractionation with limited risk of severe or permanent neurologic effects (44). Smaller volumes of the brainstem (1 to 10 mL) may be irradiated to maximum doses of 59 Gy for dose fractions ≤2 Gy. The risk appears to increase markedly at doses greater than 64 Gy.
- For single fraction SRS, maximum brainstem dose of 12.5 Gy is associated with low (less than 5%) risk. Higher doses (15 to 20 Gy) have been used with low reported incidence of complication in patient groups with poor prognosis for long-term survival (e.g., brain stem metastases) (91,127). However, the apparent safety of these higher doses may be an artifact of the poor survival.

Spinal Cord

- Extensive work has been performed by the Princess Margaret Hospital in determining the safety and efficacy of SBRT in the up-front and reirradiation settings (187,188).

Kirkpatrick et al. (189) recommend the following two irradiation treatments:
- With conventional fractionation of 2 Gy per day including the full cord cross section, a total dose of 50, 60, and approximately 69 Gy are associated with a 0.2%, 6.0%, and 50.0% rate of myelopathy. For reirradiation of the full cord cross section at 2 Gy per day after prior conventionally fractionated treatment, cord tolerance appears to increase at least 25% 6 months after the initial course of RT based on animal and human studies.
- For partial cord irradiation as part of spine radiosurgery, a maximum cord dose of 13 Gy in a single fraction or 20 Gy in three fractions appears associated with a less than 1% risk of injury.

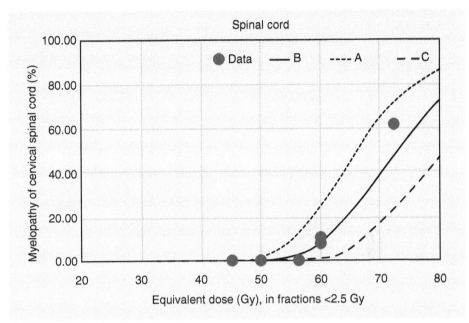

FIGURE 10-8. Myelopathy of the cervical spinal cord; QUANTEC data from Table 2 of reference 182. The curves are calculated using the same two parameter phenomenologic equation as in Figure 10-8. In this case, the inflection of the data required a much larger value for parameter $a1$ (approximately 1,000) and a much lower characteristic dose ($1/a2 \approx 10$ Gy). Detailed conclusions from these models are unwarranted given the quantity of, and scatter in, the data. However, it is clear that normal tissue damage is occurring at lower equivalent doses than with brain irradiation $1/a2$ values are: 9.1, 10, and 11.1 Gy, for curves A, B, and C.

- Figure 10-8 shows the QUANTEC data for myelopathy of the cervical spinal cord for fractionated irradiation at 3 Gy or less. The few points do not justify any serious fitting, but we have drawn probability curves using the same phenomenologic function as in Figure 10-7.

References

1. Bruner JM. Neuropathology of malignant gliomas. *Semin Oncol* 1994;21(2):126–138.
2. Louis DN, Perry A, Reifenberger G, et al. The 2016 World Health Organization classification of tumors of the central nervous system: a summary. *Acta Neuropathol* 2016;131(6):803–820.
3. Nelson DF, Nelson JS, Davis DR, et al. Survival and prognosis of patients with astrocytoma with atypical or anaplastic features. *J Neurooncol* 1985;3(2):99–103.
4. Curran WJ Jr, Scott CB, Horton J, et al. Recursive partitioning analysis of prognostic factors in three Radiation Therapy Oncology Group malignant glioma trials. *J Natl Cancer Inst* 1993;85(9): 704–710.
5. Scott CB, Scarantino C, Urtasun R, et al. Validation and predictive power of Radiation Therapy Oncology Group (RTOG) recursive partitioning analysis classes for malignant glioma patients: a report using RTOG 90-06. *Int J Radiat Oncol Biol Phys* 1998;40(1):51–55.
6. Bell EH, Pugh SL, McElroy JP, et al. Molecular-based recursive partitioning analysis model for glioblastoma in the temozolomide era: a correlative analysis based on NRG oncology RTOG 0525. *JAMA Oncol* 2017;3(6):784–792.

7. Levin VA, Silver P, Hannigan J, et al. Superiority of post-radiotherapy adjuvant chemotherapy with CCNU, procarbazine, and vincristine (PCV) over BCNU for anaplastic gliomas: NCOG 6G61 final report. *Int J Radiat Oncol Biol Phys* 1990;18(2):321–324.

8. Chang JE, Khuntia D, Robins HI, et al. Radiotherapy and radiosensitizers in the treatment of glioblastoma multiforme. *Clin Adv Hematol Oncol* 2007;5(11):894–902, 907–815.

9. Stupp R, Taillibert S, Kanner AA, et al. Maintenance therapy with tumor-treating fields plus temozolomide vs temozolomide alone for glioblastoma: a randomized clinical trial. *JAMA* 2015;314:2535–2543.

10. Stupp R, Wong ET, Kanner AA, et al. NovoTTF-100A versus physician's choice chemotherapy in recurrent glioblastoma: a randomised phase III trial of a novel treatment modality. *Eur J Cancer* 2012;48:2192–2202.

11. Wick W. TTFields: where does all the skepticism come from? *Neuro Oncol* 2016;18:303–305.

12. Loureiro LVM, da Silva Victor E, Callegaro-Filho D, et al. Minimizing the uncertainties regarding the effects of delaying radiotherapy for Glioblastoma: a systematic review and meta-analysis. *Radiother Oncol* 2016;118(1):1–8.

13. Chan JL, Lee SW, Fraass BA, et al. Survival and failure patterns of high-grade gliomas after three-dimensional conformal radiotherapy. *J Clin Oncol* 2002;20(6):1635–1642.

14. Roa W, Brasher PM, Bauman G, et al. Abbreviated course of radiation therapy in older patients with glioblastoma multiforme: a prospective randomized clinical trial. *J Clin Oncol* 2004;22(9): 1583–1588.

15. Mauch P, Loeffler J. *Radiation oncology: technology and biology*. Philadelphia, PA: WB Saunders, 1994.

16. Wallner K. Radiation treatment planning for malignant astrocytomas. *Semin Radiat Oncol* 1991;1(1):17–22.

17. Phillips MH, Stelzer KJ, Griffin TW, et al. Stereotactic radiosurgery: a review and comparison of methods. *J Clin Oncol* 1994;12(5):1085–1099.

18. Yanagihara TK, Saadatmand HJ, Wang TJ. Reevaluating stereotactic radiosurgery for glioblastoma: new potential for targeted dose-escalation. *J Neurooncol* 2016;130(3):397–411.

19. Riva P, Arista A, Franceschi G, et al. Local treatment of malignant gliomas by direct infusion of specific monoclonal antibodies labeled with 131I: comparison of the results obtained in recurrent and newly diagnosed tumors. *Cancer Res* 1995;55(23 suppl):5952s–5956s.

20. Fitzek MM, Thornton AF, Rabinov JD, et al. Accelerated fractionated proton/photon irradiation to 90 cobalt gray equivalent for glioblastoma multiforme: results of a phase II prospective trial. *J Neurosurg* 1999;91(2):251–260.

21. Hug EB, Slater JD. Proton radiation therapy for chordomas and chondrosarcomas of the skull base. *Neurosurg Clin N Am* 2000;11(4):627–638.

22. Nguyen QN, Chang EL. Emerging role of proton beam radiation therapy for chordoma and chondrosarcoma of the skull base. *Curr Oncol Rep* 2008;10(4):338–343.

23. Santoni R, Liebsch N, Finkelstein DM, et al. Temporal lobe (TL) damage following surgery and high-dose photon and proton irradiation in 96 patients affected by chordomas and chondrosarcomas of the base of the skull. *Int J Radiat Oncol Biol Phys* 1998;41(1):59–68.

24. Urtasun RC, Kinsella TJ, Farnan N, et al. Survival improvement in anaplastic astrocytoma, combining external radiation with halogenated pyrimidines: final report of RTOG 86-12, Phase I-II study. *Int J Radiat Oncol Biol Phys* 1996;36(5):1163–1167.

25. Weiss E, Krebeck M, Kohler B, et al. Does the standardized helmet technique lead to adequate coverage of the cribriform plate? An analysis of current practice with respect to the ICRU 50 report. *Int J Radiat Oncol Biol Phys* 2001;49(5):1475–1480.

26. Karlsson U, Kirby T, Orrison W, Lionberger M. Ocular globe topography in radiotherapy. *Int J Radiat Oncol Biol Phys* 1995;33(3):705–712.

27. Hochberg FH, Pruitt A. Assumptions in the radiotherapy of glioblastoma. *Neurology* 1980;30(9):907–911.

28. Halperin EC, Burger PC, Bullard DE. The fallacy of the localized supratentorial malignant glioma. *Int J Radiat Oncol Biol Phys* 1988;15(2):505–509.

29. Gilbert MR, Dignam JJ, Armstrong TS, et al. A randomized trial of bevacizumab for newly diagnosed glioblastoma. *N Engl J Med* 2014;370:699–708.

30. Chang EL, Akyurek S, Avalos T, et al. Evaluation of peritumoral edema in the delineation of radiotherapy clinical target volumes for glioblastoma. *Int J Radiat Oncol Biol Phys* 2007;68(1):144–150.

31. Cooley G, Gillin MT, Murray KJ, et al. Improved dose localization with dual energy photon irradiation in treatment of lateralized intracranial malignancies. *Int J Radiat Oncol Biol Phys* 1991;20(4):815–821.

32. Marks LB, Sherouse GW, Das S, et al. Conformal radiation therapy with fixed shaped coplanar or noncoplanar radiation beam bouquets: a possible alternative to radiosurgery. *Int J Radiat Oncol Biol Phys* 1995;33(5):1209–1219.

33. Abrey LE, Yahalom J, DeAngelis LM. Treatment for primary CNS lymphoma: the next step. *J Clin Oncol* 2000;18(17):3144–3150.

34. Ding M, Newman F, Chen C, et al. Dosimetric comparison between 3DCRT and IMRT using different multileaf collimators in the treatment of brain tumors. *Med Dosim* 2009;34(1):1–8.

35. Hermanto U, Frija EK, Lii MJ, et al. Intensity-modulated radiotherapy (IMRT) and conventional three-dimensional conformal radiotherapy for high-grade gliomas: does IMRT increase the integral dose to normal brain? *Int J Radiat Oncol Biol Phys* 2007;67(4):1135–1144.

36. MacDonald SM, Ahmad S, Kachris S, et al. Intensity modulated radiation therapy versus three-dimensional conformal radiation therapy for the treatment of high grade glioma: a dosimetric comparison. *J Appl Clin Med Phys* 2007;8(2):47–60.

37. Mackley HB, Reddy CA, Lee SY, et al. Intensity-modulated radiotherapy for pituitary adenomas: the preliminary report of the Cleveland Clinic experience. *Int J Radiat Oncol Biol Phys* 2007;67(1):232–239.

38. Narayana A, Yamada J, Berry S, et al. Intensity-modulated radiotherapy in high-grade gliomas: clinical and dosimetric results. *Int J Radiat Oncol Biol Phys* 2006;64(3):892–897.

39. Halperin EC. Concerning the inferior portion of the spinal radiotherapy field for malignancies that disseminate via the cerebrospinal fluid. *Int J Radiat Oncol Biol Phys* 1993;26(2):357–362.

40. Weller M, van den Bent M, Tonn JC, et al. European Association for Neuro-Oncology (EANO) guideline on the diagnosis and treatment of adult astrocytic and oligodendroglial gliomas. *Lancet Oncol* 2017;18(6):e315–e329.

41. Stupp R, Hegi ME, Mason WP, et al. Effects of radiotherapy with concomitant and adjuvant temozolomide versus radiotherapy alone on survival in glioblastoma in a randomised phase III study: 5-year analysis of the EORTC-NCIC trial. *Lancet Oncol* 2009;10(5):459–466.

42. Hegi ME, Diserens AC, Gorlia T, et al. MGMT gene silencing and benefit from temozolomide in glioblastoma. *N Engl J Med* 2005;352(10):997–1003.

43. Bannister R. Disorders of the spinal cord. In: Brain WR, Bannister R, eds. *Clinical neurology*, 6th ed. London, UK: Oxford University; 1985:358.

44. Barbaro NM, Gutin PH, Wilson CB, et al. Radiation therapy in the treatment of partially resected meningiomas. *Neurosurgery* 1987;20(4):525–528.

45. Desjardins A, Reardon DA, Herndon JE II, et al. Bevacizumab plus irinotecan in recurrent WHO grade 3 malignant gliomas. *Clin Cancer Res* 2008;14(21):7068–7073.

46. Kreisl TN, Kim L, Moore K, et al. Phase II trial of single-agent bevacizumab followed by bevacizumab plus irinotecan at tumor progression in recurrent glioblastoma. *J Clin Oncol* 2009;27(5):740–745.

47. Vredenburgh JJ, Desjardins A, Herndon JE II, et al. Bevacizumab plus irinotecan in recurrent glioblastoma multiforme. *J Clin Oncol* 2007;25(30):4722–4729.

48. Zuniga RM, Torcuator R, Jain R, et al. Efficacy, safety and patterns of response and recurrence in patients with recurrent high-grade gliomas treated with bevacizumab plus irinotecan. *J Neurooncol* 2009;91(3):329–336.

49. Cairncross G, Berkey B, Shaw E, et al. Phase III trial of chemotherapy plus radiotherapy compared with radiotherapy alone for pure and mixed anaplastic oligodendroglioma: Intergroup Radiation Therapy Oncology Group Trial 9402. *J Clin Oncol* 2006;24(18):2707–2714.

50. van den Bent MJ, Carpentier AF, Brandes AA, et al. Adjuvant procarbazine, lomustine, and vincristine improves progression-free survival but not overall survival in newly diagnosed anaplastic oligodendrogliomas and oligoastrocytomas: a randomized European Organisation for Research and Treatment of Cancer phase III trial. *J Clin Oncol* 2006;24(18):2715–2722.

51. Mikkelsen T, Doyle T, Anderson J, et al. Temozolomide single-agent chemotherapy for newly diagnosed anaplastic oligodendroglioma. *J Neurooncol* 2009;92(1):57–63.

52. Quon H, Abdulkarim B. Adjuvant treatment of anaplastic oligodendrogliomas and oligoastrocytomas. *Cochrane Database Syst Rev* 2008(2):CD007104.

53. Cairncross G, Wang M, Shaw E, et al. Phase III trial of chemoradiotherapy for anaplastic oligodendroglioma: long-term results of RTOG 9402. *J Clin Oncol* 2013;31:337–343.

54. Vogelbaum MA, Hu C, Peereboom DM, et al. Phase II trial of pre-irradiation and concurrent temozolomide in patients with newly diagnosed anaplastic oligodendrogliomas and mixed anaplastic oligoastrocytomas: long term results of RTOG BR0131. *J Neurooncol* 2015;124:413–420.

55. Lesser GJ, Grossman S. The chemotherapy of high-grade astrocytomas. *Semin Oncol* 1994;21(2): 220–235.

56. Stupp R, Taillibert S, Kanner A, et al. Effect of tumor-treating fields plus maintenance temozolomide vs maintenance temozolomide alone on survival in patients with glioblastoma: a randomized clinical trial. *JAMA* 2017;318:2306–2316.

57. van den Bent MJ, Baumert B, Erridge SC, et al. Interim results from the CATNON trial (EORTC study 26053-22054) of treatment with concurrent and adjuvant temozolomide for 1p/19q non-co-deleted anaplastic glioma: a phase 3, randomised, open-label intergroup study. *Lancet* 2017;390:1645–1653.

58. Zhao F, Li M, Kong L, Zhang G, Yu J. Delineation of radiation therapy target volumes for patients with postoperative glioblastoma: a review. *Onco Targets Ther* 2016;9:3197–3204.

59. Walker MD, Alexander E Jr, Hunt WE, et al. Evaluation of BCNU and/or radiotherapy in the treatment of anaplastic gliomas. A cooperative clinical trial. *J Neurosurg* 1978;49(3):333–343.

60. Walker MD, Green SB, Byar DP, et al. Randomized comparisons of radiotherapy and nitrosoureas for the treatment of malignant glioma after surgery. *N Engl J Med* 1980;303(23):1323–1329.

61. Walker MD, Strike TA, Sheline GE. An analysis of dose-effect relationship in the radiotherapy of malignant gliomas. *Int J Radiat Oncol Biol Phys* 1979;5(10):1725–1731.

62. Souhami L, Seiferheld W, Brachman D, et al. Randomized comparison of stereotactic radiosurgery followed by conventional radiotherapy with carmustine to conventional radiotherapy with carmustine for patients with glioblastoma multiforme: report of Radiation Therapy Oncology Group 93-05 protocol. *Int J Radiat Oncol Biol Phys* 2004;60:853–860.

63. Bauman GS, Gaspar LE, Fisher BJ, Halperin EC, Macdonald DR, Cairncross JG. A prospective study of short-course radiotherapy in poor prognosis glioblastoma multiforme. *Int J Radiat Oncol Biol Phys* 1994;29:835–839.

64. Malmstrom A, Gronberg BH, Marosi C, et al. Temozolomide versus standard 6-week radiotherapy versus hypofractionated radiotherapy in patients older than 60 years with glioblastoma: the Nordic randomised, phase 3 trial. *Lancet Oncol* 2012;13:916–926.

65. Roa W, Kepka L, Kumar N, et al. International Atomic Energy Agency randomized phase III study of radiation therapy in elderly and/or frail patients with newly diagnosed glioblastoma multiforme. *J Clin Oncol* 2015;33:4145–4150.

66. Keime-Guibert F, Chinot O, Taillandier L, et al. Radiotherapy for glioblastoma in the elderly. *N Engl J Med* 2007;356(15):1527–1535.

67. Minniti G, Scaringi C, Arcella A, et al. IDH1 mutation and MGMT methylation status predict survival in patients with anaplastic astrocytoma treated with temozolomide-based chemoradiotherapy. *J Neurooncol* 2014;118:377–383.

68. Brandes AA, Franceschi E, Tosoni A, et al. MGMT promoter methylation status can predict the incidence and outcome of pseudoprogression after concomitant radiochemotherapy in newly diagnosed glioblastoma patients. *J Clin Oncol* 2008;26(13):2192–2197.

69. Brandsma D, Stalpers L, Taal W, et al. Clinical features, mechanisms, and management of pseudoprogression in malignant gliomas. *Lancet Oncol* 2008;9(5):453–461.

70. Wara W, Bauman GS, Sneed PK, et al. Brain, brainstem, and cerebellum. In: Perez CA, Brady LW, eds. *Principles and practice of radiation oncology*, 3rd ed. Philadelphia, PA: Lippincott–Raven, 1998:777–828.

71. van den Bent MJ, Afra D, de Witte O, et al. Long-term efficacy of early versus delayed radiotherapy for low-grade astrocytoma and oligodendroglioma in adults: the EORTC 22845 randomised trial. *Lancet* 2005;366(9490):985–990.

72. Buckner JC, Shaw EG, Pugh SL, et al. Radiation plus procarbazine, CCNU, and vincristine in low-grade glioma. *N Engl J Med* 2016;374:1344–1355.

73. Karim AB, Maat B, Hatlevoll R, et al. A randomized trial on dose-response in radiation therapy of low-grade cerebral glioma: European Organization for Research and Treatment of Cancer (EORTC) Study 22844. *Int J Radiat Oncol Biol Phys* 1996;36(3):549–556.

74. Shaw E, Arusell R, Scheithauer B, et al. Prospective randomized trial of low- versus high-dose radiation therapy in adults with supratentorial low-grade glioma: initial report of a North Central Cancer Treatment Group/Radiation Therapy Oncology Group/Eastern Cooperative Oncology Group study. *J Clin Oncol* 2002;20(9):2267–2276.

75. Shaw EG, Scheithauer BW, O'Fallon JR. Management of supratentorial low-grade gliomas. *Oncology (Williston Park)* 1993;7(7):97–104, 107; discussion 108–111.

76. Cairncross JG, Ueki K, Zlatescu MC, et al. Specific genetic predictors of chemotherapeutic response and survival in patients with anaplastic oligodendrogliomas. *J Natl Cancer Inst* 1998;90: 1473–1479.

77. Baumert BG, Hegi ME, van den Bent MJ, et al. Temozolomide chemotherapy versus radiotherapy in high-risk low-grade glioma (EORTC 22033-26033): a randomised, open-label, phase 3 intergroup study. *Lancet Oncol* 2016;17:1521–1532.

78. Shaw EG, Evans RG, Scheithauer BW, et al. Postoperative radiotherapy of intracranial ependymoma in pediatric and adult patients. *Int J Radiat Oncol Biol Phys* 1987;13(10):1457–1462.

79. Wallner KE, Wara WM, Sheline GE, et al. Intracranial ependymomas: results of treatment with partial or whole brain irradiation without spinal irradiation. *Int J Radiat Oncol Biol Phys* 1986;12(11):1937–1941.

80. Pieters RS, Niemierko A, Fullerton BC, Munzenrider JE. Cauda equina tolerance to high-dose fractionated irradiation. *Int J Radiat Oncol Biol Phys* 2006;64:251–257.

81. Russell DS, Rubinstein LJ. Medulloblastomas. In: Russell DS, Rubinstein LJ, eds. *Pathology of tumors of the nervous system*, 5th ed. Baltimore, MD: Williams & Wilkins, 1989:251–254.

82. Chang C, Housepian E, Herbert CJ. An operative staging system and a megavoltage radiotherapeutic technique for cerebellar medulloblastomas. *Radiology* 1969;93:1351–1359.

83. Packer RJ, Goldwein J, Nicholson HS, et al. Treatment of children with medulloblastomas with reduced-dose craniospinal radiation therapy and adjuvant chemotherapy: a Children's Cancer Group Study. *J Clin Oncol* 1999;17(7):2127–2136.

84. Thomas PR, Deutsch M, Kepner JL, et al. Low-stage medulloblastoma: final analysis of trial comparing standard-dose with reduced-dose neuraxis irradiation. *J Clin Oncol* 2000;18(16): 3004–3011.

85. Wolden SL, Dunkel IJ, Souweidane MM, et al. Patterns of failure using a conformal radiation therapy tumor bed boost for medulloblastoma. *J Clin Oncol* 2003;21(16):3079–3083.

86. Prados MD, Warnick RE, Wara WM, et al. Medulloblastoma in adults. *Int J Radiat Oncol Biol Phys* 1995;32(4):1145–1152.

87. Brandes AA, Franceschi E, Tosoni A, et al. Adult neuroectodermal tumors of posterior fossa (medulloblastoma) and of supratentorial sites (stPNET). *Crit Rev Oncol Hematol* 2009;71: 165–179.

88. Brandes AA, Franceschi E, Tosoni A, Blatt V, Ermani M. Long-term results of a prospective study on the treatment of medulloblastoma in adults. *Cancer* 2007;110:2035–2041.

89. Zulch KJ. Pineal cell tumors. In: Zulch KJ, ed. *Brain tumors*, 3rd ed. Berlin: Springer-Verlag, 1986:283–292.

90. Watanabe T, Mizowaki T, Arakawa Y, et al. Pineal parenchymal tumor of intermediate differentiation: treatment outcomes of five cases. *Mol Clin Oncol* 2014;2:197–202.

91. DeAngelis LM, Seiferheld W, Schold SC, et al. Combination chemotherapy and radiotherapy for primary central nervous system lymphoma: Radiation Therapy Oncology Group Study 93-10. *J Clin Oncol* 2002;20(24):4643–4648.

92. Simpson D. The recurrence of intracranial meningiomas after surgical treatment. *J Neurol Neurosurg Psychiatry* 1957;20:22–39.

93. Goldsmith BJ, Wara WM, Wilson CB, et al. Postoperative irradiation for subtotally resected meningiomas. A retrospective analysis of 140 patients treated from 1967 to 1990. *J Neurosurg* 1994;80(2):195–201.

94. Taylor BW Jr, Marcus RB Jr, Friedman WA, et al. The meningioma controversy: postoperative radiation therapy. *Int J Radiat Oncol Biol Phys* 1988;15(2):299–304.

95. Petty AM, Kun LE, Meyer GA. Radiation therapy for incompletely resected meningiomas. *J Neurosurg* 1985;62(4):502–507.

96. Rogers L, Zhang P, Vogelbaum MA, et al. Intermediate-risk meningioma: initial outcomes from NRG Oncology RTOG 0539. *J Neurosurg* 2017;6:1–13.

97. Elia AE, Shih HA, Loeffler JS. Stereotactic radiation treatment for benign meningiomas. *Neurosurg Focus* 2007;23(4):E5.

98. Kondziolka D, Lunsford LD, Coffey RJ, et al. Stereotactic radiosurgery of meningiomas. *J Neurosurg* 1991;74(4):552–559.

99. Rogers L, Mehta M. Role of radiation therapy in treating intracranial meningiomas. *Neurosurg Focus* 2007;23(4):E4.

100. Flickinger JC, Kondziolka D, Maitz AH, Lunsford LD. Gamma Knife radiosurgery of imaging-diagnosed intracranial meningioma. *Int J Radiat Oncol Biol Phys* 2003;56:801–806.

101. Jang CK, Jung HH, Chang JH, Chang JW, Park YG, Chang WS. Long-term results of Gamma Knife radiosurgery for intracranial meningioma. *Brain Tumor Res Treat* 2015;3:103–107.

102. dos Santos MA, de Salcedo JB, Gutierrez Diaz JA, et al. Long-term outcomes of stereotactic radiosurgery for treatment of cavernous sinus meningiomas. *Int J Radiat Oncol Biol Phys* 2011;81:1436–1441.

103. Wen BC, Hussey DH, Staples J, et al. A comparison of the roles of surgery and radiation therapy in the management of craniopharyngiomas. *Int J Radiat Oncol Biol Phys* 1989;16(1):17–24.

104. Manaka S, Teramoto A, Takakura K. The efficacy of radiotherapy for craniopharyngioma. *J Neurosurg* 1985;62(5):648–656.

105. Merchant TE, Kiehna EN, Sanford RA, et al. Craniopharyngioma: the St. Jude Children's Research Hospital experience 1984–2001. *Int J Radiat Oncol Biol Phys* 2002;53(3):533–542.

106. Stripp DC, Maity A, Janss AJ, et al. Surgery with or without radiation therapy in the management of craniopharyngiomas in children and young adults. *Int J Radiat Oncol Biol Phys* 2004;58(3):714–720.

107. Zacharia BE, Bruce SS, Goldstein H, Malone HR, Neugut AI, Bruce JN. Incidence, treatment and survival of patients with craniopharyngioma in the surveillance, epidemiology and end results program. *Neuro Oncol* 2012;14:1070–1078.

108. Zhang C, Verma V, Lyden ER, et al. The role of definitive radiotherapy in craniopharyngioma: a SEER analysis. *Am J Clin Oncol* 2017. DOI: 10.1097/COC.0000000000000378.

109. Fuss M, Debus J, Lohr F, et al. Conventionally fractionated stereotactic radiotherapy (FSRT) for acoustic neuromas. *Int J Radiat Oncol Biol Phys* 2000;48(5):1381–1387.

110. Koh ES, Millar BA, Menard C, et al. Fractionated stereotactic radiotherapy for acoustic neuroma: single-institution experience at The Princess Margaret Hospital. *Cancer* 2007;109(6):1203–1210.

111. Andrews DW, Werner-Wasik M, Den RB, et al. Toward dose optimization for fractionated stereotactic radiotherapy for acoustic neuromas: comparison of two dose cohorts. *Int J Radiat Oncol Biol Phys* 2009;74:419–426.

112. Regis J, Roche PH, Delsanti C, et al. Modern management of vestibular schwannomas. *Prog Neurol Surg* 2007;20:129–141.

113. Kano H, Kondziolka D, Khan A, Flickinger JC, Lunsford LD. Predictors of hearing preservation after stereotactic radiosurgery for acoustic neuroma. *J Neurosurg* 2009;111(4):863–873.

114. Pollock BE. Vestibular schwannoma management: an evidence-based comparison of stereotactic radiosurgery and microsurgical resection. *Prog Neurol Surg* 2008;21:222–227.

115. Iwai Y, Yamanaka K, Shiotani M, Uyama T. Radiosurgery for acoustic neuromas: results of low-dose treatment. *Neurosurgery* 2003;53:282–287; discussion 287–288.

116. Ruess D, Pohlmann L, Grau S, et al. Long-term follow-up after stereotactic radiosurgery of intracanalicular acoustic neurinoma. *Radiat Oncol* 2017;12:68.

117. Morimoto M, Yoshioka Y, Kotsuma T, et al. Hypofractionated stereotactic radiation therapy in three to five fractions for vestibular schwannoma. *Jpn J Clin Oncol* 2013;43:805–812.

118. Poen JC, Golby AJ, Forster KM, et al. Fractionated stereotactic radiosurgery and preservation of hearing in patients with vestibular schwannoma: a preliminary report. *Neurosurgery* 1999;45:1299–1305; discussion 1305–1297.

119. Williams JA. Fractionated stereotactic radiotherapy for acoustic neuromas. *Acta Neurochir (Wien)* 2002;144:1249–1254; discussion 1254.

120. Williams JA. Fractionated stereotactic radiotherapy for acoustic neuromas. *Stereotact Funct Neurosurg* 2002;78:17–28.

121. Williams JA. Fractionated stereotactic radiotherapy for acoustic neuromas. *Int J Radiat Oncol Biol Phys* 2002;54:500–504.

122. Kano H, Kondziolka D, Khan A, Flickinger JC, Lunsford LD. Predictors of hearing preservation after stereotactic radiosurgery for acoustic neuroma: clinical article. *J Neurosurg* 2013;119(Suppl):863–873.

123. Kano H, Niranjan A, Mongia S, et al. The role of stereotactic radiosurgery for intracranial hemangioblastomas. *Neurosurgery* 2008;63(3):443–450; discussion 450–441.

124. Soyuer S, Chang EL, Selek U, et al. Intracranial meningeal hemangiopericytoma: the role of radiotherapy: report of 29 cases and review of the literature. *Cancer* 2004;100(7):1491–1497.

125. Grigsby PW, Simpson JR, Fineberg B. Late regrowth of pituitary adenomas after irradiation and/or surgery. Hazard function analysis. *Cancer* 1989;63(7):1308–1312.

126. Kernohan J, Sayre G. *Tumors of the pituitary gland and infundibulum. Section X, fascicle 26.* Washington, DC: Armed Forces Institute of Pathology, 1956:7.

127. Hall WA, Luciano MG, Doppman JL, et al. Pituitary magnetic resonance imaging in normal human volunteers: occult adenomas in the general population. *Ann Intern Med* 1994;120(10):817–820.

128. Poon A, McNeill P, Harper A, O'Day J. Patterns of visual loss associated with pituitary macroadenomas. *Aust N Z J Ophthalmol* 1995;23(2):107–115.

129. Schoenthaler R, Albright N, Wara W, et al. Reirradiation of pituitary adenoma. *Int J Radiat Oncol Biol Phys* 1992;24:307–314.

130. Ikeda H, Yoshimoto T. Visual disturbances in patients with pituitary adenoma. *Acta Neurol Scand* 1995;92(2):157–160.
131. Steiner E, Imhof H, Knosp E. Gd-DTPA enhanced high resolution MR imaging of pituitary adenomas. *Radiographics* 1989;9(4):587–598.
132. Hardy J, Vezina JL. Transsphenoidal neurosurgery of intracranial neoplasm. *Adv Neurol* 1976;15:261–273.
133. Grigsby PW, Simpson JR, Emami BN, et al. Prognostic factors and results of surgery and post-operative irradiation in the management of pituitary adenomas. *Int J Radiat Oncol Biol Phys* 1989;16(6):1411–1417.
134. Knosp E, Perneczky A, Kitz K, et al. The need for adjunctive focused radiation therapy in pituitary adenomas. *Acta Neurochir Suppl* 1995;63:81–84.
135. McCollough WM, Marcus RB Jr, Rhoton AL Jr, et al. Long-term follow-up of radiotherapy for pituitary adenoma: the absence of late recurrence after greater than or equal to 4500 cGy. *Int J Radiat Oncol Biol Phys* 1991;21(3):607–614.
136. Tsang RW, Brierley JD, Panzarella T, et al. Radiation therapy for pituitary adenoma: treatment outcome and prognostic factors. *Int J Radiat Oncol Biol Phys* 1994;30(3):557–565.
137. Zaugg M, Adaman O, Pescia R, et al. External irradiation of macroinvasive pituitary adenomas with telecobalt: a retrospective study with long-term follow-up in patients irradiated with doses mostly of between 40 and 45 Gy. *Int J Radiat Oncol Biol Phys* 1995;32(3):671–680.
138. Zierhut D, Flentje M, Adolph J, et al. External radiotherapy of pituitary adenomas. *Int J Radiat Oncol Biol Phys* 1995;33(2):307–314.
139. Grigsby PW. Pituitary. In: Perez CA, Brady LW, eds. *Principles and practice of radiation oncology*, 3rd ed. Philadelphia, PA: Lippincott–Raven Publishers, 1998:829–848.
140. Kovalic JJ, Grigsby PW, Fineberg BB. Recurrent pituitary adenomas after surgical resection: the role of radiation therapy. *Radiology* 1990;177(1):273–275.
141. Castinetti F, Nagai M, Morange I, et al. Long-term results of stereotactic radiosurgery in secretory pituitary adenomas. *J Clin Endocrinol Metab* 2009;94(9):3400–3407.
142. Jagannathan J, Yen CP, Pouratian N, et al. Stereotactic radiosurgery for pituitary adenomas: a comprehensive review of indications, techniques and long-term results using the Gamma Knife. *J Neurooncol* 2009;92(3):345–356.
143. Thoren M, Rahn T, Guo WY, et al. Stereotactic radiosurgery with the cobalt-60 gamma unit in the treatment of growth hormone-producing pituitary tumors. *Neurosurgery* 1991;29(5):663–668.
144. Pollock BE, Brown PD, Nippoldt TB, et al. Pituitary tumor type affects the chance of biochemical remission after radiosurgery of hormone-secreting pituitary adenomas. *Neurosurgery* 2008;62(6):1271–1276; discussion 1276–1278.
145. Loeffler JS, Shih HA. Radiation therapy in the management of pituitary adenomas. *J Clin Endocrinol Metab* 2011;96:1992–2003.
146. Wattson DA, Tanguturi SK, Spiegel DY, et al. Outcomes of proton therapy for patients with functional pituitary adenomas. *Int J Radiat Oncol Biol Phys* 2014;90:532–539.
147. Sheehan JP, Pouratian N, Steiner L, Laws ER, Vance ML. Gamma Knife surgery for pituitary adenomas: factors related to radiological and endocrine outcomes. *J Neurosurg* 2011;114:303–309.
148. Elhateer H, Muanza T, Roberge D, et al. Fractionated stereotactic radiotherapy in the treatment of pituitary macroadenomas. *Curr Oncol* 2008;15:286–292.
149. Kopp C, Theodorou M, Poullos N, et al. Fractionated stereotactic radiotherapy in the treatment of pituitary adenomas. *Strahlenther Onkol* 2013;189:932–937.
150. Li X, Li Y, Cao Y, et al. Safety and efficacy of fractionated stereotactic radiotherapy and stereotactic radiosurgery for treatment of pituitary adenomas: a systematic review and meta-analysis. *J Neurol Sci* 2017;372:110–116.
151. Jackson IM, Noren G. Gamma Knife radiosurgery for pituitary tumours. *Baillieres Best Pract Res Clin Endocrinol Metab* 1999;13(3):461–469.

152. Shin M, Kurita H, Sasaki T, et al. Stereotactic radiosurgery for pituitary adenoma invading the cavernous sinus. *J Neurosurg* 2000;93(suppl 3):2–5.

153. Beyer S, von Bueren AO, Klautke G, et al. A systematic review on the characteristics, treatments and outcomes of the patients with primary spinal glioblastomas or gliosarcomas reported in literature until March 2015. *PLoS One* 2016;11:e0148312.

154. Hernández-Durán S, Bregy A, Shah AH, Hanft S, Komotar RJ, Manzano GR. Primary spinal cord glioblastoma multiforme treated with temozolomide. *J Clin Neurosci* 2015;22:1877–1882.

155. Linstadt DE, Wara WM, Leibel SA, et al. Postoperative radiotherapy of primary spinal cord tumors. *Int J Radiat Oncol Biol Phys* 1989;16(6):1397–1403.

156. Michalski JM. Spinal canal. In: Halperin EC, Perez CA, Brady LW, eds. *Principles and practice of radiation oncology*, 5th ed. Philadelphia, PA: Lippincott Williams & Wilkins, 2008:765–777.

157. Michalski JM, Garcia DM. Spinal canal. In: Perez CA, Brady LW, eds. *Principles and practice of radiation oncology*, 3rd ed. Philadelphia, PA: Lippincott–Raven Publishers, 1998:849–866.

158. Constantini S, Eptstein FJ. Intraspinal tumors in infants and children. In: Youman JR, ed. *Neurological surgery*, 4th ed. Philadelphia, PA: WB Saunders, 1996:3123.

159. Gado M, Sartor K, Hodges FI. The spine. In: Lee JK, Sagel SS, Stanley RJ, eds. *Computed body tomography*, 2nd ed. New York, NY: Raven Press, 1989:991.

160. Sze G. Neoplastic disease of the spine and spinal cord. In: Atlas SW, ed. *Magnetic resonance imaging of the brain and spine*, 2nd ed. Philadelphia, PA: Lippincott–Raven Publishers, 1996:1339–1385.

161. McCormick PC, Stein BM. Intramedullary tumors in adults. *Neurosurg Clin N Am* 1990;1(3):609–630.

162. Sandler HM, Papadopoulos SM, Thornton AF Jr, et al. Spinal cord astrocytomas: results of therapy. *Neurosurgery* 1992;30(4):490–493.

163. Ferrante L, Mastronardi L, Celli P, et al. Intramedullary spinal cord ependymomas—a study of 45 cases with long-term follow-up. *Acta Neurochir (Wien)* 1992;119(1–4):74–79.

164. Garrett PG, Simpson WJ. Ependymomas: results of radiation treatment. *Int J Radiat Oncol Biol Phys* 1983;9(8):1121–1124.

165. Shaw EG, Evans RG, Scheithauer BW, et al. Radiotherapeutic management of adult intraspinal ependymomas. *Int J Radiat Oncol Biol Phys* 1986;12(3):323–327.

166. Whitaker S, Bessell E, Ashley S, et al. Postoperative radiotherapy in the management of spinal cord ependymomas. *J Neurosurg* 1991;74:720–728.

167. Juthani RG, Bilsky MH, Vogelbaum MA. Current management and treatment modalities for intramedullary spinal cord tumors. *Curr Treat Options Oncol* 2015;16:39.

168. Shirato H, Kamada T, Hida K, et al. The role of radiotherapy in the management of spinal cord glioma. *Int J Radiat Oncol Biol Phys* 1995;33(2):323–328.

169. Wen BC, Hussey DH, Hitchon PW, et al. The role of radiation therapy in the management of ependymomas of the spinal cord. *Int J Radiat Oncol Biol Phys* 1991;20(4):781–786.

170. Chamberlain MC. Temozolomide for recurrent low-grade spinal cord gliomas in adults. *Cancer* 2008;113(5):1019–1024.

171. Chamoun RB, Alaraj AM, Al Kutoubi AO, et al. Role of temozolomide in spinal cord low grade astrocytomas: results in two paediatric patients. *Acta Neurochir (Wien)* 2006;148(2):175–179; discussion 180.

172. Rovin RA, Winn R. Expression of O6-methylguanine-deoxyribose nucleic acid methyltransferase and temozolomide response in a patient with a malignant spinal cord astrocytoma. Case report. *J Neurosurg Spine* 2007;6(5):447–450.

173. Vaillant B, Loghin M. Treatment of spinal cord tumors. *Curr Treat Options Neurol* 2009;11(4):315–324.

174. DeLaney TF, Liebsch NJ, Pedlow FX, et al. Long-term results of Phase II study of high dose photon/proton radiotherapy in the management of spine chordomas, chondrosarcomas, and other sarcomas. *J Surg Oncol* 2014;110:115–122.

175. Rotondo RL, Folkert W, Liebsch NJ, et al. High-dose proton-based radiation therapy in the management of spine chordomas: outcomes and clinicopathological prognostic factors. *J Neurosurg Spine* 2015;23:788–797.

176. Yock TI, Yeap BY, Ebb DH, et al. Long-term toxic effects of proton radiotherapy for paediatric medulloblastoma: a phase 2 single-arm study. *Lancet Oncol* 2016;17:287–298.

177. Cohen AR, Wisoff JH, Allen JC, et al. Malignant astrocytomas of the spinal cord. *J Neurosurg* 1989;70(1):50–54.

178. Youssef B, Shank J, Reddy JP, et al. Incidence and predictors of Lhermitte's sign among patients receiving mediastinal radiation for lymphoma. *Radiat Oncol* 2015;10:206.

179. Larson D. Radiation therapy of tumors of the spine. In: Youman J, ed. *Neurological surgery*, 4th ed. Philadelphia, PA: WB Saunders, 1996:3168.

180. Wara WM, Phillips TL, Sheline GE, et al. Radiation tolerance of the spinal cord. *Cancer* 1975;35(6):1558–1562.

181. Schultheiss TE, Stephens LC, Jiang GL, et al. Radiation myelopathy in primates treated with conventional fractionation. *Int J Radiat Oncol Biol Phys* 1990;19(4):935–940.

182. Marks LB, Yorke ED, Jackson A, et al. Use of normal tissue complication probability models in the clinic. *Int J Radiat Oncol Biol Phys* 2010;76:S10–S19.

183. Lawrence YR, Li XA, el Naqa I, et al. Radiation dose-volume effects in the brain. *Int J Radiat Oncol Biol Phys* 2010;76(3 suppl):S20–S27.

184. Zaider M, Amols HI. Practical considerations in using calculated healthy-tissue complication probabilities for treatment-plan optimization. *Int J Radiat Oncol Biol Phys* 1999;44(2):439–447.

185. Mayo C, Martel MK, Marks LB, et al. Radiation dose-volume effects of optic nerves and chiasm. *Int J Radiat Oncol Biol Phys* 2010;76(3 suppl):S28–S35.

186. Mayo C, Yorke E, Merchant TE. Radiation associated brainstem injury. *Int J Radiat Oncol Biol Phys* 2010;76(3 suppl):S36–S41.

187. Sahgal A, Ma L, Weinberg V, et al. Reirradiation human spinal cord tolerance for stereotactic body radiotherapy. *Int J Radiat Oncol Biol Phys* 2012;82:107–116.

188. Sahgal A, Weinberg V, Ma L, et al. Probabilities of radiation myelopathy specific to stereotactic body radiation therapy to guide safe practice. *Int J Radiat Oncol Biol Phys* 2013;85:341–347.

189. Kirkpatrick JP, van der Kogel AJ, Schultheiss TE. Radiation dose-volume effects in the spinal cord. *Int J Radiat Oncol Biol Phys* 2010;76(3 suppl):S42–S49.

CHAPTER 11

NASOPHARYNX

ANATOMY

- The nasopharynx is an approximately cuboidal chamber at the most superior portion of the tubular pharynx; its borders are the posterior choanae anteriorly, the body of the sphenoid superiorly, the clivus and C1-2 vertebrae posteriorly, and the superior surface of the soft palate inferiorly (Fig. 11-1).

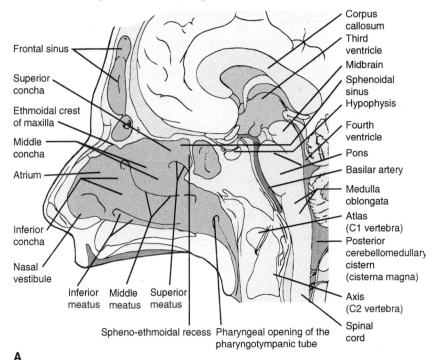

Frontal sinus
Superior concha
Ethmoidal crest of maxilla
Middle concha
Atrium
Inferior concha
Nasal vestibule
Inferior meatus   Middle meatus   Superior meatus
Spheno-ethmoidal recess   Pharyngeal opening of the pharyngotympanic tube

Corpus callosum
Third ventricle
Midbrain
Sphenoidal sinus
Hypophysis
Fourth ventricle
Pons
Basilar artery
Medulla oblongata
Atlas (C1 vertebra)
Posterior cerebellomedullary cistern (cisterna magna)
Axis (C2 vertebra)
Spinal cord

A

FIGURE 11-1. A: Midsagittal section of head shows nasopharynx and related structures. (Reprinted with permission from Agur AMR, Dalley, AF, eds. *Grant's atlas of anatomy*, 12th ed. Philadelphia, PA: Lippincott Williams & Wilkins, 2009:694. © Wolters Kluwer.)

continued

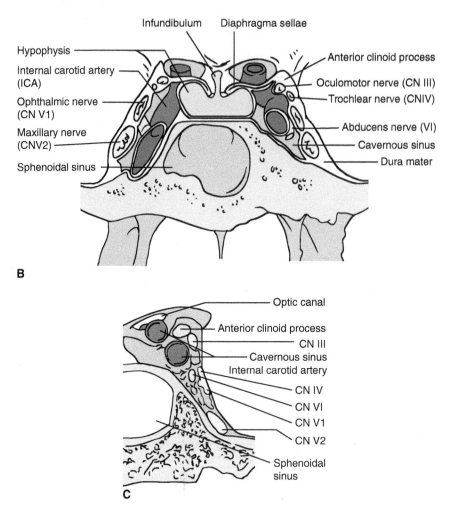

FIGURE 11-1. (*continued*) **B** and **C:** Coronal sections through the cavernous sinus. (Reprinted with permission from Agur AMR, Dalley, AF, eds. *Grant's atlas of anatomy*, 12th ed. Philadelphia, PA: Lippincott Williams & Wilkins, 2009:644. © Wolters Kluwer.)

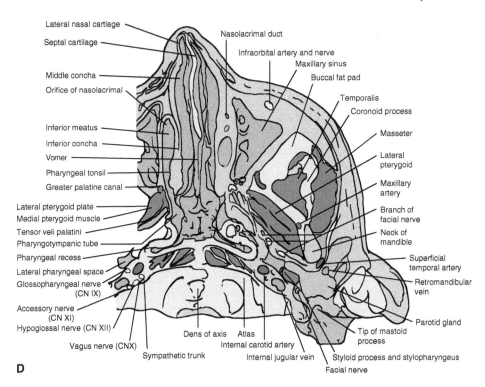

Lateral nasal cartilage
Septal cartilage
Middle concha
Orifice of nasolacrimal
Inferior meatus
Inferior concha
Vomer
Pharyngeal tonsil
Greater palatine canal
Lateral pterygoid plate
Medial pterygoid muscle
Tensor veli palatini
Pharyngotympanic tube
Pharyngeal recess
Lateral pharyngeal space
Glossopharyngeal nerve
(CN IX)
Accessory nerve
(CN XI)
Hypoglossal nerve (CN XII)
Vagus nerve (CNX)
Sympathetic trunk

Nasolacrimal duct
Infraorbital artery and nerve
Maxillary sinus
Buccal fat pad
Temporalis
Coronoid process
Masseter
Lateral
pterygoid
Maxillary
artery
Branch of
facial nerve
Neck of
mandible
Superficial
temporal artery
Retromandibular
vein
Parotid gland
Tip of mastoid
process

Dens of axis   Atlas
Internal carotid artery
Internal jugular vein
Facial nerve
Styloid process and stylopharyngeus

D

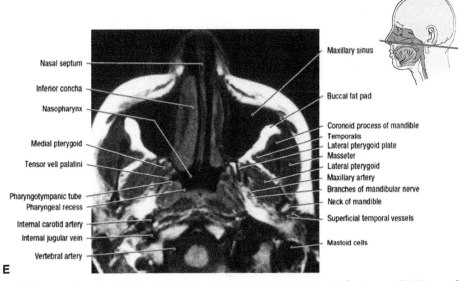

Nasal septum
Inferior concha
Nasopharynx
Medial pterygoid
Tensor veli palatini
Pharyngotympanic tube
Pharyngeal recess
Internal carotid artery
Internal jugular vein
Vertebral artery

Maxillary sinus
Buccal fat pad
Coronoid process of mandible
Temporalis
Lateral pterygoid plate
Masseter
Lateral pterygoid
Maxillary artery
Branches of mandibular nerve
Neck of mandible
Superficial temporal vessels
Mastoid cells

E

FIGURE 11-1. (*continued*) **D** and **E:** Transverse section showing anatomic features and MRI scan of the same axial slice through the nasal cavity and nasopharynx. (Reprinted with permission from Agur AMR, Dalley, AF, eds. *Grant's atlas of anatomy*, 12th ed. Philadelphia, PA: Lippincott Williams & Wilkins, 2009:720. © Wolters Kluwer.)

- The lateral and posterior walls are composed of the pharyngeal fascia, which extends outward bilaterally along the undersurface of the apex of the petrous pyramid just medial to the carotid canal. The roof of the nasopharynx slopes downward and is continuous with the posterior wall.
- The eustachian tube opens into the lateral wall, marked by the torus tubarius (an elevation of the nasopharyngeal wall formed by eustachian tube cartilage). The fossa of Rosenmüller (also known as lateral pharyngeal recess) is posterior and superolateral to the torus tubarius on axial and coronal views, respectively.
- Many foramina and fissures are located in the base of the skull, through which several structures pass (Fig. 11-2, Table 11-1). Some are potential routes of spread of nasopharyngeal carcinoma (NPC).
- Lymphatics of the nasopharyngeal mucosa run in an anteroposterior direction to meet in the midline; from there they drain into a small group of nodes lying near the base of the skull in the space lateral and posterior to the parapharyngeal or retropharyngeal space. This group lies close to cranial nerves (CNs) IX, X, XI, and XII, which run through the parapharyngeal space.
- Another lymphatic pathway from the nasopharynx leads to the deep posterior cervical node at the confluence of the spinal accessory and jugular lymph node chains.
- A third pathway leads to the jugulodigastric node, which is frequently involved in NPC.

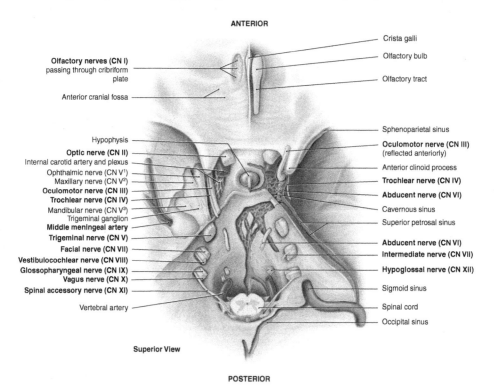

FIGURE 11-2. Anatomic drawing of base of the skull illustrates bony anatomy and foramina for cranial nerves of base of skull. (Adapted with permission from Agur AMR, Dalley, AF, eds. *Grant's atlas of anatomy*, 12th ed. Philadelphia, PA: Lippincott Williams & Wilkins, 2009:813. © Wolters Kluwer.)

Foramina of the Base of the Skull and Associated Anatomic Structures

Foramen/Fissure	Cranial Nerve	Other Structures
Cribriform plate	Olfactory nerve (I)	Anterior ethmoidal nerve
Optic foramen	Optic nerve (II)	Ophthalmic artery
Superior orbital fissure	Oculomotor (III), trochlear (IV), ophthalmic division of trigeminal (V_1) nerve, abducent (VI) nerves	Ophthalmic vein, orbital branch of middle meningeal and recurrent branch of lacrimal arteries, sympathetic plexus, filaments from carotid plexus
Foramen rotundum	Maxillary division of trigeminal (V_2) nerve	
Foramen ovale	Mandibular division of trigeminal (V_3) nerve	Accessory meningeal artery, lesser superficial petrosal nerve
Foramen lacerum		Internal carotid, sympathetic carotid plexus; vidian nerve, meningeal branch of ascending pharyngeal artery, emissary vein
Foramen spinosum	Recurrent branch of V_3 nerve	Middle meningeal artery and vein
Stylomastoid foramen	Facial (VII) nerve	
Internal acoustic meatus	Auditory (VIII) nerve	Internal auditory artery
Jugular foramen	Glossopharyngeal (IX), vagus (X), spinal accessory (XI) nerves	Inferior petrosal sinus; transverse sinus, meningeal branches from occipital and ascending pharyngeal arteries
Hypoglossal canal	Hypoglossal (XII) nerve	Meningeal branch of ascending pharyngeal artery
Foramen magnum		Spinal cord, spinal accessory nerve, vertebral vessels, anterior and posterior spinal vessels

EPIDEMIOLOGY AND NATURAL HISTORY

- Worldwide incidence of NPC is 86,000 cases, with 50,000 deaths annually. NPC demonstrates a unique racial and geographic distribution: rare in the United States and Western Europe (0.5 to 2 per 100,000) and more prevalent in southern China, Southeast Asia, North Africa, the Middle East, and the Arctic (25 per 100,000) (1).
- Incidence is 2 to 3 times higher in males. In endemic regions, peak incidence is 50 to 59 years, with a minor peak in young adults. In low-risk groups, incidence increases with age.

- Among endemic populations, risk factors include Epstein-Barr virus (EBV) infection, environmental factors (salt-cured food, smoking), and genetic factors.
- In the United States, NPC is more commonly associated with smoking and alcohol abuse (2).
- Human papillomavirus (HPV) has been identified in a subset of nonendemic patients, nearly always mutually exclusive with EBV infection (3,4); clinical significance is currently under study.
- NPC frequently arises from the lateral wall, with a predilection for the fossa of Rosenmüller and the roof of the nasopharynx.
- Tumor may involve the mucosa or grow predominantly in the submucosa, invading adjacent tissues including the nasal cavity. In approximately 5% of patients, tumor extends into the posterior or medial walls of the maxillary antrum and ethmoids (5).
- In more advanced stages, tumor may involve the oropharynx, particularly the lateral or posterior wall.
- Upward extension of tumor through the basilar foramen results in CN involvement and destruction of the middle fossa.
- The floor of the sphenoid may be involved.
- Approximately 90% of patients develop lymphadenopathy, which is present in more than 70% at initial diagnosis (5). Approximately 50% have bilateral lymph node involvement at diagnosis.
- Retropharyngeal and level II neck nodes are first sites of lymphatic drainage, and skip metastasis is rare in the lower neck without disease in the upper neck (6).
- The incidence of distant metastasis is not related to stage of the primary tumor but does correlate strongly with degree of cervical lymph node involvement. In 63 patients with N0 necks, 11 (17%) developed metastatic disease, in contrast to 69 of 93 (74%) with N3 cervical lymphadenopathy (7). The most common site of distant metastasis is bone, followed closely by lung and liver (8).

CLINICAL PRESENTATION

- Patients may remain asymptomatic initially and present with locoregional advanced disease.
- Tumor growth into the posterior nasal fossa can produce nasal stuffiness, discharge, or epistaxis. Occasionally, the voice has a nasal twang.
- The orifice of the eustachian tube can be obstructed by a relatively small tumor; ear pain or a unilateral decrease in hearing may occur. Eustachian tube dysfunction can result in middle ear effusion, and one study reported serous otitis media in up to 41% of patients (9). Rarely, tinnitus can also be observed.
- Headache or pain in the temporal or occipital region may occur. Proptosis sometimes results from direct extension of tumor into the orbit.
- Sore throat can occur when tumor involves the oropharynx.
- Although a neck mass elicits medical attention in only 18% to 66% of cases, clinical involvement of cervical lymph nodes on examination at presentation ranges from 60% to 87% (10,11).

- Some patients present with CN involvement, including diplopia. In a study of 924 patients, 82 (9%) initially presented with CN palsy. CN involvement was seen on magnetic resonance imaging (MRI) in 333 (36%) patients (12).
- Cranial nerves III through VI are involved by extension of tumor up through the foramen lacerum to the cavernous sinus. This may result in diplopia. Cranial nerves I, VII, and VIII are rarely involved.

DIAGNOSTIC WORKUP

- A complete history and physical examination includes detailed evaluation of extent of disease in the pharynx (Table 11-2). A thorough CN exam and flexible fiber-optic laryngoscopy should be completed.
- Extent of neck node metastases must be assessed, including the size and number of involved lymph nodes, the position in the neck (upper versus lower neck), and laterality. In addition, there should be an evaluation for distant metastases.
- Recommended imaging studies include MRI of the neck, CT of the neck, and positron emission tomography/computed tomography (PET/CT) scan. Some institutions may use PET/MRI, if available.

Table 11-2
Diagnostic and Staging Workup for Nasopharyngeal Carcinoma
General
Medical history
Physical examination:
Palpation of neck node (record size, laterality, and lowest extent of enlarged nodes)
Testing of cranial nerve (including assessment of vision and hearing functions)
Exclusion of gross signs of distant metastases
Endoscopic examination
Nasopharyngoscopy and biopsies
± Panendoscopy
Otologic assessment
Inspection of tympanic membranes (as clinically indicated)
Baseline audiologic testing (preferable)
Laboratory studies
Complete blood count; basic metabolic panel
Liver and renal function studies
± Baseline hormonal profile
Radiographic studies
Magnetic resonance imaging (study of choice)
Computed tomography (acceptable alternative)
Chest radiograph
Positron emission tomography (study of choice)
Computed tomography of thorax and upper abdomen, or ultrasound of liver, and bone scan (acceptable alternative)

Adapted with permission from Lee AWM, Perez CA, Law SCK, et al. Nasopharynx. In: Halperin EC, Perez CA, Brady LW. *Principles and practice of radiation oncology*, 5th ed. Philadelphia, PA, Lippincott Williams & Wilkins, 2008:820–857. © Wolters Kluwer.

NEW! **SUMMARY OF CHANGES TO AJCC STAGING**

NASOPHARYNX

* Lymph node size greater than 6 cm and lymph node involvement in supraclavicular fossa will be merged into a single N3 category (formerly N3a and N3b, respectively).
* N3 will be categorized as group stage IVA (formerly IVB).

See: Amin MB, Edge SB, Greene FL, et al., eds. *AJCC cancer staging manual*, 8th ed. New York, NY: Springer, 2017.

---

* Biopsies must be done of the nasopharynx, adjacent suspicious areas, and/or enlarged lymph nodes.
* Test for EBV and HPV, though results are unlikely to change management.

STAGING

* The multiplicity of staging systems makes comparison of results from different institutions extremely difficult.
* The most commonly used staging system is the American Joint Committee (13) tumor-node-metastasis (TNM) system.
* The box above summarizes the changes made in the eighth edition.
* However, there is evidence that the AJCC T stage is not predictive of locoregional control and overall survival (OS) with widespread adoption of intensity-modulated radiation therapy (IMRT). A recent prospective trial including 492 NPC patients aimed to establish a new T-staging standard based on MRI and IMRT (14).

PATHOLOGIC CLASSIFICATION

* The World Health Organization (WHO) classifies NPC into three histologic subtypes: keratinizing subtype (WHO type I); nonkeratinizing subdivided into differentiated (WHO type II) and undifferentiated (WHO type III); and basaloid squamous cell carcinoma (15).
* Sporadic form of NPC is typically keratinizing, whereas the endemic form is the undifferentiated subtype, which is strongly associated with EBV. Basaloid squamous cell type is rare but has an aggressive course and poor survival.
* Less frequently seen histologies include lymphoma (most common large cell non-Hodgkin's), plasmacytoma, tumors of minor salivary gland origin (most common adenoid cystic carcinoma), melanoma, rhabdomyosarcoma, chordoma, and lymphoepithelioma.

PROGNOSTIC FACTORS

* Race, age, and gender rarely have prognostic significance (16).
* Cranial nerve involvement was not significantly associated with decreased survival in several series (16); however, Sham et al. (17) found it to be the only significant prognostic factor.

- Survival decreases as cervical lymph node involvement progresses from the upper to the middle and lower cervical nodes (18).
- In 122 patients with localized NPC, histology was the most important prognostic factor for survival; the relative risk of death was 3.4 and 3.2 for nonkeratinizing and squamous cell carcinoma, respectively, compared with undifferentiated carcinoma (19).
- In 759 patients with stage I to IV tumors treated with definitive irradiation, tumor and nodal stage, size and fixation of cervical lymph nodes, gender, patient age, presence of CN involvement, and ear symptoms at presentation were significant factors affecting survival on Cox multivariate analysis of (20). Nonsignificant prognostic factors included bilateral neck lymph node involvement, histologic subtype, and irradiation dose to primary tumor and neck.

GENERAL MANAGEMENT

- Because the nasopharynx is immediately adjacent to the base of the skull, surgical resection with an acceptable margin is technically challenging. Radiation therapy (RT) is the mainstay of treatment for carcinoma of the nasopharynx.
- Rarely, radical neck dissection has been performed for treatment of neck node metastasis, but it is not superior to irradiation alone.
- A randomized phase III intergroup trial in which chemoradiotherapy was compared with radiotherapy alone in patients with stage III and IV nasopharyngeal cancers revealed the advantages of chemotherapy. Radiotherapy was administered in both arms for a total dose of 70 Gy. During radiotherapy, the investigational arm received chemotherapy with cisplatin 100 mg per m^2 on days 1, 22, and 43; postradiotherapy, chemotherapy with cisplatin 80 mg per m^2 on day 1 and fluorouracil (FU) 1,000 mg per m^2 per day on days 1 to 4 was administered every 4 weeks for 3 courses.
- The 5-year progression-free survival rate was 29% versus 58% in favor of chemotherapy arm ($p < 0.001$). The 5-year OS rate was 37% versus 67%, respectively ($p < 0.001$) (21,22).
- Because of the high likelihood of cervical metastases, most authors recommend electively treating all the cervical lymphatics in N0 patients. In 384 patients with clinically negative necks, 11% of those receiving elective neck irradiation had regional failure, compared with 40% of those not electively treated (23). These observations strongly support elective irradiation of the neck in patients with clinically negative neck nodes.

RADIATION THERAPY TECHNIQUES

NPC was previously treated using 3D conformal radiation therapy (3DCRT) technique, which has been predominantly replaced by IMRT.

Rationale for IMRT

IMRT allows for delivery of high dose to the tumor while significantly reducing adjacent normal tissue dose. A prospective phase III trial comparing IMRT to 2D treatment demonstrated superior local recurrence-free survival for IMRT (24). IMRT was significantly better than conventional 2D treatment in terms of parotid sparing and improved quality of life in another phase III randomized study (25).

IMRT Target Volume Delineation

- A dose of 70 Gy is typically prescribed to the primary tumor and involved lymph nodes.
- A dose of 50 to 60 Gy is typically prescribed to the elective neck.
- A common dosing schedule utilizing simultaneous integrated boost (SIB) is detailed here:
- Gross tumor volume (GTV):
  - Gross disease is determined from clinical exam, endoscopic findings, CT, MRI, and PET scan.
  - Grossly positive nodes are defined as any lymph node greater than 1 cm in short axis, nodes with necrotic center, or those that are FDG-PET avid.
  - Whenever possible, use MRI fusion and assistance from neuroradiology for more accurate delineation of the tumor.
- The clinical target volume (CTV) is defined as subclinical regions at risk for involvement as follows:
- CTV_{70} (high-risk clinical target volume; 2.12 Gy per fraction to 69.96 Gy):
  - Includes all primary and nodal GTV with a 5-mm margin, for microscopic extension.
  - If GTV is involving clivus or adjacent to brainstem, CTV margin can be 1 mm. May truncate air, skin, bone, and optic pathway structures if not invaded by tumor.
- $CTV_{59.4}$ (intermediate-risk clinical target volume; 1.8 Gy per fraction to 59.4 Gy):
  - Includes 5-mm margin on CTV_{70}, plus areas at risk for microscopic involvement.
  - Include entire nasopharynx, soft palate, clivus, skull base (ensure coverage of foramen ovale and foramen rotundum), pterygoid fossae, bilateral parapharyngeal space, sphenoid sinus, posterior 1/3 of maxillary sinuses (ensure coverage of pterygopalatine fossae), posterior 1/3 of nasal cavity, posterior ethmoid sinus.
  - Important to use bone window to ensure coverage of the skull base foramen noted earlier.
  - For T1/T2 disease, superior margin extends to the floor of sphenoid sinus.
  - For T3/T4 disease, superior margin extends to include complete sphenoid sinus.
  - For T3/T4 lesions ensure coverage of the cavernous sinus to Meckel's cave.
  - Include all pterygoid muscles on the involved side to mandibular ramus.
  - Split the pterygoid muscles on the uninvolved side.
  - Nodal $CTV_{59.4}$ includes bilateral retropharyngeal nodes and levels IB to V.
  - In patients with N0 neck, level IB nodal region can be omitted.
  - May truncate air, skin, and bone if not invaded by tumor.
- CTV_{54} (low-risk clinical target volume; 1.64 Gy per fraction to 54 Gy):
  - N0 neck or low neck (levels IV and VB) at discretion of treating physician.
  - Includes contralateral uninvolved nodal disease.

- Optionally excludes level IB.
- Includes medial retropharyngeal nodes to the superior edge of hyoid bone.
- Inferior margin extends to 2 cm above the sternoclavicular joint.
- May truncate air, skin, and bone if not invaded by tumor.
- PTV70, PTV59.4, and PTV54 are obtained by 3- to 5-mm expansions from respective CTVs depending on reproducibility of setup. Expansions can be as small as 1 mm when near critical normal tissues such as brainstem and spinal cord.
- Daily image guidance (IGRT) should be used if available, which can allow for smaller (3 mm) PTV margins.
- Figure 11-3 is an example of definitive IMRT target delineation in a patient with T2N1 left-sided NPC.

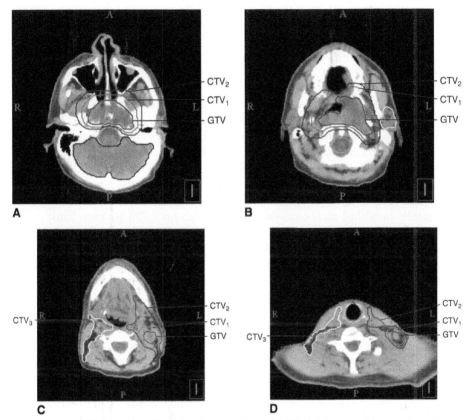

FIGURE 11-3. IMRT target delineation for a patient with T2N1 left nasopharyngeal carcinoma. Planning CT scans, axial view, at four anatomic levels: GTV, gross tumor volume (red contour); CTV, clinical target volume; CTV1, high-risk volume (contour just outside red GTV); CTV2, intermediate risk volume (contour just outside CTV1); CTV3, low-risk volume (white contour at left of sections C and D).

Brachytherapy

- Brachytherapy has been used to deliver a higher dose to a limited volume of nasopharynx; frequently it is combined with external irradiation to treat extensive primary or recurrent carcinoma (26). Different types of intracavitary applicators have been designed, and various isotopes have been implanted.
- Doses of 5 to 25 Gy (calculated at 0.5 to 1.0 cm) combined with external irradiation usually are delivered.
- A review of brachytherapy techniques for carcinoma of the nasopharynx has been published (27).

Normal Tissue Complications—QUANTEC

- Readers are referred to Chapter 10, where the QUANTEC recommendations are summarized for irradiation of the brain, optic nerve and chiasm, brainstem, and spinal cord. Incidence of xerostomia is described in Chapter 13.

CHEMOTHERAPY

- At least nine randomized trials have a shown a benefit of concurrent CRT (±adjuvant chemotherapy) over RT alone in locally advanced NPC (stages III to IVB) (22,28–34).
- Benefit was seen regardless of chemotherapy regimens, which include cisplatin, uracil plus tegafur (prodrug of fluorouracil), or oxaliplatin.
- Cisplatin given either 30 to 40 mg per m^2 once a week or 100 mg per m^2 every 3 weeks is accepted regimen. A cisplatin dose threshold of 200 mg per m^2 has been shown to be optimal (31,35,36).
- A recently published meta-analysis, reviewing data on 4,798 patients (mostly stage III to IVB NPC), found that the addition of chemotherapy is associated with a 6% absolute OS benefit at 5 years, and 8% at 10 years (37). Other meta-analyses show similar hazard ratio (HR) estimates of 0.64 to 0.79 for OS, 0.67 to 0.71 for distant metastasis-free survival, and 0.59 to 0.73 for locoregional control in favor of chemoradiation (38,39).
- The value of induction chemotherapy in addition to CRT in locally advanced NPC is not clear. A randomized phase II study by Hui et al. (40) revealed a 26.5% absolute OS improvement at 3 years with addition of induction cisplatin and docetaxel to CRT. However, this study was not powered to detect a survival difference, and subsequent phase III studies failed to report an OS advantage at 3 years (41,42). Longer follow-up and results from ongoing trials may further clarify the role of induction chemotherapy.
- A large phase III study showed that adjuvant cisplatin plus 5-FU did not improve failure-free survival after a 2-year follow-up (43). Updated results of this study, with a median follow-up of 68.4 months, also failed to demonstrate a significant survival benefit (44).

- Current focus of research is to identify subgroups that may benefit from adjuvant chemotherapy, based on elevated plasma EBV DNA following chemoradiation (45).
- A phase III trial demonstrated a considerable survival benefit for patients with stage II NPC receiving chemoradiation, with a 5-year OS of 95% versus 86% in the radiotherapy alone arm (33).
- Retrospective studies in the IMRT era predict a 5-year disease-specific survival of 94% to 97% for radiation alone in stage I to II NPC (46).

SEQUELAE OF TREATMENT

- The incidence of brainstem or cervical spine myelopathy is 0.2% to 18.0%, with a median of 2% (47).
- Mucositis usually develops because of RT and limits oral intake.
- Lhermitte's sign may occur. It is a transient demyelination of the spinal cord from RT that results in shocklike pain in the back and extremities on neck flexion.
- Radiation may damage the temporal lobe, which can result in short-term memory loss or personality changes.
- Hypothyroidism can occur as a result of RT.
- Hypopituitarism causing significant clinical signs and symptoms is not commonly reported in most series of adults but has been described in children. Sham et al. (48) concluded that shielding of the pituitary/hypothalamus is feasible in a significant proportion of patients and that this technique may improve tolerance to treatment without compromising local tumor control.
- Ophthalmologic side effects after tumor doses of 60 Gy include opacities in the lens that develop several years after irradiation, similar to radiation cataracts (49), and vision loss.
- Hearing loss may occur because the cochlea is irradiated and because cisplatin may cause ototoxicity.
- Osteonecrosis of the mandible or maxilla can be kept to a minimum (1%) by avoiding unnecessarily high doses to these structures. Avoidance of elective dental extractions before and after irradiation, a vigorous program of oral hygiene and fluoride applications, and a close working relationship between radiation oncologist and dentist are equally important in reducing this complication.
- Dental decay frequently occurs. Dental caries may be reduced with prophylactic fluoride treatment and appropriate dental care. Dental extractions or restorations should be performed before initiation of irradiation to allow adequate time for healing of the gingiva and tooth canal. If dental care is required after irradiation, coverage with antibiotics should be instituted 1 week before dental extractions, and trauma should be minimized.
- Xerostomia (moderate to severe) occurs in approximately 75% of patients treated with conventional beam arrangement. IMRT can significantly reduce this complication at 4% per Gy of mean parotid dose (50).
- Trismus may occur because the pterygoids are targeted with radiation.
- Fibrosis of subcutaneous tissues of the neck may occur.

RETREATMENT OF RECURRENT NASOPHARYNGEAL CARCINOMA

- Retrospective and prospective reports of IMRT-treated patients demonstrated that 5% to 15% of patients develop local failures, and 15% to 30% fail at distant sites (24,51–54).
- Isolated neck recurrences occur in less than 10% of cases (55). In this setting, salvage neck dissection is an effective option even for deep retropharyngeal nodes (56).
- Although surgery and reirradiation are potential options in some patients with recurrent disease, most patients are eligible to receive only palliative chemotherapy. Platinum-containing regimens with paclitaxel, FU, gemcitabine, or capecitabine have shown median OS rates of 11 to 28 months (57–59).
- Activation of programmed cell death ligand 1 (PD-L1) /PD-1 pathway may contribute to immune evasion in NPC (60,61), and there are ongoing studies of PD-1 axis inhibitors in recurrent or metastatic NPC.
- Determination of dose received at site of recurrence may differentiate a marginal miss versus a true in-field recurrence, as the latter may represent radioresistant disease.
- Small T1-2 recurrences may be more amenable to surgery, brachytherapy, or stereotactic radiosurgery; larger T3-4 tumors may best be suited for IMRT. Depending on the location of the recurrence, stereotactic body radiation therapy (SBRT) may also be a reasonable treatment option.
- Proton therapy is a good option because it can reduce dose to adjacent organs at risk (62).
- Reirradiation treatment is typically limited to a 1- to 2-cm margin around the GTV, typically smaller when adjacent to critical optic structures or spinal cord.
- In patients salvaged with IMRT, half of all mortality was related to late effects (63,64).
- Total dose depends on the initial irradiation dose given and the tolerance of adjacent critical structures. Recommended doses can vary, but 60 to 70 Gy is the general reirradiation dose delivered in protocols. It is extremely important to determine the full extent of the recurrent tumor and the possibility of extension into the base of the skull. With base of skull involvement or intracranial extension, retreatment should be given primarily with external irradiation rather than with brachytherapy. However, the latter can be used to deliver a portion of the dose (20 to 50 Gy). Because of the inverse-square law, the effective volume treated is limited.
- Some of these patients with recurrent disease may survive for several years or potentially be cured, and most experience substantial palliative benefit. This justifies an aggressive approach, although morbidity of therapy is relatively high.

NASOPHARYNGEAL CARCINOMA IN PATIENTS YOUNGER THAN 30 YEARS OF AGE

- Children or young adults should be treated aggressively with concurrent chemoradiation.

- A German NPC-2003-GPOG protocol (65) uses radiation followed by 6 months of adjuvant interferon beta (IFN-β). High-risk patients receive neoadjuvant cisplatin/5-FU and concurrent cisplatin. The CTV includes a 1-cm margin on the primary and nodal GTVs, the entire nasopharynx, retropharyngeal lymph nodes, and level II cervical nodes. In stage III and IV patients, the CTV also includes levels III, IV, and V cervical nodes. RT dose was 45 Gy (1.8-Gy fractions) to the tumor and draining lymph nodes, followed by a 14.4-Gy boost to the GTV.
- A recent protocol from The Children's Oncology Group ARAR0331 uses a dose of 61.2 Gy and 66.6 Gy for stages I and IIa, respectively. For more advanced disease, neoadjuvant cisplatin and 5-FU is employed, followed by 61.2 to 70.2 Gy, depending on response to neoadjuvant chemotherapy (66).

References

1. Ferlay J, Soerjomataram I, Ervik M, et al. GLOBOCAN 2012 v1 0, Cancer Incidence and Mortality Worldwide: IARC CancerBase No 11. 2012. Available from: http://globocan.iarc.fr, accessed on September 28, 2017.
2. Vaughan TL, et al. Nasopharyngeal cancer in a low-risk population: defining risk factors by histological type. *Cancer Epidemiol Biomarkers Prev* 1996;5(8):587–593.
3. Stenmark MH, et al. Nonendemic HPV-positive nasopharyngeal carcinoma: association with poor prognosis. *Int J Radiat Oncol Biol Phys* 2014;88(3):580–588.
4. Dogan S, et al. Human papillomavirus and Epstein-Barr virus in nasopharyngeal carcinoma in a low-incidence population. *Head Neck* 2014;36(4):511–516.
5. Lee AWM, Perez CA, Law SCK, et al. Nasopharynx. In: Halperin E, Perez C, Brady L, eds. *Principles and practice of radiation oncology*. Philadelphia, PA: Lippincott Williams & Wilkins, 2008:820–857.
6. Tang L, et al. The volume to be irradiated during selective neck irradiation in nasopharyngeal carcinoma: analysis of the spread patterns in lymph nodes by magnetic resonance imaging. *Cancer* 2009;115(3):680–688.
7. Petrovich Z, et al. Advanced carcinoma of the nasopharynx. 2. Pattern of failure in 256 patients. *Radiother Oncol* 1985;4(1):15–20.
8. Valentini V, et al. Tumors of the nasopharynx: review of 132 cases. *Rays* 1987;12(1):77–88.
9. Sham JS, et al. Serous otitis media. An opportunity for early recognition of nasopharyngeal carcinoma. *Arch Otolaryngol Head Neck Surg* 1992;118(8):794–797.
10. Fletcher GH, Million R. Nasopharynx. In: Fletcher GH, ed. *Textbook of radiotherapy*. Philadelphia, PA: Lea & Febiger, 1980:364–383.
11. Lederman M. *Cancer of the nasopharynx: its natural history and treatment*. Springfield, IL: Charles C Thomas Publisher, 1961.
12. Liu L, et al. Prognostic impact of magnetic resonance imaging-detected cranial nerve involvement in nasopharyngeal carcinoma. *Cancer* 2009;115(9):1995–2003.
13. American Joint Commission of Cancer. In: Edge S, et al., eds. *AJCC cancer staging manual*, 7th ed. New York, NY: Springer Verlag, 2009.
14. Kang M, et al. A new T staging system for nasopharyngeal carcinoma based on intensity-modulated radiation therapy: results from a prospective multicentric clinical study. *Am J Cancer Res* 2017;7(2):346–356.
15. Barnes L, Everson JW, Reichart P, et al. Pathology and genetics of head and neck tumors. In: *World Health Organization classification of tumours*. Lyon, France: IARC Press, 2005.

16. Chu AM, et al. Irradiation of nasopharyngeal carcinoma: correlations with treatment factors and stage. *Int J Radiat Oncol Biol Phys* 1984;10(12):2241–2249.

17. Sham JS, et al. Cranial nerve involvement and base of the skull erosion in nasopharyngeal carcinoma. *Cancer* 1991;68(2):422–426.

18. Qin DX, et al. Analysis of 1379 patients with nasopharyngeal carcinoma treated by radiation. *Cancer* 1988;61(6):1117-1124.

19. Kaasa S, et al. Prognostic factors in patients with nasopharyngeal carcinoma. *Acta Oncol* 1993;32(5):531–536.

20. Sham JS, Choy D. Prognostic factors of nasopharyngeal carcinoma: a review of 759 patients. *Br J Radiol* 1990;63(745):51–58.

21. Al-Sarraf M, et al. Superiority of five year survival with chemo-radiotherapy (CT-RT) vs radiotherapy in patients (pts) with locally advanced nasopharyngeal cancer (NPC). Intergroup (0099) (SWOG 8892, RTOG 8817, ECOG 2388) Phase III study: final report. Presented at 37th Annual Meeting of the American Society of Clinical Oncology, San Francisco, CA, 2001.

22. Al-Sarraf M, et al. Chemoradiotherapy versus radiotherapy in patients with advanced nasopharyngeal cancer: phase III randomized Intergroup study 0099. *J Clin Oncol* 1998;16(4):1310–1317.

23. Lee AW, et al. Retrospective analysis of 5037 patients with nasopharyngeal carcinoma treated during 1976–1985: overall survival and patterns of failure. *Int J Radiat Oncol Biol Phys* 1992;23(2):261–270.

24. Peng G, et al. A prospective, randomized study comparing outcomes and toxicities of intensity-modulated radiotherapy vs. conventional two-dimensional radiotherapy for the treatment of nasopharyngeal carcinoma. *Radiother Oncol* 2012;104(3):286–293.

25. Pow EH, et al. Xerostomia and quality of life after intensity-modulated radiotherapy vs. conventional radiotherapy for early-stage nasopharyngeal carcinoma: initial report on a randomized controlled clinical trial. *Int J Radiat Oncol Biol Phys* 2006;66(4):981–991.

26. Wang CC. Improved local control of nasopharyngeal carcinoma after intracavitary brachytherapy boost. *Am J Clin Oncol* 1991;14(1):5–8.

27. Erickson BA, Wilson JF. Nasopharyngeal brachytherapy. *Am J Clin Oncol* 1993;16(5):424–443.

28. Wu X, et al. Long-term follow-up of a phase III study comparing radiotherapy with or without weekly oxaliplatin for locoregionally advanced nasopharyngeal carcinoma. *Ann Oncol* 2013;24(8): 2131–2136.

29. Wee J, et al. Randomized trial of radiotherapy versus concurrent chemoradiotherapy followed by adjuvant chemotherapy in patients with American Joint Committee on Cancer/International Union against cancer stage III and IV nasopharyngeal cancer of the endemic variety. *J Clin Oncol* 2005;23(27):6730–6738.

30. Chen Y, et al. Progress report of a randomized trial comparing long-term survival and late toxicity of concurrent chemoradiotherapy with adjuvant chemotherapy versus radiotherapy alone in patients with stage III to IVB nasopharyngeal carcinoma from endemic regions of China. *Cancer* 2013;119(12):2230–2238.

31. Lee AW, et al. Factors contributing to the efficacy of concurrent-adjuvant chemotherapy for locoregionally advanced nasopharyngeal carcinoma: combined analyses of NPC-9901 and NPC-9902 Trials. *Eur J Cancer* 2011;47(5):656–666.

32. Lee AW, et al. Randomized trial of radiotherapy plus concurrent-adjuvant chemotherapy vs radiotherapy alone for regionally advanced nasopharyngeal carcinoma. *J Natl Cancer Inst* 2010;102(15):1188–1198.

33. Chen QY, et al. Concurrent chemoradiotherapy vs radiotherapy alone in stage II nasopharyngeal carcinoma: phase III randomized trial. *J Natl Cancer Inst* 2011;103(23):1761–1770.

34. Chan AT, et al. Overall survival after concurrent cisplatin-radiotherapy compared with radiotherapy alone in locoregionally advanced nasopharyngeal carcinoma. *J Natl Cancer Inst* 2005;97(7):536–539.

35. Tao CJ, et al. Comparison of long-term survival and toxicity of cisplatin delivered weekly versus every three weeks concurrently with intensity-modulated radiotherapy in nasopharyngeal carcinoma. *PLoS One* 2014;9(10):e110765.

36. Loong HH, et al. Prognostic significance of the total dose of cisplatin administered during concurrent chemoradiotherapy in patients with locoregionally advanced nasopharyngeal carcinoma. *Radiother Oncol* 2012;104(3):300–304.

37. Blanchard P, et al. Chemotherapy and radiotherapy in nasopharyngeal carcinoma: an update of the MAC-NPC meta-analysis. *Lancet Oncol* 2015;16(6):645–655.

38. Zhang L, et al. The role of concurrent chemoradiotherapy in the treatment of locoregionally advanced nasopharyngeal carcinoma among endemic population: a meta-analysis of the phase III randomized trials. *BMC Cancer* 2010;10:558.

39. Chen YP, et al. A Bayesian network meta-analysis comparing concurrent chemoradiotherapy followed by adjuvant chemotherapy, concurrent chemoradiotherapy alone and radiotherapy alone in patients with locoregionally advanced nasopharyngeal carcinoma. *Ann Oncol* 2015;26(1):205–211.

40. Hui EP, et al. Randomized phase II trial of concurrent cisplatin-radiotherapy with or without neoadjuvant docetaxel and cisplatin in advanced nasopharyngeal carcinoma. *J Clin Oncol* 2009;27(2):242–249.

41. Fountzilas G, et al. Induction chemotherapy followed by concomitant radiotherapy and weekly cisplatin versus the same concomitant chemoradiotherapy in patients with nasopharyngeal carcinoma: a randomized phase II study conducted by the Hellenic Cooperative Oncology Group (HeCOG) with biomarker evaluation. *Ann Oncol* 2012;23(2):427–435.

42. Tan T, et al. Concurrent chemo-radiation with or without induction gemcitabine, Carboplatin, and Paclitaxel: a randomized, phase 2/3 trial in locally advanced nasopharyngeal carcinoma. *Int J Radiat Oncol Biol Phys* 2015;91(5):952–960.

43. Chen L, et al. Concurrent chemoradiotherapy plus adjuvant chemotherapy versus concurrent chemoradiotherapy alone in patients with locoregionally advanced nasopharyngeal carcinoma: a phase 3 multicentre randomised controlled trial. *Lancet Oncol* 2012;13(2):163–171.

44. Chen L, et al. Adjuvant chemotherapy in patients with locoregionally advanced nasopharyngeal carcinoma: long-term results of a phase 3 multicentre randomised controlled trial. *Eur J Cancer* 2017;75:150–158.

45. Chan ATC, Ngan RKC, Hui EP, et al. A multicenter randomized controlled trial (RCT) of adjuvant chemotherapy (CT) in nasopharyngeal carcinoma (NPC) with residual plasma EBV DNA (EBV DNA) following primary radiotherapy (RT) or chemoradiotherapy (CRT). *J Clin Oncol* 2012;35(Suppl 15): abstract 5511.

46. Su SF, et al. Long-term outcomes of early-stage nasopharyngeal carcinoma patients treated with intensity-modulated radiotherapy alone. *Int J Radiat Oncol Biol Phys* 2012;82(1):327–333.

47. Marks JE, et al. Dose-response analysis for nasopharyngeal carcinoma: an historical perspective. *Cancer* 1982;50(6):1042–1050.

48. Sham J, et al. Radiotherapy for nasopharyngeal carcinoma: shielding the pituitary may improve therapeutic ratio. *Int J Radiat Oncol Biol Phys* 1994;29(4):699–704.

49. de Schryver A, Wachtmeister L, Baryd I. Ophthalmologic observations on long-term survivors after radiotherapy for nasopharyngeal tumours. *Acta Radiol Ther Phys Biol* 1971;10(2):193–209.

50. Chao KS, et al. A prospective study of salivary function sparing in patients with head-and-neck cancers receiving intensity-modulated or three-dimensional radiation therapy: initial results. *Int J Radiat Oncol Biol Phys* 2001;49(4):907–916.

51. Wu F, et al. Concurrent chemoradiotherapy in locoregionally advanced nasopharyngeal carcinoma: treatment outcomes of a prospective, multicentric clinical study. *Radiother Oncol* 2014;112(1):106–111.

52. Lai SZ, et al. How does intensity-modulated radiotherapy versus conventional two-dimensional radiotherapy influence the treatment results in nasopharyngeal carcinoma patients? *Int J Radiat Oncol Biol Phys* 2011;80(3):661–668.

53. Sun X, et al. Long-term outcomes of intensity-modulated radiotherapy for 868 patients with nasopharyngeal carcinoma: an analysis of survival and treatment toxicities. *Radiother Oncol* 2014;110(3):398–403.

54. Lin S, et al. Update report of nasopharyngeal carcinoma treated with reduced-volume intensity-modulated radiation therapy and hypothesis of the optimal margin. *Radiother Oncol* 2014;110(3):385–389.

55. Zeng L, et al. Comparative study on prophylactic irradiation to the whole neck and to the upper neck for patients with neck lymph node-negative nasopharyngeal carcinoma. *Head Neck* 2014;36(5):687–693.

56. Chan JY, et al. Surgical salvage for recurrent retropharyngeal lymph node metastasis in nasopharyngeal carcinoma. *Head Neck* 2013;35(12):1726–1731.

57. Chua DT, et al. Phase II trial of capecitabine plus cisplatin as first-line therapy in patients with metastatic nasopharyngeal cancer. *Head Neck* 2012;34(9):1225–1230.

58. Ngan RK, et al. Combination gemcitabine and cisplatin chemotherapy for metastatic or recurrent nasopharyngeal carcinoma: report of a phase II study. *Ann Oncol* 2002;13(8):1252–1258.

59. Tan EH, et al. Phase II trial of a paclitaxel and carboplatin combination in Asian patients with metastatic nasopharyngeal carcinoma. *Ann Oncol* 1999;10(2):235–237.

60. Fang W, et al. EBV-driven LMP1 and IFN-gamma up-regulate PD-L1 in nasopharyngeal carcinoma: implications for oncotargeted therapy. *Oncotarget* 2014;5(23):12189–12202.

61. Hsu MC, et al. Increase of programmed death-1-expressing intratumoral CD8 T cells predicts a poor prognosis for nasopharyngeal carcinoma. *Mod Pathol* 2010;23(10):1393–1403.

62. Taheri-Kadkhoda Z, et al. Intensity-modulated radiotherapy of nasopharyngeal carcinoma: a comparative treatment planning study of photons and protons. *Radiat Oncol* 2008;3:4.

63. Han F, et al. Long-term outcomes and prognostic factors of re-irradiation for locally recurrent nasopharyngeal carcinoma using intensity-modulated radiotherapy. *Clin Oncol (R Coll Radiol)* 2012;24(8):569–576.

64. Tian YM, et al. Prognostic model for survival of local recurrent nasopharyngeal carcinoma with intensity-modulated radiotherapy. *Br J Cancer* 2014;110(2):297–303.

65. Buehrlen M, et al. Multimodal treatment, including interferon beta, of nasopharyngeal carcinoma in children and young adults: preliminary results from the prospective, multicenter study NPC-2003-GPOH/DCOG. *Cancer* 2012;118(19):4892–4900.

66. Rodriguez-Galindo C. ARAR0331—Treatment of childhood nasopharyngeal carcinoma with neoadjuvant chemotherapy and concomitant chemoradiotherapy. NCI-COG protocol. Available from: https://childrensoncologygroup.org/index.php/arar0331.

CHAPTER 12

NASAL CAVITY AND PARANASAL SINUSES

- Nasal cavity and paranasal sinus cancers are twice as common in males as in females and show a bimodal age distribution (10 to 20 and 50 to 60 years of age).
- Most cancers of the nasal cavity and sinuses present at advanced stages because of early symptoms being mistaken for benign sinusitis. Patients with advanced disease may present with epistaxis, headache, and cranial neuropathies.
- Risk factors for nasal cavity and paranasal sinus cancers include smoking, alcohol consumption, and chemical/occupational exposures; however, most cases are idiopathic.
- The most common sites of these cancers are the maxillary sinus followed by the nasal cavity. Cancers of other sinuses are very rare.

ANATOMY (FIG. 12-1)

- The nasal cavity is defined by the hard palate inferiorly, by the base of the skull superiorly, by the nasal vestibule anteriorly (the skin to mucous membrane transition), and by the choanae posteriorly. Laterally, the nasal cavity is bounded by the medial walls of the maxillary sinus. The nasal cavity is divided into halves by the nasal septum.
- The nasal vestibule is the triangular space defined by the aperture of the nostril, laterally by the alae, medially by the membranous septum, distally by the end of the cartilaginous septum and columella, and inferiorly by the adjacent floor of the nasal cavity.
- There are four major paranasal sinuses: the maxillary sinuses, the ethmoid sinuses, the frontal sinuses, and the sphenoid sinus.
- The maxillary sinuses are located in the maxillary bones and are bounded medially by the nasal cavity, inferiorly by the alveolar processes, and superiorly by the orbital floors.
- The ethmoid sinuses are situated between the nasal cavity and orbit just below the anterior cranial fossa. The optic chiasm is just posterior to the ethmoid sinuses, and the optic nerves run just laterally to the sinuses. The ethmoid air cells drain fluid directly and indirectly into the nasal cavity.
- The sphenoid sinus is situated within the sphenoid bone. Superior to the sinus lie the pituitary gland and optic chiasm. Lateral to the sphenoid sinus is the cavernous sinus providing a direct route of skull invasion.
- The frontal sinuses are two paired sinuses located in the frontal bone.

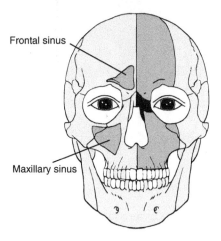

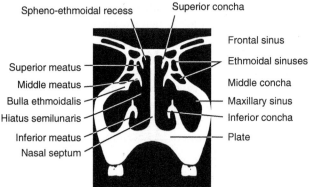

A

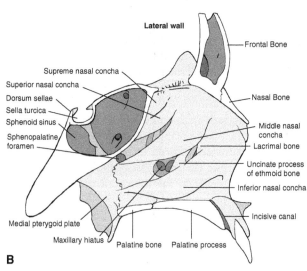

B

FIGURE 12-1. Anatomy of nasal cavity and surrounding structures. **A:** Placement in the skull, and cross section of nasal structures. **B:** Enlarged lateral view.

NATURAL HISTORY

- Most lesions are advanced and commonly involve the nasal cavity, several adjacent sinuses, and often, the nasopharynx.
- There is often orbital invasion from maxillary sinus or ethmoid sinus cancers. Orbital invasion from nasal cavity tumors occurs later.
- The anterior cranial fossa is invaded by way of the cribriform plate and roof of the ethmoid sinuses. The middle cranial fossa is invaded by way of the infratemporal fossa, pterygoid plates, or lateral extension from the sphenoid sinus.
- Lesions involving the olfactory region tend to destroy the septum and may invade through the nasal bone, producing expansion of the nasal bridge and, eventually, skin invasion.
- Lesions of the anterolateral infrastructure of the maxillary sinus commonly extend through the lateral inferior wall and appear in the oral cavity, where they erode through the maxillary gingiva or the gingivobuccal sulcus. Tumors that extend posteriorly from the maxillary sinus have immediate access to the base of the skull.
- Lymph node metastases generally do not occur until the tumor has extended to areas that contain abundant capillary lymphatics. However, in patients with node-negative large (T3-T4) maxillary sinus cancers, lymph node failure is common (35%) without elective nodal irradiation (1). The submandibular and subdigastric lymph nodes (levels IB and II) are most commonly involved.

Nasal Vestibule

- Lymph node spread from vestibule cancer is usually to a solitary ipsilateral submandibular or facial node, although bilateral spread occasionally is seen.
- The preauricular and submental nodes are at small risk.
- Approximately 5% of patients have clinically positive lymph nodes on initial presentation; lymph node metastases develop in another 15% of patients after treatment has controlled the primary tumor (2).

DIAGNOSTIC WORKUP

- A complete history and physical examination, including bimanual examination and cranial nerve assessment, is important in the workup. Fiberoptic nasal endoscopy may aid in evaluating extent of disease.
- Computed tomography (CT) scan is superior in detecting bone erosion or cribriform plate involvement, whereas T2-weighted magnetic resonance imaging (MRI) is more useful in differentiating between tumor and benign secretions. MRI is also useful in demonstrating intracranial, perineural, or leptomeningeal disease.

NEW!   **SUMMARY OF CHANGES TO AJCC STAGING**

- The 7th edition of the American Joint Committee on Cancer (AJCC) staging system (2009) groups nasal cavity and ethmoid sinus tumors together. A separate staging system applies to maxillary sinus tumors. Nasal vestibule tumors are often staged using the system for skin cancer (3). Nodal staging in the 7th edition was similar for all head and neck sites excluding nasopharynx and incorporates size, number of nodes, and laterality.
- The new 8th edition of the AJCC staging system was published in 2016 and went into effect in 2018 for nasal cavity and paranasal sinus cancers. There are no changes to the T staging for nasal cavity and paranasal sinus tumors. There is a new N staging system for nasal cavity and paranasal sinus cancers similar to other non-nasopharyngeal, nonoropharyngeal head and neck cancers. The new N staging system has been separated into clinical and pathologic nodal staging. Both clinical and pathologic nodal staging now incorporate extracapsular extension in addition to the traditional nodal staging factors of size, number of nodes, and laterality.

See: Amin MB, Edge SB, Greene FL, et al., eds. *AJCC Cancer Staging Manual*. 8th ed. New York: Springer; 2017.

- In addition to a dedicated CT/MRI of the sinus, neck imaging with CT or MRI is necessary to rule out lymphadenopathy.
- A chest x-ray, complete blood count (CBC), dental evaluation, and ophthalmologic examination should be performed to complete the pretreatment evaluation.

PATHOLOGIC CLASSIFICATION

- Squamous cell carcinoma is the most common malignancy of the nasal cavity and paranasal sinuses.
- Approximately 10% to 15% of neoplasms in this region are minor salivary gland tumors.
- Malignant melanoma accounts for 10% to 15% of cancers of the nasal cavity.
- Other histologic types are lymphoma (usually histiocytic), esthesioneuroblastoma, sarcoma, sinonasal undifferentiated carcinoma (SNUC), and inverted papilloma.
- Inverted papilloma, although usually histologically benign, is associated with squamous cell carcinoma in 10% to 15% of cases.

PROGNOSTIC FACTORS

- Massive tumor extension to the base of the skull, nasopharynx, posterior wall or roof of the sphenoid sinus, or cavernous sinus significantly increases surgical morbidity and decreases the likelihood of obtaining negative surgical margins.
- Tumor extension through the periorbita usually requires sacrifice of the eye.

GENERAL MANAGEMENT

Nasal Vestibule

- Radiation therapy is the preferred treatment. The 5-year local control rate is 87%, and overall survival rate is 77% for stages I and II and 73% for stages III and IV (4,5).
- Because excision almost always produces deformity, it can be done only if the lesion is very small and favorably located.

Nasal Cavity

- Inverted papilloma without carcinoma is treated by surgery.
- Traditional intranasal excision, Caldwell-Luc procedure, and ethmoidectomy result in a high recurrence rate for carcinoma of the nasal cavity (6).
- Primary surgery followed by postoperative irradiation (to a lesser dose than used for irradiation alone) is preferred to reduce the risk of unilateral or bilateral optic nerve injury. In most cases, postoperative doses are limited to 60 Gy; 66 to 68 Gy is administered for positive margins (7).
- Frazell and Lewis (8) observed a 5-year cure rate of 56% for 68 nasal cavity cancers treated surgically.
- In 45 patients with nasal cavity cancers (18 treated with definitive irradiation and 27 with surgery and irradiation), the 5-year disease-specific and overall survival rates were 83% and 75%, respectively (9).

Paranasal Sinuses

- In a study of 85 patients with nasal cavity and paranasal sinus tumors treated with surgical resection followed by irradiation, 5-year local control and overall survival rates were 62% and 67%, respectively (10).
- For unresectable lesions, outcomes are generally poor. Radiotherapy to a median of 70 Gy in 2 Gy daily fractions with concurrent cisplatin-based chemotherapy in a series from Memorial Sloan Kettering resulted in 5-year recurrence-free and overall survival rates of only 21% and 15%, respectively (11).

Ethmoid Sinus

- Surgical resection requires medial maxillectomy and *en bloc* ethmoidectomy. If tumor extends superiorly to involve the fovea ethmoidalis or the cribriform plate, a combined craniofacial approach is required.
- If the tumor is resectable, surgery is usually performed first. Postoperative irradiation is advisable for T3 and T4 tumors and should be considered for any T1 and T2 tumors with high-risk pathologic features. For unresectable tumors, definitive radiation therapy may be combined with chemotherapy, although overall survival remains poor (11).

Maxillary Sinus

- Most malignancies require radical maxillectomy, including the entire maxilla and ethmoid sinus, via a Weber-Fergusson incision. The globe and orbital floor are preserved for inferiorly located tumors.
- Orbital exenteration is indicated when tumor has spread through the periorbita.
- If the ethmoid roof is involved, craniofacial resection is required.
- Early infrastructure lesions are often cured by surgery alone. However, irradiation is given postoperatively in most cases of maxillary sinus cancer, even if the margins are clear.
- Massive tumor extension to the base of the skull, nasopharynx, or sphenoid sinus may contraindicate surgery.
- Borderline resectable lesions sometimes are treated with full-dose external beam irradiation, followed by surgery (if technically feasible).
- Ninety-six patients with maxillary sinus carcinomas were treated at Washington University, St. Louis, MO, from 1960 to 1976; 74 (77%) had squamous cell carcinoma (12). After preoperative irradiation (mostly 50 to 70 Gy) and surgery, 5-year disease-free survival rates were 60%, 45%, 38%, and 28% in patients with T1, T2, T3, and T4 tumors, respectively.
- It is reasonable to expect 5-year survival rates of approximately 60% to 70% for T1 and T2 lesions and 30% to 40% for T3 and T4 lesions after resection and postoperative irradiation. For advanced, unresectable disease, average 5-year survival rates of 10% to 15% are achieved with high-dose irradiation alone.

Sphenoid Sinus

- Irradiation is usually the treatment of choice.

Neck

- Patients with recurrent or poorly differentiated cancers and tumors that extend to an area with dense capillary lymphatics (nasopharynx, oropharynx, oral cavity) have a higher risk of metastasis and are often given elective neck irradiation of 50 Gy over 5 to 6 weeks, administered in 2.0 Gy daily fractions.
- Maxillary sinus cancers have increased rates of subclinical nodal metastasis when compared to other sinonasal primaries as evidenced by nodal recurrence rates upward of 38% in the non–electively irradiated neck (1). Further, data from UCSF (13) and MD Anderson have shown low nodal recurrence risks and reduced incidence of distant metastases with elective neck irradiation for T3-T4 maxillary sinus tumors. As such, we recommend nodal radiation for large (T3-T4) maxillary sinus tumors. Because most neck recurrences are reported in ipsilateral neck levels IB and II, it may be sufficient to cover these areas electively.
- Elective neck irradiation may be considered for T3-T4 tumors arising in other sinuses though data are limited.

Rare Histologies

Esthesioneuroblastoma

- Esthesioneuroblastoma is an aggressive rare neural crest malignancy with a small round blue cell appearance thought to arise from the olfactory apparatus.
- These tumors are staged using the Kadish's system by extent of involvement (Kadish A—tumor limited to the nasal cavity, Kadish B—tumor involving nasal cavity and paranasal sinuses, and Kadish C—tumor extending beyond these structures) (14).
- Similar to other sinonasal malignancies, management includes maximal surgical resection followed by radiation therapy. The role of chemotherapy remains uncertain.
- Outcomes with esthesioneuroblastoma are modest with 5-year survival estimated between 45% and 70% (15).
- Elective nodal radiation is controversial with one series reporting a 44% rate of nodal failure without elective nodal irradiation (16), whereas another series reports a rate of less than 10% without elective nodal irradiation (17).

Sinonasal Undifferentiated Carcinoma

- SNUC is another rare histology of sinonasal cancers with unknown histologic origin.
- Management remains uncertain. Most tumors have been treated with a combination of maximal surgical resection followed by radiation therapy with or without chemotherapy (18,19). Outcomes are considered to be poor with a meta-analysis reporting a disease-free survival of 26.3% and disease-specific morality of 52.7% at a median follow-up of 15 months (20).
- Because of the rarity of the tumor, the role of elective nodal irradiation is not well defined.

RADIATION THERAPY TECHNIQUES

- Patients should be simulated using CT simulation with a five-point mask to immobilize the head and shoulders. A bite block/oral stent may be used to help reduce dose to the inferior oral cavity.
- Intensity-modulated radiation therapy (IMRT) is the preferred technique for sinonasal and nasal cavity tumors. Proton radiation utilizing both conventional proton therapy and intensity-modulated proton therapy may result in better dosimetry and should be evaluated on a case-by-case basis (21–23).
- In cases of induction chemotherapy, targets should be based on prechemotherapy volumes accounting for anatomic confinement.
- Target volume delineation is outlined in Table 12-1.
- In definitive radiotherapy patients, gross disease plus an anatomically confined 5- to 10-mm margin (CTV1) should be treated to 70 Gy, with areas at high risk of subclinical spread (CTV2) receiving 60 to 63 Gy. The CTV2 should include any anatomically confined space involved by gross disease (i.e., the remainder of the ipsilateral maxillary

Table 12-1

Clinical Target Volume and Doses for Sinonasal Cancers

	Definitive Setting	Postoperative Setting
High-Risk Areas (CTV1)	Gross disease plus 0.5- to 1.0-cm margin (70 Gy)	Areas of residual disease (70 Gy), extracapsular extension, or positive margins plus 0.5- to 1.0-cm margin (60–66 Gy)
Intermediate-Risk Areas (CTV2)	Areas of subclinical spread including any involved anatomic compartment (60–63 Gy)	Postoperative tumor bed including dissected neck (60 Gy)
Low-Risk Areas (CTV3)	Elective neck nodes and nerve tracts/base of the skull (if indicated) (50–54 Gy)	Elective neck nodes and nerve tracts/base of the skull (if indicated) (50–54 Gy)

sinus if there is tumor involvement). Patients receiving definitive radiotherapy should receive concurrent chemotherapy with a similar regimen to other head and neck cancers if tolerated.

- Stereotactic body radiotherapy (SBRT) may be considered to deliver a boost in patients who have unresectable disease (24) (Fig. 12-2) or in the setting of palliation.
- In postoperative patients, the high-risk region (CTV1) includes areas of suspected positive margin, gross residual disease, or extracapsular extension from metastatic lymphadenopathy in the neck and should be treated as gross disease in the definitive patient to 66 Gy (70 Gy if gross disease remains). Postoperatively, the surgical bed (CTV2) should receive 60 Gy. Patients with high-risk postoperative features including residual disease, positive margins, or extracapsular extension should receive concurrent chemotherapy if tolerated. A sample isodose plan for a patient receiving postoperative radiation for a R0 resection of a nasal cavity cancer is shown in Figure 12-3.
- Low-risk elective volumes (CTV3) including elective nodal volumes and nerve tracts/base of the skull (if indicated) should receive 50 to 54 Gy.
- A planning target volume (PTV) margin of 3 to 5 mm for each clinical target volume (CTV) is reasonable with daily image guidance.
- Because of the proximity of sinonasal structures to the orbit, special consideration should be paid to the tolerance of critical structures to prevent ocular toxicities. Radiation dose to the optic nerves and chiasm should be limited to 54 Gy in 1.8 Gy fractions. Radiation dose to the retina should be limited to a maximum dose 45 Gy. Finally, the lacrimal gland should be contoured and limited to a mean dose of 40 Gy (25).
- Other important critical structures that should be constrained are similar to other head and neck sites and include the brainstem, spinal cord, cochlea, lenses, and parotid glands.
- Radiation therapy to the nasal vestibule may be delivered by external beam therapy using conventional radiation treatment with photons or electrons (Figs. 12-4 and 12-5), interstitial therapy, a combination of the two techniques, or more recently proton radiation (not shown).

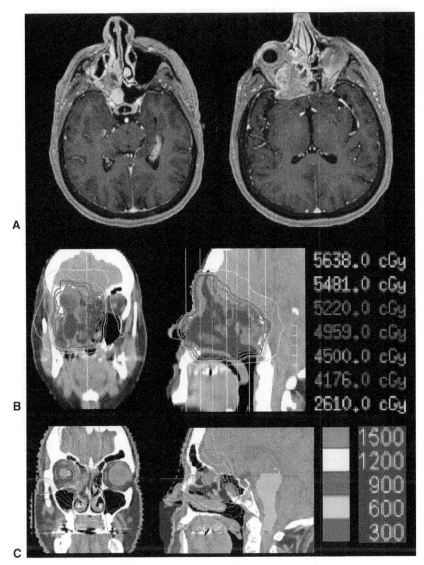

FIGURE 12-2. Treatment plan for patient receiving definitive chemoradiation for T4N0 squamous cell carcinoma of the right ethmoid sinus. The patient has a large ethmoid mass with concern for intracranial extension on MRI **(A)**. The patient received induction chemotherapy and then received an initial dose to 52.2 Gy in 1.8 Gy fractions to areas of subclinical spread including the bilateral ethmoid sinuses, the ipsilateral maxillary sinus, and the sphenoid sinus because of the proximity of the optic nerve **(B)**. Higher doses were not given to these areas of subclinical spread because of the proximity to the optic structures. Elective nodes were not treated as the tumor arose from the ethmoid sinus. The initial plan of 52.2 Gy was followed by a radiosurgical boost to the residual gross disease to a total dose of 15 Gy in three fractions **(C)**.

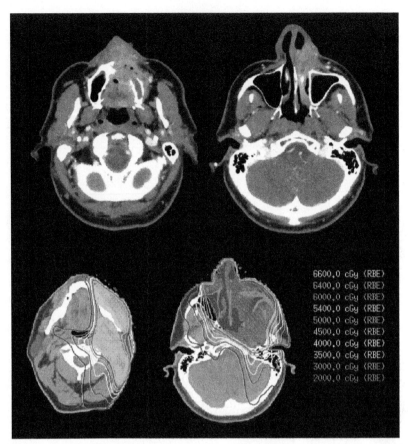

6600.0 cGy (RBE)
6400.0 cGy (RBE)
6000.0 cGy (RBE)
5400.0 cGy (RBE)
5000.0 cGy (RBE)
4500.0 cGy (RBE)
4000.0 cGy (RBE)
3500.0 cGy (RBE)
3000.0 cGy (RBE)
2000.0 cGy (RBE)

FIGURE 12-3. Treatment plan for patient receiving postoperative radiation for a gross total resection of a T4N0 squamous cell carcinoma of the anterior nasal cavity. On CT scan, one notes the extensive mass arising in the posterior left nasal cavity with extension into the maxillary sinus, hard palate, and soft palate (*top panes*). The patient had surgery with gross total resection and negative margins. The patient received 60 Gy to the entire nasal cavity, maxillary sinus, and masticator space because of involvement of this region and 54 Gy electively to the ipsilateral levels IB and II because of T4 disease.

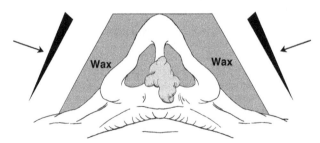

FIGURE 12-4. Treatment plan for external beam irradiation of nasal vestibule carcinoma. (Reprinted with permission from Million RR, Cassisi NJ, Wittes RE. Cancer of the head and neck. In: DeVita VT Jr, Hellman S, Rosenberg SA, eds. *Cancer: principles and practice of oncology,* 3rd ed. Philadelphia, PA: JB Lippincott Co, 1989:407–506. © Wolters Kluwer.)

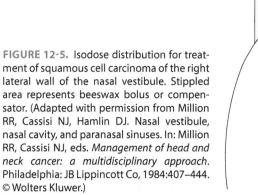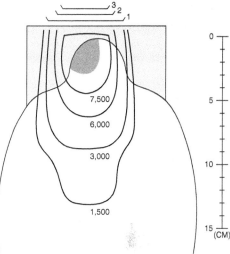

FIGURE 12-5. Isodose distribution for treatment of squamous cell carcinoma of the right lateral wall of the nasal vestibule. Stippled area represents beeswax bolus or compensator. (Adapted with permission from Million RR, Cassisi NJ, Hamlin DJ. Nasal vestibule, nasal cavity, and paranasal sinuses. In: Million RR, Cassisi NJ, eds. *Management of head and neck cancer: a multidisciplinary approach.* Philadelphia: JB Lippincott Co, 1984:407–444. © Wolters Kluwer.)

SEQUELAE OF TREATMENT

Surgery

- Complications of ethmoid sinus surgery include total blindness, loss of ocular motility, hemorrhage, meningitis, cerebrospinal fluid leak, cellulitis, pansinusitis, brain abscess, stroke, fistula between the cavernous sinus and internal carotid artery, and damage to the frontal lobe.
- Complications of maxillectomy include failure of the split-thickness graft to heal, trismus, cerebrospinal fluid leak, and hemorrhage.

Radiation Therapy

- Complications of irradiation of nasal cavity or paranasal sinus tumors include central nervous system damage, unilateral or bilateral vision loss, serous otitis media, and chronic sinusitis.
- Long-term complications after irradiation of nasal vestibule cancers have been minimal.
- The optic nerve or retina may receive a substantial amount of radiation in patients with tumor in the ethmoid or sphenoid sinuses. Radiation retinopathy is rare at 45 Gy after conventional fractions of irradiation. Nakissa et al. (26) reported decreased visual acuity only in patients receiving over 65 Gy. Monroe et al. reported a 4% rate of radiation retinopathy below 50 Gy, with escalating toxicity above 50 Gy that was minimized with hyperfractionation (27). Parsons et al. (28) reported no optic nerve injury in patients receiving less than 59 Gy (less than or equal to 1.9 Gy per day); however, the 15-year actuarial incidence of optic nerve injury reached 11% for doses above 60 Gy.

References

1. Jiang GL, Ang KK, Peters LJ, et al. Maxillary sinus carcinomas: natural history and results of postoperative radiotherapy. *Radiother Oncol* 1991;21(3):193–200. http://www.ncbi.nlm.nih.gov/pubmed/1924855. Accessed September 20, 2017.

2. Jeannon J-P, Riddle PJ, Irish J, et al. Prognostic indicators in carcinoma of the nasal vestibule. *Clin Otolaryngol* 2007;32(1):19–23. doi:10.1111/j.1365-2273.2007.01353.x.

3. Bridger MW, van Nostrand AW. The nose and paranasal sinuses—applied surgical anatomy. A histologic study of whole organ sections in three planes. *J Otolaryngol Suppl* 1978;6:1–33. http://www.ncbi.nlm.nih.gov/pubmed/282450. Accessed September 20, 2017.

4. McCollough WM, Mendenhall NP, Parsons JT, et al. Radiotherapy alone for squamous cell carcinoma of the nasal vestibule: management of the primary site and regional lymphatics. *Int J Radiat Oncol Biol Phys* 1993;26(1):73–79. http://www.ncbi.nlm.nih.gov/pubmed/8482633. Accessed September 20, 2017.

5. Wallace A, Morris CG, Kirwan J, et al. Radiotherapy for squamous cell carcinoma of the nasal vestibule. *Am J Clin Oncol* 2007;30(6):612–616. doi:10.1097/COC.0b013e31815aff1f.

6. Raveh E, Feinmesser R, Shpitzer T, et al. Inverted papilloma of the nose and paranasal sinuses: a study of 56 cases and review of the literature. *Isr J Med Sci* 1996;32(12):1163–1167. http://www.ncbi.nlm.nih.gov/pubmed/9007145. Accessed September 20, 2017.

7. Ahamad A, Ang KK. Nasal cavity and paranasal sinuses. In: Halperin EC, Perez CA, Brady LW, eds. *Principles and practice of radiation oncology*, 5th ed. Philadelphia, PA: Lippincott Williams & Wilkins, 2008:858–873.

8. Frazell EL, Lewis JS. Cancer of the nasal cavity and accessory sinuses. A report of the management of 416 patients. *Cancer* 1963;16:1293–1301. http://www.ncbi.nlm.nih.gov/pubmed/14074213. Accessed September 20, 2017.

9. Ang KK, Jiang GL, Frankenthaler RA, et al. Carcinomas of the nasal cavity. *Radiother Oncol* 1992;24(3):163–168. http://www.ncbi.nlm.nih.gov/pubmed/1410570. Accessed September 20, 2017.

10. Hoppe BS, Stegman LD, Zelefsky MJ, et al. Treatment of nasal cavity and paranasal sinus cancer with modern radiotherapy techniques in the postoperative setting—the MSKCC experience. *Int J Radiat Oncol Biol Phys* 2007;67(3):691–702. doi:10.1016/j.ijrobp.2006.09.023.

11. Hoppe BS, Nelson CJ, Gomez DR, et al. Unresectable carcinoma of the paranasal sinuses: outcomes and toxicities. *Int J Radiat Oncol Biol Phys* 2008;72(3):763–769. doi:10.1016/j.ijrobp.2008.01.038.

12. Lee F, Ogura JH. Maxillary sinus carcinoma. *Laryngoscope* 1981;91(1):133–139. http://www.ncbi.nlm.nih.gov/pubmed/7453460. Accessed September 20, 2017.

13. Le QT, Fu KK, Kaplan MJ, et al. Lymph node metastasis in maxillary sinus carcinoma. *Int J Radiat Oncol Biol Phys* 2000;46(3):541–549. http://www.ncbi.nlm.nih.gov/pubmed/10701732. Accessed September 20, 2017.

14. Kadish S, Goodman M, Wang CC. Olfactory neuroblastoma. A clinical analysis of 17 cases. *Cancer* 1976;37(3):1571–1576. http://www.ncbi.nlm.nih.gov/pubmed/1260676. Accessed September 20, 2017.

15. Dulguerov P, Allal AS, Calcaterra TC. Esthesioneuroblastoma: a meta-analysis and review. *Lancet Oncol* 2001;2(11):683–690. doi:10.1016/S1470-2045(01)00558-7.

16. Monroe AT, Hinerman RW, Amdur RJ, et al. Radiation therapy for esthesioneuroblastoma: rationale for elective neck irradiation. *Head Neck* 2003;25(7):529–534. doi:10.1002/hed.10247.

17. Ozsahin M, Gruber G, Olszyk O, et al. Outcome and prognostic factors in olfactory neuroblastoma: a rare cancer network study. *Int J Radiat Oncol Biol Phys* 2010;78(4):992–997. doi:10.1016/j.ijrobp.2009.09.019.

18. Chen AM, Daly ME, El-Sayed I, et al. Patterns of failure after combined-modality approaches incorporating radiotherapy for sinonasal undifferentiated carcinoma of the head and neck. *Int J Radiat Oncol Biol Phys* 2008;70(2):338–343. doi:10.1016/j.ijrobp.2007.06.057.

19. Al-Mamgani A, van Rooij P, Mehilal R, et al. Combined-modality treatment improved outcome in sinonasal undifferentiated carcinoma: single-institutional experience of 21 patients and review of the literature. *Eur Arch Otorhinolaryngol* 2013;270(1):293–299. doi:10.1007/s00405-012-2008-5.

20. Reiersen DA, Pahilan ME, Devaiah AK. Meta-analysis of treatment outcomes for sinonasal undifferentiated carcinoma. *Otolaryngol Head Neck Surg* 2012;147(1):7–14. doi:10.1177/0194599812440932.

21. Lomax AJ, Goitein M, Adams J. Intensity modulation in radiotherapy: photons versus protons in the paranasal sinus. *Radiother Oncol* 2003;66(1):11–18. http://www.ncbi.nlm.nih.gov/pubmed/12559516. Accessed September 20, 2017.

22. Mock U, Georg D, Bogner J, et al. Treatment planning comparison of conventional, 3D conformal, and intensity-modulated photon (IMRT) and proton therapy for paranasal sinus carcinoma. *Int J Radiat Oncol Biol Phys* 2004;58(1):147–154. http://www.ncbi.nlm.nih.gov/pubmed/14697432. Accessed September 20, 2017.

23. Zenda S, Kohno R, Kawashima M, et al. Proton beam therapy for unresectable malignancies of the nasal cavity and paranasal sinuses. *Int J Radiat Oncol Biol Phys* 2011;81(5):1473–1478. doi:10.1016/j.ijrobp.2010.08.009.

24. Lee DS, Kim YS, Cheon JS, et al. Long-term outcome and toxicity of hypofractionated stereotactic body radiotherapy as a boost treatment for head and neck cancer: the importance of boost volume assessment. *Radiat Oncol* 2012;7(1):85. doi:10.1186/1748-717X-7-85.

25. Parsons JT, Bova FJ, Mendenhall WM, et al. Response of the normal eye to high dose radiotherapy. *Oncology (Williston Park)* 1996;10(6):837–847; discussion 847–848, 851–852. http://www.ncbi.nlm.nih.gov/pubmed/8823799. Accessed September 20, 2017.

26. Nakissa N, Rubin P, Strohl R, et al. Ocular and orbital complications following radiation therapy of paranasal sinus malignancies and review of literature. *Cancer* 1983;51(6):980–986. http://www.ncbi.nlm.nih.gov/pubmed/6336990. Accessed September 20, 2017.

27. Monroe AT, Bhandare N, Morris CG, et al. Preventing radiation retinopathy with hyperfractionation. *Int J Radiat Oncol Biol Phys* 2005;61(3):856–864. doi:10.1016/j.ijrobp.2004.07.664.

28. Parsons JT, Bova FJ, Fitzgerald CR, et al. Radiation optic neuropathy after megavoltage external-beam irradiation: analysis of time-dose factors. *Int J Radiat Oncol Biol Phys* 1994;30(4):755–763. http://www.ncbi.nlm.nih.gov/pubmed/7960976. Accessed September 20, 2017.

CHAPTER 13

SALIVARY GLANDS

ANATOMY

- The salivary glands consist of three large, paired major glands (parotid, submandibular, and sublingual) and many smaller, minor glands located throughout the upper aerodigestive tract (Fig. 13-1).
- Minor salivary glands are widely distributed in the upper aerodigestive tract, palate, buccal mucosa, base of tongue, pharynx, trachea, cheek, lip, gingiva, floor of mouth, tonsil, paranasal sinuses, nasal cavity, and nasopharynx.
- The largest concentration of minor salivary glands is within the hard and soft palates.

Parotid Gland

- The parotid, the largest of the three major salivary glands, is located superficial to and partly behind the ramus of the mandible covering the masseter muscle and largely fills the space anterior to the border of the sternocleidomastoid muscle.
- Superiorly, the parotid gland extends to the zygomatic arch and inferiorly to the angle of the mandible.
- The facial nerve traverses the gland upon exiting the base of the skull at the stylomastoid foramen. It enters the deep surface of the gland as a single trunk, passing postero-laterally to the styloid process and then dividing into branches behind the ramus of the mandible.
- The gland drains into the parotid duct (also known as Stensen's duct) opposite the 2nd upper molar along the oral surface of the cheek.
- The primary lymphatic drainage of the parotid is to the lymph nodes within the gland itself. The majority of these are located in the superficial lobe. Second echelon lymph nodes include the upper cervical levels.

Submandibular Gland

- The submandibular gland fills the triangle between the two bellies of the digastric and the lower border of the mandible and extends upward deeply to the mandible.

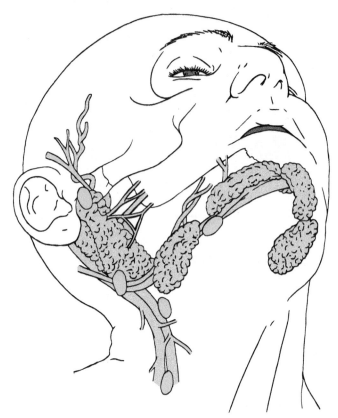

FIGURE 13-1. Anatomy of the salivary glands. (Reprinted with permission from Simpson JR, Lee HK. Salivary glands. In: Perez CA, Brady LW, eds. *Principles and practice of radiation oncology*, 3rd ed. Philadelphia, PA: Lippincott–Raven, 1998:961–980. © Wolters Kluwer.)

- It lies partly on the lower surface of the mylohyoid and partly behind the muscle against the lateral surface of the muscle of the tongue, the hypoglossus.
- The gland drains via the Wharton duct, which opens at the anterior floor of mouth lateral to the lingual frenulum.
- The marginal mandibular branch of the facial nerve runs through the fascia overlying the gland and is an important surgical landmark.
- A fairly rich lymphatic capillary network lies in the interstitial spaces of the gland and drains to submandibular or subdigastric nodes.

Sublingual Gland

- The smallest of the three major salivary glands, the sublingual gland, along with many minor salivary glands, lies between the mucous membrane of the floor of the mouth above, the mylohyoid muscle below, the mandible laterally, and the genioglossus muscles of the tongue medially.
- The sublingual gland drains directly to the floor of mouth through many small ducts.

- This is a rare site for malignant neoplasms, which often are combined with minor salivary gland tumors originating in the floor of mouth.
- The sublingual gland drains either to the submandibular lymph nodes or, more posteriorly, into the deep internal jugular chain.

NATURAL HISTORY

- The primary pattern of spread for salivary gland tumors is local invasion of adjacent structures.
- The risk of lymph node involvement increases with increasing T stage, size, and grade. Tumors arising in or involving lymphatic-rich areas and certain histologies are also associated with a greater risk of lymph node involvement.
- As many as 25% of patients with malignant parotid tumors present with lymph node metastases. Lymph node involvement at presentation is common (44%) with submandibular gland malignancies (1).
- High-grade tumors, regardless of histologic type, have a high (49%) risk of occult lymph node metastasis, compared with only a 7% risk for intermediate- or low-grade tumors (1).
- Adenoid cystic carcinoma patients have the lowest frequency of cervical node metastases—approximately 7.5% at diagnosis—and thus do not routinely require prophylactic management (2). Perineural invasion, however, is more common.
- Tumors in the minor salivary glands account for approximately 23% of all salivary gland neoplasms; 88% of them are malignant (3).
- The rate of cervical lymph node metastasis is about 40% for high-grade minor salivary gland tumors. Overall, adenocarcinoma had a 21.3% rate of metastasis, followed by mucoepidermoid tumors with a 15.8% rate (4).

CLINICAL PRESENTATION

- The most common presentation is a painless, enlarging mass.
- Patients may present with a mass for years before a sudden change in its indolent growth pattern prompts them to seek medical attention.
- Patients with perineural invasion may present with facial nerve weakness, numbness, or other cranial neuropathies.

DIAGNOSTIC WORKUP

- The diagnostic workup of major salivary gland tumors includes a careful history and physical examination, with particular attention to signs of local fixation, regional adenopathy, and potential nerve involvement.
- Computed tomography is useful in evaluating the extent of lesions involving the parotid gland, especially the deep lobe.

- Magnetic resonance imaging provides excellent anatomic detail and may be useful for detecting perineural invasion.
- Fine needle aspiration is the usual biopsy method for parotid and submandibular tumors as it has been shown to be safe and accurate (5).

STAGING SYSTEM

- The American Joint Committee on Cancer (AJCC) staging system for major (parotid, submandibular, and sublingual) salivary gland sites is based on size, extension, nodal involvement, and the presence or absence of extranodal extension (ENE) (6).
- Major changes to staging from the AJCC 7th to 8th edition of major salivary gland tumors include the addition of ENE to the clinical and pathologic N staging as follows:
  - Any nodes with clinically overt ENE are classified as N3b.
  - Metastasis in a single ipsilateral lymph node, 3 cm or smaller with ENE, is considered pN2a.
  - Metastasis in a single ipsilateral lymph node, more than 3 cm with ENE, or metastasis in multiple ipsilateral, contralateral, or bilateral nodes with ENE is considered pN3b.
- A formal staging system has not been developed for minor gland tumors, but similar to major salivary gland tumors, significant local extension or lymph node metastases confer a poor prognosis.

PATHOLOGIC CLASSIFICATION

- Salivary gland tumors show an unparalleled range of pathologic diversity.
- The latest World Health Organization (WHO) classification of salivary gland tumors incorporates key genetic translocations and gene fusions when diagnosing certain tumor types (7).
- Commonly encountered malignant histologies include acinic cell carcinoma, mucoepidermoid carcinoma, adenoid cystic carcinoma, adenocarcinoma, and carcinoma ex pleomorphic adenoma. Common benign tumors include pleomorphic adenoma, myoepithelioma, Warthin tumor, and oncocytoma.
- The most common malignant cell type of major salivary gland tumors is mucoepidermoid carcinoma. Adenoid cystic carcinoma is the most common malignant cell type of the minor salivary glands, and the palate is the most common single site.
- Primary squamous cell carcinomas of the parotid gland are rare, but lymph node metastases from skin cancer commonly present as parotid masses. The diagnosis of squamous cell carcinoma within a parotid mass should prompt an evaluation for a separate primary skin cancer.
- Most parotid masses are benign. In one series, only 21% of 231 parotid masses were malignant (8).

- Salivary gland tumors in children are rare, but the most common malignant subtype of parotid tumors in children is the mucoepidermoid tumor, accounting for almost 50% of cases. Fifty-seven percent of parotid gland tumors in children are malignant, compared with only 15% to 25% in adults (9).
- Acinic cell carcinoma usually occurs only in the parotid gland (10).

PROGNOSTIC FACTORS

- Survival is influenced most by tumor type, grade, postsurgical residual disease, tumor size, nerve invasion, and presence of lymph node or distant metastases.
- There is a growing understanding of the molecular pathogenesis of salivary gland malignancies. Mutations involving the PIK3CA and epidermal growth factor receptor (EGFR) pathways among others have recently been elucidated and may represent novel therapeutic targets for these tumors.

GENERAL MANAGEMENT

Major Salivary Gland

- General management in most patients includes surgical excision followed by radiation therapy for high-risk features.
- Postoperative irradiation should be considered for microscopic or macroscopic residual disease, recurrent cancer, intermediate- and high-grade tumors, and all adenoid cystic carcinomas. Tumors with perineural invasion, lymphovascular space invasion, lymph node metastases, and T3-4 malignancies, and low-grade tumors with tumor spillage may also benefit from adjuvant radiation.
- Low-grade tumors of the parotid are usually treated with a superficial parotidectomy, unless the lesion begins in the deep lobe.
- A neck dissection is not electively done for low-grade tumors as the rate of lymph node metastases is low (11).
- Surgical treatment includes neck dissection in patients with clinically positive nodes or high-grade, high-stage disease.
- Removal of all or part of the parotid gland demands meticulous dissection if the facial nerve is to be spared.
- If the facial nerve is not involved by tumor, a nerve-sparing operation is generally done. If the facial nerve is involved, reconstruction of the facial nerve trunk by a cable nerve graft with the sural or greater auricular nerve decreases the incidence of postoperative facial palsy.
- The benefit of radiation therapy following surgery has not been studied in a prospective, randomized manner. Several retrospective series have demonstrated a significant local control benefit to adjuvant radiation following surgery for patients with high-risk salivary gland tumors. The expected local control following surgery and radiation is approximately 50% to 90% depending on the stage and grade of the tumor (12,13,26).

- Definitive radiation therapy is indicated for medically inoperable or unresectable cancers.
- High linear energy transfer (LET) radiation, such as neutron therapy, has been advocated for advanced and recurrent neoplasms, particularly of the parotid gland. Local control rates of 67% for major and 50% for minor salivary gland tumors have been achieved (14). The adjuvant setting in which neutron therapy is most likely to be advantageous over photon therapy is in patients with gross residual disease (15).
- A small randomized trial of photon versus neutron therapy in inoperable parotid carcinoma found that neutrons provided superior locoregional control (56% versus 17%) but with more severe toxicity and no survival benefit (16).
- Review of world literature found a locoregional control rate of 67% for fast neutrons but only 25% for photons or electrons in the treatment of inoperable, unresectable, or recurrent disease (17).
- Adjuvant chemotherapy has not proven to be efficacious and should be reserved for the clinical trial or palliative setting.

Minor Salivary Gland

- Treatment of minor salivary gland tumors varies with tumor location but generally first involves an attempt at adequate surgical excision.
- Irradiation has been used in surgically inaccessible sites and has also been combined with surgery in cases of locally aggressive tumors and incomplete resection.
- Surgery alone may be adequate to treat early-stage hard palate lesions without evidence of positive margins, perineural spread, or bone invasion, especially in young patients.
- Although surgery generally is given first consideration, irradiation alone may be used as an alternative for early lesions in which surgery would cause significant functional or cosmetic morbidity.
- Small retrospective series have shown improved locoregional control for the addition of adjuvant radiation following surgery with results similar to those of major salivary gland tumors (18,19).

RADIATION THERAPY TECHNIQUES

Parotid Gland

- Two classic approaches to treating parotid tumors were used frequently in the past. The wedged pair technique used unilateral anterior and posterior wedged-pair fields, using 4- to 6-MV photons (Fig. 13-2). The second technique used homolateral fields with 12- to 16-MeV electrons, either alone or in combination with photons. Usually, 80% of the dose was delivered with electrons and 20% with ^{60}Co or 4- to 6-MV photons; this was to spare the opposite salivary gland, reduces mucositis, and decreases the skin reaction produced by electrons.

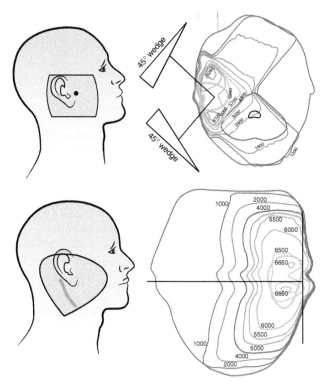

FIGURE 13-2. Unilateral wedge arrangement for parotid treatment and isodose distribution using wedged-pair oblique portals. (Reprinted with permission from Simpson JR, Lee HK. Salivary glands. In: Perez CA, Brady LW, eds. *Principles and practice of radiation oncology*, 3rd ed. Philadelphia, PA: Lippincott–Raven, 1998:961–980. © Wolters Kluwer.)

- With the advent of computed tomography (CT)-based planning, these classic techniques have largely been replaced by 3D conformal radiotherapy (3DCRT) or intensity-modulated radiation therapy (IMRT).
- IMRT with five to seven fields may allow optimal coverage while sparing critical structures such as the mandible, cochlea, spinal cord, brain, and oropharynx (see Fig. 13-3). Volumetric modulated arc therapy (VMAT) may further improve conformality and normal tissue sparing.
- In the postoperative patient, different dose levels may be used based on the risk of microscopic involvement either using a simultaneous integrated boost or a sequential boost.
- The entire surgical bed with appropriate margins for microscopic spread (clinical target volume, CTV) is treated to 60 Gy. An additional boost of 6 to 10 Gy can be considered to areas concerning for residual disease. Lower-risk areas (cervical lymphatic in the node-negative, but high-grade patient) may be treated with 50 to 54 Gy.
- Bolus should be used to ensure adequate dosing of the surgical scar or skin when involved.

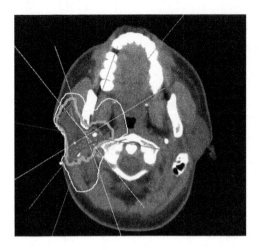

FIGURE 13-3. IMRT target delineation in a patient with parotid cancer. The inner *red* contour is the CTV showing the postoperative tumor bed. The *gray* contour just outside the CTV is the isodose line for an exposure of 60 Gy, and the outer *white* contour is the isodose curve for 50 Gy.

- Careful review of the preoperative imaging and operative report and discussion with the surgeon are imperative in determining the postoperative treatment volume.
- In tumors with a propensity for perineural invasion (adenoid cystic carcinoma), or in cases of named perineural invasion, it is important to cover the cranial nerve pathways from the parotid up to the base of the skull.
- Elective irradiation of the neck should be considered for tumors that have been incompletely excised and for any high-grade lesions, even after complete local excision. The exception to this is the adenoid cystic cell type, which has only a 5% to 10% frequency of occult nodal metastasis.
- Proton beam therapy may further improve normal tissue sparing and the acute toxicity profile for unilateral targets (20).

Submandibular Gland

- The entire ipsilateral neck and submandibular area should be irradiated, following the indications outlined for parotid tumors; technical considerations are similar.
- In cases of named perineural invasion, the dose should be escalated to 60 to 66 Gy, and the nerve path should be treated to the base of skull.

Pleomorphic Adenoma

- The pleomorphic adenoma (benign mixed tumor) is histologically benign and accounts for 65% to 75% of all parotid epithelial tumors.
- Standard therapy has been conservative (superficial) parotidectomy, with recurrence rates ranging from 0% to 5% (21).
- Indications for postoperative irradiation may include the following:
  - Involvement of the deep lobe of the parotid, which would require sacrificing the facial nerve
  - Histologically proven recurrences, with deeper infiltration in successive presentations

- Large (greater than 5 cm) lesions, which may not allow complete surgical excision with adequate margins
- Microscopically positive margins after surgical resection
- Malignant transformation within a predominantly benign tumor
- The cumulative risk of recurrence after surgery and irradiation is 8% at 20 years (22).

Minor Salivary Gland

- The radiation therapy technique for treating minor salivary gland tumors depends on the area involved and is similar to the treatment for squamous cell carcinoma in these areas, with two significant exceptions.
- For adenoid cystic carcinomas, which have a high propensity for perineural invasion and local spread for considerable distances, coverage of major nerve trunks to the base of the skull is emphasized, especially for palate lesions. IMRT may be helpful in reducing the dose to critical structures.
- Because the incidence of lymph node metastases is generally lower than that for squamous cell carcinoma of similar size, the irradiation fields are rarely extended to cover these areas if there are no palpable lymph node metastases. However, when the primary tumor arises from the oral tongue, floor of mouth, pharynx, or larynx, risk of lymph node metastasis is higher and irradiation of the undissected neck is indicated (23).
- For patients receiving postoperative irradiation after surgical resection, 60 Gy is given for negative margins and 66 Gy for microscopically positive margins.
- For gross residual disease after surgery or for lesions treated with irradiation alone, a total dose of 70 Gy is given in 2-Gy fractions.
- An improved control rate with postoperative irradiation has been demonstrated, particularly for high-grade adenoid cystic carcinoma and adenocarcinoma (24). Local tumor control rates with combined-modality therapy for these tumors approach 80% at 5 years (25).
- The University of Florida reported on 101 patients with adenoid cystic carcinoma, the majority presenting in minor salivary gland sites, and found 5-year local control rates of 56% for irradiation alone and 94% for surgery plus irradiation (23).

SEQUELAE OF TREATMENT

- The most notable complication of treatment of parotid malignancies is facial nerve paralysis, which is often caused by the initial (or a repeated) surgical procedure.
- Other postoperative sequelae, such as salivary fistulas and neuromas of the greater auricular nerve, are sometimes seen.
- Partial xerostomia after irradiation is frequently observed and may be permanent.
- Severe xerostomia (long-term salivary function less than 25% of baseline) can usually be avoided if at least one parotid gland has been spared to a mean dose of less than approximately 20 Gy or if both glands have been spared to a mean dose of less than approximately 25 Gy.

- For IMRT planning, the mean dose to each parotid gland should be kept as low as possible, consistent with the desired CTV coverage. A lower mean dose to the parotid gland usually results in better function, even for relatively low mean doses (less than 10 Gy). Similarly, the mean dose to the parotid gland should still be minimized, consistent with adequate target coverage, even if one or both cannot be kept to a threshold of less than 20 or less than 25 Gy. When it can be deemed oncologically safe, submandibular gland sparing to modest mean doses (less than 35 Gy to see any effect) might reduce xerostomia ms.

References

1. Armstrong JG, Harrison LB, Spiro RH, et al. Malignant tumors of major salivary gland origin. A matched-pair analysis of the role of combined surgery and postoperative radiotherapy. *Arch Otolaryngol Head Neck Surg* 1990;116:290–293.
2. Leafstedt SW, Gaeta JF, Sako K, et al. Adenoid cystic carcinoma of major and minor salivary glands. *Am J Surg* 1971;122(6):756–762.
3. McGregor GI, Robins RE. Submandibular and minor salivary gland carcinoma: a 15-year review. *Am Surg* 1977;43(11):737–742.
4. Lloyd S, Yu JB, Ross DA, et al. A prognostic index for predicting lymph node metastasis in minor salivary gland cancer. *Int J Radiat Oncol Biol Phys* 2010;76(1):169–175.
5. Postema RJ, van Velthuysen MF, van den Brakel MWM, et al. Accuracy of fine-needle aspiration cytology of salivary gland lesions in the Netherlands Cancer Institute. *Head Neck* 2004;26:418–424
6. AJCC: Amin MB, Edge SB, Greene FL, et al., eds. *AJCC cancer staging manual,* 8th ed. New York, NY: American Joint Committee on Cancer, 2017.
7. Seethala RR, Stenman G. Update from the 4th Edition of the World Health Organization Classification of Head and Neck Tumours: Tumors of the Salivary Gland. *Head Neck Pathol* 2017;11:55–67.
8. Byrne MN, Spector JG. Parotid masses: evaluation, analysis, and current management. *Laryngoscope* 1988;98(1):99–105.
9. Castro EB, Huvos AG, Strong EW, et al. Tumors of the major salivary glands in children. *Cancer* 1972;29(2):312–317.
10. Chong GC, Beahrs OH, Woolner LB. Surgical management of acinic cell carcinoma of the parotid gland. *Surg Gynecol Obstet* 1974;138(1):65–68.
11. Ozawa H, Tomita T, Sakamoto K, et al. Mucoepidermoid carcinoma of the head and neck: clinical analysis of 43 patients. *Jpn J Clin Oncol* 2008;38:414–418.
12. Armstrong JG, Harrison LB, Thaler HT, et al. The indications for elective treatment of the neck in cancer of the major salivary glands. *Cancer* 1992;69(3):615–619.
13. North CA, Lee DJ, Piantadosi S, et al. Carcinoma of the major salivary glands treated by surgery or surgery plus postoperative radiotherapy. *Int J Radiat Oncol Biol Phys* 1990;18:1319–1326.
14. Saroja KR, Mansell J, Hendrickson FR, et al. An update on malignant salivary gland tumors treated with neutrons at Fermilab. *Int J Radiat Oncol Biol Phys* 1987;13(9):1319–1325.
15. Douglas JG, Koh WJ, Austin-Seymour M, et al. Treatment of salivary gland neoplasms with fast neutron radiotherapy. *Arch Otolaryngol Head Neck Surg* 2003;129(9):944–948.
16. Laramore GE, Krall JM, Griffin TW, et al. Neutron versus photon irradiation for unresectable salivary gland tumors: final report of an RTOG-MRC randomized clinical trial. Radiation Therapy Oncology Group. Medical Research Council. *Int J Radiat Oncol Biol Phys* 1993;27(2):235–240.
17. Koh WJ, Laramore G, Griffin T, et al. Fast neutron radiation for inoperable and recurrent salivary gland cancers. *Am J Clin Oncol* 1989;12(4):316–319.

18. Papageorgakis N, Parara E, Petsinis V, et al. A retrospective review of malignant minor salivary gland tumors and a proposed protocol for future care. *Craniomaxillofac Trauma Reconstr* 2011;4:1–10.
19. Strick MJ, Kelly C, Soames JV, et al. Malignant tumours of the minor salivary glands—a 20 year review. *Br J Plast Surg* 2004;57:624–631.
20. Romesser PB, Cahlon O, Scher E, et al. Proton beam radiation therapy results in significantly reduced toxicity compared with intensity-modulated radiation therapy for head and neck tumors that require ipsilateral radiation. *Radiother Oncol* 2016;118:286–292.
21. Witt RL. The significance of the margin in parotid surgery for pleomorphic adenoma. *Laryngoscope* 2002;112(12):2141–2154.
22. Dawson AK, Orr JA. Long-term results of local excision and radiotherapy in pleomorphic adenoma of the parotid. *Int J Radiat Oncol Biol Phys* 1985;11(3):451–455.
23. Mendenhall WM, Morris CG, Amdur RJ, et al. Radiotherapy alone or combined with surgery for adenoid cystic carcinoma of the head and neck. *Head Neck* 2004;26(2):154–162.
24. Simpson JR, Thawley SE, Matsuba HM. Adenoid cystic salivary gland carcinoma: treatment with irradiation and surgery. *Radiology* 1984;151(2):509–512.
25. Million RR, Cassisi JN. Minor salivary gland tumors. In: Million RR, Cassisi JN, eds. *Management of head and neck cancer: a multidisciplinary approach*, 2nd ed. Philadelphia, PA: JB Lippincott Co., 1994.
26. McNaney D, McNeese MD, Guillamondegui OM, et al. Postoperative irradiation in malignant epithelial tumors of the parotid. *Int J Radiat Oncol Biol Phys* 1983;9(9):1289–1295.
27. Parsons JT, Mendenhall WM, Stringer SP, et al. Management of minor salivary gland carcinomas. *Int J Radiat Oncol Biol Phys* 1996;35(3):443–454.

CHAPTER 14

ORAL CAVITY

ANATOMY

- The oral cavity consists of the upper and lower lips, buccal mucosa, upper and lower gingiva (including alveolar ridge), retromolar trigone, hard palate, floor of the mouth, and the anterior two thirds of the mobile tongue.
- The lips are composed of orbicularis muscle, which is covered by skin and mucous membrane on the inner surface. The transitional area between the two is the vermilion border. Blood is supplied through the labial artery, a branch of the facial artery. The motor nerve branches emerge from the facial nerve. The infraorbital branch of the maxillary nerve serves as the sensory nerve to the upper lip, whereas the lower lip is served by branches of the mental nerve, which originates in the inferior alveolar nerve. The commissure is partially innervated by the buccal branch of the mandibular nerve.
- The buccal mucosa is made up of the mucous membrane that covers the internal surface of the lips and cheeks (buccinator muscle), extending from the line of attachment of the upper and lower alveolar ridges to the point of contact of the lips (posteriorly) and the orbicularis (anteriorly). The masseter muscle lies posterior and lateral to the buccinator muscle. The blood supply comes from the facial artery. Sensory fibers are supplied by the buccal nerve, which is a branch of the mandibular nerve. The motor nerve to the buccinator muscle is derived from the facial nerve.
- The upper gingiva is formed by the alveolar ridge of the maxilla, which is covered by mucosa and the teeth; it continues medially with the hard palate. The lower gingiva covers the mandible from the gingivobuccal sulcus to the mucosa of the floor of the mouth. It continues posteriorly with the retromolar trigone and above with the maxillary tuberosity. There are no minor salivary glands in the mucous membrane over the alveolar ridges.
- The retromolar trigone is a small triangular surface posterior to the third mandibular molar, overlying the ascending ramus. Its borders are the maxillary tuberosity superiorly, anterior tonsillar pillar medially, gingivobuccal sulcus laterally, and posterior aspect of the third molar tooth inferoanteriorly.
- The hard palate makes up the anterior two thirds of the palate, which forms the roof of the oral cavity and floor of the nasal cavity. It is formed by the palatine processes of the maxilla and the horizontal plates of the palatine bones and is covered by a mucous

membrane overlying the periosteum. The hard palate is bound posteriorly by the soft palate and anteriorly and laterally by the maxillary alveolar ridge and gingiva.

- The floor of the mouth is bounded by the lower gingiva anteriorly and laterally and extends to the insertion of the anterior tonsillar pillar into the tongue posteriorly. It is divided into halves by the lingual frenulum and is covered by a mucous membrane with stratified squamous epithelium. The sublingual glands lie below the mucous membrane and are separated by the midline genioglossus and geniohyoid muscles. The genial tubercles are bony protuberances occurring at the point of insertion of these two muscle groups on the mandibular symphysis. Muscles include the mylohyoid and digastric muscles. The submandibular glands are located on the external surface of the mylohyoid muscle between its insertion to the mandible. The submandibular duct (Wharton's duct) is approximately 5 cm long and courses between the sublingual gland and genioglossus muscle; its orifice is in the anterior floor of the mouth, near the midline. The sensory nerve is the lingual nerve, a branch of the submandibular nerve. The arterial supply is the lingual artery, a branch of the external carotid artery.
- The tongue is a muscular organ composed of the styloglossus, hyoglossus, and stylohyoid muscles (Fig. 14-1). It is covered by a mucous membrane with stratified squamous epithelium. The circumvallate papillae, situated posteriorly with a V-shaped configuration, separate the base of the tongue from the mobile, oral tongue. The oral tongue consists of the tip, dorsum, lateral borders, and ventral surface. The blood supply is the lingual artery, a branch of the external carotid artery. The sensory nerve is the lingual nerve, a branch of the maxillary nerve; the hypoglossal nerve is the motor nerve. The taste buds are innervated by the chorda tympani branch of the sensory root of the facial nerve.

EPIDEMIOLOGY AND RISK FACTORS

- The incidence of oral cavity cancer is 4.3 patients per 100,000 in the United States (1).
- The majority of cases occur in people aged 50 and over, and the median age of diagnosis is 62 (2).
- Oral cavity cancers are more common in men than in women.
- Risk factors include tobacco use, alcohol (in synergy with smoking), betel nut use, lip trauma, poor dental hygiene, human papillomavirus, and prior radiation exposure.

HISTOLOGY

- The overwhelming predominant histology in oral cavity malignancies is squamous cell carcinoma.
- Minor salivary gland tumors may arise in the oral cavity. Adenoid cystic and mucoepidermoid carcinomas account for 2% to 3% of the floor of mouth tumors and can also be found among hard palate primaries.
- Basal cell carcinoma can occur, most commonly, on the upper lip.
- Verrucous carcinoma can occur in the buccal mucosa.

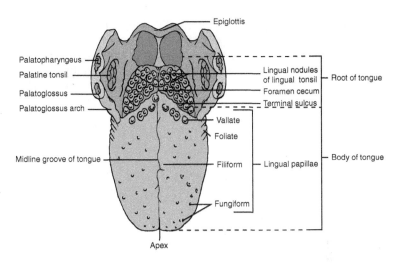

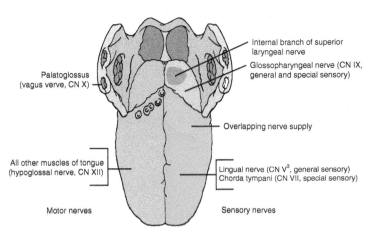

FIGURE 14-1. Musculature of the tongue and floor of the oral cavity. (Reprinted with permission from Agur AMR, Dalley AF, eds. *Grant's atlas of anatomy*, 12th ed. Philadelphia: Lippincott, Williams & Wilkins, 2009:676. © Wolters Kluwer.)

NATURAL HISTORY AND PATTERNS OF SPREAD

Lip

- Tumors commonly start on the vermilion of the lower lip, less commonly the upper lip, and rarely the commissure.
- Leukoplakia may precede carcinoma for many years.
- Lesions can invade adjacent skin, orbicularis oris muscle, lip commissures, buccal mucosa, and eventually the mandible and mental nerve.
- Lymphatics of the upper lip drain mostly to the submandibular lymph nodes, although the periauricular, parotid, and subdigastric lymph nodes also occasionally

receive lymphatic channels from the upper lip. Lower lip lymphatics drain to the submandibular, submental, and subdigastric lymph nodes.

- Lymph nodes are involved at presentation in up to 20% of patients with lip cancer, and risk increases with depth of invasion, grade, size, and involvement of the commissure (3,4). Upper lip cancers are more likely to have LN involvement than lower lip.

Buccal Mucosa

- Lymphatic drainage of the buccal mucosa is primarily to the submandibular and subdigastric lymph nodes.
- For cancers of the buccal mucosa, the incidence of positive cervical lymph nodes on presentation is 10% to 30% (5).

Gingiva

- Over 75% of gingival carcinomas arise from the lower gingiva, and the majority of these are posterior to the bicuspid (6).
- Tumors can invade the underlying bone, retromolar trigone, adjacent buccal mucosa, and floor of the mouth.
- Lymphatics of the gingiva drain to the submandibular and subdigastric lymph nodes, with up to 16% patients with clinically positive nodes at diagnosis (7).
- The incidence of lymph node metastases of the upper gingiva is 15% to 20% on presentation (7). There is approximately the same incidence of later development of clinical cervical lymph node metastases in initially clinically negative necks (8).

Retromolar Trigone

- Tumors can have bone invasion in up to 25% of cases at diagnosis (9).
- Lymphatics drain primarily to the submandibular and subdigastric nodes.

Hard Palate

- Incidence is relatively rare and are most often adenoid cystic or mucoepidermoid carcinomas arising from minor salivary glands.
- Hard palate tumors may invade into the maxillary sinus and soft palate. Adenoid cystic carcinomas can spread along V2 into the middle cranial fossa.
- Risk of lymph node involvement in hard palate cancers is 13% to 26% at diagnosis (10).

Floor of the Mouth

- Tumors can extend toward the gingiva, tongue, mandibular periosteum, and into the genioglossus/geniohyoid muscles.
- The first echelon of lymph node drainage of the floor of the mouth is to the submandibular, subdigastric, and submental lymph nodes.

- Approximately 30% to 65% of patients with cancer of the floor of the mouth and oral tongue have positive neck nodes on presentation (11). Of patients with clinically negative nodes, approximately 21% to 62% have pathologically positive nodes (12).
- Submental lymph nodes are involved in fewer than 5% of patients (11).
- Lymph node risks increase with depth of invasion, grade, lymphovascular, and perineural invasion (12).

Oral Tongue

- Tumors occur on the lateral and ventral surfaces.
- Primary lymphatic drainage in the oral tongue is to the submental, subdigastric, and submandibular lymph nodes. Rouviére (13) described the lymphatic trunks that bypass this primary lymphatic drainage and go directly to the mid-jugular lymph nodes, which probably accounts for the relative frequency of metastatic lymph nodes in these locations (Fig. 14-2).
- Fifteen to seventy-five percent of patients have clinically positive nodes at diagnosis, depending on T stage, and 5% to 10% have bilateral lymph node metastases (8).

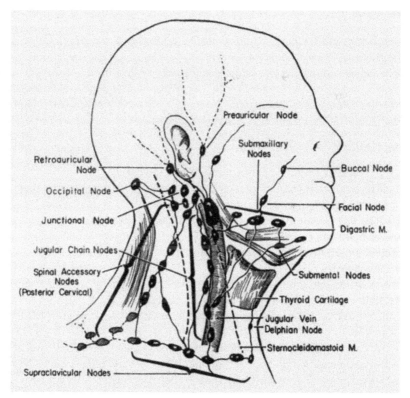

FIGURE 14-2. Lymphatic drainage of the oral cavity and nasopharynx. (Reprinted with permission from Lee AWM, et al. Nasopharynx. In: Halperin EC, Perez CA, Brady LW, eds. *Principles and practice of radiation oncology*, 5th ed. Philadelphia, PA: Lippincott Williams & Wilkins, 2008. © Wolters Kluwer.)

PRESENTATION

- Clinical presentation includes enlarging mass, pain, bleeding, foul odor, speech changes, swallowing difficulty, ear pain, trismus, loose teeth, nonhealing ulcer, ill-fitting dentures, facial numbness, and/or weakness.

WORKUP

- History and physical examination, including complete head and neck and cranial nerve exam, mirror, and/or fiberoptic examination as indicated.
- Biopsy and, if indicated, examination under anesthesia.
- CT and/or MRI with contrast, consider PET/CT for stages III to IV disease.
- Panorex can be used to assess bone invasion.
- Chest imaging as clinically indicated.
- Dental, nutrition, and speech and swallow evaluation.

STAGING

- The staging system for oral cavity lesions can be found in the *AJCC Cancer Staging Manual*.
- The box below summarizes the changes made in the 8th edition.

NEW!   **SUMMARY OF CHANGES TO AJCC STAGING**

ORAL CAVITY

- T1 will be size ≤2 cm AND ≤5 mm depth of invasion (DOI)
- T2 will be size ≤2 cm AND DOI greater than 5 mm and ≤10 mm or greater than 2 cm but ≤4 cm AND ≤10 mm DOI
- T3 will be size greater than 4 cm or *any tumor* greater than 10 mm DOI
- cN3 will be *clinical* extranodal extension (ENE)
- Positive single pathologic lymph node (ipsilateral or contralateral) size ≤3 cm AND ENE(+) will be N2a
- Positive pathologic lymph node size greater than 3 cm but ≤6 cm AND ENE(+) will be N3b
- Multiple positive pathologic lymph nodes in ipsilateral neck ≤6 cm AND ENE(+) will be N3b
- Positive pathologic contralateral lymph nodes (greater than 1) AND ENE(+) will be N3b
- Positive pathologic lymph node size greater than 6 cm and ENE(−) will be N3a
- Positive pathologic lymph node size greater than 6 cm AND ENE(+) will be N3b

See: Amin MB, Edge SB, Greene FL, et al., eds. *AJCC cancer staging manual*, 8th ed. New York, NY: Springer, 2017.

GENERAL MANAGEMENT

- A variety of therapeutic measures is available for managing carcinomas of the oral cavity, including surgery, laser excision, radiation therapy, chemotherapy, and combinations of these methods.
- Upfront surgery is typically recommended because of the acute and chronic toxicity of definitive RT to the oral cavity.
- Postoperative irradiation is recommended for pT3-4 lesions, close or positive margins, perineural invasion, lymphovascular invasion, N2-3, level IV or V lymph node, and/or extracapsular nodal spread. It is also recommended for patients with initially positive surgical margins who later have negative surgical margins on reexcision (14).
- Postoperative chemotherapy combined with radiation is indicated for patients with positive margins or extracapsular nodal spread (15).
- If the patient is medically inoperable or refuses surgery, definitive RT (often with concurrent chemotherapy) is a reasonable treatment option.
- Smoking cessation is imperative to improve chance of cure and survival.

Surgical Technique and Site-Specific Considerations

- Surgery should consist of complete tumor resection *en bloc* with at least 0.5- to 1-cm margins from invasive tumor to the specimen edge.
- Frozen section analysis of margins should be conducted intraoperatively as indicated.
- Because of the proximity of the mandible and maxilla, surgical removal of bone may be required to obtain negative margins. Reconstruction is usually performed in conjunction with these extensive surgeries.

Lip

- For less than 4-cm lesions, wide local excision can be performed with minimal reconstruction required.
- For tumors involving greater than 50% of the lip, a flap reconstruction is required following wide local excision. Although cosmetic outcome is usually good, functional outcome is poor (decreased perioral sensation, oral incontinence, and microstomia) compared to RT.

Gingiva

- Transoral resection is adequate for small gingival primaries though rim resections are needed in most cases.
- If bone is involved, then a segment of mandible/maxilla may need to be removed.

Hard Palate

- Upfront surgery is typically recommended for minor salivary gland cancers of the hard palate and other sites of the oral cavity.

Floor of the Mouth

- In the floor of mouth lesions that are tethered or fixed to the mandible, resection of the inner table is often recommended; this results in reasonable speech and swallowing.
- For advanced lesions because of bone invasion, composite resection of tumor along with segmental resection of the mandible is often followed by reconstruction of the floor of the mouth and mandible.
- For very advanced disease involving the floor of the mouth, tongue, and mandible, and for massive neck disease, the chance of cure with any aggressive treatment is low and is often associated with formidable complications. In these cases, a course of definitive chemoradiation should strongly be considered instead of upfront surgery.

Oral Tongue

- Partial glossectomy is the treatment of choice for well-circumscribed lesions that can be excised transorally with at least a 0.5- to 1-cm margin.
- Wide local excision of lesions of the posterior part of the mobile tongue can result in serious functional deficits in swallowing and speech without reconstruction. External radiation and/or interstitial implant may be used for these patients.
- The extent of surgery for larger lesions is usually hemi- or total glossectomy.

Management of Neck Nodes

- In patients with small oral tongue lesions (thickness of less than 2 mm) resected with adequate margins and no poor prognostic factors, observation can be considered if the neck is clinically and radiographically negative.
- In patients with resected primary lesions of the oral tongue that are more than 2 to 3 mm thick, or with poor prognostic factors such as perineural or lymphovascular invasion, neck dissection is recommended (16).
- A recent trial randomized patients with T1-2 oral cavity squamous cell carcinoma to elective or therapeutic neck dissection (watchful waiting followed by neck dissection at relapse) and found that elective neck dissection was associated with improved disease-free and overall survival (16).
- A retrospective study of patients with T1-2N0 oral tongue squamous cell carcinoma treated with partial glossectomy and ipsilateral neck dissection demonstrated a recurrence rate of 5.7% for tumors less than 4 mm and 24% for tumors ≥4 mm. Recurrence was contralateral in 39% of patients (17).
- If neck dissection reveals only one positive node less than 3 cm (N1) with no extracapsular extension, adjuvant radiation therapy to the neck is not indicated. If neck dissection shows more than one node involved, metastases at more than one nodal station, or extracapsular extension of a single or multiple nodes, a course of postoperative irradiation to the neck is indicated.
- In patients with clinically or radiographically positive neck nodes (by computed tomography scan with contrast and/or PET scan), treatment of choice for the neck is neck dissection followed by postoperative neck irradiation, as indicated.

- Contralateral prophylactic neck dissection is controversial in early-stage patients but is indicated in locally advanced disease.
- Sentinel lymph node biopsy is now being used for patients with early-stage oral cavity cancers in select centers (18).

RADIATION THERAPY TECHNIQUES

- Optimal oral hygiene and pretreatment dental care are of utmost importance in patients in whom radiation therapy is contemplated. All patients with teeth should be seen by a dentist or oral surgeon for dental evaluation and fluoride treatment.
- Any potential surgical procedures and tooth extractions should be carried out before initiation of irradiation. Approximately 8 to 10 days lapse-time is needed for complete recovery before initiation of radiation therapy.
- After a course of radiation, tooth extraction or any other oral procedure carries a lifelong increased risk of complications. Awareness of this issue by radiation oncologists, dentists, oral surgeons, and, especially, patients is an important factor in reducing potential complications of radiation therapy.
- Ideally, postoperative radiation therapy should be initiated 4 to 6 weeks after surgery.

External Beam Radiation Therapy

- The most commonly used technique for carcinoma of the oral cavity is intensity-modulated radiation therapy (IMRT). Advantages over conventional RT include reducing tissue toxicity including reduced dose to the parotid glands and the mandible as well as a reduction in mucositis.
- Patients are simulated supine with neck extended, immobilized with a thermoplastic head and shoulders mask. IV contrast is recommended if there are no contraindications. Bolus can be considered for disease near the skin.
- The tongue is depressed away from the palate with an individually constructed tongue "bite block" or a cork and tongue blade.
- For postoperative IMRT, clinical target volumes (CTVs) are as follows (Fig. 14-3):
  - CTV high risk, 63 to 66 Gy in 30 to 33 fractions, includes areas of positive margins or extracapsular spread. There will not be a CTV high risk if there is a negative margin and no extracapsular extension.
  - CTV intermediate risk, approximately 60 Gy in 30 fractions, includes preoperative gross disease/tumor bed and lymph nodes at substantial risk for subclinical disease.
  - CTV low risk, approximately 50 Gy, includes nodes at low risk for subclinical disease.
- For definitive IMRT (often administered with concurrent chemotherapy), CTVs are as follows:
  - CTV high risk, 66 to 70 Gy in 30 to 35 fractions, includes the gross tumor volume (GTV) + 5- to 10-mm margin for subclinical disease.

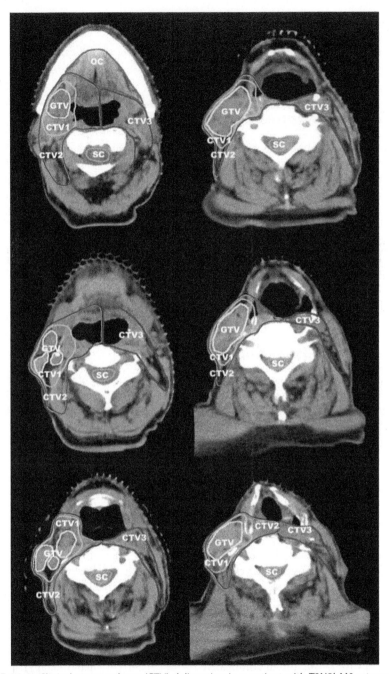

FIGURE 14-3. Clinical target volume (CTV) delineation in a patient with T3N2bM0 retromolar trigone carcinoma who received definitive IMRT. The GTV is contoured in *white*; contours for CTV1 and CTV2 surround the GTV successively. CTV3 is the contour on the right side. OC, oral cavity; SC, spinal cord. (Reprinted with permission from Chao KSC, Apisarnthanarax S, Ozyigt G. *Practical essentials of intensity modulated radiation therapy*. Philadelphia, PA: Lippincott Williams & Wilkins, 2004:163. © Wolters Kluwer.)

- CTV intermediate risk, approximately 60 to 63 Gy, includes nodes at substantial risk for subclinical disease.
- CTV low risk, approximately 50 to 56 Gy, includes nodes at low risk for subclinical disease.
- PTV includes the CTV + 3- to 5-mm margin for setup error.
- Treatment can be delivered either via simultaneous integrated boost (SIB) or sequential boost.
- The CTV intermediate risk typically includes the submandibular and subdigastric lymph nodes. The submental nodes may be included; their coverage is especially important when the lesion is located at the tip of the tongue, anterior floor of the mouth, or lower lip (see below for site-specific considerations).
- The CTV low risk typically includes the ipsilateral low neck and contralateral uninvolved neck, based on primary site and stage. If the ipsilateral low neck is involved, it will require higher doses.
- For patients with cervical nodal metastases, treatment of lower level cervical nodal stations is likely indicated.
- Omission of the contralateral neck is considered for well-lateralized cancers of the buccal mucosa, retromolar trigone, hard palate, or gingiva.
- If treated by radiation alone, larger tumors may require higher doses, potentially with the use of altered fractionation scheme.
- A low anterior neck (LAN) field may be matched to the IMRT plan to spare the larynx.
- For positive margins or extracapsular extension, concurrent chemotherapy (typically cisplatin) is recommended.
- Every attempt should be made to avoid an excessive dose of radiation to the mandible though challenging because of oral cavity primary.

Interstitial Irradiation

- Volume implants are used to cover the primary tumor volume with at least 0.5- to 1.0-cm margin.
- Brachytherapy will not target cervical lymph nodes. If brachytherapy is used alone, it should be used in cases in which lymph node risk is low. If a patient has greater than 10% to 15% risk of lymph node involvement, EBRT can be used to treat the primary tumor and lymph nodes, and a brachytherapy boost can be given to the primary tumor.
- An accepted technique is percutaneous after-loading technique with angiocatheters and iridium-192.
- Implants can be done with a classic low-dose rate (LDR), which delivers approximately 0.4 to 0.5 Gy per hour to the target volume.
  - If LDR alone, then 60 to 70 Gy total over several days.
  - If EBRT + LDR, then 40 to 50 Gy via EBRT and 20 to 35 Gy via LDR.
- High-dose rate (HDR) brachytherapy at 3 to 6 Gy per fraction is also used.
  - If HDR alone, then 45 to 60 Gy total at 3 to 6 Gy per fraction.
  - If EBRT + HDR, then 40 to 50 Gy via EBRT and 21 Gy in 3 Gy per fraction via HDR.

- Interstitial implant alone (for small T1 and T2 tumors) or after external beam irradiation yields good results.
- In patients treated with surgical resection who have microscopic tumor at the margin of resection, an interstitial implant can convert their ominous outcome in local control to that of patients with negative margins (19).

Intraoral Cone

- Intraoral cone is a localized radiation technique suitable for lesions located in the anterior tongue or anterior segment of the floor of the mouth.
- Radiation with intraoral cone uses either 250 keV or electron beams of 6 to 12 MeV.
- The cone is equipped with a device to visualize the target volume and ensure proper coverage.
- Intraoral cone will not target cervical lymph nodes. If intraoral cone is used alone, it should be used in cases in which lymph node risk is low. If a patient has greater than 10% to 15% risk of lymph node involvement, EBRT can be used to treat the primary tumor and lymph nodes, and an intraoral cone boost can be given to the primary tumor.

TREATMENT OF SPECIFIC SUBSITES

Lip

- Small cancers (less than 2 cm) can be cured with surgery or radiation alone in more than 90% of patients, with excellent cosmetic and functional results.
- Tumors of the oral commissure may be best treated with RT instead of surgery because surgery may result in oral incontinence and/or microstomia.
- Larger lesions (greater than 2 cm) also can be treated with either surgery or radiation. However, with surgery, reconstruction with a flap is often necessary. Unfortunately, the reconstructed lip is often functionally problematic. Therefore, RT may be preferred.
- Postoperative irradiation is recommended for patients with adverse postoperative features (see above).
- Regional nodes are not treated in T1-2 cases, unless adverse features are present.
- External beam radiation of 100 to 200 keV and/or electron beam of a suitable energy (6 to 9 MeV with 1.0- to 1.5-cm bolus) can be used.
- Individually designed and constructed lead shields in the gingivobuccal sulcus can be used to protect the underlying gum and mandible.
- For definitive treatment of primary site alone, recommended doses usually are 66 Gy (2.2 Gy per fraction) to 70 Gy (2 Gy per fraction) given daily over 6 to 7 weeks.
- If there is no indication for nodal irradiation, the target volume includes the primary tumor with a 1- to 1.5-cm margin if keV photons are used and a 2- to 2.5-cm margin if electrons are used.
- In smaller lesions, interstitial brachytherapy alone can be used.

- Some practitioners have used external beam irradiation of approximately 50 Gy followed by an interstitial boost of 20 to 35 Gy for tumors greater than 4 cm.

Buccal Mucosa

- Primary surgery is preferred for patients with T1 or superficial T2 lesions that do not involve the oral commissure. The procedure removes the malignancy and eradicates adjacent leukoplakia.
- For T2 lesions and for those involving the commissure, primary radiation is considered because it produces a high cure rate with good functional and cosmetic results.
- For T3 and T4 tumors with deep muscular invasion, cure rates after radiation therapy are poor. These lesions are usually treated with radical surgery, reconstruction, and postoperative radiation (possibly with concurrent chemotherapy).
- For moderately advanced lesions with or without positive nodes, appropriate radiation therapy must include the primary site and regional lymph nodes (at least ipsilateral levels I and II).

Gingiva

- Because bony involvement by carcinoma compromises results of irradiation, careful radiographic examination of the mandible, including CT and Panorex, can be extremely valuable in deciding on the upfront treatment modality.
- Small T1 exophytic lesions without bony involvement can be managed by external beam therapy alone.
- Radical surgery is preferred for advanced lesions associated with destruction of the mandible because partial mandibulectomy with radical neck dissection provides good survival rates (19).
- Postoperative radiation fields include the adjacent segment of the mandible or maxilla. If perineural invasion is present, it may be necessary to cover the entire hemimandible or hemimaxilla from the distal neural foramen to the pterygopalatine ganglion.
- The low neck is irradiated if nodes are positive or if lesions are advanced.

Floor of the Mouth

- When the tumor is small or limited to the mucosa, it is highly curable by surgery or irradiation alone. Surgery is typically preferred to prevent the toxicity associated with oral cavity radiation.
- For extensive, infiltrative T3 and T4 lesions with marked involvement of the adjacent muscle of the tongue and mandible, radical surgery is the procedure of choice, followed by plastic closure and postoperative radiation.
- Very small superficial lesions can be treated with interstitial implant (60 to 65 Gy) or intraoral cone (45 Gy over 3 weeks) alone.

- T1 and early T2 lesions can be treated with external beam radiation and various boost techniques such as interstitial implant (45 Gy external plus 25 Gy with implant) or intraoral cone (45 Gy external plus 20 Gy intraoral cone).
- Management of the neck is similar to that for the oral tongue.

Oral Tongue

- Upfront surgery is typically recommended for oral tongue cancers unless surgery would require severe functional morbidity such as in total glossectomy, in which case definitive chemoradiation may be preferred.
- Although surgery or irradiation is effective in controlling small cancers, it is not unreasonable to consider transoral surgical resection for small, well-defined lesions involving the tip and anterolateral border of the tongue (20). These lesions can be cured by resection without risk of functional morbidity.
- Radiation therapy (60 to 70 Gy in 6 to 7 weeks) can be used for small, posteriorly situated, ill-defined lesions if they are inaccessible for transoral surgical excision.
- Superficial, exophytic T1 and T2 lesions with little muscle involvement are amenable to successful treatment with irradiation (65 to 70 Gy in 7 weeks).
- Tumors with at least 2 mm of depth of invasion require neck dissection (16) and, if adverse features are present, postoperative radiation.
- For locally advanced tumors, surgical treatment may involve composite resection including partial glossectomy, partial mandibulectomy, and neck dissection.
- Advanced disease with deep muscle invasion, which often is associated with cervical lymph node metastases, is unlikely to be cured with irradiation alone and requires a combined modality approach with concurrent chemotherapy.

OUTCOMES AND FOLLOW-UP

- Five-year cause-specific survival (CSS) for lip carcinoma: less than 1 cm primary: 100%, 1 to 3 cm primary: 92%, greater than 3 cm primary: 71%, and bone invasion: 50% (21).
- Three-year CSS for buccal mucosa carcinoma: stage I: 85%, stage II: 63%, stage III: 41%, and stage IV: 15% (22).
- Five-year CSS for retromolar trigone carcinoma: stages I to III: 83% and stage IV: 61% (23).
- Five-year CSS for the floor of mouth carcinoma: stage I: 96%, stage II: 70%, stage III: 67%, and stage IVA: 44% (24).
- Five-year CSS for oral tongue carcinoma: stage I: 71% to 100%, stage II: 50% to 87%, stage III: 25% to 71%, and stage IV: 11% to 40% (25).
- Follow-up includes history and physical exam every 1 to 3 months for year 1, every 2 to 6 months for year 2, every 4 to 8 months for years 3 to 5, and every 12 months thereafter.
- Posttreatment baseline imaging of the head/neck (CT, MRI, or PET/CT) is recommended at approximately 12 weeks and as clinically indicated thereafter.

- Chest imaging is performed as clinically indicated for patients with smoking history.
- Thyroid-stimulating hormone (TSH) should be checked every 6 to 12 months if patient received neck irradiation.
- Dental evaluation at least once every 6 months.
- Speech and swallowing therapy is extremely important during and after therapy.

SEQUELAE OF TREATMENT

Surgical Complications

- Surgical complications are highly dependent on the site and extent of disease but may include infection (5%), wound slough (9.6%), orocutaneous fistula (6.1%), and carotid artery injury (1.1%) (25). Dysarthria, bleeding, aspiration, chronic pain, and eating difficulties are also possible complications.

Radiation Complications

- Major complications include osteoradionecrosis (6.2%), soft tissue necrosis (9.8%), dysphagia (1.3%), flap necrosis (0.4%), orocutaneous fistula (2.7%), carotid hemorrhage (0.4%), and radiation caries (3.1%) (25).
- Other complications include sun sensitivity, mucositis, tongue sensitivity/pain, dysgeusia, dysarthria, taste changes, difficulties with mastication, xerostomia, lymphedema, and fibrosis/trismus.

References

1. Weatherspoon DJ, Chattopadhyay A, Boroumand S, et al. Oral cavity and oropharyngeal cancer incidence trends and disparities in the United States: 2000–2010. *Cancer Epidemiol* 2015;39(4):497–504.
2. Warnakulasuriya S, et al. Global epidemiology of oral and oropharyngeal cancer. *Oral Oncol* 2009;45(4–5):309–316.
3. Cross JE, Guralnick E, Daland EM. Carcinoma of the lip. A review of 563 case records of carcinoma of the lip at the Pondville Hospital. *Surg Gynecol Obstet* 1948;81:153–162.
4. Vartanian JG, et al. Predictive factors and distribution of lymph node metastasis in lip cancer patients and their implications on the treatment of the neck. *Oral Oncol* 2004; 40(2):223–227.
5. MacComb WS, Fletcher GH, Healey JE. Intra-oral cavity. In: MacComb WS, Fletcher GH, eds. *Cancer of the head and neck.* Baltimore, MD: The Williams & Wilkins Co., 1967:89–151.
6. Soo KC, et al. Squamous carcinoma of the gums. *Am J Surg* 1988;156(4):281–285.
7. Byers RM, Newman R, Russell N, et al. Results of treatment for squamous carcinoma of the lower gum. *Cancer* 1981;47:2236–2238.
8. Lindberg R. Distribution of cervical lymph node metastases from squamous cell carcinoma of the upper respiratory and digestive tracts. *Cancer* 1972;29(6):1446–1449.
9. Byers RM, Anderson B, Schwarz EA, et al. Treatment of squamous carcinoma of the retromolar trigone. *Am J Clin Oncol* 1984;7:647–652.

10. Chung CK, Rahman SM, Lim ML, et al. Squamous cell carcinoma of the hard palate. *Int J Radiat Oncol Biol Phys* 1979;5:191–196.

11. Woolgar JA, Scott J. Prediction of cervical lymph node metastasis in squamous cell carcinoma of the tongue/floor of mouth. *Head Neck* 1995;17:463–472.

12. Hicks WJ Jr, et al. Squamous cell carcinoma of the floor of mouth: a 20-year review. *Head Neck* 1997;19(5):400–405.

13. Rouviére H. In: Tobias MJ, translator. *Anatomy of the human lymphatic system.* Ann Arbor, MI: Edwards Brothers, 1938:1–28, 44–56, 77–78.

14. Scholl P, Byers RM, Batsakis JG, et al. Microscopic cut-through of cancer in the surgical treatment of squamous carcinoma of the tongue. Prognostic and therapeutic implications. *Am J Surg* 1986;152(4):354–360.

15. Bernier J, Cooper JS, Pajak TF, et al. Defining risk levels in locally advanced head and neck cancers: a comparative analysis of concurrent postoperative radiation plus chemotherapy trials of the EORTC (#22931) and RTOG (# 9501). *Head Neck* 2005;27(10):843–850.

16. D'Cruz AK, Vaish R, Kapre N, et al.; Head and Neck Disease Management Group. Elective versus therapeutic neck dissection in node-negative oral cancer. *N Engl J Med* 2015;373(6):521–529.

17. Ganly I, et al. Long-term regional control and survival in patients with "low-risk," early stage oral tongue cancer managed by partial glossectomy and neck dissection without postoperative radiation: the importance of tumor thickness. *Cancer* 2013;119(6):1168–1176.

18. Civantos FJ, et al. Sentinel lymph node biopsy accurately stages the regional lymph nodes for T1-T2 oral squamous cell carcinomas: results of a prospective multi-institutional trial. *J Clin Oncol* 2010;28(8):1395–1400.

19. Chao KS, Emami B, Akhileswaran R, et al. The impact of surgical margin status and use of an interstitial implant on T1, T2 oral tongue cancers after surgery. *Int J Radiat Oncol Biol Phys* 1996;36(5):1039–1043.

20. Spiro RH, Spiro JD, Strong EW. Surgical approach to squamous carcinoma confined to the tongue and the floor of the mouth. *Head Neck Surg* 1986;9(1):27–31.

21. Baker SR, Krause CJ. Carcinoma of the lip. *Laryngoscope* 1980;90:19–27.

22. Nair MK, et al. Evaluation of the role of radiotherapy in the management of carcinoma of the buccal mucosa. *Cancer* 1988;61(7):1326.

23. Mendenhall WM, et al. Retromolar trigone squamous cell carcinoma treated with radiotherapy alone or combined with surgery. *Cancer* 2005;103(11):2320.

24. Rodgers LW Jr, Stringer SP, Mendenhall WM, et al. Management of squamous cell carcinoma of the floor of the mouth. *Head Neck* 1993;15:16–19.

25. Sessions DG, Spector GJ, Lenox J, et al. Analysis of treatment results for oral tongue cancer. *Laryngoscope* 2002;112(4):616–625.

CHAPTER 15

OROPHARYNX AND HYPOPHARYNX

OROPHARYNX

Anatomy

- The oropharynx is bounded by the oral cavity anteriorly, the hypopharynx and larynx inferiorly, and the nasopharynx superiorly. It is divided into four subsites: the tonsillar region, base of tongue, lateral and posterior pharyngeal walls, and soft palate (see Fig. 15-1).
- The tonsillar region contains the palatine tonsils and is bounded by the anterior and posterior tonsillar pillars, which are mucosal folds produced by the underlying palatoglossal and palatopharyngeal muscles, respectively.
- The base of tongue is bounded anteriorly by the circumvallate papillae, laterally by the glossotonsillar sulci and the glossopharyngeal sulci posteriorly. Inferiorly, the base of tongue region encompasses the vallecula and is bounded by the superior surface of the hyoid bone (see Fig. 15-2).
- The lateral and posterior walls of the oropharynx are formed by the superior pharyngeal constrictor muscles, whereas the superior border is composed of the inferior surface of the soft palate and uvula.

Etiology

- Tobacco and alcohol use were traditionally reported to be responsible for greater than 80% of oropharyngeal cancers, with the effect dependent on duration and intensity of use (1). The effect on cancer risk of the use of both substances simultaneously is reported to be synergistic (2).
- Infection with high-risk human papillomavirus (HPV) is now recognized to confer a several-fold increased risk of oropharynx cancer (3). HPV-16 is the subtype seen in 85% to 90% of HPV-associated oropharyngeal squamous cell carcinomas (OPSCCs) (4,5).
- HPV-associated and non–HPV-associated OPSCCs are now recognized as distinct clinicopathologic disease entities, with different etiology, natural history (6,7), biomolecular signature (8,9), and treatment responsiveness (10). However, treatment recommendations for these two entities remain the same, pending results of ongoing clinical trials.

291

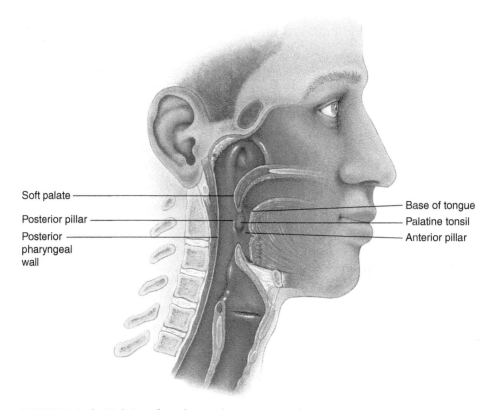

Soft palate

Posterior pillar

Posterior
pharyngeal
wall

Base of tongue

Palatine tonsil

Anterior pillar

FIGURE 15-1. Sagittal view of oropharynx demonstrating subsites.

Epidemiology

- In the United States, the number of new cases of cancers of the "oral cavity and pharynx" was estimated at 48,330 in 2016. Tumors within the oropharynx are thought to represent approximately 25% of this total, or just over 12,000 new cases per year.
- The incidence rate of OPSCC is rising, with a 28% increase from 1998 to 2004, owing to a 225% increase in the incidence of HPV-associated OPSCC despite a 50% decline in the incidence of non–HPV-associated OPSCC. The incidence of HPV-associated OPSSC now accounts for greater than 70% of newly diagnosed OPSCC in the United States (11).

Natural History and Patterns of Spread

- At diagnosis, nodal involvement is present in 69% to 74% of patients with primary tonsil tumors (12,13), 64% to 78% of patients with base of tongue primary tumors (12,14), 57% to 60% of patients with pharyngeal wall primary tumors (15), and 40% to 66% of patients with soft palate primary tumors (12,14). Tonsillar cancers

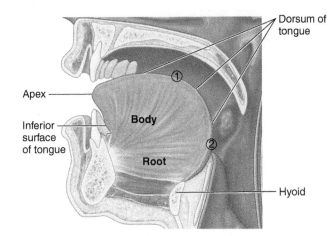

A Median section of mouth

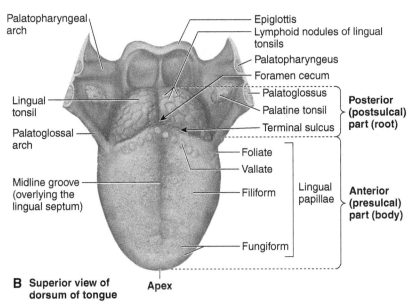

B Superior view of dorsum of tongue

FIGURE 15-2. Parts and features of tongue. **A:** The anterior free part constituting the majority of the mass of the tongue is the body of the tongue. The superior surface of the body in the oral cavity (*1*) is the dorsum. The posterior attached portion with an oropharyngeal surface (*2*) is the root of the tongue. **B:** The anterior (two thirds) and posterior (third) parts of the dorsum of the tongue are separated by the terminal sulcus (groove) and foramen cecum. (Reprinted from Tank PW, Gest TR. *Lippincott Williams & Wilkins atlas of anatomy.* Philadelphia, PA: Lippincott Williams & Wilkins, 2008; Plate 7.39A. © Wolters Kluwer.)

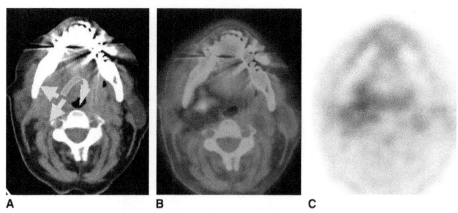

A   **B**   **C**

FIGURE 15-3. Palatine tonsil carcinoma with spread to the retromolar trigone, tongue base, and parapharyngeal space (*yellow arrows*). **A:** Unenhanced CT. **B:** FDG-PET/CT fusion. **C:** Axial FDG-PET (attenuation corrected).

not uncommonly spread locally to involve the retromolar trigone, tongue base, and/ or parapharyngeal space (see Fig. 15-3). Base of tongue cancers are insidious and when detectable clinically often demonstrate vallecular involvement and present with metastatic regional lymphadenopathy (see Fig. 15-4A and B).

- Ten percent to 15% of patients with nodal involvement will also have distant metastases (16).
- The most common location for lymph node metastasis is the ipsilateral level II neck. The pattern of metastatic progression is systematic, with next echelon drainage to levels III and IV and retropharyngeal nodes. Involvement of levels I and V is rare with T1-T2 primary tumors (17).
- Radiographic involvement of the retropharyngeal nodes is present in 16% of all OPSCC patients, rising to 23% if disease is evident in other nodal stations. Incidence of involved retropharyngeal nodes varies by subsite, with 11% of base of tongue/vallecular, 14% of tonsil, 38% of pharyngeal wall, and 56% of soft palate (18) (see Fig. 15-5).
- Patients presenting with HPV-associated OPSCCs are typically younger and more likely to have nodal involvement than their non–HPV-associated counterparts (19).

Clinical Presentation

- Presenting symptoms vary by subsite, but commonly include either local or referred pain or a painless neck mass.
  - Pain of the inner ear or temporomandibular joint is referred via the tympanic nerve of Jacobson (CN IX via the petrosal ganglion).
  - Pain of the external auditory canal is referred via the auricular nerve of Arnold (CN X).
- Symptoms of more advanced disease may include dysarthria ("hot potato voice" caused by involvement of CN XII), odynophagia, dysphagia with or without secondary weight loss, or trismus (if pterygoids are involved).

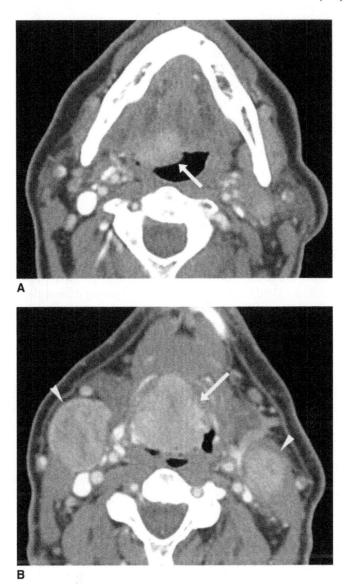

FIGURE 15-4. Squamous cell carcinoma of the right base of tongue. **A:** Axial contrast-enhanced CT image demonstrates an enhancing mass at the right base of tongue (*arrow*), causing mass effect. The involved hemitongue enhances and is not hypodense from fatty infiltration. **B:** Axial image more caudally demonstrating inferior extension into the vallecula (*arrow*). Also noted are bilateral necrotic metastatic nodes (*arrowheads*).

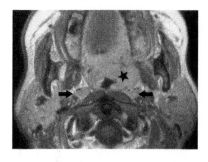

FIGURE 15-5. Axial postcontrast T1 shows carci-noma in left palatine tonsil region (*star*) and bilaterally enlarged retropharyngeal lymph nodes (*arrows*).

Diagnostic Workup

• Workup is presented in Table 15-1.

Pathologic Classification

• More than 95% are squamous cell carcinomas, approximately 60% of which are moderately differentiated, with 20% each well and poorly differentiated.
• Traditionally, tumor grade and subtype were thought to confer prognostic value; however, these factors appear to have limited prognostic value in the HPV era, particularly in comparison to clinical staging parameters (20,21).

Table 15-1
Diagnostic Workup for Malignant Tumors of the Oropharynx
General
History with emphasis on alcohol and tobacco use Physical examination, with attention to: Inspection and palpation of oral cavity and oropharynx, mirror examination and nasopharyngo-laryngoscopy as clinically indicated
Laboratory Studies
Complete blood cell count Blood chemistry profile Thyroid-stimulating hormone
Radiographic Studies
CT and/or MRI of the neck with contrast FDG-PET/CT and/or CT chest
Pathology
Biopsy of primary site and/or FNA of neck node HPV or p16 testing Dental, nutrition, speech/swallow evaluation, audiogram as clinically indicated

NEW! SUMMARY OF CHANGES TO AJCC STAGING

- The 8th edition American Joint Committee on Cancer clinical and pathologic staging system has undergone significant changes for staging of oropharyngeal cancers, highlighted by separate staging system for HPV-associated (p16+) oropharyngeal cancers.
- HPV-associated (p16+) oropharyngeal cancers: clinical and pathologic T staging is highlighted by the elimination of the T4 a/b designation. Tumors with moderate or very locally advanced disease are now simply designated T4. In clinical nodal staging, N1 now encompasses ipsilateral lymph nodes ≤ 6 cm. Bilateral or contralateral lymph nodes ≤ 6 cm are N2, and any lymph node metastasis greater than 6 cm is N3. Pathologic nodal staging focuses only on number of positive lymph nodes, with pN1 ≤ 4 LNs, and pN2 greater than 4 LNs. Overall TNM stage groupings have changed significantly with elimination of stage IV disease (with exception of distant metastases), and grouping systems differ for clinical and pathologic staging. Some illustrative examples include cT2N1 disease now stage I (previously 7th edition stage III); cT1N2 disease now stage II (previously 7th edition stage IVA); any T4 or N3 disease now stage III (previously stage IVB).
- Staging changes do not apply to HPV-associated (p16+) hypopharynx cancers. Such cases are to be staged using non–HPV-associated staging system.
- Hypopharynx and non–HPV-associated (p16−) oropharynx: in AJCC 8th edition, no changes have been made to T stage. For nodal staging, extranodal extension (ENE) has been included as an important new consideration. In clinically staged cases, the nodal staging remains largely unchanged from the 7th edition in cases without clinical evidence of extranodal extension (ENE$_c$), with exception of any lymph node metastasis greater than 6 cm now designated as cN3a (previously cN3). ENE$_c$ is defined as invasion of skin, infiltration of muscle, dense tethering, or fixation to adjacent structures, cranial nerve, brachial plexus, sympathetic trunk, or phrenic nerve invasion with dysfunction. Cases with clinical evidence of extranodal extension are to be staged as cN3b irrespective of number, size, or laterality of lymph node metastases. In pathologically staged cases, N staging remains the same in cases that are negative for extranodal extension [ENE(−)]. Any lymph node metastasis greater than 6 cm without extranodal extension is now pN3a. A single lymph node metastasis ≤ 3 cm size and ENE(+) is now pN2a. In cases with single lymph node metastasis greater than 3 cm and ENE(+) or multiple lymph nodes (ipsilateral or bilateral) with any ENE(+), N staging is now pN3b. Overall stage groupings remains the same as in the 7th edition AJCC.

See: Amin MB, Edge SB, Greene FL, et al., eds. *AJCC cancer staging manual*, 8th ed. New York, NY: Springer, 2017.

- Alternative histologies include primary lymphoid tumors, melanoma, minor salivary gland tumors, and sarcomas.
- Lymphovascular space invasion (LVI) and perineural invasion (PNI) are associated with increased rates of nodal involvement and a poorer prognosis (20).
- Evaluation of association with high-risk HPV may be performed via either p16 immunohistochemistry or in situ hybridization for high-risk HPV subtypes (HPV-ISH). Given availability, low cost, and relatively straightforward interpretation, p16 immunohistochemistry is most commonly used. There may be some discordance (less than 10%). A few studies show as high as a 15% to 20% false-positive and false-negative rate for p16 IHC testing as a surrogate for HPV infection (22,23). Cutoff for p16 positivity is typically diffuse tumor expression (≥75%) and at least moderate staining intensity. p16 staining typically localizes to nucleus and cytoplasm; cytoplasmic-only staining is considered nonspecific and should be interpreted as negative (24). In cases where p16 testing is felt to be equivocal, or if negative testing does not clinically correlate, HPV-ISH testing should be considered.

Prognostic Factors

- HPV positivity in head and neck cancer confers improved rates of OS (HR, 0.85) and DFS (HR, 0.62) in comparison to HPV-negative disease (25). This has been confirmed in the ECOG phase II trial, in which patients with HPV-associated disease were noted to have higher response rates to induction chemotherapy and after chemoradiation treatment, leading to a significant improvement in OS and a lower risk of progression (26).
- Subset analysis of patients with AJCC 7th edition stage III-IV OPC demonstrated HPV status to be the primary determinant of OS, followed by duration of tobacco use and tumor stage (10).
- In surgical patients, pathologically positive resection margins and extracapsular spread of tumor outside of neck nodes are prognostic for poor outcome (27). However, data on the prognostic significance of ECE in HPV-associated disease are conflicting (28–31).
- Number of pathologically involved nodes confers prognostic information in HPV-associated disease (32).

General Management by Stage

Early-Stage OPCs

- Although radiation therapy was historically preferred for treatment of OPSCC because of the potential functional compromise resulting from large surgical resections, newer transoral surgical techniques such as transrobotic oral surgery and transoral laser surgery have emerged as additional therapeutic options. However, such modalities are operator dependent and adequate training is essential in obtaining optimal oncologic outcomes.

T1-2 N0-1

• Definitive radiation therapy (consider chemoradiation for T2N1 BOT disease; select tonsillar cases may be treated with radiotherapy alone) OR surgery.

T3-4a N0-1

• Definitive chemoradiation OR surgery with adjuvant treatment as indicated (see "Postoperative" sections).

Any T, N2-3

• Definitive chemoradiation OR surgery followed by adjuvant treatment as indicated (see "Postoperative" sections).

Postoperative T3-4, Multiple Positive Nodes, Perineural Invasion, Lymphovascular Invasion, Level IV-V Nodes

• Consider adjuvant radiation, especially if 2 or more adverse features.

Postoperative Positive Margins or Extracapsular Extension

• Consider adjuvant platinum-based chemoradiation (27).

T4b, any N; Medically Inoperable; Unresectable Tumor

• Definitive chemoradiation (preferred) OR induction chemotherapy followed by RT OR definitive RT OR palliative intent chemoradiation.

M1

• Palliative intent chemo, RT, surgery, or supportive care.

Radiation Therapy Techniques

• IMRT is preferred, as it has been shown to be useful in reducing long-term toxicity by reducing dose to the salivary glands, auditory structures, and optic structures.
• Image guidance (when available) may be a helpful adjunct. Various imaging modalities and frequencies are utilized including daily onboard imaging, weekly or more frequent CBCT, off-board kV imaging (such as Exactrac), etc.

Volumes Treated

• For head and neck cases, it is encouraged to review contours with radiologist and head and neck surgeon for optimal target delineation, or in cases where any uncertainty exists as to the extent of involvement.

Definitive Intent Treatment Volumes

- GTV:
  - Gross primary and nodal disease based on clinical exam and imaging.
- CTV1 (high-risk volume):
  - Includes all primary and nodal GTV plus margin for subclinical disease (typically 5 to 10 mm). Can use smaller margins if gross tumor is well delineated through use of careful examination, diagnostic CT/PET/MRI image fusion, and IV contrast at time of simulation.
  - Margins on lymph nodes are typically 5 mm or less, but may be larger if evidence of extranodal extension.
  - May truncate air, skin, and bone if not invaded by tumor.
- CTV2 (intermediate-risk volume):
  - Tonsil: adjacent soft palate, glossotonsillar sulcus, base of tongue, parapharyngeal space, extend superiorly to ipsilateral pterygoid plate.
  - Base of tongue: entire uninvolved base of tongue (may include portion of oral tongue anteriorly), glossotonsillar sulci, vallecula, preepiglottic space, mucosal margin.
  - Soft palate: include entire soft palate, superior portions of tonsillar arches and fossa.
  - Pharyngeal wall: generous mucosal margin.
  - For pharyngeal wall lesions, especially posterior wall lesions, consider inclusion of medial retropharyngeal nodes bilaterally as part of the CTV2.
  - T3-4 disease superior margin extends to cover entire ipsilateral pterygoid plates.
  - Nodal CTV of the involved neck extends superiorly to the base of skull and inferiorly to the sternoclavicular junction.
  - Should include ipsilateral levels IB through V and RP nodes. Include IA if oral cavity is involved. Can consider omission of level IB in the node-negative ipsilateral neck.
  - Some practitioners only target lateral RP nodes, especially when attempting to spare pharyngeal constrictors. However, in cases of pharyngeal wall primaries, the medial RP node chain should not be ignored.
- CTV3 (low-risk volume):
  - Includes contralateral uninvolved neck nodes, typically levels II-IV or II-V and lateral RP nodes. Medial RP nodes for the uninvolved neck are often omitted, especially if attempting to spare pharyngeal constrictor dose.
  - Contralateral CTV3 coverage may be omitted in the case of a well-lateralized (less than 1 cm invasion into the soft palate or base of tongue), T1-2 N0-1 tonsillar cancer (33,34).
  - Treatment of the contralateral neck is strongly encouraged for all soft palate, base of tongue, and pharyngeal wall lesions. See Figure 15-6 for risk of nodal involvement in the N0 neck for base of tongue cancers.
- PTVs:
  - CTVs + 3 to 5 mm margin, depending on image guidance techniques and clinical judgment.
- Borderline or suspicious lymph nodes can be treated to 66 Gy, whereas grossly involved nodes should be treated as GTV.

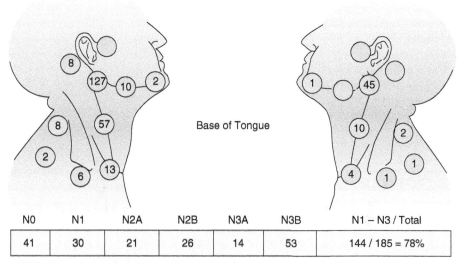

N0	N1	N2A	N2B	N3A	N3B	N1 – N3 / Total
41	30	21	26	14	53	144 / 185 = 78%

FIGURE 15-6. Distribution of nodal involvement at presentation of squamous cell carcinoma of base of the tongue (BOT). (Adapted with permission from Rubin P, Hansen JT. *TNM staging atlas with oncoanatomy*, 2nd ed. Philadelphia, PA: Lippincott Williams & Wilkins, 2012:78, as modified from Agur AMR, Dalley AF, eds. *Grant's atlas of anatomy*, 12th ed. Philadelphia, PA: Lippincott Williams & Wilkins, 2009. © Wolters Kluwer.)

Sequelae of Treatment

Acute Toxicities

- Mucositis: occurs in virtually all patients undergoing RT to the head and neck, with 85% scoring it as severe/extreme (35).
- Dermatitis
- Xerostomia
- Dysphagia
- Odynophagia
- Thickened secretions
- Taste alteration
- Candidiasis
- Secondary sequelae such as weight loss, compromised nutrition, and dehydration occasionally necessitating a feeding tube.
- The addition of concurrent chemotherapy to RT may substantially increase the risk and severity of acute toxicities, with one postoperative study noting a doubling of acute grade 3 toxicity (34 to 77%) with the addition of concurrent cisplatin (36).

Late Toxicities

- Xerostomia, predisposing to dental caries.
- Osteoradionecrosis: rare, occurs in less than 5% to 10% of patients treated with definitive radiation therapy. Risk is dependent on T stage, primary site (more common in oral cavity cancers), proximity of bone to tumor, dentition, and radiation dose (37,38).

- Dysphagia, the incidence of which is reduced in the IMRT era (39,40). The incidence and severity of dysphagia is correlated with increasing radiation dose and the volume of pharyngeal constrictors treated (41–43).
- Trismus
- Hypothyroidism
- Cervical fibrosis
- Lymphedema of the neck
- Altered taste
- Hearing loss
- Secondary radiation-induced malignancy

HYPOPHARYNX

Anatomy

- The hypopharynx is the most inferior of the three divisions of the pharynx, extending from the hyoid bone at the superior aspect to the cricoid cartilage at the inferior aspect.
- The hypopharynx is further subdivided clinically into the pyriform sinuses, the posterolateral pharyngeal wall, and the postcricoid region (Fig. 15-7).

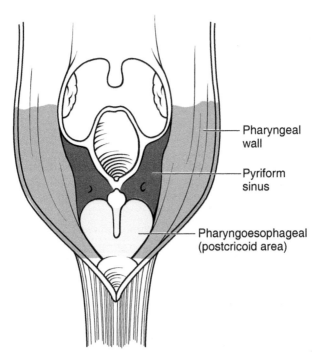

Pharyngeal wall

Pyriform sinus

Pharyngoesophageal (postcricoid area)

FIGURE 15-7. Anatomy of the hypopharynx. (Adapted with permission from Thorne CH, Gurtner GC, et al. *Grabb and Smith's plastic surgery.* Philadelphia, PA: Lippincott Williams & Wilkins, 2013:443. © Wolters Kluwer.)

- The invagination of the larynx into the hypopharynx creates two pear-shaped recesses, called the pyriform sinuses.
- The pyriform fossa lies laterally to the larynx. The medial wall is formed by the aryepiglottic fold and the lateral laryngeal wall (cricothyroid muscle). The anterior and lateral walls are formed by the thyroid ala. The posterior wall is open and communicates fully with the hypopharyngeal lumen. Its apex lies below the level of the vocal cords and occasionally below the cricoid cartilage.
- The postcricoid pharynx covers the posterior aspect of the cricoid cartilage and begins superiorly at the level of the arytenoids and ends inferiorly at the esophagus. See Figure 15-8.

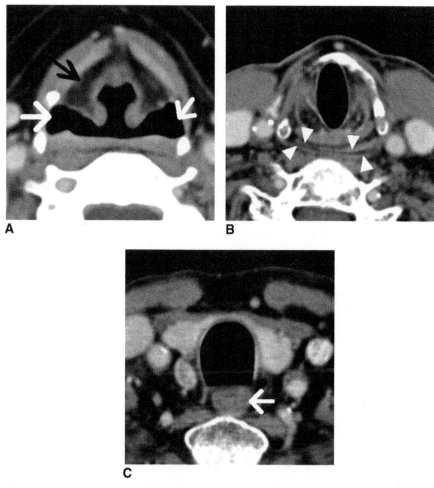

FIGURE 15-8. Axial postcontrast CT images of the hypopharynx. At the upper level of the hypopharynx **(A)** are the paired pyriform sinuses (*white arrows*). The paraglottic fat (*black arrow*) is well visualized as a low attenuation region anterior to the aryepiglottic folds. **B:** At the postcricoid level, the hypopharynx appears as a thin ellipse (*arrowheads*). **C:** Posterior to the trachea the hypopharynx has merged into the esophagus, which appears as a rounded structure (*arrow*).CT, computed tomography. (Reprinted with permission from Harrison LB, Sessions RB, Kies MS. *Head and neck cancer*, 4th ed. Philadelphia, PA: Lippincott Williams & Wilkins, 2013. © Wolters Kluwer.)

Natural History and Patterns of Spread

- Approximately 5% to 15% of presenting cases require an emergency tracheotomy.
- A major neurologic finding is referred pain to the ipsilateral ear. Pain is referred along the internal branch of the superior laryngeal nerve (sensory division to the larynx and hypopharynx) via the vagus nerve (X) to the auricular branch of the vagus nerve (Arnold's nerve).
- On rare occasions, direct tumor involvement or lymph node extension to the hypoglossal nerve may produce ipsilateral tongue paralysis.
- In the United States, tumors occur in the following decremental frequency: pyriform sinus tumors, posterior pharyngeal wall, and postcricoid region.
- Medial wall pyriform fossa tumors, the most common group, often spread along the mucosal surface to involve the aryepiglottic folds. Occasionally, they invade medially and deeply into the false vocal folds and larynx via the paraglottic space. Involvement of the paraglottic space allows a lesion to behave as a transglottic carcinoma (44). See Figure 15-9.
- Cancers of the lateral wall and apex of the pyriform fossa commonly involve the posterior hypopharyngeal wall, the thyroid cartilage, the cricoid cartilage, or directly into the thyroid gland.
- Once they penetrate the constrictor muscle, tumors can spread along the muscle and fascial planes to the base of the skull (the origin and suspension of the constrictor muscles) and along the neurovascular planes following the vagus, glossopharyngeal, and sympathetic nerves.
- Posterior hypopharyngeal wall tumors can extend superiorly to involve the oropharynx, posteriorly to involve the prevertebral fascia and retropharyngeal space, and interior to involve the cervical esophagus.
- Postcricoid area tumors commonly invade the cricoid cartilage, interarytenoid space, and posterior cricothyroid muscle to produce hoarseness (45). The esophagus, trachea, and pyriform sinuses are at risk of advanced local extension. See Figure 15-10.

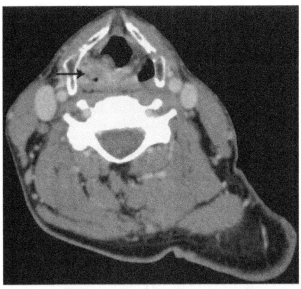

FIGURE 15-9. Axial CT image depicting a T2 hypopharynx tumor involving the right pyriform sinus.

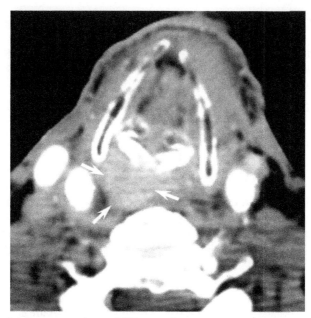

FIGURE 15-10. Axial contrast-enhanced CT image shows a tumor arising in the postcricoid region of the hypopharynx (*arrows*).

- The abundant lymphatics of the hypopharynx, coupled with extensive primary disease at presentation, account for the high incidence of metastases to the regional lymph nodes (46–49).
- There is free communication with the spinal accessory lymph nodes and retropharyngeal nodes.
- Level II and III lymph nodes most commonly are involved, and bilateral lymphadenopathy can be seen in approximately 15% of patients at presentation (50).
- Occult nodal disease occurs irrespective of T stage in pyriform fossa tumors, with an incidence of 60% for T1 and T2 and 84% for T3 and T4 disease (51).

Diagnostic Workup

- The initial history and physical examination should include indirect laryngoscopy and a flexible endoscopic examination under topical anesthesia. Posterior pharyngeal wall lesions may be missed during indirect laryngoscopy.
- Radiologic evaluation includes the following:
  - CT scan and/or MRI with contrast of the head and neck region
  - Chest CT
  - Consider FDG-PET/CT for stage III to IV disease
- Biopsy of the primary site or FNA of the neck
- EUA with endoscopy
- Nutrition, speech/swallow evaluation/therapy, audiogram as clinically indicated
- Dental evaluation
- Consider pulmonary function tests for conservation surgery candidates.

> **NEW!** **SUMMARY OF CHANGES TO AJCC STAGING**
>
> • The 8th edition American Joint Committee on Cancer staging system for hypopharynx cancer is the same as the staging used for system used for p16-negative oropharynx cancer (52). See "Oropharynx" section of this chapter.
>
> See: Amin MB, Edge SB, Greene FL, et al., eds. *AJCC cancer staging manual*, 8th ed. New York, NY: Springer, 2017.

Pathologic Classification

• Over 95% of tumors of the hypopharynx are squamous cell carcinoma.
• In general, tumor margins are infiltrating in 80% and pushing in 20% of specimens studied. Whole-organ sections of the pyriform fossa have demonstrated unsuspected submucosal tumor spread well beyond 1 cm of the visible tumor margins (50).

Prognostic Factors

• Increasing age, T stage, N stage, and size of regional metastases are all inversely correlated with survival (47,48). Male gender, black race, and lower socioeconomic status have also been shown to confer a worse prognosis (53).
• Survival decreases with involvement of lower cervical chain lymph nodes (54).
• Pathologic findings in pyriform fossa tumors that adversely affect survival include positive surgical margins, extracapsular spread, or tumor persistence in the irradiation field after initial definitive therapy (55,56).
• Tumor location influences cure rates. The decremental frequency for survival with hypopharyngeal carcinomas at different sites is as follows: pyriform fossa, pharyngeal walls, and postcricoid region (57). This is due to the fact that aryepiglottic fold and medial wall pyriform sinus tumors are typically smaller and more localized.

General Management

• Table 15-2 outlines the management of hypopharyngeal tumors.

Early-Stage Tumors

• The aim of treatment is to achieve locoregional control and survival without compromising functional outcomes (respiration, deglutition, and phonation). Whenever possible, preserving laryngeal function with definitive RT or a conservative surgical procedure is preferred.
• Although not compared directly in randomized trials, in patients with early-stage hypopharynx tumors, OS and DSS following definitive RT are comparable to radical or larynx-sparing surgery (58,59).
• Because of the high incidence (30% to 50%) of occult cervical metastases in clinically node-negative patients, initial treatment should include either bilateral elective neck dissection or RT (60).

Table 15-2

Management of Hypopharyngeal Cancer

Stage	Treatment
T1-T2 N0	Irradiation alone (70 Gy) OR partial laryngopharyngectomy, ipsilateral or bilateral neck dissection, hemithyroidectomy, pretracheal and ipsilateral paratracheal lymph node dissection (postoperative irradiation, depending on pathologic findings)
T2-3 any N; T1 N+	Induction chemotherapy OR partial/total laryngopharyngectomy + neck dissection (including level VI), thyroidectomy, pretracheal and ipsilateral paratracheal lymph node dissection OR concurrent chemoradiation
Response to induction therapy T2-3 any N, T1 N+	Primary site CR and stable/improved neck disease → definitive RT, consider systemic therapy/RT; Primary site PR and stable/improved neck disease → systemic therapy/RT OR surgery; Primary site < PR → surgery
T4a, any N	Total laryngopharyngectomy, neck dissection, hemi/total thyroidectomy, ipsilateral or bilateral paratracheal lymph node dissection OR induction chemotherapy OR concurrent CRT
Response to induction therapy for T4a, any N	Primary site CR and stable/improved neck disease → definitive RT, consider systemic therapy Primary site PR and stable/improved neck disease → systemic therapy/RT Primary site < PR or neck progression → surgery + neck dissection as indicated

- Larger lesions and neck metastases require combined surgical resection and adjuvant radiation therapy.
- When treating with RT alone, some series have shown improved outcomes with altered fractionation schemes when compared with historical control data (61,62). However, one must be mindful that improvements in RT technique and patient selection criteria may be, at least in part, responsible for these outcomes.

Locally Advanced Tumors

- Whenever feasible, a functional organ-preservation strategy is the treatment of choice for patients with T3-4 primary hypopharyngeal tumors. Treatment selection depends on a multitude of factors including tumor extent and location, patient-specific factors, physician expertise, and the availability of rehabilitation services.
- Regarding larynx preservation therapy for these patients, the same principles used for the selection of larynx cancer patients should be applied (63,64).
- Concurrent chemoradiation, induction chemotherapy followed by radiation therapy alone, and sequential trimodality therapy with surgery are all used as organ preservation techniques. Concurrent chemoradiation may be preferable in patients with

N0-N2a disease, whereas induction chemotherapy may be beneficial in patients with a higher risk of distant metastases, though a definitive survival advantage has not been confirmed in randomized trials (65,66).
- Sequential therapy may be optimal in patients with bulky T3 and select T4 tumors and/or patients with advanced nodal presentations at high risk for distant metastases.
- In patients with small primary tumors and more extensive neck disease, primary treatment minimally invasive surgery may be preferable.

Postoperative Therapy

- Adjuvant radiotherapy should be considered in patients with LVI, PNI, pT3-4 primary disease, or pathologically positive lymph nodes.
- Adjuvant chemoradiation therapy is recommended for patients with pathologically positive margins or extracapsular extension (67).

Radiation Therapy Techniques

- Image-guided IMRT (IG-IMRT) is preferred.

Volume Treated

- GTV
  - Gross disease on clinical exam and imaging.
- CTV1 (high-risk volume)
  - Includes primary and nodal GTVs plus margin for subclinical disease spread (typically 10 mm).
- CTV2 (intermediate-risk volume)
  - Should encompass the entire high-risk CTV + 5 to 10 mm margin, the entire hypopharynx subsite of the primary tumor, and adjacent structures including the remainder of the hypopharyngeal apparatus. Particular consideration should be given to potential directions of mucosal and submucosal spread. The entire larynx should be included, as well as adjacent fat spaces.
  - In the ipsilateral neck, the retropharyngeal nodes and levels IB-IV should be covered. If there is gross nodal disease, coverage of level V should be strongly considered. IB may be considered for omission in cases of the ipsilateral node-negative neck, or ipsilateral neck with small volume low neck lymph node metastasis.
  - Nodal CTV of the involved neck extends superiorly to the base of skull and inferiorly to the sternoclavicular junction.
  - Hypopharyngeal cancers involving the postcricoid region mandate coverage of the level VI nodal station as well.
  - If the primary tumor is not well lateralized, the intermediate-risk dose may be prescribed to the bilateral neck.
- CTV3 (low-risk volume)
  - Includes contralateral uninvolved nodal levels II-IV and RP nodes.
- PTV
  - CTV + 3 to 5 mm margin depending on image guidance techniques and clinical judgment.

Postoperative Treatment Volumes

- In addition to the suggested definitive volumes as noted above, post-operative volumes generally include the postoperative tumor bed, any surgical clips or markers, and dissected neck levels.
- In cases where indication for postoperative therapy is due to lymphadenopathy, some practitioners omit primary site RT if no adverse features (ie widely negative margins, etc).

Doses

- Definitive intent radiation:
  - Single course regimen commonly delivered with concurrent chemotherapy: high-risk volume: 70 Gy in 35 fx; intermediate-risk volume: 63 Gy in 35 fx; low-risk volume: 56 Gy in 35 fx. High dose concurrent platinum (100 mg/m^2 q3wk) is recommended whenever possible.
  - Single course with boost or cone-down: initial 60 Gy in 30 fractions to gross/high-risk/int-risk disease, 54 Gy in 30 fx to low-risk disease; followed by boost/cone-down 10 Gy in 5 fractions to gross/high-risk disease, cumulative 35 fractions.
  - Integrated boost regimens: (a) GTV/high-risk 69.96 Gy in 33 fx; int-risk volume 59.4 Gy in 33 fx; low-risk 54.12 Gy in 33 fx OR (b) GTV/high-risk 66 Gy in 30 fx; int-risk volume 60 Gy in 30 fx; low-risk 54 Gy in 30 fx.
  - RT Alone: 70 Gy in 2 Gy fractions; or integrated boost regimens; or hyperfractionation regimen of 81.6 Gy in 1.2 Gy fractions delivered twice daily over seven weeks. In patients with locally advanced disease who are not chemotherapy candidates, consider hyperfractionation.
- Postoperative/adjuvant radiation:
  - Typically 60 Gy in 30 fractions to the pre-operative extent of disease, postoperative bed, and/or dissected neck.
  - Consider higher doses (66 Gy in 33 fx, or 63 Gy in 30 fx) or a boost for regions of positive margins and/or nodal levels with pathologic evidence of extranodal extension.
  - Undissected and uninvolved neck can typically be treated with 50 to 54 Gy in 25 to 30 fractions.

Sequelae of Treatment

- As the dose and radiation target volumes in hypopharynx cancer are generally similar to oropharynx cancer, the early and late sequelae are also comparable.
- The incidence of pharyngocutaneous fistulas after pharyngectomy is the same whether the pharynx has been irradiated before or not, but the time required to heal a preoperatively irradiated fistula is significantly greater than for a nonirradiated fistula (69).

References

1. Negri E, La Vecchia C, Franceschi S, et al. Attributable risk for oral cancer in northern Italy. *Cancer Epidemiol Biomarkers Prev* 1993;2:189–193.
2. Hashibe M, Brennan P, Chuang S-c, et al. Interaction between tobacco and alcohol use and the risk of head and neck cancer: pooled analysis in the International Head and Neck Cancer Epidemiology Consortium. *Cancer Epidemiol Biomarkers Prev* 2009;18:541–550.

3. Mork J, Lie AK, Glattre E, et al. Human papillomavirus infection as a risk factor for squamous-cell carcinoma of the head and neck. *N Engl J Med* 2001;344:1125–1131.

4. Gillison ML, Koch WM, Capone RB, et al. Evidence for a causal association between human papillomavirus and a subset of head and neck cancers. *J Natl Cancer Inst* 2000;92:709–720.

5. Kreimer AR, Clifford GM, Boyle P, et al. Human papillomavirus types in head and neck squamous cell carcinomas worldwide: a systematic review. *Cancer Epidemiol Biomarkers Prev* 2005;14:467–475.

6. Fakhry C, Zhang Q, Nguyen-Tan PF, et al. Human papillomavirus and overall survival after progression of oropharyngeal squamous cell carcinoma. *J Clin Oncol* 2014;32:3365–3373.

7. O'Sullivan B, Huang SH, Siu LL, et al. Deintensification candidate subgroups in human papillomavirus-related oropharyngeal cancer according to minimal risk of distant metastasis. *J Clin Oncol* 2013;31:543–550.

8. Slebos RJ, Yi Y, Ely K, et al. Gene expression differences associated with human papillomavirus status in head and neck squamous cell carcinoma. *Clin Cancer Res* 2006;12:701–709.

9. Cancer Genome Atlas N. Comprehensive genomic characterization of head and neck squamous cell carcinomas. *Nature* 2015;517:576–582.

10. Ang KK, Harris J, Wheeler R, et al. Human papillomavirus and survival of patients with oropharyngeal cancer. *N Engl J Med* 2010;363:24–35.

11. Chaturvedi AK, Engels EA, Pfeiffer RM, et al. Human papillomavirus and rising oropharyngeal cancer incidence in the United States. *J Clin Oncol* 2011;29:4294–4301.

12. Jose J, Coatesworth AP, Johnston C, et al. Cervical node metastases in oropharyngeal squamous cell carcinoma: prospective analysis of prevalence and distribution. *J Laryngol Otol* 2002;116:925–928.

13. Foote RL, Schild SE, Thompson WM, et al. Tonsil cancer. Patterns of failure after surgery alone and surgery combined with postoperative radiation therapy. *Cancer* 1994;73:2638–2647.

14. Lindberg R. Distribution of cervical lymph node metastases from squamous cell carcinoma of the upper respiratory and digestive tracts. *Cancer* 1972;29:1446–1449.

15. Meoz-Mendez RT, Fletcher GH, Guillamondegui OM, et al. Analysis of the results of irradiation in the treatment of squamous cell carcinomas of the pharyngeal walls. *Int J Radiat Oncol Biol Phys* 1978;4:579–585.

16. Gunderson LL. *Clinical radiation oncology*. Elsevier Health Sciences, 2015.

17. Sanguineti G, Califano J, Stafford E, et al. Defining the risk of involvement for each neck nodal level in patients with early T-stage node-positive oropharyngeal carcinoma. *Int J Radiat Oncol Biol Phys* 2009;74:1356–1364.

18. Bussels B, Hermans R, Reijnders A, et al. Retropharyngeal nodes in squamous cell carcinoma of oropharynx: incidence, localization, and implications for target volume. *Int J Radiat Oncol Biol Phys* 2006;65:733–738.

19. Khode SR, Dwivedi RC, Rhys-Evans P, et al. Exploring the link between human papilloma virus and oral and oropharyngeal cancers. *J Cancer Res Ther* 2014;10:492–498.

20. Sternberg SS, Mills SE, Carter D. *Sternberg's diagnostic surgical pathology*. Lippincott Williams & Wilkins, 2004.

21. Begum S, Westra WH. Basaloid squamous cell carcinoma of the head and neck is a mixed variant that can be further resolved by HPV status. *Am J Surg Pathol* 2008;32:1044–1050.

22. Harris SL, Thorne LB, Seaman WT, et al. Association of p16INK4a overexpression with improved outcomes in young patients with squamous cell cancers of the oral tongue. *Head Neck* 2011;33:1622–1627.

23. Chau NG, Perez-Ordonez B, Zhang K, et al. The association between EGFR variant III, HPV, p16, c-MET, EGFR gene copy number and response to EGFR inhibitors in patients with recurrent or metastatic squamous cell carcinoma of the head and neck. *Head Neck Oncol* 2011;3:11.

24. Lydiatt WM, et al. Head and neck cancers–major changes in the American Joint Committee on cancer eighth edition cancer staging manual. *CA Cancer J Clin* 2017;67(2):122–137.

25. Ragin CC, Taioli E. Survival of squamous cell carcinoma of the head and neck in relation to human papillomavirus infection: review and meta-analysis. *Int J Cancer* 2007;121:1813–1820.

26. Fakhry C, Westra WH, Li S, et al. Improved survival of patients with human papillomavirus-positive head and neck squamous cell carcinoma in a prospective clinical trial. *J Natl Cancer Inst* 2008;100:261–269.

27. Bernier J, Cooper JS, Pajak TF, et al. Defining risk levels in locally advanced head and neck cancers: a comparative analysis of concurrent postoperative radiation plus chemotherapy trials of the EORTC (#22931) and RTOG (# 9501). *Head Neck* 2005;27:843–850.

28. Maxwell JH, Ferris RL, Gooding W, et al. Extracapsular spread in head and neck carcinoma: impact of site and human papillomavirus status. *Cancer* 2013;119:3302–3308.

29. Sinha P, Lewis JS, Piccirillo JF, et al. Extracapsular spread and adjuvant therapy in human papillomavirus-related, p16-positive oropharyngeal carcinoma. *Cancer* 2012;118:3519–3530.

30. Lewis JS, Carpenter DH, Thorstad WL, et al. Extracapsular extension is a poor predictor of disease recurrence in surgically treated oropharyngeal squamous cell carcinoma. *Mod Pathol* 2011;24:1413–1420.

31. An Y, Park HS, Kelly JR, et al. The prognostic value of extranodal extension in human papillomavirus-associated oropharyngeal squamous cell carcinoma. *Cancer.* 2017;123(14):2762–2772.

32. Haughey BH, Sinha P, Kallogjeri D, et al. Pathology-based staging for HPV-associated squamous carcinoma of the oropharynx. *Oral Oncol* 2016;62:11–19.

33. O'Sullivan B, Warde P, Grice B, et al. The benefits and pitfalls of ipsilateral radiotherapy in carcinoma of the tonsillar region. *Int J Radiat Oncol Biol Phys* 2001;51:332–343.

34. Expert Panel on Radiation O-H, Neck C, Yeung AR, et al. ACR Appropriateness Criteria(R) ipsilateral radiation for squamous cell carcinoma of the tonsil. *Head Neck* 2012;34:613–616.

35. Elting LS, Keefe DM, Sonis ST, et al. Patient-reported measurements of oral mucositis in head and neck cancer patients treated with radiotherapy with or without chemotherapy. *Cancer* 2008;113:2704–2713.

36. Cooper JS, Pajak TF, Forastiere AA, et al. Postoperative concurrent radiotherapy and chemotherapy for high-risk squamous-cell carcinoma of the head and neck. *N Engl J Med* 2004;350:1937–1944.

37. Taylor JM, Mendenhall WM, Lavey RS. Dose, time, and fraction size issues for late effects in head and neck cancers. *Int J Radiat Oncol Biol Phys* 1992;22:3–11.

38. Mendenhall WM. Mandibular Osteoradionecrosis. *J of Clin Oncol* 2004;22:4867–4868. http://ascopubs.org/doi/abs/10.1200/JCO.2004.09.959.

39. Lok BH, Setton J, Caria N, et al. Intensity-modulated radiation therapy in oropharyngeal carcinoma: effect of tumor volume on clinical outcomes. *Int J Radiat Oncol Biol Phys* 2012;82:1851–1857.

40. McBride SM, Parambi RJ, Jang JW, et al. Intensity-modulated versus conventional radiation therapy for oropharyngeal carcinoma: long-term dysphagia and tumor control outcomes. *Head Neck* 2014;36:492–498.

41. Feng FY, Kim HM, Lyden TH, et al. Intensity-modulated chemoradiotherapy aiming to reduce dysphagia in patients with oropharyngeal cancer: clinical and functional results. *J Clin Oncol* 2010;28:2732–2738.

42. Levendag PC, Teguh DN, Voet P, et al. Dysphagia disorders in patients with cancer of the oropharynx are significantly affected by the radiation therapy dose to the superior and middle constrictor muscle: a dose-effect relationship. *Radiother Oncol* 2007;85:64–73.

43. Eisbruch A, Schwartz M, Rasch C, et al. Dysphagia and aspiration after chemoradiotherapy for head-and-neck cancer: which anatomic structures are affected and can they be spared by IMRT? *Int J Radiat Oncol Biol Phys* 2004;60:1425–1439.

44. Richard JM, Sancho-Garnier H, Micheau C, et al. Prognostic factors in cervical lymph node metastasis in upper respiratory and digestive tract carcinomas: study of 1,713 cases during a 15-year period. *Laryngoscope* 1987;97:97–101.

45. Wang CC, Schulz MD, Miller D. Combined radiation therapy and surgery for carcinoma of the supraglottis and pyriform sinus. *Am J Surg* 1972;124:551–554.

46. Mendenhall WM, Parsons JT, Mancuso AA, et al. Squamous cell carcinoma of the pharyngeal wall treated with irradiation. *Radiother Oncol* 1988;11:205–212.

47. Spector JG, Sessions DG, Emami B, et al. Squamous cell carcinoma of the pyriform sinus: a nonrandomized comparison of therapeutic modalities and long-term results. *Laryngoscope* 1995;105:397–406.

48. Vandenbrouck C, Eschwege F, De la Rochefordiere A, et al. Squamous cell carcinoma of the pyriform sinus: retrospective study of 351 cases treated at the Institut Gustave-Roussy. *Head Neck Surg* 1987;10:4–13.

49. Wang CC. Carcinoma of the hypopharynx. In: Wang CC, ed. *Radiation therapy for head and neck neoplasms: indications, techniques and results.* Chicago, IL: Year Book Medical Publishers, 1990.

50. Lindberg R. Distribution of cervical lymph node metastases from squamous cell carcinoma of the upper respiratory and digestive tracts. *Cancer* 1972;29:1446–1449.

51. El Badawi SA, Goepfert H, Fletcher GH, et al. Squamous cell carcinoma of the pyriform sinus. *Laryngoscope* 1982;92:357–364.

52. AJCC. In: Edge SB, Byrd DR, Compton CC, et al., eds. *AJCC cancer staging manual,* 7th ed. New York, NY: Springer Verlag, 2009.

53. Molina MA, Cheung MC, Perez EA, et al. African American and poor patients have a dramatically worse prognosis for head and neck cancer. *Cancer* 2008;113:2797–2806.

54. Donald PJ, Hayes HR, Dhaliwal R. Combined therapy for pyriform sinus cancer using postoperative irradiation. *Otolaryngol Head Neck Surg* 1980;88:738–744.

55. Brugere JM, Mosseri VF, Mamelle G, et al. Nodal failures in patients with N0 N+ oral squamous cell carcinoma without capsular rupture. *Head Neck* 1996;18:133–137.

56. Spector JG, Sessions DG, Emami B, et al. Squamous cell carcinomas of the aryepiglottic fold: therapeutic results and long-term follow-up. *Laryngoscope* 1995;105:734–746.

57. Farrington W, Weighill J, Jones P. Postcricoid carcinoma (a 10-year retrospective study). *J Laryngol Otol* 1986;100:79–84.

58. Takes RP, Strojan P, Silver CE, et al. Current trends in initial management of hypopharyngeal cancer: the declining use of open surgery. *Head Neck* 2012;34:270–281.

59. Hall SF, Groome PA, Irish J, et al. Radiotherapy or surgery for head and neck squamous cell cancer. *Cancer* 2009;115:5711–5722.

60. Byers RM, Wolf PF, Ballantyne AJ. Rationale for elective modified neck dissection. *Head Neck Surg* 1988;10:160–167.

61. Garden AS, Morrison WH, Clayman GL, et al. Early squamous cell carcinoma of the hypopharynx: outcomes of treatment with radiation alone to the primary disease. *Head Neck* 1996;18:317–322.

62. Amdur RJ, Mendenhall WM, Stringer SP, et al. Organ preservation with radiotherapy for T1-T2 carcinoma of the pyriform sinus. *Head Neck* 2001;23:353–362.

63. Beauvillain C, Mahe M, Bourdin S, et al. Final results of a randomized trial comparing chemotherapy plus radiotherapy with chemotherapy plus surgery plus radiotherapy in locally advanced resectable hypopharyngeal carcinomas. *Laryngoscope* 1997;107:648–653.

64. Prades J-M, Lallemant B, Garrel R, et al. Randomized phase III trial comparing induction chemotherapy followed by radiotherapy to concomitant chemoradiotherapy for laryngeal preservation in T3M0 pyriform sinus carcinoma. *Acta Otolaryngol* 2010;130:150–155.

65. Posner MR, Hershock DM, Blajman CR, et al. Cisplatin and fluorouracil alone or with docetaxel in head and neck cancer. *N Engl J Med* 2007;357:1705–1715.

66. Forastiere AA, Zhang Q, Weber RS, et al. Long-term results of RTOG 91-11: a comparison of three nonsurgical treatment strategies to preserve the larynx in patients with locally advanced larynx cancer. *J Clin Oncol* 2012;31:845–852.

67. Bernier J, Cooper JS, Pajak TF, et al. Defining risk levels in locally advanced head and neck cancers: a comparative analysis of concurrent postoperative radiation plus chemotherapy trials of the EORTC (#22931) and RTOG (# 9501). *Head Neck* 2005;27:843–850.

68. Vandenbrouck C, Sancho H, Le Fur R, et al. Results of a randomized clinical trial of preoperative irradiation versus postoperative in treatment of tumors of the hypopharynx. *Cancer* 1977;39:1445–1449.

69. Cachin Y, Eschwege F. Combination of radiotherapy and surgery in the treatment of head and neck cancers. *Cancer Treat Rev* 1975;2:177–191.

CHAPTER 16

LARYNX

ANATOMY

- The larynx is divided into three regions: the supraglottic (epiglottis, false vocal cords, ventricles, aryepiglottic folds, arytenoids), glottic (true vocal cords, anterior commissure), and subglottic (located below the vocal cords) (1) (see Fig. 16-1).
- The lateral line of demarcation between the glottis and supraglottic larynx clinically is the apex of the ventricle. The demarcation between the glottis and subglottis is ill defined, but the subglottis is considered to begin 5 mm below the free margin of the vocal cord and to end at the inferior border of the cricoid cartilage and the beginning of the trachea.
- The superior and inferior laryngeal arteries are branches of the superior and inferior thyroid arteries, respectively.
- The intrinsic muscles of the larynx are innervated by the recurrent laryngeal nerve. The cricothyroid muscle, an intrinsic muscle responsible for tensing the vocal cords, is supplied by a branch of the superior laryngeal nerve. Isolated damage to this nerve causes a bowing of the true vocal cord, which continues to be mobile, although the voice may become hoarse.
- The supraglottic structures have a plexus rich with lymphatic capillaries. The trunks pass through the preepiglottic space and thyrohyoid membrane and terminate mainly in the subdigastric lymph nodes; a few drain to the middle internal jugular chain lymph nodes.
- There are essentially no lymphatic capillaries of the true vocal cords. Lymphatic spread from glottic cancer occurs only if tumor extends to the supraglottic or subglottic areas.
- The subglottic area has relatively few lymphatic capillaries. The lymphatic trunks pass through the cricothyroid membrane to the pretracheal (delphian) lymph nodes in the region of the thyroid isthmus. The subglottic area also drains posteriorly through the cricotracheal membrane, with some trunks going to the paratracheal lymph nodes and others continuing to the inferior jugular chain.

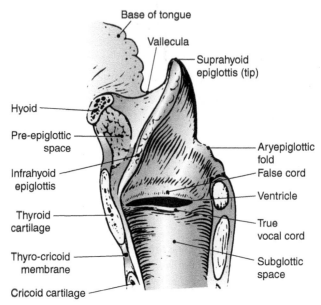

FIGURE 16-1. Diagrammatic sagittal section of the larynx. (Redrawn with permission from *Sobotta atlas of human anatomy* © Elsevier GmbH, Urban & Fischer, Munich.)

EPIDEMIOLOGY AND RISK FACTORS

- Cancer of the larynx occurs in around 13,400 people in the United States annually and accounts for approximately 3,700 deaths (2).
- The vast majority of laryngeal cancers arise from the glottis and supraglottis, with the ratio of glottic to supraglottic carcinomas approximately 3 to 1. Primary subglottic carcinomas are rare, accounting for approximately 1% of all primary laryngeal cancers.
- Cancer of the larynx is strongly related to cigarette smoking, and more than 95% of patients with laryngeal cancer have a history of tobacco use (3). The risk of tobacco-related cancers of the upper alimentary and respiratory tracts declines among ex-smokers after 5 years of abstention and approaches the risk of nonsmokers after 10 years of abstention (4).

NATURAL HISTORY

Supraglottic Larynx

- Suprahyoid epiglottic lesions tend to invade the vallecula and preepiglottic space, lateral pharyngeal walls, and the remainder of the supraglottic larynx (see Fig. 16-2).

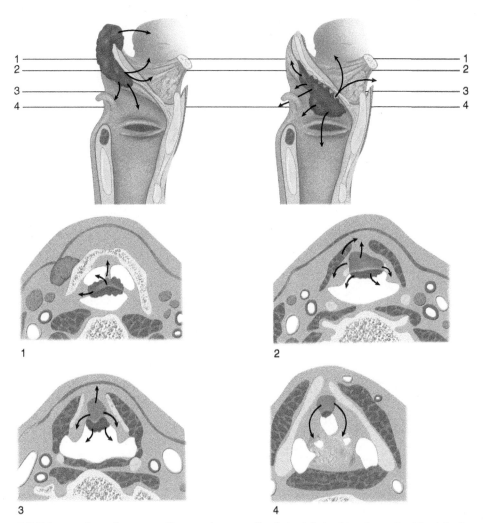

FIGURE 16-2. Spread patterns of laryngeal cancer of both the infrahyoid and suprahyoid epiglottis.

- Infrahyoid epiglottic lesions grow circumferentially to involve the false cords, aryepiglottic folds, medial wall of the pyriform sinus, and the pharyngoepiglottic fold. Invasion of the anterior commissure and cords and anterior subglottic extension usually occur only in advanced lesions (see Fig. 16-2).
- Extension of false cord tumors to the lower portion of the infrahyoid epiglottis and invasion of the preepiglottic space are common (see Fig. 16-3).
- It may be difficult to ascertain whether aryepiglottic fold/arytenoid lesions originated on the medial wall of the pyriform sinus versus the aryepiglottic fold. Advanced lesions invade the thyroid, epiglottic, and cricoid cartilages, and eventually, the pyriform sinus and postcricoid space.

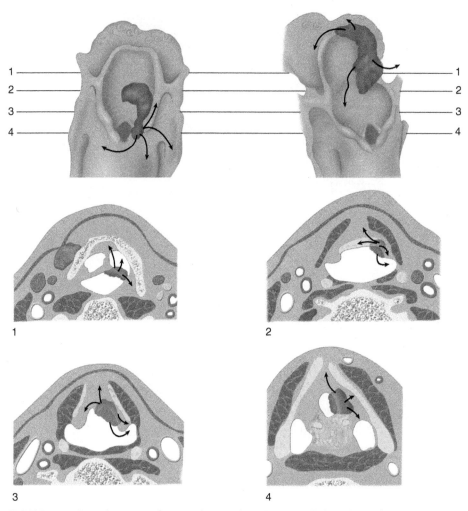

FIGURE 16-3. Spread patterns of marginal supraglottic lesions including those of the aryepiglottic fold, false cord, and laryngeal ventricle mucosa.

Glottic Larynx

- At diagnosis, approximately two thirds of tumors are confined to the cords, usually one cord. The anterior portion and upper surface of the cord is the most common site (Fig. 16-4).
- Anterior commissure involvement is common and is considered involved if no tumor-free cord can be seen anterior to lesion.
- Tumors can grow in exophytic nature or infiltrate into the intrinsic muscles of the larynx, potentially causing voice changes and respiratory obstruction.

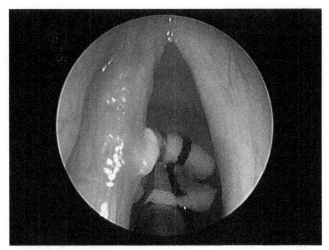

FIGURE 16-4. T1a glottic carcinoma of the left true cord.

- Subglottic extension may occur by simple mucosal surface growth, but it more commonly occurs by submucosal penetration beneath the conus elasticus (see Fig. 16-5). One centimeter of subglottic extension anteriorly or 4 to 5 mm of extension posteriorly brings the border of the tumor to the upper margin of the cricoid, exceeding the anatomic limits for conventional hemilaryngectomy.
- Infiltrative tumors can invade the paraglottic and preepiglottic spaces, and advanced glottic lesions eventually penetrate through the thyroid cartilage or via the cricothyroid space to enter the neck, where they may invade the thyroid gland.

Subglottic Larynx

- Tumors may spread inferiorly to the trachea or cricoid cartilage, or superiorly to the underside of the true vocal cords.
- Because early diagnosis is uncommon, most lesions are bilateral or circumferential at discovery.
- Tracheal extension of disease is commonly noted.

Lymphatic Spread

- Disease spreads mainly to the subdigastric nodes.
- In supraglottic carcinoma, the incidence of clinically positive nodes is 55% at the time of diagnosis; 16% are bilateral (5).
- Elective neck dissection for patients with supraglottic carcinoma reveals pathologically positive nodes in 16% of cases. Observation of initially node-negative necks eventually identifies the appearance of positive nodes in 33% of cases (6,7).
- The risk of late-appearing contralateral lymph node metastasis is 37% if the ipsilateral neck is pathologically positive (8).

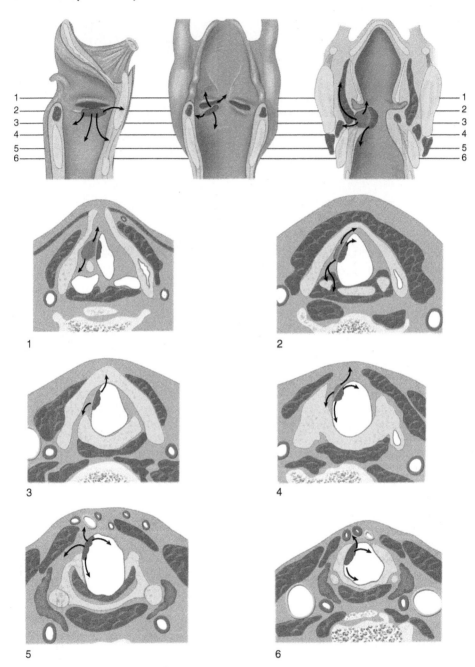

FIGURE 16-5. Spread patterns of glottic carcinoma.

- For glottis cancers, the incidence of clinically positive lymph nodes at diagnosis is approximately 5% for T1/T2 tumors, rising to approximately 20% to 30% for T3/T4 tumors (9,10) secondary to involvement of the supraglottic or subglottic larynx, and again primarily to the subdigastric basins, particularly level II and III (11).

DIAGNOSTIC WORKUP

- History and physical exam is performed including palpation of the base of tongue and cervical neck node and thyroid examination.
- Fiber-optic illuminated endoscopes (rigid and flexible) and indirect laryngoscopy with mirror examination are indicated.
- Thin-cut computed tomography (CT) with contrast and/or magnetic resonance imaging (MRI) with contrast of the primary lesion and neck should be performed prior to biopsy so that anatomic distortions or artifact from biopsy are not confused with tumor (see Fig. 16-6).
- Chest imaging, as clinically indicated, and consider positron emission tomography (PET)/CT for locally advanced disease.
- Archer et al. (12) correlated CT findings with the incidence of cartilage or bone invasion on whole-organ sections. In 12 of 14 patients with pathologic evidence of cartilage invasion, the average diameter of the tumor in two dimensions was more than 16 mm, and the lesion was located below the top of the arytenoid.
- Dental, nutrition, and speech and swallow evaluation as clinically indicated.

NEW! SUMMARY OF CHANGES TO AJCC STAGING

- In AJCC 8th edition, no changes have been made to T stage. For nodal staging, extranodal extension (ENE) has been included as an important new consideration. In clinically staged cases, the nodal staging remains unchanged from the 7th edition in cases without clinical evidence of extranodal extension (ECE_C), with exception of any lymph node metastasis greater than 6 cm is now cN3a (previously cN3). ECE_C is defined as invasion of skin, infiltration of muscle, dense tethering or fixation to adjacent structures, cranial nerve, brachial plexus, sympathetic trunk, or phrenic nerve invasion with dysfunction. Cases with clinical evidence of extranodal extension are to be staged as cN3b irrespective of number, size, or laterality of lymph node metastases. In pathologically staged cases, N staging remains the same in cases that are negative for extranodal extension [ENE(−)]. Any lymph node metastasis greater than 6 cm without extranodal extension is now pN3a. A single lymph node metastasis less than or equal to 3 m size and ENE(+) is now pN2a. In cases with single lymph node metastasis greater than 3 cm and ENE(+) or multiple lymph nodes (ipsilateral or bilateral) with any ENE(+), N staging is now pN3b. Overall staging remains the same as in 7th edition AJCC.

See Amin MB, Edge SB, Greene FL, et al., eds. *AJCC cancer staging manual*, 8th ed. New York, NY: Springer, 2017.

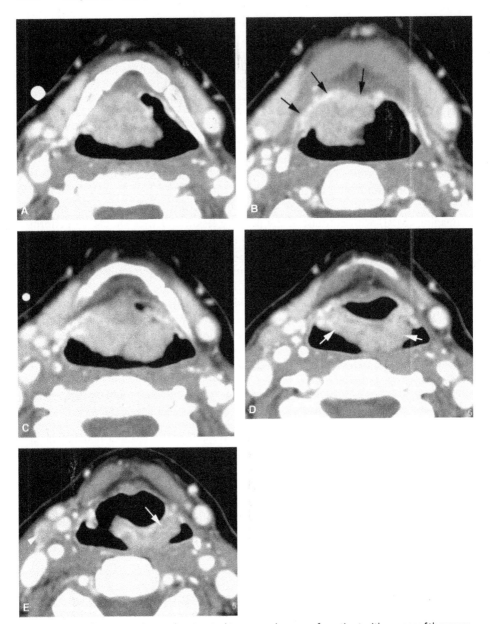

FIGURE 16-6. Contrast-enhanced computed tomography scan of a patient with cancer of the supra-hyoid epiglottis. **A:** Bulky exophytic lesion encompasses the suprahyoid epiglottis. **B:** The tumor spills superiorly from **A** into vallecula to involve but not invade the tongue base mucosa (*arrows*). **C:** Tumor extends to the base of the suprahyoid epiglottis in an exophytic plaquelike manner. **D:** Tumor continues inferiorly along the pharyngoepiglottic folds and upper aryepiglottic folds and in **E** continues inferiorly along the aryepiglottic fold (*arrows*).

MANAGEMENT

Glottic (Vocal Cord) Carcinoma

Carcinoma *In Situ* (Tis)

- Endoscopic resection with microexcision, laser ablation, or vocal cord stripping is recommended.
- Definitive radiotherapy is an effective first-line alternative, particularly for diffuse lesions, or can be used for recurrence.
- Nearly two thirds of patients will ultimately develop invasive cancer (13), and many have occult invasive disease at diagnosis (14).

Early Glottic Carcinoma (T1-T2, N0)

- Upfront management is controversial: definitive radiation and surgery have comparable control rates in large series, and have not been compared head to head prospectively.
- In some centers, definitive radiotherapy is the initial treatment for T1 and T2 lesions. In these cases, surgery can be used for salvage after radiotherapy failure (10,15,16).
- The local control rate with definitive radiotherapy is approximately 90% for T1 lesions and 70% to 80% for T2 lesions.
- Alternatively, transoral laser excision or partial laryngectomy can be performed as indicated. Partial laryngectomy procedures such as hemilaryngectomy or cordectomy demonstrate comparable control rates for selected T1 and T2 vocal cord lesions. However, radiotherapy may be associated with improved voice quality compared to surgery (17).

Moderately Advanced Glottic Carcinoma

- Fixed-cord lesions (T3) can be subdivided into tumors that are amenable to larynx-preserving surgery, or that require total laryngectomy.
- Patients with select, favorable T3 lesions that may be amenable to larynx-preserving surgery have disease confined mostly to one side of the larynx, have a good airway, and are reliable for follow-up.
- These patients may undergo primary radiation or surgery with postoperative radiation as indicated.
- T3 tumors requiring total laryngectomy are treated as locally advanced disease.

Advanced Glottic Carcinoma

- Primary treatment consists of larynx preservation therapy, typically with concurrent chemoradiation (18), or with total laryngectomy and adjuvant radiation or chemoradiation, as indicated.
- Indications for postoperative irradiation include close or positive margins, significant subglottic extension (greater than or equal to 1 cm), cartilage invasion, lymphovascular invasion, perineural invasion, extension of primary tumor into the soft tissues of

the neck, multiple positive neck nodes, N3 disease, extranodal extension, and control of subclinical disease in the opposite neck (19–21).

- Indications for postoperative concurrent chemoradiation include positive margins and/or extranodal extension (Cooper + Bernier).
- As an alternative approach, patients may be treated with induction chemotherapy, with interval response assessment. If there is response to induction therapy, can follow with radiation or concurrent chemoradiation. If minimal response or evidence of progression, consider surgery (22).
- Patients with bulky T4 disease were underrepresented in the VA larynx trial and had higher failure rates with sequential chemoradiation; these patients should be offered upfront surgery.

Surgical Treatment

- In men, the maximum cordal involvement suitable for vertical hemilaryngectomy is one full cord plus one third of the opposite cord. In general, women have smaller larynges, and usually only one vocal cord may be removed without compromising the airway.
- For consideration of vertical hemilaryngectomy, the maximum subglottic extension is 8 to 9 mm anteriorly and 5 mm posteriorly. These limits are necessary to preserve the integrity of the cricoid.
- Tumor extension to the epiglottis, false cord, or bilateral arytenoids is generally a contraindication to vertical hemilaryngectomy.

Radiation Therapy Techniques

Early-stage disease (T1-T2, N0)
- T1-T2, N0 tumors are typically treated with a pair of opposed parallel photon fields, occasionally with a tilt to avoid the shoulders.
- For T1 tumors, the field is centered on the true vocal cords (see Fig. 16-6) with field borders as follows:
  - Superior: top of the thyroid notch
  - Inferior: bottom of the cricoid cartilage
  - Anterior: flash skin at least 1 cm
  - Posterior: anterior margin of the vertebral bodies (11)
- For T1 tumors, the field size ranges from 4 × 4 cm to 5 × 5 cm (plus an additional cm of "flash" anteriorly). For T2 tumors, the field is extended to 6 × 6 cm, although can be greater for large T2 lesions.
- For anteriorly located lesions, or if evidence of anterior commissure involvement, the use of bolus should be considered.
- Recommended radiation dose-fractionation schedule is 63 Gy in 2.25 Gy fractions for T1 tumors, and 65.25 Gy in 2.25 Gy fractions or 70 Gy in 2 Gy fractions for T2 tumors. Dose-fractionation schemes are shown in Table 16-1.
- Yamazaki et al. (23) reported the results of a prospective trial in which patients with T1N0 squamous cell carcinoma of the glottic larynx were randomized to definitive radiotherapy regimens at 2 Gy per fraction or 2.25 Gy per fraction. The 5-year local

Table 16-1

External Beam Radiation Therapy Treatment Plan for Glottic Carcinoma

Tumor Stage	Total Dose (Gy)/Fractions (n)	Time (wk)
Tis	60.75 Gy/27 or 66 Gy/33	5–6
T1	63/28 or 66 Gy/33	5.5–6.5
T2a	65.25/29 or 70 Gy/35	6–7
T2b	65.25/29 or 70 Gy/35	6–7

control rates were 77% after 2 Gy per fraction regimens and 92% after 2.25 Gy per fraction regimens ($p = 0.004$); there was no difference in either acute or late toxicity.
* Patients are commonly treated in the supine position with 4- or 6-MV x-rays using equally weighted parallel-opposed lateral fields with wedges for improved dose homogeneity (Fig. 16-7).

Advanced-stage disease
* Patients with locally advanced disease and/or positive nodes are often treated with intensity-modulated radiation therapy (IMRT). The IMRT technique and design is described in detail below.
* Radiation fields typically cover the at-risk jugulodigastric, middle, and inferior jugular lymph nodes (9) (Fig. 16-1).
* If concurrent chemotherapy is being utilized, patients typically receive 70 Gy in 2 Gy fractions to gross disease, whereas intermediate-risk regions receive 63 Gy in 1.8-Gy fractions, and low-risk regions receive 56 Gy in 1.6-Gy fractions in single course of treatment. Alternative regimens include initial course of treatment to 50 to 54 Gy to sites of gross disease and intermediate- and low-risk regions, followed by a boost or cone-down plan(s) to intermediate-risk regions and gross disease to cumulative doses of 70 Gy to gross disease.
* The entire larynx, preepiglottic space, paraglottic space, vallecula, pyriform sinuses, thyroid cartilage, and tracheostomy site should be contained within the low- and/or intermediate-risk targets, as applicable.
* If treating with radiotherapy alone, accelerated fractionation per the DAHANCA regimen (70 Gy delivered 6 days per week over 6 weeks) can be used (24). Alternative fractionation schedules include 66 Gy in 2.2 Gy fractions over 6 weeks; 72 Gy in 2 Gy fractions over 7 weeks. Hyperfractionation can also be considered using a regimen of twice-daily irradiation at 1.2 Gy per fraction to total doses of 74.4 to 76.8 Gy (25,26) delivered over 7 weeks.
* For patients undergoing chemoradiation, results from a recent randomized trial suggest that PET/CT scan be performed 12 weeks following the completion of chemoradiation, with salvage surgery/neck dissection reserved for patients with incomplete or equivocal responses on imaging (27).

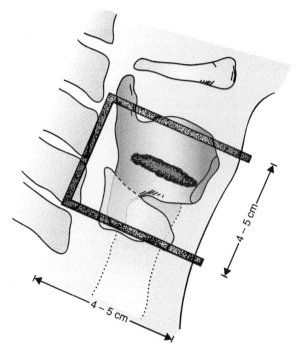

FIGURE 16-7. Early-stage glottic carcinoma radiotherapy field design. The top border is adjusted according to the lesion. The middle of the thyroid notch is the landmark for very early lesions, and the top of the notch is the marker for larger lesions or those with minimal supraglottic extension. The posterior border is 1 cm posterior to the back edge of the thyroid cartilage if the lesion is confined to the anterior two thirds of the vocal cord; if the posterior one third of the vocal cord is involved, the posterior border is placed 1.0 to 1.5 cm behind the cartilage. The inferior border is placed at the bottom of the cricoid cartilage if there is no subglottic extension. (Reprinted with permission from Million RR, Cassisi NJ, Mancuso AA. Larynx. In: Million RR, Cassisi NJ, eds. *Management of head and neck cancer: a multidisciplinary approach*, 2nd ed. Philadelphia, PA: JB Lippincott, 1994:431–497. © Wolters Kluwer.)

Treatment of Recurrence

- Radiation therapy failures may be salvaged by cordectomy, hemilaryngectomy, or total laryngectomy.
- Biller et al. (28) reported a 78% salvage rate by hemilaryngectomy for 18 selected patients in whom irradiation failed; total laryngectomy eventually was required in two patients.
- The rate of salvage by irradiation for recurrences or new tumors that appear after initial treatment by hemilaryngectomy is approximately 50%.

Supraglottic Larynx Carcinoma

Early and Moderately Advanced Supraglottic Lesions

- Tumors that are amenable to larynx-preserving surgery (most T1-2, N0, and select T3) may be treated with definitive radiotherapy, endoscopic resection, or partial supraglottic laryngectomy, with treatment of the neck as indicated.

- If a patient has early, resectable neck disease (N1 or N2a) and surgery is elected for the primary site, postoperative radiotherapy should be considered if there are adverse features (see above).

Advanced Supraglottic Lesions

- These are managed similarly to advanced vocal cord carcinomas.
- Primary treatment consists of larynx preservation with concurrent chemoradiation, or with total laryngectomy and adjuvant radiotherapy or chemoradiation, as indicated.
- Neoadjuvant chemotherapy followed by radiotherapy or chemoradiation for responders is a reasonable alternative for selected patients.

Surgical Treatment

- Supraglottic laryngectomy is a voice-sparing surgery that can be used successfully for selected lesions involving the epiglottis, a single arytenoid, the aryepiglottic fold, or the false vocal cord.
- Extension of the tumor to the true vocal cord, anterior commissure, or both arytenoids precludes supraglottic laryngectomy, as does fixation of the vocal cord or thyroid or cricoid cartilage invasion.
- Supraglottic laryngectomy can be extended to include the base of the tongue if one lingual artery is preserved.
- All patients have difficulty swallowing with a tendency to aspirate immediately after surgery, but almost all learn to swallow again within a short period of time. Motivation and the amount of tissue removed are key factors in learning to swallow again.
- Preoperatively, adequate pulmonary reserve should be confirmed through laboratory evaluation, exercise tolerance, pulmonary function testing, and imaging as indicated.
- Voice quality is generally normal after supraglottic laryngectomy.

Radiation Therapy Techniques

Radiation therapy techniques and doses are similar to those for glottic tumors. However, because of rich lymphatic plexus in the supraglottis, treatment of the bilateral neck regional lymphatics is strongly encouraged in early-stage tumors.

Postoperative treatment
- Adjuvant radiotherapy is added for close or positive margins, invasion of soft tissues of the neck, subglottic extension (greater than or equal to 1 cm), thyroid cartilage invasion, perineural invasion, lymphovascular invasion, multiple positive nodes, and extranodal (extracapsular) extension. Concurrent chemotherapy is typically utilized in cases of positive margins or extranodal extension.
- The base of the tongue and the neck are usually high-risk areas. The stoma is at risk primarily if there is evidence of subglottic extension.
- The postoperative radiotherapy dose as a function of known residual disease is as follows: negative margins, 60 Gy in 30 fractions; microscopically positive margins, 66 Gy in 33 fractions; and gross residual disease, 70 Gy in 35 fractions, with IMRT

commonly used (see detail below). For postoperative treatment of the dissected neck without extranodal extension, a dose of 60 Gy in 30 fractions should be utilized. For neck levels with extranodal extension, a dose of 66 Gy in 33 fractions should be utilized.

- All patients receive continuous-course treatment of 1 fraction per day, 5 days per week.
- Adjuvant radiotherapy should ideally commence within 6 weeks of operative treatment.
- If conventional radiotherapy is used, the undissected lower neck is treated with doses of 50 to 54 Gy in 25 to 30 fractions.
- If there is presence of subglottic extension, the stoma should be boosted with electrons (usually 10 to 14 MeV) for an additional 10 Gy in 5 fractions. Additional situations in which a stoma boost should be considered include but are not limited to emergent tracheostomy, anterior extension of primary tumor, a close or positive margin in this region, presence of extranodal extension in this region (level IV), and involvement of the apex of the pyriform sinus.

COMPARISON OF SURGERY AND RADIATION THERAPY

- The 659 patients with stage I (T1N0M0) glottic carcinoma treated with curative intent at Washington University, St. Louis, MO, were subdivided into four groups. Ninety patients received low-dose irradiation (mean dose 58 Gy; range 55 to 65 Gy; daily fractionation 1.5 to 1.8 Gy); 104 patients received high-dose irradiation (mean dose 66.5 Gy; range 65 to 70 Gy; daily fractionation 2.0 to 2.25 Gy); 404 patients underwent conservation surgery; and 61 patients had endoscopic resection. T1a (85%) and T1b (15%) disease was equally distributed among the groups (29). No significant difference in the 5-year, cause-specific survival rate was observed among the four therapeutic groups for T1 tumors ($p = 0.68$). Actuarial survival was significantly decreased in the low-dose radiation therapy group as compared with the other three therapeutic groups ($p = 0.04$). Initial local control was poorer for the endoscopic (77%) and low-dose irradiation (78%) groups as compared with the high-dose irradiation (89%) and conservation surgery (92%) groups ($p = 0.02$), but significant differences were not found for ultimate local control following salvage treatment. Unaided laryngeal voice preservation was similar for high-dose radiation therapy (89%), conservation surgery (93%), and endoscopic resection (90%), but significantly poorer for low-dose irradiation (80%; $p = 0.02$) (29).
- Among 134 patients with stage II glottic carcinomas treated with curative intent and function preservation, 47 patients were treated with low-dose radiation therapy (median dose, 58.5 Gy at 1.5- to 1.8-Gy daily fractions), 16 patients with high-dose irradiation (67.5 to 70.0 Gy) at higher daily fractionation doses (2.0 to 2.25 Gy), and 71 patients underwent conservation surgery. There were no statistical differences in local control, voice preservation, and 5-year actuarial and disease-specific cure rates between conservation surgery and high-dose irradiation ($p = 0.89$). Patients treated with low-dose irradiation had statistically lower local control, 5-year survival, and voice preservation ($p = 0.014$) (30).

CHEMORADIOTHERAPY FOR LARYNGEAL PRESERVATION

- The Veterans Affairs Larynx Trial established larynx-preservation therapy as a viable alternative to total laryngectomy in patients with advanced laryngeal carcinoma. The trial randomized patients to total laryngectomy followed by postoperative RT versus induction chemotherapy followed by definitive RT for responders. Sixty-four percent of patients in the chemotherapy and radiation arm were able to preserve their larynx at 2 years, and there was no difference in overall survival. Of note, patients with T4 tumors in the nonoperative arm had a lower larynx preservation rate of 44% (31).
- A randomized intergroup trial (Radiation Therapy Oncology Group 91-11) compared three treatment arms: Arm A, three cycles of induction cisplatin and fluorouracil followed by irradiation in complete and partial responders; Arm B, radiation therapy and concomitant cisplatin (100 mg per m^2 on days 1, 22, and 43 of radiation therapy); and Arm C, once-daily irradiation (70 Gy in 35 fractions during 7 weeks) alone (18). Five hundred forty-seven patients were randomized, and 518 patients were evaluable. The rates of larynx preservation were as follows: Arm A, 72%; Arm B, 84%; and Arm C, 67%. The rates of larynx presentation were significantly improved for Arm B; there was no significant difference between Arm A and Arm C. The 5-year survival rates were similar for the three treatment groups: Arm A, 55%; Arm B, 54%; and Arm C, 56%. The likelihood of developing distant metastases was lower for the two groups of patients that received chemotherapy. On 10-year follow-up, concurrent chemoradiation maintained an improvement in rate of larynx preservation (32).

IMRT TARGET VOLUME DELINEATION

Definitive IMRT for Laryngeal Carcinoma (Intact Larynx)

- CTV1 (high-risk volume):
  - Includes all primary and nodal GTV with 5- to 10-mm margin.
  - May truncate air, skin, and bone if not invaded by tumor.
- CTV2 (intermediate-risk volume):
  - Includes the entire CTV1 with a 0- to 5-mm margin (primary and nodal).
  - Includes the entire larynx.
  - Includes high-risk nodal regions:
    - In N1/2a/2b/3, includes ipsilateral nodal levels 1B, 2, 3, 4, and 5
    - In N2c, includes bilateral nodal levels 1B, 2, 3, 4, and 5
  - Level 6 coverage is indicated for subglottic tumor or extension, hypopharyngeal involvement, level 6 adenopathy, emergent tracheostomy, or soft tissue extension from the primary into the neck. Some practitioners routinely cover level 6.
  - Lateral retropharyngeal node coverage is indicated on the N+ side; need not include medial retropharyngeal nodes routinely.
  - Nodal CTV2 of the involved neck extends up to the base of skull (i.e., covers retrostyloid nodes).

- Between the transverse process of C1 and jugular foramen on the ipsilateral involved neck, CTV2 can optionally be defined as CTV3.
- Nodal CTV2 extends inferiorly to sternoclavicular joint when complete ipsilateral neck is treated with IMRT.
- May truncate air, skin, and bone if not invaded by tumor.
- CTV3 (low-risk volume):
  - Includes contralateral uninvolved nodes, at least levels 2 to 4.
  - Optionally excludes nodal levels 5 and IB, retropharyngeal nodes.
  - Inferior margin extends to 2 cm above sternoclavicular joint.
  - Superior margin extends to transverse process C1.
  - May truncate air, skin, and bone if not invaded by tumor.
- Typical CTV dose levels are as follows:
  - CTV1: 70 Gy
  - CTV2: 59.4 to 63 Gy
  - CTV3: 46 to 54 Gy
- Figure 16-3 is an example of definitive IMRT target delineation in a patient with T3N1 left-sided laryngeal carcinoma.

Postoperative IMRT for Laryngeal Carcinoma

- It is important that the treating physician obtain preoperative imaging, clinical exam data, and pathologic data to assist in delineation of primary and nodal disease.
- Where available, seek assistance of surgeon to help delineate extent primary and nodal tumor.
- CTV1 (high-risk volume):
  - Includes all areas of preoperative primary tumor and nodal involvement, as well as the operative bed, including any surgical clips and markers and/or drain sites.
  - Primary
    - Superior coverage to top of hyoid bone or 10 to 20 mm of margin on known primary disease.
    - Inferior coverage to sternoclavicular joint.
    - Include stoma if:
      - o Emergent tracheostomy
      - o Subglottic extension
      - o Tumor invasion into the soft tissues of neck
      - o Close or positive tracheal margin
      - o Surgical scar crosses stoma
    - Optionally exclude esophagus if no risk for tumor extension.
  - Nodal
    - Includes levels 2, 3, 4, 5, and 6; if bilateral involvement is the case then this pertains to bilateral coverage.
    - Includes level IB if positive or if level 2 involvement.
    - Optionally excludes retropharyngeal nodes.
    - Superior coverage to top of C1.

- Inferior coverage to sternoclavicular joint.
- May truncate air, skin, and bone if not invaded by tumor.
- CTV2 (intermediate-risk volume):
  - Includes contralateral undissected, uninvolved neck levels 2, 3, and 4, with 5 and 6 optional.
  - Includes bilateral level IB if dissected but uninvolved and no level 2 involvement.
  - Superior coverage to base of skull.
  - Contralateral uninvolved neck optionally ends at the transverse process of C1.
  - Inferior extension to sternoclavicular joint on uninvolved, dissected neck is optional.
  - Includes stoma if not covered by CTV1.
  - May truncate air, skin, and bone if not invaded by tumor.
- Generally, CTV1 is to 60 Gy and CTV2 is to 54 Gy.
- If positive margin, operative bed should be boosted to 66 Gy.
- If there is ECE, operative bed/areas of ECE should be boosted to 63 to 66 Gy.
- Figure 16-4 is an example of postoperative IMRT target delineation in a patient with resected T2N2b right-sided laryngeal carcinoma.

FOLLOW-UP

- Follow-up of patients with early lesions is planned for every 1 to 3 months for year 1, every 2 to 6 months for year 2, every 4 to 8 months for years 3 to 5, and then annually for life.
- Posttreatment baseline imaging is recommended within 6 months of treatment, with further surveillance imaging as clinically indicated.
- If recurrence is suspected but the biopsy is negative, patients are reexamined at 2- to 4-week intervals until resolution.

SEQUELAE OF TREATMENT

Surgical Sequelae

- Postoperative complications and sequelae of hemilaryngectomy include chondritis, wound slough, inadequate glottic closure, and anterior commissure webs (33).
- Complications associated with supraglottic laryngectomy and total laryngectomy for supraglottic carcinomas include fistula (8%), carotid artery exposure or blowout (3% to 5%), infection or wound sloughing (3% to 7%), and fatal complications (3%) (33).

Radiation Therapy Sequelae

- The voice may improve as the tumor regresses during the first 2 to 3 weeks, but it generally becomes hoarse again because of radiation-induced changes, even as the tumor continues to regress.

- The voice begins to improve approximately 3 weeks after completion of treatment, usually reaching a plateau in 2 to 3 months.
- Edema of the larynx is the most common sequela after irradiation for glottic or supra-glottic lesions. It may be accentuated by radical neck dissection and may require 6 to 12 months to subside.
- Soft tissue necrosis leading to chondritis occurs in less than 1% of patients, usually in those who continue to smoke.
- Corticosteroids such as dexamethasone have been used to reduce radiation-induced edema after recurrence has been ruled out by biopsy. If ulceration and pain occur, administration of an antibiotic, for example, tetracycline, may help.
- It is unusual for patients to require a tracheotomy before irradiation unless severe lymphedema develops at the time of direct laryngoscopy and biopsy. In patients who have recovered from direct laryngoscopy and biopsy without obstruction, a tracheotomy rarely has been required during a fractionated course of irradiation.
- Patients treated twice a day with 1.2-Gy fractions (continuous-course technique) to total doses of 74.0 to 76.8 Gy usually have brisker acute reactions than those treated once a day with 2-Gy fractions (8). Approximately 20% treated with b.i.d. irradiation require nasogastric feeding tubes because of difficulty in swallowing.

References

1. Clemente CD. *Anatomy: a regional atlas of the human body*. Philadelphia, PA: Lea & Febiger, 1975.
2. Siegel RL, Miller KD, Jemal A. Cancer Statistics, 2017. *CA Cancer J Clin* 2017;67(1):7.
3. Wydner EL, Bross IJ, Day E. Epidemiological approach to the etiology of cancer of the larynx. *JAMA* 1956;160:1384.
4. Wynder EL. The epidemiology of cancers of the upper alimentary and upper respiratory tracts. *Laryngoscope* 1978;88(1 Pt 2 Suppl 8):50–51.
5. Lindberg R. Distribution of cervical lymph node metastases from squamous cell carcinoma of the upper respiratory and digestive tracts. *Cancer* 1972;29(6):1446–1449.
6. Fletcher GH. Elective irradiation of subclinical disease in cancers of the head and neck. *Cancer* 1972;29(6):1450–1454.
7. Ogura JH, Biller HF, Wette R. Elective neck dissection for pharyngeal and laryngeal cancers. An evaluation. *Ann Otol Rhinol Laryngol* 1971;80(5):646–650.
8. Mendenhall W, Hinerman R, Amdur R, et al. Larynx. In: Halperin E, Perez C, Brady L, eds. *Principles and practice of radiation oncology*. Philadelphia, PA: Lippincott Williams & Wilkins, 2008:975–995.
9. Mendenhall WM, Million RR, Sharkey DE, et al. Stage T3 squamous cell carcinoma of the glottic larynx treated with surgery and/or radiation therapy. *Int J Radiat Oncol Biol Phys* 1984;10(3):357–363.
10. Mendenhall WM, Parsons JT, Stringer SP, et al. T1-T2 vocal cord carcinoma: a basis for comparing the results of radiotherapy and surgery. *Head Neck Surg* 1988;10(6):373–377.
11. Million RR, Cassisi NJ. *Management of head and neck cancer: a multidisciplinary approach*, 2nd ed. Philadelphia, PA: JB Lippincott Co., 1994.
12. Archer CR, Yeager VL, Herbold DR. Improved diagnostic accuracy in laryngeal cancer using a new classification based on computed tomography. *Cancer* 1984;53(1):44–57.
13. Hintz BL, Kagan AR, Nussbaum H, et al. A watchful waiting policy for in situ carcinoma of the vocal cords. *Arch Otolaryngol* 1981;107:746.

14. Pene F, Fletcher GH. Results in irradiation of the in situ carcinoma of the vocal cord. *Cancer* 1976;37:2586.
15. Fein DA, Mendenhall WM, Parsons JT, et al. T1-T2 squamous cell carcinoma of the glottic larynx treated with radiotherapy: a multivariate analysis of variables potentially influencing local control. *Int J Radiat Oncol Biol Phys* 1993;25(4):605–611.
16. Mendenhall WM, Parsons JT, Stringer SP, et al. Management of Tis, T1, and T2 squamous cell carcinoma of the glottic larynx. *Am J Otolaryngol* 1994;15(4):250–257.
17. Higgins KM, Shah MD, Ogaick MJ, et al. Treatment of early-stage glottic cancer. Meta-analysis comparison of laser excision versus radiotherapy. *J Otolaryngol Head Neck Surg* 2009;38:603–612.
18. Forastiere AA, Goepfert H, Maor M, et al. Concurrent chemotherapy and radiotherapy for organ preservation in advanced laryngeal cancer. *N Engl J Med* 2003;349(22):2091–2098.
19. Amdur RJ, Parsons JT, Mendenhall WM, et al. Postoperative irradiation for squamous cell carcinoma of the head and neck: an analysis of treatment results and complications. *Int J Radiat Oncol Biol Phys* 1989;16(1):25–36.
20. Huang DT, Johnson CR, Schmidt-Ullrich R, et al. Postoperative radiotherapy in head and neck carcinoma with extracapsular lymph node extension and/or positive resection margins: a comparative study. *Int J Radiat Oncol Biol Phys* 1992;23(4):737–742.
21. Mendenhall WM, Parsons JT, Buatti JM, et al. Advances in radiotherapy for head and neck cancer. *Semin Surg Oncol* 1995;11(3):256–264.
22. Urba S, et al. Single-cycle induction chemotherapy selects patients with advanced laryngeal cancer for combined chemoradiation: a new treatment paradigm. *J Clin Oncol* 2006;24(4):593–598.
23. Yamazaki H, Nishiyama K, Tanaka E, et al. Radiotherapy for early glottic carcinoma (T1N0M0): results of prospective randomized study of radiation fraction size and overall treatment time. *Int J Radiat Oncol Biol Phys* 2006;64(1):77–82.
24. Overgaard J, et al. Five compared with six fractions per week of conventional radiotherapy of squamous-cell carcinoma of head and neck: DAHANCA 6 and 7 randomised controlled trial. *Lancet* 2003;362:1588.
25. Parsons JT, Mendenhall WM, Cassisi NJ, et al. Hyperfractionation for head and neck cancer. *Int J Radiat Oncol Biol Phys* 1988;14(4):649–658.
26. Parsons JT, Mendenhall WM, Mancuso AA, et al. Twice-a-day radiotherapy for T3 squamous cell carcinoma of the glottic larynx. *Head Neck* 1989;11(2):123–128.
27. Mehanna H, et al. PET-CT Surveillance versus Neck Dissection in Advanced Head and Neck Cancer. *N Engl J Med* 2016;374:1444–1454.
28. Biller HF, Barnhill FR Jr, Ogura JH, et al. Hemilaryngectomy following radiation failure for carcinoma of the vocal cords. *Laryngoscope* 1970;80(2):249–253.
29. Spector JG, Sessions DG, Chao KS, et al. Stage I (T1 N0 M0) squamous cell carcinoma of the laryngeal glottis: therapeutic results and voice preservation. *Head Neck* 1999;21(8):707–717.
30. Spector JG, Sessions DG, Chao KS, et al. Management of stage II (T2N0M0) glottic carcinoma by radiotherapy and conservation surgery. *Head Neck* 1999;21(2):116–123.
31. The Department of Veterans Affairs Laryngeal Cancer Study Group. Induction chemotherapy plus radiation compared with surgery plus radiation in patients with advanced laryngeal cancer. *N Engl J Med* 1991;324:1685–1690.
32. Forastiere AA, Zhang Q, Weber RS, et al. Long-term results of RTOG 91-11: a comparison of three nonsurgical treatment strategies to preserve the larynx in patients with locally advanced larynx cancer. *J Clin Oncol* 2013;31(7):845–852.
33. Gall AM, Sessions DG, Ogura JH. Complications following surgery for cancer of the larynx and hypopharynx. *Cancer* 1977;39(2):624–631.

CHAPTER 17

RARE TUMORS OF THE HEAD AND NECK

NONEPITHELIAL TUMORS OF THE HEAD AND NECK

Glomus Tumors

Anatomy

- Glomus bodies are found in the jugular bulb and along the tympanic (Jacobson) and auricular (Arnold) branch of the tenth nerve in the middle ear or in other sites (see Fig. 17-1).
- Glomus tumors (paraganglioma) can be classified as tympanic (middle ear), jugular, or carotid vagal, or may originate from other locations such as the orbit, larynx, adventitia of thoracic aorta, abdominal aorta, or surface of the lungs (1).
- Although histologically benign, they may extend along the lumen of the vein to regional lymph nodes, but rarely to distant sites.

Clinical Presentation

- Glomus tumors of the middle ear initially may cause earache or discomfort, pulsatile tinnitus, or hearing loss; in later stages, cranial nerve paralysis results from invasion of the base of skull (10% to 15%) (2).
- If the tumor invades the middle cranial fossa, symptoms may include temporoparietal headache, retroorbital pain, proptosis, and paresis of cranial nerves V and VI. If the posterior fossa is involved, symptoms may include occipital headache, ataxia, and paresis of cranial nerves V to VII, IX, and XII; invasion of the jugular foramen causes paralysis of nerves IX to XI.
- Paraganglioma of the carotid body usually presents as a painless, slowly growing mass in the upper neck; occasionally, it may be pulsatile and have a thrill or bruit. As it enlarges, it may extend into the parapharyngeal space and be visible on examination of the oropharynx (3).
- Metastases occur in 2% to 5% of cases (4) and up to 5% are associated with symptomatic catecholamine hypersecretion (5).

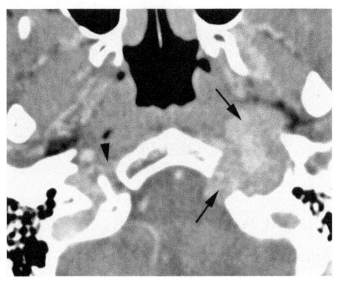

FIGURE 17-1. Contrast-enhanced computed tomography of a patient with a glomus jugulare type of paraganglioma. The enhancing mass arises in the jugular fossa and extends below the skull base and also into the hypoglossal canal (*arrows*) compared to the normal hypoglossal canal on the opposite side (*arrowhead*). The jugular vein can either be invaded or displaced (*arrowhead*); in this case, the vein is more displaced than invaded, but invasion cannot be excluded (*arrowhead*). (Reprinted with permission from Mancuso AA. *Head and neck radiology*. Philadelphia, PA: Lippincott Williams & Wilkins, 2012. © Wolters Kluwer.)

Diagnostic Workup

- Diagnostic evaluation for glomus tumors of the ear and base of skull is outlined in Table 17-1.
- High-resolution computed tomography (CT) with contrast has the highest degree of sensitivity and specificity.
- Biopsy of glomus tumors may result in severe hemorrhage.

Staging

- Prognosis is closely related to anatomic location and volume of lesion, as reflected in the Fisch and Glasscock-Jackson classification systems (Table 17-2) (6–8).

General Management

Surgery
- Surgery generally is used to treat small tumors that can be completely excised as well as catecholamine-secreting tumors, if anatomically possible (9).
- Percutaneous embolization of a low-viscosity silicone polymer has been used, frequently as preoperative preparation of the tumor to decrease intraoperative bleeding.
- Surgical treatment of a glomus tumor arising in the jugular bulb requires more complex surgical approaches involving the base of the skull. It often consists of piece-by-piece removal, which is accompanied by significant bleeding and damage to adjacent neurovascular structures.

Table 17-1

Diagnostic Workup for Glomus Tumors of the Ear and Base of Skull, Hemangiopericytoma, Esthesioneuroblastoma, Extramedullary Plasmacytoma, and Sarcoma of the Head and Neck

General
History
Physical examination

Radiographic Studies
Computed tomography scan to define tumor extent and possible central nervous system involvement
Magnetic resonance imaging with gadolinium
Arteriography to determine bilateral involvement and collateral cerebral blood flow (optional)

Laboratory Studies
Complete blood counts on admission
Blood chemistries
Urinalysis
Fractionated urinary metanephrines and catecholamines or plasma free metanephrines

Special Tests
Audiograms to establish baseline hearing loss
Histologic staining to determine presence of catecholamines

Radiation Therapy
- Irradiation frequently is used to treat glomus tumors, particularly those in the tympanicum, jugular bulb (10), or carotid body (3) where surgery poses increased risk.
- Tumors with destruction of petrous bone, jugular fossa, or occipital bone are more reliably managed with irradiation, as are patients with jugular foramen syndrome (11).
- Some reports describe successful combinations of surgery with either preoperative or postoperative irradiation (10,12).

Radiation Therapy Techniques
- Dickens et al. (13) used a three-field arrangement with a superior-inferior wedged and lateral open field, with a weighting of 1.00 to 1.00 to 0.33.
- Intensity-modulated radiation therapy (IMRT) is typically employed to limit dose to nearby structures, particularly the major salivary glands.
- A recent study of 131 patients with head and neck paragangliomas reported local control rates at 5 and 10 years were 99% and 96%, respectively, when treated to a median dose of 45 Gy in 25 fractions (14).
- Stereotactic radiosurgery has shown promise in local control of this tumor both as primary treatment as well as salvage after incomplete resection. The median dose using gamma knife radiosurgery is 15 Gy. For patients with upfront versus salvage GKS, actuarial tumor progression-free survival at 5 years is 86% versus 90% (15).

Table 17-2

Fisch and Jackson/Glasscock Classification of Head and Neck Paragangliomas

Fisch Classification	
Class A Limited to Middle Ear	Tumors that arise along the tympanic plexus on the cochlear promontory
Class B Limited to Tympanomastoid area	Tumors with invasion of hypotympanum; cortical bone over jugular bulb intact
Class C Tumors involving the infralabyrinthine and apical spaces of temporal bone with extension into the apex	C1—Tumors with encroachment of the carotid foramen, but no invasion of the carotid artery C2—Tumors with destruction of the vertical carotid canal C3—Tumors that invade the horizontal portion of the carotid canal, but do not reach the foramen lacerum C4—Tumors with growth to foramen lacerum and along the carotid artery and the cavernous sinus
Class D Tumors with intracranial extension	$De_{1/2}$—only extradural extension; De_1 with less than 2 cm displacement of the dura. De_2 with more than 2 cm displacement $Di_{1/2/3}$—intradural extension; Di_1 with <2 cm invasion into posterior cranial fossa, Di_2 with between 2 and 4 cm invasion, and Di_3 with >4 cm invasion

Jackson/Glasscock classification	
Jugular Bulb (Glomus jugulare)	Tympanicum (Glomus tympanicum)
Type I Small tumor involving jugular bulb, middle ear, and mastoid	Small tumor limited to the promontory
Type II Tumor extending under internal auditory canal with or without intracranial canal extension	Tumor completely filling middle ear space
Type III Tumor extending into petrous apex with or without intracranial canal extension	Tumor filling middle ear and extending into the mastoid
Type IV Tumor extending beyond petrous apex into clivus or infratemporal fossa with or without intracranial canal extension	Tumor filling middle ear, extending into the mastoid or through tympanic membrane to fill the external auditory canal; may extend anterior to carotid

Data from Fisch U, Mattox D. *Microsurgery of the skull base*. New York, NY: Thieme, 1988:149; Boedeker CC. Paragangliomas and paraganglioma syndromes. *GMS Curr Top Otorhinolaryngol Head Neck Surg* 2011;10:Doc03; and Jackson CG, Glasscock ME III, Harris PF. Glomus tumors. Diagnosis, classification, and management of large lesions. *Arch Otolaryngol* 1982;108:401.

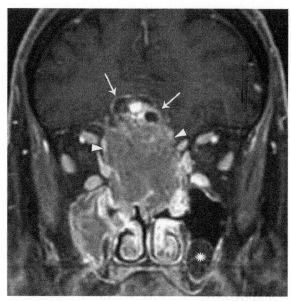

FIGURE 17-2. Esthesioneuroblastoma. Coronal-enhanced fat-saturated T1-weighted image shows a bilateral nasoethmoidal mass (*arrowheads*) with intracranial extension. Peritumoral cysts (*arrows*) are noted at the junction of the tumor and brain parenchyma. (Reprinted with permission from Hoang JK, Becker AM. Diagnostic imaging. In: Johnson J, Rosen CA, *Bailey's head and neck surgery*, 5th ed. Philadelphia, PA: Lippincott Williams & Wilkins; 2014. © Wolters Kluwer.)

- A recent meta-analysis showed that patients undergoing SRS alone for jugular paragangliomas have a tumor control rate of 95% (16).

Hemangiopericytoma

- Hemangiopericytoma is an unusual vascular tumor that is closely related to or indistinguishable from solitary fibrous tumors in the majority of cases; although it may occur anywhere in the body, the head and neck are the most common locations after the lower extremities and retroperitoneum.

Clinical Presentation

- In the head and neck, hemangiopericytoma may be a polypoid, painless, soft gray, or red mass that grows slowly and may cause nasal obstruction; epistaxis is common.
- On arteriography, hemangiopericytoma is the only vascular tumor that has characteristic angiographic features, including radially arranged or spider-like branching vessels around and inside the tumor and a long-standing, well-demarcated tumor stain.

General Management

- Complete local resection, if possible, combined with preoperative embolization of tumor, is the treatment of choice.
- More extensive surgery is required for tumors with malignant features.

- Adjuvant irradiation is associated with increased local control after subtotal and gross total resection. In a retrospective analysis from MDACC, patients with gross total resection plus adjuvant radiotherapy versus gross total resection alone had 5-year local control rates of 92% versus 57%. Radiation doses ≥60 Gy were associated with improved local control (17).
- The role of chemotherapy is not well established and not routinely recommended.

Radiation Therapy Techniques

- Use of radiation therapy alone is controversial.
- The main role of irradiation is either as an adjuvant after complete excision of the lesion or postoperatively for minimal residual disease (18).
- Tumor doses of 60 to 65 Gy in 6 to 7 weeks are required to produce local tumor control in postoperative cases (19).
- The tumor is considered relatively radioresistant; an effective dose for hemangiopericytoma is 75 to 90 Gy in 30 to 60 days (20).
- Fields and beam selection are similar to those used to treat malignant brain tumors or soft tissue sarcomas.
- Stereotactic radiosurgery has shown promise in the local control of this tumor as an adjuvant to surgery, treatment of recurrence, as well as salvage after failure of conventionally fractionated adjuvant therapy. Marginal doses greater than 14 Gy are associated with improved progression-free survival (21–23).

Chordomas

Anatomy

- Chordomas are rare neoplasms of the axial skeleton that arise from the remnant of the primitive notochord (chorda dorsalis) with about one third of tumors arising in the skull base.
- Basisphenoidal chordoma may be difficult to differentiate histologically from chondroma and chondrosarcoma, and radiographically from craniopharyngioma, pineal tumor, and hypophyseal and pontine glioma. Expression of the transcription factor brachyury can aid in diagnosis (24).

Natural History

- Lethality rests on critical location, aggressive local behavior, and extremely high local recurrence rate.
- Lymphatic spread is uncommon.
- Chordomas of the skull base generally have a low metastatic potential unless they have a dedifferentiated histologic subtype. The risk of metastasis in skull base chordomas for all subtypes is less than 10% and the most common site of distant metastasis is the lung, followed by liver and bone (2,25).

Prognostic Factors

- Aside from histology, prognostic factors that most influence choice of treatment are location, local extent of tumor, and surgical resectability.

Clinical Presentation

- In the head, extension may be intracranial or extracranial, into the sphenoid sinus, nasopharynx, clivus, and sellar and parasellar areas, with a resultant mass effect.
- In the spheno-occipital region, the most common presenting symptom is headache.
- Other presentations include symptoms of pituitary insufficiency, nasal stuffiness, bitemporal hemianopia, diplopia, and other cranial nerve deficits.
- Cranial nerve palsies are common in patients with clivus chordoma.

Diagnostic Workup

- Diagnostic workup varies with primary location of disease.
- Most patients have significant bony destruction; some have calcifications in the tumor. Plain x-ray films and CT scans are highly useful; contrast enhancement is required.
- Magnetic resonance imaging (MRI) is inferior to CT in its ability to demonstrate bony destruction and intratumoral calcification but is superior to CT in delineation of tumor extent.
- Because of its greater availability and lower cost, CT is the technique of choice for routine follow-up of previously treated patients.

General Management

- A surgical approach is preferentially recommended (when feasible), but complete surgical extirpation alone is unusual.
- Because of surgical inaccessibility, relative resistance to irradiation, and a high incidence of local recurrence, a combined surgical excision and postoperative irradiation is commonly used.

Radiation Therapy Techniques

- IMRT is a common modality given the proximity of chordoma to various critical structures. Diagnostic CT and/or MRI fusion is routinely employed in treatment planning to help delineate tumor extent.
- Frequently used doses are 55 to 70 Gy (median, 60 Gy) in 1.8- to 2.0-Gy fractions (26). Though challenging to dose escalate due to their locations, chordomas respond best to doses in the range of 70 Gy in conventional fractionation (30).
- Stereotactic irradiation has been used in some patients (27).
- Brachytherapy can be used for recurrent tumors of the base of skull or adjacent to the spine when more aggressive surgical exposure is offered (28), though there are no recent reports of brachytherapy on skull base chordomas, and would be limited to centers with experience in this technique.
- Because of the slow proliferative nature of chordomas, high linear energy transfer may be useful (29). Proton beam boosts have been employed and proton therapy alone may lead to superior local control when compared with conventionally fractionated photon irradiation though no head-to-head trials have been conducted (30).
- A prospective outcomes study of 51 patients treated with proton therapy for spinal chordoma showed a 4-year local control rate of 58%, 4-year cause-specific survival rate of 72%, and 4-year overall survival rate of 57% (31).

Sequelae of Treatment

- In patients treated with high irradiation doses or charged particles, sequelae include brain damage, spinal cord injury, bone or soft tissue necrosis, and xerostomia (2).
- Some patients experience unilateral vision loss or radiation injury to the brainstem (32).
- After high-dose proton therapy for clivus tumors, the actuarial incidence of endocrine abnormalities was 26% at 3 years and 37% at 5 years; hypothyroidism was the most frequent abnormality (33). The dose to the pituitary in patients with abnormalities was equivalent to 63.1 to 67.7 Gy.

Extranodal Nasal-Type NK/T-Cell Lymphoma

- Formerly called lethal midline granuloma or polymorphic malignant reticulosis, it is characterized by progressive, unrelenting ulceration, and necrosis of the midline facial tissues. It is associated with Epstein-Barr virus.
- *Wegener's granulomatosis* is a nonmalignant syndrome consisting of epithelioid necrotizing granulomatosis with vasculitis of small vessels. Systemic involvement of the kidneys and lungs is common. It should be considered in the differential diagnosis of patients with a nasal granuloma.
- Most patients have involvement of the nasal cavity (including destruction of septum) and paranasal sinuses (particularly maxillary antrum).
- The primary lesion may extend into the orbits, oral cavity (palate, gingiva), or even the pharynx and up to 25% of patients have primary extra nasal disease (34).

Clinical Features and Diagnostic Workup

- Clinical manifestations include progressive nasal discharge, obstruction, foul odor emanating from the nose, and, in later stages, pain in the nasal cavity, paranasal areas, and even in the orbits.
- Examination discloses ulceration and necrosis in the nasal cavity, perforation or destruction of nasal septum and turbinates, and even ulceration of the nose.
- Edema of the face and eyelids may be noted; the bridge of the nose may be sunken.
- Radiographic studies initially show soft tissue swelling, mucosal thickening, and findings consistent with chronic sinusitis.
- CT is invaluable in demonstrating the full extent of the tumor, including bone or cartilage destruction.
- Other workup includes PET scan, bone marrow biopsy, and EBV viral load (35).

General Management and Radiation Therapy Techniques

- When treatment is planned, it is extremely important to exclude the diagnosis of Wegener's granulomatosis, a benign process that is commonly treated with immunosuppressive agents and occasionally systemic chemotherapy. The treatment of choice for localized ENKTL is still under study, but recommended regimens consist of chemoradiation, if the patient can tolerate chemotherapy or radiation therapy alone for early-stage disease (36,37).

- High-dose extended field radiotherapy is recommended with doses of at least 50 Gy in 1.8 to 2 Gy fractions (38). Target volume should encompass all areas of involvement, including adjacent areas at risk (i.e., for a lesion of the anterior nasal cavity, the CTV would include the bilateral nasal cavity, frontal ethmoid sinus, and ipsilateral maxillary sinus) (37).
- Irradiation techniques are similar to those for tumors of the paranasal sinuses, nasal cavity, or nasopharynx (2).
- In a more recent series, 5-year OS and PFS rates for stage I disease treated with extended field radiotherapy alone were 80% and 69% respectively.
- The majority of treatment failures are because of systemic dissemination, and the utility of systemic chemotherapy to decrease risk of distant failure in localized disease is under study (39,40).

Myeloid Sarcoma

- Myeloid sarcoma (chloroma, granulocytic sarcoma, and myeloblastoma) is a solid extramedullary tumor composed of early myeloid precursors usually associated with AML.
- It can be seen in patients with CML, myelodysplastic, or myeloproliferative syndromes and can serve as evidence of progression into an acute phase of disease such as acute myelocytic leukemia or blast crisis.
- Myeloid sarcoma has been identified in 3% of patients with acute chronic granulocytic leukemia. It also can be seen with other myeloproliferative disorders (polycythemia vera, hypereosinophilia, and myeloid metaplasia) (2).

Clinical Presentation and Diagnostic Workup

- The most common sites of presentation are the orbit and other craniofacial bones. Intraorbital (retrobulbar) myeloid sarcoma causes insidiously progressive exophthalmos or temporal swelling.
- Central nervous system (CNS) involvement causes local pressure phenomena and elevation of intracranial pressure with consequent headaches, nausea, and vomiting.
- All patients require complete hematologic and neurologic testing, as in any patient with suspected leukemia.
- Radiographic findings include localized bone destruction with predominantly lytic lesions and associated soft tissue masses in orbital and periorbital myeloid sarcoma.
- Intracranial myeloid sarcoma may exhibit intermediate or high attenuation on unenhanced CT scans, with intense, uniform enhancement after intravenous administration of contrast material. Confusion with meningioma, hematoma, solitary metastasis, and lymphoma may occur on CT scans.
- Open biopsy is the best diagnostic tool.

General Management and Radiation Therapy Techniques

- Myeloid sarcomas are extremely radiosensitive. Responses of leukemic infiltrates have been reported with doses as low as 4 Gy; yet the need for higher doses up to 30 Gy has been reported in older studies (2).

- Radiation therapy is typically given as consolidative treatment after chemotherapy.
- A recent report from Memorial Sloan Kettering suggests an algorithm for the inclusion of radiotherapy for patients with myeloid sarcoma based several factors (marrow involvement, relapse, response to chemo, history of bone marrow transplant, and symptomatology).
- The recommended dose is 24 Gy in 12 fractions with 1 to 2 cm margins on the post-chemotherapy volume (41).
- Irradiation techniques depend on location of the infiltrate. For superficial lesions, electron beam is recommended.
- Orbital myeloid sarcoma constitutes a radiation therapy emergency, because vision loss is possible if the patient is not treated promptly.

Esthesioneuroblastoma

- Esthesioneuroblastomas are rare tumors thought to arise in the olfactory receptors in the nasal mucosa of the cribriform plate of the ethmoid bone.
- The olfactory nerves perforate grooves in the ethmoid bone in the cribriform plate and continue into the subarachnoid spaces, accounting for the high incidence of intracranial extension.

Natural History

- Lymphatic spread may be to subdigastric, posterior cervical, submaxillary, or preauricular nodes, as well as the nodes of Rouviere.
- The exact incidence of distant metastases is uncertain; it has been reported to be as high as 50%, but this rate is influenced by the use of chemotherapy in high-risk patients.

Clinical Presentation

- Epistaxis and nasal blockage are the most common clinical symptoms (42).
- Local pain or headache, visual disturbances, rhinorrhea, tearing, proptosis, anosmia, or swelling in the cheek may occur.
- Symptoms may be associated with a mass in the neck.

Diagnostic Workup and Staging

- Table 17-1 outlines the suggested diagnostic workup.
- Physical examination may reveal the inferior aspect of a nasal polypoid friable mass.
- Ocular findings or a mass in the nasopharynx may be present.
- With early lesions, radiographs or CT may show only nonspecific opacification, soft tissue swelling, and occasionally, bone destruction.
- MRI, especially with gadolinium contrast, may be used as a supplement or alternative to CT scanning (43) (see Fig. 17-2).
- A staging system has been proposed by Kadish et al. (Table 17-3) (44) and continues to be commonly used today.
- PET/CT imaging may be useful in detecting lymphatic metastasis or distant disease in patients with Kadish C or high-grade disease (45).

Table 17-3	
Kadish System for Staging of Esthesioneuroblastoma	
Stage	Characteristic
A	Disease confined to the nasal cavity
B	Disease confined to the nasal cavity and one or more paranasal sinuses
C	Disease extending beyond the nasal cavity or paranasal sinuses; includes involvement of the orbit, base of skull, or intracranial cavity
D	Tumor with neck or distant metastasis

Data from Kadish S, Goodman M, Wang CC. Olfactory neuroblastoma: a clinical analysis of 17 cases. *Cancer* 1976;37:1571–1576.

Prognostic Factors

- Extension of primary tumor based on the Kadish staging system is the most important determinant of treatment outcome.
- High-grade tumors have worse outcomes (46).

General Management

- Surgery alone appears to be adequate treatment for small, low-grade tumors confined to the ethmoids in which negative surgical margins can be obtained (2).
- An ethmoidomaxillary resection is usually necessary, with or without orbital sparing. Minimally invasive endoscopic surgery can be considered in select patients to minimize complications. Either procedure can be combined with preoperative or postoperative irradiation, though postoperative RT is more typical.
- Patients with locally advanced disease or high-grade tumors should receive aggressive treatment with combined modalities, such as surgery, irradiation, and chemotherapy (47).
- Chao et al. (42) showed that in 25 patients with esthesioneuroblastoma treated at the Mallinckrodt Institute of Radiology, the 5-year actuarial overall survival, disease-free survival, and local tumor control rates were 66.3%, 56.3%, and 73.0%, respectively. The local control rates were 87.4% for the combination of surgery and radiation therapy and 51.2% for irradiation alone. With adjuvant radiation therapy, the surgical margin status did not influence local tumor control. Among the eight patients who received neoadjuvant chemotherapy, six patients showed no response, one had partial response, and one showed a complete response.
- The role of adjuvant chemotherapy is unclear. However, a study of nine pediatric patients treated with neoadjuvant chemotherapy, surgery, and postoperative radiotherapy showed a 5 year disease-free survival rate of 91% (48).
- For advanced lesions in which disseminated disease is likely, chemotherapy may decrease the incidence of distant metastases.
- Chemotherapy regimens vary and more commonly utilize cisplatin and etoposide, whereas other regimens may employ adriamycin, vincristine, and ifosfamide or cyclophosphamide.

Elective Neck Treatment

- In a literature review of 110 patients, 24 patients (22%) with esthesioneuroblastoma had metastatic disease, with cervical lymph nodes being the most common site (49).
- A retrospective review found that the cumulative cervical metastasis rate was 27% (55 of 207 patients) (50).
- Because of the low incidence of cervical lymph node metastasis (≤10%) in early-stage disease, elective irradiation of the neck or a dissection is not indicated. However, in patients with Kadish stage C disease, the cervical lymph node metastatic rate increases significantly, with one report suggesting rates above 40% (6). In patients with Kadish stage B or C disease, or Hyams grade 3 or 4 disease, cervical nodes should be managed by irradiation, selective neck dissection, or a combination of both. The role of elective neck treatment is unclear in the setting of in the setting of chemotherapy treatment, with one series suggesting limited clinical value in neck treatment (51).

Radiation Therapy Techniques

- For intracranial or posterior extension or tumor that has spread into the maxillary sinus, a pair of perpendicular (anteroposterior and lateral) fields with wedges, or two lateral wedge fields in conjunction with an open anterior photon field, will give good coverage of the treatment volume with the dose inhomogeneity around 10% to 20% (2).
- The orbits can be spared or treated as the degree of extension dictates.
- Eye blocks must be positioned precisely to avoid undesirable side effects.
- For extensive disease, a pair of wedged lateral and anterior portals gives the best uniform coverage. This beam arrangement can be modified for disease extending into the orbit or maxillary sinus. Obturator or bolus may be needed postoperatively to compensate for tissue deficit.
- Techniques are similar to those described for treatment of paranasal sinuses (Chapter 15).
- IMRT is typically employed to limit dose to nearby structures.
- A minimum postoperative dose of 54 Gy in 1.8 Gy per fraction is recommended (52). High dose per fraction (exceeding 2 Gy) increases the possibility of late sequelae such as blindness and bone (or brain) necrosis.
- Doses of 65 to 70 Gy have been delivered with irradiation alone in patients with inoperable tumors, though survival has not been found to improve with higher radiation doses in patients receiving only radiotherapy in a large retrospective series (53).
- Contrast-enhanced CT or MRI scans before initiation of treatment are crucial to demarcate extension of the tumor. Fusion with treatment planning CT can aid significantly in target delineation. Because of the proximity of esthesioneuroblastoma to the optic nerves, optic chiasm, and brainstem, the precision of treatment setup, tumor control and treatment sequelae are dictated by target volume definition and dose homogeneity.
- Treatment techniques similar to those for paranasal sinuses may create "hot spots" along the optic tracks, and care should be taken to avoid such hot spots.
- Three-dimensional treatment planning provides an alternative technique. Incorporation of a vertex field eliminates the high inhomogeneous dose along the junction line of the conventional three-field technique.

- Meta-analysis and systematic review showed proton beam therapy had higher disease-free survival and locoregional tumor control compared with IMRT (54,55).

Extramedullary Plasmacytomas

- Solitary plasmacytomas are rare tumors of plasma cell origin; multiple myeloma occurs approximately 40 times more frequently than solitary plasmacytoma.
- The nasopharynx, nasal cavity, paranasal sinuses, and tonsils are the most common sites of extramedullary plasmacytoma in the head and neck.

Clinical Presentation and Diagnostic Workup

- Usual criteria for solitary plasmacytomas (medullary or extramedullary) are a biopsy-proven plasma cell tumor with one or two (at the most) solitary foci, absence of Bence Jones protein in the urine, bone marrow taken some distance from the primary site not involved by tumor (less than 10% of plasma cells), hemoglobin of 13 g/mL or more, and normal serum protein level or serum electrophoresis at the time of diagnosis. The diagnosis of solitary plasmacytoma is made by exclusion, by eliminating the possibility of multiple myeloma.
- Approximately 10% to 35% of solitary extramedullary cases will convert to multiple myeloma (56).
- Solitary bone plasmacytomas have a high conversion rate to multiple myeloma, with 65% to 84% of patients progressing to multiple myeloma 10 years after diagnosis (57). In contrast, the rate of patients with extramedullary plasmacytoma progressing to multiple myeloma is much lower, reported in a large study to be 16.1% (58).
- Plasmacytomas tend to be sessile in the nasal cavity and paranasal sinuses and pedunculated in the nasopharynx and larynx.
- Although some authors have reported that bone destruction adversely affects prognosis (59), it is not a particularly bad prognostic sign.
- Cervical lymph node metastases follow the same pattern of spread as squamous cell carcinoma; the incidence is 12% to 26% (2).
- Diagnostic workup for extramedullary plasmacytoma arising in the head and neck region is shown in Table 17-1.

General Management

- Pedunculated extramedullary plasmacytoma lesions may be treated by surgical excision because the chance of local recurrence is slight.
- Treatment of choice for all other lesions is radiation therapy.

Radiation Therapy Techniques

- Techniques are similar to those for primary tumors in comparable locations (nasopharynx, tonsil, and paranasal sinuses).
- Extramedullary plasmacytomas respond well to doses of 45 to 50 Gy in 1.8- to 2-Gy fractions.

- Local tumor control with irradiation alone is approximately 85%.
- A study of head and neck extramedullary plasmacytoma showed doses greater than 45 Gy improve local control (60).

Nasopharyngeal Angiofibroma

- Juvenile nasopharyngeal angiofibroma is found most frequently in young, pubertal boys. It is believed to originate from the broad area of the posterolateral wall of the nasal cavity where the sphenoidal process of the palatine bone meets the horizontal ala of the vomer and the roof of the pterygoid process (61).

Clinical Presentation

- Nasal obstruction or epistaxis followed by nasal voice or discharge, cheek swelling, proptosis, diplopia, hearing loss, and headaches are the most common complaints (62).
- Anomalous sexual development has been noted.

Diagnostic Workup

- After a history and physical examination, CT scans, with and without contrast, should be obtained. The pattern of enhancement in this highly vascular tumor is diagnostic; many authors believe carotid angiograms are unnecessary (63) after CT diagnosis of the lesion, unless embolization is contemplated (see Fig. 17-3).
- If intracranial extension is noted and radiation therapy is contemplated, no further studies are indicated.
- If the lesion is extracranial and surgery is indicated, bilateral carotid angiograms will identify the feeding vessels and delineate the boundaries of the tumor.
- Biopsies are not indicated in all patients because of the potential for severe hemorrhage. However, it is important to perform a biopsy of the lesion when the clinical picture (sex and age of patient, location and behavior of lesion) is not consistent with juvenile nasopharyngeal angiofibroma.

Staging

- Table 17-4 shows the staging system of Chandler et al. (64).
- A radiographic staging system was proposed by Sessions et al. (65):
  - Stage Ia is limited to the nasopharynx and posterior nares.
  - Stage Ib extends to the paranasal sinuses.
  - Stages IIa, b, and c extend to other extracranial locations.
  - Stage III is intracranial.

General Management

- For extracranial tumors, surgery is the treatment of choice and yields near-zero mortality or long-term morbidity.
- Newer endoscopic techniques may be the treatment of choice as opposed to open surgery (66).

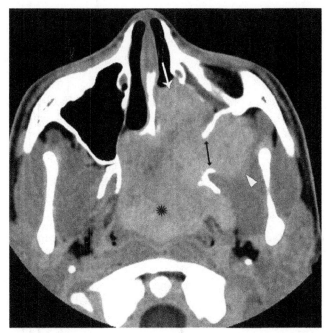

FIGURE 17-3. Juvenile nasopharyngeal angiofibroma. Enhanced axial CT shows a large enhancing mass in the nasopharynx (*asterisk*), left nasal cavity (*arrow*), left maxillary sinus, and infratemporal fossa/masticator space (*arrowhead*). There is widening of the pterygomaxillary fissure (*double headed arrow*). (Reprinted with permission from Hoang JK, Becker AM. Diagnostic imaging. In: Johnson J, Rosen CA, *Bailey's head and neck surgery*, 5th ed. Philadelphia, PA: Lippincott Williams & Wilkins; 2014. © Wolters Kluwer.)

- For intracranial tumor extension, which occurs in approximately 20% of patients, the risk of surgically related death increases. Most of these patients are best treated with irradiation though a recent systematic review of surgical outcomes for patients with intracranial involvement showed no surgical mortality and a recurrence rate of 18% with effective salvage surgery or radiation treatment (67).
- Some authors recommend preoperative intra-arterial tumor vessel embolization at the time of diagnostic bilateral carotid angiography, which may lead to a decrease in operative bleeding.

Table 17-4	
Staging of Nasopharyngeal Angiofibromas	
Stage I	Confined to the nasopharynx
Stage II	Extension to nasal cavity and/or sphenoid sinus
Stage III	Extension to one or more: antrum, ethmoid, pterygomaxillary, and infratemporal fossae, orbit, and/or cheek
Stage IV	Intracranial extension

Data from Chandler JR, Goulding R, Moskowitz L, et al. Nasopharyngeal angiofibromas: staging and management. *Ann Otol Rhinol Laryngol* 1984;93:322.

- Although radiation therapy is equally effective in extracranial tumors, the low but existing risk of secondary malignancies should limit its use to the most advanced tumors only (62,68,69).

Radiation Therapy Techniques

- Treatment techniques and fields are similar to those used in carcinoma of the nasopharynx (without irradiating the cervical lymph nodes) or carcinoma of the paranasal sinuses when these structures or the nasal cavity is involved.
- The eyes are protected in all cases.
- Recommended tumor dose ranges from 30 to 55 Gy in 1.8 to 2 Gy fractions. Doses greater than 40 Gy are recommended in larger tumors (70,71).

Sequelae of Therapy

- Surgical mortality increases with intracranial extension of the tumor.
- Delayed growth secondary to hypopituitarism and decreased bone maturation are the most common irradiation sequelae (64).
- Cataracts are seen infrequently with adequate protection of the eyes during therapy.
- There are four well-documented cases of radiation-induced sarcomas in these patients, with doses ranging from 66 Gy to more than 90 Gy (68).

Nonlentiginous Melanoma

- Malignant melanoma accounts for 11% of primary head and neck malignancies (2).
- Of all malignant melanomas, 20% to 35% are located in the head and neck area (72).
- Head and neck melanoma have higher rates of local recurrence and regional lymphatic spread than extremity or trunk melanomas.

Cutaneous Melanomas

- The superficial spreading and nodular types of malignant melanoma have a metastatic potential of 10% to 30% and 50%, respectively (72).
- A thorough evaluation with CT scans should determine whether there is intracranial or base of the skull involvement.

Mucosal Melanomas

- Primary mucosal melanomas of the head and neck area comprise less than 2% of all melanomas in the United States. Five percent of mucosal melanomas are located in the head and neck (73). Metastatic melanoma to the mucosa of the head and neck area is uncommon; the most common sites are the larynx, tongue, and tonsil.

Diagnostic Workup

- An excisional biopsy should be performed when feasible in order to determine the thickest part of the lesion and because of possible local or metastatic spread secondary to a punch or incisional biopsy, although this has not been noted in cutaneous melanomas.

Prognostic Factors

- Greater than 0.5-mm invasion is a poor prognostic factor.
- Lymph node involvement is a poor prognostic factor (74).
- Mucosal melanomas fare worse than their cutaneous counterparts.

Management

- Melanomas ≤1 mm thick should be excised with a 1 cm margin. Melanomas greater than 1 mm thick should be excised with a 2 cm if possible. Margins greater than 2 cm have not demonstrated a local recurrence or survival benefit (75,76).
- Sentinel lymph node biopsy should be performed in lesions greater than 1 mm thick.
- Adjuvant irradiation should be considered in the setting of inadequate surgical margins, clinical lymph node positivity, histologic extracapsular extension after neck dissection, or as palliation in metastatic disease (77,78).
- The recommended adjuvant or elective radiation treatment for patients with cervical disease is 48 Gy in 20 fractions administered daily or 30 Gy in 5 fractions administered twice weekly (79,80).
- Numerous dose fractionation schedules have shown efficacy in the treatment of melanomas.

Lentigo Maligna Melanoma

- Lentigo maligna (Hutchinson's melanotic freckle or circumscribed precancerous melanosis of Dubreuilh) and its invasive counterpart, lentigo maligna melanoma (LMM), are well-recognized clinicopathologic entities.
- Approximately one third of lentigo maligna lesions, if left untreated, will transform into invasive LMM.

Clinical Presentation and Diagnostic Workup

- Superficial nodularity, hyperpigmentation of the skin, and eventual ulceration may develop as lentigo maligna lesions become more invasive.
- The 10% regional and distant metastatic spread in LMM contrasts with the 25% metastatic tendency in nodular melanomas arising in superficial spreading melanomas and 50% metastatic spread in nodular melanomas arising *de novo* (2).
- Biopsies of the lesion are required to obtain histopathologic confirmation of diagnosis. Careful physical examination must rule out any areas of extension or regional or distant spread.
- Only one third of pathologically proven LMMs show clinical evidence of nodular formation.

General Management

- Usual treatment of lentigo maligna and LMM is surgery, with approximately 1-cm margin of normal skin and skin grafting (if necessary).

- Because of the low incidence of regional lymph node metastases, elective lymph node dissection is not indicated.
- In 26 patients with lentigo maligna and 19 patients with LMM treated with Mohs' microsurgery, all were free of local disease or metastases at an average of 29.2 months (81).
- Radiation therapy with various techniques has been used frequently to treat these patients, particularly those with larger lesions and in general patient outcomes are similar to surgery (82).

Radiation Therapy Techniques

- As in other skin lesions, fields should be carefully designed to include the entire tumor with adequate margin (1 cm for lesions less than 2 cm; 2 cm for larger tumors).
- Superficial x-rays (100 to 200 keVp) with adequate filtration or electrons (6 to 9 MeV) with appropriate thickness of bolus (approximately 1.5 cm) are adequate for most patients (72,83).
- Doses of 45 to 50 Gy in 15 to 25 fractions delivered in 3 to 5 weeks will control disease in most patients (84).
- We recommend delivering 3.0 to 3.5 Gy three times weekly, every other day, to a total dose of approximately 50 Gy. Elective irradiation of the regional lymphatics is unnecessary.

Sarcomas of the Head and Neck

- Sarcomas account for less than 1% of malignant neoplasms in the head and neck.
- Histologies include osteosarcoma, angiosarcoma, chondrosarcoma, hemangiosarcoma, leiomyosarcoma, liposarcoma, malignant fibrous sarcoma, rhabdomyosarcoma, malignant schwannoma, neurofibrosarcoma, and synovial sarcoma. Fibrosarcoma and rhabdomyosarcoma are the most common types.

NEW! **SUMMARY OF CHANGES TO AJCC STAGING**

- Several changes have been made in the 8th edition of the AJCC staging for melanoma. Changes include the use of T0 if no evidence of primary tumor and Tis for in-situ melanoma. Mitoses are no longer part of the T category, and T1b category now signifies a tumor greater than 0.8 to 1 mm thick with or without ulceration.
- "Microscopic" and "macroscopic" detection of tumor in lymph nodes is now referred to as "clinically occult" and "clinically detected," respectively. N1c, N2c, and N3c categories now take into account the presence of microsatellites, satellite metastases, and in-transit metastases.
- A new M1d category accounts for distant metastasis to CNS, and the M category is modified based on normal or elevated LDH.

See: Amin MB, Edge SB, Greene FL, et al., eds. *AJCC Cancer Staging Manual*. 8th ed. New York: Springer, 2017.

Clinical Presentation and Diagnostic Workup

- Clinical presentation varies with primary site of disease; distribution is 33% in the scalp or face, 26% in the orbit or paranasal sinuses, 14% in the upper aerodigestive tract including larynx, and 27% in the neck (2).
- Tumors arising from the aerodigestive tract usually present with nasal bleeding, palpable mass in the neck, or difficulty in swallowing or breathing.
- In tumors arising from the base of skull or the nerve sheath, cranial nerve deficit is the most common presentation.
- Diagnostic workup is the same as for soft tissue sarcomas of other sites in the body.
- Table 17-1 outlines the suggested diagnostic workup.
- With early lesions, radiographs or CT may show only nonspecific opacification, soft tissue swelling, and occasionally, bone destruction.
- MRI, especially with gadolinium contrast, may be used as a supplement or alternative to CT scanning (43), but a CT of the chest is mandatory for staging workup.

Prognostic Factors

- Prognostic factors for predicting local recurrence or disease-free survival include anatomic site, treatment modality, tumor histologic subtype, tumor grade, tumor size, extension of disease, and surgical margins (85,86).

General Management

- Surgery initially is the preferred treatment modality. Unfortunately, it is often difficult to achieve complete tumor resection; extracapsular enucleation of the tumor results in 90% local recurrence.
- Wide local excision, with a 5-cm margin around the pseudo capsule in extremity sarcomas, is associated with better outcome, although approximately 20% will have local recurrence.
- Criteria for surgical resection are impractical for head and neck sarcomas; wide local excision is rarely possible because tumors extend beyond the confines of origin and in the proximity of vital neurovascular structures.

NEW! SUMMARY OF CHANGES TO AJCC STAGING

- The AJCC 8th edition has a new chapter regarding staging of soft tissue sarcomas of the head and neck. The T staging has lower cutoffs than the sarcoma staging of the trunk, with T1 ≤ 2 cm, T2 > 2 cm but ≤4 cm, T3 > 4 cm, and T4 invading adjacent structures. The N category remains the same for soft tissue sarcoma of other sites, with N0 indicating no overt regional lymph node metastasis, and N1 indicating regional lymph node metastasis.

See: Amin MB, Edge SB, Greene FL, et al., eds. *AJCC Cancer Staging Manual*. 8th ed. New York: Springer, 2017.

- As in soft tissue sarcomas in other locations, wide local excision with an adequate margin and preoperative or postoperative irradiation is recommended to avoid more extensive and potentially morbid surgery (87).
- Given the rarity of head and neck sarcoma, no randomized trials exist that prove benefit to adjuvant irradiation. Adjuvant radiotherapy should be strongly considered in large, high-grade tumors and is mandatory in tumors with close or positive margins.

Radiation Therapy Techniques

- Complete coverage of the surgical bed and scar with adequate margins (3 to 5 cm) is required; however, because of the proximity of critical and radiosensitive organs (eyes, spinal cord, and brainstem), it is important to select clinical target margins without risking compromise of the functioning of these organs.
- Techniques similar to those used in epithelial tumors of the head and neck can be applied to sarcomas. IMRT is commonly employed.
- For postoperative irradiation, the recommended regimen is 50 Gy in 2 Gy fractions followed by a 10 to 16 Gy boost if negative margins, 16 to 18 Gy boost if microscopically positive margins, or a 20 to 26 Gy boost if gross residual disease.
- Some institutions prefer preoperative irradiation (88) followed by a postoperative boost for treatment of microscopic or gross residual disease, including techniques such as intraoperative RT, brachytherapy, and/or external beam radiotherapy. The initial preoperative dose is 50 Gy followed by a postoperative 16 to 18 Gy boost if microscopically positive margins, or a 20 to 26 Gy boost if gross residual disease (89).

EAR

Anatomy

- The external ear consists of the auricle (pinna), the external auditory meatus, external auditory canal (EAC), and the tympanic membrane (Fig. 17-4). The auricle is composed of several cartilaginous subunits which are continuous with the cartilaginous EAC: the helix, antihelix, tragus, and antitragus (Fig. 17-4). The outer third of the EAC is cartilaginous, whereas the inner two third is bony and slightly narrower. The tympanic membrane is composed of multiple layers of squamous epithelium and serves to separate the auditory canal from the middle ear.
- The middle ear (tympanic cavity) houses the auditory ossicles and opens into the eustachian tube to communicate with the pharynx (Fig. 17-5).
- The inner ear lies in the petrous portion of the temporal bone and contains the cochlea and the vestibular system (semicircular canals).
- The vestibulocochlear nerve (cranial nerve VIII), exits the brainstem, enters the internal acoustic meatus, and innervates the inner ear's auditory and vestibular function.
- Lymphatic vessels of the tragus and anterior portion of the auricle drain into the superficial parotid lymph nodes. The posterior and superior aspects of the auricle drain into the retroauricular lymph nodes, whereas the lobule drains into the superficial cervical group of lymph nodes.

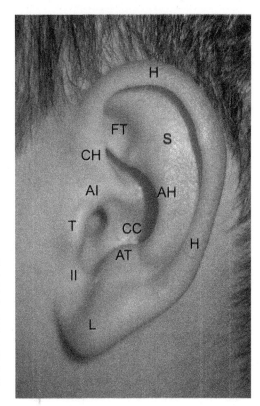

FIGURE 17-4. Anatomy of the external ear. AH, antihelix; AI, anterior incisura; AT, antitragus; CC, conchal cavum; CH, crus of helix; FT, fossa triangularis; H, helix; II, intertragic incisures; L, lobule; S, scaphoid fossa; T, tragus. (Reprinted with permission from Gidley PW. Special considerations: periauricular lesions. In: Weber RS, Moore BA, eds. *Cutaneous malignancy of the head and neck: a multidisciplinary approach*. San Diego, CA: Plural Publishing, Inc.; 2011:155–172.)

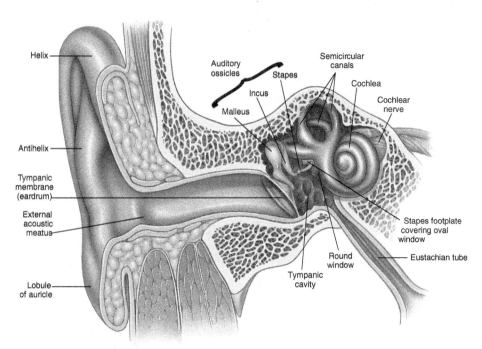

FIGURE 17-5. Cross-sectional anatomy of the external and internal ear.

- Lymphatics from the middle ear drain to the parotid nodes and the upper deep cervical lymph nodes.
- The lymphatics in the middle ear and eustachian tube are sparse.
- The inner ear has no lymphatics (90).

Clinical Presentation and Pathologic Classification

- Auricle tumors are most commonly cutaneous malignancies, whereas EAC and middle ear are extremely rare. Basal cell carcinomas are more frequently seen than squamous cell carcinomas (SCC) in the external ear (91). Tumors present as small ulcerations and tend to occur on the helix (92).
- Pruritus, pain, decreased hearing, and facial paralysis can occur for lesions of the external auditory canal. These are more often SCC.

Diagnostic Workup

- CT can help determine the operability of tumors in the EAC (93) (Fig. 17-6)
- MRI can differentiate tumor from mastoiditis or cholesteatomas, and helps better estimate tumor extent by evaluating involvement of the parotid gland, parapharyngeal space, muscle infiltration, vascular involvement, and intracranial extension (94).

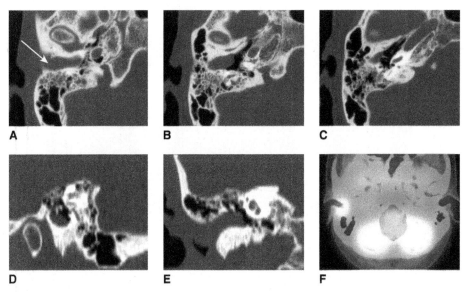

FIGURE 17-6. CT of a small external auditory canal (EAC) squamous cell carcinoma. Axial **(A–C)**, reformatted sagittal **(D)**, and coronal **(E)** CT scans show a soft tissue mass filling the right EAC (*arrow*) with minimal, if any adjacent osseous destruction. The mass invades the middle ear and abuts the ossicles. Fused PET/CT **(F)** demonstrates a focus of increase activity in the same region of the EAC and middle ear, uptake in the area consistent with a squamous cell carcinoma.

Prognostic Factors

- External ear lesions tend to have the best prognosis because of their early diagnosis, amenability to adequate surgery, and mostly cutaneous histology. Extension into the middle ear or temporal bone, cranial nerve VII palsy, and lymph node involvement are all poor prognostic signs (95).

Staging System

- The AJCC 7th edition chapter on cutaneous squamous cell carcinoma includes the primary anatomic site of the ear as a high-risk feature. Any tumor with two high risk features is staged as at least T2 regardless of size. Other high risk features include primary anatomic site of the hair-bearing lip, >2 mm depth, Clark level ≥IV, or perineural invasion.
- Arriaga et al. (96) have proposed a staging system for carcinoma of the EAC based on clinical and radiographic findings, also referred to as the Pittsburgh staging system (Table 17-5).

Treatment

Auricle and Early EAC Involvement

- Tumors of the auricle are most often are treated with limited surgery, with definitive radiotherapy reserved for anatomy preservation or in poor surgical candidates.

Table 17-5

Proposed Staging System for Tumors of the External Auditory Canal (Pittsburgh System)

T1	Tumor limited to the EAC without bony erosion or evidence of soft tissue involvement.
T2	Tumor with limited EAC bone erosion (not full thickness) or limited (<0.5 cm) soft tissue involvement.
T3	Tumor eroding the osseous EAC (full thickness) with limited (<0.5 cm) soft tissue involvement, or tumor involving the middle ear and/or mastoid.
T4	Tumor eroding the cochlea, petrous apex, medial wall of the middle ear, carotid canal, jugular foramen, or dura, or with extensive soft tissue involvement (>0.5 cm), such as involvement of the TMJ or styloid process, or evidence of facial paresis.

N status
Involvement of lymph nodes is a poor prognostic finding and automatically places the patient in and advanced stage (i.e., stage III (T1N1) or stage IV (T2, 3, and 4, N1) disease).

M status
Distant metastasis indicates a very poor prognosis and immediately places the patient in the stage IV category

Reprinted with permission from Arriaga M, Curtin H, Takahashi H, et al. Staging proposal for external auditory meatus carcinoma based on preoperative clinical and computed tomography findings. *Ann Otol Rhinol Laryngol* 1990;99(9 Pt 1):714–721.

- Irradiation treatment in early stages is usually with orthovoltage or electron beam therapy (97). Most techniques have been fairly successful in the treatment of lesions in this area, with local control rates of around 80% to 90%.
- Of note, invasion into cartilage or medial extension into the EAC makes surgery a more optimal definitive treatment choice.
- Surgery is beneficial if the lesion has invaded the cartilage of the ear or extends medially into the auditory canal.
- Afzelius et al. (92) indicated that lesions over 4 cm, as well as those with cartilage invasion, have an increased risk of nodal spread. Prophylactic neck dissection in this setting remains controversial (98). A retrospective review of advanced auricular squamous or basal cell carcinoma patients undergoing total auriculectomy and parotidectomy showed that the incidence of pathologic lymph node metastasis was 0% (99)
- Interstitial irradiation using afterloading ^{192}Iris also an effective method of treatment for tumors smaller than 4 cm, affording excellent local control with good cosmesis

Middle Ear and Temporal Bone Involvement

- Radical surgery (temporal bone resection and mastoidectomy) and postoperative irradiation are the accepted methods of treatment for more advanced lesions of the external auditory canal and lesions in the middle ear and mastoid.
- When the tumor involves the bony auditory canal and impinges on the tympanic membrane, but does not involve the middle ear or the mastoid, a partial temporal bone resection may be necessary. Some groups favor a more limited surgery with postoperative radiation because of the morbidity associated with subtotal temporal bone resection (100).
- Depending on tumor extent, surgical options are mastoidectomy, lateral temporal bone resection, subtotal temporal bone resection, and total temporal bone resection.
- Postoperative irradiation is essential to increase the chance of local tumor control when tumors extensively involve the EAC or middle ear (100).

Outcomes

- Madsen et al. (95) reviewed 68 cases (47 squamous and 10 basal cell carcinoma) in the external auditory canal or middle ear and reported on 50 patients treated with radiation to 60 to 70 Gy in 30 to 35 fractions, with or without primary surgery. Middle ear involvement reduced locoregional control from 70% to less than 30% at 5 years. 5-year overall survival for the whole cohort was just under 50%.
- Caccialanza et al. (101) reported 5-year local control of 78% with a mean follow-up of 2.4 years in 115 cases of basal cell and squamous cell carcinoma of the pinna treated with definitive kilovoltage radiation to a total dose of 45 to 70 Gy in 2.5- to 5-Gy fractions given 2 to 3 times per week. No long-term complications were observed.
- Silva et al. (97) reported on 334 cases of basal cell and squamous cell carcinoma of the pinna treated with definitive orthovoltage or megavoltage electrons to doses of 35 to 65 Gy in 2- to 7-Gy fractions with a median follow-up of 3.3 years. Five-year local control was 79%. Late grade 4 toxicity was 7% and was associated with larger fraction size.

- Pfreundner et al. (102) reported on 27 patients with carcinoma of the external auditory canal and middle ear treated primarily with surgical resection followed by postoperative external beam radiotherapy to a dose of 50 to 75 Gy in 2 to 3 Gy fractions with a brachytherapy boost given for incompletely resected tumors or local recurrences. Five-year survival for T1/T2 tumors was 86%; for T3, 50%; and for T4, 41%.
- Yeung et al. (103) reported 5-year cause-specific survival of 90%, 45%, 40%, and 19% in 51 patients with stages 1 through 4 carcinoma, respectively, that involved the EAC or temporal bone. These patients were treated with primary surgery and postoperative radiotherapy for unfavorable features. Survival was improved with the attainment of negative margins.
- Moody et al. (104) reported 2-year survival rates in 32 patients with SCC of the EAC treated with surgery and radiotherapy for unfavorable features according to stage: T1 100%, T2 80%, T3 50%, and T4 7%. Adjuvant radiation was associated with improved survival in patients with T3 disease.
- Ogawa et al. (105) reported 5-year disease-free survival rates of 83% in early-stage invasive squamous cell carcinoma of the EAC treated with definitive radiotherapy and improved DFS with the addition of surgery to radiotherapy for more advanced disease in a retrospective review of 87 cases of SCC of the EAC.
- Moore et al. (106) reported 5-year disease-free survival of 52% in 35 patients with malignancies of the ear or temporal bone treated with lateral temporal bone resection and either pre- or postoperative radiotherapy, mostly for T3 and T4 tumors.

Radiation Therapy Techniques

- Tumors involving the auricle can be treated with electrons or with superficial/orthovoltage irradiation. The fields can be round or polygonal with margins of 1 cm adequate for small superficial tumors. More extensive lesions require portals which may encompass the entire pinna or external canal, with 2- to 3-cm margins around the clinically apparent tumor. Lesions involving the pinna must be treated with conventional fractionation (1.8 to 2.0 Gy daily) to prevent cartilage necrosis. Doses of 66 Gy over 6.5 weeks are recommended.
- Large lesions of the external auditory canal may be treated with irradiation alone or combined with surgery. Treatment fields should encompass the entire ear and temporal bone with an adequate margin. The volume treated should include the ipsilateral preauricular, postauricular, and subdigastric lymph nodes. Treatment of lymphatics below level II is usually not necessary. IMRT can improve target coverage and is necessary when nodal coverage is indicated. Doses of 60 to 70 Gy over 6 to 7 weeks are required. Doses higher than this may produce osteoradionecrosis of the temporal bone.
- Most patients receiving radiation therapy to the middle ear and temporal bone regions will benefit from immobilization devices, such as the Aquaplast system.

Normal Tissue Complications (QUANTEC)

- "For conventionally fractionated RT, to minimize the risk for sensorineural hearing loss (SNHL), the mean dose to the cochlea should be limited to ≤45 Gy (or more conservatively ≤35 Gy). Because a threshold for SNHL cannot be determined from the present data, to prevent SNHL the dose to the cochlea should be kept as low as possible." See Ref. (107).

Sequelae of Treatment

- Possible sequelae of surgery include hemorrhage, infection, loss of facial nerve function, and, rarely, carotid artery thrombosis.
- Radiation therapy sequelae include cartilage necrosis of the external auditory canal and osteoradionecrosis of temporal bone (96).
- An overall 4% to 10% incidence of bone necrosis can be expected after administration of 60 to 65 Gy. Risk of necrosis increases for lesions larger than 4 cm (108).

EYE

Anatomy

- The anterior structures consist of eyelids, cilia, lacrimal glands, drainage apparatus, and conjunctiva (see Figs. 17-7 and 17-8).
- The globe is composed of three tunicae: the outer fibrous coat (cornea and sclera), the middle vascular coat (iris, ciliary body, and choroid), and the inner nervous layer (the retina) (see Fig. 17-9).
- The vascular supply to the orbit is provided by the ophthalmic artery which is derived from the internal carotid artery. The retina is supplied by the central retinal artery and short posterior ciliary arteries.
- The lens forms the boundary between the anterior structures (anterior chamber and iris) and the posterior structures (vitreous body and retina).

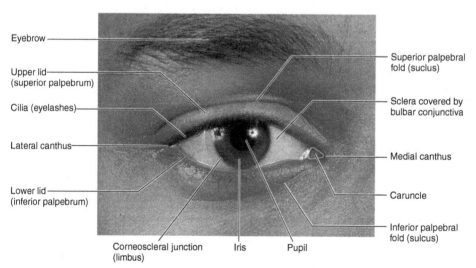

FIGURE 17-7. Anatomy of the eyelid and visible eye.

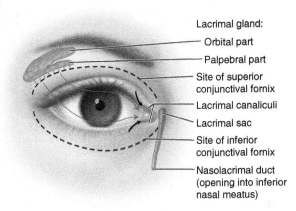

[*Black arrows* indicate lacrimal punctae (opening onto lacrimal papillae)]

Lacrimal gland:
- Orbital part
- Palpebral part
- Site of superior conjunctival fornix
- Lacrimal canaliculi
- Lacrimal sac
- Site of inferior conjunctival fornix
- Nasolacrimal duct (opening into inferior nasal meatus)

FIGURE 17-8. Overview of lacrimal glands and drainage apparatus.

Ocular Malignancies

Basal and Squamous Cell Carcinomas of Eyelid

- Basal cell carcinomas make up 90% of eyelid skin cancers, with the rest being SCC (109) (see Fig. 17-10).

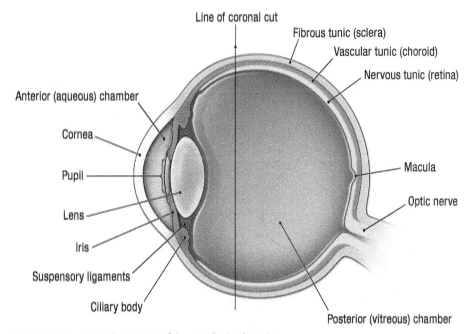

Line of coronal cut
Fibrous tunic (sclera)
Vascular tunic (choroid)
Nervous tunic (retina)
Anterior (aqueous) chamber
Cornea
Pupil
Macula
Lens
Optic nerve
Iris
Suspensory ligaments
Ciliary body
Posterior (vitreous) chamber

FIGURE 17-9. Internal anatomy of the eye. Sagittal section.

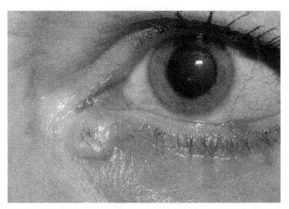

FIGURE 17-10. Basal cell carcinoma in medial canthus area. Well-circumscribed, pearly gray tumor of the epithelium, with raised, rolled edges and central ulceration. An independent vascular pattern is also visible. Lesions of the medial canthal area can easily involve the lacrimal drainage system and orbit. (Reprinted with permission from Tasman W, Jaeger E. *The Wills Eye Hospital atlas of clinical ophthalmology*, 2nd ed. Philadelphia, PA: Lippincott Williams & Wilkins; 2001.)

- Though Mohs surgery and excision with frozen-section control are considered front line treatments (110), radiation therapy is effective and results in acceptable cosmesis when tumors are extensive, unamenable to surgery, or recurrent (111, 112,113).
- Overall cure rates of 90% or better are achieved by delivering up to 60 Gy using conventional low energy x-rays, with appropriate shielding of the lens (112).

Meibomian Gland Carcinoma

- Meibomian gland carcinomas are sebaceous gland carcinomas that may be multicentric, resulting in local recurrences (see Fig. 17-11).
- Radiation therapy is an equivalent alternative to surgery, with acceptable cosmesis for both primary and recurrent disease.

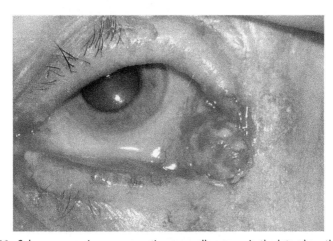

FIGURE 17-11. Sebaceous carcinoma presenting as a yellow mass in the lateral canthus.

- High radiation doses of 60 to 65 Gy in 6 to 7 weeks are highly recommended. Doses of around 60 Gy in conventional fractionation led to local progression-free rates over 90% at 5 years in a cohort of patients with mostly sebaceous carcinoma of the eyelid (114).

Uveal Tumors

Metastatic Tumors of Posterior Uvea

- Metastatic carcinoma to the eye is the most common malignant disease involving the eye (115).
- Metastatic uveal lesions account for 15% of all cases. The most common primary sites are the breast or lung in women and the lung or gastrointestinal tract in men (116).
- Uveal metastases are most commonly unifocal, although multifocal disease within the same eye is not uncommon.
- Metastatic uveal tumors can cause visual symptoms that should be treated. The aim of therapy is to return visual function to patients.
- Observation for small lesions may be appropriate if the patient is undergoing systemic therapy; however, lack of response to systemic therapy mandates local treatment to the involved eye with radiation therapy.
- For patients with active systemic disease, palliative irradiation to 30 to 40 Gy in 2 to 2.5 Gy fractions to the entire ocular structure is recommended (117), with potentially improved tumor response and visual acuity with doses higher than 35.5 Gy (118).
- In the absence of active systemic disease, and in patients with projected long-term survival, a more aggressive approach, delivering 45 to 50 Gy in 4.5 to 5.5 weeks, is required.
- Radiation therapy can be delivered with lateral portals, with shielding of the lens and cornea.
- Treatment can be delivered with 15- to 18-MeV electrons or with low-energy photons (4 to 6 MV).
- The lateral field should be tilted posteriorly 5 to 10 degrees to avoid irradiation of the contralateral lens and cornea, and parallel to the base of the skull (when possible) to avoid the brain.
- Plaque radiation therapy is an option for treating solitary uveal metastasis, particularly when external-beam irradiation fails to control the disease.

Malignant Melanoma of Uvea

- Arise from melanocytes in the uvea with molecular pathogenesis distinct from cutaneous melanoma.
- Uveal melanoma is not characterized by frequent BRAF mutations as seen in cutaneous melanoma, but other mutations that lead to downstream activation of signaling pathways like the mitogen-activated protein kinases (MAPK) pathway are seen (119).
- The predominant site of metastatic disease for uveal melanoma is the liver.
- Compared to uveal melanoma, BRAF mutation is relatively more common in iris (nearly half) and conjunctival melanomas (~25%) (120,121).

- Malignant melanoma represents 75% of primary malignant tumors involving the eye (2,500 new cases annually).
- Melanoma of the anterior uvea usually is detected earlier than posterior tumors.
- Anterior uveal melanoma may be removed by iridectomy or iridocyclectomy.
- Posterior uveal melanoma is more likely to present with visual symptoms, especially when the tumor is large or associated with retinal detachment.
- Management depends on the tumor size/location, presence of metastatic disease, extraocular extension, and functionality of the eye (117). Radiotherapy appears to achieve local tumor control with similar survival to those who undergo enucleation (122).
- Brachytherapy techniques using various sources, including cobalt 60, iodine 125 (^{125}I), iridium 192, ruthenium 109, and gold 198 seeds, have been used (123) (see Fig. 17-12).
- Indications for plaque radiation therapy are: (a) selected small melanomas that are growing, (b) potential for preservation of vision with medium-sized choroidal and ciliary body melanomas, or (c) actively growing tumor that occurs in the patient's only useful eye.
- For tumors that exceed 15 mm in diameter and 10 mm in thickness, radiation therapy can cause significant morbidity, and enucleation is preferred.
- The visual outcome of eye treatment with radiation therapy depends on tumor size and location relative to the fovea or optic disc. Large tumors and tumors in proximity to the fovea or optic disc place patients at high risk of radiation retinopathy and papillopathy after treatment.
- Studies have shown increased risk of visual loss when doses higher than 50 Gy are delivered to the fovea or optic disc (124).
- Combined plaque irradiation and laser photocoagulation, transpupillary thermotherapy (125), or chemotherapy have been used to increase local control, particularly in tumors close to the optic disc.
- There is general agreement that large ocular melanomas and tumors with extrascleral extension at diagnosis are not readily amenable to radiation therapy. In this group of patients, enucleation or exenteration is the preferred option.
- There is a controversial theory that enucleation may induce dissemination of tumor cells and affect survival.
- The Collaborative Ocular Melanoma Study (COMS) is a prospective randomized study that, among other aims, was designed to compare survival in patients treated with either brachytherapy or enucleation. 1,317 patients with medium-sized choroidal melanoma (height 2.5 to 10.0 mm and size ≤16.0 mm) accrued from 1987 to 1998 and were randomly assigned to enucleation ($n = 660$) or to ^{125}I plaque brachytherapy ($n = 657$). Mortality rates following ^{125}I brachytherapy did not differ from those following enucleation through 12 years of follow-up (126). The 12-year overall survival with enucleation was 59% versus 57% with brachytherapy (p = NS). The risk of death from metastatic disease was 17% versus 21%, respectively.
- Two randomized trials using particle therapy for uveal melanoma have been published. A randomized trial of protons using 50 cGE versus 70 cGE in the treatment of choroidal melanoma concluded that the lower dose resulted in similar local and

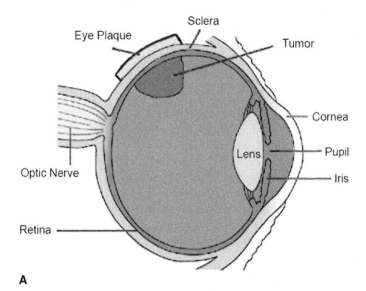

A

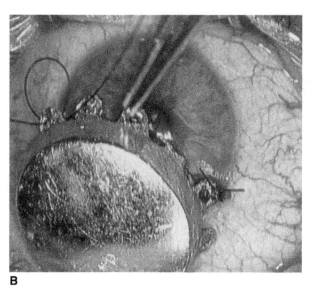

B

FIGURE 17-12. **A:** Eye anatomy and plaque placement in location of tumor. (Adapted with permission from Chaudhari S, Deshpande S, Anand V, et al. Dosimetry and treatment planning of Occu-Prosta I-125 seeds for intraocular lesions. *J Med Phys* 2008;33:14–18.) **B:** Plaque brachytherapy for melanoma of the iris. (Reprinted with permission from Khan MK, Khan N, et al. Future of radiation therapy for malignant melanoma in an era of newer, more effective biological agents. *Onco Targets Ther* 2011;4:137–148. © Khan MK & Dove Medical Press Ltd.)

distant control but had an improved toxicity profile with respect to visual field loss (127). A randomized trial of helium ion therapy versus ^{125}I plaque brachytherapy for uveal melanoma reported improved local control with helium ion treatment but no difference in overall survival (128).

- The prognostic factors associated with poor visual acuity or vision loss include increasing tumor thickness, proximity of the plaque to foveola of less than 5 mm, and patient age over 60 years (129).

Retinoblastoma

- Retinoblastoma is the most common intraocular malignancy in children (130).
- There are approximately 250 new cases diagnosed in the United States each year, and retinoblastoma is bilateral in one third of patients.
- Retinoblastoma is hereditary in approximately 40% of diagnosed cases and is transmitted as an autosomal-recessive trait (131). The genetic abnormality involves deletion or mutation of tumor suppressor gene (RB gene) on the long arm of chromosome 13 (13q).
- In general, the hereditary form is diagnosed earlier than the nonhereditary form of the disease. Most patients with the hereditary form have bilateral disease.
- A small proportion of tumors appear to develop in the context of normal RB1. In these cases, amplification of N-MYC has been described (132).
- Most children with this tumor are diagnosed before 3 to 4 years of age.
- Leukocoria (white papillary reflex), strabismus (squint), and a mass in the fundus are the common presenting signs and symptoms, which are commonly noticed at 6 to 24 months of age.
- Diagnostic workup of retinoblastoma requires a history, a physical examination (including a complete ophthalmologic examination with retinal drawings and photographs), ultrasound for documentation of tumor location and size, and a cranial CT scan.
- Routine cerebrospinal fluid study and bone marrow examination are not recommended, except when there are signs and symptoms suggestive of extraocular extension.
- Factors that carry a poor prognosis include orbital invasion, involvement of the optic nerve, central nervous system dissemination, and heritable bilateral tumors. Tumor parameters such as size, growth pattern (endophytic or exophytic), and differentiation do not significantly influence the systemic prognosis (133).
- Historically, the most widely used grouping system for retinoblastoma was the Reese-Ellsworth classification system (Table 17-6). More recently, the International Classification System (ICS) (134) has been employed for risk stratification and is used in current Children's Oncology Group (COG) protocols (Table 17-7).
- The goal of therapy is both cure and preservation of vision.
- There is a trend away from enucleation and external-beam radiotherapy and toward focal conservative treatments for small tumors (135).
- For patients with unilateral tumors without subretinal or vitreous seeding, focal techniques including cryotherapy, laser photocoagulation, and plaque radiotherapy can be used. If the tumor involves the macula, chemotherapy (systemic or local) is used to shrink the tumor before local therapy.
- Moderate and high-risk tumors (ICS groups C and D) are treated with chemotherapy (either systemic or intra-arterially in the ophthalmic artery) (117) as a means of potentially eliminating the need for enucleation or external-bream radiation therapy (136).
- Enucleation is indicated in unilateral tumor in which the eye is blind (ICS group E), or when the retinoblastoma fills most of the eye, especially when there is a concern

Table 17-6

Reese-Ellsworth Classification System for Retinoblastoma

Group I

Very favorable for preserving eye
Solitary tumor, <4 dd in size, at or behind the equator
Multiple tumors, none >4 dd in size, all at or behind the equator

Group II

Favorable for preserving eye
Solitary lesion 4–10 dd in size, at or behind the equator
Multiple tumors, 4–10 dd in size, behind the equator

Group III

Doubtful if eye can be preserved
Any lesion anterior to the equator
Solitary tumors >10 dd, behind the equator

Group IV

Unfavorable for eye preservation
Multiple tumors, some >10 dd
Any lesions extending anteriorly to the ora

Group V

Very unfavorable for eye preservation
Massive tumors involving over half the retina
Vitreous seeding

dd, optic disc diameter, normally about 1.5 mm.
Adapted from Reese AB, Ellsworth FM. The evaluation and current concept of retinoblastoma therapy. *Trans Am Acad Ophthalmol Otolaryngol* 1963;67:164 and Eye prognosis from American Cancer Society.

for tumor invasion into the optic nerve or choroid. External-beam radiotherapy continues to be an important method of treating less advanced retinoblastoma, especially when there is diffuse vitreous or subretinal seeding (135).
- Other indications for enucleation include glaucoma following rubeosis iridis with vision loss, and tumor recurrence not amenable to more conservative therapy.
- In bilateral disease, enucleation of the more severely affected eye is indicated only when the eye is blind, with systemic or local chemotherapy used in an attempt to salvage the second eye.
- Trilateral retinoblastoma consists of unilateral or bilateral retinoblastoma associated with an intracranial primitive neuroectodermal tumor (PNET). It is treated with neurosurgical resection, chemotherapy and cranial/craniospinal radiotherapy but is almost uniformly fatal (137,138).
- Chemoreduction has been used successfully to reduce the size of Reese-Ellsworth group V retinoblastoma: There was 78% ocular salvage; of this group, 25% avoided external-beam radiation therapy. Vitreous seeds and subretinal seeds showed initial

Table 17-7

International Classification System for Retinoblastoma

Group	Tumor Characteristics
Group A Very low risk; small discrete tumors away from critical structures	≤3 mm across, ≥3 mm from fovea, ≥1.5 mm from optic nerve; confined to retina; no vitreous seeding
Group B Low risk; discrete tumors of any size or place on the retina	>3 mm size or small but close to fovea; clear subretinal fluid ≤3 mm from tumor margin; no vitreous or subretinal seeding
Group C Moderate risk; retinal tumors any size or place with only focal vitreous or subretinal seeding	Fine, limited localized vitreous seeding (C1), subretinal seeding ≤3 mm from tumor margin (C2), or both (C3)
Group D High risk; diffuse vitreous or subretinal seeding	Diffuse vitreous (D1) or subretinal seeding >3 mm from tumor margin (D2), or both (D3). Subretinal fluid >3 mm from tumor margin. More than one quadrant of retinal detachment
Group E Very high risk: eye anatomically or functionally destroyed by tumor; retina may be detached	No visual potential, or presence of ≥1 of the following: tumor in anterior segment, tumor in ciliary body, neovascular glaucoma, vitreous hemorrhage, phthisical eye, orbital cellulitis-like presentation, involvement of optic nerve, and extraocular disease on neuroimaging

Data from Linn Murphree A. Intraocular retinoblastoma: the case for a new group classification. *Opthamol Clin North Am* 2005;18:41–53, and the American Cancer Society.

regression and often complete disappearance with chemoreduction. Seed recurrence also was decreased, by approximately 70% (133,135,139,140).

- Though radiation therapy was historically a primary modality for patients with bilateral disease with excellent disease control (enucleation of the more advanced eye and full orbital irradiation to the contralateral eye in most cases; irradiation of both eyes when possible), the high incidence of second malignancy has prompted techniques to avoid external-beam radiation when possible.
- The most important complication of external beam radiation is the induction of in-field second malignancies. One study revealed that patients receiving external-beam radiotherapy for retinoblastoma die of second tumors more than of retinoblastoma itself (141).
- Preservation of vision with external-beam radiation therapy in more advanced tumors drops to 79% in group III, 70% in group IV, and 29% in group V (131).
- Radioactive plaque therapy offers another option for local treatment of retinoblastoma. Historically, various sources have been used, including ^{60}Co, ^{125}I, ^{192}Ir, and ^{109}Ru (see Fig. 17-13).
- The advantage of ^{125}I plaque therapy is its physical properties of low energy, adequate dose distribution, and ease of shielding, which contribute to decreased radiation exposure to the opposite side of the eye and epiphyseal centers of the eye.

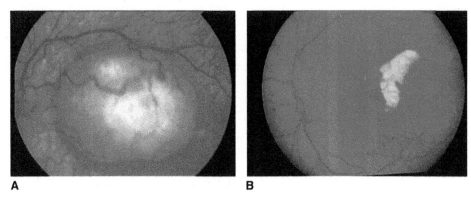

FIGURE 17-13. Plaque radiotherapy. **A:** Macular retinoblastoma before plaque radiotherapy. **B:** Regressed retinoblastoma after plaque radiotherapy.

- The Wills Eye Tumor Group recommends doses of 40 to 45 Gy to the tumor apex (extended to include vitreous seeds if present) using ^{125}I The dose to the tumor base approximates 120 Gy (142).
- Shields et al. (142) reported 5-year local control of 79% in 208 tumors managed with plaque brachytherapy in a retrospective case series from the Wills Eye Hospital. About 71% had received some form of prior therapy. Toxicity was reported as non-proliferative retinopathy in 27%, proliferative retinopathy in 15%, maculopathy in 25%, papillopathy in 26%, cataract in 31%, glaucoma in 11%, and scleral necrosis in 0% at 5 years.

Radiation Therapy Techniques

- The goal of external-beam irradiation is to provide a homogeneous tumoricidal dose to the tumor with minimal normal tissue toxicity.
- IMRT was found to best spare the bony orbit, lacrimal gland, and temporal lobe, whereas ensuring adequate dose to the target (138,143).
- It is necessary to treat the entire retina to avoid tumor recurrence in the anterior part of the eye. Studies have shown that whole-eye irradiation of retinoblastoma results in recurrence in the anterior retina in only 1.4% of cases in which the anterior retina has received a full radiation dose. This certainly allows for better tumor control as compared to lens-sparing techniques, which result in tumor recurrences in 19% of patients (141).
- There are several options for irradiation fields, including a single lateral field, a single anterior field, or a combination of both anterior and lateral fields.
- The best technique to avoid anterior failures is a lateral field with a sufficient anterior field border (with or without an equally weighted anterior beam) or a single anterior field that encompasses the entire eye.
- It is important to encompass the entire retinal anlage when designing the anterior half-beam block of the lateral field.

- Retinoblastoma can be adequately treated with 45 Gy in 1.8 Gy daily fractions if external beam alone is used.
- The volume of ipsilateral bony orbit receiving doses ≥20 Gy should be minimized to prevent midface hypoplasia with retardation of bone growth (117).

Optic Glioma

- Optic nerve glioma is more common in children younger than 15 years of age.
- The incidence is approximately 1% of all central nervous system tumors; more than 50% of cases involve the optic chiasm. A quarter to a third of patients with optic pathway gliomas have neurofibromatosis type 1, and a similar proportion of children with neurofibromatosis type 1 have an optic glioma (144).
- These tumors grow slowly and can cause visual defects, proptosis, optic atrophy, and nystagmus, but may also be asymptomatic depending on their location.
- Very young patients with neurofibromatosis can be observed, as this subset of patients tends to have a low rate of progression before the age of 6 (145).
- Surgical resection can result in a considerable risk of infarction, especially in chiasmatic low-grade gliomas (146).
- Radiation therapy is indicated when intracranial extension (progression into the optic canal) or progressive symptoms (i.e., evidence of vision loss) are present.
- Radiation therapy can be delivered with bilateral temporal or multiportal beam arrangements for lesions involving both the posterior optic nerve and chiasm, using three-dimensional techniques.
- Doses of 50 to 54 Gy in 1.8- to 2.0-Gy fractions 5 times per week are recommended for adults; for children younger than 15 years of age, recommended dose is 45 Gy in 1.8-Gy daily fractions.
- Proton therapy leads to significant normal tissue sparing compared to 3D conformal radiotherapy, and should be considered in this young patient cohort (147).
- Chemotherapy is an option, especially for very young patients, when there is a high likelihood of neurocognitive damage. Though relapse rate is high, it can delay the need for radiation (148).
- Optic gliomas are indolent tumors, and long-term survival ranging from 80% to 100% is achieved with radiation therapy.

Orbital Tumors

Rhabdomyosarcoma

- Rhabdomyosarcoma of the orbit is a favorable site for disease and is most often seen in young children. It has a rapid onset with marked proptosis and swelling of the adnexal tissue (see Fig. 17-14).
- The optimal dose for orbital rhabdomyosarcoma is controversial, though recent data suggests that reducing the dose to 45 Gy at 1.8 Gy/fraction does not result in inferior local control when cyclophosphamide is given as part of the treatment regimen. In COG D9602, the cumulative incidence of local/regional failure was 14% in orbital tumors (149).

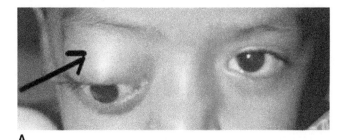

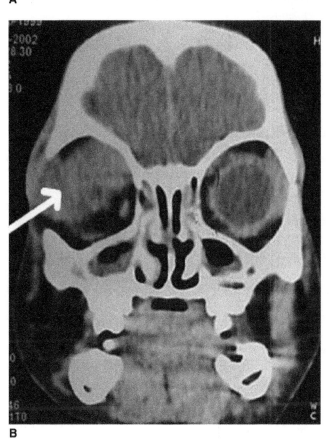

FIGURE 17-14. A: Orbital rhabdomyosarcoma with proptosis. **B:** Coronal computed tomography scan of patient with orbital rhabdomyosarcoma. (Reprinted with permission from Das JK, Tiwary BK, Paul SB, et al. Primary orbital rhabdomyosarcoma with skeletal muscle metastasis. *Oman J Ophthalmol* 2010;3:91–93. © Wolters Kluwer Medknow Publications.)

Malignant Lymphoma of the Orbit

- Orbital lymphoma may be the only manifestation of lymphoma or may be part of a generalized lymphoma.
- Primary adnexal lymphoma (involving the conjunctiva, lacrimal gland, or orbital soft tissues) is primarily MALT (mucosa-associated lymphoid tissue) lymphoma whereas

diffuse large B-cell lymphoma (DLBCL) is more commonly seen in ocular involvement in primary CNS lymphoma (which occurs in up to ¼ of this subset of patients).

- The staging workup is the same as that used for non-Hodgkin's lymphoma at other sites.
- For indolent lymphomas of the orbit, primary radiotherapy is the standard of care, with the CTV including the entire orbit; partial orbital irradiation is associated with a higher likelihood of local failure. An exception may be those tumors confined to the conjunctiva. A whole orbital radiation technique that avoids the contralateral orbit is a superior-inferior wedge pair, though IMRT is also effective (150).
- For indolent lymphomas of the orbit, doses of 24 to 25 Gy in smaller daily fractions (1.5 to 1.8 Gy) can reduce toxicity and provide high rates of local control (151).
- For DLBCL with a complete response to chemotherapy, the radiation dose can be limited to 30 Gy, with doses over 36 Gy confined to sites of gross disease using advanced planning techniques (150).
- Radiation therapy alone results in excellent local tumor control (greater than 85% at 5 years) (152,153).

Lacrimal Gland Tumors

- The most common epithelial neoplasms of the lacrimal gland are adenoid cystic carcinoma and mucoepidermoid carcinoma (154).
- Primary therapy is surgical resection with adjuvant external-beam radiotherapy required for close margins, perineural invasion, or adenoid cystic histology (155). The mortality associated with these tumors makes radiation therapy an important part of the treatment program to reduce postoperative recurrences.
- Doses of radiotherapy approaching 60 Gy are required (156).

Normal Tissue Complications/Sequelae of Treatment

- The most sensitive structure in the eye is the lens, which can develop cataracts characteristically presenting first as a posterior, subcapsular opacification. Emami data are used to provide a constraint of V10 Gy less than 100% of the lens to reduce the risk of cataracts to 5%. Total fractionated doses under 5 Gy have not produced significant lens opacifications (117).
- Fractionated radiation to the conjunctiva to over 40 Gy can produce edema with punctate keratitis (157), with ulcerations reported as the dose approaches 48 Gy.
- Skin changes resulting from radiation therapy include erythema, depigmentation, atrophy, and telangiectasia.
- Loss of eyebrows or eyelashes may or may not be permanent (transient at 30 to 40 Gy and permanent over 50 Gy).
- Hair loss from the scalp may occur at the exit area of an external-beam portal. Loss may be transient and followed by hair regrowth, although hair may have a different texture.
- Radiation-induced retinopathy and retinal atrophy can result in gradual vision loss.
- Significant retinal damage will not occur at doses below 50 Gy with conventional fractionation, but the risk of radiation retinopathy is increased in patients with diabetes.

- Optic nerve damage may result from either ischemic injury because of small vessel changes or retrobulbar optic neuropathy because of proximal nerve injury.
- Doses of 60 Gy or higher are associated with increased risk of optic nerve atrophy, particularly when fraction sizes are larger than 1.9 Gy (48), though recent clinical trial protocols constrain the optic nerve to 54 to 55 Gy point doses.
- In a study where plaque radiotherapy (median apex dose of 91.2 Gy) was used to treat 630 patients with choroidal melanoma visually significant maculopathy developed at 5 years in 40% of the patients, cataract in 32%, papillopathy in 13%, and tumor recurrence in 9%. Vision decrease by 3 or more Snellen lines was found in 40% of the patients at 5 years. Sixty-nine eyes (11%) were enucleated because of radiation complications and recurrence (158).
- Cranial irradiation in children with optic glioma, particularly with high radiation doses, can result in hypothalamic or pituitary dysfunction.
- Growth hormone deficiency and precocious puberty may result at doses above 45 to 55 Gy.

References

1. Michaels L. Jugulotympanic paraganglioma. In: Barnes L, Eveson JW, Reichart P, et al., eds. *World Health Organization Classification of Tumours. Pathology & Genetics Head and Neck Tumours.* Lyon, France: IARCPress, 2005:362.
2. Perez CA, Thorstad WL. Unusual nonepithelial tumors of the head and neck. In: Halperin EC, Perez CA, Brady LW, eds. *Principles and Practice of Radiation Oncology.* Philadelphia, PA: Lippincott Williams & Wilkins, 2008:996–1034.
3. Mendenhall WM, Million RR, Parsons JT, et al. Chemodectoma of the carotid body and ganglion nodosum treated with radiation therapy. *Int J Radiat Oncol Biol Phys* 1986;12(12): 2175–2178. doi:0360-3016(86)90017-9 [pii].
4. Konefal JB, Pilepich MV, Spector GJ, et al. Radiation therapy in the treatment of chemodecto-mas. *Laryngoscope* 1987;97(11):1331–1335. doi:10.1288/00005537-198711000-00016.
5. van Duinen N, Steenvoorden D, Kema IP, et al. Increased urinary excretion of 3-methoxytyramine in patients with head and neck paragangliomas. *J Clin Endocrinol Metab* 2010;95(1):209–214. doi:10.1210/jc.2009-1632.
6. Boedeker CC. Paragangliomas and paraganglioma syndromes. *GMS Curr Top Otorhinolaryngol Head Neck Surg* 2011;10:Doc03. doi:10.3205/cto000076.
7. Fisch U. *Microsurgery of the skull base.* Stuttgart, Germany: Thieme, 1988.
8. Jackson CG, Glasscock ME III, Harris PF. Glomus tumors. Diagnosis, classification, and man-agement of large lesions. *Arch Otolaryngol* 1982;108(7):401–410.
9. Glasscock ME, Jackson CG. Glomus tumors: diagnosis and surgery. *Rev Laryngol Otol Rhinol (Bord)* 1979;100(1–2):131–136.
10. Spector GJ, Compagno J, Perez CA, et al. Glomus jugulare tumors: effects of radiotherapy. *Cancer* 1975;35(5):1316–1321.
11. Powell S, Peters N, Harmer C. Chemodectoma of the head and neck: results of treatment in 84 patients. *Int J Radiat Oncol Biol Phys* 1992;22(5):919–924.
12. Mitchell DC, Clyne CA. Chemodectomas of the neck: the response to radiotherapy. *Br J Surg* 1985;72(11):903–905.
13. Dickens WJ, Million RR, Cassisi NJ, et al. Chemodectomas arising in temporal bone structures. *Laryngoscope* 1982;92(2):188–191.
14. Gilbo P, Morris CG, Amdur RJ, et al. Radiotherapy for benign head and neck paragangliomas: a 45-year experience. *Cancer* 2014;120(23):3738–3743. doi:10.1002/cncr.28923.

15. Sheehan JP, Tanaka S, Link MJ, et al. Gamma Knife surgery for the management of glomus tumors: a multicenter study. *J Neurosurg* 2012;117(2):246–254. doi:10.3171/2012.4. jns11214.

16. Ivan ME, Sughrue ME, Clark AJ, et al. A meta-analysis of tumor control rates and treatment-related morbidity for patients with glomus jugulare tumors. *J Neurosurg* 2011;114(5): 1299–1305. doi:10.3171/2010.9.jns10699.

17. Ghia AJ, Chang EL, Allen PK, et al. Intracranial hemangiopericytoma: patterns of failure and the role of radiation therapy. *Neurosurgery* 2013;73(4):624–630; discussion 630–621. doi:10.1227/ neu.0000000000000064.

18. Jha N, McNeese M, Barkley HT Jr, et al. Does radiotherapy have a role in hemangiopericytoma management? Report of 14 new cases and a review of the literature. *Int J Radiat Oncol Biol Phys* 1987;13(9):1399–1402.

19. Jaaskelainen J, Servo A, Haltia M, et al. Intracranial hemangiopericytoma: radiology, surgery, radiotherapy, and outcome in 21 patients. *Surg Neurol* 1985;23(3):227–236.

20. Friedman M, Egan JW. Irradiation of hemangiopericytoma of Stout. *Radiology* 1960;74:721–730.

21. Kano H, Niranjan A, Kondziolka D, et al. Adjuvant stereotactic radiosurgery after resection of intracranial hemangiopericytomas. *Int J Radiat Oncol Biol Phys* 2008;72(5):1333–1339. doi:10.1016/j.ijrobp.2008.03.024.

22. Spina A, Boari N, Gagliardi F, et al. The current role of Gamma Knife radiosurgery in the management of intracranial haemangiopericytoma. *Acta Neurochir (Wien)* 2016;158(4):635–642. doi:10.1007/s00701-016-2742-3.

23. Veeravagu A, Jiang B, Patil CG, et al. CyberKnife stereotactic radiosurgery for recurrent, metastatic, and residual hemangiopericytomas. *J Hematol Oncol* 2011;4:26. doi:10.1186/1756-8722-4-26.

24. Gunderson LL. Spinal cord tumors. *Clinical Radiation Oncology.* Philadelphia, PA: Elsevier, 2016:535.

25. Gay E, Sekhar LN, Rubinstein E, et al. Chordomas and chondrosarcomas of the cranial base: results and follow-up of 60 patients. *Neurosurgery* 1995;36(5):887–896; discussion 896–887.

26. Fuller DB, Bloom JG. Radiotherapy for chordoma. *Int J Radiat Oncol Biol Phys* 1988;15(2):331–339.

27. Kondziolka D, Lunsford LD, Flickinger JC. The role of radiosurgery in the management of chordoma and chondrosarcoma of the cranial base. *Neurosurgery* 1991;29(1):38–45; discussion 45-36.

28. Gutin PH, Leibel SA, Hosobuchi Y, et al. Brachytherapy of recurrent tumors of the skull base and spine with iodine-125 sources. *Neurosurgery* 1987;20(6):938–945.

29. Fagundes MA, Hug EB, Liebsch NJ, et al. Radiation therapy for chordomas of the base of skull and cervical spine: patterns of failure and outcome after relapse. *Int J Radiat Oncol Biol Phys* 1995;33(3):579–584. doi:0360301695020143 [pii]

30. Amichetti M, Cianchetti M, Amelio D, et al. Proton therapy in chordoma of the base of the skull: a systematic review. *Neurosurg Rev* 2009;32(4):403–416. doi:10.1007/s10143-009-0194-4.

31. Indelicato DJ, Rotondo RL, Begosh-Mayne D, et al. A prospective outcomes study of proton therapy for chordomas and chondrosarcomas of the spine. *Int J Radiat Oncol Biol Phys* 2016;95(1):297-303. doi:10.1016/j.ijrobp.2016.01.057.

32. Berson AM, Castro JR, Petti P, et al. Charged particle irradiation of chordoma and chondrosarcoma of the base of skull and cervical spine: the Lawrence Berkeley Laboratory experience. *Int J Radiat Oncol Biol Phys* 1988;15(3):559–565.

33. Slater JD, Austin-Seymour M, Munzenrider J, et al. Endocrine function following high dose proton therapy for tumors of the upper clivus. *Int J Radiat Oncol Biol Phys* 1988;15(3):607–611.

34. Au WY. Current management of nasal NK/T-cell lymphoma. *Oncology (Williston Park)* 2010;24(4):352–358.

35. NCCN. T-cell Lymphomas (version 2.2017). 2017. Available from https://www.nccn.org/professionals/physician_gls/pdf/t-cell.pdf

36. Kim TH, Kim JS, Suh YG, et al. The roles of radiotherapy and chemotherapy in the era of multi-modal treatment for early-stage nasal-type extranodal natural killer/T-cell lymphoma. *Yonsei Med J* 2016;57(4):846–854. doi:10.3349/ymj.2016.57.4.846.

37. Li YX, Wang H, Jin J, et al. Radiotherapy alone with curative intent in patients with stage I extranodal nasal-type NK/T-cell lymphoma. *Int J Radiat Oncol Biol Phys* 2012;82(5):1809–1815. doi:10.1016/j.ijrobp.2010.10.040.

38. Huang MJ, Jiang Y, Liu WP, et al. Early or up-front radiotherapy improved survival of localized extranodal NK/T-cell lymphoma, nasal-type in the upper aerodigestive tract. *Int J Radiat Oncol Biol Phys* 2008;70(1):166–174. doi:10.1016/j.ijrobp.2007.05.073.

39. Kim SJ, Kim K, Kim BS, et al. Phase II trial of concurrent radiation and weekly cisplatin followed by VIPD chemotherapy in newly diagnosed, stage IE to IIE, nasal, extranodal NK/T-Cell Lymphoma: Consortium for Improving Survival of Lymphoma study. *J Clin Oncol* 2009;27(35):6027–6032. doi:10.1200/jco.2009.23.8592.

40. Yamaguchi M, Tobinai K, Oguchi M, et al. Phase I/II study of concurrent chemoradiotherapy for localized nasal natural killer/T-cell lymphoma: Japan Clinical Oncology Group Study JCOG0211. *J Clin Oncol* 2009;27(33):5594–5600. doi:10.1200/jco.2009.23.8295.

41. Bakst R, Wolden S, Yahalom J. Radiation therapy for chloroma (granulocytic sarcoma). *Int J Radiat Oncol Biol Phys* 2012;82(5):1816–1822. doi:10.1016/j.ijrobp.2011.02.057.

42. Chao KS, Kaplan C, Simpson JR, et al. Esthesioneuroblastoma: the impact of treatment modality. *Head Neck* 2001;23(9):749–757. doi:10.1002/hed.1107 [pii].

43. Schroth G, Gawehn J, Marquardt B, et al. MR imaging of esthesioneuroblastoma. *J Comput Assist Tomogr* 1986;10(2):316–319.

44. Kadish S, Goodman M, Wang CC. Olfactory neuroblastoma. A clinical analysis of 17 cases. *Cancer* 1976;37(3):1571–1576.

45. Broski SM, Hunt CH, Johnson GB, et al. The added value of 18F-FDG PET/CT for evaluation of patients with esthesioneuroblastoma. *J Nucl Med* 2012;53(8):1200–1206. doi:10.2967/jnumed.112.102897.

46. Van Gompel JJ, Giannini C, Olsen KD, et al. Long-term outcome of esthesioneuroblastoma: hyams grade predicts patient survival. *J Neurol Surg B Skull Base* 2012;73(5):331–336. doi:10.1055/s-0032-1321512.

47. Weiden PL, Yarington CT Jr, Richardson RG. Olfactory neuroblastoma. Chemotherapy and radiotherapy for extensive disease. *Arch Otolaryngol* 1984;110(11):759–760.

48. El Kababri M, Habrand JL, Valteau-Couanet D, et al. Esthesioneuroblastoma in children and adolescent: experience on 11 cases with literature review. *J Pediatr Hematol Oncol* 2014;36(2):91–95. doi:10.1097/mph.0000000000000095.

49. Bailey BJ, Barton S. Olfactory neuroblastoma. Management and prognosis. *Arch Otolaryngol* 1975;101(1):1–5.

50. Davis RE, Weissler MC. Esthesioneuroblastoma and neck metastasis. *Head Neck* 1992;14(6):477–482.

51. Noh OK, Lee SW, Yoon SM, et al. Radiotherapy for esthesioneuroblastoma: is elective nodal irradiation warranted in the multimodality treatment approach? *Int J Radiat Oncol Biol Phys* 2011;79(2):443–449. doi:10.1016/j.ijrobp.2009.10.067.

52. Ozsahin M, Gruber G, Olszyk O, et al. Outcome and prognostic factors in olfactory neuroblastoma: a rare cancer network study. *Int J Radiat Oncol Biol Phys* 2010;78(4):992–997. doi:10.1016/j.ijrobp.2009.09.019.

53. Benfari G, Fusconi M, Ciofalo A, et al. Radiotherapy alone for local tumour control in esthesioneuroblastoma. *Acta Otorhinolaryngol Ital* 2008;28(6):292–297.

54. Lucas JT Jr, Ladra MM, MacDonald SM, et al. Proton therapy for pediatric and adolescent esthesioneuroblastoma. *Pediatr Blood Cancer* 2015;62(9):1523–1528. doi:10.1002/pbc.25494.

55. Patel SH, Wang Z, Wong WW, et al. Charged particle therapy versus photon therapy for paranasal sinus and nasal cavity malignant diseases: a systematic review and meta-analysis. *Lancet Oncol* 2014;15(9):1027–1038. doi:10.1016/s1470-2045(14)70268-2.

56. Galieni P, Cavo M, Pulsoni A, et al. Clinical outcome of extramedullary plasmacytoma. *Haematologica* 2000;85(1):47–51.

57. Kilciksiz S, Karakoyun-Celik O, Agaoglu FY, et al. A review for solitary plasmacytoma of bone and extramedullary plasmacytoma. *Scientific World Journal* 2012;2012:895765. doi:10.1100/2012/895765.

58. Alexiou C, Kau RJ, Dietzfelbinger H, et al. Extramedullary plasmacytoma: tumor occurrence and therapeutic concepts. *Cancer* 1999;85(11):2305–2314.

59. Ahmad K, Fayos JV. Role of radiation therapy in the treatment of olfactory neuroblastoma. *Int J Radiat Oncol Biol Phys* 1980;6(3):349–352.

60. Tournier-Rangeard L, Lapeyre M, Graff-Caillaud P, et al. Radiotherapy for solitary extramedullary plasmacytoma in the head-and-neck region: a dose greater than 45 Gy to the target volume improves the local control. *Int J Radiat Oncol Biol Phys* 2006;64(4):1013–1017. doi:10.1016/j.ijrobp.2005.09.019.

61. Antonelli AR, Cappiello J, Di Lorenzo D, et al. Diagnosis, staging, and treatment of juvenile nasopharyngeal angiofibroma (JNA). *Laryngoscope* 1987;97(11):1319–1325. doi:10.1288/00005537-198711000-00014.

62. Cummings BJ, Blend R, Keane T, et al. Primary radiation therapy for juvenile nasopharyngeal angiofibroma. *Laryngoscope* 1984;94(12 Pt 1):1599–1605.

63. Bremer JW, Neel HB III, DeSanto LW, et al. Angiofibroma: treatment trends in 150 patients during 40 years. *Laryngoscope* 1986;96(12):1321–1329.

64. Chandler JR, Goulding R, Moskowitz L, et al. Nasopharyngeal angiofibromas: staging and management. *Ann Otol Rhinol Laryngol* 1984;93(4 Pt 1):322–329.

65. Sessions RB, Bryan RN, Naclerio RM, et al. Radiographic staging of juvenile angiofibroma. *Head Neck Surg* 1981;3(4):279–283.

66. Khoueir N, Nicolas N, Rohayem Z, et al. Exclusive endoscopic resection of juvenile nasopharyngeal angiofibroma: a systematic review of the literature. *Otolaryngol Head Neck Surg* 2014;150(3):350–358. doi:10.1177/0194599813516605.

67. Leong SC. A systematic review of surgical outcomes for advanced juvenile nasopharyngeal angiofibroma with intracranial involvement. *Laryngoscope* 2013;123(5):1125–1131. doi:10.1002/lary.23760.

68. Spagnolo DV, Papadimitriou JM, Archer M. Postirradiation malignant fibrous histiocytoma arising in juvenile nasopharyngeal angiofibroma and producing alpha-1-antitrypsin. *Histopathology* 1984;8(2):339–352.

69. Wiatrak BJ, Koopmann CF, Turrisi AT. Radiation therapy as an alternative to surgery in the management of intracranial juvenile nasopharyngeal angiofibroma. *Int J Pediatr Otorhinolaryngol* 1993;28(1):51–61.

70. McAfee WJ, Morris CG, Amdur RJ, et al. Definitive radiotherapy for juvenile nasopharyngeal angiofibroma. *Am J Clin Oncol* 2006;29(2):168–170. doi:10.1097/01.coc.0000203759.94019.76.

71. McGahan RA, Durrance FY, Parke RB Jr, et al. The treatment of advanced juvenile nasopharyngeal angiofibroma. *Int J Radiat Oncol Biol Phys* 1989;17(5):1067–1072.

72. Harwood AR, Cummings BJ. Radiotherapy for mucosal melanomas. *Int J Radiat Oncol Biol Phys* 1982;8(7):1121–1126.

73. Chang AE, Karnell LH, Menck HR. The National Cancer Data Base report on cutaneous and noncutaneous melanoma: a summary of 84,836 cases from the past decade. The American College of Surgeons Commission on Cancer and the American Cancer Society. *Cancer* 1998;83(8):1664–1678.

74. Shashanka R, Smitha BR. Head and neck melanoma. *ISRN Surg* 2012;2012:948302. doi:10.5402/2012/948302.

75. Gillgren P, Drzewiecki KT, Niin M, et al. 2-cm versus 4-cm surgical excision margins for primary cutaneous melanoma thicker than 2 mm: a randomised, multicentre trial. *Lancet* 2011;378(9803):1635–1642. doi:10.1016/S0140-6736(11)61546-8.

76. Veronesi U, Cascinelli N, Adamus J, et al. Thin stage I primary cutaneous malignant melanoma. Comparison of excision with margins of 1 or 3 cm. *N Engl J Med* 1988;318(18):1159–1162. doi:10.1056/nejm198805053181804.

77. Ballo MT, Garden AS, Myers JN, et al. Melanoma metastatic to cervical lymph nodes: can radiotherapy replace formal dissection after local excision of nodal disease? *Head Neck* 2005;27(8): 718–721. doi:10.1002/hed.20233.

78. Henderson MA, Burmeister BH, Ainslie J, et al. Adjuvant lymph-node field radiotherapy versus observation only in patients with melanoma at high risk of further lymph-node field relapse after lymphadenectomy (ANZMTG 01.02/TROG 02.01): 6-year follow-up of a phase 3, randomised controlled trial. *Lancet Oncol* 2015;16(9):1049–1060. doi:10.1016/s1470-2045(15)00187-4.

79. Burmeister BH, Henderson MA, Ainslie J, et al. Adjuvant radiotherapy versus observation alone for patients at risk of lymph-node field relapse after therapeutic lymphadenectomy for melanoma: a randomised trial. *Lancet Oncol* 2012;13(6):589–597. doi:10.1016/s1470-2045(12)70138-9.

80. Gunderson LL. Malignant melanoma. *Clinical Radiation Oncology*. Philadelphia, PA: Elsevier, 2016:785.

81. Cohen LM, McCall MW, Hodge SJ, et al. Successful treatment of lentigo maligna and lentigo maligna melanoma with Mohs' micrographic surgery aided by rush permanent sections. *Cancer* 1994;73(12):2964–2970.

82. Barker CA, Lee NY. Radiation therapy for cutaneous melanoma. *Dermatol Clin* 2012;30(3): 525–533. doi:10.1016/j.det.2012.04.011.

83. Dancuart F, Harwood AR, Fitzpatrick PJ. The radiotherapy of lentigo maligna and lentigo maligna melanoma of the head and neck. *Cancer* 1980;45(9):2279–2283.

84. Harwood AR. Conventional fractionated radiotherapy for 51 patients with lentigo maligna and lentigo maligna melanoma. *Int J Radiat Oncol Biol Phys* 1983;9(7):1019–1021.

85. Huber GF, Matthews TW, Dort JC. Soft-tissue sarcomas of the head and neck: a retrospective analysis of the Alberta experience 1974 to 1999. *Laryngoscope* 2006;116(5):780–785. doi:10.1097/01.mlg.0000206126.48315.85.

86. Le Vay J, O'Sullivan B, Catton C, et al. An assessment of prognostic factors in soft-tissue sarcoma of the head and neck. *Arch Otolaryngol Head Neck Surg* 1994;120(9):981–986.

87. Lindberg RD, Martin RG, Romsdahl MM, et al. Conservative surgery and postoperative radiotherapy in 300 adults with soft-tissue sarcomas. *Cancer* 1981;47(10):2391–2397.

88. Barkley HT Jr, Martin RG, Romsdahl MM, et al. Treatment of soft tissue sarcomas by preoperative irradiation and conservative surgical resection. *Int J Radiat Oncol Biol Phys* 1988;14(4): 693–699.

89. NCCN *Soft Tissue Sarcoma*. 2017.

90. Wang TJC, Chao KSC. Ear. In: Halperin EC, Perez CA, Brady LW, eds. *Principles and Practice of Radiation Oncology*. 6th ed. Philadelphia, PA: Lippincott Williams & Wilkins, 2013: 712–717.

91. Ahmad I, Das Gupta AR. Epidemiology of basal cell carcinoma and squamous cell carcinoma of the pinna. *J Laryngol Otol* 2001;115:85–86.

92. Afzelius LE, Gunnarsson M, Nordgren H. Guidelines for prophylactic radical lymph node dissection in cases of carcinoma of the external ear. *Head Neck Surg* 1980;2(5):361–365.

93. Arriaga M, Curtin HD, Takahashi H, et al. The role of preoperative CT scans in staging external auditory meatus carcinoma: radiologic-pathologic correlation study. *Otolaryngol Head Neck Surg* 1991;105:6–11.

94. Wang Z, Zheng M, Xia S. The contribution of CT and MRI in staging, treatment planning and prognosis prediction of malignant tumors of external auditory canal. *Clin Imaging* 2016;40(6):1262–1268.

95. Madsen AR, Gundgaard MG, Hoff CM, et al. Cancer of the external auditory canal and middle ear in Denmark from 1992 to 2001. *Head Neck* 2008;30(10):1332–1338.

96. Arriaga M, Curtin H, Takahashi H, et al. Staging proposal for external auditory meatus carcinoma based on preoperative clinical examination and computed tomography findings. *Ann Otol Rhinol Laryngol* 1990;99(9 Pt 1):714–721.

97. Silva JJ, Tsang RW, Panzarella T, et al. Results of radiotherapy for epithelial skin cancer of the pinna: the Princess Margaret Hospital experience, 1982-1993. *Int J Radiat Oncol Biol Phys* 2000;47(2):451–459.

98. Ariyan S, Sasaki CT, Spencer D. Radical en bloc resection of the temporal bone. *Am J Surg* 1981;142(4):443–447.

99. Osborne RF, Shaw T, Zandifar H, et al. Elective parotidectomy in the management of advanced auricular malignancies. *Laryngoscope* 2008;118(12):2139–2145.

100. Zhang B, Tu G, Xu G, et al. Squamous cell carcinoma of temporal bone: reported on 33 patients. *Head Neck* 1999;21(5):461–466.

101. Caccialanza M, Piccinno R, Kolesnikova L, et al. Radiotherapy of skin carcinomas of the pinna: a study of 115 lesions in 108 patients. *Int J Dermatol* 2005;44(6):513–517.

102. Pfreundner L, Schwager K, Willner J, et al. Carcinoma of the external auditory canal and middle ear. *Int J Radiat Oncol Biol Phys* 1999;44(4):777–788.

103. Yeung P, Bridger A, Smee R, et al. Malignancies of the external auditory canal and temporal bone: a review. *ANZ J Surg* 2002;72(2):114–120.

104. Moody SA, Hirsch BE, Myers EN. Squamous cell carcinoma of the external auditory canal: an evaluation of a staging system. *Am J Otol* 2000;21(4):582–588.

105. Ogawa K, Nakamura K, Hatano K, et al. Treatment and prognosis of squamous cell carcinoma of the external auditory canal and middle ear: a multi-institutional retrospective review of 87 patients. *Int J Radiat Oncol Biol Phys* 2007;68(5):1326–1334.

106. Moore MG, Deschler DG, McKenna MJ, et al. Management outcomes following lateral temporal bone resection for ear and temporal bone malignancies. *Otolaryngol Head Neck Surg* 2007;137(6):893–898.

107. Bhandare N, Jackson A, Eisbruch A, et al. Radiation therapy and hearing loss. *Int J Radiat Oncol Biol Phys* 2010;76(3 Suppl):S50–S57.

108. Mazeron JJ, Ghalie R, Zeller J, et al. Radiation therapy for carcinoma of the pinna using iridium 192 wires: a series of 70 patients. *Int J Radiat Oncol Biol Phys* 1986;12(10):1757–1763.

109. Cook BE Jr, Bartley GB. Epidemiologic characteristics and clinical course of patients with malignant eyelid tumors in an incidence cohort in Olmsted County, Minnesota. *Ophthalmology* 1999;106(4):746.

110. Cook BE Jr, Bartley GB. Treatment options and future prospects for the management of eyelid malignancies: an evidence-based update. *Ophthalmology* 2001;108(11):2088.

111. Fitzpatrick PJ. Organ and functional preservation in the management of cancers of the eye and eyelid. *Cancer Invest* 1995;13(1):66–74.

112. Avril MF, Auperin A, Margulis A, et al. Basal cell carcinoma of the face: surgery or radiotherapy? Results of a randomized study. *Br J Cancer* 1997;76(1):100.

113. Petsuksiri J, Frank SJ, Garden AS, et al. Outcomes after radiotherapy for squamous cell carcinoma of the eyelid. *Cancer* 2008;112(1):111.

114. Hata M, Koike I, Maegawa J, et al. Radiation therapy for primary carcinoma of the eyelid: tumor control and visual function. *Strahlenther Onkol* 2012;188(12):1102–1107.

115. Fahmy P, Heegaard S, Jensen OA, et al. Metastases in the ophthalmic region in Denmark 1969-98. A histopathological study. *Acta Ophthalmol Scand.* 2003;81(1):47–50.

116. Shields CL, Shields JA, Gross NE, et al. Survey of 520 eyes with uveal metastases. *Ophthalmology.* 1997;104(8):1265–1276.

117. Gunderson LL, Tepper JE. *Clinical Radiation Oncology.* 4th ed. Philadelphia, PA: Elsevier Saunders, 2016.

118. Rosset A, Zografos L, Coucke P, et al. Radiotherapy of choroidal metastases. *Radiother Oncol* 1998;46:263–268.

119. Van Raamsdonk CD, Bezrookove V, Green G, et al. Frequent somatic mutations of GNAQ in uveal melanoma and blue naevi. *Nature* 2009;457(7229):599.

120. Henriquez F, Janssen C, Kemp EG, et al. The T1799A BRAF mutation is present in iris melanoma. *Invest Ophthalmol Vis Sci* 2007;48(11):4897–4900.

121. Gear H, Williams H, Kemp EG, et al. BRAF mutations in conjunctival melanoma. *Invest Ophthalmol Vis Sci* 2004;45(8):2484–2488.

122. Augsburger JJ, Corrêa ZM, Freire J, et al. Long-term survival in choroidal and ciliary body melanoma after enucleation versus plaque radiation therapy. *Ophthalmology* 1998;105(9):1670.

123. Karlsson UL, Augsburger JJ, Shields JA, et al. Recurrence of posterior uveal melanoma after ⁶⁰Co episcleral plaque therapy. *Ophthalmology* 1989;96(3):382–388.

124. Cruess AF, Augsburger JJ, Shields JA, et al. Visual results following cobalt plaque radiotherapy for posterior uveal melanomas. *Ophthalmology* 1984;91(2):131–136.

125. Shields CL, Shields JA. Transpupillary thermotherapy for choroidal melanoma. *Curr Opin Ophthalmol* 1999;10(3):197–203.

126. Collaborative Ocular Melanoma Study Group. The COMS randomized trial of iodine 125 brachytherapy for choroidal melanoma: V. Twelve-year mortality rates and prognostic factors: COMS report No. 28. *Arch Ophthalmol* 2006;124(12):1684–1693.

127. Gragoudas ES, Lane AM, Regan S, et al. A randomized controlled trial of varying radiation doses in the treatment of choroidal melanoma. *Arch Ophthalmol* 2000;118(6):773–778.

128. Char DH, Quivey JM, Castro JR, et al. Helium ions versus iodine 125 brachytherapy in the management of uveal melanoma. A prospective, randomized, dynamically balanced trial. *Ophthalmology* 1993;100(10):1547–1554.

129. Shields CL, Shields JA, Cater J, et al. Plaque radiotherapy for uveal melanoma: long-term visual outcome in 1106 consecutive patients. *Arch Ophthalmol* 2000;118(9):1219–1228.

130. Holladay DA, Holladay A, Montebello JF, et al. Clinical presentation, treatment, and outcome of trilateral retinoblastoma. *Cancer.* 1991;67(3):710.

131. Retinoblastoma: genetics, diagnosis, treatment and sequelae. 39th Annual Meeting of American Society for Therapeutic Radiology and Oncology (ASTRO); 1997; Orlando, FL.

132. Malik RK, Friedman HS, Djang WT, et al. Treatment of trilateral retinoblastoma with vincristine and cyclophosphamide. *Am J Ophthalmol.* 1986;102(5):650.

133. Singh AD, Shields CL, Shields JA. Prognostic factors in retinoblastoma. *J Pediatr Ophthalmol Strabismus* 2000;37(3):134–141; quiz 168–139.

134. Linn Murphree A. Intraocular retinoblastoma: the case for a new group classification. *Ophthalmol Clin North Am* 2005;18(1):41–53, viii.

135. Shields CL, Shields JA. Recent developments in the management of retinoblastoma. *J Pediatr Ophthalmol Strabismus* 1999;36(1):8–18; quiz 35–16.

136. Friedman DL, Himelstein B, Shields CL, et al. Chemoreduction and local ophthalmic therapy for intraocular retinoblastoma. *J Clin Oncol* 2000;18(1):12–17.

137. Abramson DH, Frank CM. Second nonocular tumors in survivors of bilateral retinoblastoma: a possible age effect on radiation-related risk. *Ophthalmology* 1998;105(4):573.

138. Reisner ML, Viegas CM, Grazziotin RZ, et al. Retinoblastoma—Comparative analysis of external radiotherapy techniques, including an IMRT technique. *Int J Radiat Oncol Biol Phys* 2007;67:933–941.

139. Gunduz K, Shields CL, Shields JA, et al. The outcome of chemoreduction treatment in patients with Reese-Ellsworth group V retinoblastoma. *Arch Ophthalmol* 1998;116(12):1613–1617.

140. Shields CL, Shields JA, Needle M, et al. Combined chemoreduction and adjuvant treatment for intraocular retinoblastoma. *Ophthalmology* 1997;104(12):2101–2111.

141. Perez CA, Brady LW, Becker A, et al. *Principles and Practice of Radiation Oncology*. 6th ed. Philadelphia, PA: Lippincott Williams & Wilkins, 2013.

142. Shields CL, Shields JA, Cater J, et al. Plaque radiotherapy for retinoblastoma: long-term tumor control and treatment complications in 208 tumors. *Ophthalmology* 2001;108(11):2116–2121.

143. Krasin MJ, Crawford BT, Zhu Y, et al. Intensity-modulated radiation therapy for children with intraocular retinoblastoma: Potential sparing of the bony orbit. *Clin Oncol* 2004;16:215–222.

144. Czyzk E, Jóźwiak S, Roszkowski M, et al. Optic pathway gliomas in children with and without neurofibromatosis. *J Child Neurol*. 2003;18(7):471–478.

145. Grill J, Laithier V, Rodriguez D, et al. When do children with optic pathway tumors need treatment? An oncological perspective in 106 patients treated in a single centre. *Eur J Pediatr* 2000;159:692–696.

146. Hupp M, Falkenstein F, Bison B, et al. Infarction following chiasmatic low grade glioma resection. *Childs Nerv Syst* 2012;28(3):391–398.

147. Fuss M, Hug EB, Schaefer RA, et al. Proton radiation therapy (PRT) for pediatric optic pathway gliomas: comparison with 3D planned conventional photons and a standard photon technique. *Int J Radiat Oncol Biol Phys* 1999;45(5):1117.

148. Janss AJ, Grundy R, Cnaan A, et al. Optic pathway and hypothalamic/chiasmatic gliomas in children younger than age 5 years with a 6-year follow-up. *Cancer*. 1995;75(4):1051.

149. Breneman J, Meza J, Donaldson SS, et al. Local control with reduced-dose radiotherapy for low-risk rhabdomyosarcoma: a report from the Children's Oncology Group D9602 study. *Int J Radiat Oncol Biol Phys* 2012;83(2):720.

150. Yahalom J, et al. "Modern radiation therapy for extranodal lymphomas: field and dose guidelines from the International Lymphoma Radiation Oncology Group." *Int J Radiat Oncol Biol Phys* 2015;92(1):11–31.

151. Tran KH, Campbell BA, Fua T, et al. Efficacy of low dose radiotherapy for primary orbital marginal zone lymphoma. *Leuk Lymphoma* 2013;54:491–496.

152. Chao CK, Lin HS, Devineni VR, et al. Radiation therapy for primary orbital lymphoma. *Int J Radiat Oncol Biol Phys* 1995;31(4):929–934.

153. Bolek TW, Moyses HM, Marcus RB, et al. Radiotherapy in the management of orbital lymphoma. *Int J Radiat Oncol Biol Phys* 1999;44(1):31–36.

154. Simmerman LE, Saners TE, Ackerman LV. Epithelial tumors of the lacrimal gland: prognostic and therapeutic significance of histologic types. *Int Ophthalmol Clin* 1962;2:337–367.

155. Esmaeli B, Golio D, Kies M, et al. Surgical management of locally advanced adenoid cystic carcinoma of the lacrimal gland. *Ophthal Plast Reconstr Surg* 2006;22(5):366–370.

156. El-Sawy T, Frank SJ, Hanna E, et al. Multidisciplinary management of lacrimal sac/nasolacrimal duct carcinomas. *Ophthal Plast Reconstr Surg* 2013;29:454–457.

157. Merriam GR, Jr. The effects of B-irradiation on the eye. *Radiology*. 1956;66(2):240–245.

158. Gunduz K, Shields CL, Shields JA, et al. Radiation complications and tumor control after plaque radiotherapy of choroidal melanoma with macular involvement. *Am J Ophthalmol* 1999;127(5):579–589.

CHAPTER 18

THYROID

ANATOMY

- The thyroid gland is made up of the right and left lobes, which are joined by an isthmus that crosses the trachea at the second or third cartilaginous ring. A pyramidal lobe may extend superiorly from the isthmus or one of the thyroid lobes (Figs. 18-1 and 18-2).
- The parathyroid glands are situated on the posterior aspect of the thyroid lobes.
- The recurrent laryngeal nerves are branches of the vagus nerve. They course posteriorly to the thyroid lobes and are located in a groove between the trachea and esophagus.
- Lymph node drainage includes the periglandular nodes, then the prelaryngeal (Delphian), pretracheal, and paratracheal nodes along the recurrent laryngeal nerve, and then to cervical and mediastinal lymph nodes.

NATURAL HISTORY

- Thyroid cancer represents approximately 2% of all malignancies and accounts for less than 1% of cancer deaths in the United States (1). In 2015, there were estimated to be 62,450 new cases and 1,950 thyroid cancer deaths in the United States (2).
- The incidence has recently increased by varying degrees across all cancer stages and age groups (3).
- The peak incidence is approximately age 50 years.
- Thyroid exposure to radiation, particularly before puberty, is the only well-documented environmental factor. Studies of the Chernobyl incident demonstrated a linear relationship between risk of thyroid cancer and dose of iodine isotopes, especially ^{131}I. For a dose of 1 Gy, the estimated odds ratio varied from 5 to 8 (4). Similar risk has been found in children who received EBRT to the neck for pediatric malignancies. The risk of thyroid cancer started to increase at a dose as low as 0.1 Gy. At radiation doses of 20 to 29 Gy, the odds ratio reached 10. At doses greater than 30 Gy, a downturn in the dose-response relation was observed (5). The median interval from the time of radiation therapy until the recognition of thyroid disease was 13 years (6).

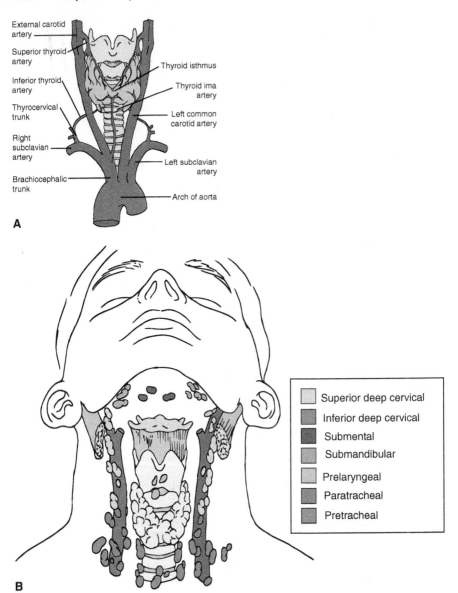

FIGURE 18-1. Anatomy **(A)** and lymphatic drainage **(B)** of the thyroid. (**A:** Adapted from Agur AMR, Dalley AF, eds. *Grant's atlas of anatomy*, 12th ed. Philadelphia, PA: Lippincott Williams & Wilkins, 2009:770.)

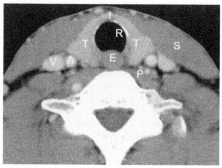 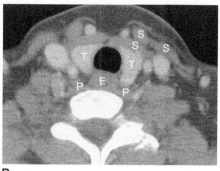

A   **B**

FIGURE 18-2. Important anatomic relations of the normal thyroid gland in two separate patients on CT imaging. **A:** Section at the level of the isthmus (I). **B:** Section just about the isthmus. Note that the thyroid gland (T) overlies the tracheal ring (R), and the lobes are in direct contact with the strap muscles (S) anteriorly and anterolaterally. The lobes also abut the prevertebral muscles (P) posteriorly, the esophagus (E) posteromedially, and the common carotid artery (A) and the internal jugular vein (V) laterally. (Reprinted with permission from Chao KSC, Apisarnthanarax S, Ozyigt G. *Practical essentials of intensity modulated radiation therapy*. Philadelphia, PA: Lippincott Williams & Wilkins, 2003:211. © Wolters Kluwer.)

DIAGNOSTIC WORKUP

- Most thyroid cancers are asymptomatic for long periods and commonly present as a solitary thyroid nodule. However, evaluating all nodules is difficult because benign nodules are so prevalent and because malignant thyroid cancer is present in only 4% to 7% of all thyroid nodules.
- A patient with a thyroid nodule of any size should be evaluated for clinical features, TSH level, and ultrasound-guided FNA.
- *Radionuclide imaging*: Patients with thyroid nodules and low TSH should have radio-iodine ^{123}I imaging or technetium ^{99}Tm imaging. Hyperfunctioning nodules (hot) have low risk of malignancy and do not warrant further FNA. Only cold nodules are considered for FNA. On the other hand, all nodules with elevated or normal TSH are considered for FNA without additional assessment with radioiodine imaging.
- *Ultrasonography and fine needle aspiration biopsy*: For all the nodules considered for FNA, only those with suspicious sonographic features will be selected for biopsy. Sonographic features of low predictive values include simple cyst of any size, spongiform nodules less than 2 cm, and solid or cystic-solid nodules less than 1 cm. These thyroid nodules are not required for FNA, but surveillance using ultrasound every 6 to 12 months is required (7).

STAGING

- The staging system for carcinoma of the thyroid can be found in the *AJCC Cancer Staging Manual* (8).

NEW!   **SUMMARY OF CHANGES TO AJCC STAGING**

THYROID

- T3 will be subdivided into T3a (greater than 4 cm limited to the thyroid) and T3b (gross extrathyroidal extension invading only strap muscles)
- N0a will be 1 or more cytologic or histologically confirmed benign lymph node
- N0b will be no radiologic or clinical evidence of lymph node metastasis
- N1a will be metastasis to level VI or VII (unilateral or bilateral)
- N1b will be metastasis to unilateral, bilateral, or contralateral neck lymph node levels I, II, III, IV, V, or retropharyngeal nodes

See: Amin MB, Edge SB, Greene FL, et al., eds. *AJCC cancer staging manual*, 8th ed. New York, NY: Springer, 2017.

PATHOLOGIC CLASSIFICATION

Differentiated Thyroid Cancer

- Differentiated thyroid cancer consists of papillary, follicular, and Hürthle cell histology.
- It arises from thyroid follicular cells (endodermal origin).
- Papillary cancer (including mixed papillary-follicular) represents 90% of diagnosed malignant thyroid lesions and 90% of thyroid neoplasms found incidentally at autopsy.
- It occurs mostly in the third to fifth decades and is two to four times more common in women than in men.
- Follicular and Hürthle cell cancer represents 7% of primary thyroid tumors and affects women two to three times more frequently than men. Average age at diagnosis is 50 to 58 years; it rarely is seen in children.

Medullary Thyroid Cancer

- Medullary thyroid cancer is derived from parafollicular or C cells that arise from neuroectoderm.
- It accounts for 2% of all thyroid cancers.

Anaplastic Thyroid Cancer

- Anaplastic cancer likely develops from more differentiated tumors as a result of dedifferentiation, because approximately half of anaplastic cancer have either a prior or coexistent differentiated cancer. Fifty percent of patients with anaplastic thyroid cancer have a history of goiter.
- It represents approximately less than 1% of all malignant thyroid lesions.
- Mean age of diagnosis is 70 years old. Women outnumber men three to one.

PROGNOSTIC FACTORS

- Anaplastic thyroid cancer has dismal outcome, with a disease-specific mortality approaching 100%. All anaplastic thyroid cancers are considered stage IV.
- For differentiated tumors, age is the most important prognostic variable. Thyroid cancer is more lethal in patients older than 40 years of age.
- Women typically have better outcomes than men, especially in those older than 40 years.
- Other high-risk factors include Hürthle cell variety, tumor size exceeding 4 cm, extra-thyroidal extension, and distant metastases.
- Lymph node involvement is not a significant factor.

GENERAL MANAGEMENT

Differentiated Thyroid Cancer

- *Surgery:* Recommended initial therapy is thyroid resection. But the extent of resection, either ipsilateral lobectomy or total thyroidectomy, is controversial, depending on cancer stage and other prognostic factors. Lobectomy may be followed by completion thyroidectomy if pathology from lobectomy shows high-risk features.
- *Radioactive ^{131}iodine (RAI) therapy:* After total thyroidectomy, postoperative RAI as part of the initial therapy functions to treat persistent macroscopic disease, to eliminate suspected micrometastases, or to ablate the remnant normal thyroid to help surveillance. Multiple studies showed decreased tumor recurrence, distant metastasis, and disease-specific mortality rates when postoperative RAI was used, compared with surgery alone (9).
- RAI is recommended for any of the following high-risk clinicopathologic features: residual disease, gross extrathyroidal extension, distant metastases, and postoperative unstimulated Tg exceeding 5 to 10 ng/mL.
- RAI is considered in patients with intermediate-risk factors: greater than 4-cm tumor size, involved lymph nodes, vascular invasion, aggressive histologic subtypes (tall cell, columnar cell, insular, poorly differentiated), and microscopic extrathyroidal extension.
- RAI is not typically recommended for low-risk disease (gross total resection with tumor size less than 4 cm, without involved LNs or metastases).
- Administration of an empiric fixed ^{131}I dose is the most widely practiced method. In general, 30 to 50 mCi is used for thyroid remnant, 75 to 150 mCi for subclinical micrometastatic disease, and 100 to 200 mCi for gross residual disease or distant metastases.
- To enable maximum stimulation of ^{131}I uptake, patients are prepared prior to RAI. Either recombinant human TSH (rhTSH) stimulation or thyroid hormone withdrawal is used. In addition, dietary iodine should be restricted and iodine-containing medications or IV contrast should be avoided for at least 1 week prior to RAI treatment.

- *Thyroid hormone–suppressive therapy:* Because TSH is a trophic hormone that can stimulate the growth of differentiated thyroid cancer cells arising from follicular cells, it is optimal to use postoperative levothyroxine to decrease TSH level as a treatment of differentiated thyroid cancers after subtotal thyroidectomy. Decreased recurrence and disease-specific mortality rates have been reported (10). In addition, patients treated with RAI should be maintained on suppressive doses of levothyroxine between RAI treatments.
- *EBRT* is rarely used in the management of differentiated thyroid cancer. Its main indication is for palliation of an unresectable mass that does not take up ^{131}I. Other indications include inoperable macroscopic disease after thyroidectomy or patients with very high risk of residual microscopic disease that is nonradioiodine avid. A series from MD Anderson reported durable locoregional control in patients with high-risk features undergoing postoperative EBRT for differentiated thyroid cancers (11). Intensity-modulated radiation therapy (IMRT) has been shown safe, effective, and less morbid (12).
- *Systemic therapy:* Kinase inhibitors can be considered for metastatic diseases refractory to RAI. Lenvatinib is the preferred agent based on an improved progression-free survival (PFS) of 18.3 m compared with 3.6 m using placebo (13).

Medullary Thyroid Cancer

- *Surgery:* Optimal management is early removal of the tumor, especially because medullary thyroid cancer can metastasize early regardless of whether the patient develops a virulent form of the disease.
- *RAI therapy:* RAI treatment is not effective because medullary thyroid cancer does not concentrate iodine.
- *Thyroid hormone–suppressive therapy:* TSH suppression is not appropriate because C cells lack TSH receptors. Thus, TSH should be kept in the normal range by adjusting levothyroxine dose.
- *EBRT:* Postoperative RT to the neck and mediastinum may be considered for gross extrathyroidal extension with positive margins or extracapsular extension in dissected neck lymph nodes (14).
- *Systemic therapy:* Kinase inhibitors such as vandetanib or cabozantinib can be used to improve PFS in recurrent or persistent medullary thyroid cancers (15,16).

Anaplastic Thyroid Cancer

- *Surgery:* This is usually used for airway management because most patients with anaplastic thyroid cancer have unresectable or metastatic disease.
- *RAI therapy:* It is not effective because anaplastic thyroid cancer is poorly differentiated and therefore does not concentrate iodine.
- *EBRT:* Radiotherapy can be used for local control and palliation.
- *Systemic therapy:* Doxorubicin is the only agent approved.
- A combination of surgery, irradiation, and chemotherapy (doxorubicin) produces the best results. An SEER database analysis (17) concluded that combined surgery and

radiotherapy improves survival in these patients. Hyperfractionated radiotherapy may be associated with improved outcomes (18).

- All patients with anaplastic thyroid cancer should be considered for clinical trials. RTOG 0912 is a randomized phase II trial of concurrent IMRT, paclitaxel, and pazopanib for anaplastic thyroid cancer. The grossly involved disease is to receive 66 Gy and subclinical disease receives 59.4 Gy, in 33 daily fractions.

RADIATION THERAPY TECHNIQUES

- Definitive EBRT requires careful treatment planning because high doses are needed and serious injuries may occur.
- IMRT is recommended to minimize toxicity to adjacent critical structures.
- 66 to 70 Gy to gross residual disease and 50 to 60 Gy to at-risk regions including cervical lymph nodes (levels III to VI). This can be achieved with either sequential boost or simultaneous integrated boost (SIB) techniques.

SEQUELAE OF TREATMENT

- Regarding RAI therapy, acute radiation sickness (fatigue, headache, nausea, vomiting) may occur within 12 hours after ^{131}I administration.
- Sialadenitis (swelling and pain in salivary glands, reductions in salivary flow, and altered sense of taste) is dose related and occurs shortly after ^{131}I administration or hospital discharge in 5% to 10% of patients and may last for a few days.
- Transient hyperthyroidism may occur after massive thyroid tissue destruction and release into circulation of large amounts of thyroid hormone.
- Radiation pneumonitis and pulmonary fibrosis have been associated with ^{131}I therapy, especially if there were diffuse functioning lung metastases.
- Gonadal dysfunction may occur, including transient oligospermia and decrease in ovarian function.
- Secondary malignancies that occur with significantly increased relative risk (RR) include bone and soft tissue (RR 4.0), leukemia (RR 2.5), and female genital organs (RR 2.2) (19). Although the RR is increased, the magnitude of the risk is quite small with an excess absolute risk of 6 cases of second malignancies per 10,000 person-years (20).
- Acute side effects of EBRT may include dermatitis, mucositis, dysphagia, odynophagia, weight loss, and fatigue. Late effects of EBRT may include skin changes, neck fibrosis/edema, esophageal stricture, tracheal stenosis, xerostomia, and dysphagia.
- Thyroidectomy may result in hypoparathyroidism or hoarseness.

References

1. Weiss TE, Grigsby PW. Thyroid. In: Halperin EC, Perez CA, Brady LW, eds. *Principles and practice of radiation oncology*. Philadelphia, PA: Lippincott Williams & Wilkins, 2008:1055–1075.
2. Siegel RL, Miller KD, Jemal A. Cancer statistics, 2015. *CA Cancer J Clin* 2015;65(1):5–29.

3. Enewold L, Zhu K, Ron E, et al. Rising thyroid cancer incidence in the United States by demographic and tumor characteristics, 1980–2005. *Cancer Epidemiol Biomarkers Prev* 2009; 18(3):784–791.

4. Cardis E, Kesminiene A, Ivanov V, et al. Risk of thyroid cancer after exposure to 131I in childhood. *J Natl Cancer Inst* 2005;97(10):724–732.

5. Sigurdson AJ, Ronckers CM, Mertens AC, et al. Primary thyroid cancer after a first tumour in childhood (the Childhood Cancer Survivor Study): a nested case-control study. *Lancet* 2005; 365(9476):2014–2023.

6. Acharya S, Sarafoglou K, LaQuaglia M, et al. Thyroid neoplasms after therapeutic radiation for malignancies during childhood or adolescence. *Cancer* 2003;97(10):2397–2403.

7. Haugen BR, Alexander EK, Bible KC, et al. 2015 American Thyroid Association Management Guidelines for Adult Patients with Thyroid Nodules and Differentiated Thyroid Cancer: The American Thyroid Association Guidelines Task Force on Thyroid Nodules and Differentiated Thyroid Cancer. *Thyroid* 2016;26(1):1–133.

8. AJCC. In: Edge SB, Byrd DR, Compton CC, et al., eds. *AJCC cancer staging manual*, 7th ed. New York, NY: Springer Verlag, 2009.

9. Tsang RW, Brierley JD, Simpson WJ et al. The effects of surgery, radioiodine, and external radiation therapy on the clinical outcome of patients with differentiated thyroid carcinoma. *Cancer* 1998;82(2):375–388.

10. Cooper DS, Specker B, Ho M, et al. Thyrotropin suppression and disease progression in patients with differentiated thyroid cancer: results from the National Thyroid Cancer Treatment Cooperative Registry. *Thyroid* 1998;8(9):737–744.

11. Schwartz DL, Lobo MJ, Ang KK, et al. Postoperative external beam radiotherapy for differentiated thyroid cancer: outcomes and morbidity with conformal treatment. *Int J Radiat Oncol Biol Phys* 2009;74(4):1083–1091.

12. Lee EK, Lee YJ, Jung YS, et al. Postoperative simultaneous integrated boost-intensity modulated radiation therapy for patients with locoregionally advanced papillary thyroid carcinoma: preliminary results of a phase II trial and propensity score analysis. *J Clin Endocrinol Metab* 2015;100(3):1009–1017.

13. Schlumberger M, Tahara M, Wirth LJ, et al. Lenvatinib versus placebo in radioiodine-refractory thyroid cancer. *N Engl J Med* 2015;372(7):621–630.

14. Wells SA Jr, Asa SL, Dralle H, et al. Revised American Thyroid Association guidelines for the management of medullary thyroid carcinoma. *Thyroid* 2015;25(6):567–610.

15. Wells SA Jr, Robinson BG, Gagel RF, et al. Vandetanib in patients with locally advanced or metastatic medullary thyroid cancer: a randomized, double-blind phase III trial. *J Clin Oncol* 2012;30(2):134–141.

16. Elisei R, Schlumberger MJ, Müller SP, et al. Cabozantinib in progressive medullary thyroid cancer. *J Clin Oncol* 2013;31(29):3639–3646.

17. Chen J, Tward JD, Shrieve DC, et al. Surgery and radiotherapy improves survival in patients with anaplastic thyroid carcinoma: analysis of the surveillance, epidemiology, and end results 1983–2002. *Am J Clin Oncol* 2008;31(5):460–464.

18. Wang Y, Tsang R, Asa S, et al. Clinical outcome of anaplastic thyroid carcinoma treated with radiotherapy of once- and twice-daily fractionation regimens. *Cancer* 2006;107(8):1786–1792.

19. Rubino C, de Vathaire F, Dottorini ME, et al. Second primary malignancies in thyroid cancer patients. *Br J Cancer* 2003;89(9):1638–1644.

20. Brown AP, Chen J, Hitchcock YJ, et al. The risk of second primary malignancies up to three decades after the treatment of differentiated thyroid cancer. *J Clin Endocrinol Metab* 2008;93(2):504–515.

CHAPTER 19

LUNG

ANATOMY

- The right lung is composed of the upper, middle, and lower lobes, which are separated by the oblique (or major) and horizontal (or minor) fissures.
- The left lung is composed of two lobes separated by a single fissure.
- The lingular portion of the left upper lobe corresponds to the middle lobe on the right.
- The trachea enters the superior mediastinum and bifurcates approximately at the level of the fifth thoracic vertebra.
- The hila contain the bronchi, pulmonary arteries and veins, various branches from the pulmonary plexus, bronchial arteries and veins, and lymphatics.
- The lung has a rich network of lymphatic vessels that ultimately drain into various lymph node stations: the intrapulmonary lymph nodes, along the secondary bronchi or in the bifurcation of branches of the pulmonary artery; the bronchopulmonary lymph nodes, situated either alongside the lower portions of the main bronchi (hilar lymph nodes) or at the bifurcations of the main bronchi into lobar bronchi (interlobar nodes) (1); and the mediastinal lymph nodes. Lymph node stations have been designated by the International Association for the Study of Lung Cancer with mediastinal lymph node stations making up stations 1 to 9, whereas the hilar and peripheral nodal stations were labeled as stations 10 to 14 (Table 19-1; Fig. 19-1) (2).
- Lymph from the right upper lobe flows to the hilar and tracheobronchial lymph nodes. Lymph from the left upper lobe flows to the venous angle of the same side and to the right superior mediastinum.
- The right and left lower lobe lymphatics drain into the inferior mediastinal and the subcarinal nodes and from there to the right superior mediastinum (the left lower lobe also may drain into the left superior mediastinum) (3).

Table 19-1

Mediastinal Lymph Node Stations as Classified by the International Association for the Study of Lung Cancer (IASLC)

Station	Nodal Group	Separation	Superior Border	Inferior Border
1	Lower cervical Supraclavicular Sternal notch	Right vs left (separated at midline of trachea)	Inferior aspect of cricoid cartilage	Lateral: clavicles Medial: superior aspect of manubrium
2	Upper paratracheal	Right vs left (separated at left border of trachea)	Lateral: apex of lung and pleural space Medial: superior aspect of manubrium	Right: superior aspect of where left innominate vein crosses trachea Left: superior aspect of aortic arch
3	Prevascular Retrotracheal	Anterior (anterior to SVC and left carotid) vs. posterior (posterior to posterior aspect of trachea)	Apex of chest	Carina
4	Lower paratracheal	Right vs left (separated at left border of trachea) Note: lateral border of 4 L is at the ligamentum arteriosum	Right: superior aspect of where left innominate vein crosses trachea Left: superior aspect of aortic arch	Right: inferior aspect of azygous vein Left: superior aspect of left pulmonary artery
5	Subaortic	None Note: lateral to the ligamentum arteriosum	Inferior aspect of aortic arch	Superior aspect of left pulmonary artery
6	Paraaortic	None Note: anterior and lateral to the ascending aorta and arch	Superior aspect of aortic arch	Inferior aspect of aortic arch
7	Subcarinal	None	Carina	Right: inferior aspect of the bronchus intermedius Left: superior aspect of the left lower lobe bronchus

Table 19-1

Mediastinal Lymph Node Stations as Classified by the International Association for the Study of Lung Cancer (IASLC) *(continued)*

Station	Nodal Group	Separation	Superior Border	Inferior Border
8	Paraesophageal	None Note: adjacent to esophageal wall	Right: inferior aspect of the bronchus intermedius Left: superior aspect of the left lower lobe bronchus	Diaphragm
9	Pulmonary ligament	None Note: within the pulmonary ligament	Inferior pulmonary vein	Diaphragm
10	Hilar	Right vs left Note: adjacent to mainstem bronchi and hilar vessels	Right: inferior aspect of azygous vein Left: superior aspect of main pulmonary artery	Bifurcation of the mainstem bronchi
11	Interlobar	Right vs left Note: distal to bifurcation of the mainstem bronchi	Not applicable	Not applicable
12	Lobar	Right vs left Note: adjacent to lobar bronchi	Not applicable	Not applicable
13	Segmental	Right vs left Note: adjacent to segmental bronchi	Not applicable	Not applicable
14	Subsegmental	Right vs left Note: adjacent to subsegmental bronchi	Not applicable	Not applicable

NATURAL HISTORY

- The pattern of spread may be local (intrathoracic), regional (lymphatic), or distant (hematogenous).
- Small cell carcinomas have a higher incidence of distant metastasis than non–small cell cancers; of the latter, adenocarcinoma has the highest potential for distant metastasis.

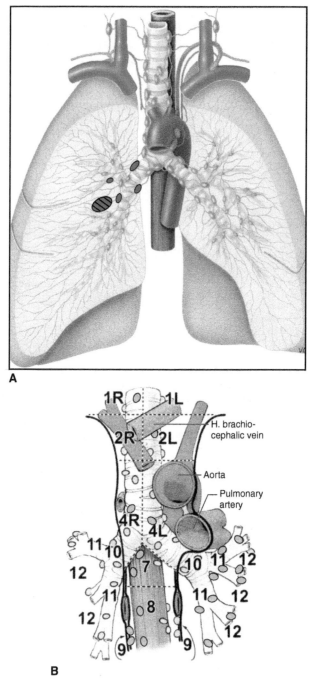

A

B

FIGURE 19-1. A and **B:** Regional lymph node stations for lung cancer staging as classified by the International Association for the Study of Lung Cancer (IASLC). (Reprinted with permission from Rubin P, Hansen JT. *TNM staging atlas with oncoanatomy*. 2nd ed. Philadelphia, PA: Wolters Kluwer Health/Lippincott Williams &Wilkins; 2012.) Labels correlate with Table 19-1.

- The incidence of nodal involvement is lowest in lobectomy series (37%) and highest in necropsy series (94%).
- Hilar lymph node metastases from lung cancer occur in approximately 60% of right upper lobe and middle lobe lesions and 75% of lower lobe tumors.
- Mediastinal nodal involvement, which has been studied in both surgical (early cases) and autopsy series, occurs in 40% to 50% of operative specimens (1).
- The incidence of scalene (supraclavicular) nodal involvement is 2% to 15%, predominantly from ipsilateral upper lobes or in patients with superior mediastinal metastases.
- Hematogenous spread with multiple-organ involvement is frequent. The most common metastatic sites are the lung, liver, brain, and bone.
- Adrenal metastasis has been reported in 27% of patients with epidermoid (squamous cell) carcinoma, 35% to 40% of patients with small or large cell undifferentiated carcinoma, and 43% of patients with adenocarcinoma (4).
- Abdominal lymph nodes are involved in over 50% of patients with small cell undifferentiated carcinoma.

CLINICAL PRESENTATION

- Cough is a major symptom in 75% of patients and is severe in 40%.
- Hemoptysis occurs in 57% of patients.
- Dyspnea and chest pain also are common symptoms, resulting from involvement of the pleura, chest wall, or mediastinal structures.
- Nonspecific, initial symptoms such as weight loss, weakness, anorexia, and malaise occur in 10% to 15% of patients. Febrile respiratory episodes are less common (5).
- Tumors located in the apex of the lungs may involve the cervical and thoracic nerves, resulting in Pancoast's or superior sulcus tumor syndrome (shoulder pain, brachial plexopathy, or Horner's syndrome) (6).
- Sympathetic nerve involvement results in Horner's syndrome (enophthalmos, ptosis, meiosis, and ipsilateral loss of sweating).
- Involvement of the recurrent laryngeal nerve may lead to hoarseness; this is more common with tumors of the left lung and with aorticopulmonary window lymphadenopathy.
- Involvement of the phrenic nerve can result in dyspnea and paralysis of the hemidiaphragm.
- Dysphagia may result from compression of the tumor on the esophagus.
- Primary tumors located in the right lung or metastatic tumors in the right mediastinal lymph nodes may cause superior vena cava syndrome.
- Secondary tumor effects (paraneoplastic syndromes) are sometimes seen, the two most common of which are humoral hypercalcemia of malignancy in squamous cell carcinoma and the syndrome of inappropriate antidiuretic hormone (SIADH) secretion in small cell lung cancer.

DIAGNOSTIC WORKUP

- Routine chest x-ray is the most common radiologic examination.
- Computed tomography (CT) of the chest with upper abdomen (to assess for liver, adrenal involvement) is the most valuable radiologic study for evaluation, staging, and therapeutic planning of lung cancer, but it cannot differentiate inflammatory disease from neoplasia.
- Mediastinal nodes less than 1 cm in diameter in short axis are considered unlikely to contain metastatic disease. Nodes 1 to 2 cm are intermediate, and those larger than 2 cm in a patient with bronchogenic carcinoma almost certainly are metastatic (7).
- Positron emission tomography (PET) scanning is routinely used to determine the malignant nature of suspicious lesions, to more accurately define tumor extent, including lymph node involvement (8–11), and to aid in three-dimensional conformal radiation therapy (3DCRT) treatment planning (12).
- Studies have uniformly shown improvements in sensitivity and specificity for staging of individual patients ranging from approximately 60% to more than 85%, particularly if the PET scans were read in conjunction with the CT scans (13).
- Kalff et al. (14) prospectively studied 105 patients with non–small cell lung cancer to assess the impact of 18F-fluorodeoxyglucose PET on clinical management. PET influenced the radiation delivery in 22 (65%) of 34 patients receiving definitive radiotherapy. Twelve patients considered probably inoperable on conventional imaging studies were downstaged by PET and underwent potentially curative surgery. CT and PET understaged 3 of 20 surgical patients, and PET missed one small intrapulmonary metastasis apparent on CT. No pathologic N2 disease was missed on PET.
- A brain CT or magnetic resonance imaging (MRI) scan is frequently used in the workup of small cell carcinoma and advanced non–small cell carcinoma.
- Pulmonary function tests (which yield parameters such as FEV1, FEV1/FVC, DLCO) are important predictors of the patient's ability to undergo surgical resection or withstand irradiation.
- Sputum cytology can diagnose malignancy in 65% to 75% of patients, but with lower yield for peripheral tumors.
- Bronchoscopic examination provides important data, even in the presence of preoperative cytologic proof of cancer; endobronchial ultrasonography permits visualization of suspicious lymph nodes for needle sampling.
- In patients with suspicious, undiagnosed peripheral lung lesions seen on x-ray or CT imaging, radiographically guided percutaneous biopsy can be performed.
- Other procedures used in establishing the diagnosis/staging are mediastinoscopy (to assess level 2, 4, 7 nodes), thoracoscopy, anterior mediastinotomy/Chamberlain procedure (to assess level 5, 6 nodes), thoracotomy, and biopsy of scalene/supraclavicular lymph nodes or distant metastatic sites.

STAGING

- Staging of non–small cell lung cancer was updated in January 2018 as the eighth edition of American Joint Committee on Cancer staging was incorporated into clinical use.

- Changes from the AJCC 7th to 8th editions consist of inclusion of a T1mi category for adenocarcinoma with less than 5 mm of invasion, altered size cutoffs for T stages, addition of a T1c category, allowance of bronchial invasion to be T2 regardless of distance from the carina, allowance of whole lung atelectasis to be considered T2 as opposed to T3, designating diaphragmatic invasion at T4, and separation of M1 disease into three categories instead of two with M1b now comprising patients with a single extrathoracic metastasis and M1c being patients with multiple extrathoracic metastases.
- Since the seventh edition of its staging system, the American Joint Committee on Cancer adopted the tumor-node-metastasis system proposed by the International Association for the Study of Lung Cancer (2).
- Small cell lung carcinomas are generally staged more simply as limited or extensive. Limited stage includes stage I to III (T any, N any, M0) (AJCC 7th edition) that can be safely treated with definitive radiation doses, excluding T3-T4 because of multiple lung nodules that are too extensive or have tumor/nodal volume that is too large to be encompassed in a tolerable radiation plan.

NEW!   SUMMARY OF CHANGES TO AJCC STAGING

LUNG[a]

- This staging system is now recommended for the classification of both non–small cell and small cell lung carcinomas and for carcinoid tumors of the lung.
- The T classifications have been redefined:
- T1 has been subclassified into T1a (≤1 cm in size), T1b (>1 to ≤2 cm), and T1c (>2 cm to ≤3 cm).
- T2a has been subclassified into T2a (>3 to ≤4 cm in size) and T2b (>4 to ≤5 cm).
- Bronchial involvement is now T2 regardless of distance to the carina.
- Tumor-associated atelectasis of the entire lung has been reclassified from T3 to T2.
- T2b (greater than 5 cm in size) has been reclassified as T3.
- Diaphragmatic involvement has been reclassified from T3 to T4.
- No changes have been made to the N classification.
- The M classifications have been redefined.
- M1 has been subdivided into M1a, M1b, and M1c.
- Malignant pleural and pericardial effusions have been reclassified from T4 to M1a.
- Separate tumor nodules in the contralateral lung are considered M1a.
- M1b designates a solitary distant metastasis to a single organ.
- M1c designates multiple extrathoracic metastases.

[a]Carcinoid tumors are included. Sarcomas and other rare tumors are not included.

See: Staging from Edge SB, Greene FL, Byrd DR, et al., eds. *AJCC cancer staging manual*, 8th ed. New York, NY: Springer Verlag, 2017.

PATHOLOGIC CLASSIFICATION

- Primary lung carcinoma is divided into non–small cell carcinoma (including adenocarcinoma, squamous cell (epidermoid) carcinoma, adenosquamous carcinoma, large cell carcinoma, and sarcomatoid carcinoma) and small cell carcinoma.
- Bronchoalveolar carcinoma (BAC) is now an obsolete term used to describe a heterogeneous subtype of adenocarcinoma that commonly presents in nonsmokers. What was previously classified as BAC is now categorized into adenocarcinoma in situ (AIS), minimally invasive adenocarcinoma (MIA), lepidic predominant adenocarcinoma (LPA), predominantly invasive adenocarcinoma with some nonmucinous lepidic component, and invasive mucinous adenocarcinoma, better reflecting the pathologic, radiologic, and clinical correlation of lung adenocarcinomas.

PROGNOSTIC FACTORS

- Tumor size, stage, histologic type, performance status (Karnofsky score), and weight loss are the most important prognostic factors related to survival.
- Genetic prognostic factors include mutations in the *EGFR*, *K-ras* oncogene, deletion of tumor suppressor genes (e.g., *p53* gene), presence of *N-cam* expression, and elevated serum levels of neuron-specific enolase.

GENERAL MANAGEMENT

Non–Small Cell Lung Cancer

- The first management step for non–small cell lung cancer is to decide whether the treatment aim is definitive or palliative and whether the tumor is resectable or unresectable.

Resectable Tumors

- Non–small cell carcinoma of the lung should be treated surgically, if resectable.
- Lobectomy is preferred over pneumonectomy; wedge resection is associated with a high local failure rate (15).
- Alternatively, stereotactic body radiation therapy (SBRT) can be considered as an option in patients who wish to forgo surgical intervention as combined analysis of two randomized controlled trials, both of which completed early because of poor accrual, revealed similar relapse-free survival (80% versus 86%), and significantly improved 3-year overall survival (95% versus 79%) for SBRT as compared to lobectomy (16).

Preoperative Irradiation, Chemotherapy, or Chemoradiation
- Several collaborative studies failed to show significant improvement in survival with use of preoperative irradiation (17).

- Preoperative chemotherapy has been associated with improved survival versus surgery alone for patients with N2 disease (18,19).
- Preoperative high-dose RT (60 to 66.7 Gy) is safe for pulmonary resection with significantly higher complete pathologic response rate (28%) comparing to lower dose (10%) (35 to 50.4 Gy) (20).
- Trimodality preoperative chemoradiation for N2 patients proved to be an encouraging approach in the SWOG 8805 trial (21).
- INT 0139/RTOG 9309 trial demonstrated that preoperative chemoradiation to 45 Gy is associated with improved progression-free survival versus definitive chemoradiation to 61 Gy (5 year: 22% versus 11%) and better 5-year overall survival; pN0 disease was associated with improved survival, indicating the prognostic importance of mediastinal sterilization by preoperative chemoradiation; trimodality therapy may not be appropriate if pneumonectomy is required, because of a high rate of treatment-related deaths (22). This observation of mortality risk of pneumonectomy was not seen in ESPATUE trial although the study design has difference (23).
- High-dose thoracic radiotherapy (approximately 60 Gy or higher) as a component of preoperative chemoradiation can be delivered safely and offers favorable outcomes (16,24,25).

Postoperative Radiation Therapy

- Postoperative irradiation has been advocated for patients with pN2 disease (approximately 50 to 54 Gy), positive surgical margins (approximately 54 to 60 Gy), or nodal extracapsular extension (approximately 54 to 60 Gy).
- The PORT meta-analysis demonstrated lower survival in patients receiving postoperative irradiation; this was related to greater irradiation sequelae due likely in part to poor radiation technique in many included studies (e.g., high doses, large fraction sizes, use of lateral fields, use of spinal cord blocks, use of ^{60}Co, lack of CT-based planning). Although there was an absolute reduction in 2-year overall survival from 55% to 48%, subgroup analyses indicated that this adverse effect was greatest for patients with stage I or II, N0 to N1 disease, whereas for those with stage III, N2 disease, there was no evidence of an adverse effect (26,27).
- Subsequent studies have confirmed a survival benefit of postoperative irradiation for pN2 patients (28–30).

Postoperative Chemotherapy or Chemoradiation

- Adjuvant postoperative chemotherapy—generally cisplatin based—has been associated with an absolute survival benefit of approximately 5% at 5 years versus surgery alone (23,28,31,32).
- Postoperative chemotherapy is generally reserved for patients with pathologic stage more advanced than pT1N0 (although there is debate if pT2N0 patients benefit from chemotherapy).
- Postoperative concurrent chemoradiation did not offer a survival gain versus postoperative irradiation alone in the ECOG 3590/INT 0115 trial (33).

Medically Inoperable Patients

- Stereotactic body radiotherapy (SBRT) is indicated for medically inoperable node-negative patients with primary lesions up to about 5 cm in size, offering 80% to 95% local control (34).
- Alternatively, definitive radiation therapy (±chemotherapy) can be considered if SBRT is unable to be performed, with 5-year overall survival of approximately 15% (35).

Unresectable Tumors

- Lack of tumor resectability is primarily because of inability to resect all known disease at the time of surgery and may be a result of local invasion of the primary tumor into or near critical structures or the presence of pathologic lymphadenopathy in the contralateral mediastinum.
- The standard of care radiation dose for conventional radiation fractionation was established through multiple Radiation Therapy Oncology Group (RTOG) trials. RTOG 73-01 dose-escalation trial utilized radiation without concurrent systemic therapy and reported the incidence of clinically apparent local failure to be lower in patients treated to 60 Gy (33%) versus 50 Gy (39%) versus 40 Gy (44% to 49%) (36). The radiation dose was further safely escalated using three-dimensional conformal techniques to 83.8 Gy for patients with V(20) values of <25% and to 77.4 Gy for patients with V(20) values between 25% and 36%, using fraction sizes of 2.15 Gy in RTOG 93-11 studies. The 90.3-Gy dose level was too toxic, resulting in dose-related deaths (37). RTOG 0617 revealed that delivery of 74 Gy versus 60 Gy with concurrent carboplatin and paclitaxel resulted in higher rates of severe esophageal toxicity (grade 3 or worse) (21% versus 7%), worse quality of life 3 months following treatment (45% decline versus 30% decline), and worse median overall survival (20 months versus 29 months) (38,39). Addition of cetuximab to concurrent chemoradiation and consolidation treatment provided no benefit in overall survival for these patients (38).

Accordingly, current guidelines suggest that patients receiving conventional definitive radiotherapy are being treated with doses of 60 to 70 Gy (40).

Chemoradiation

- Combined chemotherapy and irradiation is the treatment of choice for locally advanced, inoperable non–small cell lung cancer patients with good performance status and absence of significant weight loss or those without other medical contraindications to chemotherapy (41).
- Sequential cisplatin/vinblastine chemotherapy for two cycles, followed by irradiation (60 Gy in 6 weeks) has shown 11% to 13% absolute improvement in 2-year overall survival compared with 60 Gy alone (42,43).
- Chemotherapy regimens used with radiation include cisplatin/vinblastine, cisplatin/etoposide, carboplatin/paclitaxel, cisplatin/gemcitabine, and cisplatin/pemetrexed (for nonsquamous histology).
- Cisplatin-based concurrent chemoradiation has been associated with 11% to 14% absolute improvement in 3-year overall survival compared with irradiation alone (44).

- A number of trials have demonstrated superior overall survival for concurrent chemo-radiation versus sequential chemoradiation (45,46). RTOG 94-10 demonstrated improved median overall survival with concurrent chemoradiation (cisplatin/vinblastine/60 Gy daily thoracic RT) versus sequential chemoradiation (cisplatin/vinblastine → 60 Gy daily thoracic RT): 17.0 versus 14.6 months (45).

Novel Systemic Therapies

- Durvalumab, an antiprogrammed death ligand 1 (anti-PD1) antibody, has been shown to significantly improve progression-free survival as consolidation therapy comparing with placebo in patients with unresectable stage III NSCLC treated with definitive current chemoradiotherapy (47).
- Recent years have led to many exciting developments in novel systemic therapies in non–small cell carcinoma of the lung.
- Everolimus may be used in patients with nonfunctional neuroendocrine tumors of the lung that are locally advanced, unresectable, or metastatic at diagnosis (48).
- Erlotinib a tyrosine kinase inhibitor that targets EGFR may be used as second-line therapy in nonmetastatic disease, first-line therapy in metastatic disease, and maintenance therapy following platinum-based first-line chemotherapy in all stages as long as patients have specific EGFR mutations present (8).
- Avastin (anti-VEGF) may be used in combination with carboplatin/paclitaxel in patients with lung adenocarcinoma that is unresectable, locally advanced, metastatic, or recurrent (49).
- In the metastatic setting, pembrolizumab (anti-PD-L1) is currently approved in the first-line and second-line settings, whereas atezolizumab (anti-PD-L1) and nivolumab (anti-PD1) are approved in the second-line setting alone. The anti-EGFR monoclonal antibody necitumumab can be used as first-line therapy in metastatic squamous cell carcinoma of the lung when used in combination with gemcitabine and cisplatin (50). Additionally, various tyrosine kinase inhibitors, including crizotinib, ceritinib, brigatinib, and the combination of dabrafenib/trametinib, may be used in the metastatic setting depending on the specific mutational status of the patient's malignancy (48).
- The additions of targeted therapies to radiation treatment in patients with brain metastases in an attempt to improve treatment efficacy have been investigated with encouraging results when newer generation TKIs are used. Further, there is increasing interest in utilization of targeted therapy that can cross the blood-brain barrier as primary treatment for small volume, minimally symptomatic intracranial metastatic disease in an effort to defer brain radiation to a later time (51,52).

Small Cell Lung Cancer

- Small cell lung carcinoma is sensitive to many chemotherapeutic agents; multiagent drug combinations are more effective than single agents (53).
- Initial chemotherapy induces complete response in about 40% to 68% of patients with limited disease and 18% to 40% with extensive disease (53).

Limited Stage Disease

- A meta-analysis of 13 prospective randomized trials showed that thoracic irradiation combined with chemotherapy resulted in a 5.4% absolute increase in 3-year overall survival compared with chemotherapy alone (54). Cisplatin/etoposide is a regimen commonly combined with radiotherapy for small cell lung carcinoma.
- There has been interest in the inclusion of surgery in the multidisciplinary management of limited stage small cell carcinoma; however, prospective studies have shown that few patients are candidates for thoracotomy before or after chemotherapy (55), although surgery may be a reasonable option for very early-stage patients (e.g., T1-T2, N0), followed by adjuvant chemotherapy (±radiotherapy).
- Dose escalation to greater than 50 Gy have shown to have favorable outcome than lower dose in limited stage SCLC (56).
- INT 0096 demonstrated superior survival for 45 Gy b.i.d. versus 45 Gy q.d. in limited stage patients receiving cisplatin/etoposide concurrent with thoracic irradiation (5-year overall survival: 26% versus 16%) but with increased rate of grade 3 esophagitis (27% versus 11%) (57).
- CALGB 8837 attempted to determine the maximum tolerated dose (MTD) of radiation therapy in patients with limited stage small cell lung cancer undergoing concurrent chemoradiotherapy through a dose escalation study using both daily and BID fractionation. For BID fractionation, the MTD was determined to be 45 Gy over 30 fractions though was as high as 70 Gy if patients were treated daily for 35 fractions (58). The tolerance of 70 Gy over 30 fractions with concurrent chemotherapy was further validated in CALGB 39808 with a grade 3+ esophagitis rate of only 16% and 90% of patients completing therapy (59).
- The single-arm phase II RTOG 0239 study revealed favorable outcomes compared to those noted in INT 0096 (2-year overall survival: 37%; 2-year local control: 80%) when treating to a dose of 61.2 Gy using daily fractions at first but transitioning to BID fractionation following the 16th treatment (60).
- Currently, RTOG 0538 is underway comparing the radiation therapy regimens delineated in INT 0096, RTOG 0239, and CALGB 39808 to better assess optimal radiation treatment.
- CONVERT trial, a phase III superiority trial, demonstrated that overall survival outcomes did not differ between twice-daily (45 Gy in 30 fractions BID) and once-daily (66 Gy in 33 fractions) concurrent chemoradiotherapy in patients with limited stage small cell lung cancer, and toxicity was similar and lower than expected with both regimens (61). Grade 3 to 4 esophagitis is similar between the groups (19% in both arms) and so is grade 3 to 4 radiation pneumonitis (RP) (3% versus 2%). Because the trial was designed to show superiority of once-daily radiotherapy and was not powered to show equivalence, twice-daily radiotherapy should continue to be considered as the standard of care currently.
- Similar to non–small cell carcinoma, SBRT can be considered in the treatment of early-stage (T1-2N0) small cell lung cancer with current retrospective evidence showing very favorable outcomes (local control: 82% to 100%; overall survival: 48% to

76%; disease-specific survival: 79% to 86%) (22). Importantly, in this setting, it appears that patients derive significant added benefit to the addition of chemotherapy following SBRT (median disease-free survival: 61.3 months versus 9.0 months; median overall survival: 31.4 versus 14.3 months) (62).

Sequence of Irradiation and Chemotherapy

- Concurrent chemoradiation is standard and preferred to sequential chemo/RT.
- Limited stage patients benefit from early thoracic irradiation (i.e., early in the course or concurrently with chemotherapy). RT should start with cycle 1 or 2 of chemotherapy (4,63).
- A shorter time from the start of any therapy to the end of RT (SER) is associated with significantly improved overall survival (64).

Extensive Stage Disease

- Chemotherapy is the primary treatment modality utilized in extensive stage small cell lung cancer.
- Consolidative radiation treatment to the initial area of intrathoracic disease has been shown to improve both 6-month progression-free survival (24% versus 7%) and 2-year overall survival (13% versus 3%) in patients with partial or complete response to induction chemotherapy (65).

Elective Cranial Irradiation

- The incidence of brain metastasis in small cell carcinoma of the lung is as high as 50%. The actuarial incidence has been projected to be as high as 80% in patients surviving for 5 years.
- Elective whole brain irradiation decreases the cumulative incidence of intracranial metastasis by about 50% and provides approximately a 5% absolute 3-year overall survival increase in patients in complete remission (66).
- The utility of prophylactic cranial irradiation (PCI) in patients with extensive stage disease is unclear. Past studies have indicated that it is associated with an increase in 1-year overall survival from 13.3% to 27.1% in patients with a response to chemotherapy without mandated brain imaging confirmation of negative brain metastases prior to PCI (67). More recently, however, a Japanese trial studying PCI in patients with extensive stage small cell lung cancer who responded to chemotherapy and a confirmed absence of brain metastases on MRI revealed that the elective treatment did not result in longer overall survival compared with observation (median overall survival: 11.6 months versus 13.7 months, $p = 0.094$) (68).
- A 25 Gy in 10 fractions is an appropriate dose for PCI; there does not appear to be a benefit to dose escalation (69).

RADIATION THERAPY TECHNIQUES

Volumes, Portals, Beam Arrangements, and Planning

- The volume to be treated and the configuration of the irradiation portals are determined by size and location of the primary tumor/involved lymph nodes, areas of lymphatic drainage (if elective nodal irradiation is delivered), prescription dose, and equipment/beam energies available.
- Treatment portals are generally designed with a 1.5- to 2.0-cm margin around the gross tumor volume (GTV) of primary tumor plus involved lymph nodes determined by CT size (short axis diameter greater than 1.0 to 1.5 cm), PET avidity, and/or pathologic sampling positivity.
- A significant problem in defining GTV is distinguishing between actual tumor and postobstructive atelectasis or pneumonitis. Significant interclinician variability in contouring target volumes has been reported (70). Consultation with a diagnostic radiologist is invaluable. Imaging modalities such as PET scanning may further improve tumor definition (12).
- In a study of lung cancer surgical specimens, Giraud et al. (71) concluded that margins of 6 mm for adenocarcinoma and 8 mm for squamous cell carcinoma around the gross tumor are necessary to include microscopic tumor in 95% patients.
- Classic radiotherapy portals incorporate elective nodal irradiation. However, the merit of elective mediastinal (±supraclavicular) nodal irradiation is highly questionable given an elective nodal failure rate of only 5% to 10% in a number of non–small cell lung cancer series omitting elective nodal irradiation in both early-stage inoperable and locally advanced patients (65,72). Indeed, involved-field radiotherapy may facilitate dose escalation to gross disease without unacceptable toxicity (Fig. 19-2). Accordingly, the trend has been to move away from elective nodal irradiation.

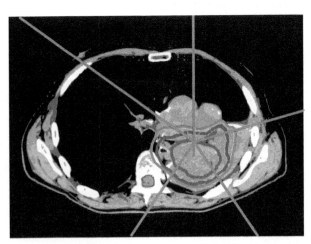

FIGURE 19-2. An illustration of IMRT plan for a patient with locally advanced non–small cell lung carcinoma (NSCLC). *Innermost gray contour* depicts GTV. *Solid red line* represents CTV, which includes nodal regions adjacent to left of the GTV. *Outer orange line* represents 60-Gy isodose coverage.

- For postoperative radiotherapy, the target volume is generally the mediastinum and the ipsilateral hilum, with boost fields to areas of extracapsular nodal extension or positive margins.
- 3DCRT allows for more precise targeting of tumor volumes while limiting dose to normal structures, when compared with 2D techniques (73,74). Intensity-modulated radiation therapy (IMRT) may further enhance the therapeutic ratio, especially for relatively large or irregularly shaped tumor volumes (34).
- Classic irradiation technique generally begins with an anteroposterior/postero-anterior beam arrangement, followed by use of oblique portals in order to keep the spinal cord dose below 45 Gy while minimizing irradiation of normal lung tissue. Examples of anterior-posterior and oblique portal MLC fields are shown in Figure 19-3.
- Radiotherapy planning and/or treatment techniques that account for tumor motion should be used; for example, use of a maximum intensity projection CT simulation method to allow for definition of an internal target volume that incorporates tumor temporal motion data, breath-hold/control methods, and respiratory gating techniques (49,75,76).
- Organs at risk that must be contoured during treatment planning generally include the lungs, heart, spinal cord, esophagus, liver, and brachial plexuses.
- In the analysis of dose distributions and dose-volume histograms, special attention is paid to coverage of the target volumes and the volumes of normal tissues receiving specific doses.
- In a seminal analysis, Graham et al. (77) reported that the most important prognostic factors in predicting for pneumonitis in patients treated with 3DCRT were percentage of total lung volume receiving greater than 20 Gy ($V_{20\text{ Gy}}$), total lung mean dose, and location of the primary tumor (upper versus lower lobe). Generally, minimum planning goals are $V_{20\text{ Gy}}$ less than 35% to 37% (but ideally even lower, especially in the preoperative setting or when delivering chemoradiation) and mean lung dose (MLD) less than 20 to 21 Gy.

Tumor Doses

- In patients with non–small cell carcinoma, the goal is to deliver at least 60 Gy to gross disease. However, dose escalation to higher than 70 Gy has been achieved safely; the highest doses have generally been reported in the protocol setting (38,78). If elective mediastinal irradiation is performed although in general not recommended, typically 40 to 45 Gy is delivered to this volume, followed by cone-down to gross disease to a final dose of at least 60 Gy.
- In the preoperative setting for non–small cell lung cancer, although INT 0139/RTOG 9309 utilized 45 Gy, doses of greater than 60 Gy can be safely delivered (16,24,25).
- In the postoperative setting for non–small cell lung cancer, the typical dose is approximately 50 to 54 Gy, with a boost to 54 to 60 Gy for patients with positive surgical margins or nodal extracapsular extension.
- Single or multiple fractionation regimens have been used for SBRT delivery with best current data suggesting that a biologically equivalent dose of at least 100 Gy is

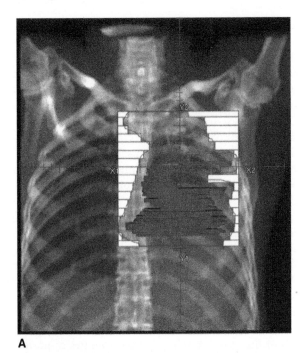

A

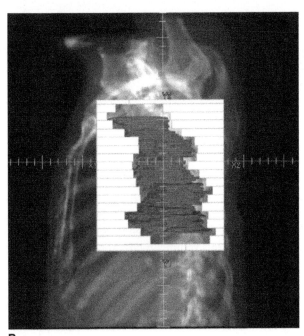

B

FIGURE 19-3. A and **B:** Examples of anterior-posterior and oblique multileaf collimator configuration.

required to achieve a local control rate of greater than 85% (79). SBRT doses that have been described in literature include 34 Gy in single fraction, 54 to 60 Gy in 3 fractions over 1.5 to 2 weeks, 48 Gy in 4 daily consecutive fractions, and 50 to- 60 Gy in 5 daily consecutive fractions for patients who are clinically node negative by CT and/or PET with early-stage tumors (less than 5 cm) in a peripheral loca- tion (greater than 2 cm in all directions around the proximal bronchial tree, see Fig. 19-4). More centrally located tumors require a more protracted SBRT course such as 4 to 5 fractions, 60 Gy delivered over 8 consecutive daily fractions or 70 Gy over 10 daily fractions, whereas 54 to 60 Gy in 3 fractions is unsafe and should be avoided.

- Thoracic irradiation for small cell lung cancer can be delivered as 45 Gy b.i.d. (1.5-Gy fractions twice daily) or 60 to 70 Gy q.d. (1.8 to 2.0-Gy daily fractions).

Brachytherapy

- Brachytherapy has been used as an alternative treatment for localized unresectable cancers or as a boost (three 5-Gy fractions or one 10-Gy fraction) in combination with external irradiation (80–82).
- Indications include thoracic symptoms (dyspnea because of endobronchial tumor or obstructive pneumonia), previous high-dose irradiation to the chest, and endobron- chial or endotracheal lesion as determined by bronchoscopy.
- Brachytherapy may be administered by permanent ^{125}I interstitial implants performed intraoperatively, removable ^{192}Ir implants through intraoperative insertion of cath- eters in the tumor, or intrabronchial low- or high-dose rate ^{192}Ir sources (83).

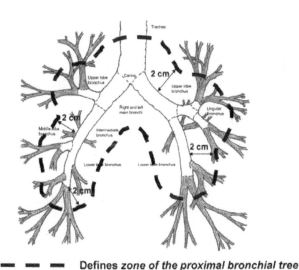

■ ■ ■ ■ **Defines** *zone of the proximal bronchial tree*

A

FIGURE 19-4. **A:** The *dashed line* defines the zone of the proximal bronchial tree. Patients with medi- cally inoperable stage I NSCLC outside this boundary can be treated with SBRT.

continued

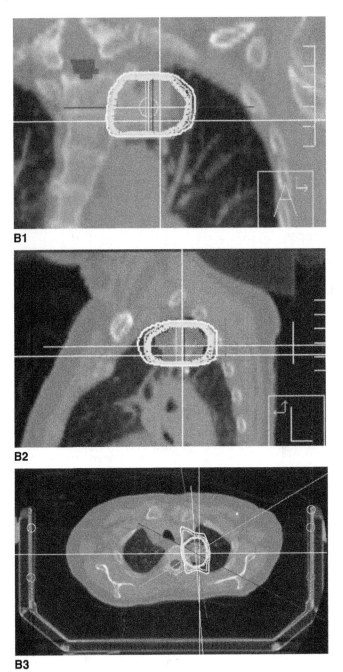

FIGURE 19-4. (*continued*) **B1, B2,** and **B3:** A patient with T1N0M0 left upper lobe NSCLC was treated with SBRT. GTV was in *gray color wash*, gray contour line surrounding GTV represents ITV. Outer white contour line represents isodose line of 48 Gy in 4 fractions.

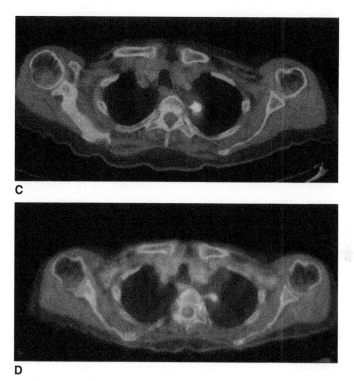

FIGURE 19-4. *(continued)* **C:** CT and PET before. **D:** CT and PET 3 months after SBRT. Notice the substantial reduction in the size of the lesion detected by PET (white object slightly to right of vertebral column).

SUPERIOR SULCUS LUNG CARCINOMA

- These tumors were traditionally treated by preoperative irradiation with doses of 30 to 50 Gy, followed by *en bloc* resection (6).
- INT 0160 defined a new standard of care for these patients: induction chemoradiation followed by resection (84). Patients were treated with cisplatin/etoposide and concurrent 45-Gy thoracic irradiation, then resection (for patients who had stable/responsive disease after chemoradiation), followed by adjuvant cisplatin/etoposide. The 5-year overall survival was 44%, which compared favorably with an approximate 30% rate historically.
- For patients who have inoperable tumors (even after neoadjuvant therapy) or are medically inoperable, radical irradiation (with chemotherapy for those patients who can tolerate it) is a reasonable management approach.
- Particular attention must be paid to spinal cord and brachial plexus doses when conducting radiotherapy treatment planning for patients with superior sulcus tumors.

SUPERIOR VENA CAVA SYNDROME

- Superior vena cava syndrome is a medical emergency occasionally seen in patients with malignant neoplasia; it requires immediate therapeutic action.
- Most cases (80%) of superior vena cava syndrome result from bronchogenic carcinoma. Malignant lymphoma represents 10% to 18% of the cases, and benign causes, such as goiter, account for 2% to 3%.
- Radiation therapy should be initiated as soon as possible.
- Patients initially should be given high-dose fractions (3 Gy or higher) for 2 or 3 days, followed by additional daily doses of 1.8 to 2.0 Gy to complete definitive irradiation; patients who are not candidates for definitive therapy can be treated with a regimen such as 3 Gy × 10 fractions.
- In patients with small cell carcinoma presenting with superior vena cava syndrome, the mode of initial therapy is controversial; both irradiation and chemotherapy are effective, and often chemotherapy is attempted first.
- Irradiation techniques are similar to those described for primary bronchogenic carcinoma.

SEQUELAE OF THERAPY

Acute Sequelae

- Acute toxicities (occurring during the course of irradiation or within 1 month after its completion) include esophagitis, cough, skin reaction, and fatigue.
- Acute radiation esophagitis usually begins in the third week of radiotherapy. The combination of irradiation and chemotherapy may increase the incidence of esophageal sequelae.
- Treatment for acute esophagitis includes mucosal anesthetics (viscous lidocaine) and agents that coat the irritated surfaces (suspension or liquid antacids). Liquid analgesics sometimes are required, especially with combined chemotherapy and thoracic irradiation. If symptoms do not improve and nutritional status is compromised, a nasogastric tube, temporary gastrostomy, or intravenous hyperalimentation may be necessary. Superimposed candidias should be ruled out; if present, it should be treated with appropriate medication.
- Cough is common (probably secondary to bronchial mucosal irritation) but usually not severe. Antitussive therapy with or without codeine is usually effective.
- Treatment of the acute phase of RP includes bed rest, use of bronchodilators, and/or corticosteroid therapy (e.g., prednisone 1 mg/kg/day). In severe cases, it may be necessary to use positive pressure oxygen. Antibiotics are not indicated unless there is associated secondary infection. After control of acute symptoms, corticosteroid use should be tapered over a period of several weeks; abrupt discontinuation of steroids may result in activation of subclinical radiation injuries in the lung.
- Lhermitte's syndrome, observed in 10% to 15% of patients, is transient and not of long-term clinical significance.

- With megavoltage therapy, skin reaction is mild to moderate; topical moisturizing creams or ointments may relieve itching and dryness.

Late Sequelae

- Late sequelae include pneumonitis/pulmonary fibrosis (both symptomatic and radiographic), esophageal stricture, cardiac sequelae (e.g., pericardial effusion, constrictive pericarditis, and cardiomyopathy), spinal cord myelopathy, and brachial plexopathy.
- The most frequently reported sequelae in RTOG trials were pneumonitis (approximately 10% grade 2 and 4.6% grade 3) and pulmonary fibrosis (approximately 20% grade 2 and 8% grade 3 or greater) (85). Using new technology with IMRT has been shown to be associated with less ≥grade 3 pneumonitis than 3DCRT (3.5% versus 7.9%) with a secondary analysis from RTOG 0617 (86).
- The threshold MLD for RP is approximately 20 to 22 Gy. The incidence and the degree of RP depend on the total dose, fractionation, and volume of lung irradiated (77). Additionally, the risk of RP appears to be greater if the patient receives carboplatin/paclitaxel versus cisplatin/etoposide concurrent with their radiation therapy (OR 3.33) (87).
- Long-term esophageal problems such as stenosis, ulceration, perforation, and fistula formation are seen in 5% to 15% of patients. Graham et al. (unpublished data) showed that the volume of esophagus receiving doses higher than 55 Gy correlated with an increased incidence of esophageal sequelae (i.e., strictures) in patients treated with 3DCRT. The estimated dose is 63 Gy in 30 fractions for 5% incidence of esophageal injury and 66.5 Gy (30 fractions) for a 50% incidence (88). Late esophageal complications increase with cisplatin-based chemotherapy given concurrently with brachytherapy (89).
- Radiation-induced cardiac disease after irradiation for lung cancer is relatively rare; pericarditis is most common. Certain chemotherapeutic agents, such as doxorubicin, have synergistic cardiotoxicity with radiation. Caution is required when irradiation is combined with such drugs.
- Spinal cord myelopathy may occur with doses higher than 45 Gy in 1.8- to 2.0-Gy fractions; factors important in its causation are total irradiation dose, length of the irradiated cord, and fractionation schedule.

MEDIASTINUM AND TRACHEA

Anatomy

- The boundaries of the mediastinum are the thoracic inlet superiorly (at level of first thoracic vertebra and first rib), diaphragm inferiorly, sternum anteriorly, vertebral column posteriorly, and parietal pleura laterally.
- The mediastinum is divided into anterior, middle, and posterior compartments. Some suggest that the superior mediastinum is a separate compartment, whereas others include it in the anterior mediastinum.

Table 19-2

Classification of Mediastinal Structures and Tumors/Cysts by Anatomic Location

Anterosuperior Mediastinum	Middle Mediastinum	Posterior Mediastinum
Anatomic Structures		
Aorta and great vessels	Heart and pericardium	Sympathetic chain vagus
Thymus gland	Trachea and major bronchi	Esophagus
Lymph glands	Pulmonary vessels	Thoracic duct
	Lymph nodes	Descending aorta
		Lymph nodes
Mediastinal Tumors and Cysts		
Thymic tumors	Lymphomas	Neurogenic tumors
Lymphomas	Sarcoidosis	Lymphomas
Germinal cell tumors	Cardiac and pericardial tumors	Esophageal tumors
Endocrine tumors	Tracheal tumors	Endocrine tumors
Thyroid tumors	Vascular tumors	Tumors of spinal column
Parathyroid tumors	Lung cancers	Lung cancers
Mesenchymal tumors	Cysts	Cysts
Lung cancers		
Cysts		

Reprinted with permission from Graham MV, Emami B. Mediastinum and trachea. In: Perez CA, Brady LW, eds. *Principles and practice of radiation oncology*, 3rd ed. Philadelphia, PA: Lippincott–Raven, 1998:1221–1239.

- Tumors arising in the mediastinal compartments are listed in Table 19-2.
- In adults, most thyroid tumors, thymomas, mediastinal germ cell tumors, and teratomas are located in the superior and anterior mediastinum. Eighty percent of neurogenic tumors are located in the posterior mediastinum, and 50% of mediastinal lymphomas are in the middle mediastinum.
- In adults, the incidence of anterosuperior, middle, and posterior mediastinal tumors is approximately 54%, 20%, and 26%, respectively. In children, the posterior mediastinum contains 63% of lesions, the anterior mediastinum 26%, and the middle mediastinum 11% (90).
- Primary mediastinal tumors are relatively rare. In adults, the ratio of benign to malignant tumors is approximately 3 to 2; the relative incidence of malignant mediastinal tumors in children is approximately 50%.

Thymomas

- Thymomas are the most common tumors of the anterior mediastinum, accounting for approximately 20% of all mediastinal tumors in adults.

Natural History

- From 39% to 64% of thymomas in surgical series are noninvasive (90). The predominant pattern of spread is direct invasion of the capsule surrounding the thymus.
- In more advanced cases, invasion into the superior vena cava, brachiocephalic vein, lung, and pericardium is observed frequently. Superior vena cava syndrome as a presenting symptom is not unusual.
- The most frequent area of dissemination is the pleural cavity, although pericardial effusions also are reported.
- Although rare, distant metastases to liver, lung, and bone have been reported.
- Thymoma is frequently associated with myasthenia gravis, an autoimmune disease characterized by antiacetylcholine receptor antibodies resulting in an acetylcholine receptor deficiency at the motor end plate. The most common clinical feature is neuromuscular fatigue. Ocular muscles are involved in 90% of patients. Next in frequency of involvement are facial and pharyngeal muscles, progressing to fatigue of proximal limb girdle muscles and respiratory suppression. Of patients with myasthenia gravis, approximately 25% have a normal-sized thymus and 75% have thymic abnormalities; 15% of these abnormalities are associated with thymoma, and the remaining are due to thymic lymphoid hyperplasia.

Clinical Presentation

- Approximately 30% to 40% of thymomas are asymptomatic; the tumor is usually an incidental finding on chest x-ray.
- Symptoms may include chest pain, dyspnea, hoarseness, and superior vena cava syndrome.
- Dysphagia, fever, weight loss, and anorexia may also be present.
- Approximately 33% to 50% of thymomas are associated with myasthenia gravis, 5% with red cell aplasia, and 5% with hypogammaglobulinemia (91).

Diagnostic Workup

- The diagnostic workup for mediastinal tumors is outlined in Table 19-3.
- CT of the chest is the most valuable radiologic technique. It defines size, contour, tissue density, and homogeneity of the lesion, as well as the lesion's relationship to other structures—data that are critical for planning irradiation portals.
- CT is well suited for staging of many of these tumors and is helpful for monitoring response to irradiation and/or chemotherapy.
- MRI of the chest sometimes offers supplementary information to CT scan.
- Because most mediastinal tumors are surgically removed, tissue diagnosis is most often done at thoracotomy.
- Bronchoscopy, mediastinoscopy, or anterior mediastinotomy may yield the diagnosis, especially if enlarged lymph nodes are present.

Staging

- The most widely accepted classification of thymomas has two categories: invasive and noninvasive.

Table 19-3
Diagnostic Workup for Mediastinal Tumors

General
History
Physical examination—for male patients with mediastinal germ cell tumors, this should include a thorough examination of the testes

Radiographic Studies
Standard
Chest x-ray
CT chest
Supplementary
MRI chest
PET scan
Barium swallow
Angiogram/arteriography
Ultrasonography of testes (in mediastinal germ cell tumors)

Laboratory Studies
Complete blood cell count, blood chemistries, urinalysis
Germ cell tumors: AFP, β-hCG, LDH, CEA
Thymoma: radioimmunoassay for acetylcholine receptors

Special Tests/Procedures
Mediastinoscopy
Anterior mediastinotomy with biopsy
Bronchoscopy
Esophagoscopy
Biopsy of palpable supraclavicular lymph nodes

Adapted from Graham MV, Emami B. Mediastinum and trachea. In: Perez CA, Brady LW, eds. *Principles and practice of radiation oncology*, 3rd ed. Philadelphia, PA: Lippincott–Raven, 1998:1221–1239.

- Staging of thymomas is based on degree of invasiveness.
- The pathologic staging system of Masaoka et al. (92) is the most widely used (Table 19-4).
- The American Joint Committee on Cancer has released their own staging for thymoma for the first time in their 8th edition staging manual.

Pathologic Classification

- Rosai and Levine (93) divided thymomas into three types based on histopathology, depending on the predominant tumor cell type: lymphocytic, epithelial, and mixed (lymphoepithelial). Some authors have suggested spindle cell type as a fourth group, but it is often considered a variant of the epithelial type.

Table 19-4
Modified Masaoka Thymoma Staging System

Stage I	Macroscopically and microscopically completely encapsulated
Stage II	A. Microscopic transcapsular invasion or B. Macroscopic invasion into surrounding fatty tissue or grossly adherent to but not through mediastinal pleura or pericardium
Stage III	Invasive growth into neighboring intrathoracic organs (ie, pericardium, great vessels, lung) A. Without invasion of great vessels B. With invasion of great vessels
Stage IVA	Pleural or pericardial implants
Stage IVB	Lymphogenous or hematogenous metastases

Source: Masaoka A, Monden Y, Nakahara K, et al. Follow-up study of thymomas with special reference to their clinical stages. *Cancer* 1981;48:2485–2492. This staging system has been modified by Koga K et al. and is sometimes referenced as Masaoka-Koga staging system.

- The World Health Organization classification is currently the advocated system although with debates. Classification is based on "organotypical" features (i.e., histologic characteristics mimicking those observed in the normal thymus) including growth pattern (encapsulation and a "lobular architecture") and cellular composition. The five main subtypes (A, AB, B1, B2, and B3) can be broadly divided into thymomas containing spindled neoplastic epithelial cells (A, AB) and thymomas composed of epithelioid neoplastic epithelial cells (B1–3).
- Most series report no correlation between histopathology and malignant potential (93) and no correlation between histopathologic subtype of thymoma and the associated systemic syndromes.
- The more recent histologic classification of Marino and Muller-Hermelink (94) showed prognostic significance independent of tumor stage. Medullary and mixed thymomas were benign tumors even with capsular invasion and showed no risk of recurrence. Organoid and cortical thymomas had intermediate invasiveness and low but significant risk of late relapse. Well-differentiated carcinoma was always invasive and had a significant risk of relapse and death, even in stage II patients.

Prognostic Factors

- Invasiveness of the tumor is the most important prognostic factor.
- Patients with complete or radical excision have significantly better survival than those with subtotal resection or biopsy only (92,95).
- Although older series reported that the presence of myasthenia gravis resulted in a poor prognosis, more recent series have found no influence of coexisting myasthenia gravis on prognosis (12,96,97).

General Management

- Complete surgical resection is the treatment of choice for all thymomas regardless of invasiveness, except in rare cases with extrathoracic or extensive intrathoracic metastasis (98).
- Survival is excellent for encapsulated, noninvasive thymomas, and adjuvant (postoperative) irradiation is not indicated for Masaoka stage I thymomas because of the very low likelihood of recurrence (99–101).
- Radiation therapy is excellent adjuvant therapy for invasive thymomas, which are generally radioresponsive.
- Long-term follow-up data suggest that postoperative irradiation reduced the recurrence rate and prolonged DFS even after complete resection of thymoma. Type B2 or type B3 encapsulated thymoma and invasive thymoma are recommended with adjuvant radiotherapy after complete resection (102).
- For invasive thymomas (Masaoka stage II or higher), postoperative irradiation is generally delivered to decrease the likelihood of recurrence (95,97–100,103–105). In a classic series by Curran et al. (99), the 5-year actuarial mediastinal relapse rates for stage II to III patients who did versus did not receive adjuvant radiotherapy after total resection were 0% versus 53%, respectively. However, other reports suggest that adjuvant radiotherapy can be safely deferred without incurring a prohibitively high relapse rate, especially for stage II patients (106,107).
- Irradiation is indicated for patients with postoperative gross residual disease and those with unresectable thymomas.
- For large, invasive thymomas thought to be marginally resectable, preoperative irradiation has been advocated (96).
- An alternative strategy for locally advanced thymomas is preoperative chemotherapy (generally cisplatin based) with postoperative irradiation (108,109). Kim et al. (108) reported 7-year progression-free and overall survival rates of 77% and 79%, respectively, for Masaoka stage III, IVA, IVB patients treated with induction chemotherapy (cisplatin, doxorubicin, cyclophosphamide, and prednisone), resection, postoperative irradiation, and consolidation chemotherapy.
- Others have demonstrated favorable results with induction chemoradiation, then resection for locally advanced thymoma patients (61).

Radiation Therapy Techniques

- Although some advocate that the volume treated should include the entire mediastinum, it is common practice to treat the postoperative tumor bed plus any gross residual disease (or the thymus itself for unresected disease) + 1.0- to 1.5-cm margin, with demarcation of the treatment volume guided by preoperative/postoperative imaging, surgical clips, and pathology/operative reports.
- Treatment can be delivered using anteroposterior/posteroanterior portals or oblique portals with wedges. Although 2D planning techniques were the historical standard, 3D conformal radiotherapy should be employed in the modern era to optimize dose distributions. Complex beam arrangements using intensity-modulated radiotherapy can also be helpful, especially for large and/or irregularly shaped target volumes intimately associated with critical normal tissues (34).

- The recommended irradiation dose range for malignant thymomas after resection is 45 to 54 Gy, with stage II patients receiving doses at the lower end of this range and stage III patients receiving doses at the higher end; in fact, even higher doses have been used (104), with excellent local tumor control with all doses over 40 Gy. Increased rate of local recurrence has been reported with doses less than 40 Gy.
- For inoperable cases or patients with postoperative gross residual disease, doses in the range of 60 Gy (or higher) are often employed.

Sequelae of Treatment

- Late sequelae are unusual in reported studies.
- RP, cardiotoxicity such as pericarditis, and, rarely, myelopathy have been reported.

Malignant Mediastinal Germ Cell Tumors

- Malignant mediastinal germ cell tumors are significantly more common in males.
- Pure seminomas are most common in the third decade of life, followed by the fourth and second decades.
- Nonseminomatous germ cell tumors (NSGCTs) (pure or mixed histology) occur in young adults (15 to 35 years).

Natural History

- Most mediastinal germ cell tumors are located in the anterosuperior mediastinum.
- Mediastinal germ cell tumors have the same morphologic appearance as that of germinal tumors of the testes.
- If anterior mediastinal metastases are present, middle and posterior mediastinal lymph nodes, as well as retroperitoneal nodes, are frequently involved.

Clinical Presentation

- Patients with mediastinal germ cell tumors may be entirely asymptomatic, particularly when the tumor is a benign teratoma or seminoma.
- Some tumors may produce substernal pressure and pain radiating to the neck and the arms.
- Tumors produce superior vena cava syndrome in 10% of patients (99).
- Embryonal cell carcinoma, teratocarcinoma, and choriocarcinoma are more aggressively infiltrating neoplasms, resulting in substernal pleuritic pain that occasionally is associated with dyspnea, cough, and hemoptysis.
- Approximately 40% of patients with choriocarcinoma show gynecomastia.

Diagnostic Workup

- CT of the chest is the radiologic method of choice (Table 19-4).
- If testicular abnormalities are present, appropriate radiologic examinations should be obtained for a testicular or retroperitoneal neoplasm (ultrasonography, CT of the abdomen/pelvis).

- Germ cell tumors elaborate β-subunit of human chorionic gonadotropin (β-hCG), which is elevated in the serum of 60% of patients with NSGCTs and 7% of patients with pure seminomas (90). All patients with choriocarcinoma have elevated urinary and serum β-hCG levels.
- Alpha-fetoprotein (AFP) is elevated in approximately 70% of patients with NSGCT. The presence of an elevated AFP level indicates that a presumed seminomatous germ cell tumor actually has some NSGCT component.
- Over 90% of patients with germ cell tumors have elevated levels of AFP, β-hCG, or both. These biomarkers are helpful in monitoring the response of the tumor to therapy and can be used to detect recurrences.
- In most mediastinal tumors, a thoracotomy is needed to establish histopathologic diagnosis. When surgical removal of the tumor is not indicated or possible, an open biopsy can be done.

Pathologic Classification

- Rosai and Levine (93) divided mediastinal germ cell tumors into germinomas (seminomas), adult (mature) teratomas, embryonal carcinomas, teratocarcinomas, choriocarcinomas, yolk sac tumors (endodermal sinus tumors), and mixed tumors.
- A simpler system of classification divides tumors into pure seminomas or nonseminomatous carcinomas.

Staging

- No staging system exists for mediastinal germ cell tumors.

Prognostic Factors

- Histologic type is the most important prognostic factor in anterior mediastinal extragonadal germinal tumors. Mature teratomas and seminomas are highly curable and have a better prognosis than immature teratomas and NSGCTs.

General Management

Seminomas
- Thoracotomy with radical intent has been performed in approximately 50% of patients who had surgery. Complete tumor removal was possible in only 40% to 50% of patients undergoing radical surgery (4).
- If radical resection is not performed, excellent results still may be obtained with radical postoperative irradiation, or even irradiation after biopsy alone (110,111).
- Chemotherapy usually is reserved for locally extensive tumors, failures of surgery or irradiation, or metastatic disease (112).

Nonseminomatous Germ Cell Neoplasms
- Because of their propensity for distant metastasis, primary treatment for nonseminomatous malignant tumors is chemotherapy and radical resection, if possible (4).

- Mediastinal NSGCT does not respond as well to chemotherapy as other extragonadal or testicular presentations. Relapses are more frequent, and survival is worse.
- For better local tumor control, resection of postchemotherapy residual disease may be necessary (112).
- The role of irradiation in NSGCT has been highly debated. Because of a poor resectability rate and frequent residual masses after chemotherapy, radiation therapy has been mainly used to increase local tumor control.
- Irradiation given before chemotherapy may adversely affect the patient's ability to tolerate full cytotoxic doses.

Radiation Therapy Techniques

- The treatment technique for seminoma is similar to that for thymoma.
- Both supraclavicular areas may be irradiated, although this is not uniformly practiced.
- Doses of 20 to 60 Gy have been used; Cox suggested that 30 Gy given in 15 fractions is adequate (99). However, Bagshaw et al. (110) recommended 40 to 50 Gy to the mediastinum and supraclavicular lymph nodes. Bush et al. (111) reported that no patient receiving greater than 47 Gy of definitive irradiation had local or systemic relapse.
- One potential therapeutic approach is approximately 30 Gy for minimal disease. For gross tumors, 40 Gy can be delivered with large fields encompassing the mediastinum (±supraclavicular areas), followed by an additional 10 Gy with reduced portals to GTV (visible on CT scan).

Sequelae of Treatment

- Fatigue, dysphagia, cough, and mild skin reaction are early (acute) sequelae of thoracic irradiation.
- In the 30- to 50-Gy range used for seminomas, late effects might be expected to be similar to those of patients with Hodgkin's disease treated with mediastinal irradiation.
- Late sequelae of thoracic irradiation for mediastinal NSGCT are generally overshadowed by the high local and systemic failure rate.

Tracheal Tumors

- Primary malignant tumors of the trachea are rare.

Natural History

- Squamous cell cancer has a predilection for the distal third of the trachea; over 60% of cases originate in the posterior or the lateral wall.
- Approximately one third of patients have mediastinal spread or pulmonary metastases when first seen.
- Tumor first involves adjacent lymph nodes and, by direct extension, the mediastinal structures. Metastases to distant organs (lungs, liver, and bone) are common.

- Adenoid cystic carcinomas and adenocarcinomas tend to appear in the upper third of the trachea; they may extend for a greater distance in the tracheal wall, with only a portion of tumor presenting intratracheally. With both surgery and irradiation, larger margins of clearance are needed. Neutron irradiation has offered some promising results for adenoid cystic tumors (113,114).
- Extension beyond the trachea occurs 3 times more frequently with adenoid cystic carcinomas (58%) than with squamous cell carcinomas (90).

Clinical Presentation

- Hemoptysis (60%), dyspnea (56%), hoarseness (40%), and cough (36%) were the most common symptoms in a series from Washington University, St. Louis (115).
- Other potential signs and symptoms include recurrent pneumonia and vocal cord palsy.

Diagnostic Workup

- Patients with nonspecific symptoms may have a normal chest x-ray film.
- Bronchoscopy can be helpful in determining resectability and relief of obstruction in occasional life-threatening situations. A rigid bronchoscope is usually used, although laser resection is being used more frequently.
- CT of the chest is the radiologic study of choice for delineation of tumor extent.

Pathologic Classification

- The World Health Organization revised the classification of laryngeal, hypopharyngeal, and tracheal tumors in 1993 (116). This histologic typing includes epithelial tumors and precancerous lesions (from benign to malignant), soft tissue tumors, tumors of bone and cartilage, lymphomas, and tumor-like lesions.
- Malignant lesions include adenocarcinoma, squamous cell carcinoma, adenosquamous carcinoma, adenoid cystic carcinoma, mucoepidermoid carcinoma, and neuroendocrine carcinoma, grades 1 through 3.
- The most common primary carcinomas of the trachea are squamous cell and adenoid cystic carcinomas; the other malignant entities are rare.

Staging

- No staging system exists for primary tracheal tumors.

Prognostic Factors

- Major prognostic factors include histologic type, location (upper versus lower), and resectability, which is related to the first two factors.
- Lymph node involvement and positive surgical margins after resection also appear to have prognostic significance.
- In reported series, adenoid cystic carcinoma has had improved survival and relatively indolent progression of disease.

General Management

- Treatment of choice for tracheal carcinomas is primary resection and reanastomosis of the involved airway; sleeve resection is often required (117).
- Postoperative irradiation is routinely recommended, although it has not been studied in a formal prospective manner (118–121).
- In patients who cannot undergo resection, external beam irradiation and/or endotracheal brachytherapy may be used (120,122–125).
- Chemotherapy alone is not generally useful, but it has been recommended in conjunction with other modalities.

Radiation Therapy Techniques

- Because of the high incidence of mediastinal nodal involvement, classically almost the entire mediastinum (low border at least 5 to 6 cm below the carina) and both supraclavicular regions were included in the initial irradiation portals up to a dose of at least 45 Gy in tumors of the upper or mid trachea, with the value of elective supraclavicular lymph node irradiation for carinal or lower tracheal tumors unknown. However, some institutions have now moved away from routine large-field elective nodal irradiation.
- Because of a predilection for longitudinal (perineural) spread, the initial treatment volume for adenoid cystic histology should include wide superior-inferior tracheal margins.
- A portion of the treatment for tracheal tumors can be delivered with an anteroposterior/posteroanterior technique while respecting spinal cord tolerance dose.
- An additional boost dose (to a total tumor dose of about 60 to 70 Gy, with higher doses for gross disease) can be delivered through anterior oblique portals with wedges.
- 3D conformal radiotherapy should be used for treatment planning; intensity-modulated radiotherapy may be of benefit, especially for cases with large volume disease burden and/or irregularly shaped target volumes in critical locations (34).
- If there is massive tumor extension through the tracheal wall and if surgery is ruled out, high risk of fistula may preclude a radical dose of radiation therapy. In this situation, as well as in any scenario in which the patient cannot tolerate a high dose of irradiation, a protracted palliative irradiation course such as 45 Gy in 5 weeks can be used.
- Endobronchial high-dose rate afterloading treatment using an ^{192}Ir source was described by Schraube et al. (124) in four patients treated with megavoltage external beam irradiation (46 to 60 Gy). Brachytherapy consisted of five 3- to 4-Gy fractions, two high-dose rate placements per week, calculated at 10 mm from the source center.
- Use of fast neutron radiation therapy for tracheal tumors was reported by Saroja and Mansell (126) in six patients, most with recurrent tumors after surgery. Dose ranged from 18 Gy in 12 fractions over 26 days to 26.6 Gy in 12 fractions over 39 days, delivered primarily with anterior and oblique beams. Favorable results with neutron irradiation have been reported by Bittner et al. (114), who observed 5-year actuarial locoregional control and overall survival rates of 54.1% and 89.4%, respectively, for a series of 20 tracheal adenoid cystic carcinoma patients treated with neutron irradiation (median dose, 19.2 Gy) ± endobronchial high-dose rate brachytherapy boost at the University of Washington.

NORMAL TISSUE COMPLICATIONS—QUANTEC RESULTS

The recommendations of the QUANTEC review by Marks et al. (127) include the following:

- The rate of symptomatic pneumonitis is related to many dosimetric parameters, and there are no evident threshold "tolerance dose-volume" levels. There are strong volume and fractionation effects.
- Despite these caveats, it is prudent to limit V_{20} to ≤30% to 35% and MLD to ≤20 to 23 Gy (with conventional fractionation) if one wants to limit the risk of RP to ≤20% in definitively treated patients with non–small cell lung cancer. Similar guidelines for other parameters can be extracted from the figures. Limiting the dose to the central airways to ≤80 Gy may reduce the risk of bronchial stricture. In patients treated after pneumonectomy for mesothelioma, it is prudent to limit the V_5 to less than 60%, the V_{20} to less than 4% to 10%, and the MLD to less than 8 Gy.
- We have presented plots based on fits to V_{20} data from Yorke et al. (128) in Figure 19-5. As noted in the above recommendations, the incidence of severe complications rises sharply above 20% when total lung volume irradiated exceeds 35% to 40%.

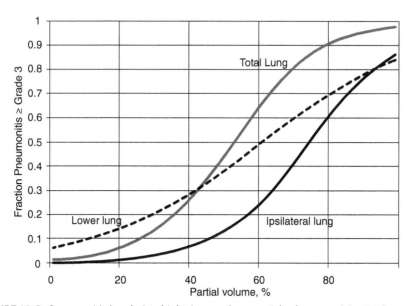

FIGURE 19-5. Pneumonitis (grade 3 or higher) versus lung partial volume receiving 20 Gy or more. (Curves are from data reported by Yorke ED, Jackson A, Rosenzweig KE, et al. Correlation of dosimetric factors and RP for non-small-cell lung cancer patients in a recently completed dose escalation study. *Int J Radiat Oncol Biol Phys* 2005;63[3]:672–682 for total lung, ipsilateral and lower subvolumes. Their V_{20} data were fit using a "probit" function of the form: $P(x) = \exp(b0 + b1 \times x)/(1+ \exp(b0 + b1 \times x))$, where $b0$ and $b1$ are adjustable parameters.)

Sequelae of Treatment

- Side effects to the tracheal cartilage and esophagus with irradiation doses of 60 to 70 Gy or higher are described in most series.
- Most patients develop acute odynophagia/dysphagia, cough, and local irritation.
- Late effects include softening of the cartilage, tracheitis, and tracheal stenosis.
- Esophageal stricture has been reported.
- Esophageal and mediastinal fistulas, vocal cord paralysis as a result of laryngeal nerve damage, and other complications (including infection, pulmonary edema, and even death) have been observed, particularly in surgically treated patients.

References

1. Baird JA. The pathways of lymphatic spread of carcinoma of the lung. *Br J Surg* 1965;52(11): 868–875.
2. Goldstraw P, Crowley J, Chansky K, et al. The IASLC Lung Cancer Staging Project: proposals for the revision of the TNM stage groupings in the forthcoming (seventh) edition of the TNM Classification of malignant tumours. *J Thorac Oncol* 2007;2(8):706–714.
3. Nohl-Oser HC. An investigation of the anatomy of the lymphatic drainage of the lungs as shown by the lymphatic spread of bronchial carcinoma. *Ann R Coll Surg Engl* 1972;51(3):157–176.
4. Dulmet EM, Macchiarini P, Suc B, et al. Germ cell tumors of the mediastinum. A 30-year experience. *Cancer* 1993;72(6):1894–1901.
5. Muers MF, Round CE. Palliation of symptoms in non-small cell lung cancer: a study by the Yorkshire Regional Cancer Organisation Thoracic Group. *Thorax* 1993;48(4):339–343.
6. Paulson D. Management of superior sulcus carcinomas. In: Choi N, Grillo H, eds. *Thoracic oncology*. New York, NY: Raven Press, 1983.
7. Grenier P, Dubray B, Carette M. Preoperative thoracic staging of lung cancer: CT and MR evaluation. *Diagnost Int Radiol* 1989;1:23–28.
8. Faivre-Finn C, Snee M, Ashcroft L, et al. Concurrent once-daily versus twice-daily chemoradiotherapy in patients with limited-stage small-cell lung cancer (CONVERT): an open-label, phase 3, randomised, superiority trial. *Lancet Oncol* 2017;18(8):1116–1125.
9. Lowe VJ, Naunheim KS. Positron emission tomography in lung cancer. *Ann Thorac Surg* 1998;65(6):1821–1829.
10. Marom EM, McAdams HP, Erasmus JJ, et al. Staging non-small cell lung cancer with whole-body PET. *Radiology* 1999;212(3):803–809.
11. Sura S, Gupta V, Yorke E, et al. Intensity-modulated radiation therapy (IMRT) for inoperable non-small cell lung cancer: the Memorial Sloan-Kettering Cancer Center (MSKCC) experience. *Radiother Oncol* 2008;87(1):17–23.
12. Munley MT, Marks LB, Scarfone C, et al. Multimodality nuclear medicine imaging in three-dimensional radiation treatment planning for lung cancer: challenges and prospects. *Lung Cancer* 1999;23(2):105–114.
13. Vanuytsel LJ, Vansteenkiste JF, Stroobants SG, et al. The impact of (18)F-fluoro-2-deoxy-D-glucose positron emission tomography (FDG-PET) lymph node staging on the radiation treatment volumes in patients with non-small cell lung cancer. *Radiother Oncol* 2000;55(3):317–324.
14. Kalff V, Hicks RJ, MacManus MP, et al. Clinical impact of (18)F fluorodeoxyglucose positron emission tomography in patients with non-small-cell lung cancer: a prospective study. *J Clin Oncol* 2001;19(1):111–118.
15. Ginsberg RJ, Rubinstein LV. Randomized trial of lobectomy versus limited resection for T1 N0 non-small cell lung cancer. Lung Cancer Study Group. *Ann Thorac Surg* 1995;60(3):615–622; discussion 622–613.

16. Chang JY, Senan S, Paul MA et al. Stereotactic ablative radiotherapy versus lobectomy for operable stage I non-small-cell lung cancer: a pooled analysis of two randomized trials. *Lancet* 2015;16(6):630–637.

17. Trakhtenberg A, Kiseleva ES, Pitskhelauri VG, et al. Preoperative radiotherapy in the combined treatment of lung cancer patients. *Neoplasma* 1988;35(4):459–465.

18. Rosell R, Gomez-Codina J, Camps C, et al. Preresectional chemotherapy in stage IIIA non-small-cell lung cancer: a 7-year assessment of a randomized controlled trial. *Lung Cancer* 1999;26(1):7–14.

19. Roth JA, Atkinson EN, Fossella F, et al. Long-term follow-up of patients enrolled in a randomized trial comparing perioperative chemotherapy and surgery with surgery alone in resectable stage IIIA non-small-cell lung cancer. *Lung Cancer* 1998;21(1):1–6.

20. Cerfolio RJ, Bryant AS, Spencer SA, et al. Pulmonary resection after high-dose and low-dose chest irradiation. *Ann Thorac Surg* 2005;80(4):1224–1230; discussion 1230.

21. Albain KS, Rusch VW, Crowley JJ, et al. Concurrent cisplatin/etoposide plus chest radiotherapy followed by surgery for stages IIIA (N2) and IIIB non-small-cell lung cancer: mature results of Southwest Oncology Group phase II study 8805. *J Clin Oncol* 1995;13(8):1880–1892.

22. Alongi F, Arcangeli S, De Bari B, et al. Stage-I small cell lung cancer: a new potential option for stereotactic ablative radiation therapy? A review of literature. *Crit Rev Oncol Hematol* 2017;112: 67–71.

23. Winton T, Livingston R, Johnson D, et al. Vinorelbine plus cisplatin vs. observation in resected non-small-cell lung cancer. *N Engl J Med* 2005;352(25):2589–2597.

24. Sonett JR, Suntharalingam M, Edelman MJ, et al. Pulmonary resection after curative intent radiotherapy (>59 Gy) and concurrent chemotherapy in non-small-cell lung cancer. *Ann Thorac Surg* 2004;78(4):1200–1205; discussion 1206.

25. Vora SA, Daly BD, Blaszkowsky L, et al. High dose radiation therapy and chemotherapy as induction treatment for stage III non-small cell lung carcinoma. *Cancer* 2000;89(9):1946–1952.

26. METAGROUP. Meta-Analysis Group. Postoperative radiotherapy for non-small cell lung cancer: PORT Meta-Analysis Trialists Group. *Cochrane Database Syst Rev* 2000;(2):CD002142.

27. POST. Postoperative radiotherapy in non-small-cell lung cancer: systematic review and meta-analysis of individual patient data from nine randomised controlled trials. PORT Meta-analysis Trialists Group. *Lancet* 1998;352(9124):257–263.

28. Douillard JY, Rosell R, De Lena M, et al. Impact of postoperative radiation therapy on survival in patients with complete resection and stage I, II, or IIIA non-small-cell lung cancer treated with adjuvant chemotherapy: the Adjuvant Navelbine International Trialist Association (ANITA) Randomized Trial. *Int J Radiat Oncol Biol Phys* 2008;72(3):695–701.

29. Lally BE, Zelterman D, Colasanto JM, et al. Postoperative radiotherapy for stage II or III non-small-cell lung cancer using the surveillance, epidemiology, and end results database. *J Clin Oncol* 2006;24(19):2998–3006.

30. Sawyer TE, Bonner JA, Gould PM, et al. Effectiveness of postoperative irradiation in stage IIIA non-small cell lung cancer according to regression tree analyses of recurrence risks. *Ann Thorac Surg* 1997;64(5):1402–1407; discussion 1407–1408.

31. Arriagada R, Bergman B, Dunant A, et al. Cisplatin-based adjuvant chemotherapy in patients with completely resected non-small-cell lung cancer. *N Engl J Med* 2004;350(4):351–360.

32. CHEMO. Chemotherapy in non-small cell lung cancer: a meta-analysis using updated data on individual patients from 52 randomised clinical trials. Non-small Cell Lung Cancer Collaborative Group. *BMJ* 1995;311(7010):899–909.

33. Keller SM, Adak S, Wagner H, et al. A randomized trial of postoperative adjuvant therapy in patients with completely resected stage II or IIIA non-small-cell lung cancer. Eastern Cooperative Oncology Group. *N Engl J Med* 2000;343(17):1217–1222.

34. Timmerman RD, Herman J, Cho LC. Emergence of Stereotactic Body Radiation Therapy and Its Impact on Current and Future Clinical Practice . *J Clin Oncol.* 2014;32(26):2847-2854.

35. Sibley GS. Radiotherapy for patients with medically inoperable Stage I nonsmall cell lung carcinoma: smaller volumes and higher doses—a review. *Cancer* 1998;82(3):433–438.

36. Perez CA, Stanley K, Rubin P, et al. A prospective randomized study of various irradiation doses and fractionation schedules in the treatment of inoperable non-oat-cell carcinoma of the lung. Preliminary report by the Radiation Therapy Oncology Group. *Cancer* 1980;45(11):2744–2753.

37. Bradley J, Graham MV, Winter K, et al. Toxicity and outcome results of RTOG 9311: a phase I-II dose-escalation study using three-dimensional conformal radiotherapy in patients with inoperable non-small-cell lung carcinoma. *Int J Radiat Oncol Biol Phys* 2005;61(2):318–328.

38. Bradley JD, Paulus R, Komaki R, et al. Standard-dose versus high-dose conformal radiotherapy with concurrent and consolidation carboplatin plus paclitaxel with or without cetuximab for patients with IIIA or IIIB non-small-cell lung cancer (RTOG 0617): a randomized two-by-two factorial phase 3 study. *Lancet Oncol* 2015;16(2): 187-199.

39. Movsas B, Hu C, Sloan J, et al. Quality of life analysis of radiation dose escalation study of patients with non-small cell lung cancer: a secondary analysis of the Radiation Therapy Oncology Group 0617 randomized clinical trial. *JAMA Oncol* 2016;2(3):359–367

40. National Comprehensive Cancer Network. Non-small cell lung cancer (Version 4.2016). https://www.nccn.org/professionals/physician_gls/pdf/nscl.pdf. Accessed July 24, 2017.

41. Johnson DH. Locally advanced, unresectable non-small cell lung cancer: new treatment strategies. *Chest* 2000;117(4 suppl 1):123S–126S.

42. Dillman RO, Herndon J, Seagren SL, et al. Improved survival in stage III non-small-cell lung cancer: seven-year follow-up of cancer and leukemia group B (CALGB) 8433 trial. *J Natl Cancer Inst* 1996;88(17):1210–1215.

43. Sause WT, Scott C, Taylor S, et al. Radiation Therapy Oncology Group (RTOG) 88-08 and Eastern Cooperative Oncology Group (ECOG) 4588: preliminary results of a phase III trial in regionally advanced, unresectable non-small-cell lung cancer. *J Natl Cancer Inst* 1995;87(3): 198–205.

44. Schaake-Koning C, van den Bogaert W, Dalesio O, et al. Effects of concomitant cisplatin and radiotherapy on inoperable non-small-cell lung cancer. *N Engl J Med* 1992;326(8):524–530.

45. Curran WJ Jr, Paulus R, Langer CJ, et al. Sequential vs. concurrent chemoradiation for stage III non-small cell lung cancer: randomized phase III trial RTOG 9410. *J Natl Cancer Inst* 2011;103(19):1452–1460.

46. Furuse K, Fukuoka M, Kawahara M, et al. Phase III study of concurrent versus sequential thoracic radiotherapy in combination with mitomycin, vindesine, and cisplatin in unresectable stage III non-small-cell lung cancer. *J Clin Oncol* 1999;17(9):2692–2699.

47. Antonia SJ, Villegas A, Daniel D, et al. Durvalumab after chemoradiotherapy in stage III non-small-cell lung cancer. *N Engl J Med* 2017;377(20):1919–1929.

48. Hematology/Oncology (Cancer) Approvals & Safety Notifications. https://www.fda.gov/Drugs/InformationOnDrugs/ApprovedDrugs/ucm279174. Accessed July 21, 2017.

49. Ezhil M, Vedam S, Balter P, et al. Determination of patient-specific internal gross tumor volumes for lung cancer using four-dimensional computed tomography. *Radiat Oncol* 2009;4:4.

50. Necitumumab full prescribing information. https://www.asseccdata.fda.gov/drugsatfda_docs/label/2015/125547s000lbl.pdf. Accessed July 21, 2017.

51. Rancoule C, Vallard A, Guy JB, Espenel S, Diao P, Chargari C, Magne N. Brain metastases from non-small cell lung carcinoma: changing concepts for improving patients' outcome. *Crit Rev Oncol Hematol* 2017;116: 32–37.

52. Shonka N, Venur VA, Ahluwalia MS. Targeted Treatment of Brain Metastases. *Curr Neurol Neurosci Rep* 2017;17(4): 37.

53. Goodman G, Livingston R. Small cell lung cancer. *Curr Probl Cancer* 1989;13:7–55.
54. Pignon JP, Arriagada R, Ihde DC, et al. A meta-analysis of thoracic radiotherapy for small-cell lung cancer. *N Engl J Med* 1992;327(23):1618–1624.
55. Graham BL Jr, Balducci L, Khansur T, et al. Surgery in small cell lung cancer. *Ann Thorac Surg* 1988;45(6):687–692.
56. Roof KS, Fidias P, Lynch TJ, et al. Radiation dose escalation in limited-stage small-cell lung cancer. *Int J Radiat Oncol Biol Phys* 2003;57(3):701–708.
57. Turrisi AT III, Kim K, Blum R, et al. Twice-daily compared with once-daily thoracic radiotherapy in limited small-cell lung cancer treated concurrently with cisplatin and etoposide. *N Engl J Med* 1999;340(4):265–271.
58. Choi NC, Herndon JE II, Rosenman J, et al. Phase I study to determine the maximum-tolerated dose of radiation in standard daily and hyperfractionated-accelerated twice-daily radiation schedules with concurrent chemotherapy for limited-stage small-cell lung cancer. *J Clin Oncol* 1998;16(11):3528–3536.
59. Bogart JA, Herndon JE II, Lyss AP, et al. 70 Gy thoracic radiotherapy is feasible concurrent with chemotherapy for limited-stage small-cell lung cancer: analysis of Cancer and Leukemia Group B study 39808. *Int J Radiat Oncol Biol Phys* 2004;59(2):460–468.
60. Komaki R, Paulus R, Ettinger DS, et al. Phase II study of accelerated high-dose radiotherapy with concurrent chemotherapy for patients with limited stage small-cell lung cancer: Radiation Therapy Oncology Group protocol 0239. *Int J Radiat Oncol Biol Phys* 2012;83(4):e531–e536.
61. Wright CD, Choi NC, Wain JC, et al. Induction chemoradiotherapy followed by resection for locally advanced Masaoka stage III and IVA thymic tumors. *Ann Thorac Surg* 2008;85(2):385–389.
62. Verma V, Simone CB 2nd, Allen PK, Lin SH. Outcomes of Stereotactic Body Radiotherapy for T1-T2N0 Small Cell Carcinoma According to Addition of Chemotherapy and Prophylactic Cranial Irradiation: A Multicenter Analysis. Clin Lung Cancer 2017; epub ahead of print.
63. Fried DB, Morris DE, Poole C, et al. Systematic review evaluating the timing of thoracic radiation therapy in combined modality therapy for limited-stage small-cell lung cancer. *J Clin Oncol* 2004;22(23):4837–4845.
64. De Ruysscher D, Pijls-Johannesma M, Bentzen SM, et al. Time between the first day of chemotherapy and the last day of chest radiation is the most important predictor of survival in limited-disease small-cell lung cancer. *J Clin Oncol* 2006;24(7):1057–1063.
65. Slotman BJ, van Tinteren H, Praag JO, et al. Use of thoracic radiotherapy for extensive stage small-cell lung cancer: a phase 3 randomized controlled trial. *Lancet* 2015;385(9962): 36-42.
66. Auperin A, Arriagada R, Pignon JP, et al. Prophylactic cranial irradiation for patients with small-cell lung cancer in complete remission. Prophylactic Cranial Irradiation Overview Collaborative Group. *N Engl J Med* 1999;341(7):476–484.
67. Slotman B, Faivre-Finn C, Kramer G, et al. Prophylactic cranial irradiation in extensive small-cell lung cancer. *N Engl J Med* 2007;357(7):664–672.
68. Takahashi T, Yamanaka T, Seto T, et al. Prophylactic cranial irradiation versus observation in patients with extensive-disease small-cell lung cancer: a multicenter, randomized, open-label, phase 3. *Lancet Oncol* 2017;18(5): 663-671.
69. Le Pechoux C, Dunant A, Senan S, et al. Standard-dose versus higher-dose prophylactic cranial irradiation (PCI) in patients with limited-stage small-cell lung cancer in complete remission after chemotherapy and thoracic radiotherapy (PCI 99-01, EORTC 22003-08004, RTOG 0212, and IFCT 99-01): a randomised clinical trial. *Lancet Oncol* 2009;10(5):467–474.
70. Senan S, van Sornsen de Koste J, Samson M, et al. Evaluation of a target contouring protocol for 3D conformal radiotherapy in non-small cell lung cancer. *Radiother Oncol* 1999;53(3): 247–255.

71. Giraud P, Antoine M, Larrouy A, et al. Evaluation of microscopic tumor extension in non-small-cell lung cancer for three-dimensional conformal radiotherapy planning. *Int J Radiat Oncol Biol Phys* 2000;48(4):1015–1024.

72. Rosenzweig KE, Sura S, Jackson A, et al. Involved-field radiation therapy for inoperable non small-cell lung cancer. *J Clin Oncol* 2007;25(35):5557–5561.

73. Armstrong J, McGibney C. The impact of three-dimensional radiation on the treatment of non-small cell lung cancer. *Radiother Oncol* 2000;56(2):157–167.

74. Graham MV, Purdy JA, Emami B, et al. 3-D conformal radiotherapy for lung cancer: the Washington University experience. In: Meyer JA, Purdy JA, eds. *Frontiers of radiation therapy and oncology: 3-D conformal radiotherapy.* Basel, Switzerland: Karger, 1996:188–198.

75. Mah D, Hanley J, Rosenzweig KE, et al. Technical aspects of the deep inspiration breath-hold technique in the treatment of thoracic cancer. *Int J Radiat Oncol Biol Phys* 2000;48(4):1175–1185.

76. Shirato H, Shimizu S, Kunieda T, et al. Physical aspects of a real-time tumor-tracking system for gated radiotherapy. *Int J Radiat Oncol Biol Phys* 2000;48(4):1187–1195.

77. Graham MV, Purdy JA, Emami B, et al. Clinical dose-volume histogram analysis for pneumonitis after 3D treatment for non-small cell lung cancer (NSCLC). *Int J Radiat Oncol Biol Phys* 1999;45(2):323–329.

78. Kong FM, Ten Haken RK, Schipper MJ, et al. High-dose radiation improved local tumor control and overall survival in patients with inoperable/unresectable non-small-cell lung cancer: long-term results of a radiation dose escalation study. *Int J Radiat Oncol Biol Phys* 2005;63(2):324–333.

79. Park S, Urm S, Cho H. Analysis of biologically equivalent dose of stereotactic body radiotherapy for primary and metastatic lung tumors. *Cancer Res Treat* 2014;46(4):403–410.

80. Marsiglia H, Baldeyrou P, Lartigau E, et al. High-dose-rate brachytherapy as sole modality for early-stage endobronchial carcinoma. *Int J Radiat Oncol Biol Phys* 2000;47(3):665–672.

81. Muto P, Ravo V, Panelli G, et al. High-dose rate brachytherapy of bronchial cancer: treatment optimization using three schemes of therapy. *Oncologist* 2000;5(3):209–214.

82. Timmerman RD, McGarry R, Yiannoutsos C, et al. Excessive toxicity when treating central tumors in a phase II study of stereotactic body radiation therapy for medically inoperable early-stage lung cancer. *J Clin Oncol* 2006;24(30):4833–4839.

83. Speiser BL. Brachytherapy in the treatment of thoracic tumors. Lung and esophageal. *Hematol Oncol Clin North Am* 1999;13(3):609–634.

84. Rusch VW, Giroux DJ, Kraut MJ, et al. Induction chemoradiation and surgical resection for superior sulcus non-small-cell lung carcinomas: long-term results of Southwest Oncology Group Trial 9416 (Intergroup Trial 0160). *J Clin Oncol* 2007;25(3):313–318.

85. Perez CA, Azarnia N, Cox JD, et al. Sequelae of definitive irradiation in the treatment of carcinoma of the lung. In: Motta G, ed. *Lung cancer: advanced concepts and present status.* Genoa, Italy: G. Motta Publishing, 1989.

86. Chun SG, Hu C, Choy H, Komaki RU, et al. Impact of intensity-modulated radiation therapy technique for locally advanced non-small-cell lung cancer: a secondary analysis of the NRG Oncology RTOG 0617 Randomized Clinical Trial. *J Clin Oncol* 2017;35(1):56–62.

87. Palma DA, Senan S, Tsujino K, et al. Predicting radiation pneumonitis after chemoradiation therapy for lung cancer: an international individual patient data meta-analysis. *Int J Radiat Oncol Biol Phys* 2013;85(2): 444–450.

88. Graham MV. Carcinoma of the lung and esophagus. In: Levitt SH, Khan FM, Potish RA, et al., eds. *Levitt and Tapley's technological basis of radiation therapy: practical clinical applications,* 3rd ed. Philadelphia, PA: Lippincott Williams & Wilkins, 1999:315–333.

89. Gaspar LE, Winter K, Kocha WI, et al. A phase I/II study of external beam radiation, brachytherapy, and concurrent chemotherapy for patients with localized carcinoma of the esophagus (Radiation Therapy Oncology Group Study 9207): final report. *Cancer* 2000;88(5):988–995.

90. Graham MV, Emami B. Mediastinum and trachea. In: Perez CA, Brady LW, eds. *Principles and practice of radiation oncology*, 3rd ed. Philadelphia, PA: Lippincott–Raven, 1998:1221–1239.

91. Kersh CR, Eisert DR, Hazra TA. Malignant thymoma: role of radiation therapy in management. *Radiology* 1985;156(1):207–209.

92. Masaoka A, Monden Y, Nakahara K, et al. Follow-up study of thymomas with special reference to their clinical stages. *Cancer* 1981;48(11):2485–2492.

93. Rosai J, Levine G. *Tumors of the thymus. Atlas of tumor pathology, second series, fascicle 13.* Washington, DC: Armed Forces Institute of Pathology, 1977.

94. Marino M, Muller-Hermelink HK. Thymoma and thymic carcinoma. Relation of thymoma epithelial cells to the cortical and medullary differentiation of thymus. *Virchows Arch A Pathol Anat Histopathol* 1985;407(2):119–149.

95. Pollack A, Komaki R, Cox JD, et al. Thymoma: treatment and prognosis. *Int J Radiat Oncol Biol Phys* 1992;23(5):1037–1043.

96. Ohara K, Okumura T, Sugahara S, et al. The role of preoperative radiotherapy for invasive thymoma. *Acta Oncol* 1990;29(4):425–429.

97. Urgesi A, Monetti U, Rossi G, et al. Role of radiation therapy in locally advanced thymoma. *Radiother Oncol* 1990;19(3):273–280.

98. Nakahara K, Ohno K, Hashimoto J, et al. Thymoma: results with complete resection and adjuvant postoperative irradiation in 141 consecutive patients. *J Thorac Cardiovasc Surg* 1988;95(6):1041–1047.

99. Curran WJ Jr, Kornstein MJ, Brooks JJ, et al. Invasive thymoma: the role of mediastinal irradiation following complete or incomplete surgical resection. *J Clin Oncol* 1988;6(11):1722–1727.

100. FDA approval for Erlotinib Hydrochloride. https://www.cancer.gov/about-cancer/treatment/drugs/fda-erlotinib-hydrocholide#Ancor-First-6524. Accessed July 21, 2017.

101. Maggi G, Giaccone G, Donadio M, et al. Thymomas. A review of 169 cases, with particular reference to results of surgical treatment. *Cancer* 1986;58(3):765–776.

102. Yuan ZY, Gao SG, Mu JW, et al. Long-term outcomes of 307 patients after complete thymoma resection. *Chin J Cancer* 2017;36(1):46.

103. Krueger JB, Sagerman RH, King GA. Stage III thymoma: results of postoperative radiation therapy. *Radiology* 1988;168(3):855–858.

104. Mornex F, Resbeut M, Richaud P, et al. Radiotherapy and chemotherapy for invasive thymomas: a multicentric retrospective review of 90 cases. The FNCLCC trialists. Federation Nationale des Centres de Lutte Contre le Cancer. *Int J Radiat Oncol Biol Phys* 1995;32(3):651–659.

105. Park HS, Shin DM, Lee JS, et al. Thymoma. A retrospective study of 87 cases. *Cancer* 1994;73(10):2491–2498.

106. Korst RJ, Kansler AL, Christos PJ, et al. Adjuvant radiotherapy for thymic epithelial tumors: a systematic review and meta-analysis. *Ann Thorac Surg* 2009;87(5):1641–1647.

107. Rena O, Papalia E, Oliaro A, et al. Does adjuvant radiation therapy improve disease-free survival in completely resected Masaoka stage II thymoma? *Eur J Cardiothorac Surg* 2007;31(1):109–113.

108. Kim ES, Putnam JB, Komaki R, et al. Phase II study of a multidisciplinary approach with induction chemotherapy, followed by surgical resection, radiation therapy, and consolidation chemotherapy for unresectable malignant thymomas: final report. *Lung Cancer* 2004;44(3):369–379.

109. Macchiarini P, Chella A, Ducci F, et al. Neoadjuvant chemotherapy, surgery, and postoperative radiation therapy for invasive thymoma. *Cancer* 1991;68(4):706–713.

110. Bagshaw MA, McLaughlin WT, Earle JD. Definitive radiotherapy of primary mediastinal seminoma. *Am J Roentgenol Radium Ther Nucl Med* 1969;105(1):86–94.

111. Bush SE, Martinez A, Bagshaw MA. Primary mediastinal seminoma. *Cancer* 1981;48(8): 1877–1882.

112. Lemarie E, Assouline PS, Diot P, et al. Primary mediastinal germ cell tumors. Results of a French retrospective study. *Chest* 1992;102(5):1477–1483.

113. Azar T, Abdul-Karim FW, Tucker HM. Adenoid cystic carcinoma of the trachea. *Laryngoscope* 1998;108(9):1297–1300.

114. Bittner N, Koh WJ, Laramore GE, et al. Treatment of locally advanced adenoid cystic carcinoma of the trachea with neutron radiotherapy. *Int J Radiat Oncol Biol Phys* 2008;72(2):410–414.

115. FDA approval for Bevacizumab. https://www.cancer.gov/about-cancer/treatment/drugs/fda-bevacizumab#Ancor-NSCLC. Accessed July 21, 2017.

116. Farrell MA, McAdams HP, Herndon JE, et al. Non-small cell lung cancer: FDG PET for nodal staging in patients with stage I disease. *Radiology* 2000;215(3):886–890.

117. Grillo HC, Mathisen DJ. Primary tracheal tumors: treatment and results. *Ann Thorac Surg* 1990;49(1):69–77.

118. Cheung AY. Radiotherapy for primary carcinoma of the trachea. *Radiother Oncol* 1989;14(4):279–285.

119. Chow DC, Komaki R, Libshitz HI, et al. Treatment of primary neoplasms of the trachea. The role of radiation therapy. *Cancer* 1993;71(10):2946–2952.

120. Harms W, Latz D, Becker H, et al. Treatment of primary tracheal carcinoma. The role of external and endoluminal radiotherapy. *Strahlenther Onkol* 2000;176(1):22–27.

121. Maziak DE, Todd TR, Keshavjee SH, et al. Adenoid cystic carcinoma of the airway: thirty-two-year experience. *J Thorac Cardiovasc Surg* 1996;112(6):1522–1531; discussion 1531–1522.

122. Chao MW, Smith JG, Laidlaw C, et al. Results of treating primary tumors of the trachea with radiotherapy. *Int J Radiat Oncol Biol Phys* 1998;41(4):779–785.

123. Green N, Kulber H, Landman M, et al. The experience with definitive irradiation of clinically limited squamous cell cancer of the trachea. *Int J Radiat Oncol Biol Phys* 1985;11(7):1401–1405.

124. Schraube P, Latz D, Wannenmacher M. Treatment of primary squamous cell carcinoma of the trachea: the role of radiation therapy. *Radiother Oncol* 1994;33(3):254–258.

125. Thotathil ZS, Agarwal JP, Shrivastava SK, et al. Primary malignant tumors of the trachea - the Tata Memorial Hospital experience. *Med Princ Pract* 2004;13(2):69–73.

126. Saroja KR, Mansell J. Treatment of tracheal tumors with high energy fast neutron radiation. *Oncology (Williston Park)* 1993;7(1):16, 21–22.

127. Marks LB, Bentzen SM, Deasy JO, et al. Radiation dose-volume effects in the lung. *Int J Radiat Oncol Biol Phys* 2010;76(3 suppl):S70–S76.

128. Yorke ED, Jackson A, Rosenzweig KE, et al. Correlation of dosimetric factors and RP for non-small-cell lung cancer patients in a recently completed dose escalation study. *Int J Radiat Oncol Biol Phys* 2005;63(3):672–682.

CHAPTER 20

ESOPHAGUS

ANATOMY

- The esophagus is a thin-walled, hollow tube with an average length of 25 cm.
- The normal esophagus is lined with stratified squamous epithelium.
- There are many methods of subdividing the esophagus. The American Joint Committee on Cancer divides the esophagus into four regions: cervical, upper thoracic, midthoracic, and lower thoracic.
- The cervical esophagus begins at the cricopharyngeal muscle (C7) and extends to the thoracic inlet (T3). The thoracic esophagus represents the remainder of the organ, going from T3 to T10 or T11, ending at the gastroesophageal junction. Figure 20-1 correlates the basic anatomy of the esophagus with the subdivision schemes described above.
- The esophagus has a dual longitudinal interconnecting system of lymphatics. As a result, lymph fluid can travel the entire length of the esophagus before draining into the lymph nodes, so that the entire esophagus is at risk for lymphatic metastatic spread.
- In "skip areas," up to 8 cm of normal tissue can exist between gross tumor and micrometastasis in the esophagus (1).
- Lymphatics of the esophagus drain into nodes that usually follow arteries, including the inferior thyroid artery, the bronchial and esophageal arteries from the aorta, and the left gastric artery (celiac axis) (2). Figure 20-2 illustrates the major lymph node groups draining the esophagus.

NATURAL HISTORY

- The estimated incidence of squamous cell cancer in each third of the esophagus is as follows: upper third, 10% to 25%; middle third, 40% to 50%; and lower third, 25% to 50% (3,4).

- Achalasia of long duration (≥25 years) is associated with a 5% incidence of squamous cell carcinoma of the esophagus (5). Caustic burns, especially lye corrosion, are related to the development of esophageal cancer (6,7).
- Adenocarcinoma has now surpassed squamous cell carcinoma as the most common histology (8). The incidence of adenocarcinoma has increased 350% since 1970 and now accounts for 75% of all esophageal cancers in Caucasian males.
- The condition most commonly associated with adenocarcinoma of the esophagus is Barrett's esophagus. Dietary and lifestyle habits likely also contribute to the increasing incidence of adenocarcinoma.

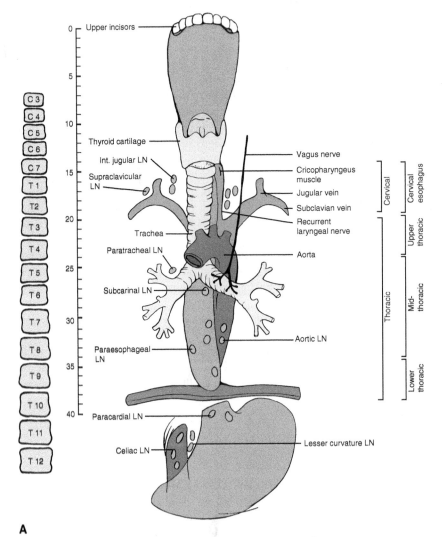

A

FIGURE 20-1. **A:** Basic anatomy of the esophagus. Note the lengths of the various segments of the esophagus from the upper central incisors and the two classification schemes for subdividing the esophagus. LN, lymph node.

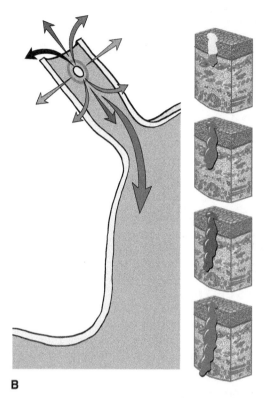

B

FIGURE 20-1. (*continued*) **B:** Esophagus tissue cross section with various T1-4 stage tumors shown. T1 is at top; T4 is at bottom. (Reprinted with permission from Rubin P, Hansen JT. *TNM staging atlas.* Philadelphia, PA: Lippincott Williams & Wilkins, 2008:179. © Wolters Kluwer.)

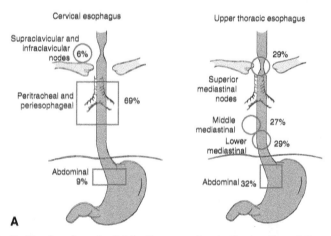

A

FIGURE 20-2. Positive lymph node distribution according to the location of the primary tumor. (Adapted from Akiyama H, Tsurumaru M, Kawamura T, et al. Principles of surgical treatment for carcinoma of the esophagus: analysis of lymph node involvement. *Ann Surg* 1981;194:438; Dormans E. Das Oesophaguscarcinom. Ergebnisse der unter Mitarbeit von 39 pathologischen instituten Deutschlands durchgeführten Erhebung über das Oesophaguscarcinom (1925–1933). *Z Krebforsch* 1939;49:86.)

continued

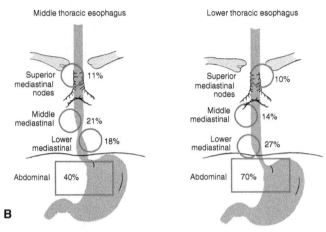

FIGURE 20-2. (*continued*)

CLINICAL PRESENTATION

- Symptoms of esophageal cancer usually start 3 to 4 months before diagnosis.
- Dysphagia and weight loss are seen in over 90% of patients.
- Odynophagia (pain on swallowing) is present in up to 50% of patients.

DIAGNOSTIC WORKUP

- All patients with suspected esophageal cancer should have a workup similar to that outlined in Figure 20-3.
- Computed tomography (CT) (9) has an accuracy of 51% to 70% (based on a threshold for malignancy of 10 mm) in the detection of mediastinal nodes in patients with esophageal cancer and 79% (based on a threshold of 8 mm) in the detection of left-sided gastric or celiac nodes (10). Understaging of disease with CT occurs more frequently than overstaging.
- Endoscopic ultrasound is superior for T staging (sensitivity, 81%; specificity, 67%) and for N staging (sensitivity, 63%; specificity, 88%) (9).
- Fluorodeoxyglucose positron emission tomography (FDG-PET) imaging is superior to CT imaging for evaluating distant metastases (sensitivity, 74%; specificity, 90%) (9). PET-CT imaging also can be helpful for staging and radiation treatment planning.

STAGING SYSTEMS

- A number of staging systems have been proposed.

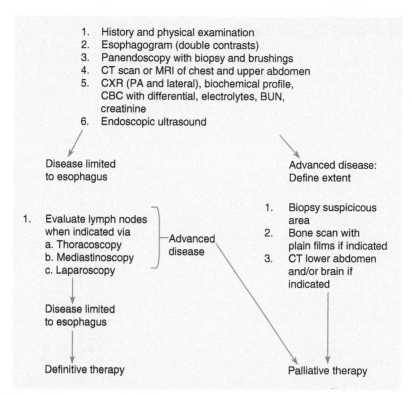

1. History and physical examination
2. Esophagogram (double contrasts)
3. Panendoscopy with biopsy and brushings
4. CT scan or MRI of chest and upper abdomen
5. CXR (PA and lateral), biochemical profile, CBC with differential, electrolytes, BUN, creatinine
6. Endoscopic ultrasound

Disease limited to esophagus

Advanced disease: Define extent

1. Evaluate lymph nodes when indicated via
   a. Thoracoscopy
   b. Mediastinoscopy
   c. Laparoscopy

Advanced disease

1. Biopsy suspicicous area
2. Bone scan with plain films if indicated
3. CT lower abdomen and/or brain if indicated

Disease limited to esophagus

Definitive therapy

Palliative therapy

FIGURE 20-3. Diagnostic workup for patients with esophageal cancer. CBC, complete blood count; CT, computed tomography; CXR, chest X-ray; MRI, magnetic resonance imaging; PA, posterior-anterior.

NEW! SUMMARY OF CHANGES TO AJCC STAGING

ESOPHAGUS AND ESOPHAGOGASTRIC JUNCTION

- T1 subcategorized (11).
- T4a includes invasion of peritoneum.
- G4 eliminated.
- cTNM not shared with pTNM. Separate stage grouping for adenocarcinoma and squamous cell carcinoma.
- Location of cancer based on epicenter, previously upper edge of cancer.
- Tumors with epicenters greater than 2 cm distal to the esophagogastric junction are staged as gastric cancers even if esophagus is involved.
- Stage IV subgrouped into IVA and IVB.

See: Amin MB, Edge SB, Greene F, et al., eds. *AJCC cancer staging manual*, 8th ed. New York, NY: Springer International, 2017.

PROGNOSTIC FACTORS

- Esophageal cancer usually manifests as advanced-stage disease. According to Pearson (13), most tumors are not localized to the esophagus, and the majority have locally extensive or distant disease at the time of diagnosis. Seventy-five percent of patients have lymph node involvement at initial presentation.
- Approximately 18% of patients will have distant metastases, typically to abdominal lymph nodes (45% of cases), liver (35%), lung (20%), supraclavicular nodes (18%), bone (9%), or adrenal glands (5%).
- Upper one-third lesions do better than the lower one third.
- Tumors 5 cm or smaller are 40% resectable, whereas tumors larger than 5 cm have a 75% chance of distant metastasis (3).
- Patients who are male, are older than 65 years of age, and have poor performance status and excessive weight loss have the worst prognosis.
- Although survival rates are improving, prognosis remains poor, with a 5-year survival rate of 22% (14).

GENERAL MANAGEMENT

- Carcinoma of the esophagus remains a difficult disease to treat and often requires multimodality management in the nonmetastatic setting.
- With single-modality therapy, locoregional failure occurs in approximately 20% to 80% of patients.
- With chemoradiation alone, locoregional failure ranges from 35% to 45%.
- With preoperative chemoirradiation followed by surgery, according to recent clinical trials, locoregional failure occurs in less than 10% of patients.
- The rate of distant metastasis is high with any therapeutic approach and exceeds 50% with long-term follow-up. Distal recurrence remains the most common site of recurrence after multimodality treatment.
- In patients who are medically and surgically fit, either chemoradiation alone or preoperative concurrent chemoradiation (41.4 to 50.4 Gy) followed by surgery should be considered a standard of care treatment.
- Many patients are not able to tolerate adjuvant therapy after surgical resection; therefore, neoadjuvant chemoradiation followed by surgical resection may be the best tolerated sequence.
- For stage IV patients, palliation with single- or multiple-modality therapy, tailored to a patient's specific symptoms, should be used.

Single-Modality Therapy

Surgery

- Surgery (endoscopic resection or esophagectomy) is the standard approach for early-stage lesions, but curative resection is feasible in only 50% of patients at the time of surgery because of more extensive disease than clinically judged.

- Surgical mortality is now less than 10% in experienced centers.
- Median survival of patients with resectable tumors treated with surgery alone is 21 to 24 months in recent randomized trials (15,16).
- Esophagogastrostomy is the most widely used surgical approach. Common approaches are transthoracic resection or transhiatal resection. Colon interposition, preferably with the left colon, can also be used (17).
- Squamous cell carcinoma of the cervical esophagus presents a very difficult situation. If surgery is performed, it usually requires removal of portions of the pharynx, the entire larynx and thyroid gland, and the proximal esophagus. Radical neck dissection may also be performed (18).
- Postoperative chemoradiation should be used for patients with early-stage esophageal cancer with positive margins or positive nodes at the time of surgery.

Radiation Therapy

- Radiotherapy is mainly used for palliation or for medically inoperable patients.
- Overall survival after irradiation alone is approximately 18% at 1 year and 6% at 5 years. A general assessment of radiation as the sole treatment indicates median survival of 6 to 12 months with survival at 5 years less than 10% (19).
- Two prospective, randomized trials were launched to compare radiation therapy with surgery in early-stage lesions, but they were aborted because of poor accrual.
- Intracavitary brachytherapy for local control or durable palliation of dysphagia can be used but does not improve survival (20,21).

Chemotherapy

- Chemotherapy is not effective as a single modality.
- Cisplatin (cis-diamminedichloroplatinum, CDDP)-based combination chemotherapy can achieve response rates of 30% to 50%, but there are rarely complete responses.

Multimodality Therapy

Radiation Therapy and Surgery

- A European Organization for Research and Treatment of Cancer trial involving 192 patients receiving either 33 Gy in 10 fractions preoperatively or immediate surgery demonstrated no survival benefit to radiation therapy (10% versus 9% 5-year overall survival), but a longer median time to recurrence was noted in the irradiation group (22).
- Postoperative radiation therapy after curative therapy, regardless of surgical margins, has shown a slight reduction of local relapse (85% down to 70% at 5 years), especially in node-negative patients; however, no survival benefit has been observed (23).

Chemotherapy and Surgery

- The US Intergroup 113/RTOG 8911 study randomized 467 patients (57% adenocarcinoma) to surgery alone versus 5-fluorouracil (5-FU)/CDDP followed by surgery. No improvement was seen in R0 resection rate, disease-free survival, or overall survival. Long-term follow-up shows that R0 resection is the only determinant of substantial long-term survival (24). The Medical Research Council Trial (European Intergroup) randomized 802 patients (66% adenocarcinoma) to 5-FU/CDDP followed by surgery versus surgery alone. This study demonstrated a 6% increase in R0 resection rate in the preoperative chemotherapy arm, as well as a 9% increase in 2-year survival (25).

- Perioperative chemotherapy has been used with success in tumors of the gastroesophageal junction (26).
- Postoperative chemotherapy has not been investigated adequately.

Definitive Chemoradiation

- The combination of chemotherapy and irradiation suggests a benefit for both local control and overall survival duration that is superior to radiation alone in inoperable disease.
- In an Eastern Cooperative Oncology Group study, 119 patients were randomized to receive radiation therapy of 60 Gy with or without 5-FU/mitomycin-C (27). The 2-year survival rate was 27% versus 12% in favor of combined modality therapy; median survival was 14.8 months versus 9.2 months, respectively.
- In the Radiation Therapy Oncology Group study 85-01, 129 patients were randomized to receive 50 Gy and 5-FU/CDDP versus 64 Gy alone (28). The 5-year survival rate was 26% versus 0%; median survival was 14.1 months versus 9.3 months, respectively.
- In Intergroup 0123/RTOG 9405, 239 patients were randomized to receive combined modality therapy of concurrent high-dose radiation of 64.8 Gy and 5-FU/CDDP versus standard dose 50.4 Gy and concurrent 5-FU/CDDP. No significant difference in median survival (13.0 months versus 18.1 months), 2-year survival (31% versus 40%), or locoregional failure and locoregional persistence of disease was seen between the high-dose arm and the standard-dose arm. Higher radiation did not increase survival or locoregional control (29). As there were unexpected early deaths on the dose-escalated arm, interpretation of this study remains unclear.

Postoperative Chemoradiation

- In Intergroup 0116, 556 patients with resected adenocarcinoma of the stomach or gastroesophageal junction were randomized to receive surgery plus postoperative chemoradiotherapy of 5-FU/leucovorin with radiation of 45 Gy versus surgery alone. Approximately 20% of patients had GEJ cancer. There was a significant improvement in median survival (36 months versus 27 months) with 3-year survival of 50% versus 41% in the chemoradiotherapy group compared to surgery alone (30).

Preoperative Chemoradiation

- In the important, practice-changing CROSS trial, 366 patients with resectable esophageal or esophagogastric junction cancer were randomized to receive surgery alone or carboplatin and paclitaxel concurrent with radiation of 41.4 Gy in 23 fractions followed by surgery. Median overall survival was significantly improved in the chemoradiotherapy group compared to the surgery alone group (49.4 months versus

24.0 months) (16). There was a 29% pathologic complete response rate in chemo-radiation and surgery arm. The CROSS study has established multimodality management (neoadjuvant chemoradiation followed by surgery) as a standard of care treatment option in localized esophageal cancer.

- Similar to the CROSS trial, the CALGB 9781 study randomized fifty-six patients to concurrent cisplatin/5-FU and radiation of 50.4 Gy followed by esophagectomy versus esophagectomy alone (15). The trial was closed because of poor accrual but demonstrated a significant increase in median survival for the preoperative chemoradiation arm versus surgery alone (4.48 years versus 1.79 years).
- In the French FFCD 9102 trial, 259 patients with operable thoracic esophageal cancer were treated with 5-FU/cisplatin and concurrent conventional or split-course radiotherapy (46 Gy in 4.5 weeks or 15 Gy, days 1 to 5 and 22 to 26). Patients were then randomized to surgery or continuation of chemoradiation to 20 or 15 Gy. There was no difference in 2-year survival rate (34% versus 40%) (31).
- The POET trial randomized 119 patients with locally advanced GE junction adenocarcinoma to chemotherapy followed by surgery or induction chemotherapy and chemoradiotherapy followed by surgery. There was a significant 5-year local progression-free survival benefit and a trend to 5-year survival benefit (39.5% versus 24.4%) in the chemoradiotherapy arm. Although the trial did not meet its accrual target, it suggests that neoadjuvant chemoradiation is superior to neoadjuvant chemotherapy as a treatment strategy (32).

Palliative Treatment

- The best surgical palliation involves resection and reconstruction, if possible. This removes the bulk of the disease and can potentially prevent abscess and fistula formation, as well as bleeding.
- Intraluminal intubation is good for extremely debilitated patients with tracheoesophageal fistula or invasion of vital structures.
- Dilation is another reasonable alternative. When the lumen of the esophagus is dilated to 15 mm, dysphagia is no longer experienced. Attempts should be made to get 17 mm of dilation and to maintain this with weekly or monthly dilations thereafter (18).
- Both neodymium:yttrium-aluminum-garnet (Nd:YAG) laser and photoirradiation with an argon laser, together with presensitization of tumor with intravenous hematoporphyrin derivative, have provided palliation with minimal risk (33).
- Palliative treatment regimens range from 30 Gy over 2 weeks (4) to 50 Gy over 5 weeks or up to 60 Gy over 6 weeks, with up to 80% relief of pain and dysphagia (17).

RADIATION THERAPY TECHNIQUES

- Consider 4D simulation and fiducial marker placement for motion management and more precise targeting of the radiotherapy fields.

- A field margin of 4 to 5 cm, above and below the tumor, is generally recommended, in addition to 1 to 2 cm radially around the tumor (34). This is because of the nodal drainage pattern—mucosal lymphatics drain to muscularis propria lymphatics in a largely longitudinal pattern.
- Lesions in the upper cervical or postcricoid esophagus are usually treated from the laryngopharynx to the carina.
- Supraclavicular nodes are irradiated electively for cervical and upper thoracic tumors. Mediastinal lymph nodes may be included in the CTV of proximal tumors. This can be achieved with 3D conformal fields or intensity-modulated radiation therapy (IMRT).
- For tumors in the distal third and large lesions (5 cm) in the middle or upper third of the thoracic esophagus, the clinical target volume includes the celiac axis lymph nodes because of their frequent metastatic involvement (19,35).
- Other radiographically positive nodes should be included with margin.
- A recent single institution retrospective study demonstrated improved survival outcomes and decreased toxicity using IMRT compared to historical reports using 3D conformal methods (36).
- Figure 20-4 illustrates several different dose distributions using CT-based dosimetry.

Radiation Dose

- Based on data from squamous cell carcinoma of the upper aerodigestive tract, 50.4 Gy at 1.8 Gy per fraction over 5 weeks should control more than 90% of subclinical disease.
- If treating according to the CROSS study, the clinical target volume, including radiographically suspicious nodes, should be treated to 41.4 Gy in 23 fractions with concurrent carboplatin/taxol.
- In addition to external beam therapy, intracavitary therapy can be used as part of a radical or palliative treatment plan.
- Selection of a high dose rate, intermediate dose rate, or low dose rate technique is operator dependent. These techniques are roughly defined as more than 12 Gy per hour, 2 to 12 Gy per hour, and 0.4 to 2.0 Gy per hour, respectively. High dose rate treatment can be given quickly but may require two or three placements; low dose rate takes 1 to 2 days with only one placement. Local control with any technique ranges from 40% to 95%, with a 4% to 20% risk of stricture and 2% to 10% risk of fistula formation (5).

NORMAL TISSUE COMPLICATIONS: QUANTEC RESULTS

Werner-Wasik et al. (37) presented recommendations for radiation dosage, based on a review of reported side effects in patients treated for thoracic tumors.

- At present, it is not possible to identify a single best threshold volumetric parameter for esophageal irradiation, because a wide range of V_{dose} parameters correlate significantly with severe acute esophagitis. In particular, the studies we analyzed illustrate a clear trend demonstrating that volumes receiving greater than 40 to 50 Gy correlated significantly with acute esophagitis.

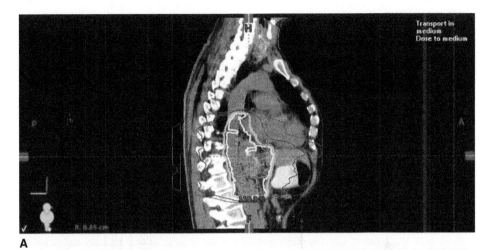

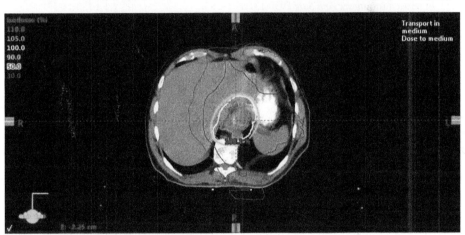

FIGURE 20-4. Dose distributions for a midesophageal cancer IMRT plan.

SEQUELAE OF TREATMENT

Surgery

- Operative mortality is generally less than 10% (38).
- The overall complication rate can exceed 75%, including pulmonary and cardiac complications, anastomotic leak (5% to 10%), and recurrent laryngeal nerve paralysis (5% to 10%).
- Stricture formation occurs in 14% to 27% of cases (19).
- The addition of preoperative radiation therapy and chemotherapy can significantly increase complications.
- Perioperative mortality of 17% has been reported (39).

Radiation Therapy

- The acute complications of radiation therapy include esophagitis, modest skin tanning, fatigue, and, in most patients, weight loss.
- Pneumonitis is a potentially serious complication, although it rarely occurs.
- A perforated esophagus is characterized by substernal chest pain, a high pulse rate, fever, and hemorrhage. If it is confirmed with an esophagogram, treatment should be stopped (3).
- The most common chronic complication from radiation therapy is stenosis and stricture formation. When this occurs, recurrence should be ruled out. Stenosis can occur in more than 60% of patients receiving additional chemotherapy (40).

References

1. Goodner JT, Miller TP, Pack GT. Torek esophagectomy; the case against segmental resection for esophageal cancer. *J Thorac Surg* 1956;32:347–359.
2. Shapiro AL, Robillard GL. The esophageal arteries their configurational anatomy and variations in relation to surgery. *Ann Surg* 1950;131:171–185.
3. Hussey DH, Barakley T, Bloedorn F. Carcinoma of the esophagus. In: Fletcher GH, ed. *Textbook of radiotherapy*, 3rd ed. Philadelphia, PA: Lea & Febiger, 1980.
4. Moertel CG. The esophagus. In: Holland JF, Frei E III, eds. *Cancer medicine*, 2nd ed. Philadelphia, PA: Lea & Febiger, 1982.
5. Gaspar LE. Radiation therapy for esophageal cancer: improving the therapeutic ratio. *Semin Radiat Oncol* 1994;4:192–201.
6. Appelqvist P, Salmo M. Lye corrosion carcinoma of the esophagus: a review of 63 cases. *Cancer* 1980;45:2655–2658.
7. Hopkins RA, Postlethwait RW. Caustic burns and carcinoma of the esophagus. *Ann Surg* 1981;194:146–148.
8. Enzinger PC, Mayer RJ. Esophageal cancer. *N Engl J Med* 2003;349:2241–2252.
9. Flamen P, Lerut A, Van Cutsem E. Utility of positron emission tomography for the staging of patients with potentially operable esophageal carcinoma. *J Clin Oncol* 2000;18:3202–3210.
10. Rankin S. Oesophageal cancer. In: Husband J, Reznek R, eds. *Imaging in oncology*, 1st ed. Oxford, UK: Isis Medical Media, 1998:93–110.
11. Rice TW, Ishwaran H, Ferguson MK, et al. Cancer of the esophagus and esophagogastric junction: an eighth edition staging primer. *J Thorac Oncol* 2017;12:36–42.
12. Amin MB, Edge S, Greene F, et al., eds. *AJCC cancer staging handbook*, 8th ed. New York, NY: Springer International, 2017.
13. Pearson JG. The present status and future potential of radiotherapy in the management of esophageal cancer. *Cancer* 1977;39:882–890.
14. Dubecz A, Gall I, Solymosi N, et al. Temporal trends in long-term survival and cure rates in esophageal cancer: a SEER database analysis. *J Thorac Oncol* 2012;7:443–447.
15. Tepper J, Krasna MJ, Niedzwiecki D, et al. Phase III trial of trimodality therapy with cisplatin, fluorouracil, radiotherapy, and surgery compared with surgery alone for esophageal cancer: CALGB 9781. *J Clin Oncol* 2008;26:1086–1092.
16. van Hagen P, Hulshof MCCM, van Lanschot JJB, et al. Preoperative chemoradiotherapy for esophageal or junctional cancer. *N Engl J Med* 2012;366:2074–2084.
17. Rosenberg JC, Franklin R, Steiger Z. Squamous cell carcinoma of the thoracic esophagus: an interdisciplinary approach. *Curr Probl Cancer* 1981;5:1–52.
18. Rosenberg JC, Lichter AS, Leichman LP. Cancer of the esophagus. In: DeVita V, Hellman S, Rosenberg S, eds. *Cancer: principles and practice of oncology*, 3rd ed. Philadelphia, PA: JB Lippincott Co., 1989:725.

19. Czito BG, Denittis AS, Palta M, et al. Esophageal cancer. In: Halperin E, Perez CA, Brady LW, eds. *Principles and practice of radiation oncology*, 6th ed. Philadelphia, PA: Lippincott Williams & Wilkins, 2013.

20. Earlam RJ, Johnson L. 101 oesophageal cancers: a surgeon uses radiotherapy. *Ann R Coll Surg Engl* 1990;72:32–40.

21. Sur RK, Levin CV, Donde B, et al. Prospective randomized trial of HDR brachytherapy as a sole modality in palliation of advanced esophageal carcinoma—an International Atomic Energy Agency study. *Int J Radiat Oncol Biol Phys* 2002;53:127–133.

22. Gignoux M, Buyse M, Segol P. Multicenter randomized study comparing preoperative radiotherapy with surgery only in cases of resectable oesophageal cancer (author's transl). *Acta Chir Belg* 1982;82:373–379.

23. Teniere P, Hay JM, Fingerhut A. Postoperative radiation therapy does not increase survival after curative resection for squamous cell carcinoma of the middle and lower esophagus as shown by a multicenter controlled trial. *Surg Gynecol Obstet* 1991;173:123–130.

24. Kelsen DP, Winter KA, Gunderson LL. Long-term results of RTOG trial 8911 (USA Intergroup 113): a random assignment trial comparison of chemotherapy followed by surgery compared with surgery alone for esophageal cancer. *J Clin Oncol* 2007;25:3719–3725.

25. Medical Research Council Oesophageal Cancer Working Group. Surgical resection with or without preoperative chemotherapy in oesophageal cancer: a randomised controlled trial. *Lancet* 2002;359:1727–1733.

26. Cunningham D, Allum WH, Stenning SP. Perioperative chemotherapy versus surgery alone for resectable gastroesophageal cancer. *N Engl J Med* 2006:11–20.

27. Smith TJ, Ryan LM, Douglass HO, et al. Combined chemoradiotherapy vs. radiotherapy alone for early stage squamous cell carcinoma of the esophagus: a study of the Eastern Cooperative Oncology Group. *Int J Radiat Oncol Biol Phys* 1998;42:269–276.

28. Herskovic A, Martz K, al-Sarraf M. Combined chemotherapy and radiotherapy compared with radiotherapy alone in patients with cancer of the esophagus. *N Engl J Med* 1992;326:1593–1598.

29. Minsky BD, Pajak TF, Ginsberg RJ. INT 0123 (Radiation Therapy Oncology Group 94-05) phase III trial of combined-modality therapy for esophageal cancer: high-dose versus standard-dose radiation therapy. *J Clin Oncol* 2002:1167–1174.

30. Macdonald JS, Smalley SR, Benedetti J, et al. Chemoradiotherapy after surgery compared with surgery alone for adenocarcinoma of the stomach or gastroesophageal junction. *N Engl J Med* 2001;345:725–730.

31. Bedenne L, Michel P, Bouché O, et al. Chemoradiation followed by surgery compared with chemoradiation alone in squamous cancer of the esophagus: FFCD 9102. *J Clin Oncol* 2007;25:1160–1168.

32. Stahl M, Walz MK, Riera-Knorrenschild J, et al. Preoperative chemotherapy versus chemoradiotherapy in locally advanced adenocarcinomas of the oesophagogastric junction (POET): long-term results of a controlled randomised trial. *Eur J Cancer* 2017;81:183–190.

33. Karlin DA, Fisher RS, Krevsky B. Prolonged survival and effective palliation in patients with squamous cell carcinoma of the esophagus following endoscopic laser therapy. *Cancer* 1987; 59:1969–1972.

34. Wu AJ, Bosch WR, Chang DT, et al. Expert consensus contouring guidelines for IMRT in esophageal and gastroesophageal junction cancer. *Int J Radiat Oncol Biol Phys* 2015;92:911–920.

35. Fisher SA, Brady L. Esophagus. In: Perez CA, Brady L, eds. *Principles and practice of radiation oncology*, 3rd ed. Philadelphia, PA: Lippincott–Raven Publishers, 1998.

36. Shi A, Liao Z, Allen PK, et al. Long-term survival and toxicity outcomes of intensity modulated radiation therapy for the treatment of esophageal cancer: a large single-institutional cohort study. *Adv Radiat Oncol* 2017;2:316–324.

37. Werner-Wasik M, Yorke E, Deasy J. Radiation dose-volume effects in the esophagus. *Int J Radiat Oncol Biol Phys* 2010:86–93.

38. Tsutsui S, Moriguchi S, Morita M. Multivariate analysis of postoperative complications after esophageal resection. *Ann Thorac Surg* 1992:1052–1056.

39. Forastiere AA, Orringer MB, Perez-Tamayo C. Concurrent chemotherapy and radiation therapy followed by transhiatal esophagectomy for local-regional cancer of the esophagus. *J Clin Oncol* 1990:119–127.

40. Araujo CM, Souhami L, Gil RA. A randomized trial comparing radiation therapy versus concomitant radiation therapy and chemotherapy in carcinoma of the thoracic esophagus. *Cancer* 1991:2258–2261.

CHAPTER 21

BREAST

STAGE TIS, T1, AND T2 TUMORS

EPIDEMIOLOGY

- Breast cancer is the most frequently diagnosed cancer among American women. Approximately 1 in 8 women will be diagnosed with breast cancer during their lifetime.
- It is estimated that there will be 266,120 new cases of invasive breast cancer and 63,960 new cases of *in situ* breast cancer among women in the United States in 2018. Because of increased screening and awareness, breast cancer incidence rates continue to rise from the 1980s (1).
- An estimated 41,400 people will die of breast cancer in 2018. Second to lung cancer, breast cancer remains a leading cause of cancer death in women (1).

RISK FACTORS

- The most important risk factor for breast cancer is being female, as only 1% of breast cancers are diagnosed in men.
- Age is the second-most important risk factor, with 95% of breast cancers developing in women 40 years or older. The annual risk of developing breast cancer increases exponentially beginning at the age of 40 and then slows considerably at menopause (2).
- Estrogen exposure over an individual's lifetime also influences the risk of breast cancer. Increased estrogen exposure because of young age at menarche, use of hormonal contraception, nulliparity, older age at first pregnancy, lack of breastfeeding, older age at menopause, postmenopausal estrogen replacement, and obesity may all increase breast cancer risk (3).
- Family history of breast cancer in first-degree relatives, personal history of atypical ductal hyperplasia, lobular or ductal carcinoma *in situ* (DCIS), or benign breast biopsies are other known risk factors.
- Germ-line mutations in the *BRCA1/BRCA2*, *PTEN*, *TP53*, and *CDH1* genes are associated with an inherited susceptibility to breast cancer.
- Prior radiation treatment to the thorax, such as for Hodgkin's lymphoma, increases risk of breast cancer and has implications for prevention, screening, and treatment.
- Lifestyle factors such as higher alcohol consumption and lack of exercise may also increase breast cancer risk.

443

ANATOMY

- The breast lies on the anterior chest wall superficial to the pectoralis major muscle. Its borders are the midline medially, the midaxillary line laterally, the anterior second rib cranially, and the anterior sixth rib caudally.
- The upper outer quadrant of breast tissue that extends into the low axilla is the *axillary tail of Spence* (4).
- The breast parenchyma is composed of lobules, which function to produce milk, and ducts, which serve as a connection between lobules and the nipple. These ductal lobular units are suspended in fat, as well as a rich network of connective tissue, lymphatics, and vasculature.
- The fibrous septa, which run between the superficial fascia of the breast skin and the deep fascia of the chest wall, are called *Cooper's ligament*. Patients may present with skin dimpling when there is involvement of these suspensory structures by tumor (4).
- The primary lymphatic drainage of the breast is the axillary lymph nodes, which passes from the upper and lower halves of the breast to the chain of nodes between the second and third intercostal space. The axillary lymph nodes are divided into three levels based on relation to the pectoralis minor muscle. Level I is inferolateral to the muscle, level II beneath the muscle, and level III craniomedial to the pectoralis muscle.
- The breast may also drain to the internal mammary nodes as well as the supraclavicular lymph nodes (Fig. 21-1).

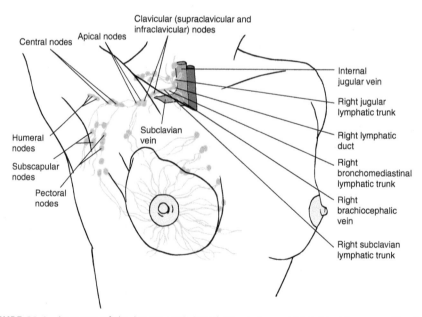

FIGURE 21-1. Anatomy of the breast, with lymphatic drainage highlighted in *green*. (Reprinted with permission from Agur AMR, Dalley AF., eds. *Grant's atlas of anatomy*, 14th ed. Philadelphia, PA: Lippincott Williams & Wilkins, 2017:198 (Plate 3.7). © Wolters Kluwer.)

CLINICAL PRESENTATION

- Most patients with carcinoma *in situ*, T1, or T2 breast cancers present with an abnormal screening mammogram or have a painless or slightly tender breast mass.
- About 10% to 40% of newly diagnosed T1 and T2 breast cancers have pathologic evidence of axillary nodal metastases; the incidence is strongly correlated with tumor size (Table 21-1), as well as other factors such as high-grade, lymphatic vascular invasion and young age (4,5).
- Metastases to the internal mammary nodes are more frequent from medial or central primary lesions and more often when there is axillary node involvement.

DIAGNOSTIC WORKUP

- The workup of a patient with an abnormal mammogram or breast mass, including complete clinical and family history and physical exam, is summarized in Table 21-2.
- Mammography is invaluable in the detection of over 90% of breast cancers (6).
- Ultrasonography, which has a sensitivity of 73% and specificity of 95%, is helpful in differentiating cysts from solid tumors (7).
- Magnetic resonance imaging may be used for both staging and preoperative evaluation, as well as to assess response to systemic therapy. False-positive findings are common and surgical decisions should not be based solely on MRI findings alone. There is no evidence that demonstrates improved local control or survival with the use of MRI (8).

Table 21-1

Incidence of Metastatic Axillary Lymph Nodes in Carcinoma of Breast Correlated with Primary Tumor Size

Study (Reference)	Tumor Size[a] (cm)				
	≤0.5	0.6–1.0	1.0–2.0	2.1–3.0	3.1–5.0
Washington University[b]	3/55 (5%)	25/203 (12%)	59/294 (20%)	38/113 (34%)	9/31 (29%)
Tinnemans et al. (9)	1/13 (7.7%)	3/24 (12.5%)	13/44 (29.5%)	—	—
Silverstein et al. (10)	3/96 (3%)	27/156 (17%)	115/357 (32%)	145/330 (44%)[c]	—
Kambouris (11)	—	—	13/357 (32%)	15/25 (60%)	1/7 (14%)
Greco et al. (12)	—	40/306 (13%)	—	49/69 (71%)	
Fein et al. (13)	6/68 (9%)	7/48 (15%)	16/50 (32%)	—	—

[a]Number of patients with axillary metastasis/total number of patients with tumor size indicated.
[b]Unpublished data.
[c]T2 tumors (2 to 5 cm).
Source: Table 53.4 in Haffty B, Buchholz TA, Perez CA. Early stage breast cancer. In: Halperin EC, Perez CA, Brady LW, eds. *Principles and practice of radiation oncology*, 5th ed. Philadelphia, PA: Lippincott Williams & Wilkins, 2008.

Table 21-2
Diagnostic Workup for Carcinoma of the Breast, Stages T1 and T2

General
History with emphasis on presenting symptoms, menstrual status, parity, family history of cancer, and other risk factors
Physical examination with emphasis on the breast, axilla, supraclavicular area, and abdomen

Special Tests
Biopsy (core biopsy directed by physical examination, ultrasound, or mammography as indicated or needle localization)

Radiologic Studies
Before biopsy
Mammography/ultrasonography
Chest radiographs
Magnetic resonance imaging of the breast (selected cases)
After positive biopsy
Bone scan (when clinically indicated, for stage II or III disease or elevated serum alkaline phosphatase levels)
CT of the chest, abdomen, and pelvis for stage II or III disease and/or abnormal liver function tests

Laboratory Studies
Complete blood cell count and blood chemistry
Urinalysis

Other Studies
Hormone receptor status (ER, PR)
HER2/neu status
Consider genetic counseling/BRCA testing in selected cases

ER, estrogen receptor; PR, progesterone receptor.
Source: Table 53.8 in Haffty B, Buchholz TA, Perez CA. Early stage breast cancer. In: Halperin EC, Perez CA, Brady LW, eds. *Principles and practice of radiation oncology*, 5th ed. Philadelphia, PA: Lippincott Williams & Wilkins, 2008.

- In patients with stage 0, I, or II disease, the incidence of abnormal bone scan is approximately 2%; it is not routinely obtained in these patients and may be considered if there is localized bone pain or elevated alkaline phosphatase.
- Patient should undergo genetic counseling if they are less than 50 years of age at presentation or at high risk for hereditary breast cancer.

PATHOLOGIC STUDIES

- Histopathologic diagnosis is obtained by fine-needle aspiration, stereotactic core biopsy, or excisional biopsy of solid masses. Needle localization and radiographic techniques may be employed for nonpalpable lesions.

- Estrogen receptor (ER) and progesterone receptor (PR) assays are routinely performed on tissue obtained from patients with both invasive and noninvasive breast cancer. These parameters correlate with prognosis and tumor response to chemotherapeutic and hormonal agents.
- The *her-2-neu* (*c-erbB-2*) proto-oncogene encodes a transmembrane protein tyrosine kinase receptor called the human epidermal growth factor receptor 2 (HER2) and is over-expressed and/or amplified in 15% to 20% of primary breast cancers. Overexpression is correlated with poorer prognosis and should therefore also be routinely tested (14).

PATHOLOGIC CLASSIFICATION

- The World Health Organization classification of breast tumors was updated in 2012 to include neoplastic and preneoplastic lesions, incorporating molecular and genetic data into their morphologically defined system (15).
- The American Joint Committee on Cancer has developed an alternative system mainly comprised of two main categories: *in situ* carcinomas and invasive carcinomas (16).
- Ductal carcinoma *in situ* (DCIS) is a noninvasive clonal proliferative process confined to the ducts of the breast. It is a precursor to invasive disease. There exist five sub-types of DCIS: comedo, solid, cribriform, micropapillary, and papillary, which may be present in combination within a single lesion.
- Lobular carcinoma *in situ* (LCIS) is a noninvasive abnormal proliferation of epithelial cells in the lobules of the breast that confers an increased risk of subsequent invasive breast cancer in either breast. It is considered a benign entity. Loss of *E-cadherin* (CDH1) gene expression is characteristic.
- Paget's disease is characterized by presence of Paget's cells involving the nipple-areola complex. The prevailing *epidermotropic theory* states that the malignant Paget's cells originate from underlying *in situ* or invasive disease of the breast, which is found in more than 95% of cases.
- Microinvasive carcinoma is defined as invasive carcinoma with no focus measuring greater than 1 mm, nearly always encountered in a setting of DCIS, where small foci of tumor cells have invaded through the basement membrane into the surrounding stroma.
- Invasive ductal carcinoma, the most common type of breast cancer, accounts for more than 80% of all cases.
- Invasive lobular carcinoma (ILC) may be interspersed with LCIS; it is often "mammograph-ically silent" and is much more commonly ER positive than invasive ductal carcinoma.
- Tubular carcinoma has a nonaggressive growth pattern; axillary lymph node involve-ment is reported in approximately 10% of patients.
- Medullary carcinoma is well circumscribed, with infrequent lymph node metastases.
- Mucinous carcinoma, also called mucoid or colloid carcinoma, is most often observed in older women. It is slow growing with a low frequency of axillary lymph node metastasis. Survival is appreciably better than with infiltrating ductal carcinoma.
- Cystosarcoma phyllodes is usually benign, however, may be considered borderline or malignant depending on grade, proliferative index, and surgical margins. While tumors may be large, they are often well encapsulated without invasion of the adjacent breast. A few cases of metastases to the contralateral breast, axillary lymph nodes, mediastinum, and lungs have been reported (7).

- Other unusual tumors occasionally described in the breast include primary mammary lymphomas, primary neuroendocrine small cell carcinoma, sarcoma, squamous cell carcinoma, basal cell carcinoma, and adenocystic carcinoma.

STAGING

- The American Joint Committee on Cancer (AJCC) staging system (17) is the most widely used system in the United States.

NEW!   SUMMARY OF CHANGES TO AJCC STAGING

STAGING GROUPS

- Introduced two new stage groupings including an anatomic stage grouping based solely on the anatomic extent of cancer defined by the traditional TNM categories as well as a prognostic stage grouping, which includes additional prognostic information of tumor grade and ER, PR, and HER2 status in the staging of patients.
- The prognostic stage grouping is preferred, but the anatomic stage grouping may be used in regions where biomarkers cannot be routinely obtained.

Breast

- Lobular carcinoma *in situ* (LCIS) was removed under the T category as Tis (LCIS), as it is a benign entity.
- Invasive tumors measuring 1.0 to 1.9 mm should be reported rounding to 2 mm and should be classified as T1a and not T1mi.
- Confirmed that the maximum invasive tumor size is a reasonable estimate of tumor volume alone. Small microscopic satellite foci around the primary tumor do not appreciably alter tumor volume and are not added to the maximum tumor size.
- In the scenario of multiple synchronous tumors identified clinically and/or pathologically, their presence is documented using the (m) modifier for the T category. The maximum dimension of the largest tumor is used to determine cT and pT; the size of multiple tumors is not added together.
- Clarified that satellite tumor nodules in the skin must be separated from the primary tumor and macroscopically identified to be categorized as T4b. Skin and dermal tumor satellite nodules identified only on microscopic examination and in the absence of epidermal ulceration or skin edema do not qualify as T4b and should be categorized based on tumor size.

Nodes (N)

- The dimension of the area containing several or multiple tumor deposits is not used to determine pN category, only the largest contiguous tumor deposit is used. Adjacent satellite deposits are not added to the final dimension of the largest tumor deposit.
- Affirmed that cNX is not a valid category unless the node basin has been removed and cannot be examined by imaging or clinical examination. A cN0 category is to be assigned when any evaluation of the nodes is possible, such as by physical examination or imaging, and is negative.

Metastases (M)

- Affirmed that pM0 is not a valid category. All cases should be categorized as either cM0 or cM1; however, if cM1 is subsequently microscopically confirmed, pM1 is used.

Postneoadjuvant Therapy (yc or ypTNM)

- Clarified that the postneoadjuvant therapy pathologic T category (ypT) is based on the largest focus of residual tumor present. Treatment-related fibrosis that may be adjacent to residual invasive carcinoma is not included in the ypT maximum dimension. When multiple foci of residual tumor are present, the (m) modified is included. When possible, the pretreatment cT category should be documented.
- Clarified that the largest focus of residual tumor in the lymph nodes is used for the ypN categorization. Again, treatment-related fibrosis adjacent to residual nodal tumor deposits is not included in the ypN dimension and classification.
- Affirmed that any residual invasive carcinoma detected by pathologic examination in the breast or lymph nodes precludes the posttreatment classification of a complete pathologic response (pCR).
- If a cancer is categorized as cM1 or pM1 prior to therapy, the cancer is categorized as M1 following neoadjuvant therapy regardless of the observed response to therapy.

Collection of Biomarkers

- Determined that all invasive carcinomas should have estrogen receptor, progesterone receptor, and human epidermal growth factor receptor 2 (HER2) status determined by appropriate assays whenever possible.

Inclusion of Multigene Panels

- For patients with hormone receptor–positive, HER2-negative, and lymph node-negative tumors, a 21-gene (Oncotype Dx) recurrence score less than 11, regardless of T size, places the tumor into the same prognostic category as T1a-T1b N0 M0 and staged using the AJCC prognostic stage table as stage I.
- For patients with hormone receptor–positive, HER2-negative, and lymph node-negative tumors, a MammaPrint low-risk score, regardless of T size, places the tumor into the same prognostic category as T1a-T1b N0 M0.
- For patients with hormone receptor–positive, HER2-negative, and lymph node-negative tumors, a 12-gene (EndoPredict) low-risk score, regardless of T size, places the tumor into the same prognostic category as T1a-T1b N0 M0.
- For patients with hormone receptor–positive, HER2-negative, and lymph node-negative tumors, a PAM50 risk of recurrence (ROR) score in the low range, regardless of T size, places the tumor into the same prognostic category as T1a-T1b N0 M0.
- For patients with hormone receptor–positive, HER2-negative, and lymph node-negative tumors, a Breast Cancer Index in the low-risk range, regardless of T size, places the tumor into the same prognostic category as T1a-T1b N0 M0.

See: Amin MB, Edge SB, Greene FL, et al. *AJCC cancer staging manual*, 8th ed. New York, NY: Springer Verlag, 2017.

PROGNOSTIC FACTORS FOR RELAPSE AND SURVIVAL

- Available literature supports the concept that local control influences overall survival in breast cancer patients. A meta-analysis combining information on 42,000 women from 78 randomized trials comparing radiotherapy versus no radiotherapy, more versus less surgery, and more surgery versus radiotherapy helped to relate the impact of locoregional recurrence on breast cancer mortality. The study authors conclude that differences in local treatment, which substantially affect local recurrence rates, in the absence of other causes of death, avoid one breast cancer death at 15 years for every four local recurrences (18).
- It is important to appreciate that while locoregional recurrence may affect survival, prognostic factors for distant relapse and overall survival may not also be prognostic for local relapse (19).
- In 1999, the College of American Pathologists presented a consensus statement summarizing prognostic factors for distant metastasis and overall survival (20). Category I factors proven to be of prognostic importance and useful in clinical patient management included tumor size, lymph node status, micrometastases, histologic grade, mitotic count, and hormonal receptor status.
- Prognostic factors of distant relapse and survival are discussed below. Prognostic factors for local relapse will be discussed later in this chapter.

Patient Factors

- In a consecutive series of 1,703 premenopausal patients, young age was associated with significantly lower survival rates and higher distant relapse rates than older patients. This observation was independent of other factors such as clinical tumor size, clinical node status, histologic grade, hormone status, and adjuvant systemic therapy (21).
- Black women are commonly diagnosed with more advanced stages of breast cancer than white women and, in general, have lower 5-year breast cancer survival rates. When adjusted for income, in addition to stage and age, the effect of race on survival is reduced (22).

Axillary Nodal Status

- Axillary nodal status is the strongest predictor of relapse and survival. The importance of the presence as well as the extent of nodal involvement is reflected in the current AJCC staging system.
- Outcomes continue to improve as systemic therapies advance. Based on older NSABP trials, 5-year survival in node-negative women is 82.8%, for 1 to 3 positive nodes 73%, for 4 to 12 positive nodes 45.7% and for greater than 13 positive nodes 28.4% (5).
- The prognostic significance of micrometastases is controversial. Several retrospective studies found the prognosis of patients with isolated micrometastases in axillary nodes to be the same as node-negative patients, whereas other studies have suggested that these patients may have worse prognosis.
- The detection of micrometastases in clinically node-negative patients is 15% to 20% with the use of immunohistochemistry (20).

Tumor Size

- Tumor size is one of the strongest predictors of distant metastasis and disease-free and overall survival. Although it correlates strongly with the presence and number of axillary lymph nodes involved, it still serves as an independent prognostic factor alone.
- In a population of mastectomy patients for T1 N0 breast cancers, Rosen et al. reported recurrence-free survival of 88% for tumor size less than 1 cm, 72% for tumors 1.1 to 3 cm, and 59% for tumors 3.1 to 5 cm (23).

Histologic Type

- The histologic type of invasive cancer has been shown to be prognostic in several studies. The tubular, mucinous, and medullary subtypes have more favorable prognosis compared to invasive ductal carcinoma (5,23). Invasive lobular tumors have similar prognosis to invasive ductal tumors.
- Subtypes associated with poorer prognosis include metaplastic, undifferentiated, and other rare subtypes (24).

Histologic Grade

- Various grading systems exist; however, the Nottingham grading system (Elston-Ellis modification of Scarff-Bloom-Richardson grading system) is recommended by the College of American Pathologists (20,25).
- In a population of 1,831 patients, Elston found a strong correlation between histologic grade and prognosis. Patients with grade I tumors had statistically better survival than those with grade II/III tumors (25).

Proliferation Index

- There are a number of techniques to evaluate the proliferative rate of tumor cells including thymidine labeling index (TLI), mitotic index, and quantification of Ki-67 and/or the proliferating cell nuclear antigen (PCNA) using immunohistochemistry.
- Ki-67 positivity is associated with higher probability of relapse and worse survival in early-stage breast cancers (26) and can be used to distinguish luminal A from luminal B tumors, which have poorer prognosis (27).

Lymphatic and Vascular Invasion

- Lymphatic and vascular invasion (LVI) in the peritumoral region has been demonstrated to be of independent prognostic significance in several studies (23,28).

Hormonal Receptor and HER2 Status

- Patients with ER-positive tumors have significantly higher survival rates than ER-negative tumors (29), and these patients derive the greatest benefit from hormonal therapy.

- Overexpression or gene amplification of HER2/neu is seen in up to 20% of breast cancers and is associated with an aggressive phenotype with shorter disease-free survival (30). Amplification of the oncogene identified by fluorescent *in situ* hybridization (FISH) has been found to be of more prognostic value with better interobserver reproducibility compared to immunohistochemistry techniques (31).

LOBULAR CARCINOMA *IN SITU*

- LCIS is a benign proliferative lesion. It was included in prior editions of the AJCC Cancer Staging Manual but was removed from the recent 8th edition.
- It is found in a multicentric distribution in up to 90% of mastectomy specimens, with bilateral involvement in up to 60% (32).
- The presence of LCIS is considered a marker of increased risk for subsequent development of invasive ductal or lobular carcinoma in either breast. The risk appears to be nearly equal for both breasts (33).

Treatment of Lobular Carcinoma *In Situ*

- If LCIS is the sole histologic diagnosis, treatment recommendations range from conservative to radical.
- Observation with close surveillance and regular physical examinations is commonly practiced.
- More aggressive variants of LCIS, such as pleomorphic LCIS or LCIS associated with necrosis carry similar risk for invasive cancer as DCIS and may be managed with surgical excision.
- Studies have shown that the presence of more than 4 foci of LCIS increases the risk for upstaging at surgical excision. Therefore, surgical excision of LCIS found on core biopsy to exclude associated DCIS or invasive disease may also be reasonable (34).
- The common involvement of the bilateral breasts with LCIS makes a unilateral mastectomy illogic and inadequate (4). Prophylactic bilateral total mastectomies may be considered in highly anxious and/or high-risk patients with a strong family history of breast cancer.
- Endocrine therapy such as tamoxifen has demonstrated efficacy in reducing the risk of invasive carcinoma, in the context of LCIS, by 56% (35).

DUCTAL CARCINOMA *IN SITU*

- DCIS is a precursor lesion to invasive carcinoma with low propensity for nodal spread.
- The University of Southern California/Van Nuys Prognostic Index (USC/VNPI) quantified 5 measurable prognostic factors in predicting local recurrence including tumor size, margin width, nuclear grade, age, and the presence of comedonecrosis (36).
- The histologic diversity of DCIS with variable propensity for local recurrence suggests that some patients may be treated with breast-conserving surgery alone (without adjuvant whole-breast radiation therapy).

Treatment of Ductal Carcinoma *In Situ*

Surgical Management

- The surgical options for DCIS include total mastectomy or breast-conserving surgery. Although studies suggest lower rates of locoregional recurrence with mastectomy, there is no difference in overall survival (37).
- Mastectomy should be considered in the case of large extent of disease, multifocal disease, and/or inability to obtain negative margins.
- Sentinel lymph node dissection (SLND) is not routinely performed for DCIS given the low reported rates of axillary spread. Predictors for positive SLND in DCIS include larger lesion size (greater than 2 cm), palpability, occult invasive disease, and multiple prior ipsilateral breast biopsies (38). SLND should be performed at the time of planned total mastectomy.
- Surgical excision alone without radiation was studied in the prospective ECOG-ACRIN E5194 trial including patients with either low-intermediate grade DCIS measuring less than 2.5 cm (cohort 1) or high-grade DCIS measuring less than 1 cm (cohort 2). Tamoxifen was given in an optional, nonrandomized fashion in 30% of patients. Twelve-year ipsilateral breast events were 14.4% for cohort 1 patients compared 24.6% ($p = 0.003$) (39).
- In a single-institution, prospective trial of 158 patients with predominantly low-intermediate grade DCIS measuring less than 2.5 cm, the outcomes of wide local excision alone (margin ≥1 cm) were evaluated. Tamoxifen was not permitted. The rate of ipsilateral breast local recurrence was 12% at 5 years (40).
- The 2016 Society of Surgical Oncology-American Society for Radiation Oncology-American Society of Clinical Oncology (SSO/ASTRO/ASCO) Consensus Guidelines recommend use of a 2-mm excision margin for DCIS treated with whole-breast therapy (41).

Adjuvant Radiation Therapy

- Three prospective randomized trials (NSABP B-17, EORTC 10853, UKCCCR) demonstrated the benefit of adjuvant whole-breast radiation following breast-conserving surgery for DCIS (42–44).
- In the EBCTCG meta-analysis of these studies, radiotherapy reduced the absolute 10-year risk of any ipsilateral breast event by 15.2% (12.9% versus 28.1%, $p < 0.00001$) regardless of age, extent of BCS, use of tamoxifen, method of DCIS detection, margin status, focality, grade, presence of necrosis, tumor size, or architecture (45). Whole-breast therapy remains the standard of care in the management of DCIS after breast-conserving surgery (46).
- Pooled retrospective analysis demonstrated a 15-year reduction of in-breast tumor recurrences with the use of a lumpectomy boost independent of age and tamoxifen use (47).
- The RTOG 98-04 prospective randomized trial determined the benefit of adjuvant whole-breast radiation therapy in good-risk DCIS defined as screen detected, low-intermediate grade, size ≤2.5 cm, and ≥3 mm margins. Tamoxifen use (62%) was

optional, and at 7 years, the local failure rate was 0.9% in the RT arm compared to 6.7% without RT ($p < 0.001$) (48).
* Good-risk DCIS as defined by RTOG 98-04 was recently included in updated ASTRO Accelerated Partial Breast Irradiation (APBI) consensus guidelines as "suitable" (49).

Adjuvant Endocrine Therapy

* Results of NSABP-B24 demonstrated that tamoxifen reduced the risk of subsequent invasive tumor recurrence in estrogen receptor–positive DCIS by (11.1% versus 7.7%, $p = 0.02$) 44% (50).
* The UKCCCR trial performed a 2 × 2 factorial randomization of DCIS patients to radiotherapy, tamoxifen, or both. In patients who received tamoxifen alone without radiation therapy after lumpectomy, tamoxifen had no effect on the incidence of invasive recurrence, but did significantly reduce risk (10% versus 6%, $p = 0.03$) of DCIS recurrence (44). The role of tamoxifen in the absence of whole-breast radiotherapy remains to be defined in DCIS.
* The NSABP B-35 study randomized postmenopausal women to tamoxifen or anastrozole for 5 years after whole-breast radiotherapy. Anastrozole resulted in a significant decrease in breast cancer-free survival compared to tamoxifen (HR 0.73, $p = 0.02$), and thus, anastrozole should be used in the adjuvant treatment of postmenopausal women with hormone receptor–positive DCIS (51).

Future Direction

* Current trials (COMET, LORIS, LORD) examine the feasibility of active surveillance of low-risk DCIS treated with endocrine therapy alone compared to standard BCS and adjuvant radiation and endocrine therapy.

MANAGEMENT OF INVASIVE BREAST CANCER

Breast Conservation

* Breast-conserving surgery (BCS) and mastectomy are both reasonable options for patients with stage I and II breast cancer. Breast-conserving therapy consisting of BCS and adjuvant whole-breast radiation therapy provides equivalent overall survival to that of total mastectomy while preserving the breast (52–54).
* The benefit of whole-breast radiotherapy after BCS was reported by the EBCTCG meta-analysis on over 10,000 women in 17 randomized trials. Radiation was found to half the rate of ipsilateral breast tumor recurrence (IBTR) and reduced the breast cancer death rate by a sixth (55). Adjuvant whole-breast therapy remains the standard of care after BCS.
* The Society of Surgical Oncology-American Society for Radiation Oncology (SSO-ASTRO) consensus guideline on margins defined a negative margin as no tumor on ink. Wider margins did not minimize the risk of an ipsilateral breast recurrence, and it is not routine practice to obtain wider negative margin widths than no tumor on ink (56).

- Mastectomy may be warranted in patients with high-risk disease or in patients who have absolute/relative contraindications to radiation.
- Absolute contraindications to breast-conserving therapy include pregnancy, diffuse suspicious or malignant calcifications, diffusely positive pathologic margins, and homozygosity for the ATM mutation. Relative contraindications include prior radiation therapy to the chest wall or breast, large ratio of tumor to breast size, active connective tissue disease, and Li-Fraumeni syndrome.

Surgical Management of Axillary Lymph Nodes

- The contents of the axilla are divided into three levels defined by relation to the pectoralis minor muscle. Traditionally, a complete axillary lymph node dissection (ALND) involves dissection of levels I and II, with removal of ≥10 lymph nodes. Previous studies have shown routine dissection of level III to be associated with increased morbidity without a survival benefit and should only be performed in the presence of gross level II and/or III disease (5).
- Sentinel lymph node dissection (SLND) has been developed as a means to stage the axilla in patients with early-stage, clinically node-negative breast cancer given the lower risk of involvement and increased morbidity with full ALND. Upfront ALND is usually reserved for patients with clinically apparent involvement of the axilla.
- The NSABP B32 and Milan trials evaluated the outcomes in early-stage, clinically node-negative patients managed with SLND alone. Patients were randomized to either SLND and ALND or SLND with completion of ALND only if a sentinel lymph node was found to be involved. They found no significant difference in axillary failure or disease-free and overall survival between the two arms. With the use of dual tracers (radioisotope and isosulfan blue dye), the overall accuracy of SLND was approximately 97% with a false-negative rate of 9.8% (57,58).
- The ACOSOG Z0011 randomized trial examined the outcomes in clinically node-negative women found to have sentinel node metastases at the time of breast-conserving surgery if treated with SLND alone. At 10 years, there was no difference in disease-free survival (80.2% versus 78.2%, $p = 0.32$) between patients who underwent SLND alone versus ALND. Overall survival was noninferior in the SLND arm (86.3% versus 83.6%, $p = 0.02$) (59).

Irradiation of Regional Lymph Nodes

- In patients with a pathologically confirmed negative axilla, irradiation of the regional nodes is not routine but may be considered in the presence of additional high-risk clinical and/or pathologic features.
- Retrospective review of available radiation records from the ACOSOG Z0011 trial (228 patients, 29%) revealed the use of high tangents in 52.6% of patients in the SLND arm and a third directed nodal field in 16.9% (60). High tangents therefore may be considered in clinically node-negative patients found to have a low burden of axillary disease on SLND.

- The EORTC 10981-22023 AMAROS trial compared axillary radiation therapy to standard ALND in patients with T1-2 lesions, and no apparent clinical lymphade-nopathy was found to have a positive sentinel lymph node. Patients underwent a complete ALND or received no further dissection followed by radiotherapy directed to the axilla and medial supraclavicular fossa. Five-year axillary recurrence rates were found to be comparable between the two groups with significantly less lymphedema (23% versus 11%, $p < 0.0001$) in the radiation arm (61).
- Three major studies have examined the benefit of comprehensive regional nodal irradiation in women with early-stage breast cancer including the MA.20, EORTC 22922/10925, and French study (62–64).
- The MA.20 trial examined the benefit of comprehensive nodal irradiation (axilla, supraclavicular, and internal mammary) in addition to standard adjuvant whole-breast therapy for early-stage patients (clinical T1-3, N1) found to have positive axil-lary lymph nodes at the time of surgery or with high-risk features (tumor measuring 5 cm or more or 2 cm or more with fewer than 10 axillary nodes removed and at least one of the following: high-grade disease, estrogen receptor negativity, lymphovascular invasion). At 10 years, nodal irradiation reduced the rate of breast recurrence signifi-cantly (82% versus 77%, $p = 0.01$) but did not improve overall survival (62).
- The EORTC 22922/10925 trial examined the effect of internal mammary and medial supraclavicular nodal irradiation in patients with central or medially located tumors, irrespective of axillary involvement, or externally located tumors with axillary involve-ment. At 10 years, there was no difference in overall survival; however, disease-free survival (72.1% versus 69.1%, $p = 0.04$) was improved with nodal irradiation (63).
- The French performed a randomized trial to evaluate the benefit of internal mam-mary nodal (IMN) irradiation in central or medial tumors without or without nodal involvement and lateral tumors with axillary spread. No benefit of IMN irradiation on overall survival was seen at a median follow-up of 11.3 years (64).
- An absolute 10-year overall survival benefit with regional nodal irradiation (1% in MA.20, 1.6% in EORTC, 3.3% in the French study) was apparent in a meta-analysis of these three trials (65).
- To determine the possible survival benefit of nodal irradiation that may be offset by radiation-induced heart disease, a Dutch study randomized women with early-stage node-positive breast cancer to IMN irradiation for patients with right-sided disease, and no IMN irradiation for left-sided disease. Eight-year overall survival rates were 75.9% with IMN irradiation versus 72.2% ($p = 0.005$), with the benefit more pro-nounced in patients at high risk of IMN metastasis (46). A management summary of early-stage breast cancers is presented in Table 21-3.

Use of a Lumpectomy Boost

- The EORTC 22881-10882 "boost or no boost" study investigated the benefit of a 16-Gy lumpectomy boost following BCS in stage I and II patients. Although there was no overall survival benefit, the 20-year cumulative incidence of IBTR was significantly reduced (13% versus 9%, $p < 0.0001$) with a boost. The cumulative incidence of severe fibrosis at 20 years was 5.2% versus 1.8% ($p < 0.0001$) in the no boost group (66).

Table 21-3

Treatment Policy for Conservative Management of Early-Stage Breast Cancer

Treatment Volume	Indication	Fraction Size/Technique	Total Dose	Comment
Early-Stage Breast Cancer				
Whole breast	Routinely following BCS	200 (prefer) or 180 cGy/tangents with wedges or dynamic wedges to optimize homogeneity	4,500–5,040 cGy	Consider omission of RT in elderly with stage I (ER positive) and comorbidities
Boost	Routinely following whole breast	200 or 180 cGy (prefer 200)/En face electrons	1,000–1,600 cGy to bring total dose to >6,000	May consider no boost for widely negative margins in women over 60
Accelerated whole breast	Patient convenience	266 cGy tangents with no nodal fields/no boost	4,250 cGy	
Accelerated partial breast	On protocol	3.4–3.8 Gy/external beam conformal interstitial, or MammoSite	3,400–3,850 cGy	
Treatment Policy for Regional Nodes				
Supraclavicular	• Clinical N2 or N3 disease • >4 + LN after axillary dissection • 1–3 + LN with high-risk features • Node + sentinel lymph node with no dissection unless risk of additional axillary disease is very small • High risk* with no dissection	180–200 (prefer 200)/AP or AP/PA	4,500–5,040 cGy	May omit with 1–3 positive nodes in select cases
Axilla	• N+ with extensive ECE • SN+ with no dissection • Inadequate axillary dissection • High risk with no dissection	180–200/AP—consider posterior axillary boost if suboptimal coverage with AP only	4,500–5,040 cGy	Axilla may be intentionally included with use of "high tangents"

continued

Table 21-3
Treatment Policy for Conservative Management of Early-Stage Breast Cancer (continued)

Treatment Volume	Indication	Fraction Size/Technique	Total Dose	Comment
Internal mammary	Individualized but consider for: • Positive axillary nodes with central and medial lesions • Stage III breast cancer • +SLN in the IM chain • +SLN in axilla with drainage to IM on lymphoscintigraphy	180–200/partially wide tangents or separate IM electron/photon	4,500–5,040 cGy	

AP/PA, anteroposterior/posteroanterior; BCS, breast-conserving surgery; ECE, extranodal tumor extension; IM, internal mammary; LN, lymph nodes; N+, node positive; SLN+, sentinel lymph node.

[a]High risk defined as estimated probability of nodal involvement greater than 10% to 15%.

Source: Table 53.27 in Haffty B, Buchholz TA, Perez CA. Early stage breast cancer. In: Halperin EC, Perez CA, Brady LW, eds. *Principles and practice of radiation oncology*, 5th ed. Philadelphia, PA: Lippincott Williams & Wilkins, 2008.

- The Lyon randomized boost trial reported similar results to EORTC but utilized a boost dose of 10 Gy with less toxicity. The boost group experienced higher rates of telangiectasia; however, based on self-assessment scores, there was no significant difference in cosmetic results between treatment arms (67).
- Although the relative benefit of boost is similar among all age groups, the largest absolute benefit is in patients younger than 51 years who have a higher baseline risk for local recurrence. Factors that have a negative impact on local control and that are associated with higher IBTR include high-grade disease, hormone receptor–negative disease, HER2 overexpression disease, and adjacent DCIS (68,69).
- The use of a boost or systemic therapy does not compensate for involved surgical margins. The EORTC found higher rates of severe fibrosis and no local control benefit with a 26-Gy boost compared to 10 Gy in patients with positive margins. Positive margins are associated with a 2.4-fold increased risk of local recurrence; therefore, these patients should undergo re-excision if possible (70,71).

ACCELERATED PARTIAL BREAST IRRADIATION

- Accelerated partial breast irradiation (APBI) is a localized form of radiotherapy delivered to the lumpectomy cavity after BCS using various techniques such as multicatheter interstitial brachytherapy, MammoSite balloon brachytherapy, or external beam radiotherapy.
- Three randomized trials have compared APBI to standard whole-breast irradiation (GEC-ESTRO, Budapest, and Livi) demonstrating that APBI is a feasible option in selected low-risk women with early-stage breast cancer (72–74).
- Results from the prospective MammoSite brachytherapy trial reported a 5-year IBTR rate of 3.8% with excellent cosmetic results and few late toxicities beyond 2 years (75).
- Two randomized trials assessed the efficacy of intraoperative radiation therapy compared to standard whole-breast therapy and reported favorable results (ELIOT and TARGIT). The use of these techniques is currently recommended on clinical trial and/or a prospective registry (76,77).
- ASTRO published updated clinical guidelines for APBI in 2016, providing an outline of clinical and pathologic suitability criteria in the selection of patients for APBI summarized in Table 21-4 (49).
- Results are pending from the prospective randomized NSABP-39/RTOG 0413 trial comparing partial breast irradiation (allowing the use of multicatheter brachytherapy, MammoSite, or other single-entry intracavitary devices as well as 3D conformal external beam radiotherapy) to whole-breast irradiation.

Omission of Radiation Therapy

- The NSABP B-21 trial explored the rate of IBTR for T1 breast cancers treated with tamoxifen, radiation therapy, or both following lumpectomy. Twenty percent of women were less than 50 years, and 82% of women treated with tamoxifen alone were estrogen receptor positive. At 8 years, the cumulative rate of IBTR was 16.5% (tamoxifen alone), 9.3% (radiation alone), and 2.8% with both therapies (78).

Table 21-4

Patient Groups for APBI with Original and Updated Consensus Guidelines

Patient Group	Risk Factor	Original	Update
Suitable	Age	≥60 y	≥50 y
	Margins	Negative by at least 2 mm	No change
	T stage	T1	Tis or T1
	DCIS	Not allowed	If all of the below: • Screen detected • Low to intermediate grade • Size ≤ 2.5 cm • Resected with margins negative at ≥3 mm
Cautionary	Age	50–59 y	• 40–49 y if all other criteria for "suitable" are met • ≥50 y if patient has at least 1 of the pathologic factors below and does not have any "unsuitable" factors *Pathologic factors:* • Size 2.1–3 cm[a] • T2 • Close margins (<2 mm) • Limited/focal LVSI • ER negative • Clinically unifocal with total size 2.1–3 cm[b] • Invasive lobular histology • Pure DCIS ≤ 3 cm if criteria for "suitable" not fully met • EIC ≤ 3 cm
	Margins	Close (<2 mm)	No change
	DCIS	≤3 cm	≤3 cm and does not meet criteria for "suitable"
Unsuitable	Age	<50 y	• <40 y • 40–49 y and do not meet criteria for "cautionary"
	Margins	Positive	No change
	DCIS	>3 cm	No change

[a]The size of the invasive tumor component.
[b]Microscopic multifocality allowed, provided the lesion is clinically unifocal (a single discrete lesion by physical examination and ultrasonography/mammography) and the total lesion size (including foci of multifocality and intervening normal breast parenchyma) falls between 2.1 and 3.0 cm.
Source: Correa C, Harris EE, Leonardi MC, et al. Accelerated partial breast irradiation: executive summary for the update of an ASTRO Evidence-Based Consensus Statement. *Pract Radiat Oncol* 2017;7:73–79.

- Radiation alone reduces IBTR by 50% compared to tamoxifen alone. Radiation and tamoxifen together reduce IBTR by 63% compared to radiation alone and by 81% compared to tamoxifen alone (78).
- Three randomized studies have examined the omission of radiation therapy in older women with early-stage breast cancers including the CALGB 9343 (age ≥ 70 years), the PRIME II (age ≥ 65 years), and the Princess Margaret Experience (age ≥ 50 years). Although there was a significant reduction of IBTR with the addition of radiation in all these studies, the 5-year local relapse rates were acceptably low at approximately 5% to 8%, with no impact on overall survival or distant relapse rates (79–81).
- Certain subsets of women have a very low baseline risk of recurrence for which radiation can be safely omitted. There are currently three prospective, single-arm trials that examine the omission in low-risk, luminal A breast cancers including PRECISION (luminal A by PAM50), LUMINA (T1 with Ki-67 less than 13.25%), and the IDEA trial (T1 with Oncotype score ≤ 18).

Adjuvant Systemic Therapy

- Adjuvant endocrine therapy is appropriate in all women with estrogen and/or progesterone-positive tumors given the clear benefit in reducing rates of local and/or distant relapse and improving overall survival.
- Premenopausal women should be offered single-agent tamoxifen; however, the addition of ovarian suppression with tamoxifen or an aromatase inhibitor should be considered in women with a high risk for recurrence given the disease-free survival benefit demonstrated by the SOFT and TEXT trials (82).
- An aromatase inhibitor should be the first-line recommendation in postmenopausal women (83).
- Among patients treated with tamoxifen, the ATLAS and aTTom trials demonstrated a disease-free and overall survival benefit with extended endocrine therapy, continuing therapy for an additional 5-year course for a total of 10 years (84,85).
- The MA.17R trial demonstrated a disease-free survival benefit with extended aromatase inhibitor therapy to 10 years; however, this was preceded in most patients by tamoxifen therapy. The optimal duration to extend endocrine therapy in women taking an aromatase inhibitor remains to be clearly defined. Preliminary results from the ABCSG-16 trial suggest an additional 2 years of anastrozole therapy may be as effective as 5 additional years of therapy (86,87).
- There is a significant rate of discontinuation and nonadherence to adjuvant hormonal therapy in women with early-stage hormone-sensitive breast cancer. At 4.5 years, about 32% of women discontinued therapy with 72% of the remaining women fully adherent to therapy. Nonadherence has been associated with increased mortality and is more commonly seen in women of younger age, those who have undergone breast-conserving surgery versus mastectomy, or those who have multiple comorbidities (88).
- Genomic assays have been increasingly used to determine the benefit of chemotherapy in early-stage hormone receptor–positive breast cancers. The use of the Oncotype DX 21-gene recurrence score was validated in the prospective TAILORx trial, and MammaPrint was shown in the MINDACT trial to improve prediction of clinical outcome in high-risk early-stage breast cancers (89,90).

- Adjuvant paclitaxel and trastuzumab in HER2-positive small (T1-2) node-negative cancers have been shown to effectively decrease the rate of relapse (less than 2% at 3 years) with few serious toxicities and should be considered in even early-stage patients (91).
- Adjuvant chemotherapy should be considered in small early-stage, node-negative triple-negative breast tumors measuring 0.5 cm or greater, as these patients have a higher risk of relapse compared to other breast tumor phenotypes.

RADIATION THERAPY TECHNIQUES FOR WHOLE-BREAST IRRADIATION

- Whole-breast irradiation is classically delivered in the supine position, but more recently, prone techniques have been shown to reduce dose to the underlying heart and lung, as well as reduce skin toxicity and respiratory motion, especially in women with large pendulous breasts (92).
- Although traditionally tumor doses of 50 Gy delivered at 2 Gy daily were common, hypofractionated schedules such as 42.56 Gy in 16 fractions have been shown to have little difference in local control and survival and are the preferred course for whole-breast therapy according to NCCN Guidelines (93).
- Radiation should be delivered ideally within 8 weeks of surgery, with a detriment to local control with longer delays (94).
- In vitro studies suggest tumor cells may be less sensitive to radiation in the presence to tamoxifen because of the cytostatic effect of tamoxifen on cells; however, retrospective studies that examine sequencing of tamoxifen with radiotherapy (concurrent versus sequential) do not report any difference in outcomes (95).

Beam Arrangement

- The entire breast and chest wall should be included in the irradiated volume, along with a small portion of underlying lung to account for motion during treatment because of normal breathing as shown in Figure 21-2.
- The tangent beams should be collimated to follow the curvature of the chest wall. Special attention should be paid to minimize the volume of lung and heart irradiated.
- The lateral/posterior margin should be placed 2 cm beyond all palpable breast tissue (usually near the midaxillary line), and the inferior margin is drawn 2 to 3 cm below the inframammary fold.
- Wedges (dynamic or static) or compensating filters must be used for a portion of the treatment to achieve a uniform dose distribution within the breast as shown in Figure 21-3.
- When treatment is delivered with 6-MV or lower-energy photons in patients with wide separation (greater than 22 cm), significant dose inhomogeneity may exist within the breast; this has been correlated with less-than-satisfactory cosmetic results. The problem can be minimized by using higher-energy photons (10 to 18 MV) to deliver a portion of the breast irradiation (approximately 50%), as determined with prospective treatment planning, to maintain inhomogeneity throughout the entire breast to 10% or less.
- Details regarding irradiation of the regional lymphatics and postmastectomy radiation are covered in Chapter 22.

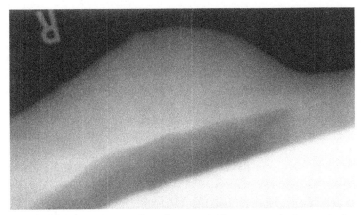

FIGURE 21-2. Example of localization film of tangential breast portals demonstrating amount of lung to be included in the field. (Reprinted with permission from Perez CA, Taylor ME. Breast: Tis, T1, and T2 tumors. In: Perez CA, Brady LW, eds. *Principles and practice of radiation oncology*, 3rd ed. Philadelphia, PA: Lippincott–Raven, 1998:1269–1414. © Wolters Kluwer.)

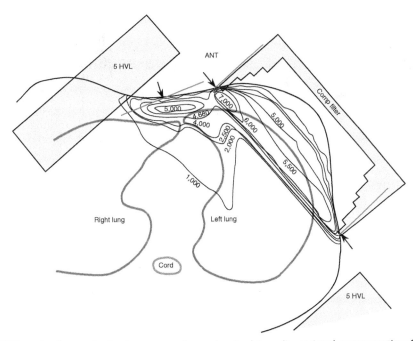

FIGURE 21-3. Composite isodose curves for customized two-dimensional compensating filters, beam splitter for tangential fields, and internal mammary portal treated with 4-MV photons (16 Gy) and 12-MeV electrons (30 Gy) or anterior oblique medial breast field. ANT, anterior. (Reprinted with permission from Perez CA, Taylor ME. Breast: Tis, T1, and T2 tumors. In: Perez CA, Brady LW, eds. *Principles and practice of radiation oncology*, 3rd ed. Philadelphia, PA: Lippincott–Raven, 1998:1269–1414. © Wolters Kluwer.)

Normal Tissue and Late Complications

- The primary organs at risk in the delivery of whole-breast radiation include the underlying lung, heart, and contralateral breast for which dose should be minimized.
- Hot spots in the treated breast should be minimized to 5% to 7% if possible. The total dose and irradiated volume receiving a boost dose have been correlated with the development of fibrosis (96).
- Rates of major coronary events increase linearly with the mean dose to the heart by 7.5% per gray with no apparent threshold (97).
- The volume of the left ventricle receiving 5 Gy (LV-V5) has also been shown to be a significant parameter in the prediction of acute coronary events, increasing by 16.5% per Gy (98).
- The risk of lymphedema following ALND or axillary irradiation was prospectively collected in the AMAROS trial. Lymphedema was observed significantly more often after ALND than axillary radiotherapy at 1-, 3-, and 5-year time points. At 5 years, the rate of lymphedema was 23% versus 11%, $p < 0.0001$ (61). Clinically significant lymphedema was defined as an increase in arm circumference by at least 10%.
- Apical pulmonary fibrosis is occasionally noted when the regional lymph nodes are irradiated. Symptomatic pneumonitis is infrequent and is related to the volume of lung irradiated. It may be enhanced by systemic therapies such as tamoxifen or Adriamycin-based regimens (99,100).

Follow-Up of Patients Treated with Conservation Surgery and Irradiation

- Monthly breast self-examinations should be emphasized, in addition to clinical examinations every 3 to 4 months for the first 3 years, every 6 months through the fifth year, and yearly thereafter.
- In patients with DCIS or invasive lesions, a baseline mammogram should be obtained 4 to 6 months after completion of treatment. Bilateral mammograms should be obtained every 6 months to 1 year for the first 2 or 3 years (as dictated by findings), and yearly thereafter.
- When there is strong evidence of suspicious microcalcifications, masses, or architectural distortions of the breast after conservation surgery and irradiation, a biopsy should be obtained to rule out a recurrence.
- Both mammography and periodic, careful physical examination are critical in the posttreatment evaluation of patients treated with breast conservation therapy. Posttreatment evaluation is mandatory at least once a year because of the possibility of late breast relapses and occasional distant metastases, even as late as 10 years after therapy.

References

1. Siegel RL, Miller KD, Jemal A. Cancer statistics, 2018. *CA Cancer J Clin* 2018;68:7–30.
2. Murthy RK, Valero V, Buchholz TA. Breast: overview. In: Gunderson L, Tepper J, eds. *Clinical radiation oncology*, 4th ed. Philadelphia, PA: Elsevier, 2016:1284–1302.

3. Morch LS, Skovlund CW, Hannaford PC, et al. Contemporary hormonal contraception and the risk of breast cancer. *N Engl J Med* 2017;377:2228–2239.

4. Wazer DE, Arthur DW. Breast: stage Tis. In: Halperin EC, Perez CA, Brady LW, eds. *Principles and practice of radiation oncology*, 5th ed. Philadelphia, PA: Lippincott Williams & Wilkins, 2008:1162–1174.

5. Haffty BG, Buchholz TA, Perez CA. Early stage breast cancer. In: Halperin EC, Perez CA, Brady LW, eds. *Principles and practice of radiation oncology*, 5th ed. Philadelphia, PA: Lippincott Williams & Wilkins, 2008:1175–1291.

6. Dershaw DD. Mammography in patients with breast cancer treated by breast conservation (lumpectomy with or without radiation). *Am J Roentgenol* 1995;164(2):309–316.

7. Perez CA, Taylor ME. Breast: Tis, T1, and T2 tumors. In: Perez CA, Brady LW, eds. *Principles and practice of radiation oncology*, 3rd ed. Philadelphia, PA: Lippincott–Raven, 1998:1269–1414.

8. Houssami N, Ciatto S, Macaskill P, et al. Accuracy and surgical impact of magnetic resonance imaging in breast cancer staging: systematic review and meta-analysis in detection of multifocal and multicentric cancer. *J Clin Oncol* 2008;26:3248–3258.

9. Tinnemans JG, Wobbes T, Holland R, et al. Treatment and survival of female patents with non palpable breast carcinoma. *Ann Surg* 1989;209(2):249–253.

10. Silverstein MJ, Skinner KA, Lomis TJ. Predicting axillary nodal positivity in 2282 patients with breast carcinoma. *World J Surg* 2001;25(6):767–772.

11. Kambouris AA. Axillary node metastases in relation to size and location of breast cancers: analysis of 147 patients. *Am Surg* 1996;62(7):519–524.

12. Greco M, Crippa F, Agresti R, et al. Axillary lymph node staging in breast cancer by 2-fluoro-2-deoxy-D-glucose-positron emission tomography: clinical evaluation and alternative management. *J Natl Cancer Inst* 2001;93(8):630–635.

13. Fein DA, Fowble BL, Hanon AL, et al. Identification of women with T1-T2 breast cancer at low risk of positive axillary nodes. *J Surg Oncol* 1997;65(1):34–39.

14. Wolff AC, Hammond EH, Hicks DG, et al.; American Society of Clinical Oncology/College of American Pathologists. Recommendations for human epidermal growth factor receptor 2 testing in breast cancer: American Society of Clinical Oncology/College of American Pathologists clinical practice guideline update. *J Clin Oncol* 2013;31(31):3997–4013.

15. Lakhani S, Ellis I, Schnitt S, et al. *WHO classification of tumours of the breast*, 4th ed. Lyon, France: IARC Press, 2012.

16. Amin MB, Edge SB, Greene FL, et al. *AJCC cancer staging manual*, 8th ed. New York, NY: Springer Verlag, 2017.

17. Edge SB, Byrd DR, Compton CC, eds. *AJCC cancer staging manual*, 7th ed. New York, NY: Springer Verlag, 2009.

18. Clarke M, Collins R, Darby S, et al. Effects of radiotherapy and differences in the extent of surgery for early breast cancer on local recurrence and 15-year survival: an overview of the randomized trials. *Lancet* 2005;366:2087–2106.

19. Veronesi U, Marubini E, Del Vecchio M, et al. Local recurrences and distant metastases after conservative breast cancer treatments: partly independent events. *J Natl Cancer Inst* 1995;87:19–27.

20. Fitzgibbons PL, Page DL, Weaver D, et al. Prognostic factors in breast cancer. College of American Pathologists Consensus Statement 1999. *Arch Pathol Lab Med* 2000;124:966–978.

21. de la Rochefordiere A, Asselain B, Campana F, et al. Age as prognostic factor in premenopausal breast carcinoma. *Lancet* 1993;341(8852):1039–1043.

22. Ansell D, Whitman S, Lipton R, et al. Race, income, and survival from breast cancer at two public hospitals. *Cancer* 1993;72(10):2974–2978.

23. Rosen PR, Groshen S, Saigo PE, et al. A long-term follow-up study of survival in stage I (T1N0M0) and stage II (T1N1M0) breast carcinoma. *J Clin Oncol* 1989;7:355–366.

24. Harris J, Lippman M, Morrow M, et al. *Diseases of the breast*. Philadelphia, PA: Lippincott Williams & Wilkins, 2004.

25. Elston CW, Ellis JO. Pathological prognostic factors in breast cancer: experience from a long study with long-term follow up. *Histopathology* 1991;19:403–410.

26. de Azambuja E, Cardoso F, de Castro G Jr, et al. Ki-67 as prognostic marker in early breast cancer: a meta-analysis of published studies involving 12,155 patients. *Br J Cancer* 2007;96(10):1504–1513.

27. Cheang MCU, Chia SK, Voduc D, et al. Ki67 index, HER2 status, and prognosis of patients with luminal B breast cancer. *J Natl Cancer Inst* 2009;101(10):736–750

28. Truong PT, Yong CM, Abnousi F, et al. Lymphovascular invasion is associated with reduced locoregional control and survival in women with node-negative breast cancer treated with mastectomy and systemic therapy. *J Am Coll Surg* 2005;200:912–921.

29. Crowe JP Jr, Gordon NH, Hubay CA, et al. Estrogen receptor determination and long term survival of patients with carcinoma of the breast. *Surg Gynecol Obstet* 1991;173:273–278

30. Sjogren S, Inganas M, Lindgren A, et al. Prognostic and predictive value of c-erbB-2 overexpression in primary breast cancer, alone and in combination with other prognostic markers. *J Clin Oncol* 1998;16:462–469.

31. Hoang MP, Sahin AA, Ordonez NG, et al. HER-2/neu gene amplification compared with HER-2/neu protein overexpression and interobserver reproducibility in invasive breast carcinoma. *Am J Clin Pathol* 2000;113:852–859.

32. Page DL, Kidd TE, Dupont WD, et al. Lobular neoplasia of the breast: higher risk for subsequent invasive cancer predicted by more extensive disease. *Hum Pathol* 1991;22:1232–1239.

33. Chuba PJ, Hamre MR, Yap J, et al. Bilateral risk for subsequent breast cancer after lobular carcinoma-in-situ: analysis of surveillance, epidemiology, and end results data. *J Clin Oncol* 2005;23:5534–5541.

34. Rendi MH, Dintzis SM, Lehman CD, et al. Lobular in-situ neoplasia on breast core needle biopsy: imaging indication and pathologic extent can identify which patients require excisional biopsy. *Ann Surg Oncol* 2012;19:914–921.

35. Vogel VG, Costantino JP, Wickerham DL, et al. National surgical adjuvant breast and bowel project update: prevention trials and endocrine therapy of ductal carcinoma in situ. *Clin Cancer Res* 2003;9:495–501.

36. Silverstein MJ, Lagio MD. Treatment selection for patients with ductal carcinoma in situ (DCIS) of the breast using the University of Southern California/Van Nuys (USC/VNPI) prognostic index. *Breast J* 2015;21:127–132.

37. Fisher ER, Leeming R, Anderson S, et al. Conservative management of intraductal carcinoma (DCIS) of the breast. *J Surg Oncol* 1991;47:139–147.

38. Francis AM, Haugen CE, Grimes LM, et al. Is sentinel lymph node dissection warranted for patients with a diagnosis of ductal carcinoma in situ? *Ann Surg Oncol* 2016;22:4270.

39. Solin LJ, Gray R, Hughes LL, et al. Surgical excision without radiation for ductal carcinoma in situ of the breast: 12-year results from the ECOG-ACRIN E5194 study. *J Clin Oncol* 2015;33(33): 3938–3944.

40. Wong JS, Kaelin CM, Troyan SL. Prospective study of wide excision alone for ductal carcinoma in situ of the breast. *J Clin Oncol* 2006;24(7):1031–1036.

41. Morrow M, Van Zee KJ, Solin LJ, et al. Society of Surgical Oncology-American Society for Radiation Oncology-American Society of Clinical Oncology Consensus Guideline on margins for breast-conserving surgery with whole-breast irradiation in ductal carcinoma in situ. *J Clin Oncol* 2016;34(33):4040–4046.

42. Wapnir IL, Dignam JJ, Fisher B, et al. Long-term outcomes of invasive ipsilateral breast tumor recurrences after lumpectomy in NSABP B-17 and B-24 randomized clinical trials for DCIS. *J Natl Cancer Inst* 2011;103(6):478–488.

43. Donker M, Litière S, Werutsky G, et al. Breast-conserving treatment with or without radiotherapy in ductal carcinoma in situ: 15-year recurrence rates and outcome after a recurrence, from the EORTC 10853 randomized phase III trial. *J Clin Oncol* 2013;31(32):4054–4059.

44. Cuzick J, Sestak I, Pinder SE, et al. Effect of tamoxifen and radiotherapy in women with locally excised ductal carcinoma in situ: long-term results from the UK/ANZ DCIS trial. *Lancet Oncol* 2010;12(1):21–29.

45. Early Breast Cancer Trialists' Collaborative Group (EBCTCG). Overview of the randomized trials of radiotherapy in ductal carcinoma in situ of the breast. *J Natl Cancer Inst Monogr* 2010;2010(41):162–177.

46. Thorsen LBJ, Offersen BV, Dano H, et al. DBCG-IN: a population-based cohort study on the effect of internal mammary node irradiation in early-node positive breast cancer. *J Clin Oncol* 2016;34(4):314–320.

47. Moran MS, Zhao Y, Ma S, et al. Association of radiotherapy boost for ductal carcinoma in situ with local control after whole-breast radiotherapy. *JAMA Oncol* 2017;3(8):1060–1068.

48. McCormick B, Winter K, Hudis C, et al. RTOG 9804: a prospective randomized trial for good-risk ductal carcinoma in situ comparing radiotherapy with observation. *J Clin Oncol* 2015;33(7):709–715.

49. Correa C, Harris EE, Leonardi MC, et al. Accelerated partial breast irradiation: executive summary for the update of an ASTRO evidence-based consensus statement. *Pract Radiat Oncol* 2017;7(2):73–79.

50. Allred DC, Anderson SJ, Paik S, et al, Adjuvant tamoxifen reduces subsequent breast cancer in women with estrogen receptor-positive ductal carcinoma in situ: a study based on NSABP protocol B-24. *J Clin Oncol* 2012;30(12):1268–1273.

51. Margolese R, Cecchini RS, Julian TB, et al. Primary results, NSABP B-35/NRG oncology: a clinical trial of anastrozole vs tamoxifen in postmenopausal patients with DCIS undergoing lumpectomy plus radiotherapy: a randomized clinical trial. *Lancet* 2016;387(10021):849–856.

52. Fisher B, Anderson S, Bryant J, et al. Twenty-year follow-up of a randomized trial comparing total mastectomy, lumpectomy, and lumpectomy plus irradiation for the treatment of invasive breast cancer. *N Engl J Med* 2002;347:1233–1241.

53. Veronesi U, Cascinelli N, Mariani L, et al. Twenty-year follow-up of a randomized study comparing breast-conserving surgery with radical mastectomy for early breast cancer. *N Engl J Med* 2002;347:1227–1232.

54. Poggi MM, Danforth DN, Sciuto LC, et al. Eighteen-year results in the treatment of early breast carcinoma with mastectomy versus breast conservation therapy: the National Cancer Institute Randomized Trial. *Cancer* 2003;98:697–702.

55. Early Breast Cancer Trialists' Collaborative Group (EBCTCG). Effect of radiotherapy after breast-conserving surgery on 10-year recurrence and 15-year breast cancer death: meta-analysis of individual patient data for 10,801 women in 17 randomised trials. *Lancet* 2011;378(9804):1707–1716.

56. Moran MS, Schnitt SJ, Giuliano AE, et al. SSO-ASTRO consensus guideline on margins for breast-conserving surgery with whole breast irradiation in stage I and II invasive breast cancer. *Int J Radiat Oncol Biol Phys* 2014;88(3):553–564.

57. Krag DN, Anderson SJ, Julian TB, et al. Sentinel-lymph-node resection compared with conventional axillary-lymph-node dissection in clinically node-negative patients with breast cancer: overall survival findings from the NSABP B-32 randomised phase 3 trial. *Lancet Oncol* 2010;11(10):927–933.

58. Veronesi U, Paganelli G, Viale G, et al. A randomized comparison of sentinel-node biopsy with routine axillary dissection in breast cancer. *N Engl J Med* 2003;349:546–553.

59. Giuliano AE, Ballman KV, McCall L, et al. Effect of axillary dissection vs no axillary dissection on 10-year overall survival among women with invasive breast cancer and sentinel node metastasis: the ACOSOG Z0011 (Alliance) randomized clinical trial. *JAMA* 2017;318(10):918–926.

60. Jagsi R, Chadha M, Moni J, et al. Radiation field design in the ACOSOG Z0011 (Alliance) trial. *J Clin Oncol* 2014;32(32):3600–3606.

61. Donker M, van Tienhoven G, Straver ME, et al. Radiotherapy or surgery of the axilla after a positive sentinel node in breast cancer (EORTC 10981-22023 AMAROS): a randomised, multicentre, open-label, phase 3 non-inferiority trial. *Lancet Oncol* 2014;15(12):1303–1310.

62. Whelan TJ, Olivotto IA, Parulekar WR, et al. Regional nodal irradiation in early-stage breast cancer. *N Engl J Med* 2015;373:307–316.

63. Poortmans PM, Collette S, Kirkove C, et al. Internal mammary and medial supraclavicular irradiation in breast cancer. *N Engl J Med* 2015;373:317–327.

64. Hennequin C, Bossard N, Servagi-Vernat S, et al. Ten-year survival results of a randomized trial of irradiation of internal mammary nodes after mastectomy. *Int J Radiat Oncol Biol Phys* 2013;86(5):860–866.

65. Budach W, Bölke E, Kammers K, et al. Adjuvant radiation therapy of regional lymph nodes in breast cancer—a meta-analysis of randomized trials—an update. *Radiat Oncol* 2015;10:258.

66. Bartelink H, Maingon P, Poortmans P, et al. Whole-breast irradiation with or without a boost for patients treated with breast-conserving surgery for early breast cancer: 20-year follow-up of a randomised phase 3 trial. *Lancet Oncol* 2015;16(1):47–56.

67. Romestaing P, Lehingue Y, Carrie C, et al. Role of a 10-Gy boost in the conservative treatment of early breast cancer: results of a randomized clinical trial in Lyon, France. *J Clin Oncol* 1997;15(3):963–968.

68. Vrieling C, van Werkhoven E, Maingon P, et al. Prognostic factors for local control in breast cancer after long-term follow-up in the EORTC boost vs no boost trial. *JAMA Oncol* 2017;3(1):42–48.

69. Lowery AJ, Kell MR, Glynn RW, et al. Locoregional recurrence after breast cancer surgery: a systematic review by receptor phenotype. *Breast Cancer Res Treat* 2012;133:831–841.

70. Poortmans PM, Collette L, Horiot J, et al. Impact of the boost dose of 10 Gy versus 26 Gy in patients with early stage breast cancer after a microscopically incomplete lumpectomy: 10-year results of the randomized EORTC boost trial. *Radiother Oncol* 2009;90:80–85.

71. Houssami N, Macaskill P, Marinovich ML, et al. The association of surgical margins and local recurrence with women with early-stage invasive breast cancer treated with breast-conserving therapy: a meta-analysis. *Ann Surg Oncol* 2014;21:717–730.

72. Strnad V, Ott OJ, Hildebrandt G, et al. 5-Year results of accelerated partial breast irradiation using sole interstitial multicatheter brachytherapy versus whole-breast irradiation with boost after breast-conserving surgery for low-risk invasive and in-situ carcinoma of the female breast: a randomised, phase 3, non-inferiority trial. *Lancet* 2016;387(10015):229–238.

73. Polgar C, Fodor J, Major T, et al. Breast-conserving therapy with partial or whole breast irradiation: ten-year results of the Budapest randomized trial. *Radiother Oncol* 2013;108(2): 197–202.

74. Livi L, Meattini I, Marrazzo L, et al. Accelerated partial breast irradiation using intensity-modulated radiotherapy versus whole breast irradiation: 5-year survival analysis of a phase 3 randomised controlled trial. *Eur J Cancer* 2015;51(4):451–463.

75. Shah C, Badiyan S, Wilkinson JB, et al. Treatment efficacy with accelerated partial breast irradiation (APBI): final analysis of the American Society of Breast Surgeons Mammosite® breast brachytherapy registry trial. *Ann Surg Oncol* 2013;20(10):3279–3285.

76. Veronesi U, Orecchia R, Maisonneuve P, et al. Intraoperative radiotherapy versus external radiotherapy for early breast cancer (ELIOT): a randomised controlled equivalence trial. *Lancet Oncol* 2013;14(13):1269–1277.

77. Vaidya JS, Wenz FW, Bulsara M, et al. Risk-adapted targeted intraoperative radiotherapy versus whole-breast radiotherapy for breast cancer: 5-year results for local control and overall survival from the TARGIT—a randomised trial. *Lancet* 2014;383(9917):603–613.

78. Fisher B, Bryant J, Dignam JJ, et al. Tamoxifen, radiation therapy, or both for prevention of ipsilateral breast tumor recurrence after lumpectomy in women with invasive breast cancers of one centimeter or less. *J Clin Oncol* 2002;20(20):4141–4149.

79. Hughes KS, Schnaper LA, Bellon JR, et al. Lumpectomy plus tamoxifen with or without irradiation in women age 70 years or older with early stage breast cancer: long-term follow-up of CALGB 9343. *J Clin Oncol* 2013;31(19):2382–2387.

80. Fyles AW, McCready DR, Manchul LA, et al. Tamoxifen with or without breast irradiation in women 50 years of age or older with early breast cancer. *N Engl J Med* 2004;351(10):963–970.

81. Kunkler IH, Wlliams LJ, Jack WJL, et al. Breast-conserving surgery with or without irradiation in women aged 65 years or older with early breast cancer (PRIME II): a randomised controlled trial. *Lancet Oncol* 2015;16(3):266–273.

82. Francis PA, Regan MM, Fleming GF, et al. Adjuvant ovarian suppression in premenopausal breast cancer. *N Engl J Med* 2015;372:436–446.

83. Early Breast Cancer Trialists' Collaborative Group (EBCTCG). Aromatase inhibitors versus tamoxifen in early breast cancer: patient-level meta-analysis of the randomised trials. *Lancet* 2015;386:1241–1252.

84. Davies C, Pan H, Godwin J, et al. Long-term effects of continuing adjuvant tamoxifen to 10 years versus stopping at 5 years after diagnosis of oestrogen receptor-positive breast cancer: ATLAS, a randomised trial. *Lancet* 2013;381(9869):805–816.

85. Gray RG, Rea DW, Handley K. ATTom: randomized trial of 10 versus 5 years of adjuvant tamoxifen among 6,934 women with estrogen receptor-positive (ER+) or ER untested breast cancer—preliminary results. *J Clin Oncol* 2008;26(Suppl. 10); abstr 513.

86. Goss PE, Ingle JN, Pritchard NJ, et al. Extending aromatase-inhibitor adjuvant therapy to 10 years. *N Engl J Med* 2016;375:209–219.

87. Gnant M, Steger G, Greil R, et al. A prospective randomized multi-center phase-III trial of additional 2 versus additional 5 years of anastrozole after initial 5 years of adjuvant endocrine therapy—results from 3,484 postmenopausal women in the ABCSG-16 trial. *Presented at 2017 San Antonio Breast Cancer Symposium*, December 5–9, 2017, San Antonio, TX, 2017; Abstract GS3-01.

88. Hershman DL, Shao T, Kushi LH, et al. Early discontinuation and non-adherence to adjuvant hormonal therapy are associated with increased mortality in women with breast cancer. *Breast Cancer Res Treat* 2011;126(2):529–537.

89. Cardoso F, van't Veer LJ, Bogaerts J, et al. 70-Gene signature as an aid to treatment decisions in early-stage breast cancer. *N Engl J Med* 2016;375:717–729.

90. Sparano JA, Gray RJ, Makower DF, et al. Prospective validation of a 21-gene expression assay in breast cancer. *N Engl J Med* 2015;373(21):2005–2014.

91. Tolaney SM, Barry WT, Dang CT, et al. Adjuvant paclitaxel and trastuzumab for node-negative, HER2-positive breast cancer. *N Engl J Med* 2015;372:134–141.

92. Huppert N, Jozsef G, DeWyngaert K, et al. The role of a prone setup in breast radiation therapy. *Front Oncol* 2011;1:31.

93. Smith BD, Bentzen SM, Correa CR, et al. Fractionation for whole breast irradiation: an American Society for Radiation Oncology (ASTRO) evidence-based guideline. *Int J Radiat Oncol Biol Phys* 2011;81(1):59–68.

94. Huang J, Barbera L, Brouwers M, et al. Doses delay in starting treatment affect the outcomes of radiotherapy? A systematic review. *J Clin Oncol* 2003;21(3):555–563.

95. Harris EER, Christensen VJ, Hwang W, et al. Impact of concurrent versus sequential tamoxifen with radiation therapy in early-stage breast cancer patients undergoing breast conservation treatment. *J Clin Oncol* 2005;23(1):11–16.

96. Borger JH, Kemperman H, Smitt HS, et al. Dose and volume effects on fibrosis after breast conservation therapy. *Int J Radiat Oncol Biol Phys* 1994;30(5):1073–1081.

97. Darby SC, Ewertz M, McGale P, et al. Risk of ischemic heart disease in women after radiotherapy for breast cancer. *N Engl J Med* 2013;368(11):987–998.

98. Van den Bogaard VAB, Ta BDP, van der Schaaf A, et al. Validation and modification of a prediction model for acute cardiac events in patients with breast cancer treated with radiotherapy based on three-dimensional dose distributions to cardiac substructures. *J Clin Oncol* 2017;35:1171–1178.

99. Bentzen SM, Skoczylas JZ, Overgaard M, et al. Radiotherapy-related lung fibrosis enhanced by tamoxifen. *J Natl Cancer Inst* 1996;88(13):918–922.

100. Rotstein S, Lax I, Svane G. Influence of radiation therapy on the lung-tissue in breast cancer patients: CT-assessed density changes and associated symptoms. *Int J Radiat Oncol Biol Phys* 1989;16(3):629–639.

CHAPTER 22

BREAST

LOCALLY ADVANCED (T3 AND T4), INFLAMMATORY, AND RECURRENT TUMORS

- Clinical or pathologic findings of locally advanced carcinoma at presentation include the following: tumor size greater than 5 cm, clinically or pathologically positive axillary lymph nodes, tumor of any size with direct extension to ribs, intercostal muscles, or skin; edema (including *peau d'orange*), ulceration of the breast skin, or satellite skin nodules confined to the same breast; inflammatory carcinoma (T4d); and metastases to ipsilateral internal mammary lymph nodes or ipsilateral axillary lymph nodes fixed to one another or other structures.

NATURAL HISTORY AND CLINICAL PRESENTATION

Locally Advanced (T3 and T4) Tumors

- Locally advanced breast cancer often arises from a tumor that has been present for a long period of time thereby allowing growth within the breast and spread to nearby areas including lymph nodes, skin, and muscle. Infiltration of the deep lymphatics of dermis causes edema of the skin and increased breast size. More pronounced edema (*peau d'orange*) can indicate superficial and deep lymphatic involvement. Often, localized erythema is apparent throughout the breast. If left untreated, this will result in ulceration and ultimately breast contraction, through tumor infiltration of Cooper's ligament. Further extensive involvement includes satellite nodules and carcinoma *en cuirasse*, as if the patient were wearing a coat of armor in which the skin becomes plaquelike, thick and yellowish, red, or gray.
- Less commonly, patients will report rapid onset and rapid enlargement of the breast with no specific palpable abnormality accompanied by redness and swelling. This is commonly referred to as inflammatory breast cancer. Often, biopsy of the skin covering the breast confirms tumor infiltration in the dermal lymphatics, or lymphatic tumor emboli, the hallmark of inflammatory breast cancer.

- Metastatic spread can occur through lymphatic or hematogenous spread; the former involving the axillary, internal mammary, or supraclavicular nodes and the latter causing spread to bone, lung, pleura, liver, and brain.
- Although their tumor characteristics may be different, inflammatory and locally advanced breast cancer are treated the same.

DIAGNOSTIC WORKUP

- A thorough physical exam must be performed paying particular attention to appearance of the breast, fixation to the chest wall, evident lymphadenopathy, and checking potential sites of spread. Radiographic evaluation of the breast will include mammogram and possibly ultrasound and magnetic resonance imaging (MRI). A repeat MRI may be particularly useful in evaluating response to neoadjuvant chemotherapy and to plan subsequent surgery.
- Laboratory studies include a complete blood cell count, serum chemistry profile, including full liver function tests. Some clinicians find breast tumor markers such as CEA, CA 15-3, or CA 27-29 useful in monitoring response to treatment.
- If liver function values are abnormal, a computed tomography (CT) scan of the abdomen should be obtained.
- If anemia, leukopenia, or thrombocytopenia is present, bone marrow biopsy is necessary.
- Radiographic studies include CT scan of chest, abdomen, and pelvis. Alternatively, some institutions utilize positron emission tomography (PET) (1) scans with or without CT to evaluate extent of disease.
- Bone scans are generally used less frequently but may be recommended for stage III or IV disease to further delineate abnormalities on the above studies and should always be included if CT or PET is not performed.
- If neurologic symptoms suggest cerebral metastases, a contrast-enhanced CT scan or gadolinium-enhanced MRI scan of the brain should be obtained; MRI is preferred if leptomeningeal spread of tumor is suspected.

PROGNOSTIC FACTORS

- One of the most important prognostic factors is response to neoadjuvant treatment (1–5). Patients who achieve a pathologic complete response to neoadjuvant therapy have been found to have improved overall and relapse-free survival, as illustrated in Figure 22-1. Other factors associated with increased poor prognosis include larger, more diffuse tumors, presence of edema, and number of involved axillary nodes.
- As with early-stage disease, tumors that are estrogen and progesterone negative and have *HER-2* overexpression signify more aggressive disease.

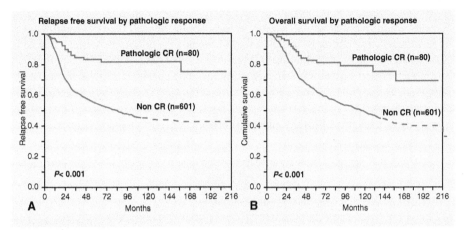

FIGURE 22-1. Pathologic response for a cohort of patients (*n* = 681; 91 not surgically resected). **A:** Correlation with relapse-free survival. **B:** Correlation with overall survival. (Reprinted with permission from Harris JR, Lippman ME, Morrow M, et al. *Diseases of the breast*, 3rd ed. Philadelphia, PA: Lippincott Williams & Wilkins, 2004:962. © Wolters Kluwer.)

GENERAL MANAGEMENT

- Because of a compelling need for systemic therapy, multiagent chemotherapy plays a primary role in the treatment of locally advanced breast tumors and therefore diagnosis is usually obtained by core biopsy and not surgical excision.
- Biopsy of any palpable lymph nodes should also be performed prior to initiation of chemotherapy to document malignancy.
- Neoadjuvant chemotherapy before surgical resection remains the cornerstone of treatment. The EORTC 10902 and NSABP B-18 compared pre- or postoperative chemotherapy and found there was no difference in overall survival; however, more patients were downstaged to allow lesser surgery, for example, lumpectomy (4,6,7,8).
- Subsequently, NSABP-27 demonstrated that the addition of a taxane (T) to doxorubicin and cyclophosphamide (AC) preoperatively versus AC alone followed by T postoperatively results in better complete pathologic response and disease-free survival (9,10).
- Studies have also shown a significant response using neoadjuvant hormone therapy (2,11).
- Radiation therapy and surgery each have important roles in optimizing locoregional tumor control.

Surgery

- Surgery should be performed on all patients with technically resectable disease. Borderline resectable and unresectable locally advanced breast cancers should be treated with definitive radiation therapy to the breast and regional lymph nodes prior to surgery (12).

- In marginal cases, it is important to have the patient evaluated by both the surgeon and the radiation oncologist so a joint decision about the next phase of treatment can be formulated. If a course of initial radiation therapy is chosen, the patient should be evaluated at 5,000 cGy. If the tumor is resectable, then surgery should be performed.
- At present, breast conservation therapy is an option for patients with locally advanced breast carcinoma (i.e., in women whose tumors respond significantly to neoadjuvant chemotherapy) (9).
- The treatment schema of locally advanced breast cancers is shown in Figure 22-2.

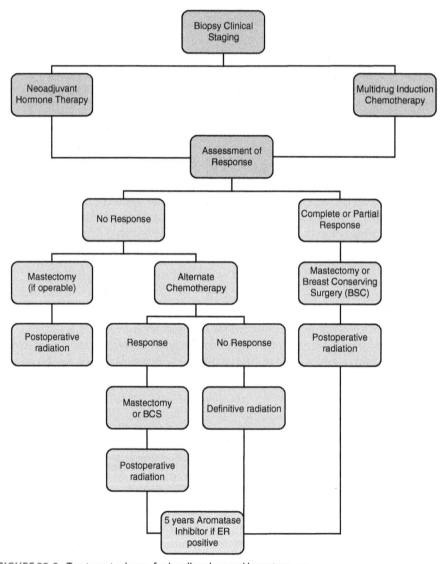

FIGURE 22-2. Treatment schema for locally advanced breast cancer.

Management of the Axilla After Neoadjuvant Therapy

- The application of sentinel lymph node dissection (SLND) following neoadjuvant therapy was explored by the American College of Surgeons Oncology Group (ACOSOG) Z1071 trial. Women with cT0-4 cN1-2 disease underwent SLND followed by a full axillary node dissection. SLND resulted in a false-negative rate (FNR) of 12.6%; this was significantly decreased when mapping was performed with the combination of both blue dye and radiolabeled colloid (10.8% vs. 20.3%, $p = 0.05$) and with the examination of at least 3 lymph nodes (FNR 9.1% for ≥ 3 SLNs vs. 21.1% for 2 SLNs, $p = 0.007$) (13).

- The Alliance A011202 trial is currently open to enrollment, and will help guide management of the axilla in women with upfront cN1 disease treated with neoadjuvant therapy. Patients with a positive SLN following neoadjuvant therapy are randomized to completion of an axillary lymph node dissection or axillary and regional nodal irradiation alone.

- Retrospective analysis of patients enrolled in NSAPB B-18 and B-27 identified predictors of locoregional recurrence (LRR) following neoadjuvant therapy. These patients were treated with neoadjuvant chemotherapy alone, with no adjuvant regional nodal irradiation following surgery. Independent predictors of LRR included age, clinical nodal status prior to neoadjuvant therapy, and pathologic nodal status/breast tumor response (14).

- The NRG Oncology/NSABP B-51/RTOG 1304 trial will examine the role for regional nodal irradiation in cN1 patients who achieve a complete pathologic response in the axilla following either mastectomy or breast-conserving surgery. These patients are randomized to comprehensive regional nodal irradiation or whole breast irradiation alone following breast-conserving surgery.

POSTMASTECTOMY RADIATION THERAPY

- In general, postmastectomy irradiation is recommended for lesions that were, at diagnosis, initially larger than 5 cm in diameter; any skin, fascial, or skeletal muscle involvement; poorly differentiated tumors, positive or close surgical margins, lymphatic permeation or inflammatory breast cancers, matted lymph nodes, two or more positive axillary lymph nodes, or gross extracapsular tumor extension.

- In an EBCTCG meta-analysis of 8,135 women who underwent mastectomy and axillary dissection, radiation to the chest wall and regional nodes reduced both recurrence (RR 0.68, $2p = 0.00006$) and breast cancer mortality (RR 0.78, $2p = 0.01$) in women with one to three positive lymph nodes (15).

- In most patients, the chest wall is irradiated with tangential photon beams, and the supraclavicular, axillary, and, as required, internal mammary lymph nodes are irradiated with techniques similar to those described in Figure 22-3.

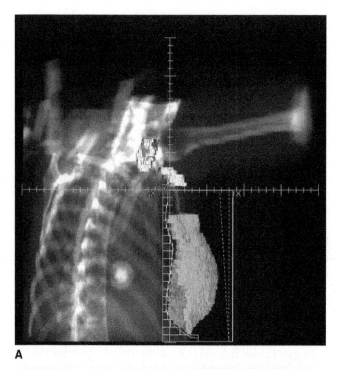

A

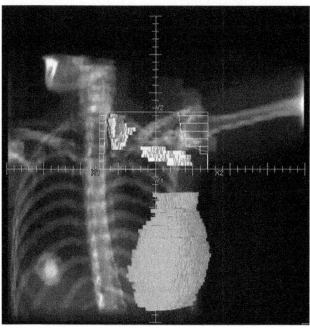

B

FIGURE 22-3. IMRT treatment planning for breast cancer. **A** and **B:** Beam's eye three-dimensional view of locoregional breast/chest wall irradiation.

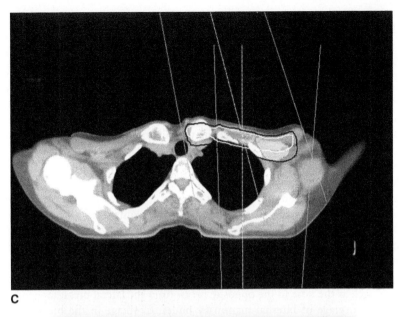

C

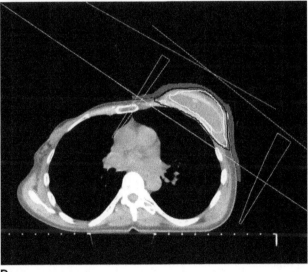

D

FIGURE 22-3. (*Continued*) **C:** Field setup for axillary supraclavicular irradiation. **D:** Field setup for breast/chest wall tangential irradiation.

RADIATION THERAPY TECHNIQUES

Irradiation of the Inoperable Breast

- Patients with technically inoperable tumors should be irradiated to the breast, supra-clavicular nodes, internal mammary nodes, and axillary nodes if clinically indicated.
- The breast is treated with photons through tangential fields with borders similar to those used in early breast cancer, ensuring that all potential tumor-bearing tissues are adequately covered.
- Treatment of the intact breast and draining lymphatics in patients with advanced breast cancer presents several technical challenges.
- Homogeneous irradiation of the breast tissue.
- Adequate skin and dermal dose, with bolus usually required for a significant portion of the treatment (50%).
- Precise matching between the plane of the inferior border of the supraclavicular field with the plane of the superior border of the medial and lateral breast tangential fields.
- Minimal beam divergence into the lung from the medial and lateral breast tangential fields as well as the dose to the opposite breast from the lateral breast tangential.
- Adequate coverage of internal mammary nodes. Coverage in the breast tangential fields often results in irradiation of additional lung volume. Various techniques including intensity-modulated radiation therapy (IMRT), field within a field, and partial treatment using electron fields may all be used to lower the ipsilateral lung dose. Successful plans allow less than 30% of the lung to receive 20 Gy; use of a sepa-rate, single electron field may lower the heart and lung dose (1).

Irradiation of the Chest Wall

- Irradiation of the chest wall after mastectomy can be accomplished with tangential photon fields (as in the intact breast) or with appositional electron beams.
- Bolus may be necessary over the entire field for part of the treatment.
- Several electron beam techniques can be used as an alternative to tangential photon treatment, the simplest is a single appositional field using 6- to 12-MeV electrons. CT scans assist in determining the thickness of the chest wall to select the optimal electron beam energy. Bolus should be used for part of the treatment to increase the surface dose beyond the 80% to 90% typically given with these beams, and to mini-mize the lung dose.

Field Borders

- Anatomic landmarks defining the field borders for treatment of breast/chest wall tan-gentials, supraclavicular nodes, internal mammary nodes, and axilla are similar to those used to treat early breast cancer and are outlined on the treatment planning CT by using the following guidelines:
  - The breast: duct tissue begins anywhere from midline up to 2 cm laterally and extends roughly to the midaxillary line. It is visible cranially caudally from 1 to 2 cm beneath the clavicle to the inframammary fold.

- The clinically significant internal mammary nodes at levels 1, 2, and 3 are found immediately lateral to the manubrium sternum inferiorly to the level of the carina.
- The supraclavicular nodal drainage area begins behind the medial clavicle extending to the medial two thirds of the clavicle and superiorly 5 cm.
- Examples of field arrangements for irradiation of the chest wall and regional lymphatics are shown in Figure 22-3.

Matchline Technique

- Many methods have been used to achieve an ideal match of the anterior-oblique supraclavicular-field caudal edge and the cephalad edge of the tangential field.
- A nondivergent supraclavicular-field edge is achieved by blocking the inferior half of the field.
- Various methods achieve a nondivergent edge from the tangential beams, including blocking and table angulation with collimator angulation combined.
- Multiple reports describe techniques using custom cerrobend blocking for the cephalad-tangential border (1).
- Another technique uses a gravity-orbited block to achieve a nondivergent edge independent of gantry angle. Use of a half-beam block that can be rotated is another matching technique.
- Precision in daily setup requires careful technical attention.
- Many use an asymmetric-jaws technique to beam-split all portals along the central axis plane. This technique uses one isocenter to treat the opposed tangential breast field, supraclavicular portal, and posterior axillary field. With the precision match line, the patient does not have to move in any direction on the treatment couch (16).

Doses

- Total dose to the entire breast or chest wall and regional nodes is 50 Gy in 1.8- to 2.0-Gy daily fractions.
- Internal mammary nodes, supraclavicular fossa nodes, and axillary nodal areas should receive 45 to 50 Gy if no macroscopic tumor is present.
- If surgery is not feasible, the breast should be given an additional 20 to 25 Gy with external irradiation (electrons or photons). This should be performed with shrinking fields. The boost dose is determined by extent of residual disease.
- In patients with close or positive margins, a boost of 10 to 15 Gy is given to a reduced volume with "mini tangential" photon or appositional electron beam portals. Any gross nodal disease should also be boosted with an additional 10 to 15 Gy.
- Khan et al. recently demonstrated in a prospective phase II trial that hypofractionation of postmastectomy radiation therapy (PMRT) is safe and effective at a dose of 36.63 Gy in 11 fractions (17).
- The safety of treating regional nodes, as well as complications in the reconstructed chest wall when delivering hypofractionated PMRT is the focus of the ongoing Alliance A221505 trial.

LOCOREGIONAL RECURRENCE AFTER MASTECTOMY

- LRR after mastectomy is recurrent cancer in the bone, muscle, skin, or subcutaneous tissue of the chest wall.
- Regional involvement may include lymph nodes in the axilla, supraclavicular, or infraclavicular region; ipsilateral internal mammary lymph nodes; or retropectoral lymph nodes.
- LRRs may be isolated or concomitant with distant metastases; complete restaging workup is mandatory.
- Patients developing LRR may be treated with a combination of irradiation, surgery, or systemic therapy.
- The CALOR trial demonstrated a disease-free and overall survival benefit with the use of adjuvant chemotherapy for locally recurrent breast cancer. The benefit was greatest in women with estrogen receptor–negative disease (18).
- Surgical management may consist of local excision for purposes of debulking, or may be extensive as in chest wall resection.
- In the treatment of chest wall recurrences with irradiation, results from Washington University, St. Louis, Missouri, documented the importance of treating the entire chest wall, and not merely a small local field, to reduce subsequent locoregional failures (19). Other series have confirmed this observation (20).
- A second issue in the treatment of isolated LRRs is elective irradiation of the chest wall and regional lymphatics to prevent second recurrences in these sites.
- Irradiation doses of 50 Gy are given to electively treated areas and to areas where recurrent tumors have been completely excised.
- For unresected lesions smaller than 3 cm, 60 to 65 Gy should be given; larger masses require 65 to 75 Gy (19). Several series have demonstrated a dose response for local tumor control (18).
- The decision to treat the dissected axilla in a chest wall recurrence will depend on the extent of tumor present and extracapsular spread.
- Patients with chest wall recurrence after breast reconstruction generally have local tumor control and disease-free and overall survival similar to those of patients not having surgical reconstruction (21).
- Breast reconstruction and irradiation are not incompatible, but complications and cosmetic failures do occur (22).

SEQUELAE OF THERAPY

- Radiation sequelae are related to irradiated volume, total dose, and concurrent chemotherapy.
- After definitive irradiation for advanced carcinoma of the breast at M.D. Anderson Cancer Center, 20% of patients developed severe subcutaneous fibrosis; 5% to 10% had rib fractures and symptomatic pneumonitis; and a lower percentage had soft tissue and skin necrosis and ulceration (23). Patients treated with three weekly fractions had a higher incidence of late complications than those who received five weekly fractions.

- At the Joint Center in Boston, 1.4% of 565 patients developed symptomatic brachial plexopathy; most patients received adjuvant chemotherapy (24).
- When treating the chest wall and regional draining lymphatics, by using CT-based planning and conformal treatment techniques, the complications to the lung are 1% (8). The risk of heart complications is slightly higher at 4% to 5% but can be kept to a minimum by keeping the maximum distance from field edge to heart (maximum heart distance) at 1 cm (25).

References

1. Buchholz TA, Haffty BG. Breast cancer: locally advanced and recurrent disease, postmastectomy radiation, and systemic therapies. In: Halperin EC, Perez CA, Brady LW, eds. *Principles and practice of radiation oncology.* Philadelphia, PA: Lippincott Williams & Wilkins, 2008:1292–1317.
2. Hortobagyi G, Singletary S, Strom E. Locally advanced breast cancer. In: Harris, JR, Lippman ME, Morrow M, et al., eds. *Diseases of the breast,* 3rd ed. Philadelphia, PA: Lippincott Williams & Wilkins, 2004:951–969.
3. Perez CA, Graham ML, Taylor ME, et al. Management of locally advanced carcinoma of the breast. I. Noninflammatory. *Cancer* 1994;74(1 suppl.):453–465.
4. Singletary SE, McNeese MD, Hortobagyi GN. Feasibility of breast-conservation surgery after induction chemotherapy for locally advanced breast carcinoma. *Cancer* 1992;69(11):2849–2852.
5. Valagussa P, Zambetti M, Bonadonna G, et al. Prognostic factors in locally advanced noninflammatory breast cancer. Long-term results following primary chemotherapy. *Breast Cancer Res Treat* 1990;15(3):137–147.
6. Fisher B, Bryant J, Wolmark N, et al. Effect of preoperative chemotherapy on the outcome of women with operable breast cancer. *J Clin Oncol* 1998;16(8):2672–2685.
7. Fisher ER, Wang J, Bryant J, et al. Pathobiology of preoperative chemotherapy: findings from the National Surgical Adjuvant Breast and Bowel (NSABP) protocol B-18. *Cancer* 2002;95(4):681–695.
8. van der Hage JA, van de Velde CJ, Julien JP, et al. Preoperative chemotherapy in primary operable breast cancer: results from the European Organization for Research and Treatment of Cancer trial 10902. *J Clin Oncol* 2001;19(22):4224–4237.
9. Bear HD, Anderson S, Brown A, et al. The effect on tumor response of adding sequential preoperative docetaxel to preoperative doxorubicin and cyclophosphamide: preliminary results from National Surgical Adjuvant Breast and Bowel Project Protocol B-27. *J Clin Oncol* 2003;21(22):4165–4174.
10. Rastogi P, Anderson SJ, Bear HD, et al. Preoperative chemotherapy: updates of National Surgical Adjuvant Breast and Bowel Project Protocols B-18 and B-27. *J Clin Oncol* 2008;26(5):778–785.
11. Krainick-Strobel UE, Lichtenegger W, Wallwiener D, et al. Neoadjuvant letrozole in postmenopausal estrogen and/or progesterone receptor positive breast cancer: a phase IIb/III trial to investigate optimal duration of preoperative endocrine therapy. *BMC Cancer* 2008;8:62.
12. Touboul E, Buffat L, Lefranc JP, et al. Possibility of conservative local treatment after combined chemotherapy and preoperative irradiation for locally advanced noninflammatory breast cancer. *Int J Radiat Oncol Biol Phys* 1996;34(5):1019–1028.
13. Boughey JC, Suman VJ, Mittendorf EA, et al. Sentinel lymph node surgery after neoadjuvant chemotherapy in patients with node-positive breast: the ACOSOG Z1071 (Alliance) clinical trial. *JAMA* 2013;310(14):1455–1461.
14. Mamounas EP, Anderson SJ, Dignam JJ, et al. Predictors of locoregional recurrence after neoadjuvant chemotherapy: results from combined analysis of National Surgical Adjuvant Breast and Bowel Project B-18 and B-27. *J Clin Oncol* 2012;30(32):3960–3966.

15. Early Breast Cancer Trialists' Collaborative Group (EBCTCG) Meta-Analysis. Effect of radiotherapy after mastectomy and axillary surgery on 10-year recurrence and 20-year breast cancer mortality: meta-analysis of individual patient data for 8135 women in 22 randomised trials. *Lancet* 2014;383:2127–2135.

16. Klein EE, Taylor M, Michaletz-Lorenz M, et al. A mono isocentric technique for breast and regional nodal therapy using dual asymmetric jaws. *Int J Radiat Oncol Biol Phys* 1994;28(3):753–760.

17. Khan AJ, Poppe MM, Goyal S, et al. Hypofractionated postmastectomy radiation therapy is safe and effective: first results from a prospective phase II trial. *J Clin Oncol* 2017;35(18):2037–2043.

18. Aebi S, Gelber S, Anderson SJ, et al. Chemotherapy for isolated locoregional recurrence of breast cancer: the CALOR randomised trial. *Lancet Oncol* 2014;15(3):156–163.

19. Halverson KJ, Perez CA, Kuske RR, et al. Isolated local-regional recurrence of breast cancer following mastectomy: radiotherapeutic management. *Int J Radiat Oncol Biol Phys* 1990;19(4):851–858.

20. Stadler B, Kogelnik HD. Local control and outcome of patients irradiated for isolated chest wall recurrences of breast cancer. *Radiother Oncol* 1987;8(2):105–111.

21. Chu FC, Kaufmann TP, Dawson GA, et al. Radiation therapy of cancer in prosthetically augmented or reconstructed breasts. *Radiology* 1992;185(2):429–433.

22. Kuske RR, Schuster R, Klein E, et al. Radiotherapy and breast reconstruction: clinical results and dosimetry. *Int J Radiat Oncol Biol Phys* 1991;21(2):339–346.

23. Spanos WJ Jr, Montague ED, Fletcher GH. Late complications of radiation only for advanced breast cancer. *Int J Radiat Oncol Biol Phys* 1980;6(11):1473–1476.

24. Salner AL, Botnick LE, Herzog AG, et al. Reversible brachial plexopathy following primary radiation therapy for breast cancer. *Cancer Treat Rep* 1981;65(9–10):797–802.

25. Hurkmans CW, Borger JH, Bos LJ, et al. Cardiac and lung complication probabilities after breast cancer irradiation. *Radiother Oncol* 2000;55(2):145–151.

CHAPTER 23

STOMACH

ANATOMY

- The stomach begins at the gastroesophageal junction (GEJ) and ends at the pylorus. The region immediately adjacent to the GEJ is the cardia, and the remainder can be further divided (from proximal to distal) into the fundus, the body, and the antrum. A plane passing through the incisura angularis on the lesser curvature divides the body and the antrum.
- There is variable visceral peritoneal (serosa) covering at the most proximal portion of the GEJ.
- The stomach's vascular supply is derived from the celiac axis, which originates at or below T12 in about 75% of patients and at or above L1 in 25% of patients.
- Lymphatic drainage follows the arterial supply. Although most lymphatics drain ultimately to the celiac nodal area, lymph drainage sites can include the splenic hilum, suprapancreatic nodal groups, porta hepatis, and gastroduodenal areas.

EPIDEMIOLOGY

- In the United States, there were an estimated 26,000 new cases in 2016 and 10,000 deaths (1). Globally, stomach cancer was the most common malignancy in the 1970s and 1980s, but now is fifth most common behind lung, breast, colorectum, and prostate with 952,000 cases in 2012 (2).
- The highest incidence rates are in Eastern Asia (which may represent a molecularly distinct malignancy), Eastern Europe, and South America.
- Risk factors include smoked and salted foods, nitrates, low intake of fruit and vegetables, obesity, smoking, alcohol, chronic gastritis/GERD, atrophic gastritis, *Helicobacter pylori* infection, and prior gastric surgery or RT.
- Gastric ulcer *per se* may not carry increased risk above and beyond the shared risk factor of *H. pylori* infection, although previous distal gastrotomy for benign disease confers a 1.5- to 3.0-fold relative risk of developing gastric cancer with a latency period of 15 to 20 years (3).

- *H. pylori* is associated with an approximately 6-fold greater risk of gastric cancer. This association may be confined to those with distal gastric cancer and intestinal-type malignancy (4).

NATURAL HISTORY

- Cancer of the stomach may extend directly into the omenta, pancreas, diaphragm, transverse colon or mesocolon, and duodenum.
- Peritoneal contamination is possible after a lesion extends beyond the gastric wall to a free peritoneal (serosal) surface (5).
- The liver and lungs are common sites of distant metastases for GEJ lesions. With gastric lesions that do not extend to the esophagus, the initial site of distant metastasis is usually the liver.
- It is difficult to perform a complete node dissection because of the numerous pathways of lymphatic drainage from the stomach (Fig. 23-1). Initial drainage is to perigastric lymph nodes along the lesser and greater curvatures (gastric and gastroepiploic nodes), and drainage continues to the celiac axis (left gastric, splenic, porta hepatis, suprapancreatic, and pancreaticoduodenal nodes), adjacent paraaortics, and distal paraesophageal system.

CLINICAL PRESENTATION

- The most common presenting symptoms are loss of appetite, abdominal discomfort, weight loss, weakness (from anemia), nausea and vomiting, and melena.

DIAGNOSTIC WORKUP

- A thorough history and physical examination is standard.
- Diagnosis is usually confirmed by upper gastrointestinal imaging and esophagogastroduodenoscopy (EGD). Endoscopy with direct vision, cytology, and biopsy yields the diagnosis in 90% or more of exophytic lesions.
- Endoscopic ultrasound is the most accurate method of assessing tumor (T) and nodal (N) stage.
- Abdominal computed tomography (CT) with contrast can be useful in determining suspicion for involvement of locoregional lymph nodes. CT of the chest, abdomen, and pelvis can also be useful to detect metastatic lesions.
- Traditionally, positron emission tomography (PET)/CT imaging was considered to be less sensitive for gastric cancer, especially for signet ring cancers (6), and especially for T and N staging. It still plays a useful role in detecting metastatic disease (7).
- Diagnostic laparoscopy to rule out peritoneal seeding is recommended for cT3-T4 and/or cN+ tumors. Positive findings are considered M1.

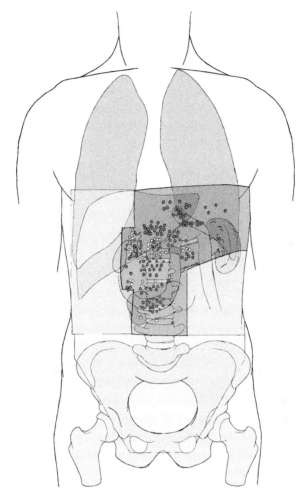

FIGURE 23-1. Patterns of failure in 82 evaluable patients in the University of Minnesota Reoperation series. *Large solid circles* indicate local failures in surrounding organs or tissues; *large open circles* indicate lymph node failures. (Adapted with permission from Gunderson LL, Sosin H. Adenocarcinoma of the stomach: areas of failure in a reoperation series (second or symptomatic looks): clinicopathologic correlation and implications of adjuvant therapy. *Int J Radiat Oncol Biol Phys* 1982;8:1–11.)

STAGING SYSTEMS

- Siewert Classification of GEJ tumors (8)
  - Type I: adenocarcinoma of distal esophagus; may infiltrate the GEJ from above
  - Type II: carcinoma of the cardia arising immediately at the GEJ
  - Type III: subcardial carcinoma that infiltrates the GEJ from below
- The updated 8th edition AJCC TNM groups with the main differences from the 7th edition are shown below (9).

NEW! **SUMMARY OF CHANGES TO AJCC STAGING**

STOMACH[a]

- Distinction between esophageal and stomach cancers has been refined: tumors involving the GEJ with the tumor epicenter no more than 2 cm into the proximal stomach are staged as esophageal cancers. GEJ tumors with their epicenter greater than 2 cm into the proximal stomach are staged as stomach cancers. Tumors less than 2 cm into the proximal stomach that do not involve the GEJ are staged as stomach cancers.
- Stage groupings have been changed:
  - There is now a separate stage grouping for cTNM compared to pTNM.
  - The division of N3 into N3a and N3b, while present in the 7th edition, is now being incorporated into pTNM stage grouping.
  - pT4aN2M0 and pT4bN0M0 were moved from stage IIIB to IIIA. pT4bN2M0 was moved from stage IIIC to IIIB.

[a]Lymphomas, sarcomas, and carcinoid tumors (low-grade neuroendocrine tumors) are not included.

See Amin MA, Greene FL, Edge S, et al. *AJCC cancer staging manual*, 8th ed. New York, NY: Springer, 2017 (9).

PATHOLOGIC CLASSIFICATION

- Adenocarcinoma accounts for 90% to 95% of all gastric malignancies. The two main histologic types of gastric adenocarcinoma are "intestinal type" and "diffuse type."
  - "Intestinal type": more differentiated, distal, older, male, associated with environmental risk factors listed above
  - "Diffuse type": less differentiated, proximal, younger, women, associated with genetic risk factors such as E-cadherin (*CDH1*) loss of function mutations and type A blood group
- Lymphoma, usually with unfavorable histology, is the second most common malignancy.

PROGNOSTIC FACTORS

- Important prognostic indicators include tumor extent, lymph node involvement, and the number and location of nodes affected.
- CEA and CA 19-9 levels are not prognostic, but may be useful for monitoring.
- It is controversial if HER2 status is prognostic, but if positive, HER2-directed therapy should be considered based on an overall survival (OS) benefit seen in the ToGA trial (10).
- Microsatellite instability high patients appear to have a better prognosis.

GENERAL MANAGEMENT

- The primary treatment modality in the management of gastric cancer is surgery. Operative attempts are highly successful if disease is limited to the mucosa, but the incidence of such early lesions at diagnosis is less than 5% in most United States series.
- Endoscopic mucosal resection may be considered for favorable early-stage disease: Tis-T1a, ≤3 cm, nonulcerated, low grade, N0.
- For lesions arising in the body or antrum, the preferred treatment is radical subtotal gastrectomy, if satisfactory margins can be achieved. This operation removes approximately 80% of the stomach with the node-bearing tissue, the gastrohepatic and gastrocolic omenta, and the first portion of the duodenum. Total gastrectomy does not offer improved locoregional control, and leads to increased morbidity and mortality. Proximal lesions, however, often require total gastrectomy to achieve adequate margins.
- The propensity for gastric carcinoma to spread by means of submucosal lymphatics suggests that a 3- to 5-cm margin of normal tissue proximally and distally may be optimal.
- The increasing incidence of T3 and T4 GEJ tumors has resulted in a greater incidence of microscopically positive radial margins. The peri-gastric tissue surrounding the GEJ and distal esophagus has no serosa, so lesions that extend to the margin at this site often represent "true" positive margins.
- The optimal extent of lymph node dissection is controversial. Two prospective randomized trials of lymphadenectomies showed no survival advantage with more extensive lymph node dissection (11,12). Sixteen or more lymph nodes removed is considered an adequate dissection.
  - D0: no nodes removed
  - D1: peri-gastric nodes less than 3 cm from stomach
  - D2: D1 + nodes of the celiac axis, splenic artery, left gastric artery, omentum, and peri-gastric nodes greater than 3 cm from stomach
  - D3: D2 + hepatoduodenal, peripancreatic, mesenteric axes, portocaval, and P-A nodes
- Disease progression within the abdomen is approximately 57%. Abdominal treatment should also address peritoneal seeding, which occurs in 23% to 43% of postgastrectomy patients (3).
- Surgery alone without adjuvant therapy is likely adequate for T1N0 and T2N0 disease without high-risk factors.

Multimodality Management

- Combination radiation therapy and chemotherapy are capable of sterilizing residual disease. Multimodality management is recommended with involved nodes, T3 or T4 primary lesions, or with close/+ margins. Other risk factors (e.g., LVI, bulky disease) should also be considered.
- Currently, there are two primary standards of care approaches to locally advanced gastric cancer: adjuvant concurrent chemoradiation therapy or perioperative chemotherapy.

- The US GI Intergroup Gastric Adjuvant Trial (INT-0116) evaluated the benefit of adjuvant combined modality therapy in the postoperative setting for patients with disease extension through the gastric wall and/or nodes positive for tumor. Five hundred and fifty-six patients with stage IB to IV M0 adenocarcinoma of the stomach or GEJ underwent R0 resection of adenocarcinoma of the stomach and were then randomized to surgery plus postoperative chemoradiation or surgery alone. Combined modality therapy (bolus 5-fluorouracil [5-FU]/leucovorin × 1 → 45 Gy + 5-FU/leucovorin × 2 → 5-FU/leucovorin × 2) increased median survival to 36 months compared to 27 months in the surgery-only arm (p = 0.005). Both 3-year relapse-free survival (RFS) and 3-year OS were improved with combined modality therapy (13). Updated results with 10-year follow-up confirmed persistent benefit for OS and RFS (14).
- The UK MRC phase III MAGIC trial randomized 503 patients with resectable stage II to IV M0 carcinoma of the stomach (74%), GEJ (11.5%), and esophagus (14.5%) to either surgery alone or surgery with perioperative chemotherapy consisting of epirubicin, cisplatin, and continuous infusion 5-FU. Perioperative chemotherapy was seen to improve both 5-year OS (36% versus 23%, p = 0.009) and progression-free survival (15).
- To date, it is uncertain whether either of these two evidence-based approaches should be preferred. More recent and ongoing studies are attempting to address this. Neoadjuvant chemoradiation therapy is also currently under investigation in gastric adenocarcinoma based on promising results from esophageal and GEJ studies (16,17), given the potential to downstage patients and increase the chance of R0 resection.
  - ARTIST I: 458 patients with T3-4 or N+ gastric adenocarcinoma after R0 gastrectomy and D2 lymphadenectomy were randomized to capecitabine + cisplatin (XP) versus XP → CRT 45 Gy with capecitabine → XP. There was no DFS or OS difference at 7-year follow-up, except the CRT arm was superior in DFS for node-positive and intestinal-type disease (18,19).
  - CRITICS: 788 patients with stage Ib to IVa resectable gastric cancer were treated with neoadjuvant triple-agent chemotherapy (ECX/EOX) followed by surgery, and were then randomized to postoperative chemotherapy (ECX/EOX) versus CRT (45 Gy with cisplatin and capecitabine). Preliminary results showed no difference in OS at 5 years (41.3% for chemotherapy versus 40.9% for CRT, p = 0.99) (20).
  - RTOG 99-04: Phase II trial of 43 localized resectable gastric adenocarcinoma patients treated with neoadjuvant chemotherapy followed by preoperative CRT. Pathologic complete response rate was 26% (21).
- In patients that are either not technically resectable or medically inoperable, definitive treatment can be given with radiation therapy, usually administered with concomitant 5-FU-based chemotherapy. Cisplatin + 5-FU/capecitabine, as well as carboplatin + paclitaxel are common combinations.
- In a Gastrointestinal Tumor Study Group randomized trial of patients with localized gastric cancer whose disease was not resected for cure, combined RT and chemotherapy was associated with increased early treatment-related morbidity and mortality but longer follow-up showed improved OS (18% versus 7% at 4 years) (22).
- In a European Organization for Research and Treatment of Cancer trial among patients with incompletely resected tumors, all long-term survivors received both concomitant and post-RT chemotherapy (23).

Table 23-1			
Patterns of Locoregional Failure after Resection of Gastric Cancer			
Failure Area	Clinical[a]	Incidence (%) Reoperation[b]	Autopsy[c]
Gastric bed	21	54	52–68
Anastomosis or stumps	25	26	54–60
Abdominal or stab wound	—	5	—
Lymph node(s)	8	42	52

[a]130 patients at risk (5).
[b]107 patients at risk (24).
[c]92 patients at risk (25) and 28 patients at risk (12).

RADIATION THERAPY TECHNIQUES

- Based on the sites of locoregional failure (Table 23-1), the gastric tumor bed, anastomosis and stump, and regional lymphatics should be included in all patients. Major nodal chains at risk include lesser and greater curvature, celiac axis, pancreaticoduodenal, splenic, suprapancreatic, and porta hepatis. With proximal gastric lesions or those at the G-E junction, a 3- to 5-cm margin of distal esophagus should be included.
- Traditionally, parallel-opposed anteroposterior-posteroanterior fields were commonly used, with an average field size of 15 × 15 cm. With single daily fractions, the usual dose is 45 to 50.4 Gy delivered in 1.8-Gy fractions. Boost fields to small areas of residual disease can sometimes be carried to doses of 55 to 60 Gy.
- Given the proximity of nearby organs at risk, toxicity from RT is a significant concern. This has been borne out with the low rates of patients able to complete planned therapy in many of the important studies in gastric cancer (e.g., only 52% in the chemo-RT arm in the CRITICS trial).
- IMRT, IGRT, and potentially magnetic resonance imaging (MRI)-guided RT provide technologically sophisticated methods of improving radiation dose delivery while sparing adjacent structures.
- Respiratory motion management should be considered when organ motion is significant.

NORMAL TISSUE COMPLICATIONS—QUANTEC RESULTS

Kavanagh et al. (26) present recommendations from the QUANTEC study, published in the special supplement of the *International Journal of Radiation Oncology Biology Physics*:

- Literature on RT-induced stomach toxicity is relatively sparse, with insufficient data to arrive at firm dose-volume constraints for partial volume irradiation. Doses of RT on the order of 45 Gy to the whole stomach are associated with late effects (primarily ulceration) in approximately 5% to 7% of patients. Data suggest that the maximum point dose might be an important predictor of toxicity, but corroborating data are needed to confirm this hypothesis. For stereotactic body radiation therapy (SBRT), the volume of stomach receiving greater than 22.5 Gy should be minimized and ideally constrained to less than 4% of the organ volume, or approximately 5 mL, with maximum point dose less than 30 Gy for 3-fraction SBRT.

- The absolute volume of small bowel receiving ≥15 Gy should be held to less than 120 mL when possible to minimize severe acute toxicity, if delineating the contours of bowel loops themselves. Alternatively, if the entire volume of peritoneal space in which the small bowel can move is delineated, the volume receiving greater than 45 Gy should be less than 195 mL when possible. Such a limit likely also reduces late toxicity risk, although this correlation is not established. The volume of small bowel receiving higher doses should also be minimized. For SBRT, the small bowel volume receiving greater than 12.5 Gy in a single fraction should ideally be kept to less than 30 mL with avoidance of circumferential coverage above that dose; for a 3- to 5-fraction regimen, the maximum point dose should be less than 30 Gy.

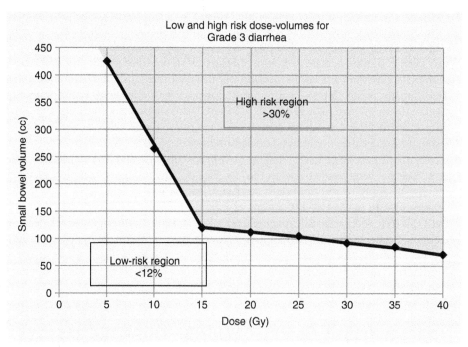

FIGURE 23-2. Delineation of high- and low-risk dose-volume regions for radiation-induced grade 3 small bowel toxicity (diarrhea). The region above the two straight lines is associated with greater than 30% incidence of grade 3 diarrhea in high-risk patients, with the incidence rising to over 40% as the total dose increases. The incidence in low-risk patients is 12% or less. If the treatment planning dose-volume histogram exceeds the threshold volumes indicated by the straight lines at any dose point, then the plan is considered high risk. (Data from Robertson JM, Lockman D, Yan D, et al. The dose-volume relationship of small bowel irradiation and acute grade 3 diarrhea during chemoradiotherapy for rectal cancer. *Int J Radiat Oncol Biol Phys* 2008;70[2]:413–418. Reference 24, replotted with a two-segment linear regression.)

- Figure 23-2 presents a dose-volume plot for bowel toxicity (grade 3 or higher) caused by radiation of bowel tissue. The dose-volume plane divides into two regions, the upper carrying a risk of complications greater than 30%. Notice that the irradiated bowel volume in the low-risk region falls rapidly as the dose is raised to 15 Gy.

SEQUELAE OF TREATMENT

- Anorexia, nausea, and fatigue are common complaints during gastric irradiation.
- The Gastrointestinal Tumor Study Group reported a minimum 13% treatment-related mortality from nutritional problems or septic events (22).
- Moderate doses of 16 to 36 Gy reduce secretion of pepsin and hydrochloric acid (24,27–29). For this reason, radiation therapy was once a common and successful therapy for peptic ulcer disease.
- Gastric late effects are rare with doses of 40 to 52 Gy using conventional fractionation.
- There is a relatively low risk of gastric late effects with doses less than 50 Gy when radiation therapy is used for locally advanced gastric cancer (with or without chemotherapy). However, at doses of 50 to 55 Gy, there is up to a 9% risk of variable gastric late effects.
- Doses of 60 Gy carry a 5% to 15% risk of gastric late effects.
- In the ARTIST I trial, in the arm with RT delivered with concomitant cisplatin and capecitabine, the most common nonhematologic adverse events were nausea (G1-2 77.0%, G3+ 12.3%), vomiting (G1-2 37.8%, G3+ 3.1%), hand-foot syndrome (G1-2 46.1%, G3+ 3.1%), and diarrhea (G1-2 44.0%, G3+ 0.9%). Grade 3 neutropenia occurred in 43.6% and grade 4 neutropenia in 4.8% (18).

References

1. Siegel RL, Miller KD, Jemal A. Cancer statistics, 2016. *CA Cancer J Clin* 2016;66:7–20.
2. Torre LA, Bray F, Siegel RL, et al. Global Cancer Statistics, 2012. *CA Cancer J Clin* 2015;65(2): 87–108.
3. Willett CG, Gunderson LL. Stomach. In: Halperin EC, Perez CA, Brady LW, eds. *Principles and practice of radiation oncology*, 5th ed. Philadelphia, PA: Lippincott Williams & Wilkins, 2008:1318–1335.
4. Fuchs CS, Mayer RJ. Gastric carcinoma. *N Engl J Med* 1995;333(1):32–41.
5. Nakajima T, Harashima S, Hirata M, et al. Prognostic and therapeutic values of peritoneal cytology in gastric cancer. *Acta Cytol* 1978;22(4):225–229.
6. Alakus H, Batur M, Schmidt M, et al. Variable 18F-fluorodeoxyglucose uptake in gastric cancer is associated with different levels of GLUT-1 expression. *Nucl Med Commun* 2010;31(6):532–538.
7. Hopkins S, Yang GY. FDG PET imaging in the staging and management of gastric cancer. *J Gastrointest Oncol* 2011;2(1):39–44.
8. Siewert JR, Feith M, Werner M, et al. Adenocarcinoma of the esophagogastric junction. *Ann Surg* 2000;232(3):353–361.
9. Amin MA, Greene FL, Edge S, et al. *AJCC cancer staging manual*, 8th ed. New York, NY: Springer, 2017.
10. Bang YJ, Van Cutsem E, Feyereislova A, et al. Trastuzumab in combination with chemotherapy versus chemotherapy alone for treatment of HER2-positive advanced gastric or gastro-oesophageal junction cancer (ToGA): a phase 3, open-label, randomised controlled trial. *Lancet* 2010;376(9742):687–697.

11. Cuschieri A, Weeden S, Fielding J, et al. Patient survival after D1 and D2 resections for gastric cancer: long-term results of the MRC randomized surgical trial. Surgical Co-operative Group. *Br J Cancer* 1999;79(9–10):1522–1530.

12. Songun I, Putter H, Kranenbarg EM, et al. Surgical treatment of gastric cancer: 15-year follow-up results of the randomised nationwide Dutch D1D2 trial. *Lancet Oncol* 2010;11(5):439–449.

13. Macdonald JS, Smalley SR, Benedetti J, et al. Chemoradiotherapy after surgery compared with surgery alone for adenocarcinoma of the stomach or gastroesophageal junction. *N Engl J Med* 2001;345(10):725–730.

14. Smalley SR, Benedetti JK, Haller DG, et al. Updated analysis of SWOG-directed intergroup study 0116: a phase III trial of adjuvant radiochemotherapy versus observation after curative gastric cancer resection. *J Clin Oncol* 2012;30(19):2327–2333.

15. Cunningham D, Allum WH, Stenning SP, et al. Perioperative chemotherapy versus surgery alone for resectable gastroesophageal cancer. *N Engl J Med* 2006;355(1):11–20.

16. van Hagen P, Hulshof MC, van Lanschot JJ, et al. Preoperative chemoradiotherapy for esophageal or junctional cancer. *N Engl J Med* 2012;366(22):2074–2084.

17. Walsh TN, Noonan N, Hollywood D, et al. A comparison of multimodal therapy and surgery for esophageal adenocarcinoma. *N Engl J Med* 1996;335(7):462–467.

18. Lee J, Lim DH, Kim S, et al. Phase III trial comparing capecitabine plus cisplatin versus capecitabine plus cisplatin with concurrent capecitabine radiotherapy in completely resected gastric cancer with D2 lymph node dissection: the ARTIST trial. *J Clin Oncol* 2012;30(3):268–273.

19. Park SH, Sohn TS, Lee J, et al. Phase III trial to compare adjuvant chemotherapy with capecitabine and cisplatin versus concurrent chemoradiotherapy in gastric cancer: final report of the adjuvant chemoradiotherapy in stomach tumors trial, including survival and subset analyses. *J Clin Oncol* 2015;33(28):3130–3136.

20. Verheij M, Jansen EP, Cats A, et al. A multicenter randomized phase III trial of neo-adjuvant chemotherapy followed by surgery and chemotherapy or by surgery and chemoradiotherapy in resectable gastric cancer: first results from the CRITICS study. *J Clin Oncol* 2016;34(15 suppl):4000.

21. Ajani JA, Winter K, Okawara GS, et al. Phase II trial of preoperative chemoradiation in patients with localized gastric adenocarcinoma (RTOG 9904): quality of combined modality therapy and pathologic response. *J Clin Oncol* 2006;24(24):3953–3958.

22. Schein P, Novak J. A comparison of combination chemotherapy and combined modality therapy for locally advanced gastric carcinoma. Gastrointestinal Tumor Study Group. *Cancer* 1982;49(9):1771–1777.

23. Bleiberg H, Goffin JC, Dalesio O, et al. Adjuvant radiotherapy and chemotherapy in resectable gastric cancer. A randomized trial of the gastro-intestinal tract cancer cooperative group of the EORTC. *Eur J Surg Oncol* 1989;15(6):535–543.

24. Goldgraber MB, Rubin CE, Palmer WL, et al. The early gastric response to irradiation; a serial biopsy study. *Gastroenterology* 1954;27(1):1–20.

25. Robertson JM, Lockman D, Yan D, et al. The dose-volume relationship of small bowel irradiation and acute grade 3 diarrhea during chemoradiotherapy for rectal cancer. *Int J Radiat Oncol Biol Phys* 2008;70(2):413–418.

26. Kavanagh BD, Pan CC, Dawson LA, et al. Radiation dose-volume effects in the stomach and small bowel. *Int J Radiat Oncol Biol Phys* 2010;76(3 suppl):S101–S107.

27. Carpender JW, Levin E, Clayman CB, et al. Radiation in the therapy of peptic ulcer. *Am J Roentgenol Radium Ther Nucl Med* 1956;75(2):374–379.

28. Rubin P, Casarett G. *Clinical radiation pathology*. Philadelphia, PA: WB Saunders, 1968.

29. Smalley S, Evans R. Radiation morbidity to the gastrointestinal tract and liver. In: Plowman P, McElwain T, Meadows A, eds. *The complications of cancer management*. London, UK: Butterworth-Heinemann, 1989.

CHAPTER 24

PANCREAS AND HEPATOBILIARY TRACT

PANCREATIC CANCER

Anatomy

The pancreas lies in the retroperitoneal space of the upper abdomen at approximately the level of the first two lumbar vertebrae.

- Tumors in the head of the pancreas commonly invade or compress the common bile duct, causing jaundice and dilatation of the bile ducts and gallbladder.
- The pancreatic head lies to the right of the superior mesenteric-portal vein confluence. The pancreatic body lies between the left border of the superior mesenteric artery and the left border of the aorta. The tail of the pancreas lies to the left of the left border of the aorta.
- Primary lymphatic drainage of pancreatic head and neck tumors includes lymph nodes along the common bile duct, common hepatic artery, portal vein, pyloric, posterior and anterior pancreaticoduodenal arcades, superior mesenteric vein, and superior mesenteric artery.
- Primary lymphatic drainage of the body and tail of the pancreas includes the common hepatic artery, celiac axis, splenic artery and splenic hilum.

Clinical Presentation

- Jaundice, pain, anorexia, new-onset diabetes, and weight loss are the most common presenting symptoms.
- Generalized peritoneal involvement is more common with carcinoma of the body and tail than with carcinoma of the head.
- The pancreatic head accounts for 60% to 70% of pancreatic adenocarcinomas, whereas 20% to 25% arise in the body and tail and 10% to 20% diffusely involve the pancreas.

Diagnostic Workup

- For diagnostic purposes and staging, a computed tomography (CT) scan and an endoscopic ultrasound (EUS) are used to best characterize the primary tumor, whereas preoperative staging laparoscopy can be used to evaluate for intraperitoneal metastases.

- Multidetector CT angiography with pancreas protocol obtains thin sections through the pancreas, with multiphase IV contrast in the arterial and portal venous phases, and is the preferred imaging modality. Coronal and sagittal reconstruction allows for further visualization of the relationship between tumor and vessels (1).
- Guidelines for reporting imaging findings have been developed to assist with standardized tumor assessment (2).
- MRI with contrast has similar sensitivity and specificity as CT, though respiratory motion is more likely to degrade image quality than on CT, and cost is significantly higher. MRI is particularly useful for characterization of CT-indeterminate liver lesions (3).
- MR cholangiopancreatography without IV contrast is not recommended for staging, unless patient is unable to receive IV contrast because of renal failure or other contraindication.
- PET/CT is of unclear utility in staging, and cannot replace pancreas protocol CT for assessment of primary tumor.
- The tumor marker CA 19-9 is also helpful in the diagnosis and follow-up of patients with pancreatic cancer. CA 19-9 levels above the upper normal limit of 37 U per mL have 80% accuracy in identifying patients with pancreatic cancer. The accuracy improves to up to 95% when the cutoff value is increased to 200 U per mL.
- Staging laparoscopy is useful in revealing imaging-occult peritoneal and liver metastases in patients who appear to have resectable disease, and can demonstrate occult metastatic disease in approximately 10% of cases involving the pancreatic head. In the setting of elevated CA 19-9, yield of staging laparoscopy is increased (4).

Staging System

- Nodal staging is N0 for no regional lymph nodes present and N1 for regional lymph node metastases. For patients who undergo resection, at least 12 nodes should be assessed to accurately stage N0 disease.
- Metastatic staging is M0 for no distant metastases present and M1 for distant metastases.
- Primary tumors are typically classified as resectable, borderline resectable, or unresectable (locally advanced). Resectability is heavily influenced by surgeon expertise and ability to perform vascular reconstruction, and should be determined in multidisciplinary tumor board (5).
- Resectable tumors have no involvement of the celiac axis, common hepatic artery, or superior mesenteric artery and either no involvement of the superior mesenteric vein and portal vein or less than 180-degree contact without vein irregularity.
- Borderline resectable tumors classically can have less than 180-degree involvement of the celiac axis or superior mesenteric artery, or reconstructable involvement of the common hepatic artery, superior mesenteric vein, or portal vein. Variant anatomy such as replaced right hepatic artery or an intact gastroduodenal artery that is amenable to the Appleby procedure may be considered borderline resectable.
- Unresectable tumors have unreconstructable involvement of the superior mesenteric vein or portal vein, or greater than 180-degree involvement of the celiac axis or superior mesenteric artery.

- The AJCC 8th edition changes T staging to a predominantly size-based one. T1 is tumors ≤ 2 cm; T2 is tumors greater than 2 cm but ≤4 cm; T3 is tumors greater than 4 cm; and T4 is tumors involving the celiac axis or superior mesenteric artery.

See: Amin MB, Edge SB, Greene FL, et al., eds. *AJCC cancer staging manual*, 8th ed. New York: Springer, 2017.

General Management

- Standard surgical treatment for pancreatic ductal adenocarcinoma of the head or neck of the pancreas is the pancreatoduodenectomy, first described by Whipple et al. in 1935. Body and tail tumors can be addressed with distal pancreatectomy, and patients with diffuse involvement can require total pancreatectomy (6).
- Completeness of resection is graded by grossly and microscopically negative margins (R0), grossly negative but microscopically positive margins (R1), or grossly and microscopically positive margins (R2). The nonuncinate posterior surface, anterior surface, and vascular groove are not considered true resection margins by the College of American Pathologists and AJCC. Tumor within 1 mm of the margin is considered a positive margin (7).
- For patients with unresectable tumors or metastatic disease, death usually results from hepatic failure because of biliary obstruction by local tumor extension or hepatic replacement by metastases.
- For the small number of patients (10% to 20%) undergoing a potentially curative pancreatoduodenectomy, the three major sites of disease relapse are the bed of the resected pancreas (local recurrence), the peritoneal cavity, and the liver.
- High local failure rates of 50% to 86% occur despite resection. This is due to frequent cancer invasion into the retroperitoneal soft tissue, as well as the inability to achieve wide retroperitoneal soft tissue margins because of anatomic constraints to wide posterior excision (superior mesenteric artery and vein, portal vein, and inferior vena cava) (7).
- For resectable tumors, the Gastrointestinal Tumor Study Group showed that adjuvant 40-Gy split course over 6 weeks with 5-fluorouracil (5-FU) could prolong median survival from 10.9 to 21.0 months (2-year survival, 18% to 46%). For unresectable pancreatic cancer, the Gastrointestinal Tumor Study Group (23) also showed that a similar chemoirradiation regimen yielded median survival of 9.6 versus 5.2 months with 60 Gy in 10 weeks alone (8).
- The European Organization for Research and Treatment of Cancer (EORTC) performed a subsequent study, randomizing 218 patients with resected adenocarcinoma of the pancreas or periampullary cancers to 40 Gy of external beam radiation therapy (EBRT) in a split-dose fashion with continuous infusional 5-FU or observation alone. No significant improvement was seen in median survival (24 versus 19 months

$p = 0.208$). Median survival for pancreatic adenocarcinoma was 17.1 versus 12.6 months ($p = 0.09$) (9,10).

- The European Study Group for Pancreatic Cancer trial allowed physicians to enroll patients with resected adenocarcinoma of the pancreas onto one of three parallel randomized studies. (a) Chemoradiation versus no chemoradiation ($n = 69$), with 40-Gy EBRT in split-dose fashion and bolus 5-FU. (b) Chemotherapy versus no chemotherapy ($n = 192$), with the treatment arm receiving bolus 5-FU and leucovorin, or (c) a 2 by 2 factorial design ($n = 289$) of chemoradiation, chemotherapy, chemoradiation with maintenance chemotherapy, or observation alone. After pooling all three trials, analysis showed no survival difference between adjuvant chemoradiation versus no therapy (median survival, 15.5 and 16.1 months, $p = 0.24$). A survival benefit was seen, however, in those patients who received chemotherapy compared to those who did not (median survival, 19.7 versus 14 months, $p = 0.0005$). Additionally, for margin-positive tumors, a survival benefit was seen for adjuvant chemotherapy but not chemoradiotherapy (11,12).

- In the Radiation Therapy Oncology Group and GI Intergroup Trial 9704, 538 patients received protracted infusion 5-FU and postoperative radiation (50.4 Gy) in 28 fractions and were then randomized to multiple cycles of either infusion 5-FU or gemcitabine hydrochloride. There was a trend toward survival advantage seen in the patients with resected pancreatic head carcinomas who received maintenance gemcitabine. Median survival was 20.6 versus 16.9 months in the 5-FU/chemoRT alone arm (13,14).

- The ESPAC-3 trial randomized 1,088 patients with completely resected pancreatic adenocarcinoma to 6 months of adjuvant gemcitabine or 5-fluorouracil. The median survival was 23.6 and 23 months, respectively ($p = 0.39$), signifying no benefit to adjuvant gemcitabine versus 5-fluorouracil (15).

- The ESPAC-4 trial randomized 732 patients with resected (R0 or R1) pancreatic cancer to six cycles of adjuvant gemcitabine monotherapy or in combination with capecitabine. The median survival for gemcitabine monotherapy was 25.5 versus 28 months for gemcitabine combined with capecitabine ($p = 0.032$) (16).

- The role for adjuvant chemoradiotherapy remains under investigation in the RTOG 0848 randomized trial.

- For borderline resectable pancreatic cancer, conversion to resectability with ability to achieve negative margins is paramount. Katz and colleagues reported a phase II trial of neoadjuvant FOLFIRINOX chemotherapy followed by 50.4 Gy of conventionally fractionated external beam radiation with concurrent capecitabine, followed by evaluation for surgical resection, to be performed 4 to 10 weeks after completion of chemoradiation. Sixty-eight percent of patients underwent pancreatectomy, with 93% of patients undergoing surgery having resection with negative margins. Thirteen percent of specimens had a pathologic complete response. The median survival was 21.7 months (17).

- A retrospective analysis from the Moffitt Cancer Center of 110 patients treated with induction chemotherapy followed by stereotactic body radiation therapy for borderline resectable pancreatic cancer (30 Gy in 5 fractions to GTV, with dose painting to the tumor/vessel interface to 40 Gy) showed that at a median of 14 months' follow-up, median overall survival was 19.2 months. Fifty-one percent of patients underwent resection, with negative margins achieved in 96% of resections. Median overall survival was 34.2 months for those undergoing resection versus 14 months for those who did not have resection ($p < 0.001$). Toxicity was low, with a grade 3+ toxicity rate of 7%. This highlights the safety of this approach, as well as the value of resection in improving overall survival (18).

- The benefit of neoadjuvant radiotherapy for borderline resectable pancreatic cancer is being evaluated on the phase III ALLIANCE A021501 trial, which randomizes patients to eight cycles of preoperative FOLFIRINOX or seven cycles of FOLFIRINOX plus stereotactic body radiation therapy to a dose of 33 to 40 Gy (19).
- For locally advanced pancreatic cancer, radiotherapy has been shown to improve local disease control, with conflicting data regarding its effect on survival.
- The Gastrointestinal Tumor Study Group published results of a randomized trial in 1981 evaluating 60 Gy of radiation versus 40 Gy with 5-fluorouracil versus 60 Gy with 5-fluorouracil. The concurrent chemoradiotherapy arms resulted in a median survival of 10 months, compared to 5.5 months with radiation alone. One-year overall survival was 40% in the chemoradiation arms, versus 10% with radiation alone (20).
- A meta-analysis of 15 randomized trials of chemoradiotherapy, radiotherapy alone, and chemotherapy alone for locally advanced pancreatic cancer showed that chemoradiotherapy had superior survival to radiotherapy alone, though survival was not statistically different for chemoradiotherapy versus chemotherapy alone (21).
- The GERCOR cooperative group performed a retrospective analysis of 181 patients with locally advanced pancreatic cancer treated on phase II and III trials who had received at least 3 months of chemotherapy and then either continued chemotherapy or were treated with chemoradiotherapy at the investigator's discretion. Among patients who did not progress during initial chemotherapy, those who subsequently were treated with chemoradiotherapy had significantly improved progression-free and overall survival (10.8 and 15 months, respectively) compared to those who received continued chemotherapy alone (7.4 and 11.7 months, respectively) (22).
- The Eastern Cooperative Oncology Group (ECOG) performed a randomized study of gemcitabine versus gemcitabine plus 50.4 Gy of radiation. Although only 74 patients were accrued, the chemoradiotherapy arm had a significantly improved overall survival (11.4 months), compared to chemotherapy alone (9.2 months) ($p = 0.17$) (23).
- The LAP07 trial was a phase III trial evaluating the effect of chemoradiotherapy (54 Gy with concurrent capecitabine) after 4 months of gemcitabine with or without erlotinib. No benefit was seen with erlotinib. Chemoradiotherapy was associated with decreased local progression (32% versus 46%) and no increase in grade 3 to 4 toxicity, but no difference was seen in overall survival compared to chemotherapy (15.2 versus 16.5 months, respectively) (24).
- Stereotactic body radiation therapy for locally advanced pancreatic cancer has been evaluated in multiple prospective and retrospective analyses (25). A phase II trial of three cycles of gemcitabine followed by 33 Gy SBRT and maintenance gemcitabine until progression or toxicity showed that at a median follow-up of 13.9 months, 2% of patients had grade 2+ acute toxicity and 11% had grade 2+ late toxicity. Median overall survival was 13.9 months, and freedom from local progression at 1 year was 78% (26).

Radiation Therapy Techniques

- Endoscopic placement of fiducial markers into the tumor or periphery is recommended prior to treatment of nonmetastatic pancreatic cancer. Biliary stents can assist in targeting, but can also shift from day-to-day and are therefore less reliable.
- For simulation, patient should be placed in the supine position with the arms up in a vac-fix or alpha cradle. IV and oral contrast should be used whenever not contraindicated. If an allergy to IV contrast is present, premedication should be considered. Otherwise, fusion with recent diagnostic CT or MRI is acceptable.
- Respiratory motion should be accounted for through the use of a 4D-CT scan, breath hold with active breathing control, and/or abdominal compression. Use of respiratory gating can allow for decreased dose to organs at risk and increased target coverage (27).
- For conventionally fractionated or mildly hypofractionated courses, both 3D conformal and intensity-modulated radiation therapy (IMRT) can produce acceptable plans. IMRT is associated with decreased toxicity compared to 3D conformal plans, particularly grade 3 to 4 nausea and diarrhea (28).
- Radiation techniques vary depending on whether radiation is given in the adjuvant, preoperative, or definitive setting, and whether conventionally fractionated or hypofractionated, stereotactic body radiation therapy (SBRT) is used.
- For adjuvant treatment of resected head of pancreas cancer, the RTOG published consensus guidelines for target volume delineation, taking into account the multiple anastomoses and vascular/lymphatic regions at risk for locoregional recurrence (29).
- In the adjuvant setting, there is no GTV. CTV includes the postoperative bed, pancreaticojejunostomy, portal vein to the portosplenic confluence, proximal 1 to 1.5 cm of the celiac artery, proximal 2.5 to 3 cm of the superior mesenteric artery, and aorta. These volumes are expanded by 1 cm, with the exception of the aorta, which is expanded 2.5 cm to the right, 1 cm to the left, 2 cm anteriorly, and posteriorly to the vertebral body. Surgical clips can be placed for a variety of reasons, and should be included in the CTV after appropriate discussion with the surgeon. Overlap of the CTV with the kidneys should be avoided. For tumors of the pancreatic body and tail, the porta hepatis lymph nodes may be excluded from the CTV, and the splenic hilar remnant should be covered. The PTV is a 0.5 cm expansion from the CTV.
- In the definitive or neoadjuvant setting, delineation of the intact pancreatic tumor and grossly enlarged lymph nodes without elective nodal irradiation is recommended.
- The CTV traditionally covered from the top of T11 to the bottom of L2, including pancreaticoduodenal, suprapancreatic, porta hepatis, celiac, superior mesenteric and para-aortic lymph nodes for pancreatic head and neck lesions; treatment fields for body and tail lesions excluded the porta hepatis, and covered the splenic hilar nodal region. Per the RTOG 1201 protocol for definitive treatment of pancreatic adenocarcinoma, these elective volumes were no longer included, with the CTV being an expansion of 1 to 1.5 cm on the primary tumor and any involved regional lymph nodes. PTV expansion is 0.5 cm radially and 0.5 to 1.5 cm cranio-caudally, depending on extent of target motion assessed by 4D CT scan.

- Normal tissue dose constraints for the adjuvant, definitive and neoadjuvant settings are as follows:

  Liver: mean < 28 Gy

  Duodenum (definitive and neoadjuvant): Dmax < 54 Gy; V45 < 30 cc

  Bowel: Dmax < 54 Gy; V45 < 135cc

  Stomach: Dmax < 54 Gy; V50< 5cc; V45<75cc

  Spinal cord: Dmax < 45 Gy

  Kidneys: 90% of the volume equivalent of one kidney < 18 Gy.

- If SBRT techniques are used, minimal expansion (3 mm) from the gross tumor (taking into account respiratory motion) to PTV is frequently used. Use of simultaneous integrated boost technique to escalate the dose to the tumor/vessel interface, as well as simultaneous integrated protection techniques to de-escalate the dose to the interface between tumor and bowel planning risk volume (PRV) is used on some protocols. SBRT is not recommended for cases in which tumor invasion into the stomach or bowel is noted on endoscopy (25). See Figure 24-1 for a representative plan of neoadjuvant SBRT for pancreatic cancer.

- At Columbia University Medical Center, the GTV is expanded by 3 mm to create at PTV1, which receives 25 Gy in 5 fractions. PTV2 is the PTV1 less the bowel PRV, and receives 33 Gy in 5 fractions. PTV3 is the tumor/vessel interface outside of the bowel PRV, and receives 36 Gy in 5 fractions. This simultaneous integrated boost SBRT is currently being utilized on the Alliance A021501 protocol.

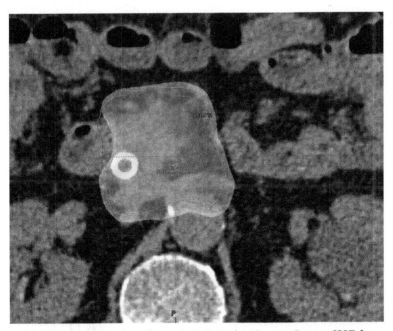

FIGURE 24-1. Representative plan of a patient treated with neoadjuvant SBRT for pancreatic adenocarcinoma. Patient received 33 Gy in 5 fractions to the pancreas tumor with 3 mm margin, and 36 Gy in 5 fractions to the tumor-vessel interface.

- For pancreas SBRT, normal tissue organ constraints are as follows:
  Duodenum: V35 Gy < 1cc; V20 Gy < 20cc
  Bowel: V35 Gy < 1cc; V20 Gy < 20cc
  Stomach: V35 Gy < 1cc; V20 Gy < 20cc
  Liver: V12<50%; at least 700 cc of liver receives < 15 Gy
  Kidneys: V12 Gy < 25 %
  Spinal cord: V20 Gy < 1 cc

BILIARY TRACT CANCER

Anatomy

- The bile ducts originate within the liver, with the left and right hepatic ducts joining to form the common hepatic duct.
- At the origin of the cystic duct, it becomes the common bile duct. The cystic duct drains bile from the gallbladder into the common duct.
- The gallbladder is adjacent to the undersurface of the liver.
- Primary lymphatic drainage of the biliary tract is to nodes within the porta hepatis and pancreaticoduodenal groups.

Clinical Presentation

- Patients often present with painless obstructive jaundice, weight loss, or Courvoisier's gallbladder.
- Liver metastases are common; the next most frequent sites of distant involvement are peritoneal and pulmonary, with less frequent spread to ovaries, spleen, bones, and other distant organs.
- Gallbladder cancer is frequently, up to 45% of the time, identified at time of cholecystectomy for presumed benign gallbladder disease.

Diagnostic Workup

- In patients with jaundice, ultrasonography or CT can distinguish between obstructive and nonobstructive etiology. Obstruction causes dilated intrahepatic ducts.
- CT body scans and ultrasound have been used in gallbladder lesions to delineate tumor extent, liver invasion, liver metastases, and retroperitoneal adenopathy. MRI and MRCP can also be used to diagnose biliary tract tumors.
- Image-guided thin-needle percutaneous biopsy with a transhepatic catheter in position is successful in achieving a tissue diagnosis in approximately 90% of patients.
- CEA and CA 19-9 can both be elevated in cases of biliary tract cancer.

Staging System

- Tumors of the intrahepatic bile ducts are staged as solitary tumor without vascular invasion (T1), either ≤ 5 cm (T1a) or greater than 5 cm (T1b); solitary tumor with intrahepatic vascular invasion or multiple tumors (T2); tumor perforating the visceral peritoneum (T3); tumor directly invading the local extrahepatic structures (T4).

- Regional lymph node metastases from intrahepatic bile duct tumors are N1, and have differences based on laterality. Left liver preferentially drains to inferior phrenic nodes, hilar, and gastrohepatic nodes. Right liver drains in a similar pattern to gallbladder cancers, primarily to right-sided hilar lymph nodes and subsequently to the portocaval nodes. Periduodenal and peripancreatic tumors can also be involved. Importantly, nonregional lymph nodes include celiac, periaortic, and pericaval regions, and these represent M1 status.

- Gallbladder cancer primary tumor staging depends not only on depth on invasion but also on location within the gallbladder. Tumors invading the lamina propria are T1a, and invasion of the muscular layer is T1b; tumor invading the perimuscular connective tissue on the peritoneal side, without involvement of the serosa are T2a, and tumor invading the perimuscular connective tissue on the hepatic side without extension to the liver is T2b; tumor perforation of the serosa visceral peritoneum and/or invasion into the liver or adjacent organs is T3; and tumor invasion of the main portal vein or hepatic artery or two or more extrahepatic organs or structures is T4.

- Regional lymph nodes for gallbladder cancer include the common bile duct, hepatic artery, portal vein, and cystic duct. A total of 1 to 3 involved regional lymph nodes are N1, 4 or more regional lymph node metastases are N2.

- Staging of perihilar bile duct tumors, including Klatskin tumors, depends on depth of invasion and extent of biliary invasion. T1 tumors are confined to the bile duct, with extension up to the muscle layer or fibrous tissue. T2 tumors have invasion of the periductal adipose tissue (T2a) or the hepatic parenchyma (T2b). T3 tumors invade unilateral branches of the portal vein or hepatic artery. T4 tumors invade the portal vein or its branches bilaterally, or secondary biliary radicals with contralateral portal vein or hepatic artery involvement.

- Regional lymph nodes for perihilar bile duct tumors include the common bile duct, hepatic artery, portal vein, and cystic duct. A total of 1 to 3 involved regional lymph nodes are N1, 4 or more regional lymph node metastases are N2.

- The Bismuth-Corlette classification of perihilar bile duct tumors lists tumor limited to the common hepatic duct, below the level of the confluence of the right and left hepatic ducts as type I; tumor involving the confluence of left and right hepatic ducts is type II; type II tumors additionally involving either the right or left second order ducts are type IIIa and IIIb, respectively; and tumor involving both right and left secondary order ducts are type IV. Type IV tumors are significantly associated with positive surgical margins and poorer survival after resection.

- Distal bile duct tumors are staged by depth of invasion. T1 tumors invade the bile duct wall with a depth less than 5 mm. T2 tumors invade the bile duct wall with depth of 5 to 12 mm. T3 tumors have greater than 12 mm of invasion of the bile duct wall. T4 tumors involve the celiac axis, superior mesenteric artery, or common hepatic artery.

- Regional lymph nodes for extrahepatic bile duct tumors include the common bile duct, hepatic artery, portal vein, and cystic duct. A total of 1 to 3 involved regional lymph nodes are N1, 4 or more regional lymph node metastases are N2.

Prognostic Factors

- Nodal status and degree of local extension are the main prognostic factors.
- Tumors of the distal common bile duct plus ampulla of Vater are the most resectable and have the best prognosis. Gallbladder plus mid-ductal lesions (cystic duct, proximal common bile duct) are prone to early regional spread and have poor prognoses.
- Klatskin's tumors (hilar or common hepatic duct lesions) have the lowest resectability rate.

General Management

- Lesions in the periampullary region or distal common duct carry a uniformly better prognosis; resection with a Whipple procedure is usually feasible and yields long-term survival in 30% to 40% of these patients.
- Radical cholecystectomy, including en bloc hepatic resection, lymphadenectomy, and bile duct excision, is recommended for management of gallbladder cancer.
- For patients with locally advanced gallbladder cancer, neoadjuvant chemotherapy or chemoradiotherapy can downstage disease and allow for identification of patients most likely to benefit from radical resection (30).
- The Southwest Oncology Group (SWOG) conducted a phase II trial of adjuvant capecitabine followed by chemoradiotherapy (45 Gy to lymphatics and 54 to 59.4 Gy to tumor bed) for patients with pT2-4 or N-positive gallbladder or extrahepatic cholangiocarcinoma. Grade 3 adverse events were seen in 52% of patients and grade 4 adverse events were seen in 11% of patients. The median overall survival was 35 months, with no differences seen between patients who got R0 and R1 resections. This compared favorably to historical controls (31). See Figure 24-2 for a representative plan of a patient treated with adjuvant chemoradiation as per SWOG S0809.
- Neoadjuvant hyperfractionated chemoradiation and liver transplantation has been evaluated for patients with unresectable perihilar cholangiocarcinoma, with 1/3 of patients who started treatment undergoing liver transplant. One- and 2-year overall survival was 70.6% and 35.5%, respectively, with 1- and 2-year posttransplant survival 83.3% and 55.6%, respectively (32).
- A 12 center analysis of neoadjuvant chemoradiation followed by liver transplantation for per, using external beam radiation with or without a brachytherapy boost, showed an 11.5% 3-month dropout. A 65% rate of recurrence-free survival was seen at 5 years, showing the therapy to be an effective strategy (33).
- Complete resection is the recommended treatment for intrahepatic cholangiocarcinoma, with R0 resection being the most important factor for survival.
- Locoregional therapies are effective in small trials of unresectable cholangioncarcinoma, though no randomized data support any particular modality over another.
- A multi-institutional trial of proton beam radiotherapy for intrahepatic cholangiocarcinoma showed 46.5% 2-year overall survival, and 94.1% local control at 2 years (34).
- Increased dose of radiation to a BED of 80.5 Gy or more is associated with a significantly increased rate of control and survival in intrahepatic cholangiocarcinoma (35).

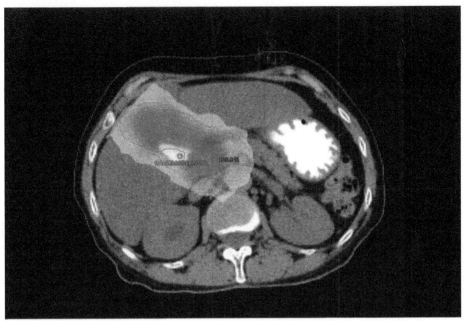

FIGURE 24-2. Representative plan of a patient treated with adjuvant chemoradiotherapy for T2N1M0 gallbladder cancer. The patient received 45 Gy to the regional lymphatics, with a simultaneous integrated boost to 52.5 Gy to the tumor bed.

LIVER CANCER

Anatomy

- The liver has a dual blood supply from the hepatic artery and the portal vein, with tumors fed predominately from the arterial system.
- The liver is divided into right and left hemilivers along the Rex-Cantlie line, which projects between the gallbladder fossa and the vena cava, and is defined by the middle hepatic vein.
- The liver is divided into eight segments, along vertical and oblique planes (scissurae) defined by the three main hepatic veins, and a transverse plane along a line through the right and left portal branches. The eight segments are numbered clockwise in the coronal plane.
- Histologically, the liver is divided into lobules, drained by central veins. Portal triads between the lobules consist of branches of the hepatic artery, portal vein, and intrahepatic lymphatic channels.

Clinical Presentation

- Malaise, anorexia, and abdominal pain are common presenting signs.
- Mass effect and ascites can result in abdominal fullness.
- Acute abdominal pain and distension from spontaneous rupture may be fatal.

Diagnostic Workup

- CT and MRI with intravenous contrast are both sensitive and specific for diagnosing and staging hepatocellular carcinoma. Multiphase imaging is essential, and arterial enhancement with delayed washout and pseudocapsule is pathognomonic of hepatocellular carcinoma.
- Ultrasound with Doppler imaging can be useful in evaluating vascular invasion, though it has lower sensitivity for detection of HCC than do CT or MRI. Ultrasound is recommended every 6 months for patients at risk for hepatocellular carcinoma.
- Lesions with abnormal imaging characteristics should undergo biopsy, which is usually well tolerated.
- Assessment for etiology is essential. Hepatitis serologic studies for hepatitis B and C are routine, with additional consideration of alcoholic cirrhosis, nonalcoholic fatty liver disease (NAFLD), Wilson's disease, and hemochromatosis as necessary.
- Assessment of degree of cirrhosis and liver function is essential with Child-Pugh scoring system commonly used. The Model for End-stage Liver Disease (MELD) is used for prioritizing for receipt of a liver transplant, using serum bilirubin, serum creatinine, and INR to predict survival.
- Alpha-fetoprotein is generally elevated in the setting of HCC.

Staging System

- Primary tumors in the AJCC staging system are evaluated by size and invasion of critical structures. T1 tumors are solitary lesions ≤2 cm (T1a) or greater than 2 cm without vascular invasion. T2 tumors are solitary tumors greater than 2 cm with vascular invasion or multiple tumors, all ≤5 cm. T3 tumors have multiple tumors, with at least 1 greater than 5 cm. T4 tumors involve major branches of the portal vein or hepatic vein, or directly invade adjacent organs (besides the gallbladder), or with perforation of the visceral peritoneum.
- Lymph node staging is defined by presence of regional lymph node metastases (N1). Regional lymph nodes are the hilar, hepatoduodenal ligament, inferior phrenic, and caval lymph nodes. The most commonly involved are the hepatic artery and portal nodes.

General Management

- Resection is the treatment of choice for primary liver tumors and solitary metastatic lesions, if technically feasible.
- Partial hepatectomy can be curative for solitary tumors without vascular invasion, if there is preserved liver function (Child-Pugh A) and appropriate functional liver reserve, with 5-year survival rates over 50% (36,37).
- Portal hypertension and low albumin are associated with significantly worse outcome after surgical resection (38–40).
- After resection or ablation, no benefit has been found with adjuvant sorafenib (41).

- Liver transplantation is potentially curative for patients with early HCC, with 4-year overall survival of 85% and relapse-free survival of 92% among cirrhotic (Child Pugh B-C) patients with tumors meeting the following criteria: single tumor ≤ 5 cm or no more than three nodules ≤ 3 cm (42,43).
- Because of the lack of available livers for transplantation, bridge therapy to reduce tumor progression and lower the dropout rate from the liver transplant list has gained in popularity. Multiple approaches have been used, including radiofrequency ablation, transarterial embolization (TAE) or transarterial chemoembolization (TACE), yttrium-90 radioembolization, sorafenib, and external beam radiotherapy. Sandroussi and colleagues reported on hypofractionated radiotherapy (median dose of 33 Gy in 1 to 6 fractions) for patients with HCC listed for liver transplantation. At a median follow-up of 14 months, all tumors were locally controlled, with 50% of patients eventually undergoing liver transplantation and 30% remaining on the list at time of publication. The treatment was deemed safe and efficacious for those on the transplant list (44).
- For patients with tumors outside of the Milan criteria for transplantation, downstaging therapies can improve disease-free survival and recurrence after transplantation (45).
- For patients unable to have resection or transplantation, nonsurgical locoregional therapy is recommended. Many modalities exist, including percutaneous alcohol injection radiofrequency ablation, microwave ablation, cryoablation, TAE, TACE, yttrium-90 radioembolization, and external beam radiation therapy.
- There is growing evidence supporting SBRT for the treatment of inoperable HCC. A phase II trial of 50 patients with HCC treated with SBRT after incomplete TACE showed 2-year local control of 94.6%, and 2-year overall survival of 68.7%.
- A combined analysis of two trials of SBRT for inoperable HCC, treating with 6 fractions to a dose of 24 to 54 Gy depending on ability to achieve normal tissue constraints, demonstrated a 1-year local control of 87% and a median survival of 17 months (46).
- A retrospective comparison of RFA and SBRT in 224 patients with inoperable HCC showed similar rates of 1- and 2-year overall survival. For tumors greater than 2 cm, SBRT was associated with a 3-fold improvement in freedom from local progression (47).
- Charged particle therapy, mostly proton beam therapy, has been evaluated for inoperable HCC. Forty-four patients treated on a phase II trial open for HCC and intrahepatic cholangiocarcinoma were treated to a median dose of 58 GyE. Local control was 94.8% at 2 years, with an overall survival of 63.2% at 2 years (34).

Radiation Therapy Techniques

- For simulation, patient should be placed in the supine position with the arms up in a vac-fix or alpha cradle. IV and oral contrast should be used whenever not contraindicated. Multiphase scans should be performed in order to capture the arterial and portal venous phases of enhancement. If an allergy to IV contrast is present, premedication should be considered. Otherwise, fusion with recent diagnostic CT or MRI is acceptable.

- Respiratory motion should be accounted for through the use of a 4D-CT scan, breath hold with active breathing control, and/or abdominal compression. Use of respiratory gating can allow for decreased dose to organs at risk and increased target coverage (27).
- Stereotactic body radiation therapy plans should be made with small expansions from GTV to PTV, with exact margin depending on target motion.

NORMAL TISSUE COMPLICATIONS—QUANTEC RESULTS

Pan et al. (48) present a review of radiation damage to the liver. Of note is Figure 2 in their paper, which shows an LQ model of the dose response for radiation-induced liver disease (RILD). The curves are quite sharp, as shown by the following values estimated from the graph (based on data from Dawson and Ten Haken (49)):

NTCP	Mean Liver Dose (Gy)	
	Primary Tumor	Metastatic Tumor
20%	31.9	35.2
50%	34.3	39.7
80%	38.1	44.3

Pan et al. present guidelines for liver dose constraints to keep the RILD rate at 5% or less (48):

Palliative Whole-Liver Doses
Liver metastases
    Less than or equal to 30 Gy, in 2 Gy per fraction
    21 Gy in 7 fractions
Primary liver cancers
    Less than or equal to 28 Gy, in 2 Gy per fraction
    21 Gy in 7 fractions

Therapeutic Partial Liver RT (Standard Fractionation)
Mean normal liver dose (liver minus gross tumor volume)
    Less than 28 Gy in 2-Gy fractions for primary liver cancer
    Less than 32 Gy in 2-Gy fractions for liver metastases

Nonuniform Liver Recommendations (SBRT, 3 to 6 Fractions)
Mean normal liver dose (liver minus gross tumor volume)
    Less than 13 Gy for primary liver cancer, in 3 fractions
    Less than 18 Gy for primary liver cancer, in 6 fractions
    Less than 15 Gy for liver metastases, in 3 fractions
    Less than 20 Gy for liver metastases, in 6 fractions
    Less than 6 Gy for primary liver cancer, Child-Pugh B, in 4 to 6 Gy per fraction (for classic or nonclassic RILD) Critical volume model based ≥700 mL of normal liver receives ≤15 Gy in 3 to 5 fractions

SEQUELAE OF TREATMENT

- Analysis of predictors of liver toxicity after SBRT for HCC showed that baseline Child-Pugh score, as well as higher liver doses (mean liver dose, effective volume, and dose to 700 to 900 cc of liver) were significantly associated with decrease in liver function at 3 months. Presence of portal vein thrombosis and thrombocytopenia were also associated with a significantly increased risk of toxicity (50,51).

Biliary Duct Tolerance

- The central hepatobiliary tract can be injured during stereotactic body radiation therapy. A dosimetric analysis from Stanford yielded a recommended constraint of V40<21cc and V37<24cc for 5 fractions (52,53).

References

1. Valls C, et al. Dual-phase helical CT of pancreatic adenocarcinoma: assessment of resectability before surgery. *AJR Am J Roentgenol* 2002;178(4):821–826.
2. Al-Hawary MM, Francis IR, Chari ST, et al. Pancreatic ductal adenocarcinoma radiology reporting template: consensus statement of the Society of Abdominal Radiology and the American Pancreatic Association. *Radiology* 2014;270(1):248–260.
3. Motosugi U, et al. Detection of pancreatic carcinoma and liver metastases with gadoxetic acid-enhanced MR imaging: comparison with contrast-enhanced multi-detector row CT. *Radiology* 2011;260(2):446–453.
4. Maithel SK, et al. Preoperative CA 19-9 and the yield of staging laparoscopy in patients with radiographically resectable pancreatic adenocarcinoma. *Ann Surg Oncol* 2008;15(12):3512–3520.
5. Vauthey JN, Dixon E. AHPBA/SSO/SSAT Consensus Conference on Resectable and Borderline Resectable Pancreatic Cancer: rationale and overview of the conference. *Ann Surg Oncol* 2009;16(7):1725–1726.
6. Evans DB, et al. Surgical treatment of resectable and borderline resectable pancreas cancer: expert consensus statement. *Ann Surg Oncol* 2009;16(7):1736–1744.
7. Campbell F, et al. Classification of R1 resections for pancreatic cancer: the prognostic relevance of tumour involvement within 1 mm of a resection margin. *Histopathology* 2009;55(3):277–283.
8. Kalser MH, Ellenberg SS. Pancreatic cancer. Adjuvant combined radiation and chemotherapy following curative resection. *Arch Surg* 1985;120(8):899–903.
9. Klinkenbijl JH, et al. Adjuvant radiotherapy and 5-fluorouracil after curative resection of cancer of the pancreas and periampullary region: phase III trial of the EORTC gastrointestinal tract cancer cooperative group. *Ann Surg* 1999;230(6):776–782; discussion 782–4.
10. Smeenk HG, et al. Long-term survival and metastatic pattern of pancreatic and periampullary cancer after adjuvant chemoradiation or observation: long-term results of EORTC trial 40891. *Ann Surg* 2007;246(5):734–740.
11. Neoptolemos JP, et al. A randomized trial of chemoradiotherapy and chemotherapy after resection of pancreatic cancer. *N Engl J Med* 2004;350(12):1200–1210.
12. Neoptolemos JP, et al. Influence of resection margins on survival for patients with pancreatic cancer treated by adjuvant chemoradiation and/or chemotherapy in the ESPAC-1 randomized controlled trial. *Ann Surg* 2001;234(6):758–768.
13. Regine WF, et al. Fluorouracil-based chemoradiation with either gemcitabine or fluorouracil chemotherapy after resection of pancreatic adenocarcinoma: 5-year analysis of the U.S. Intergroup/RTOG 9704 phase III trial. *Ann Surg Oncol* 2011;18(5):1319–1326.

14. Regine WF, et al. Fluorouracil vs gemcitabine chemotherapy before and after fluorouracil-based chemoradiation following resection of pancreatic adenocarcinoma: a randomized controlled trial. *JAMA* 2008;299(9):1019–1026.

15. Neoptolemos JP, et al. Adjuvant chemotherapy with fluorouracil plus folinic acid vs gemcitabine following pancreatic cancer resection: a randomized controlled trial. *JAMA* 2010;304(10): 1073–1081.

16. Neoptolemos JP, et al. Comparison of adjuvant gemcitabine and capecitabine with gemcitabine monotherapy in patients with resected pancreatic cancer (ESPAC-4): a multicentre, open-label, randomised, phase 3 trial. *Lancet* 2017;389(10073):1011–1024.

17. Katz MH, et al. Preoperative modified FOLFIRINOX treatment followed by capecitabine-based chemoradiation for borderline resectable pancreatic cancer: alliance for clinical trials in oncology trial A021101. *JAMA Surg* 2016;151(8):e161137.

18. Mellon EA, et al. Long-term outcomes of induction chemotherapy and neoadjuvant stereotactic body radiotherapy for borderline resectable and locally advanced pancreatic adenocarcinoma. *Acta Oncol* 2015;54(7):979–985.

19. Katz MHG, et al. Alliance for clinical trials in oncology (ALLIANCE) trial A021501: preoperative extended chemotherapy vs. chemotherapy plus hypofractionated radiation therapy for borderline resectable adenocarcinoma of the head of the pancreas. *BMC Cancer* 2017;17(1):505.

20. Moertel CG, et al. Therapy of locally unresectable pancreatic carcinoma: a randomized comparison of high dose (6000 rads) radiation alone, moderate dose radiation (4000 rads + 5-fluorouracil), and high dose radiation + 5-fluorouracil: the Gastrointestinal Tumor Study Group. *Cancer* 1981;48(8):1705–1710.

21. Chen Y, et al. Combined radiochemotherapy in patients with locally advanced pancreatic cancer: a meta-analysis. *World J Gastroenterol* 2013;19(42):7461–7471.

22. Huguet F, et al. Impact of chemoradiotherapy after disease control with chemotherapy in locally advanced pancreatic adenocarcinoma in GERCOR phase II and III studies. *J Clin Oncol* 2007;25(3):326–331.

23. Loehrer PJ Sr, et al. Gemcitabine alone versus gemcitabine plus radiotherapy in patients with locally advanced pancreatic cancer: an Eastern Cooperative Oncology Group trial. *J Clin Oncol* 2011;29(31):4105–4112.

24. Hammel P, et al. Effect of chemoradiotherapy vs chemotherapy on survival in patients with locally advanced pancreatic cancer controlled after 4 months of gemcitabine with or without erlotinib: the LAP07 Randomized Clinical Trial. *JAMA* 2016;315(17):1844–1853.

25. Kim SK, Wu CC, Horowitz DP. Stereotactic body radiotherapy for the pancreas: a critical review for the medical oncologist. *J Gastrointest Oncol* 2016;7(3):479–486.

26. Herman JM, et al. Phase 2 multi-institutional trial evaluating gemcitabine and stereotactic body radiotherapy for patients with locally advanced unresectable pancreatic adenocarcinoma. *Cancer* 2015;121(7):1128–1137.

27. Keall PJ, et al. The management of respiratory motion in radiation oncology report of AAPM Task Group 76. *Med Phys* 2006;33(10): 3874–3900.

28. Yovino S, et al. Intensity-modulated radiation therapy significantly improves acute gastrointestinal toxicity in pancreatic and ampullary cancers. *Int J Radiat Oncol Biol Phys* 2011;79(1):158–162.

29. Goodman KA, et al. Radiation Therapy Oncology Group consensus panel guidelines for the delineation of the clinical target volume in the postoperative treatment of pancreatic head cancer. *Int J Radiat Oncol Biol Phys* 2012;83(3):901–908.

30. Agrawal S, et al. Radiological downstaging with neoadjuvant therapy in unresectable gall bladder cancer cases. *Asian Pac J Cancer Prev* 2016;17(4):2137–2140.

31. Ben-Josef E, et al. SWOG S0809: a phase II intergroup trial of adjuvant capecitabine and gemcitabine followed by radiotherapy and concurrent capecitabine in extrahepatic cholangiocarcinoma and gallbladder carcinoma. *J Clin Oncol* 2015;33(24):2617–2622.

32. Loveday BPT, et al. Neoadjuvant hyperfractionated chemoradiation and liver transplantation for unresectable perihilar cholangiocarcinoma in Canada. *J Surg Oncol* 2018;117(2):213–219.

33. Darwish Murad S, et al. Efficacy of neoadjuvant chemoradiation, followed by liver transplantation, for perihilar cholangiocarcinoma at 12 US centers. *Gastroenterology* 2012;143(1):88e3–98e3; quiz e14.

34. Hong TS, et al. Multi-institutional phase II study of high-dose hypofractionated proton beam therapy in patients with localized, unresectable hepatocellular carcinoma and intrahepatic cholangiocarcinoma. *J Clin Oncol* 2016;34(5):460–468.

35. Tao R, et al. Ablative radiotherapy doses lead to a substantial prolongation of survival in patients with inoperable intrahepatic cholangiocarcinoma: a retrospective dose response analysis. *J Clin Oncol* 2016;34(3):219–226.

36. Chok KS, et al. Impact of postoperative complications on long-term outcome of curative resection for hepatocellular carcinoma. *Br J Surg* 2009;96(1):81–87.

37. Truty MJ, Vauthey JN. Surgical resection of high-risk hepatocellular carcinoma: patient selection, preoperative considerations, and operative technique. *Ann Surg Oncol* 2010;17(5):1219–1225.

38. Berzigotti A, et al. Portal hypertension and the outcome of surgery for hepatocellular carcinoma in compensated cirrhosis: a systematic review and meta-analysis. *Hepatology* 2015;61(2):526–536.

39. Ribero D, et al. Selection for resection of hepatocellular carcinoma and surgical strategy: indications for resection, evaluation of liver function, portal vein embolization, and resection. *Ann Surg Oncol* 2008;15(4):986–992.

40. Wei AC, et al. Risk factors for perioperative morbidity and mortality after extended hepatectomy for hepatocellular carcinoma. *Br J Surg* 2003;90(1):33–41.

41. Bruix J, et al. Adjuvant sorafenib for hepatocellular carcinoma after resection or ablation (STORM): a phase 3, randomised, double-blind, placebo-controlled trial. *Lancet Oncol* 2015;16(13):1344–1354.

42. Mazzaferro V, et al. Liver transplantation for hepatocellular carcinoma. *Ann Surg Oncol* 2008;15(4):1001–1007.

43. Mazzaferro V, et al. Liver transplantation for the treatment of small hepatocellular carcinomas in patients with cirrhosis. *N Engl J Med* 1996;334(11):693–699.

44. Sandroussi C, et al. Radiotherapy as a bridge to liver transplantation for hepatocellular carcinoma. *Transpl Int* 2010;23(3):299–306.

45. Parikh ND, Waljee AK, Singal AG. Downstaging hepatocellular carcinoma: a systematic review and pooled analysis. *Liver Transpl* 2015;21(9):1142–1152.

46. Bujold A, et al. Sequential phase I and II trials of stereotactic body radiotherapy for locally advanced hepatocellular carcinoma. *J Clin Oncol* 2013;31(13):1631–1639.

47. Wahl DR, et al. Outcomes after stereotactic body radiotherapy or radiofrequency ablation for hepatocellular carcinoma. *J Clin Oncol* 2016;34(5):452–459.

48. Pan CC, et al. Radiation-associated liver injury. *Int J Radiat Oncol Biol Phys* 2010;76(3 Suppl):S94–S100.

49. Dawson LA, Ten Haken RK. Partial volume tolerance of the liver to radiation. *Semin Radiat Oncol* 2005;15(4):279–283.

50. Velec M, et al. Predictors of liver toxicity following stereotactic body radiation therapy for hepatocellular carcinoma. *Int J Radiat Oncol Biol Phys* 2017;97(5):939–946.

51. Barry A, et al. Dosimetric analysis of liver toxicity after liver metastasis stereotactic body radiation therapy. *Pract Radiat Oncol* 2017;7(5):e331–e337.

52. Pollom EL, et al. Normal tissue constraints for abdominal and thoracic stereotactic body radiotherapy. *Semin Radiat Oncol* 2017;27(3):197–208.

53. Toesca DA, et al. Central liver toxicity after SBRT: an expanded analysis and predictive nomogram. *Radiother Oncol* 2017;122(1):130–136.

CHAPTER 25

COLON AND RECTUM

ANATOMY

Rectum

- The rectum begins where the large bowel loses its mesentery, at the level of the body of the third sacral vertebra.
- Peritoneum covers the upper portion laterally and anteriorly near its junction with the sigmoid colon and only anteriorly near the peritoneal reflection. The peritoneum is reflected anteriorly onto the seminal vesicles and bladder in males and onto the upper vagina and uterus in females, leaving the lower half of the rectum without a peritoneal covering.
- Three transverse folds, two on the left and one on the right, divide the rectum topographically into thirds. The middle transverse fold, approximately 11 cm from the anal verge, provides a landmark for the peritoneal reflection.
- The portion below the middle valve is the rectal ampulla; if it is resected, stool frequency is often increased markedly (important to consider when choosing between a "radical" sphincter-sparing procedure, such as coloanal anastomosis, and a "conservative" sphincter-sparing procedure, such as endocavitary irradiation).
- Lymphatic drainage follows the superior rectal vessels, which empty into the inferior mesenteric nodes.
- Lymphatic drainage of the middle and lower rectum also occurs along the middle rectal vessels, terminating in the internal iliac nodes.
- The lowest part of the rectum and upper part of the anal canal share a plexus that drains to the lymphatics that accompany the inferior rectal and internal pudendal blood vessels and ultimately drain to the internal iliac nodes.
- Carcinomas of the lower rectum or those extending into the anal canal may occasionally metastasize to superficial inguinal nodes via connections to efferent lymphatics draining the lower anus (Fig. 25-1) (1).

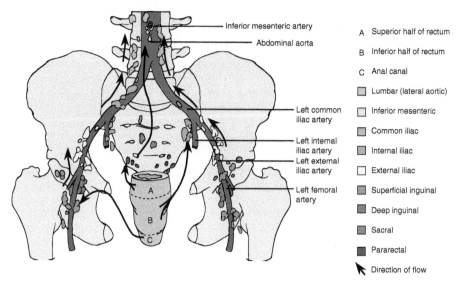

FIGURE 25-1. Lymphatic drainage of large bowel and colon wall. (Adapted from Agur AMR, Dalley AF, eds. *Grant's atlas of anatomy*, 12th ed. Philadelphia, PA: Lippincott Williams & Wilkins, 2009:213.)

Colon

- Ascending and descending colon and splenic and hepatic flexures lack mesentery and are immobile because of their retroperitoneal location.
- Cecum lacks a true mesentery but may have some mobility because of short folds of the peritoneum that are variably present.
- Lymphatic drainage follows the inferior mesenteric vessels for the left colon and superior mesenteric vessels for the right colon.
- If tumor involves adjacent organs in the true or false pelvis, iliac nodes may be at risk.
- Periaortic lymph nodes may be at risk when cancer invades the retroperitoneum.

NATURAL HISTORY

- Discontinuous spread of colon and rectal cancer occurs by peritoneal seeding, lymphatic spread, hematogenous spread, and surgical implantation.
- Peritoneal spread is rare in rectal cancer because most of the rectum is below the peritoneal reflection.
- Extension within the bowel usually occurs only for short distances.
- Primary venous and lymphatic channels originate in submucosal layers of bowel; cancers limited to the mucosa are at little risk for dissemination.
- Lymph node involvement occurs in nearly 50% of patients with deeper tumors.
- Skip metastasis or retrograde spread occurs in 1% to 3% of node-positive patients and is thought to be due to lymphatic blockage.

CLINICAL PRESENTATION

- Hematochezia is the most common presenting feature in rectal and lower sigmoid cancer.
- Abdominal pain is common in patients with colon cancer.
- Other presenting symptoms include change in bowel habit, nausea, vomiting, anemia, or abdominal mass.
- Although colorectal cancer has seen steady decline in both incidence and mortality in recent decades (2), there is, however, a significant increase in the incidence of colorectal cancers among individuals younger than 50 years of age (3). An SEER database study has concluded that colon cancer and rectal cancer for young adults between 20 and 40 years of age have increased by 17% and 75%, respectively (4). Around 75% of early colorectal cancer occurs in individuals between 40 and 49 years of age (5). There is currently no consensus on the cause of the increased incidence of colorectal cancers in younger patients; however, prior studies have shown correlation between obesity (6), diabetes (7), smoking (7), and alcohol consumptions (8) with colorectal cancer risk.

DIAGNOSTIC WORKUP

- Diagnostic procedures include detailed history, physical examination, and endoscopic, radiographic, and laboratory studies (Table 25-1).

Table 25-1
Diagnostic Workup for Colorectal Cancer

General
Complete history
Physical examination, including digital rectal examination (DRE)
Pelvic examination in female patients to assess vaginal involvement

Radiographic and Endoscopic Studies
Barium enema or colonoscopy
Proctosigmoidoscopy (if colonoscopy not done)
Chest radiography
Computed tomography to identify lymphadenopathy and metastasis outside of the pelvis
Endoscopic ultrasound (EUS)
Pelvic magnetic resonance imaging (MRI)
Positron emission tomography (PET) for evaluation of oligometastatic disease

Routine Laboratory Studies
Complete blood cell count
Blood chemistry profile, including liver and renal function studies
Carcinoembryonic antigen
Molecular biologic markers

Source: Palta M, Willett CG, Czito BG. Cancer of the colon and rectum. In: Perez CA, Brady LW, eds. *Principles and practice of radiation oncology*, 6th ed. Philadelphia, PA: Lippincott-Raven, 2013:1216–1231.

- In patients with rectal cancer, a digital rectal examination and an endoscopy are mandatory.
- For colon and rectal tumors, attention should be paid to palpation of any extra rectal mass that may suggest peritoneal spread.
- In women, a complete pelvic examination, including rectovaginal examination, is mandatory.
- Potential areas of metastatic spread, including inguinal lymph nodes (particularly with rectal lesions near the dentate line), supraclavicular lymph nodes, liver, abdominal mass, or ascites, should be evaluated.
- Barium enema and proctosigmoidoscopy or colonoscopy should be performed to rule out second primary large bowel cancers and to biopsy any suspicious lesions.
- For rectal cancer, barium enema performed before resection, including a cross-table lateral view, can assist greatly in planning radiation therapy.
- Endoscopic ultrasound (EUS) is limited to tumors of the upper rectum, and it is useful in evaluating layers of the rectal wall as well as perirectal lymph nodes.
- If liver and renal function studies are abnormal, computed tomography scan or ultrasonography is indicated.
- Preoperative carcinoembryonic antigen (CEA) value is an independent prognostic factor in large bowel cancer; serial measurement postoperatively is used to identify disease progression in asymptomatic patients.
- Magnetic resonance imaging (MRI) acquired using an endorectal coil has been shown to demonstrate similar accuracy as EUS in assessing depth of invasion (81.1% with EUS versus 81% with MRI) and staging of lymph node metastasis (63.5% with EUS versus 63% with MRI) (9).

STAGING SYSTEMS

- Dukes described a staging system based on extent of disease penetration through the bowel wall and presence or absence of nodal metastasis (10).
- The Astler-Coller staging system allows specification of both tumor penetration and nodal involvement; its modification also permits specification of tumor adherence to surrounding organ structures (11).
- The Dukes, Astler-Coller, and modified Astler-Coller systems are postoperative pathologic staging systems and cannot be used preoperatively.
- The tumor-node-metastasis system of the American Joint Committee on Cancer can be used as a clinical (preoperative) or postoperative pathologic staging system (12).

PATHOLOGY

- Most malignant tumors of the large bowel are adenocarcinomas; most are moderately to well differentiated histologically.
- Other histology includes squamous cell carcinoma, melanoma, small cell carcinoma, carcinoid, sarcoma, and lymphoma.

COLON AND RECTUM[a]

- In AJCC 8th edition, notable changes compared to AJCC 7th edition include subdivision of M1 as M1a, M1b, and M1c. M1a is defined as metastasis confined to one organ without peritoneal metastases, M1b is defined as metastasis to more than one organ, and M1c is defined as metastasis to the peritoneum with or without other organ involvement. Similarly, stage group IV was also split into IVA, IVB, and IVC corresponding to each subcategory of M1 stage.

[a]Sarcomas, lymphomas, and carcinoid tumors of the large intestine are not included.
See: Amin M, Edge S, Green F, et al., eds. *AJCC cancer staging manual*, 8th ed. New York, NY: Springer Verlag, 2017.

PROGNOSTIC FACTORS

- Tumor penetration of the bowel wall and lymph node involvement are important prognostic factors; both are associated with increased risk of local recurrence.
- Absolute number and proportion of involved lymph nodes are important predictors of outcome (13).
- Presence of both lymph node involvement and extension of disease beyond the bowel wall is more ominous than the presence of either alone (13).
- In patients with low rectal cancer being considered for sphincter-sparing treatment, clinical mobility, size, and morphology of the lesion are predictors of outcome (14).
- Aneuploidy and high proliferative index (measured by adding percentage of cells in S phase to those in G2 and M phases) are associated with worse survival in colorectal cancer (15).
- Right-sided colon cancer consisting of the cecum, ascending, hepatic flexure, and transverse colon has been shown to result in higher mortality compared to left-sided colon cancer consisting of splenic flexure, descending, sigmoid, and rectosigmoid colon (16). The mechanism behind higher mortality of right-sided colon cancer is unclear at the time; however, the higher prevalence of microsatellite instability (MSI) among right-sided colon cancer may contribute to the disparity in mortality between right- and left-sided colon cancers (17).

GENERAL MANAGEMENT

Patterns of Failure after Curative Resection

- Of 74 patients with rectal cancer treated surgically who underwent elective or symptomatic "second-look" operations because they were thought to be at high risk for local recurrence, 52 (70%) had metastatic or locally recurrent cancer. Locoregional recurrence in the pelvis or paraaortic nodes was the only failure in 24 of 52 patients (46%) and occurred as a component of failure in 48 (92%) (18).

- Patients with disease extension beyond the bowel wall, with nodal involvement, or both generally have local recurrence rates of 20% to 70% (1). Distant metastasis occurs in approximately 30% of patients who undergo curative resection of rectal cancer; the most common sites of involvement are the liver, lung, and peritoneum (1).
- Local failure in colon cancer is highest among patients with tumors adhering to surrounding structures and those with both tumor extension beyond the bowel wall and metastatically involved lymph nodes (19,20). The local recurrence rate among these patients is 30% to 49% (21).
- Approximately 20% of patients who undergo curative resection of colon cancer develop distant metastasis; most common sites are the liver, lung, and peritoneum (20).

Colon

- Intergroup 0130 randomized 187 patients with resected T4 or T3N+ to either adjuvant chemoradiation therapy (CRT) or chemotherapy alone. The trial closed due to poor accrual (goal of 700 patients). There were no differences in 5-year overall survival of 62% (chemo) versus 58% (CRT) and no differences in 5-year disease-free survival (DFS), 51% versus 51% (22).
- Postoperative irradiation can be considered in patients with close or positive surgical margins or in patients with T4 lesions adherent to the pelvic structure.
- Adjuvant radiation therapy can be properly delivered if we know what volumes need to be treated and requires proper imaging to delineate the region of interest or clip placement by the surgeon during operation.

Rectum

- Surgical resection is the treatment of choice for most patients, and surgical options include transanal excision, abdominoperineal resection, or low anterior resection.
- Low anterior resections are technically feasible in patients with tumors at least 6 to 8 cm above the anal verge; survival rates are similar to those for abdominoperineal resection.
- Neoadjuvant CRT attempting for sphincter sparing for mid- to low rectal cancer should be discussed with patients.

Preoperative Versus Postoperative Adjuvant Therapy

- Patients with rectal lesions larger than 2 cm, particularly if the lesions are sessile and not well differentiated, are candidates for a short course of preoperative irradiation (20 to 25 Gy in 5 fractions) (23–27).
- Patients with T3, tethered, or poorly differentiated tumors are frequently treated with higher doses of preoperative irradiation (45 to 46 Gy, 1.8- to 2.0-Gy fractions), frequently combined with chemotherapy (5-FU), followed by surgery 4 to 6 weeks later (28).

- MRC CR07 and NCIC-CTG C016 compared short-course preoperative radiotherapy (RT) (25 Gy in 5 fractions) to surgery with selective postoperative CRT (45 Gy in 25 fractions with concurrent 5-FU).
- Local recurrence was 4.4% versus 10.6% and DFS 77.5% versus 71.5% in preoperative RT and postoperative CRT, respectively, with no difference noted in OS (29).
- Preoperative CRT (50.4 Gy in 28 fractions with concurrent 5-FU) improved local control and was associated with reduced toxicity but did not improve overall survival when compared to postoperative CRT. The German Rectal Cancer Study demonstrated an 8% pathologic complete response rate in preoperative CRT group with 6% LR rate as compared with 13% in postoperative CRT group. Fewer acute (27% versus 40%) and late toxicities (14% versus 24%) as well as increased rate of sphincter-preserving surgery (39% versus 19%) were noted in the preoperative CRT group (30). Ten-year OS was not statistically significant with 59.6% in the preoperative CRT group and 59.9% in the postoperative CRT group (31).

RADIATION THERAPY TECHNIQUES

External Beam Radiation Therapy

- Shrinking field technique should be used, with initial irradiation fields designed to treat the primary tumor volume and regional lymph nodes.
- Smaller fields can be used to treat the primary tumor bed to higher doses, as clinically indicated.
- The width of posteroanterior portals (Fig. 25-2) should cover the pelvic inlet with a 2-cm margin; the superior margin is usually 1.5 cm above the level of the sacral promontory.
- In patients who have had anterior resection, the usual inferior margin is below the obturator foramen.
- If the pelvis is treated, lateral fields should be used for a portion of the treatment to avoid as much of the small bowel as possible. Bladder distention and prone position are useful techniques for displacing the small bowel out of the pelvis.
- The posterior field margin for lateral fields is critical because the rectum and the perirectal tissues lie just anterior to the sacrum and the coccyx; the posterior field margin should be at least 1.5 to 2.0 cm behind the anterior bony sacral margin (Fig. 25-2).
- The entire sacral canal should be included for locally advanced disease to avoid sacral recurrence from tumor spread along nerve roots (1).
- Mobile or slightly tethered lesions can be treated with 20 to 25 Gy in 4 to 5 fractions of preoperative RT. More advanced disease should be treated with 45 Gy in 25 fractions.
- When internal iliac and presacral nodes are at risk for metastases, they are not dissected and should be included in the initial irradiation volume treated to 45 Gy.
- External iliac nodes are not a primary lymph node drainage site and are not included unless pelvic organs with external iliac drainage (prostate, upper vagina, bladder, and uterus) are involved by direct extension (T4 disease).

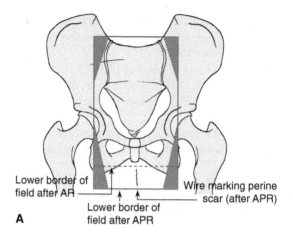

Lower border of
field after AR
Lower border of
field after APR
Wire marking perine
scar (after APR)
A

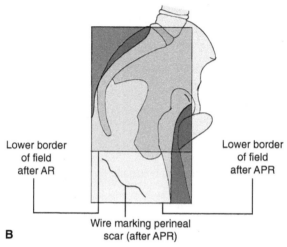

Lower border
of field
after AR

Lower border
of field
after APR

Wire marking perineal
scar (after APR)
B

FIGURE 25-2. Initial posteroanterior **(A)** and lateral **(B)** irradiation fields used in adjuvant treatment of rectal cancer. In patients with tumor adherence to the prostate, bladder, vagina, or uterus, the anterior border of lateral field is modified so that it is anterior to the symphysis pubis to provide coverage of the external iliac nodes. APR, abdominoperineal resection; AR, anterior resection. (Adapted from Martenson JA Jr, Schild SE, Haddock MG. Cancers of the gastrointestinal tract. In: Khan FM, Potish RA, eds. *Treatment planning in radiation oncology.* Baltimore, MD: Williams & Wilkins, 1997.)

- Radiopaque markers can be used to outline the extent of the perineal scar at simulation for posterior and lateral fields.
- Anteriorly, the lower third of the rectum abuts the posterior vaginal wall or prostate, which should be included in patients with distal lesions. In females, this can be verified by placing a contrast-soaked tampon in the vagina during radiation therapy simulation.
- Irradiation of the perineum after abdominoperineal resection decreases perineal recurrences. At the Mayo Clinic, the perineal failure rate was 2% at 5 years for patients receiving postoperative irradiation in whom the perineum was included in

the irradiation field for the initial 40 Gy, in contrast to 23% if the entire perineum was not treated ($p = 0.01$) (13).

- Temporary, acute, and moderate-to-moderately severe perineal discomfort can be mitigated with the use of three-field technique (posteroanterior and laterals, with wedges on lateral fields, and heels posterior). The incidence of late complications has not increased as a result of perineal irradiation.
- Bolus applied to the perineal scar during posteroanterior treatment ensures adequate dose to this site.
- Dose to the large fields, including tumor bed and regional lymph nodes, should be 45 Gy in 5 weeks.
- After this, a boost to the primary tumor bed and immediately adjacent lymph nodes should be considered. Boost fields are defined by barium enema, computed tomography scan, or clip placement. Doses greater than 50.4 Gy generally should not be administered unless there is complete shift of the small bowel out of the final boost field.
- The RTOG consensus panel contouring atlas for elective CTV in anorectal cancer provided guidelines for the contours of CTV-A, CTV-B, and CTV-C in rectal cancer (32) for intensity-modulated radiation therapy (IMRT) planning. CTV-A represents internal iliac, presacral, and perirectal nodal regions. The caudal border of CTV-A should cover the entire mesorectum to the pelvic floor or at a minimum of 2 cm inferior to gross disease. In the midpelvis, CTV-A should cover the rectum and its mesentery, the internal iliac region, and a 1-cm margin into the posterior bladder. The superior border of the perirectal component of CTV-A should extend to the rectosigmoid junction or at least 2 cm superior to the gross disease, whichever is more superior. The superior border of the entire CTV-A should be at the level of bifurcation of the common iliac vessels. CTV-A should extend at least 1 cm anterior to the sacrum. CTV-B represents external iliac nodal region for T4 disease extending into gynecologic or genitourinary structures. Some of the experts on the consensus panel also recommended including CTV-B for rectal cancers that extend into the anal canal. CTV-C represents inguinal nodal region. The consensus panel was divided on whether to include CTV-C for rectal adenocarcinomas that extend to the anal verge, perianal skin, and lower one third of the vagina. The inferior border of CTV-C should be 2 cm inferior to the saphenous/femoral junction. The transition from CTV-B to CTV-C should be at the level of the inferior border of the internal obturator vessels.
- If irradiation is used for locally advanced extra pelvic colon cancer, the tumor bed should be covered with a 3- to 5-cm margin.
- Adjuvant irradiation for colon cancer is usually given in the context of a formal prospective clinical trial.
- A combination of external and intraoperative irradiation has been used (33).

Sphincter Preservation

Endocavitary Radiation Therapy

- Indications for endocavitary radiation therapy were described by Papillon (14).
- When the suitability of a patient for this technique is assessed, intrarectal ultrasonography is helpful for determining tumor confinement to the rectal wall (34).

- Treatment is performed on an outpatient basis.
- Local anesthesia in the anal canal is occasionally required for introducing the 3-cm diameter applicator into the rectum.
- The radiation oncologist verifies the position of the applicator and coverage of the lesion. A lead apron and gloves are worn by the radiation oncologist, who holds the applicator firmly in place during the x-ray exposure.
- Treatment usually consists of four 30-Gy treatments separated by intervals of approximately 2 weeks.
- A short focal distance (contact) x-ray unit is used at 50 kVp at a dose rate of approximately 10 Gy per minute.
- If tumor size exceeds the diameter of the applicator, several overlapping fields must be used (35,36).

Local Excision with or without Postoperative Irradiation

- Limited surgical resection has been used in selected patients with superficial tumors (limited to submucosa or muscularis mucosa) (37).
- To minimize local recurrence, postoperative irradiation (45 to 50 Gy) has been used (38,39).

NORMAL TISSUE COMPLICATIONS—QUANTEC RESULTS

Michalski et al. (40) present the QUANTEC review recommendations, including the following:
- The available dose/volume/outcome data for rectal injury were reviewed. The volume of rectum receiving ≥ 60 Gy is consistently associated with the risk of grade ≥ 2 rectal toxicity or rectal bleeding.

Dose-Volume Constraints for Conventional Fractionation up to 78 Gy

- The following dose-volume constraints are provided as a conservative starting point for 3-D treatment planning: $V_{50} < 50\%$, $V_{60} < 35\%$, $V_{65} < 25\%$, $V_{70} < 20\%$, and $V_{75} < 15\%$. However, they have yet to be validated as "relatively safe." For typical DVHs, the NTCP models predict that following these constraints should limit grade ≥ 2 late rectal toxicity to less than 15% and the probability of grade ≥ 3 late rectal toxicity to less than 10% for prescriptions up to 79.2 Gy in standard 1.8- to 2-Gy fractions.
- Higher doses in the V_{dose} parameter have more impact on the complication probability. Clinicians should strive to minimize the V_{70} and V_{75} volumes below the recommended constraints without compromising tumor coverage. Reducing the V_{75} by just 5% from 15% to 10% has a significant impact in the predicted complication probability, whereas reducing the V_{50} from 50% to 45% makes relatively little difference.
- Intensity-modulated RT (IMRT) planning yields distinctly different shaped DVH curves than forward-planned 3D conformal RT (3DCRT), with considerably

decreased rectal volume receiving low-to-intermediate radiation doses. Although the parameters above provide a safe starting point for both 3DCRT and IMRT, it is likely that because IMRT can achieve better low-to-intermediate dose-volume constraints, the observed rectal toxicity will be lower (41). The Memorial Sloan-Kettering IMRT experience suggests that doses in the intermediate range of 40 to 60 Gy may become important in patients who are receiving radiation prescriptions in excess of 78 Gy. The Slovenia phase 2 trial for operable stage II to III rectal adenocarcinoma with preoperative IMRT to the pelvis and simultaneous integrated boost to rectal primary demonstrated only 2 cases of grade 3 or higher toxicity among 51 patients (42).

- RTOG 0822 is a phase 2 study of preoperative chemoradiation for T3-4N0-2 rectal cancer using IMRT to 45 Gy in 25 fractions followed by a 3D boost to the gross disease for 5.4 Gy in 3 fractions with concurrent capecitabine and oxaliplatin. Grade 2 or higher gastrointestinal (GI) toxicity was observed in 51.5% of the patients (43). This GI toxicity rate not only exceeded the target of 28% but also exceeded the rate of 40% as reported from RTOG 0247, which was a phase 2 study investigating preoperative chemoradiation for rectal cancer using 2D or 3D planning (44). Although RTOG 0822 failed to show decreased GI toxicity with IMRT, however, the role of IMRT for rectal cancer remains to be answered. IMRT may still play a role in the patient population for whom the QUANTEC bowel dose constraint cannot be satisfied with 3D planning.

- Figure 25-3 presents an adaptation of the isocomplication curves given in Figure 1 of Michalski et al. (40) for grade 2 or higher rectal toxicity. We have taken the most

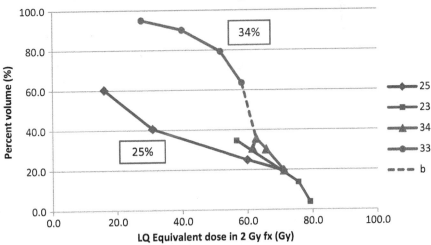

FIGURE 25-3. Simplification of QUANTEC dose-volume histogram threshold data. The individual line segments from Figure 1 of Michalski et al. (40) have been redrawn, combining those for 23% and 25% and also 33% and 34%, respectively. We have removed the threshold lines for the lower complication rates to give a worst-case scenario, but one where the 25% and 33% line segments actually bracket the V_{dose} recommendations noted in (40).

conservative approach, selecting the line segments for 23% and 25% complication and also those for 33% and 34%. These have been used to indicate the approximate threshold lines for 25% and 33% complication rates, that is, where one quarter or one third of patients will experience significant distress. Not surprisingly, the complication curves all converge at high dosage.

SEQUELAE OF TREATMENT

- Diarrhea is the most common acute toxicity during pelvic irradiation; approximately 24% of patients developed severe or life-threatening diarrhea when pelvic irradiation was used in combination with protracted 5-FU infusion (45).
- Gastrointestinal toxicity is more prevalent with 5-FU delivered via continuous infusion, whereas hematologic toxicity is more common with bolus administration of 5-FU (46).
- Hand-foot syndrome has been associated with capecitabine; however, the symptom can usually be managed with vitamin B6 and supportive care (47).
- Consistently worse bowel function was found in patients who received irradiation and chemotherapy (56% reported occasional fecal incontinence in comparison with only 7% of those not receiving adjuvant treatment) ($p < 0.001$) (48).
- Endocavitary irradiation is well tolerated; approximately 35% of patients have minor rectal bleeding; rectal urgency occurs in approximately 20%. These symptoms usually improve.
- Ulcers develop in approximately 75% of patients after intracavitary radiation therapy, but this condition is usually asymptomatic and resolves in most patients (49).

TARGETED THERAPIES

- KRAS mutation in colorectal cancer is associated with the lack of response to anti-EGFR therapy, and approximately 40% to 60% of wild-type KRAS colorectal cancers have been shown to respond to anti-EGFR therapy (50). Improved survival in metastatic or advanced colorectal cancer patients treated with panitumumab (51) or cetuximab (52) has been observed but only with wild-type KRAS.
- Immune checkpoint inhibitors in the form of monoclonal antibodies (mAbs) targeting the cytotoxic T-lymphocyte–associated protein-4 (CTLA-4) and programmed cell death (PD-1) receptors have shown promise in the treatment of colorectal cancer.
- Tremelimumab is a human immunoglobulin (Ig) G2 mAb that binds to CTLA-4 receptor, and a phase 2 study of tremelimumab for refractory metastatic colorectal cancer showed limited response with only 1 out of 49 patients experiencing a partial response (53).
- Nivolumab is a humanized IgG4 mAb that inhibits PD-1. Long-term follow-up from a phase I trial of nivolumab showed an isolated case of a patient with refractory colorectal cancer with sustained complete response lasting 3 years, and the tumor's

molecular status was notable for MSI-H and membranous PD-L1 expression on tumor-infiltrating macrophages and lymphocytes (54).

- Pembrolizumab is an IgG4 mAb that inhibits PD-1. A multicenter phase 2 study of refractory metastatic colorectal cancer patients treated with pembrolizumab showed significantly higher median PFS and OS in patients with MSI versus those without (55).

References

1. Halperin EC, et al. *Perez and Brady's principles and practice of radiation oncology*, 6th ed. Philadelphia, PA: Wolters Kluwer Health/Lippincott Williams & Wilkins, 2013:xxxii, 1936 p.
2. Ferlay J, et al. Cancer incidence and mortality worldwide: sources, methods and major patterns in GLOBOCAN 2012. *Int J Cancer* 2015;136(5):E359–E386.
3. Bailey CE, et al. Increasing disparities in the age-related incidences of colon and rectal cancers in the United States, 1975–2010. *JAMA Surg* 2015;150(1):17–22.
4. O'Connell JB, et al. Rates of colon and rectal cancers are increasing in young adults. *Am Surg* 2003;69(10):866–872.
5. You YN, et al. Young-onset colorectal cancer: is it time to pay attention? *Arch Intern Med* 2012;172(3):287–289.
6. Karahalios A, English DR, Simpson JA. Weight change and risk of colorectal cancer: a systematic review and meta-analysis. *Am J Epidemiol* 2015;181(11):832–845.
7. Yuhara H, et al. Is diabetes mellitus an independent risk factor for colon cancer and rectal cancer? *Am J Gastroenterol* 2011;106(11):1911–1921; quiz 1922.
8. Fedirko V, et al. Alcohol drinking and colorectal cancer risk: an overall and dose-response meta-analysis of published studies. *Ann Oncol* 2011;22(9):1958–1972.
9. Kim NK, et al. Comparative study of transrectal ultrasonography, pelvic computerized tomography, and magnetic resonance imaging in preoperative staging of rectal cancer. *Dis Colon Rectum* 1999;42(6):770–775.
10. Dukes CE. The classification of cancer of the rectum. *J Pathol Bacteriol* 1932;35(3):323–332.
11. Astler VB, Coller FA. The prognostic significance of direct extension of carcinoma of the colon and rectum. *Ann Surg* 1954;139(6):846–852.
12. Amin MB, et al. The Eighth Edition AJCC Cancer Staging Manual: continuing to build a bridge from a population-based to a more "personalized" approach to cancer staging. *CA Cancer J Clin* 2017;67(2):93–99.
13. Schild SE, et al. Long-term survival and patterns of failure after postoperative radiation therapy for subtotally resected rectal adenocarcinoma. *Int J Radiat Oncol Biol Phys* 1989;16(2):459–463.
14. Papillon J. *Rectal and anal cancers: conservative treatment by irradiation—an alternative to radical surgery.* Berlin/New York: Springer-Verlag, 1982:xvi, 201 p.
15. Witzig TE, et al. DNA ploidy and cell kinetic measurements as predictors of recurrence and survival in stages B2 and C colorectal adenocarcinoma. *Cancer* 1991;68(4):879–888.
16. Benedix F, et al. Right- and left-sided colonic cancer—different tumour entities. *Zentralbl Chir* 2010;135(4):312–317.
17. Hansen IO, Jess P. Possible better long-term survival in left versus right-sided colon cancer—a systematic review. *Dan Med J* 2012;59(6):A4444.
18. Gunderson LL, Sosin H. Areas of failure found at reoperation (second or symptomatic look) following "curative surgery" for adenocarcinoma of the rectum: clinicopathologic correlation and implications for adjuvant therapy. *Cancer* 1974;34(4):1278–1292.
19. Gunderson LL, Sosin H, Levitt S. Extrapelvic colon—areas of failure in a reoperation series: implications for adjuvant therapy. *Int J Radiat Oncol Biol Phys* 1985;11(4):731–741.

20. Russell AH, et al. Adenocarcinoma of the colon: an autopsy study with implications for new therapeutic strategies. *Cancer* 1985;56(6):1446–1451.
21. Willett CG, et al. Failure patterns following curative resection of colonic carcinoma. *Ann Surg* 1984;200(6):685–690.
22. Martenson JA, et al. Phase III study of adjuvant chemotherapy and radiation therapy compared with chemotherapy alone in the surgical adjuvant treatment of colon cancer: results of intergroup protocol 0130. *J Clin Oncol* 2004;22(16):3277–3283.
23. Cedermark B, Johansson H, Rutqvist LE. The Stockholm I trial of preoperative short term radiotherapy in operable rectal carcinoma. *Cancer* 1995;75(9):2269–2275.
24. Gérard A, et al. Preoperative radiotherapy as adjuvant treatment in rectal cancer. *Ann Surg* 1988;208(5):606–614.
25. Myerson RJ, et al. Five fractions of preoperative radiotherapy for selected cases of rectal carcinoma: long-term tumor control and tolerance to treatment. *Int J Radiat Oncol Biol Phys* 1999;43(3):537–543.
26. Myerson RJ, et al. Adjuvant radiation therapy for rectal carcinoma: predictors of outcome. *Int J Radiat Oncol Biol Phys* 1995;32(1):41–50.
27. Swedish Rectal Cancer Trial, Cedermark B, Dahlberg M, Glimelius B, et al. Improved survival with preoperative radiotherapy in resectable rectal cancer. *N Engl J Med* 1997;336(14):980–987.
28. Janjan NA, et al. Tumor downstaging and sphincter preservation with preoperative chemoradiation in locally advanced rectal cancer: the M.D. Anderson Cancer Center experience. *Int J Radiat Oncol Biol Phys* 1999;44(5):1027–1038.
29. Sebag-Montefiore D, et al. Preoperative radiotherapy versus selective postoperative chemoradiotherapy in patients with rectal cancer (MRC CR07 and NCIC-CTG C016): a multicentre, randomised trial. *Lancet* 2009;373(9666):811–820.
30. Sauer R, et al. Preoperative versus postoperative chemoradiotherapy for rectal cancer. *N Engl J Med* 2004;351(17):1731–1740.
31. Sauer R, et al. Preoperative versus postoperative chemoradiotherapy for locally advanced rectal cancer: results of the German CAO/ARO/AIO-94 randomized phase III trial after a median follow-up of 11 years. *J Clin Oncol* 2012;30(16):1926–1933.
32. Myerson RJ, et al. Elective clinical target volumes for conformal therapy in anorectal cancer: a radiation therapy oncology group consensus panel contouring atlas. *Int J Radiat Oncol Biol Phys* 2009;74(3):824–830.
33. Gunderson LL, et al. Intraoperative and external beam irradiation for locally advanced colorectal cancer. *Ann Surg* 1988;207(1):52–60.
34. Wang KY, et al. Colorectal neoplasms: accuracy of US in demonstrating the depth of invasion. *Radiology* 1987;165(3):827–829.
35. Myerson RJ, Walz BJ, Kodner IJ. Endocavitary radiation therapy for rectal carcinoma: results with and without external beam. *Endoc Hypertherm Oncol* 1989;5:195–200.
36. Schild SE, Martenson JA, Gunderson LL. Endocavitary radiotherapy of rectal cancer. *Int J Radiat Oncol Biol Phys* 1996;34(3):677–682.
37. Biggers OR, Beart RW, Ilstrup DM. Local excision of rectal cancer. *Dis Colon Rectum* 1986;29(6):374–377.
38. Minsky BD, et al. Sphincter preservation in rectal cancer by local excision and postoperative radiation therapy. *Cancer* 1991;67(4):908–914.
39. Rich TA, et al. Sphincter preservation in patients with low rectal cancer treated with radiation therapy with or without local excision or fulguration. *Radiology* 1985;156(2):527–531.
40. Michalski JM, et al. Radiation dose–volume effects in radiation-induced rectal injury. *Int J Radiat Oncol Biol Phys* 2010;76(3):S123–S129.

41. Zelefsky MJ, et al. Incidence of late rectal and urinary toxicities after three-dimensional conformal radiotherapy and intensity-modulated radiotherapy for localized prostate cancer. *Int J Radiat Oncol Biol Phys* 2008;70(4):1124–1129.

42. But-Hadzic J, et al. Acute toxicity and tumor response in locally advanced rectal cancer after preoperative chemoradiation therapy with shortening of the overall treatment time using intensity-modulated radiation therapy with simultaneous integrated boost: a phase 2 trial. *Int J Radiat Oncol Biol Phys* 2016;96(5):1003–1010.

43. Hong TS, et al. NRG Oncology Radiation Therapy Oncology Group 0822: a phase 2 study of preoperative chemoradiation therapy using intensity modulated radiation therapy in combination with capecitabine and oxaliplatin for patients with locally advanced rectal cancer. *Int J Radiat Oncol Biol Phys* 2015;93(1):29–36.

44. Wong SJ, et al. Radiation Therapy Oncology Group 0247: a randomized Phase II study of neoadjuvant capecitabine and irinotecan or capecitabine and oxaliplatin with concurrent radiotherapy for patients with locally advanced rectal cancer. *Int J Radiat Oncol Biol Phys* 2012;82(4):1367–1375.

45. O'Connell MJ, et al. Improving adjuvant therapy for rectal cancer by combining protracted-infusion fluorouracil with radiation therapy after curative surgery. *N Engl J Med* 1994;331(8):502–507.

46. Smalley SR, et al. Phase III trial of fluorouracil-based chemotherapy regimens plus radiotherapy in postoperative adjuvant rectal cancer: GI INT 0144. *J Clin Oncol* 2006;24(22):3542–3547.

47. Liu GC, et al. Effect of neoadjuvant chemoradiotherapy with capecitabine versus fluorouracil for locally advanced rectal cancer: a meta-analysis. *Gastroenterol Res Pract* 2016;2016:1798285.

48. Kollmorgen CF, et al. The long-term effect of adjuvant postoperative chemoradiotherapy for rectal carcinoma on bowel function. *Ann Surg* 1994;220(5):676–682.

49. Lavery IC, et al. Definitive management of rectal cancer by contact (endocavitary) irradiation. *Dis Colon Rectum* 1987;30(11):835–838.

50. Wilson PM, Labonte MJ, Lenz HJ. Molecular markers in the treatment of metastatic colorectal cancer. *Cancer J* 2010;16(3):262–272.

51. Amado RG, et al. Wild-type KRAS is required for panitumumab efficacy in patients with metastatic colorectal cancer. *J Clin Oncol* 2008;26(10):1626–1634.

52. Karapetis CS, et al. K-ras mutations and benefit from cetuximab in advanced colorectal cancer. *N Engl J Med* 2008;359(17):1757–1765.

53. Chung KY, et al. Phase II study of the anti-cytotoxic T-lymphocyte-associated antigen 4 monoclonal antibody, tremelimumab, in patients with refractory metastatic colorectal cancer. *J Clin Oncol* 2010;28(21):3485–3490.

54. Lipson EJ, et al. Durable cancer regression off-treatment and effective reinduction therapy with an anti-PD-1 antibody. *Clin Cancer Res* 2013;19(2):462–468.

55. Le DT, Uram JN, Wang H. Programmed death-1 blockade in mismatch repair deficient colorectal cancer. *J Clin Oncol* 2016;34:103.

CHAPTER 26

ANAL CANAL

ANATOMY

- The anal canal is approximately 3 to 4 cm long, and extends from the level of the pelvic floor to the anal verge. The posterior wall is longer than the anterior (1)
- The superior margin is determined clinically by the palpable upper border of the anal sphincter and puborectalis muscle of the anorectal ring. The distal end of the canal at the anal verge approximates the palpable groove between the lower edge of the internal sphincter and the subcutaneous part of the external sphincter (Fig. 26-1).
- Perianal carcinomas are arbitrarily considered to be cancers arising from the skin within a 5-cm radius of the anal verge.
- The major lymphatic pathways predominately drain to the following lymph node systems. Tumors above the dentate line drain primarily to the mesorectal and internal iliac nodes. Tumors below the dentate line can additionally spread to the superficial inguinal and external iliac (deep inguinal) lymph nodes. The perianal skin and anal verge drain predominantly to the superficial inguinal nodes, with some communications to the femoral nodes, and to the external iliac system.

NATURAL HISTORY

- Women have a significantly higher risk of developing anal cancer than do men (2).
- Human papillomavirus (HPV) was present in 88% of the tumors from 394 patients with anal cancer; HPV was absent in 20 of the tumors from patients with rectal adenocarcinoma (3). Interestingly, 73% of the anal cancer patients with HPV detected in their tumors had HPV-16, the same strain as linked to the development of cervical cancer. HPV-18 is found in 10% of anal cancer (4–6).
- Squamous cancers of the anal canal spread most commonly by direct extension and lymphatic pathways. Hematogenous metastases are less common.
- Direct invasion from the anal mucosa into the sphincter muscles and perianal connective tissue spaces occurs early.
- Invasion of the vaginal septum and mucosa is more common than is invasion of the prostate gland.

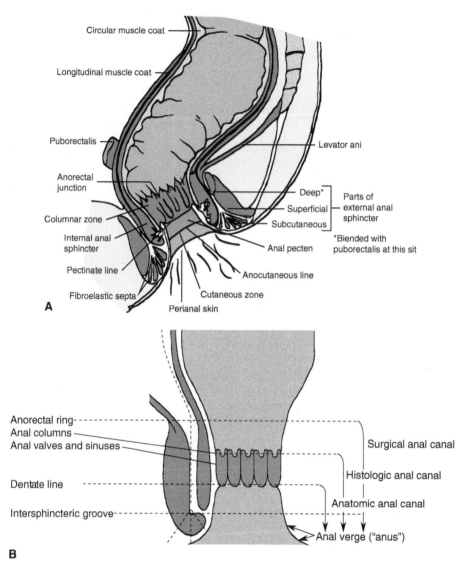

FIGURE 26-1. A: Medial view of rectum and anus. (Adapted with permission from Agur AMR, Dalley AF, eds. *Grant's atlas of anatomy*, 14th ed. Philadelphia, PA: Lippincott Williams & Wilkins; 2017:407. © Wolters Kluwer.) **B:** Detailed schematic drawing of structures in anal region.

- Extensive tumors may infiltrate the sacrum and the coccyx or the pelvic side walls.
- Lymphatic invasion occurs relatively early. Pelvic lymph node metastases are found in approximately 30% of patients treated by abdominoperineal resection. Lymphatic metastases increase in frequency with progressive enlargement of the primary cancer
- Inguinal metastases are clinically detectable in approximately 20% of patients at the time of initial diagnosis and are usually unilateral.

- Nodal metastases are seen in 30% of superficial tumors and 63% of deeply infiltrating or poorly differentiated tumors
- Extrapelvic visceral metastases are identified at the time of presentation in approximately 10% of patients and are found most frequently in the liver and the lungs (2).
- Relapse after initial treatment is more common in the area of the primary tumor and the regional lymph nodes than in extrapelvic organs.

CLINICAL PRESENTATION

- Bleeding and anal discomfort are the most common symptoms (reported by 50% of patients); other complaints include awareness of an anal mass, pruritus, anal discharge, and less frequently pain.
- With proximal anal canal tumors, there may be an alteration in bowel habits, but this symptom is unusual with distal carcinomas.
- Occasionally, asymptomatic tumors are found during physical examination, and unsuspected microinvasive carcinoma is sometimes found in mucosa removed at hemorrhoidectomy.
- Gross fecal incontinence resulting from sphincter destruction occurs in less than 5% of patients, although some fecal soiling is common.
- Synchronous inguinal node metastases are found in approximately 20% of patients.

DIAGNOSTIC WORKUP

- The history and physical examination should stress features that delineate the extent of the primary tumor, including anal sphincter competence (Table 26-1).
- A biopsy of the primary tumor is necessary to establish the diagnosis and the histologic type.
- General anesthesia may be needed to permit detailed pelvic and anorectal examination, which should include anoscopy and sigmoidoscopy.
- Because lymph node enlargement may be caused by reactive hyperplasia in as many as half of those with palpable inguinal nodes, clinically suspicious nodes should be considered for needle biopsy or simple excision.
- Transanorectal ultrasonography may help to identify the depth of tumor penetration into the anal wall.
- Female patients should have gynecologic examination to assess for extension of disease into the vaginal, as well as synchronous cervical or vulvar cancers.
- Computed tomography (CT) of the chest, abdomen, and pelvis with intravenous and oral contrast is recommended for clinical staging.
- Positron emission tomography (PET)/CT is a complementary test to the diagnostic CT for staging purposes. HIV-positive patients may have falsely positive nodes on PET imaging.
- Magnetic resonance imaging (MRI) of the pelvis can be useful, especially if there is concern for tumor invasion into adjacent organs.
- Full blood count, renal and liver function tests, and HIV testing (if unknown HIV status) (7).

Table 26-1

Diagnostic Workup for Cancer of the Anal Canal

Essential

History
Physical examination
 Regional lymph nodes
 Adjacent organs for direct invasion
 Anogenital areas for concurrent malignancies
Anoscopy
Biopsy of primary tumor
Fine needle aspiration biopsy of enlarged inguinal nodes
Computed tomography of chest, abdomen and pelvis
PET/CT
Liver and renal chemistry
Complete blood cell count
HIV testing, if HIV status unknown

Useful

MRI, if concerned about tumor invasion of adjacent organs

Source: *National Comprehensive Cancer Network Clinical Practice Guidelines in Oncology, Anal Carcinoma, Version 1, 2018.* Fort Washington, PA: National Comprehensive Cancer Network.

STAGING

- With the emergence of treatment strategies designed to preserve anorectal function, staging systems based on pathologic parameters have been replaced by clinical staging systems.
- The American Joint Committee on Cancer (AJCC), 8th edition maintains the same T staging criteria as the 7th edition. High-grade squamous intraepithelial lesions are Tis; tumors ≤ 2 cm are T1; tumors greater than 2 cm but ≤5 cm are T2; tumors greater than 5 cm are T3; and tumors invading adjacent organs (e.g., prostate, bladder, vagina, and uterus) is T4. Notably, tumor invading rectal wall, perirectal skin, subcutaneous tissue, or the sphincter muscle(s) is not classified as T4 (8).
- Nodal staging in the AJCC 8th edition has changed. Tumors without regional lymph node metastases are N0. Metastases in inguinal, mesorectal, internal iliac, or external iliac lymph nodes are N1. Involvement of inguinal, mesorectal, or internal iliac nodes is N1a; involvement of external iliac nodes is N1b; involvement of external iliac and N1a nodes is N1c.
- Nonregional lymph nodes metastases or distant metastases are M1.

PATHOLOGIC CLASSIFICATION

- The World Health Organization pathologic classification is the most commonly used.
- Squamous cell carcinomas (cloacogenic carcinomas), representing approximately 80% of all malignant tumors of the anal canal, are historically subdivided into

NEW!   SUMMARY OF CHANGES TO AJCC STAGING

ANUS[a]

- The definitions of TNM and the stage groupings for this chapter have changed from the Seventh Edition.
- Nodal staging is now delineated as N0 or N1, with N1 subdivided into N1a for lymph node metastases in inguinal, mesorectal, or internal iliac nodes; N1b for lymph node metastases in external iliac nodes; and N1c for lymph node metastases in both N1a and N1b nodes.
- Stage groups have been revised in the 7th Edition to account for changes to N staging. T1N0M0 is stage I, T2N0M0 is stage IIA, T3N0M0 is stage IIB, T1-2N1M0 is stage IIIA, T4N0M0 is stage IIIB, T3-4N1M0 is stage IIIC, and Any T Any N M1 is stage IV.
- The descriptions of both the boundaries of the anal canal and anal carcinomas have been clarified.

[a]The classification applies to carcinomas only; melanomas, carcinoid tumors, and sarcomas are not included.

See: Amin MB, Edge SB, Greene FL, Byrd DR, et al., eds. *AJCC cancer staging manual*, 8th ed. New York, NY: Springer Verlag, 2017.

---

large cell keratinizing, large cell nonkeratinizing, and basaloid. The World Health Organization (WHO) recommends the generic term *squamous cell carcinoma* for all squamous tumors of the anal canal (8).

- Some nonkeratinizing tumors resemble transitional cell cancers of the urinary bladder.
- Approximately 70% of squamous cell cancers are keratinizing or nonkeratinizing and 30% are basaloid.
- Mucoepidermoid cancers are rare.
- The remaining cancers arising in the canal include adenocarcinomas of rectal type or from anal glands or fistulas, small cell cancers, and undifferentiated cancers.

PROGNOSTIC FACTORS

- When anal cancer is confined to the pelvis, the size of the primary tumor is the most useful indicator for local control, preservation of anorectal function, and survival.
- Involvement of regional lymph nodes is a moderately adverse factor for survival but not for primary tumor control.
- Presence of extrapelvic metastases is the most adverse factor for survival (2).
- Women have a better prognosis than men, as demonstrated in multiple randomized trials (9–11).
- Age at diagnosis has no independent prognostic significance.
- Histologic subtype of squamous cell carcinoma is not an independent prognostic factor when corrected for stage. Poorly differentiated tumors are associated with a worse

prognosis than moderately or well-differentiated tumors, although this significance was lost in some series when adjusted for stage.
- HIV-positive patients may tolerate treatment less well than HIV-negative patients. However, patients whose HIV is well controlled with highly active antiretroviral therapy appear to do as well as HIV-negative patients (12).
- Palpable lymphadenopathy is prognostic for locoregional failure (13).
- Lower hemoglobin is associated with worse overall survival (13).

GENERAL MANAGEMENT

- Multiple randomized trials have established that the combination of radiation therapy, 5-fluorouracil, and mitomycin C is the standard against which other treatments should be compared (1,2,4,12).
- Nonrandomized comparisons of radical resection with this radiation-chemotherapy combination, or with radiation alone, have shown that radiation-based regimens produce survival rates at least equal to those of surgical series, while allowing the preservation of anorectal function in most patients (3).
- Wide local excision with sphincter sparing has been used in selected patients with limited, superficial tumors.
- Extensive tumors, which have destroyed the anal sphincter or have resulted in a fistula, likely require abdominoperineal resection.

Combined-Modality Therapy

Primary Tumor

- Interest in combined-modality therapy has grown steadily since Nigro reported complete tumor regression in patients treated with a combination of 30 Gy radiation, 5-FU, and mitomycin C or porfiromycin before abdominoperineal resection. The effectiveness of this combination as a radical treatment rather than as an adjuvant to surgery was demonstrated in many nonrandomized studies and was confirmed in randomized trials (3,14,15).
- The Anal Cancer Trial Working Party of the United Kingdom Coordination Committee on Cancer Research randomized 585 patients to receive either radiation therapy alone (45 Gy of external-beam irradiation with either a 15-Gy external-beam boost or a 25-Gy brachytherapy boost) or similar radiation therapy with concurrent 5-FU and mitomycin. Patients assigned to receive chemoradiation had a reduced likelihood of local failure (61% versus 39%, $p = 0.0001$) and of dying from anal cancer (28% versus 39%, $p = 0.02$) (16).
- The European Organization for the Research and Treatment of Cancer randomized 110 patients with T3–4N0–3 or T1–2N1–3 anal cancer to receive either radiation therapy (45 Gy with a 15- or 20-Gy boost) with concurrent chemotherapy (5-FU and mitomycin) or irradiation alone. The chemoradiation group experienced a higher pathologic complete remission rate (80% versus 54%), an 18% higher 5-year

locoregional control rate (p = 0.02), a 32% higher colostomy-free rate (p = 0.002), and improved progression-free survival (61% versus 43%, p = 0.05) (17).

- A randomized Radiation Therapy Oncology Group trial established that the combination of mitomycin C, 5-FU, and irradiation is more effective than 5-FU and radiation, with statistically significant improvement in disease-free survival after 5 years (67% versus 50%, p = 0.006) (10).
- In a further trial by the RTOG (98-11), induction 5-FU and cisplatin followed by 5-FU and cisplatin concurrent with radiation failed to improve disease-free survival compared to 5-FU and mitomycin with radiation. Cisplatin-based therapy also resulted in significantly worse colostomy rates (9).
- The UK ACT II trial of mitomycin or cisplatin chemoradiation with or without maintenance chemotherapy was a phase III, 2 × 2 factorial trial. At a median follow-up of 5.1 years, 90.5% of patients in the mitomycin group and 89.6% of patients in the cisplatin group had a complete response at 26 weeks. Overall toxicity was the same between groups, with 71% of patients receiving mitomycin C and 72% of patients receiving cisplatin having grade 3 to 4 toxicity. Hematologic toxicity was more prominent in patients receiving mitomycin C (26%) versus cisplatin (16%). Maintenance chemotherapy offered no benefit for progression-free survival (18).
- The UNICANCER ACCORD 03 factorial trial that treated patients with N1-3M0 anal cancer and evaluated induction chemotherapy (two cycles of cisplatin and 5-fluorouracil), as well as dose escalated radiotherapy (45 Gy plus a 15 Gy boost versus a 20- to 25-Gy boost). No difference in colostomy-free survival was seen, although the induction chemotherapy and high dose radiation arm had the highest colostomy-free survival rate at 82.4% (19).
- Oral capecitabine with bolus mitomycin C, base chemotherapy is also an effective treatment option (20).
- Tumor regression can be seen up to 26 weeks after completion of chemoradiation. For persistent disease or local recurrence, abdominoperineal resection is recommended, with reirradiation considered for patients who are not surgical candidates (7).

Lymph Node Metastases

- Lymph node metastases can be eradicated by the same radiation and chemotherapy doses effective against primary anal cancer.
- Dose to clinically involved lymph node metastases depends on size, as defined in the RTOG 0529 trial. Lymph nodes up to 3 cm in size are treated to 50.4 Gy, whereas lymph nodes greater than 3 cm in size are treated to 54 Gy (21).
- Subclinical disease in lymph node regions receives 42 Gy in 28 fractions for T1-2N0M0 disease, and 45 Gy in 28 fractions for T3-4 or N1 disease.
- Elective irradiation, with or without chemotherapy, of clinically normal inguinal node areas causes little morbidity and reduces the risk of late node failure in that area to less than 5% (33).

Extrapelvic Metastases

- Metastatic disease is identified in 13% of cases at diagnosis, per SEER data (2).
- The median survival after the diagnosis of extrapelvic metastases is 8 to 12 months.

- Platinum-based doublet chemotherapy is recommended for first-line treatment of metastatic disease (7).
- Immunotherapy with anti-PD-1 antibodies, such as nivolumab and pembrolizumab, has shown efficacy in metastatic, unresectable anal cancer.

Radiation Therapy

- Radiation therapy alone has been restricted largely to patients unable to receive combined radiation and chemotherapy as described above. Concurrent therapy is recommended by the American College of Radiology even for T1N0M0 anal cancer (22).

RADIATION THERAPY TECHNIQUES

- Intensity-modulated radiation therapy (IMRT) is the recommended treatment modality over 2D or 3D, per NCCN guidelines (7).
- RTOG 0529 was a phase II trial of dose-painted IMRT with 5-FU and mitomycin C, with T2N0 patients receiving 50.4 Gy to the primary tumor and 42 Gy to elective nodes in 28 fractions; T3-4 or N+ patients received 54 Gy to the primary tumor, involved lymph nodes 50.4 Gy if ≤3 cm and 54 Gy if greater than 3 cm, and elective nodes 45 Gy in 30 fractions (21). See Figure 26-2 for a representative plan.
- Compared to historical toxicity rates from RTOG 9811, RTOG 0529 significantly reduced acute grade 2+ hematologic toxicity (73% versus 85%, $p = 0.032$), grade 3+ gastrointestinal toxicity (21% versus 36%, $p = 0.082$), and grade 3+ dermatologic toxicity (23% versus 49%, $p < 0.001$).

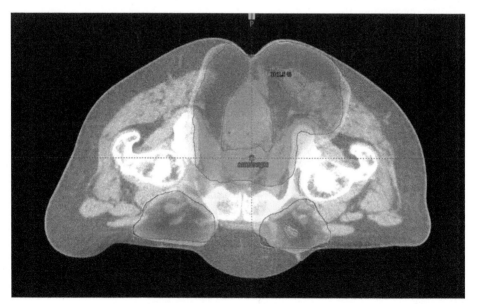

FIGURE 26-2. Axial section of a radiation plan for a patient with T4N1M0 anal cancer.

- Target delineation and normal tissue contours are particularly challenging in anal cancer, with RTOG 0529 noting 81% of cases requiring replanning on initial review. The RTOG consensus panel contouring atlas is essential for review of clinical target volumes.
- Gross tumor volume of the anal primary (GTV_A) is contoured using examination, imaging, and endoscopy data. Clinical target volume (CTV) for the primary is a 2.5-cm expansion, edited to avoid bone and non-infiltrated muscle. Planning target volume (PTV) is defined as a 1-cm expansion, per RTOG 0529, but can be reduced to 0.5-0.7 cm with daily CBCT imaging.
- Gross tumor volume for involved lymph nodes (GTV_N) is defined by clinical examination and imaging, with CTV for nodes defined as a 1-cm expansion, edited to avoid bone and noninfiltrated muscle. PTV is defined as a 1-cm expansion, per RTOG 0529, but can be reduced to 0.5-0.7 cm with daily CBCT imaging.
- Elective nodal CTVs include the mesorectum, presacrum, and bilateral internal and external iliac and bilateral inguinal regions.
- The Australasian Gastrointestinal Trials Group additionally has defined contouring and planning guidelines, which complement the RTOG-defined contouring atlas. A 2-cm CTV margin is recommended for the primary tumor, 1- to 2-cm CTV margin for involved lymph nodes, and 0.7-cm CTV margin for elective lymph node regions is recommended. A 0.5- to 1-cm PTV margin is recommended (23).
- Use of bolus on the primary tumor is often necessary, given frequent extension of disease to and through the anus and skin. Bolus is not routinely recommended for inguinal lymph nodes, unless clinically involving the skin.

Normal Tissue Complications

The recently published QUANTEC guidelines offer the most up-to-date clinical guidance on the potential damage to normal tissues that may be affected by irradiation of tumor sites (see *International Journal of Radiation Oncology Biology Physics*, special supplement, vol. 76, 2010).
- RTOG 0529 used rigorous normal tissue constraints
- Bowel V45Gy < 20cc, V35 Gy < 150 cc, V30 Gy < 200 cc
- Femoral heads V44 Gy < 5%, V40 Gy < 35%, V30 Gy < 50%
- Iliac crest V50 Gy < 5%, V40 Gy < 35%, V30 Gy < 50%
- External genitalia V40 Gy < 5%, V30 Gy < 35%, V20 Gy < 50%
- Bladder V50 Gy < 5%, V40 Gy < 35%, V35 Gy < 50%.

Perianal

- T1N0, well-differentiated perianal tumors can be locally excised with adequate margins and then observed.
- If unable to achieve negative margins, if poorly differentiated, or if larger or node positive, patients should be treated with chemoradiation as per anal cancer recommendations.

SEQUELAE OF THERAPY

- With IMRT, acute grade 3+ dermatologic, and grade 2+ gastrointestinal toxicity are seen in approximately 20% of patients (21).
- Acute hematologic toxicity is seen in 70% to 85% of patients, and is significantly greater with mitomycin C than with cisplatin.
- Acute gastrointestinal toxicity is associated with increasing patient age, tumor size greater than 4 cm, worse performance status, and dose to small bowel and anterior pelvic contents (24).
- With IMRT, treatment-related complications requiring abdominoperineal resection is seen in approximately 1% of cases (25).
- Vaginal dilator use is recommended for female patients after therapy to reduce risk of vaginal stenosis.
- With potential for pelvic fractures and decreased bone density, bone density monitoring should be considered (7).

References

1. Surabhi VR, et al. Tumors and tumorlike conditions of the anal canal and perianal region: MR imaging findings. *Radiographics* 2016;36(5):1339–1353.
2. Anal Cancer, Key statistics 2018. Accessed February 6, 2018. Available from: https://www.cancer.org/cancer/anal-cancer/about/what-is-key-statistics.html.
3. Buroker TR, et al. Combined therapy for cancer of the anal canal: a follow-up report. *Dis Colon Rectum* 1977;20(8):677–678.
4. Baricevic I, et al. High-sensitivity human papilloma virus genotyping reveals near universal positivity in anal squamous cell carcinoma: different implications for vaccine prevention and prognosis. *Eur J Cancer* 2015;51(6):776–785.
5. de Martel, C, et al. Global burden of cancers attributable to infections in 2008: a review and synthetic analysis. *Lancet Oncol* 2012;13(6):607–615.
6. Parkin DM, Bray F, Chapter 2: The burden of HPV-related cancers. *Vaccine* 2006;24Suppl 3:S3/11–S3/25.
7. *Network NCC NCCN Clinical Practice Guidelines in Oncology: Anal Carcinoma, Version 1, 2018.* 2018.
8. *AJCC cancer staging manual, 8th ed.* New York, NY: Springer Verlag, 2017.
9. Ajani JA, et al. Fluorouracil, mitomycin, and radiotherapy vs fluorouracil, cisplatin, and radiotherapy for carcinoma of the anal canal: a randomized controlled trial. *JAMA* 2008;299(16): 1914–1921.
10. Flam M, et al. Role of mitomycin in combination with fluorouracil and radiotherapy, and of salvage chemoradiation in the definitive nonsurgical treatment of epidermoid carcinoma of the anal canal: results of a phase III randomized intergroup study. *J Clin Oncol* 1996;14(9):2527–2539.
11. Northover J, et al. Chemoradiation for the treatment of epidermoid anal cancer: 13-year follow-up of the first randomised UKCCCR Anal Cancer Trial (ACT I). *Br J Cancer* 2010;102(7): 1123–1128.
12. Marcus JL, et al. Survival among HIV-infected and HIV-uninfected individuals with common non-AIDS-defining cancers. *Cancer Epidemiol Biomarkers Prev* 2015;24(8):1167–1173.
13. Glynne-Jones R, et al. Prognostic factors for recurrence and survival in anal cancer: generating hypotheses from the mature outcomes of the first United Kingdom Coordinating Committee on Cancer Research Anal Cancer Trial (ACT I). *Cancer* 2013;119(4):748–755.

14. Nigro ND, Vaitkevicius VK, ConsidineB, Jr., Combined therapy for cancer of the anal canal: a preliminary report. *Dis Colon Rectum* 1974;17(3):354–356.

15. Nigro ND, et al. Combined preoperative radiation and chemotherapy for squamous cell carcinoma of the anal canal. *Cancer* 1983;51(10):1826–1829.

16. Epidermoid anal cancer: results from the UKCCCR randomised trial of radiotherapy alone versus radiotherapy, 5-fluorouracil, and mitomycin. UKCCCR Anal Cancer Trial Working Party. UK Co-ordinating Committee on Cancer Research. *Lancet* 1996;348(9034):1049–1054.

17. Bartelink H, et al. Concomitant radiotherapy and chemotherapy is superior to radiotherapy alone in the treatment of locally advanced anal cancer: results of a phase III randomized trial of the European Organization for Research and Treatment of Cancer Radiotherapy and Gastrointestinal Cooperative Groups. *J Clin Oncol* 1997;15(5):2040–2049.

18. James RD, et al. Mitomycin or cisplatin chemoradiation with or without maintenance chemotherapy for treatment of squamous-cell carcinoma of the anus (ACT II): a randomised, phase 3, open-label, 2 x 2 factorial trial. *Lancet Oncol* 2013;14(6):516–524.

19. Peiffert D, et al. Induction chemotherapy and dose intensification of the radiation boost in locally advanced anal canal carcinoma: final analysis of the randomized UNICANCER ACCORD 03 trial. *J Clin Oncol* 2012;30(16):1941–1948.

20. Thind G, et al. Chemoradiation with capecitabine and mitomycin-C for stage I-III anal squamous cell carcinoma. *Radiat Oncol* 2014;9:124.

21. Kachnic LA, et al. RTOG 0529: a phase 2 evaluation of dose-painted intensity modulated radiation therapy in combination with 5-fluorouracil and mitomycin-C for the reduction of acute morbidity in carcinoma of the anal canal. *Int J Radiat Oncol Biol Phys* 2013;86(1):27–33.

22. Expert Panel on Radiation Oncology-Rectal/Anal Cancer, et al. ACR Appropriateness Criteria(R)-Anal Cancer. *Gastrointest Cancer Res* 2014;7(1):4–14.

23. Ng M, et al. Australasian Gastrointestinal Trials Group (AGITG) contouring atlas and planning guidelines for intensity-modulated radiotherapy in anal cancer. *Int J Radiat Oncol Biol Phys* 2012;83(5):1455–1462.

24. Olsen JR, et al. Predictors of Radiation Therapy-Related Gastrointestinal Toxicity From Anal Cancer Dose-Painted Intensity Modulated Radiation Therapy: Secondary Analysis of NRG Oncology RTOG 0529. *Int J Radiat Oncol Biol Phys* 2017;98(2):400–408.

25. Mitra, D., et al. Long-term outcomes and toxicities of a large cohort of anal cancer patients treated with dose-painted IMRT per RTOG 0529. *Adv Radiat Oncol* 2017;2(2):110–117.

CHAPTER 27

UPPER URINARY TRACT

KIDNEY, RENAL PELVIS, AND URETER

Anatomy

- The kidneys are located in the retroperitoneal space between the eleventh rib and the transverse process of the third lumbar vertebral body; the right kidney is slightly more inferior than the left because of its relationship to the right hepatic lobe.
- The kidney is enveloped by a fibrous capsule and surrounded by perinephric fat, which is surrounded by Gerota's fascia.
- The kidneys move vertically within the retroperitoneum as much as 4 cm during normal respiration (1).
- The ureters course posteriorly and inferiorly, paralleling the lateral border of the psoas muscle until they curve anteriorly to join the bladder at the trigone.
- The lymphatics of the kidney and renal pelvis drain along the renal vessels. The right kidney drains predominantly into the paracaval and the interaortocaval lymph nodes (LNs); the left kidney drains exclusively to the paraaortic lymph nodes (LNs) (2).
- Lymphatic drainage of the ureter is segmented and diffuse and may involve any of the renal hilar, abdominal paraaortic, paracaval, common iliac, internal iliac, or external iliac LNs.

NATURAL HISTORY

Renal Cell Carcinoma

- Primary renal cell tumors may spread by local infiltration through the renal capsule to involve the perinephric fat and Gerota's fascia.
- The tumor may directly grow along the venous channels to the renal vein or the vena cava.
- The renal vein is invaded by tumor in 21% of cases and the inferior vena cava (IVC) in approximately 4% (3). The incidence of LN metastases is 9% to 27%; they most frequently involve the renal hilar, paraaortic, and paracaval LNs (4).

- Approximately 45% of patients with renal cell carcinoma (RCC) have localized disease; 25% have regional disease; and approximately 30% have evidence of distant metastases at the time of diagnosis (4).
- Approximately one half of the patients with RCC will eventually develop metastatic disease. Metastatic sites include lung (75%), soft tissue (36%), bone (20%), liver (18%), skin (8%), and central nervous system (8%) (5). Needle tract relapses along biopsy tracts may occur.

Renal Pelvis and Ureter Carcinoma

- Upper urinary tract carcinoma is frequently multifocal; patients have a significant risk of developing tumors at several sites along the urothelium, particularly in those with large tumors or carcinoma *in situ*.
- Ureteral tumors tend to occur in the distal third of the ureter (5).
- Urothelial carcinoma of the upper tract may spread by both direct extension and hematologic and lymphatic metastasis.
- Recurrence of upper tract urothelial carcinoma in the bladder occurs in up to 50% of cases, presumably because of either urinary distribution or a "field cancerization effect."
- Grade of disease is correlated with lymph node metastasis risk, as well as prognosis (6). In a retrospective review of 1,363 patients, LN positivity also increased incrementally with advancing pathologic stage—less than 1% for T0/Ta/Tis, 2% for T1, 8% for T2, 17% for T3, and 46% for T4 ($p < 0.001$). High-grade tumors again were more likely to have positive LN (15% high grade versus 2% low grade, $p < 0.001$) (7).

CLINICAL PRESENTATION

Renal Cell Carcinoma

- Gross or microscopic hematuria is the most frequent symptom associated with RCC.
- Patients with RCC may be asymptomatic (with tumor being an incidental finding), or there may be signs and symptoms related to a local mass or systemic paraneoplastic syndromes.
- Paraneoplastic syndromes associated with RCC involve parathyroid-like hormones, erythropoietin, renin, gonadotropins, placental lactogen, prolactin, enteroglucagon, insulin-like hormones, adrenocorticotropic hormone, and prostaglandins (5).
- Gross hematuria, palpable flank mass, and pain describe a classic triad that occurs in only 5% to 10% of patients and suggest advanced disease.

Renal Pelvis and Ureter Carcinoma

- Gross or microscopic hematuria occurs in 70% to 95% of patients with renal pelvic or ureteral tumors (8).
- Other less common symptoms include pain (8% to 40%), bladder irritation (5% to 10%), or other constitutional symptoms (5%).
- Approximately 10% to 20% of patients present with a flank mass secondary to tumor or hydronephrosis (5).

DIAGNOSTIC WORKUP

Renal Cell Carcinoma

- Diagnostic and staging workup for RCC is given in Table 27-1.
- After radiographic evaluation, in most cases, pathologic confirmation is often made at the time of nephrectomy.
- Staging evaluation should include a complete history and physical examination, complete blood cell count, and liver and kidney function tests. A metastatic workup includes a chest x-ray and computed tomography (CT) or magnetic resonance imaging (MRI) scan of the abdomen and pelvis.
- A bone scan should be obtained in patients with symptoms suggestive of bony metastases or an elevated alkaline phosphatase level.
- Positron emission tomography (PET) scanning may be useful in the detection of LN or distant metastasis.

Table 27-1

Diagnostic Workup for Renal Cell, Renal Pelvis, or Ureter Carcinoma

General

History
Physical examination

Radiographic Studies

Standard
  Chest radiograph
  Intravenous pyelogram
  Retrograde pyelogram (renal pelvis or ureter)
  CT or MRI scan of abdomen and pelvis
  Bone scan
Complementary
  Renal ultrasound with color-flow Doppler
  Renal arteriogram with or without epinephrine
  Inferior venacavogram
  CT and digital subtraction angiogram
  CT of chest, brain, or other suspected organs

Laboratory Studies

Complete blood cell count
Blood chemistry profile
Urinalysis

Special Tests

Renal cyst puncture with fluid cytology (if no echinococcosis is suspected)
Endoscopic ureteroscopy
Percutaneous nephroscopy
CT of chest, brain, or other suspected organs
Urine cytology (endoscopically obtained)
Retrograde brush cytology or biopsy

- If metastatic lesions are detected, histologic confirmation should be made by biopsy of either the metastatic focus or the primary tumor.
- If renal vein or IVC invasion is suspected, ultrasound with color-flow Doppler may help define the extent of the tumor thrombus.
- Renal arteriography is sometimes helpful in planning surgery.

Renal Pelvis and Ureter Carcinoma

- The diagnostic workup for renal pelvis and ureter carcinoma is listed in Table 27-1.
- Intravenous urography is frequently used to evaluate patients with renal pelvis carcinoma; a filling defect in the renal pelvis or collecting system is common.
- Retrograde pyelography can be used to define the lower margin of a ureteral lesion, especially if there is significant proximal obstruction to flow of contrast from the renal pelvis.
- CT or MRI of the abdomen and pelvis before and after contrast administration gives useful information about possible extension of tumor outside the collecting system.
- An accurate cytologic diagnosis can be made in more than 80% of cases.

STAGING

- In the United States, the staging system used most commonly by clinicians is the Robson modification (9) of the Flocks and Kadesky system.
- Extension of tumor outside the renal capsule increases the stage of the cancer and worsens the prognosis.

PATHOLOGIC CLASSIFICATION

- The predominant histopathologic type of renal cancer is adenocarcinoma; subtypes include clear cell carcinoma (approximately 75%) and papillary RCC type I (*MET* alterations frequent) and type II (formerly known as granular cell carcinoma). Rarer variants include sarcomatoid.
- More than 90% of malignant tumors arising from the renal pelvis and ureter are urothelial.
- Squamous cell carcinomas account for only 7% to 8% of tumors arising from the renal pelvis or ureters; they are often locally advanced and associated with a high local relapse rate (10).
- Hereditary RCC includes von Hippel-Lindau syndrome, hereditary papillary renal carcinoma, and familial renal oncocytoma (Birt-Hogg-Dubé syndrome).

PROGNOSTIC FACTORS

Renal Cell Carcinoma

- Tumor stage at initial presentation is the most important prognostic factor.
- The prognostic significance of renal vein or vena cava invasion has been debated; a worse prognosis has been reported by some authors (4,11), with lower survival and

increased metastasis rates, but the opposite conclusion was reached by Skinner et al. (12) in a review of 309 cases treated by nephrectomy.

- Renal vein or vena cava invasion is often associated with perinephric extension of the primary tumor (about 5% to 10% of RCCs extend into the venous system as tumor thrombi, often ascending the IVC as high as the right atrium) (13).
- LN metastases are associated with increased local recurrence and distant metastasis rates (12,14,15).
- Higher pathologic grade or spindle cell or sarcomatoid variants lead to poor 5-year disease-free survival (12).
- High nuclear grade is associated with an increased incidence of advanced tumor stage, LN involvement, distant metastases, renal vein involvement, tumor size, and perirenal fat involvement.

Renal Pelvis and Ureter Carcinoma

- Initial stage and grade of the tumor are the major prognostic factors.
- LN metastases are associated with distant dissemination and lower survival (16).
- In 126 patients treated surgically (45 receiving postoperative irradiation), significant prognostic factors were tumor location, stage, Karnofsky index, nodal metastasis, and residual tumor after surgery (17).
- On a multivariate analysis, although stage and grade were the most important prognostic factors, DNA pattern (diploid versus nondiploid) and the number of lesions (unifocal versus multifocal) identified at initial diagnosis also determined prognosis. Patients with diploid tumors had a 79% survival rate, compared with only 46% in those with nondiploid tumors ($p = 0.0003$) (18).
- Genomic analyses suggest a distinct profile of urothelial carcinoma of the upper tract compared to of the bladder, with enrichment in *FGFR3* alterations (19).

GENERAL MANAGEMENT

Renal Cell Carcinoma

- Standard therapy for nonmetastatic RCC is radical nephrectomy with 5-year disease survival rate of 80% to 90%.
- Elective removal of lymphatics that may contain microscopic disease may be curative for patients at risk (20,21). Partial nephrectomy, or renal parenchyma–sparing surgery, has been used in patients with early-stage tumors with poor renal reserve or absence of a normal functioning contralateral kidney. Increased early diagnosis has led to a rise in these procedures and ablation techniques (i.e., thermal). Institution-specific practice currently determines choice of nephrectomy versus sparing procedures in those with normal function in contralateral kidneys (5,22).
- Patients with local symptoms (hematuria, pain, hypertension, or other paraneoplastic syndromes) may benefit from palliative nephrectomy.

- Cytoreductive surgery performed to facilitate the regression of extrarenal disease in response to systemic therapy remains controversial (23), with most benefit suggested in those with low-burden extrarenal disease (i.e., resected/radiated pulmonary disease only) and good performance status, and good risk (according to various stratification schemes) in the targeted therapy era (24).
- Primary surveillance is recommended in the first 2 to 3 years when the risk of recurrence is the greatest. Trials assessing efficacy of novel targeted therapies and immunotherapies as adjuvants after nephrectomy in high-risk nonmetastatic disease are in progress, with conflicting results from early assessments of anti-vascular endothelial growth factor (VEGF) therapy (i.e., ASSURE and S-TRAC trials) (25).

Radiation Therapy

- Historically, renal cell cancer was perceived to be "radioresistant" to conventionally fractionated radiotherapy and the competing risk of distant relapse too high to justify adjuvant therapy (26). Further, although some retrospective series suggest a benefit with adjuvant irradiation in high-risk disease after nephrectomy, methodologic drawbacks limited acceptance of radiotherapy in RCC.
- Early studies of preoperative irradiation demonstrated improved tumor resectability and local tumor control (27,28) but no impact on survival or overall disease control. More recently, at least one ongoing trial investigates the specific role of preoperative radiotherapy before resection of IVC tumor thrombus-associated disease (NCT02 473536), to focus the locoregional benefit of radiotherapy on those who would otherwise not be resectable/curable.
- Postoperative irradiation has not been associated with survival benefit in now dated randomized studies (29) but may be considered in select cases of gross residual disease after nephrectomy or in the setting of metastatic lymph nodes (30).
- Stereotactic radiotherapy (SBRT/SAbR) techniques incorporating higher doses per fraction along increased targeted/immune therapies improving systemic control have contributed to a recent evolution of the role of radiotherapy in RCC primarily in the oligometastatic/oligoprogressive setting. For instance, one retrospective review of a contemporary cohort (2005 to 2015) demonstrated greater than 90% local control of extracranial metastases with dosage regimens of 40 to 60 Gy in 5 fractions, 30 to 54 Gy in 3 fractions, or 20 to 40 Gy in a 1 fraction, at the cost of a favorable 2.9% late grade 3 toxicity rate (31).
- For small primary renal lesions not amenable to resection or ablation, SBRT/SAbR is being assessed in multiple ongoing clinical trials for treatment of primary RCC (i.e., NCT021 41919, TROG 15.03 FASTRACK II) and has been reported in phase I and retrospective series (32,33,34). Renal dysfunction related to this treatment has been related to sparing of remnant functional kidney from high-dose regions (35).
- Use of SAbR or stereotactic radiosurgery (SRS) for extrarenal metastases has become widely accepted on the basis of large retrospective and primarily single arm prospective series demonstrating safety and efficacy. Particular attention is being paid to use of these techniques to control oligometastatic progression at a few number of sites of disease, in conjunction with novel systemic therapies, to extend disease-free survival.

Systemic Therapy

- Conventional cytotoxic therapies have limited efficacy and use in RCC.
- Interferon-alpha has shown activity in metastatic RCC, with objective response rates of 10% to 20%.
- Interleukin-2, a lymphokine produced by activated T cells, has produced complete response rates in 5% to 10% of selected patients with metastatic renal cell cancer; another 10% to 15% have achieved objective partial responses, some lasting for as long as 2 years (5). Treatment often requires ICU admission because of cytokine release effects.
- Recent clinical trials of targeted molecular therapies and checkpoint blockade immunotherapy have yielded encouraging results in patients with advanced renal cell cancer. Examples currently include the following nonexhaustive list:
  - Nivolumab and other antiprogrammed cell death-1 (PD-1) antibodies have shown promising results in RCC. A phase III trial of RCC patients using nivolumab improved overall survival compared to everolimus in patients progressing after antiangiogenic therapy. Nivolumab administration yielded an improved overall survival of 25 versus 19.6 months in patients using everolimus. There was no difference in progression-free survival (36).
  - PD-1 ligand (PD-L1) blocking antibodies such as atezolizumab have also been investigated in metastatic RCC. In a phase I trial, 41% of patients had stable disease for 24 weeks (37). Another phase 1 study showed median overall survival and progression-free survival of 28.9 and 5.6 months, respectively (38).
  - Ipilimumab is cytotoxic T-lymphocyte–associated antigen 4 (CTLA-4) inhibitor. A phase II trial resulted in 12.5% response in higher-dose versus 5% response in the lower-dose group (39). Sunitinib, a tyrosine kinase inhibitor, targets both VEGF and platelet-derived growth factor (PDGF) receptors. In a phase II trial, the oral administration of sunitinib yielded a 40% response rate with a median time to progression of 8.7 months. Sunitinib-treated patients had a median overall survival of 26.4 versus 21.8 months for interferon-treated patients ($p = 0.051$) (13).
  - Sorafenib is an oral inhibitor of both the Raf kinase and the VEGF receptor; 50% of patients on the study drug showed no progression of disease compared to only 18% of patients who were receiving placebo ($p = 0.0077$) (40). Bevacizumab, an anti-VEGF antibody, has been investigated in a randomized phase II trial in patients with metastatic RCC. Patients receiving bevacizumab had a 4.8-month interval to progression compared to 2.5 months in patients receiving placebo (41).
- Combination therapy of antiangiogenic and checkpoint inhibitors such as bevacizumab and atezolizumab is currently being investigated in phase III trials in untreated metastatic RCC. Combination therapies are, however, more likely to result in toxicities, mainly gastrointestinal and hepatic (42,43). The latest class of agents includes the mTOR inhibitors such as temsirolimus (Torisel).

Palliation

- For patients with metastatic RCC, palliative nephrectomy can relieve pain, hemorrhage, hypertension, or hypercalcemia induced by the primary tumor.

- Palliative irradiation is effective at relieving symptoms from metastatic cancer, particularly bone metastasis. Hypofractionated courses are perceived to offer better local control, though randomized proof for an ideal regimen is lacking. With this acknowledged, SRS and SBRT/SAbR has been successful at controlling and palliating metastatic sites from RCC in multiple series, beyond the scope of this chapter (44).

Renal Pelvis and Ureter Carcinoma

- Radical nephroureterectomy is appropriate initial therapy for most patients with transitional cell carcinoma of the renal pelvis or ureter, including removal of the contents of Gerota's fascia and the ipsilateral ureter with a cuff of bladder at its distal extent.
- Conservative surgical excision should be considered only in patients with low-grade, low-stage, solitary tumors in whom radical nephrectomy is not indicated because of poor kidney function or an absent contralateral kidney.
- Neoadjuvant chemotherapy is being trialed in urothelial upper tract disease (NCT02 412670).
- The role of LN dissection and the optimal template are unclear.
- Radiation therapy may be beneficial in selected cases of high-stage (T3 or T4) carcinoma of the renal pelvis or ureter or in patients with LN metastases (45) but is controversial.
- The regimen of methotrexate, vinblastine, doxorubicin, and cisplatin has yielded objective response rates of nearly 70% in patients with metastatic transitional cell carcinoma of the bladder, ureter, and kidney.

RADIATION THERAPY TECHNIQUES (TABLE 27-2)

Renal Cell Carcinoma

- Postoperative therapy remains controversial and reserved for gross residual disease. Multiple-field (3D or intensity-modulated radiation therapy) techniques should be considered in patients receiving preoperative treatment. CT-based planning is needed to allow delineation of nephrectomy bed (surgical clips helpful), residual disease, and optionally LN drainage sites (46), while prioritizing sparing of the contralateral kidney. Total postoperative irradiation doses of 45 to 50 Gy in 1.8- to 2.0-Gy daily fractions to the nephrectomy bed and regional LNs with a boost (additional 10 to 15 Gy) to gross residual disease are appropriate. The incision site should be included in the target volume (47).
- SAbR/SBRT techniques employ 3D coordinate system–based localization of treatment targets/patient positioning, imaging verification, multiple beam angles, and careful target delineation of tumor without elective volume treatment, in order to facilitate high dose per fraction treatment safely. This technique is now increasingly utilized and favored for treatment of RCC metastases, especially those that are limited in number (oligometastasis) or focal in progression on an otherwise effective systemic therapy (oligoprogression). Because of possible long survival particularly in good risk patients, aggressive treatment for palliation should be considered in patients with good performance status.

Table 27-2

Table 27-2

Summary of Radiation Therapy/Management

Renal Cell Carcinoma/Renal Pelvis and Ureter Carcinoma

If technically feasible: total nephrectomy and elective lymphadenectomy
Unresectable tumors:
   Preoperative irradiation may improve resectability. Dose: 40–50 Gy in 2-Gy fractions
   Resected tumors: Indications for postoperative irradiation (controversial)
      Residual gross of microscopic tumor
      Perinephric fat invasion
      Adrenal gland invasion
      Metastatic regional LNs
      Dose: 45–50 Gy in 1.8–2.0-Gy fractions
      Boost: 5–10 Gy (extensive positive margins, multiple positive LNs)
Palliation: Dependent on location and reason for palliation. Consider use of stereotactic ablative radiotherapy (SAbR) to achieve more durable local control in selected cases, such as those with oligometastases.

- SAbR/SBRT courses are given in 1 to 5 treatments, with cumulative dose depending on anatomic site while respecting normal tissue tolerances. For instance, a rib metastasis might receive 40 Gy in 5 fractions, while such therapy to a spinal lesion would require careful delineation with MR/CT simulation or CT myelogram to keep the spinal cord within tolerances (often requiring compromise of target coverage).

Renal Pelvis and Ureter Carcinoma

- For post-operative elective radiation therapy, the clinical tumor volume should include the renal fossa, the course of the ureter to the bladder wall at the ipsilateral trigone. The field encompassing these sites can be easily extended to cover the paracaval and paraaortic LNs at risk of harboring metastatic disease.
- CT-based planning may facilitate dosimetric coverage of the regions at risk while minimizing dose to normal tissues.
- Irradiation doses of 45 to 50 Gy (1.8 to 2.0 Gy daily) are appropriate to treat subclinical and microscopic disease.
- For more extensive disease, such as multiple positive nodes or extensive positive margins, a boost of 5 to 10 Gy should be considered.
- For unresectable or gross residual disease, higher doses may be necessary. Multiple-field arrangements, including oblique and lateral fields with field reductions, are important to minimize toxicity to surrounding normal structures.
- CT-based simulation, three-dimensional treatment planning, and contrast-enhanced radiographs are helpful in defining the irradiation target volume.

NORMAL TISSUE COMPLICATIONS—QUANTEC RESULTS

Dawson et al. (48) note that all dose-volume recommendations are associated with substantial uncertainty, because few studies are available of patients who have been followed for ≥10 years. However, some broad guidelines can be useful and will hopefully be tested in future studies. Their summary in Table 5 of reference 48 indicates that to keep toxicity risk below 5%, bilateral irradiation of the kidneys should have a mean dose below 18 Gy and the partial organ volumes at 28 and 23 Gy should be 20% and 30%, respectively. They also provide a dose-response plot for non-total body irradiation (TBI) radiation-induced kidney toxicity, presented here in adapted form as Figure 27-1.

SAbR/SBRT dose and normal tissue constraints follow those based on anatomic site and often have institution-specific modifications. A full listing of these is beyond the scope of this chapter.

SEQUELAE OF THERAPY

- Sequelae of radiation therapy for cancer of the kidney, renal pelvis, and ureters are similar to those from irradiation of the upper abdomen and pelvis; they include nausea, vomiting, diarrhea, and abdominal cramping.
- Because patients with right-sided tumors may have significant portions of the liver irradiated, radiation-induced liver damage is possible.

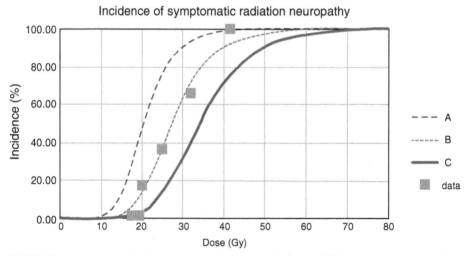

FIGURE 27-1. Incidence of radiation-induced kidney toxicity for non-TBI. Data points are taken from Figure 4 of Cassady and modeled with the empirical binomial function of Zaider and Amols (48). This is a two-parameter equation: $F(D) = 100 \times \exp[a1 \times \exp(-a2 \times D)]$, where D is the dose in Gy. The parameter $a2$ is the inverse characteristic dose, which for the three curves A, B, and C are 5, 6.7, and 8.3 Gy, respectively. Note that the threshold dose is rather small—only 15 Gy.

NEW! SUMMARY OF CHANGES TO AJCC STAGING

KIDNEY

The following changes in the American Joint Committee on Cancer staging system 8th edition for this chapter have been made since the seventh edition:

* Invasion of pelvicalyceal system added as T3a.

See: Edge SB, Byrd DR, Compton CC, et al., eds. *AJCC cancer staging manual*, 8th ed. New York, NY: Springer Verlag, 2017 (50).

NEW! SUMMARY OF CHANGES TO AJCC STAGING

RENAL PELVIS AND URETER

* N3 category (greater than 5 cm) is included in N2 category.

See: Edge SB, Byrd DR, Compton CC, et al., eds. *AJCC cancer staging manual*, 8th ed. New York, NY: Springer Verlag, 2017 (50).

References

1. Schwartz LH, Richaud J, Buffat L, et al. Kidney mobility during respiration. *Radiother Oncol* 1994;32(1):84–86.
2. Marshall FF, Powell KC. Lymphadenectomy for renal cell carcinoma: anatomical and therapeutic considerations. *J Urol* 1982;128(4):677–681.
3. Waters WB, Richie JP. Aggressive surgical approach to renal cell carcinoma: review of 130 cases. *J Urol* 1979;122(3):306–309.
4. Giuliani L, Giberti C, Martorana G, et al. Radical extensive surgery for renal cell carcinoma: long-term results and prognostic factors. *J Urol* 1990;143(3):468–473; discussion 473–464.
5. Michalski JM. Kidney, renal pelvis and ureter. In: Halperin EC, Perez CA, Brady LW, eds. *Principles and practice of radiation oncology*, 5th ed. Philadelphia, PA: Lippincott Williams & Wilkins, 2008:1397–1411.
6. Cozad SC, Smalley SR, Austenfeld M, et al. Transitional cell carcinoma of the renal pelvis or ureter: patterns of failure. *Urology* 1995;46(6):796–800.
7. Margulis V, Shariat SF, Matin SF, et al. Outcomes of radical nephroureterectomy: a series from the Upper Tract Urothelial Carcinoma Collaboration. *Cancer* 2009;115(6):1224–1233.
8. Reitelman C, Sawczuk IS, Olsson CA, et al. Prognostic variables in patients with transitional cell carcinoma of the renal pelvis and proximal ureter. *J Urol* 1987;138(5):1144–1145.
9. Robson CJ, Churchill BM, Anderson W. The results of radical nephrectomy for renal cell carcinoma. *J Urol* 1969;101(3):297–301.
10. Blacher EJ, Johnson DE, Abdul-Karim FW, et al. Squamous cell carcinoma of renal pelvis. *Urology* 1985;25(2):124–126.
11. Ljungberg B, Stenling R, Osterdahl B, et al. Vein invasion in renal cell carcinoma: impact on metastatic behavior and survival. *J Urol* 1995;154(5):1681–1684.

12. Skinner DG, Colvin RB, Vermillion CD, et al. Diagnosis and management of renal cell carcinoma. A clinical and pathologic study of 309 cases. *Cancer* 1971;28(5):1165–1177.

13. Rini BI, Campbell SC, Escudier B. Renal cell carcinoma. *Lancet* 2009;373(9669):1119–1132.

14. Golimbu M, Joshi P, Sperber A, et al. Renal cell carcinoma: survival and prognostic factors. *Urology* 1986;27(4):291–301.

15. Rabinovitch RA, Zelefsky MJ, Gaynor JJ, et al. Patterns of failure following surgical resection of renal cell carcinoma: implications for adjuvant local and systemic therapy. *J Clin Oncol* 1994;12(1):206–212.

16. Charbit L, Gendreau MC, Mee S, et al. Tumors of the upper urinary tract: 10 years of experience. *J Urol* 1991;146(5):1243–1246.

17. Ozsahin M, Zouhair A, Villa S, et al. Prognostic factors in urothelial renal pelvis and ureter tumours: a multicentre Rare Cancer Network study. *Eur J Cancer* 1999;35(5):738–743.

18. Corrado F, Ferri C, Mannini D, et al. Transitional cell carcinoma of the upper urinary tract: evaluation of prognostic factors by histopathology and flow cytometric analysis. *J Urol* 1991;145(6):1159–1163.

19. Sfkakianos JP, Cha EK, Iyer G, et al. Genomic characterization of upper tract urothelial carcinoma. *Eur Urol* 2015;68(6):970–977.

20. Gershman P, Thompson RH, Moreira DM, et al. Radical nephrectomy with or without lymph node dissection for nonmetastatic renal cell carcinoma: a propensity score-based analysis. *Eur Urol* 2017;71(4):560–567.

21. Whitson JM, Harris CR, Reese AC, Meng MV. Lymphadenectomy improves survival of patients with renal cell carcinoma and nodal metastases. *J Urol* 2011;185(5):1615–1620.

22. Manikandan R, Srinivasan V, Rane A. Which is the real gold standard for small-volume renal tumors? Radical nephrectomy versus nephron-sparing surgery. *J Endourol* 2004;18(1):39–44.

23. Montie JE, Stewart BH, Straffon RA, et al. The role of adjunctive nephrectomy in patients with metastatic renal cell carcinoma. *J Urol* 1977;117(3):272–275.

24. Biswas B, Dabkara D, Ganguly S, et al. Cytoreductive nephrectomy in metastatic renal cell carcinoma in the era of targeted therapy: scientifically relevant or natural selection? *J Clin Oncol* 2017;35(11):1265–1266.

25. Ravaud A, Motzer RJ, Pandha HS, et al. Adjuvant sunitinib in high-risk renal cell carcinoma after nephrectomy. *N Engl J Med* 2016;375(23):2246–2254.

26. Makarewicz R, Zarzycka M, Kulinska G, et al. The value of postoperative radiotherapy in advanced renal cell cancer. *Neoplasma* 1998;45(6):380–383.

27. Juusela H, Malmio K, Alfthan O, et al. Preoperative irradiation in the treatment of renal adenocarcinoma. *Scand J Urol Nephrol* 1977;11(3):277–281.

28. van der Werf-Messing B, van der Heul RO, Ledeboer RC. Renal cell carcinoma trial. *Strahlentherapie Sonderb* 1981;76:169–175.

29. Kjaer M, Frederiksen PL, Engelholm SA. Postoperative radiotherapy in stage II and III renal adenocarcinoma. A randomized trial by the Copenhagen Renal Cancer Study Group. *Int J Radiat Oncol Biol Phys* 1987;13(5):665–672.

30. Kortmann RD, Becker G, Classen J, et al. Future strategies in external radiation therapy of renal cell carcinoma. *Anticancer Res* 1999;19(2C):1601–1603.

31. Wang CJ, Christie A, Lin MH, et al. Safety and efficacy of stereotactic ablative radiation therapy for renal cell carcinoma extracranial metastases. *Int J Radiat Oncol Biol Phys* 2017;98(1):91–100.

32. Kothari G, Louie AV, Pryor D, et al. Stereotactic body radiotherapy for primary renal cell carcinoma and adrenal metastases. *Chin Clin Oncol* 2017;6(Suppl 2):S17.

33. Ponsky L, Lo SS, Zhang Y, et al. Phase I dose-escalation study of stereotactic body radiotherapy (SBRT) for poor surgical candidates with localized renal cell carcinoma. *Radiother Oncol* 2015;117(1):183–187.

34. Siva S, Pham D, Kron T, et al. Stereotactic ablative body radiotherapy for inoperable primary kidney cancer: a prospective clinical trial. *BJU Int* 2017;120(5):623–630.

35. Siva S, Jackson P, Kron T, et al. Impact of stereotactic radiotherapy on kidney function in primary renal cell carcinoma: establishing a dose-response relationship. *Radiother Oncol* 2016;118(3):540–546.

36. McDermott DF, Drake CG, Sznol M, et al. Survival, durable response, and long-term safety in patients with previously treated advanced renal cell carcinoma receiving nivolumab. *J Clin Oncol* 2015;33(18):2013–2020.

37. Weinstock M, McDermott D. Targeting PD-1/PD-L1 in the treatment of metastatic renal cell carcinoma. *Ther Adv Urol* 2015;7:365–377.

38. McDermott DF, Sosman JA, Sznol M, et al. Atezolizumab, an anti-programmed death-ligand 1 antibody, in metastatic renal cell carcinoma: long-term safety, clinical activity, and immune correlates from a phase Ia study. *J Clin Oncol* 2016;34:833–842.

39. Yang JC, Haworth L, Sherry RM, et al. A randomized trial of bevacizumab, an anti-vascular endothelial growth factor antibody, for metastatic renal cancer. *N Engl J Med* 2003;349(5):427–434.

40. Ratain MJ, Eisen T, Stadler WM, et al. Phase II placebo-controlled randomized discontinuation trial of sorafenib in patients with metastatic renal cell carcinoma. *J Clin Oncol* 2006;24(16):2505–2512.

41. Yang JC, Hughes M, Kammula U, et al. Ipilimumab (anti-CTLA4 antibody) causes regression of metastatic renal cell cancer associated with enteritis and hypophysitis. *J Immunother* 2007;30:825–830.

42. Buonerba C, Di Lorenzo G, Sonpavde G. Combination therapy for metastatic renal cell carcinoma. *Ann Transl Med* 2016;4:100.

43. Pal SK, Vogelzang NJ. Sequential treatment strategies and combination therapy regimens in metastatic renal cell carcinoma. *Clin Adv Hematol Oncol* 2013;11:146–155.

44. Wronski M, Maor MH, Davis BJ, et al. External radiation of brain metastases from renal carcinoma: a retrospective study of 119 patients from the M. D. Anderson Cancer Center. *Int J Radiat Oncol Biol Phys* 1997;37(4):753–759.

45. Brookland RK, Richter MP. The postoperative irradiation of transitional cell carcinoma of the renal pelvis and ureter. *J Urol* 1985;133(6):952–955.

46. Kao GD, Malkowicz SB, Whittington R, et al. Locally advanced renal cell carcinoma: low complication rate and efficacy of postnephrectomy radiation therapy planned with CT. *Radiology* 1994;193(3):725–730.

47. Stein M, Kuten A, Halpern J, et al. The value of postoperative irradiation in renal cell cancer. *Radiother Oncol* 1992;24(1):41–44.

48. Dawson LA, Kavanagh BD, Paulino AC, et al. Radiation-associated kidney injury. *Int J Radiat Oncol Biol Phys* 2010;76(3 suppl):S108–S115.

49. Zaider M, Amols HI. Practical considerations in using calculated healthy-tissue complication probabilities for treatment-plan optimization. *Int J Radiat Oncol Biol Phys* 1999;44(2):439–447.

50. Edge SB, Byrd DR, Compton CC, et al., eds. *AJCC cancer staging manual*, 8th ed. New York, NY: Springer Verlag, 2017.

CHAPTER 28

BLADDER

ANATOMY

- The urinary bladder lies within the true pelvis.
- The triangular superior surface of the bladder is covered with peritoneum; in females, the body of the uterus usually overhangs this surface.
- The apex of the bladder is directed toward the pubic symphysis and is joined to the umbilicus by the urachal remnant.
- The posterior surface, the base of the bladder, faces downward and backward; in females, it is closely related to the anterior wall of the vagina. In males, the upper part of the bladder base is separated from the rectum by the rectovesical pouch; the lower part is separated from the rectum by the seminal vesicles and the deferent duct.
- As the bladder fills, it becomes rounded or ovoid, and it lies directly against the anterior abdominal wall without any intervening peritoneum.
- The ureters pierce the wall of the bladder base obliquely; the orifices of the ureters and the urethral orifice define the bladder trigone, the sides of which are approximately 2.5 cm long in the contracted state and up to 5.0 cm when distended.
- In males, the bladder neck rests on the prostate; in females, it is related to the pelvic fascia surrounding the upper urethra (1).
- The bladder wall is composed of mucosa, lamina propria, muscularis propria, and perivesicle fat. Invasion of the muscularis propria (also known as detrusor muscle) or beyond is highly prognostic for lethality of disease.

NATURAL HISTORY

- Approximately 75% of bladder cancers present as localized superficial (Tis, Ta, or T1), and approximately 10% to 20% progress to muscle-invasive (≥T2) disease (1,2).
- Grade, diffuse *in situ* disease and recurrent disease are prognostic for risk of progression in superficial disease.
- Approximately 20% demonstrate muscle invasion (muscularis propria or beyond, MIBC). Untreated MIBC results in death in a majority of patients within 1 to 2 years.

- Local progression occurs by direct extension into or through the bladder wall. In some cases, the tumor spreads submucosally under intact, normal-appearing mucosa, especially *in situ*.
- Perineural invasion and lymphatic or blood vessel invasion are common after tumor has invaded muscle.
- Frequent recurrence after transurethral resection of bladder tumor (TURBT) argues for multifocality, either because of a "field effect" of exposure to carcinogens or because of urine spread (3).
- Lymphatic drainage is by the external and internal iliac and presacral lymph nodes.
- The most common sites of distant metastases are lung, bone, and liver.

CLINICAL PRESENTATION

- Between 75% and 80% of patients with bladder cancer have gross, painless, total (throughout urination) hematuria. Age, persistence of hematuria, and exposure (tobacco) influence the likelihood of bladder cancer as the etiology.
- More than 95% of patients with biopsy-proven carcinoma *in situ* have positive urine cytology results. Use of cytogenetic testing (primarily fluorescence *in situ* hybridization) improves sensitivity but has limited specificity at current (4).
- Simultaneous presentations of bladder and prostate cancer are not uncommon (1).

DIAGNOSTIC WORKUP

- Patients with bladder cancer should have a complete clinical history, physical examination, complete blood cell count, liver function tests, complete cystoscopic evaluation with mapping of tumors (number, size, patency of ureteral orifices if adjacent), and bimanual examination under anesthesia (typically during TURBT). Uteroscopy is appropriate to rule out concurrent upper tract lesions if there is suspicion from imaging.
- Cystoscopy may make use of traditional white light cystoscopy; however, emerging use of blue-light cystoscopy (identifying malignant cells due to selective retention of photoactive porphyrins) and/or narrow band imaging appear to improve staging but are not yet standard.
- Imaging should include (particularly for MIBC) CT chest and CT urography with abdomen/pelvis and excretory phases of IV contrast to evaluate the upper tract, bladder, and lymph nodes. However, note that after TURBT, inflammation may complicate assessment of perivesicle invasion.
  - MR urography is appropriate for those with poor renal function or contrast allergy contraindicating iodinated contrast. US/CT without contrast is a substitute in those with absolute contrast allergy.
  - PET for MIBC may be performed in those with high suspicion for metastatic disease but is not a substitute for CT or MR urography for urothelial tract evaluation.

Table 28-1		
Diagnostic Workup for Carcinoma of the Bladder		
Routine		
Clinical history and physical examination Pelvic/rectal examination		
Laboratory studies		
Complete blood cell count, blood chemistry profile Liver function tests Urinalysis Urine cytology (+/− FISH testing)		
Radiographic imaging		
CT or magnetic resonance imaging scan of pelvis and abdomen with urography CT chest (particularly for muscle-invasive disease) Cystourethroscopy Bimanual pelvic/rectal examination under anesthesia (EUA) Biopsies of bladder and urethra (prostate if low tumor in trigone/urethra) w/ mapping Transurethral resection		

Data from Spiess PE, Agarwal N, Bangs R, et al. Bladder Cancer, Version 5.2017, NCCN Clinical Practice Guidelines in Oncology. *J Natl Compr Canc Netw* 2017;15(10):1240–1267.

- All superficially invasive disease should be repeat sampled with TURBT/cystoscopy at 4 to 6 weeks, because of an approximately 70% chance of residual disease and approximately 30% chance of understaging (particularly if no muscularis propria was present in original TURBT specimen) (5).
- The diagnostic workup is summarized in Table 28-1.

STAGING SYSTEMS

- Clinical staging commonly differs from final pathologic staging in bladder cancer, making comparison of outcomes between series highly dependent on treatment modality and choice of staging systems.
- Clinical staging relies upon exam under anesthesia (i.e., palpable tumor indicates at least T3 disease, fixed disease indicates T4), imaging, and TURBT. Pathologic staging requires information from cystectomy and lymph node sampling/dissection. TURBT is typically insensitive in establishing depth of invasion beyond whether muscle invasion has occurred.
- Clinical understaging in terms of underestimating depth of disease or extent is common (1).
- Although multiple clinical staging systems were used historically (i.e., Jewett-Strong), the most widely used current clinical staging systems is the tumor-node-metastasis staging system of the American Joint Committee on Cancer (6). Recent updates to the system seek to further substratify advanced disease to reflect its heterogeneity (i.e., subdivision of IIIA versus IIIB and IVA versus IVB according to nodal burden and site of metastatic disease, respectively).

NEW!   **SUMMARY OF CHANGES TO AJCC STAGING**

URINARY BLADDER

* Primary staging: stage III divided into IIIa (T3a/3b/4a, N0, M0; or T1-T4a, N1, M0) and IIIb (T1-T4a, N2, N3, M0). Stage IV divided into IVA (Any T, Any N, M1a) and IVB (Any T, Any N, M1b)
* N staging system change:
* N1: perivesical lymph node involvement added
* M1 is subdivided into M1a (only nonregional lymph node) and M1b (non–lymph node distant metastases)

See: Amin MB, Edge SB, Greene FL, et al., eds. *AJCC cancer staging manual*, 8th ed. New York, NY: Springer, 2017. Ref. 7.

PATHOLOGIC CLASSIFICATION

* WHO/ISUP Consensus 2004 classification recognizes a multitude of histology subtypes and differentiation. Reports should specify the presence/invasion of lamina propria or muscularis propria, lymphovascular space invasion, carcinoma *in situ* and its extent, and grade of disease.
* In the United States, approximately 90% of bladder cancers are urothelial carcinomas, 6% to 7% are squamous cell carcinomas, and 1% to 2% are adenocarcinomas (associated with urachal remnants). Small cell carcinoma/neuroendocrine carcinomas occur rarely as well (8–10).
* Urothelial carcinoma associated with variant histology is also common, such as in 20% to 30% of urothelial carcinoma cases showing squamous and/or glandular differentiation; however, their clinical behavior appears similar to pure urothelial carcinoma (8).
* In regions with endemic *Schistosoma* parasitic infection, SCCA histology accounts for up to 75% of disease.
* Micropapillary differentiation is a negative prognostic feature, with some favoring even radical cystectomy for T1 disease.
* Papillary tumors when superficial are less commonly high grade.
* Sarcomas, pheochromocytomas, lymphomas, and carcinoid tumors account for most of the remaining 2%; because of their rarity, they are not discussed here.

PROGNOSTIC FACTORS

* Depth of tumor invasion (stage) and grade are the most important prognostic factors for bladder-confined disease.
* Presence of blood vessel or lymphatic vessel invasion is also significant, even in the absence of positive lymph nodes and even if the tumor is confined to the lamina propria (11).

- Carcinoma *in situ*, solid tumor morphology, large tumor size, multiplicity of tumors, muscle invasion, histologically positive lymph nodes, and obstructive uropathy are indicators of a poor prognosis (12).
- Treatment-specific prognosticators include hydronephrosis (adverse for triple modality therapy [TMT]) and inability to tolerate platinum therapy (for neoadjuvant chemotherapy)

GENERAL MANAGEMENT

Superficial Bladder Cancer

- Ta and T1 tumors are usually treated by TURBT and fulguration, with or without intravesical therapy (adjuvant +/– maintenance).
  - Some of the most commonly used intravesical agents are thiotepa, mitomycin C, doxorubicin, and BCG.
  - Although induction intravesical therapy in high-risk superficial disease is standard, the application of maintenance intravesical therapy is often institution specific.
- Patients with diffuse high-grade T1 disease or involvement of the prostatic urethra or ducts not amenable to conservative management are sometimes treated by cystectomy up front.
- For carcinoma *in situ*, prompt radical cystectomy is usually curative, but most patients and urologists prefer more conservative initial management; the initial treatment is TURBT and fulguration of visible lesions.
- A randomized trial of unifocal T1 G3 patients receiving TURBT +/– radiotherapy showed no difference in PFS or OS (13). Although an ongoing RTOG trial seeks to assess the role of chemoradiation in T1 high-risk disease, chemoradiation is not at present standard in non–muscle-invasive bladder cancer (13).
- Radical cystectomy is used when conservative management is unsuccessful.

Muscle-Invasive Bladder Cancer

- MIBC accounts for most disease-related morbidity and death in bladder cancer whether from initial disease or progression to metastasis. Given the common presence of comorbidities and advanced age in MIBC patients, multidisciplinary care is needed for optimal care.
- Radical cystectomy (RC) remains the most common local therapy and to most the "gold standard," though a randomized trial has never successfully been completed to compare RC to bladder preservation therapies, such as chemoradiation.
  - RC involves the removal of the bladder (+prostatectomy for men, +hysterectomy for women) with creation of a urinary diversion.
  - Advances in diversions throughout the 1980s, 1990s, and 2000s have led to options of ileal conduit diversion (cutaneous incontinent ostomy) and orthotopic diversions, including neobladders with cutaneous or primary (urethral) drainage. Detubularized bowel is used to create low-pressure reservoirs in either reconstruction.

- Pelvic lymph dissection and yield appears prognostic and therapeutic, and extended dissections above the common iliacs may further reduce recurrence risk. The latter is under investigation in the ongoing SWOG S1011 trial.
- Perioperative therapy
  - Preoperative irradiation has not demonstrated clear OS benefit in prior studies (14–16), and thus outside special palliative scenarios is not indicated.
  - Level 1 data support the use of neoadjuvant cisplatin-containing chemotherapy (MVAC or GC) prior to radical cystectomy (6,17). Importantly, as there is no clear substitute for cisplatin, for the approximately 50% of patients who are cisplatin eligible, there is no clear role for NAC.
  - Adjuvant chemotherapy benefit is less clear with methodologic issues to trials studying it and poor compliance following RC.
  - Adjuvant radiotherapy has suggested benefit based on retrospective data in ≥pT3 or R1/R2 resections; however, a randomized trial assessing its benefit failed to accrue (NRG GU-001), limiting its acceptance.
  - Perioperative immunotherapy (checkpoint inhibitors of the programmed death ligand axis) is under investigation.
- Bladder preservation is an option for select patients seeking an alternative to RC or for those who are medically inoperable. The most validated strategy is TMT, employing chemoradiation following maximum safe TURBT. Individual elements of TMT are considered necessary but not sufficient in themselves for optimal therapy:
  - TURBT alone and chemotherapy alone (SWOG S0219) are not felt adequate for bladder preservation (18).
  - Radiation alone similarly results in inferior locoregional control and is reserved for palliative treatments, in light of the many radiosensitizing chemotherapy regimens available (Table 28-2).
- A large body of retrospective and prospective data has evaluated varying chemoradiation regimens, as recently reviewed (19).
  - In the United States, investigators primarily from the Massachusetts General Hospital and the Radiation Therapy Oncology Group (RTOG) have assessed primarily cisplatin-based regimens following TURBT (Table 28-3).
    - Although a mix of chemotherapy regimens was used and altered fractionation without split course favored in more recent trials, a common tenet is to reserve RC for those with incomplete response, while those with complete response would proceed selectively to boost phase of treatment.
    - Neoadjuvant chemotherapy before TMT did not demonstrate benefit in RTOG 89-03 (20); however, as this trial was limited by high hematologic toxicity rates with MCV in the era before growth factor support, this does not preclude the use of TMT after neoadjuvant chemotherapy, as may occur when a patient decides upon bladder preservation after undergoing NAC.
  - Concurrent chemoradiation is standard of care for TMT based upon the aforementioned studies and level I data from the phase III RCT BC2001 (21), in which 5-FU/MMC–based chemoradiation demonstrated superior locoregional control (67% versus 54% at 2 years) without OS benefit (possibly due to salvage RC, which was more common in RT-alone arm) and without increased late adverse events.

Table 28-2

Summary of Radiation Therapy/Management

Urinary Bladder	
Carcinoma *in situ* (Tis, Ta) and T1:	• TURBT, fulguration with or without intravesical chemotherapy or BCG. Less frequently cystectomy, unless conservative management is unsuccessful

T2-4:	• Radical cystectomy with urinary diversion with postoperative radiotherapy 45–50.5 Gy for gross residual disease or extensive perivesicle disease
	• Bladder preservation in selected patients (no diffuse CIS, no hydronephrosis, cN0, baseline urinary function, able to receive chemotherapy, cT2-T4a), including maximum safe TURBT, concurrent chemoradiation (preferred regimens include CDDP or 5FU/MMC).
	   ◦ Radiotherapy may be delivered as a continuous course or as a split course with interim assessment after an initial phase (40–45 Gy), followed by restaging biopsies, which if negative are followed by boost phase to >64–66 Gy in conventional fractionation.
	   ◦ Contemporary trends forgo split course assessment and allow for cone down of the boost volume to a tumor bed boost, utilizing bladder mapping, imaging, or even fiducial markers. Pelvic nodal radiotherapy is of unclear benefit but commonly included given the benefit of pelvic lymphadenectomy during RC.

Target volumes	
Initial:	• Pelvic nodes including common iliacs, bladder, and prostate (men)
Boost:	• Initial gross tumor volume with 2-cm margin
Palliation:	• 40–50 Gy to involved volumes with adequate margins. • Concurrent chemotherapy may be considered, such as lower toxicity twice-weekly gemcitabine. However, radiation alone should be given when hypofractionating >3 Gy per fraction. For palliation of those with poor performance status primarily for hemostasis, short high-dose regimens, such as 7 Gy × 3 may be considered.

- Roughly equivalent survival rates compared with historic controls treated with radical cystectomy alone are reported (5-year OS approximately 50%, approximately 40% to 50% survival with intact bladder) (19,22–24). Direct comparison is limited by failure to accrue of the randomized SPARE trial in the United Kingdom and the fundamental differences in clinical versus pathologic staging and age/comorbidities of patients enrolled on TMT versus RC trials (i.e., median age on BC2001 (21) was 72 years versus median age of US Intergroup trial of RC +/– NAC of 63 years old) (17).

Table 28-3					
Summary of Selected Trimodality Therapy Trials					
Protocol	N	Regimen	Complete Response	5 yr LC	5 yr OS
RTOG 85-12	42	TURBT → RT + CDDP	66%	39%	52%
RTOG 88-02	91	TURBT → MCV × 2 · RT + CDDP	75%	57%	51%
RTOG 89-03	123	TURBT → RT + CDDP +/– neoadjuvant MCV × 2	61% vs. 55% NS	39% vs. 45% NS	48% vs. 49% NS
RTOG 95-06	34	TURBT → alt frac RT+ 5FU/CDDP	67%	55%	83% at 3 yr
RTOG 97-06	52	TURBT → alt frac RT + CDDP → MCV × 3	74%	80% at 2 yr	61% at 3 yr
RTOG 99-06	80	TURBT → alt frac RT + CDDP/taxol → CDDP/ gemcitabine × 4	81%	70%	56%
BC2001	360	+/– neoadjuvant chemotherapy → RT alone vs. RT + 5FU/MMC	NR	2 yr 54% vs. 67% $p = 0.03$	35% vs. 48% NS

- Salvage after failure of bladder preservation:
  - Up to 25% to 40% of patients will suffer an in-bladder failure after TMT, of which approximately one third of these are muscle invasive (23). RC is standard for medically operable patients with ≥T2 relapse, with thus an estimated approximately 25% to 30% long-term salvage RC rate in bladder preservation cohorts. Although more difficult because of prior radiation, salvage RC in experienced hands is feasible and associated with acceptable morbidity only slightly higher than reported RC series (25).
  - Non–muscle-invasive relapse may be managed conservatively with TURBT and adjuvant intravesical therapies but remain at risk for requiring RC, without an apparent effect on disease-specific survival (19).

CHEMOTHERAPY

- Methotrexate, vinblastine, doxorubicin (Adriamycin), and cisplatin (MVAC) toxicity is significant; Sternberg et al. (26) reported a 20% incidence of nadir sepsis and 4% mortality. Tannock et al. (27) reported septic neutropenia in 18 of 41 patients and one drug-related death.
- The toxicity of cisplatin, methotrexate, and vinblastine is similar (mortality, 4%; nadir sepsis, 26%) (1).
- Gemcitabine with cisplatin (GC) has shown similar activity and less toxicity than MVAC. Septic neutropenia was reported in 71% of patients receiving GC versus 82% with MVAC (28). Patients unable to receive cisplatin have shown similar

effects with gemcitabine and carboplatin. Compared to methotrexate, carboplatin, and vinblastine (MCAVI), carboplatin plus gemcitabine had higher although not significant objective response rate. Gemcitabine and carboplatin also had less toxicity (29).

- Combination of paclitaxel, gemcitabine, and cisplatin (PGS) reported a significant objective response rate over GC (p = 0.003) but increased incidence of grade 3/4 toxicities (30).

Targeted Therapies

- Programmed cell death-1 protein (PD-1)/PD-1 ligand (PD-L1) checkpoint inhibitors have been investigated in patients unable to tolerate cisplatin-based chemotherapy and as second-line therapy. For instance, pembrolizumab, a PD-1 checkpoint inhibitor, has shown an objective response rate of 29% with complete and partial responses of 7% and 22%, respectively, in patients not eligible for the cisplatin-based regimen (31,32). As a second-line therapy, pembrolizumab has shown significantly better overall survival and higher response rate compared with chemotherapy (33).
- Nivolumab, a PD-1 antibody, was FDA approved for use in patients with advanced metastatic urothelial cancer refractory to platinum-based therapy. A single-arm study in 270 patients had ORR of 19.6% with 7 complete response and 46 partial responses (34).
- Ipilimumab, a cytotoxic T-lymphocyte–associated antigen-4 (CTLA-4) blocker, with gemcitabine and cisplatin has shown ORR of 64% in a phase II trial (22).
- Ramucirumab, a vascular endothelial growth factor (VEGF) antibody, has shown improved progression-free survival in combination with docetaxel compared to docetaxel alone (35).

RADIOTHERAPY TECHNIQUES

- Traditional bladder preservation radiotherapy fields utilized in most reported trials utilized 3D-conformal radiotherapy with four-field box technique in the supine position (example in Fig. 28-1):
  - Initial field encompassed the entire bladder, pelvic nodes (at least internal and external iliacs), prostate in men, or proximal urethra in women. Setup included immobilization in supine position with empty bladder. AP/PA fields extended from mid-sacroiliac joint at top of S2 to bottom of obturator foramen and 2 cm laterally of pelvic brim, with femoral head blocking. Lateral fields retained the craniocaudal borders of the AP/PA field but encompassed a 2-cm margin on anterior and posterior bladder walls and internal and external iliacs, with corner block under the pubic symphysis (for genitalia shielding) and corner block ant/sup to block bowel anterior to the external iliacs lymph nodes. Posteriorly, the rectum and anal canal were blocked. A small amount of contrast in the bladder and bowels could aid this delineation.

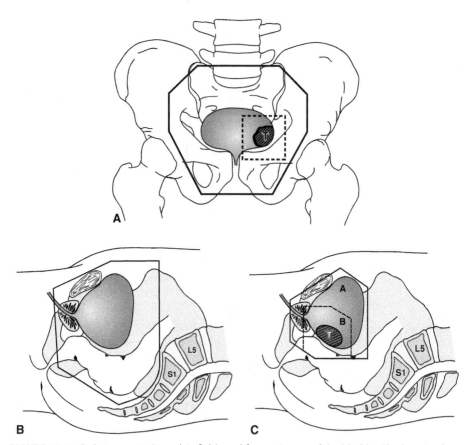

FIGURE 28-1. A: Anteroposterior pelvic field used for carcinoma of the bladder. The boost volume is outlined with *dashed lines*. **B:** Lateral pelvic field encompasses the bladder and the pelvic lymph nodes. **C:** Reduced portals after 50 Gy (*A*) and 55 or 60 Gy (*B*). T, residual primary tumor. (Reprinted with permission from Perez CA, Gerber RL, Manolis JM. Male reproductive and genitourinary tumors. In: Washington CM, Leaver DT, eds. *Principles and practice of radiation therapy: practical applications.* St. Louis, MO: Mosby–Year Book, 1997:244–289. © Elsevier.)

- Boost portals after 39.6 to 45 Gy would then be implemented in same immobilization/supine positioning but now with full bladder to allow sparing of areas beyond the immediate tumor region. Using bladder mapping/imaging and CT simulation, a 2-cm margin around the tumor would be delineated for the cone down to a dose of 60 to 66 Gy, as allowed by bowel tolerance in particular for dome of bladder lesions.
- IMRT with image-guidance (even using tumor bed intra-vesical fiducials) may improve sparing of bowel, rectum and bladder distant from the tumor site (36). An example regimen is as follows:
  - Initial phase: Empty bladder, supine positioning. CTV delineation of bladder + 1.5-cm margin, prostate in men or proximal urethra in women + 1-cm margin, and pelvic nodes (7-mm boundary around vessels of internal/external iliacs and presacrals). PTV = 7 mm depending on the use of kV only versus CBCT image guidance (latter preferred). Dose 40 to 45 Gy in conventional fractionation.

- Boost phase: Full bladder, supine positioning. CTV delineation of GTV using fiducials with 1.5-cm margin; PTV 5 to 7 mm with CBCT guidance matching on bladder fill, fiducials, and soft tissue of bladder to boost. Care particularly taken to note cumulative small bowel dose, which is typically the limiting constraint, and thus to delineate it within a generous bowel bag, so as to avoid underestimation. Boost dose to 64 to 66 Gy.
- Postoperative radiotherapy is controversial but when used should be based upon the consensus contours recommended for the now closed NRG GU-001 trial. In brief, the CTV would encompass the bed up to 2 cm superior to pubic symphysis, be bounded anteriorly by the plane created by the pubic rami, encompass the anterior one-third surface of the anorectum without actually extending inside of the anorectum, and inferiorly end 1 CT slice above the penile bulb in males or 1 cm below obturator foramen in females. Dose would be 45 to 50.4 Gy with gross disease boost as feasible, constrained by small bowel tolerance.

NORMAL TISSUE COMPLICATIONS

- Bladder constraints are not well defined, in part because of low certainty in bladder distension/volume across a typical length of fractionated radiotherapy.
- Example dose constraints for use as follows:
  - RTOG 07-12:
    - Rectum V30 less than 50%, V55 less than 10%
    - Femoral heads V50 less than 20%
  - Institution-specific example for IMRT:
    - Small bowel composite D0.03cc less than 54 Gy, D5% less than 50 Gy. Initial plan care taken to limit any hot spots in small bowel that may complicate subsequent boost.
    - Large bowel D5% less than 60 Gy
    - Bladder V66.6 Gy less than 60%
    - Rectal wall D5% less than 60 Gy

SEQUELAE OF THERAPY

- Acute side effects of cystitis and diarrhea, which are frequent, are treated with phenazopyridine (Pyridium) and diphenoxylate/atropine sulfate (Lomotil) or loperamide (Imodium).
- Patients are encouraged to drink plenty of fluids.
- The morbidity of radical irradiation is mainly associated with complications of the bladder (8% to 10%), rectum (3% to 4%), or small bowel (1% to 2%) (37).
- The mortality rate attributable to delayed irradiation complications is 1% (37).
- Radiation cystitis develops in 10% of patients receiving irradiation, and bladder contracture develops in 1% of patients.

References

1. Parsons JT, Zlotecki RA. Bladder. In: Perez CA, Brady LW, eds. *Principles and practice of radiation oncology*, 3rd ed. Philadelphia, PA: Lippincott–Raven, 1998:1543–1571.

2. Tolley DA, Hargreave TB, Smith PH, et al. Effect of intravesical mitomycin C on recurrence of newly diagnosed superficial bladder cancer: interim report from the Medical Research Council Subgroup on Superficial Bladder Cancer (Urological Cancer Working Party). *Br Med J (Clin Res Ed)* 1988;296(6639):1759–1761.

3. Oldbring J, Glifberg I, Mikulowski P, et al. Carcinoma of the renal pelvis and ureter following bladder carcinoma: frequency, risk factors and clinicopathological findings. *J Urol* 1989;141(6):1311–1313.

4. Gopalakrishna A, et al. Anticipatory positive urine tests for bladder cancer. *Ann Surg Oncol* 2017;24(6):1747–1753.

5. Herr HW. The value of a second transurethral resection in evaluating patients with bladder tumors. *J Urol* 1999;162(1):74–76.

6. Advanced Bladder Cancer Meta-analysis Collaboration. Neoadjuvant chemotherapy in invasive bladder cancer: update of a systemic review and meta-analysis of individual patient data advanced bladder cancer (ABC) meta-analysis collaboration. *Eur Urol* 2005;48:202–205.

7. Amin MB, Edge SB, Greene FL et al., eds. *AJCC cancer staging manual*, 8th ed. New York, NY: Springer, 2017.

8. Grignon DJ, Ro JY, Ayala AG, et al. Primary adenocarcinoma of the urinary bladder. A clinico-pathologic analysis of 72 cases. *Cancer* 1991;67(8):2165–2172.

9. Oblon DJ, Parsons JT, Zander DS, et al. Bladder preservation and durable complete remission of small cell carcinoma of the bladder with systemic chemotherapy and adjuvant radiation therapy. *Cancer* 1993;71(8):2581–2584.

10. Grignon DJ, Ro JY, Ayala AG, et al. Small cell carcinoma of the urinary bladder. A clinicopatho-logic analysis of 22 cases. *Cancer* 1992;69(2):527–536.

11. Greven KM, Solin LJ, Hanks GE. Prognostic factors in patients with bladder carcinoma treated with definitive irradiation. *Cancer* 1990;65(4):908–912.

12. Shipley WU, Rose MA, Perrone TL, et al. Full-dose irradiation for patients with invasive bladder carcinoma: clinical and histological factors prognostic of improved survival. *J Urol* 1985;134(4):679–683.

13. Harland SJ, Kynaston H, Grigor K, et al. A randomized trial of radical radiotherapy for the management of pT1G3 NXM0 transitional cell carcinoma of the bladder. *J Urol* 2007;178(3 Pt 1):807–813; discussion 813.

14. Reisinger SA, Mohiuddin M, Mulholland SG. Combined pre- and postoperative adjuvant radiation therapy for bladder cancer—a ten year experience. *Int J Radiat Oncol Biol Phys* 1992;24(3):463–468.

15. Sell A, Jakobsen A, Nerstrom B, et al. Treatment of advanced bladder cancer category T2, T3 and T4a. A randomized multicenter study of preoperative irradiation and cystectomy versus radical irradiation and early salvage cystectomy for residual tumor. DAVECA protocol 8201. Danish Vesical Cancer Group. *Scand J Urol Nephrol Suppl* 1991;138:193–201.

16. Spera JA, Whittington R, Littman P, et al. A comparison of preoperative radiotherapy regimens for bladder carcinoma. The University of Pennsylvania experience. *Cancer* 1988;61(2):255–262.

17. Grossman HB, et al. Neoadjuvant chemotherapy plus cystectomy compared with cystectomy alone for locally advanced bladder cancer. *N Engl J Med* 2003;349:859–866.

18. deVere White RW, et al. A sequential treatment approach to myoinvasive urothelial carcinoma: a phase II Southwest Oncology Group trial (S0219). *J Urol* 2009;181(6):2476–2480.

19. Ploussard G, et al. Critical analysis of bladder sparing with trimodal therapy in muscle-invasive bladder cancer: a systematic review. *Eur Urol* 2014;66(1):120–137.

20. Shipley WU, Winter KA, Kaufman DS, et al. Phase III trial of neoadjuvant chemotherapy in patients with invasive bladder cancer treated with selective bladder preservation by combined radiation therapy and chemotherapy: initial results of Radiation Therapy Oncology Group 89-03. *J Clin Oncol* 1998;16(11):3576–3583.

21. James ND, et al. Radiotherapy with or without chemotherapy in muscle-invasive bladder cancer. *N Engl J Med* 2012;366(16):1477–1488.

22. Galsky MD, Hahn N, Albany C, et al. Phase II trial of gemcitabine+cisplatin+ipilimumab in patients with metastatic urothelial cancer. *J Clin Oncol* 2016;34(Suppl 2S):abstr 357.

23. Giacalone NJ, et al. Long-term outcomes after bladder-preserving tri-modality therapy for patients with muscle-invasive bladder cancer: an updated analysis of the massachusetts general hospital experience. *Eur Urol* 2017;71(6):952–960.

24. Housset M, Maulard C, Chretien Y, et al. Combined radiation and chemotherapy for invasive transitional-cell carcinoma of the bladder: a prospective study. *J Clin Oncol* 1993;11(11):2150–2157.

25. Eswara JR, et al. Complications and long-term results of salvage cystectomy after failed bladder sparing therapy for muscle invasive bladder cancer. *J Urol* 2012;187(2):463–468.

26. Sternberg CN, Yagoda A, Scher HI, et al. M-VAC (methotrexate, vinblastine, doxorubicin and cisplatin) for advanced transitional cell carcinoma of the urothelium. *J Urol* 1988;139(3):461–469.

27. Tannock I, Gospodarowicz M, Connolly J, et al. M-VAC (methotrexate, vinblastine, doxorubicin and cisplatin) chemotherapy for transitional cell carcinoma: the Princess Margaret Hospital experience. *J Urol* 1989;142(2 Pt 1):289–292.

28. von der Maase H, Hansen SW, Roberts JT. Gemcitabine and cisplatin versus methotrexate, vinblastine, doxorubicin, and cisplatin in advanced or metastatic bladder cancer: results of a large, randomized, multinational, multicenter, phase III study. *J Clin Oncol* 2000;18(17):3068–3077.

29. De Santis M, Bellmunt J, Mead G. Randomized phase II/III trial assessing gemcitabine/carboplatin and methotrexate/carboplatin/vinblastine in patients with advanced urothelial cancer who are unfit for cisplatin-based chemotherapy: EORTC study 30986. *J Clin Oncol* 2012;30(2):191–199.

30. Bellmunt J, von der Maase H, Mead GM, et al. Randomized phase III study comparing paclitaxel/cisplatin/gemcitabine (PCG) and gemcitabine/cisplatin (GC) in patients with locally advanced (LA) or metastatic (M) urothelial cancer without prior systemic therapy: EORTC Intergroup Study 30987. *J Clin Oncol* 2012;30(10):1107–1113.

31. Balar AV, Castellano D, O'Donnell PH, et al. First-line pembrolizumab in cisplatin-ineligible patients with locally advanced and unresectable or metastatic urothelial cancer a multicentre, single-arm, phase 2 study. *Lancet Oncol* 2017;18(11):1483–1492.

32. Bellmunt J, de Wit R, Vaughn DJ, et al. Pembrolizumab as second-line therapy for advanced urothelial carcinoma. *N Engl J Med* 2017;376:1015–1026.

33. Bajorin DF, De Wit R, Vaughn DJ, et al. Plans survival analysis from KEYNOTE-045: phase 3, open-label study of pembrolizumab versus paclitaxel, docetaxel, or vinflunine in recurrent, advanced urothelial cancer (abstract 4501). *2017 annual meeting of the American Society for Clinical Oncology.*

34. Galsky MD, Retz MM, Siefker-Radtke A, et al. Efficacy and safety of nivolumab monotherapy in patients with metastatic urothelial cancer (mUC) who have received prior treatment: results from the phase II CheckMate-275 study. Presented at: 2016 ESMO Congress; 7–11 October 2016. Copenhagen, Denmark, 2016:abstr LBA31.

35. Petrylak DP, de Wit R, Chi KN, et al. Ramucirumab plus docetaxel versus placebo plus docetaxel in patients with locally advanced or metastatic urothelial carcinoma after platinum-based therapy (RANGE): a randomised, double-blind, phase 3 trial. *Lancet* 2017;390(10109):2266–2277.

36. Della Biancia C, et al. Image guided radiation therapy for bladder cancer: assessment of bladder motion using implanted fiducial markers. *Pract Radiat Oncol* 2014;4(2):108–115.

37. Duncan W, Quilty PM. The results of a series of 963 patients with transitional cell carcinoma of the urinary bladder primarily treated by radical megavoltage X-ray therapy. *Radiother Oncol* 1986;7(4):299–310.

CHAPTER 29

PROSTATE

ANATOMY

- The prostate gland surrounds the male urethra between the bladder base and the urogenital diaphragm (Fig. 29-1A).
- The prostate is attached anteriorly to the pubic symphysis by the puboprostatic ligament and is separated from the rectum posteriorly by Denonvilliers' fascia (recto-vesical septum), which attaches above to the peritoneum and below to the urogenital diaphragm.
- The seminal vesicles and the vas deferens pierce the posterosuperior aspect of the gland and enter the urethra at the verumontanum (Fig. 29-1B).
- The prostate is divided into the anterior, median, posterior, and two lateral lobes.
  - The posterior lobe is felt on rectal examination.
- Others divide the glandular prostate into an inner and outer portion.
  - The inner portion contains the transitional zone and the periurethral glands.
    - The transitional zone is initially 5% of gland volume.
    - But, it can grow into the largest part of the gland in benign prostatic hypertrophy.
  - The outer portion includes the central and peripheral zones.
    - They make up about 25% and 70% of the gland volume, respectively.
    - The peripheral zone is the most likely site of cancer.
- The nonglandular prostate includes the urethra and anterior fibromuscular stroma (1).

NATURAL HISTORY

- 1 in 6 men will eventually be diagnosed with prostate cancer.
- Today, most prostate cancers are asymptomatic at diagnosis.
  - Most are found due to elevated prostate-specific antigen (PSA) levels.
- Digital rectal examination (DRE) palpates tumors in only 30% to 40% of patients (2).
  - DRE feels extracapsular extension (ECE) in less than 10% of patients.
- Estimating risk of disease progression beyond prostate at diagnosis:

567

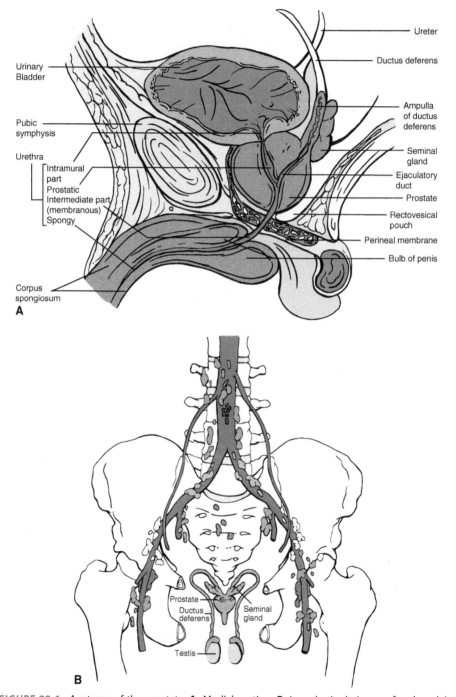

FIGURE 29-1. Anatomy of the prostate. **A:** Medial section. **B:** Lymphatic drainage of male pelvis.

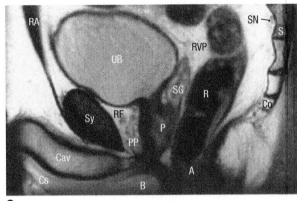

A	Anus
B	Bulb of penis
Co	Coccyx
Cav	Corpus cavernosum penis
Cs	Corpus spongiosum penis
P	Prostate
PP	Prostatic venous plexus
R	Rectum
RA	Rectus abdominis
RF	Retropubic fat
RVP	Rectovesical pouch
S	Sacrum
SG	Seminal gland
SN	Sacral nerves
Sy	Pubic symphysis
UB	Urinary bladder

C

FIGURE 29-1. (*Continued*) **C:** Medial MRI scan. (Reprinted with permission from Agur AMR, Dalley AF, eds. *Grant's atlas of anatomy*, 14th ed. Philadelphia, PA: Lippincott Williams & Wilkins, 2017:411,434,456. © Wolters Kluwer.)

- "Partin tables" developed at Hopkins (3)
- Roach formulas
  - % risk of seminal vesicles involved approximately (1) * PSA + 10*(Gleason – 6) (4).
  - % risk of regional nodes involved approximately (2/3) * PSA + 10*(Gleason – 6) (5,6).
  - % risk of capsule breached approximately (3/2) * PSA + 10*(Gleason – 3) (7).
  - Formulas apply for risk estimates less than 13% to 15% and may underestimate risk.
  - Validated nomograms estimate risk of regional nodal involvement (8).
- Today, most patients are diagnosed with local disease in prostate and seminal vesicles.
  - 67 years old is the median age of diagnosis.
  - Approximately 70% of new cancers are confined to the prostatic capsule (≤pT2N0M0) (9).
  - Less than 1% of new cancers invade the seminal vesicle (pT3b) (9).
  - Less than 1% of new cancers invade the bladder neck (pT4) (9).
  - Less than 5% to 10% of patients with T1c have positive regional lymph nodes (5,9).
  - Regional lymph nodes include:
    - External iliac and its subdivisions (23% to 39% of node-positive cases):
      ○ Lateral group (lateral to the external iliac artery)
      ○ Middle group (medial to the artery but lateral to the vein)
      ○ Medial group (medial to both artery and vein)
        • Obturator nodes are part of this group (another 17% of cases) (10).
    - Internal iliac and its subdivisions (27% to 51% of node-positive cases):
      ○ Lateral sacral (tracks lateral sacral artery)
      ○ Presacral
      ○ Anterior sacral (tracks anterior branch of the internal iliac artery)
      ○ Hypogastric
    - Perivisceral pelvic nodes:
      ○ Perirectal nodes in mesorectal fat (4% to 8% of node-positive cases)
      ○ Perivesical (bladder) nodes
      ○ Periprostatic nodes

- Other lymph nodes are considered metastatic M1 disease, including the:
  - Common iliac
  - Para-aortic lymph nodes
  - Inguinal lymph nodes
- Patients rarely have metastatic disease at diagnosis.
- Patients that fail primary treatment may eventually develop metastatic disease to the bones (common) or the liver or lungs (less common).

CLINICAL PRESENTATION

- Again, most patients are asymptomatic in the era of PSA and DRE screening.
  - Most are found due to elevated prostate-specific antigen (PSA) levels.
  - Transurethral resection of the prostate (TURP) incidentally finds a handful of new cancers. Diagnosis by TURP is staged as T1a or T1b.
- Larger tumors may present with symptoms (often because of urethral obstruction).
  - Frequency, nocturia, hesitancy, and narrow stream.
  - Isolated hematuria or hematospermia is extremely rare.
  - Rarely, patients present with pain or stiffness from bony metastatic disease (11,12).

DIAGNOSTIC WORKUP

- Screening for prostate cancer in average-risk patients is controversial (13–15).
  - Average-risk if (16):
    - No first-degree relative with prostate cancer at age less than 60
    - No African American ancestry
    - No family history of BRCA2 mutation or Lynch syndrome
    - No history of pelvic radiotherapy
    - Consider also screening if with history of prophylactic hormonal ablation
  - ACS offers annual PSA/DRE if average-risk, age ≥50, and life expectancy greater than 10 years.
  - AUA screens "well-informed" men if average-risk and age ≥50.
  - USPSTF in 2011 "recommends against the [screening] service. There is moderate or high certainty that the service has no net benefit or that the harms outweigh the benefits." (17)
  - Consider biopsy if screening PSA greater than 4 ng/mL or PSA doubling time less than 2 years (18,19).
    - But, these thresholds are controversial and unvalidated (20).
- If concerned for cancer, do a complete clinical history and physical examination.
  - Always include PSA.
  - Always include DRE. 50% of palpated nodules confirmed malignant on biopsy.
- Perineal or transrectal core needle biopsy is done if suspicious DRE or PSA.
  - 12-core biopsy has better sensitivity of 51% versus 38% of a 6-core biopsy (21).
  - Transrectal ultrasound (TRUS) guidance is routinely used.

- Bone scan is performed if any of these are present (16):
  - T1 and PSA greater than 20 ng/mL
  - T2 and PSA greater than 10 ng/mL
  - Gleason score ≥8
  - T3 and T4
  - Symptomatic
- Pelvic CT or MRI is performed if any of these are present (16):
  - T3 and T4
  - T1, T2, and nomogram risk of lymph node involvement greater than 10% (8)

STAGING

- Prostate cancer is staged according to the American Joint Committee (AJCC) system.
- AJCC 8 was adopted in January 2018, replacing the AJCC 7 adopted in 2009 (22).
- Obsolete staging systems include the Jewett-Whitmore system.
  - Used in older, mostly irrelevant studies (e.g., RTOG 7506 and 7706).

PROGNOSTIC FACTORS

Tumor-Related Factors

- Most important prognostic indicators:
  - Metastatic (or M-) stage
  - Nodal (or N-) stage (12,23)

NEW! **SUMMARY OF CHANGES TO AJCC STAGING**

- Major changes in the AJCC 8 system include (22):
  - pT2 now simply refers to organ-confined disease.
    - Unlike AJCC 7, there are no pT2a, pT2b, or pT2c subdivisions.
  - Stage Groups now depend on T, N, M, PSA, and Gleason Grade Group.
    - AJCC 7 Stage Groups depended on Gleason scores, not Grade Groups.
    - Gleason scores and Grade Groups are discussed in the Pathology section.
  - Stage III is now subdivided into IIIA, IIIB, and IIIC.
    - IIIA covers T1-2, N0, M0, PSA greater than 20, and Gleason Grade Group 1 to 4.
    - IIIB covers T3-4, N0, M0, any PSA, and Gleason Grade Group 1 to 4.
    - IIIC covers any T, N0, M0, any PSA, and Gleason Grade Group 5.
    - Unlike AJCC 7, purely organ-confined disease can be stage III(A).

See: Amin MB, Edge SB, Greene FL, et al., eds. *AJCC cancer staging manual*, 8th ed. New York, NY: Springer, 2017.

- Risk group (in patients without nodal or distant metastatic disease):
  - Very low risk (the "Epstein criteria"):
    - T1c
    - Gleason score ≤ 6
    - Gleason Grade Group 1
    - PSA less than 10 ng/mL
    - Less than 3 positive prostate biopsy cores (ideally out of a 12-core biopsy)
    - ≤50% cancer in any positive biopsy core
    - PSA density less than 0.15 ng/mL/g
  - Low risk:
    - T1-T2a
    - Gleason score ≤6
    - Gleason Grade Group 1
    - PSA less than 10 ng/mL
  - Intermediate risk:
    - T2b-T2c
    - Gleason score 7 and Gleason Grade Group 2 or 3
    - PSA 10 to 20 ng/mL
    - Unfavorable intermediate-risk disease if (24–26):
      - 2 or more intermediate-risk factors
      - Gleason 4 + 3 (instead of 3 + 4) disease
      - ≥50% positive cores on biopsy
  - High risk:
    - T3a
    - Gleason score ≥8 and Gleason Grade Group 4 or 5
    - PSA greater than 20 ng/mL
  - Very high risk:
    - T3b and T4
    - Any Gleason pattern 5 (i.e., 5 + 5, 5 + 4, 5 + 3, etc.)
    - Greater than 4 positive biopsy scores with Gleason score 8, 9, or 10
- As noted earlier, several nomograms, tables, and formulae exist that divide patients into prognostic groups and predict the probability of extracapsular tumor extension, seminal vesicle involvement, or lymph node metastases (3,4,6–8,27–29).
- Other factors that may inform patient prognosis:
  - DNA ploidy: Aneuploid lesions more aggressive than diploid ones.
  - S-phase fraction.
  - p53 mutations are rare (30) and may predict relative radioresistance.

Host-Related Factors

- Black men may have worse stage-adjusted survival than white men (12,31).
  - But not everyone agrees. If true, possible reasons include:
    - Larger tumor volume (higher pretreatment PSA)
    - Lower immune competence
    - More biologically aggressive tumors

- Testosterone level
- Environmental or socioeconomic conditions
- Genetic or other unknown factors
- Obesity may predict for higher-grade and higher-stage tumors (32).
- Finasteride chemoprevention may reduce the incidence of new prostate cancer.
  - But later, cancers in such men may, possibly, be more aggressive (33).

Radiographic Versus Surgical Staging

- NCCN advocates pelvic lymph node dissection (PLND) if metastatic risk is ≥2% (16).
  - This threshold avoids 48% of PLNDs while missing 12% of positive nodes (8).
- Validated nomograms help estimate risk of positive nodes (8).

PATHOLOGY

- Glandular adenocarcinomas are the most common tumor in the prostate.
  - They often, but not exclusively, arises from peripheral acinar glands.
- Gleason et al. created a pathologic grading system (34,35).
  - AJCC 7 formally incorporated Gleason scoring into prostate cancer staging.
  - Even in a given patient, prostate cancer differentiation is heterogeneous.
  - A Gleason *pattern* from 1 (well differentiated) to 5 (dedifferentiated) is assigned to each heterogeneous clump of cancer cells.
  - A Gleason *score* from 2 to 10 is obtained by summing the Gleason patterns of the two largest (primary and secondary) clumps of cancer cells.
  - Some places upstage patients with tertiary clumps with Gleason pattern of 5.
    - For example, Gleason 3 + 4, tertiary 5 might be treated as high (instead of intermediate) risk at some institutions. This is controversial (36).
  - In AJCC 8, the binary sums of Gleason patterns are binned into *Grade* Groups (22).
    - Gleason Grade Group 1: Binary sum of Gleason patterns ≤3 + 3.
    - Gleason Grade Group 2: Binary sum of Gleason patterns 3 + 4.
    - Gleason Grade Group 3: Binary sum of Gleason patterns 4 + 3.
    - Gleason Grade Group 4: Binary sum of Gleason patterns 4 + 4.
    - Gleason Grade Group 5: Binary sum of Gleason patterns 4 + 5, 5 + 4, and 5 + 5.
- Other, nonglandular and nonadenocarcinoma histologies exist but are rare.
  - Ductal adenocarcinomas:
    - Thought to arise from the prostatic utricle, a müllerian remnant
    - Unclear if more or less aggressive than glandular adenocarcinomas
  - Transitional cell cancers:
    - Uncommon histology that typically arises in the periurethral ducts.
    - Even more rarely, this histology can arise from the prostate stroma.
    - Node metastases more common in stromal (54%) versus ductal (24%) disease (37).
    - Less likely than adenocarcinoma to show perineural invasion.
  - Neuroendocrine tumors are a rare variant small-cell or carcinoid-like cells.
    - These tumors are positive of stain for serotonin, enolase, chromogranin, and calcitonin.

- Prostatic acid phosphatase and PSA can help confirm prostatic origin.
- Mucinous carcinomas are rare and may stain for prostatic acid phosphatase.
- Sarcomas (leiomyosarcoma, rhabdomyosarcoma, or fibrosarcoma) are vanishingly rare primary prostate neoplasms (less than 0.1% of cases).
  - Leiomyosarcoma is more common in middle-aged or older men.
  - Rhabdomyosarcoma is found more frequently in younger patients.
- Sarcomatoid carcinomas are also rare.
  - They are difficult to distinguish from a true sarcoma.
  - They are considered much more aggressive than adenocarcinoma variants.
- Adenoid cystic carcinomas are likewise rare (less than 0.1% of all tumors of this gland).
- Other epithelial tumors, such as carcinoid, have been reported in the prostate.
- Squamous cell carcinomas originating primarily in the prostate are extremely rare.
- Metastatic malignant tumors from other locations to the prostate are rare (12).
- Primary prostate lymphomas are exceedingly rare.
  - Fewer than 100 cases have been reported (38).
  - Lesions vary from diffuse small noncleaved to diffuse large cell lymphomas.
  - Per the Ann Arbor staging system, these are staged as an extranodal site:
    - Stage IE if local disease
    - Stage IVE if the lymph nodes or bone marrow is involved.
  - Prognosis is generally poor.
- Mostofi published an excellent review of prostate cancer pathology (39).

GENERAL MANAGEMENT

- Multiple consensus guidelines exist outlining current thinking on management.
  - Differing guidelines are broadly similar with some (often minor) differences.
  - Most guidelines hinge on patient risk group and life expectancy.
- The algorithm below is drawn from the NCCN 2017 guidelines (16).
  - Very low-risk local disease without nodal or distant metastatic disease:
    - Life expectancy of less than 10 years: watchful waiting (WaWa)
    - Life expectancy of 10 to 20 years: active surveillance (AS)
    - Life expectancy of ≥20 years:
      - Active surveillance (AS)
      - Definitive therapy without androgen deprivation therapy (ADT) via:
        - External beam radiotherapy (EBRT) and/or brachytherapy
        - Radical prostatectomy (RP) ± pelvic lymph node dissection (PLND) (recommend PLND if nomogram risk of involved nodes is ≥2%) (16)
  - Low-risk local disease without nodal or distant metastatic disease:
    - Life expectancy of less than 10 years: WaWa
    - Life expectancy of ≥10 years:
      - AS
      - Definitive therapy without ADT via:
        - EBRT and/or brachytherapy
        - RP ± PLND

- Intermediate-risk local disease without nodal or distant metastatic disease:
  - Life expectancy of less than 10 years:
    - WaWa
    - Definitive therapy via:
      - EBRT ± ADT (4 to 6 months) ± brachytherapy
      - Brachytherapy alone
  - Life expectancy of ≥10 years:
    - Definitive therapy via:
      - EBRT ± ADT (4 to 6 months) ± brachytherapy
      - Brachytherapy alone
      - RP ± PLND
- High-risk local disease without nodal or distant metastatic disease:
  - Definitive therapy via:
    - EBRT + ADT (1.5 to 3 years)
    - EBRT + brachytherapy ± ADT (1.5 to 3 years)
    - RP + PLND
- Very high-risk local disease without nodal or distant metastatic disease:
  - Definitive therapy via:
    - EBRT + ADT (1.5 to 3 years)
    - EBRT + brachytherapy ± ADT (1.5 to 3 years)
    - RP + PLND (in select patients)
  - If unable to tolerate definitive therapy, best supportive care via:
    - ADT
    - Observation
- Nodal metastatic disease (any T, N1, M0):
  - EBRT + ADT (1.5 to 3 years)
  - ADT alone
- Distant metastatic disease (any T, any N, M1): ADT and/or systemic therapy
- Salvage for biochemical recurrence after surgery: EBRT ± ADT

NATURAL COURSE OF DISEASE

- Patients with local prostate cancer tend to do well.
- For T1-2N0 M0 disease given radiotherapy, 8-year cause-specific survival is (40):
  - 93% across all risk groups
  - 99% in the low-risk group
  - 95% in the intermediate-risk group
  - 87% in the high-risk group
- Albertsen tracked for 20 years men treated with observation or ADT alone (41):
  - 3.3% risk of death/year from prostate cancer in the first 15 years in all men
  - 1.8% risk of death/year from prostate cancer after the first 15 years in all men
  - 0.6% risk of death/year from Gleason 2 to 4 prostate cancer over 20 years
  - 12% risk of death/year from Gleason 8 to 10 prostate cancer over first 10 years

- A Swedish trial tracked for 15 years men treated with watchful waiting (42):
  - 37% of deaths over that period were related to prostate cancer.
  - T0-2 disease had an 81% overall survival rate (without treatment).
  - T3-4 disease had a 57% overall survival rate.
  - Metastatic disease had a 6% overall survival rate.
- Radiotherapy and surgery survival outcomes are typically considered equivalent in local prostate cancer. The ProtecT phase 3 randomized prospective trial in men with local prostate cancer reported statistically *similar prostate cancer mortality* at a median of 10 years of follow-up in the men that received active surveillance, radical prostatectomy, and external beam radiotherapy (43).
- But the Grimm meta-analysis reported *superior biochemical-free progression* with brachytherapy alone in low-risk, brachytherapy ± EBRT in intermediate-risk, and brachytherapy + EBRT ± ADT in high-risk disease (44).

HORMONE ANDROGEN DEPRIVATION THERAPY

- This section discusses ADT agent classes and their mechanism of action.
  - The next section will discuss current thinking on the use of ADT for therapy.
- Physiology
  - Hypothalamus secretes gonadotropin-releasing hormone (GnRH).
    - GnRH acts on the anterior pituitary.
    - In normal physiologic settings, GnRH levels oscillate up and down.
    - Oscillating GnRH levels stimulate sustained, elevated androgen levels.
    - Sustained, elevated GnRH gives an initial androgen flare and then sustained nadir.
    - Sustained, depressed GnRH gives a sustained depression in androgen levels.
    - GnRH agonists may, slowly, inhibit androgen production.
      - Example of an agonist: leuprolide (Lupron).
      - Agonists trigger sustained, elevated GnRH levels.
      - Elevated (nonoscillating) GnRH causes a brief, initial androgen flare.
      - The initial androgen flare is followed by a sustained androgen nadir.
    - GnRH antagonists may, quickly, inhibit androgen production.
      - Example of an antagonist: degarelix (Firmagon).
      - Antagonists cause a rapid, sustained drop in GnRH levels.
      - Suppressed (nonoscillating) GnRH suppresses androgen levels.
  - Anterior pituitary secretes luteinizing hormone (LH) and follicle-stimulating hormone (FSH) that act on the testis.
  - Testis secretes androgens that act on peripheral receptors (in the prostate).
  - Androgen uptake in the prostate can fuel prostate cancer growth.
    - Peripheral androgen blockade (e.g., with bicalutamide) may slow growth.
    - Dedifferentiated (i.e., high Gleason) cancers may lack androgen receptors.
      - Unclear if such cancers are resistant to ADT (45).
- Many kinds of blockade exist to inhibit androgenic stimulation of prostate carcinoma.

- Orchiectomy promptly and durably removes 95% of circulating testosterone.
  - (Central acting) gonadotropin-releasing hormone agonists.
  - Also known as luteinizing hormone–releasing hormone (LHRH) agonists.
  - For example, goserelin, leuprolide, and buserelin.
  - They cause an initial rise in gonadotropin levels and then a sharp decline in 2 to 3 weeks.
  - For this reason, they are temporarily started with peripheral androgen blockers.
    - For example, bicalutamide (Casodex), discussed below.
- (Central acting) gonadotropin-releasing hormone antagonists:
  - For example, degarelix (Firmagon)
  - Unlike GnRH agonists, antagonists do not cause a temporary androgen flare.
    - They do not need concurrent peripheral androgen receptor blockade.
- (Peripheral acting) androgen receptor blockade:
  - Bicalutamide (Casodex) (50 mg qd)
  - A steroid antiandrogen that binds to cytosol androgen receptors.
  - This decreases testosterone and elevates gonadotropin levels (46).
  - Monotherapy with bicalutamide 150 mg qd is equivalent to surgical castration (47).
- Other less commonly used or obsolete agents:
  - Nonsteroidal estrogens:
    - Diethylstilbestrol (3 mg/d) reduces serum testosterone to castrate levels (48).
    - But diethylstilbestrol is no longer commercially available in the United States.
  - Progestational agents (49):
    - For example, megestrol (Megace)
    - Suppresses gonadotropin release
    - May also directly interfere with hormone synthesis
    - (Global) antisteroids:
      - For example, aminoglutethimide (Cytadren)
      - Blocks conversion of cholesterol to pregnenolone
        - This blocks sex steroid production.
          - This reduces androgen levels (to fight prostate cancer) (50).
          - This reduces estrogen levels (to fight metastatic breast cancer).
        - This blocks glucocorticoid production (to fight Cushing's syndrome).
        - This blocks mineralocorticoid production.
  - Nonsteroidal antiandrogens:
    - For example, flutamide (Eulexin), typically 250 mg po tid
      - Compared to other antiandrogens, less likely to produce impotence (51).
      - Diarrhea is a common side effect.
    - Does not suppress gonadotropin or testicular testosterone levels
    - But does block 5α-reductase
      - This inhibits dihydrotestosterone formation, which inhibits androgen uptake and nuclear binding in the prostate cell.
- ADT toxicities (16,52):
  - Osteoporosis/increase bone fracture risk (52):
    - Baseline DEXA scan prior to starting ADT; repeat q1-2y or if symptomatic:

- Ca 1,200 mg po qd
- Vitamin D 400 to 800 IU/d, titrating to serum level greater than 50 to 75 nmol/L
- If 10-year risk of hip or osteoporosis-related fracture is ≥3% or ≥20%, consider:
  - Denosumab 60 mg sq q6m.
  - Zoledronic acid 5 mg IV q1y.
  - Alendronate 70 mg po q1w.
  - Assess fracture risk via the WHO's FRAX algorithm (53).
- Lifestyle changes:
  - Weight-bearing exercises
  - Moderate alcohol
  - Smoking cessation
- Hepatotoxicity:
  - Order baseline liver function panel prior to starting ADT.
- Nephrotoxicity:
  - Order baseline renal function panel prior to starting ADT.
- Increased risk of cardiovascular disease
- Gynecomastia (52,54):
  - Consider prophylactic breast irradiation.
  - Consider prophylactic tamoxifen.
  - Strategic selection of hormonal agent can reduce risk of gynecomastia.
    - Approximately 90% incidence with antiandrogens like bicalutamide (Casodex).
    - Approximately 30% incidence with GnRH agonists like leuprolide (Lupron).
- Hot flashes
- Libido loss/impotence
- Sarcopenic obesity (i.e., concurrent lipid mass increase and muscle mass decrease)
- Fatigue
- Depression
- Hair loss
- Increased risk of diabetes
- Increased risk of metabolic syndrome, a nebulous clinical entity that may present with dyslipidemia, hypertension, and/or diabetes (52)

Irradiation and Adjuvant or Neoadjuvant Endocrine Therapy

- Overview of current ADT management thinking:
  - Cancer prophylaxis: Controversial
    - ADT may reduce overall incidence of later prostate cancer.
    - *But* ADT may, possibly, increase relative incidence of aggressive disease.
  - Low or favorable intermediate risk: No ADT with either radiation or surgery
  - Unfavorable intermediate risk: Short-course (4 to 6 months) ADT with radiation
  - High risk: Long-course (2 to 3 years) ADT with radiation
  - Salvage after biochemical (i.e., local) surgical failure: EBRT ± ADT
  - Before surgery: No benefit
  - After surgery: Immediate, continuous ADT if nodal disease found
- Optimal time to begin ADT therapy relative to radiotherapy start date?

- This is controversial.
- Seminal ADT studies are described later in this section, below.
  - Some trials begin ADT 1 to 2 months prior to radiotherapy start.
  - Other trials begin ADT with radiotherapy.
- Zelefsky reported that preradiation PSA nadirs of ≤0.3 ng/mL had better (55):
  - 10-year biochemical progression-free survival (74% versus 58%),
  - 10-year distant metastatic-free survival (86% versus 79%), and
  - 10-year prostate cancer-specific survival (92% versus 86%).
  - These findings suggest patients may benefit from starting neoadjuvant ADT and delaying radiotherapy until PSA values dip below 0.3 ng/mL (or until patient has had 6 months of ADT, whichever comes first).
    - But, further study is needed to confirm this.
- Nanda identified possible ADT contraindications in JAMA in 2009 (56):
  - Avoid ADT in patients with any primary heart disease:
    - Known coronary artery disease (CAD)
    - Prior myocardial infarction (MI)
    - Known congestive heart failure
    - ADT versus no ADT 5-year overall survival hazard ratio of 1.96
  - Consider avoiding ADT in patients with 2+ CAD risk factors:
    - Diabetes
    - Hypertension
    - Dyslipidemia
  - Impact of smoking or family history on ADT use remains unclear.
- Intermediate risk: Short-course (i.e., 6 months) ADT with radiation may help.
- Many studies showed ADT helps with older era, low-dose radiation (≤70 Gy).
  - RTOG 9408 (57):
    - 66.6 Gy ± 4 months ADT in T1b-2b, PSA ≤ 20
      - ADT began 2 months prior to radiation start.
    - 10-year overall survival was 62% versus 57% in the ADT versus no ADT arms.
    - On subset analysis, intermediate- (versus low-) risk disease benefits mostly.
  - DFCI 95096 (58):
    - 70 Gy ± 6-month ADT in T1-2b cancers and at least 1 unfavorable factor:
      - Gleason 7 to 10
      - PSA 10 to 40
      - Extracapsular or seminal vesicle involvement seen on MRI
    - 8-year overall survival was 74% versus 61% in the ADT versus no ADT arms.
    - On subset analysis, patients with few comorbidities benefited most.
  - TROG 9601 (59):
    - 66 Gy + 0 months or 3 months or 6 months of ADT in T2b-T4 cancers
      - ADT began either never, 2 months, or 5 months prior to radiation start.
    - 10.6-year median follow-up.
    - Compared to radiation alone, 6-month ADT had a:
      - 0.49 hazard ratio for prostate cancer–specific survival ($p < 0.01$)
      - 0.63 hazard ratio for overall survival ($p < 0.01$)
    - Compared to radiation alone, 3-month ADT had no survival advantage.

- RTOG 9910 showed short-course ADT sufficient with low-dose radiation (60).
  - 70.2 Gy + 16 weeks or 36 weeks of ADT in intermediate-risk prostate cancers
    - ADT began 8 weeks prior to radiation start.
  - Short- and long-course ADT had the same prostate cancer survival.
- Pending RTOG 0815 will see if ADT is needed with high-dose radiation (greater than 70 Gy).
- High-risk disease:
  - Older trials, like EORTC 22863 ("Bolla I") and EORTC 22961 ("Bolla II"), showed that long-course (36 months) ADT improved survival in patients treated with older era, low-dose radiation (≤70 Gy) (61,62).
  - The DART 01/05 trial confirmed that long-course (28 months) ADT improves survival in men that received modern era, high-dose radiation (63).
    - 76 to 82 Gy + 4 months or 28 months of ADT in intermediate- or high-risk T1c-3b cancers.
      - ADT began 2 months prior to radiation start.
    - 5-year overall survival was 95% versus 86% in the short versus long ADT arms.
  - In a recent abstract, Nabid reported that 18 months (versus 36 months) of ADT may be sufficient (64).
    - These results were presented at ASCO in 2017.
    - But, a paper detailing these findings remains pending.
    - Accordingly, 28+ months of ADT remains the standard of care.
  - Pending RTOG 0924 will see if ADT obviates the need for nodal radiation.
- Salvage: Early salvage radiotherapy with short-course ADT may improve outcomes.
  - GETUG-AFU 16 (65):
    - 66 Gy ± 24 months of ADT in pT2-4a cancer with post-op PSA of 0.2 to 2.0 μg/L
      - ADT began the same day as radiotherapy.
    - 5-year biochemical-free survival was 80% versus 62% in the ADT versus no ADT arms.
  - RTOG 96-01 (66):
    - 64.8 Gy ± 24 months of ADT in T2-3 cancer with post-op PSA of 0.2 to 4.0 ng/mL.
      - ADT began the same day as radiotherapy.
    - 13-year overall survival was 76% versus 71% (p = 0.04) in the ADT versus no ADT arms.
    - In subset analysis, the following groups benefited most from salvage ADT:
      - Gleason 7 (HR 0.69 for ADT versus no ADT)
        - Salvage did not benefit the subset of high-risk Gleason 8+ disease.
        - Maybe the high-risk subcohort is too small (and underpowered)
        - It is dedifferentiated, lacking androgen receptors for ADT to suppress.
        - These explanations are speculative.
      - PSA ≥ 0.7 ng/mL (HR 0.45 to 0.61 for ADT versus no ADT)
      - Positive margins (HR 0.73 for ADT versus no ADT).
  - Pending RTOG 0534 will see if ADT obviates the need for nodal radiation.

IRRADIATION OF THE BREAST BEFORE HORMONAL THERAPY

- Prophylactic breast radiation can reduce incidence of gynecomastia.
  - Glandular hyperplasia cannot be reversed with radiotherapy after-the-fact.
  - Radiotherapy, if used, must precede orchiectomy or start of estrogen therapy.
- Technique (54,67,68):
  - 12 Gy in 3 fractions prescribed to the 90% isodose line using 6-MeV electrons
  - To a circle with 5-cm radius around each nipple
- Efficacy (54):
  - Up to 90% incidence of gynecomastia in patients treated with bicalutamide alone.
  - (For comparison, up to 30% incidence of gynecomastia with leuprolide alone.)
  - With prophylactic radiotherapy, this incidence drops to around 50%.
  - With concurrent tamoxifen, this incidence further drops to around 15%.

RADIATION THERAPY TECHNIQUES

External Irradiation

- In recent years, intensity-modulated radiation therapy (IMRT) has essentially supplanted older 3D conformal and 2D techniques (69–71).
- After TURP (e.g., for relief of obstructive lower urinary tract symptoms) or other pelvic surgery, at least 4 weeks should elapse before irradiation is begun to decrease sequelae (urinary incontinence, urethral stricture).
  - This delay will give sufficient time for surgical wound healing.
  - This delay will also allow patient's urinary function to return to baseline.
  - Can wait greater than 4 weeks if post-op urinary function recovery has not plateaued.
    - Depending on risk group, consider neoadjuvant ADT during recovery.

Volume Treated

- Prostate ± seminal vesicles (SV) for intact low- and intermediate-risk prostate cancer.
- Prostate + proximal seminal vesicles ± pelvic nodes for intact high-risk cancer.
- Prostate surgical bed for postprostatectomy patients.
- Prostate, seminal vesicle, and surgical bed delineation are discussed in a later section.
- Elective pelvic nodal irradiation in high-risk patients is controversial.
  - Many institutions electively cover pelvic nodes in high-risk men.
    - But some institutions do not because there is little good evidence for it.
  - Pending RTOG 0924 will see if ADT obviates the need for elective nodal radiation.
    - Unlike older trials, long-course ADT and high-dose radiation will be used.
  - A number of older trials showed no benefit with elective nodal irradiation.
    - GETUG 01 (72): No benefit in T1b-T3N0/xM0 men.
    - RTOG 9413 (73,74): No benefit in T1c-T4N0M0 men with PSA ≤ 100 ng/mL.
    - RTOG 7506 (75): No benefit with pelvic/para-aortic radiation in N0-N1 men.
    - RTOG 7706 (76): Similar null results as RTOG 7506.

- But these trials shared all or some of the following limitations:
    - Used 3D conformal (instead of modern IMRT) technique.
        - Thus, all patients got (at least 40 to 45 Gy) pelvic nodal irradiation.
    - Patients got older, low-dose, 66 to 70 Gy (instead of modern greater than 75 Gy).
    - Some included patients with (pelvic) N1 or (para-aortic) M1 disease.
    - High-risk patients received no or short-course hormonal ablation.
    - Used obsolete Jewett-Whitmore staging system.
- Delineating the pelvic nodes for elective treatment via 3D imaging.
    - RTOG Consensus Guidelines describe how to contour pelvic nodes (77).
    - Small published an excellent guide to contouring pelvic nodes (78).
        - The guide is for gynecologic cancers.
        - But, it is applicable to prostate cancers.
    - Track external and internal iliacs with a 5- to 7-mm expansion.
    - Superior margin: L5-S1 interspace.
    - Inferior margin.
    - Lateral/medial margins:
        - 5- to 7-mm margin around vessels respecting anatomic boundaries

Simulation Procedure

- Refer for (≥3) radiopaque fiducial marker placement 1 or more weeks prior to sim.
- Supine simulation on evacuated vacuum bag, with hands folded on the chest.
- Full bladder (to move portion of bladder and bowel up and out of radiation field).
- Drink oral contrast 15 minutes prior to simulation to demarcate bowel.
- NPO and bowel preparation the night before and morning of simulation.
    - Patients may prefer early morning simulation to shorten NPO/prep window.
- Consider rectal immobilization:
    - Rectal balloon filled with approximately 90 cc of water at simulation and during daily treatment (79).
    - Hydrogel (e.g., SpaceOAR) injected between the rectum and prostate prior to sim (80).
- If irradiating pelvic nodes, consider IV contrast during simulation.
- If simulating for SBRT, consider Foley catheter placement to demarcate the urethra.

Beam Energy and Dose Distribution

- 6-MV or higher-energy photon beams are used for IMRT therapy.
    - Higher-energy beams (e.g., 10 + MV) can reduce hot spots in larger patients.
- Dose constraints are used to minimize toxicity in organs at risk (OARs).
    - Different trials use different (though roughly similar) constraints.
    - RTOG Consensus Guidelines list a typical set of constraints (77).

Tumor Doses

- Multiple studies show dose escalation improves local control.
    - MRC RT01 British 2007 study (81): 64 to 74 Gy improved 5-year biochemical control.
    - Dutch 2008 study (82): 68 to 78 Gy improved 7-year biochemical control.
    - MDACC 2008 study (83): 70 to 78 Gy improved 8-year biochemical control.

- On post hoc analysis, gastrointestinal toxicity correlated with rectal V70:
  - Rectal V70 ≤ 25% had 16% rate of grade 2 GI toxicity.
  - Rectal V70 greater than 25% had 46% rate of grade 2 GI toxicity.
- MSKCC 2008 study (84): 86.4-Gy point dose improved local and distant control.
- Table 29-1 summarizes the major dose escalation trials.
- Dose to intact prostate:
  - Conventional fractionation (16):
    - 75.6 to 79.2 or even 81.0 Gy in 1.8 to 2.0 Gy/fraction, 5 times per week.
    - Target prostate ± proximal seminal vesicles.
    - If pelvic nodes are treated, they often receive 45 to 50 Gy.
  - Hypofractionation:
    - A variety of regimens exist (16,85,86).
    - For example, 28 or 20 fractions in 2.5 or 4.0 Gy/fraction, respectively.
  - Ultrahypofractionation (or SBRT):
    - Again, multiple regimens exist (16,87).
    - For example, 5 fractions in 6.5 Gy/fraction given twice weekly.
  - Protons: same as photons (88,89).
- Radiation failure set by the "Phoenix" definition of (PSA) biochemical failure (90).
  - Occurs when PSA rises 2.0 ng/mL over the PSA nadir.

Table 29-1

Randomized Control Trials (RCTs) Showing that Dose Escalation Improves Local Control in Early Prostate Cancer in Every Risk Group

Study	Inclusion	Arms	5-Year bFFFa	F/U
Al-Mamgani et al. (82) IJROBP'08	• T1b-T4N0 • PSA < 60	• 68 P ± SV • 78 P ± SV	• Med + Hi: 45% • Med + Hi: 56%	70 mo
Beckendorf IJROBP'11	• T1b-T3a; no ADT • PSA < 50	• 70 P + SV 3D • 80 P + SV 3D	• 28% vs. 39% (AS-TRO, $p = 0.04$) • 24% vs. 32% (Phoenix, $p = 0.09$)	61 mo
Dearnaley et al. (81) Lancet Onc'07	• T1b-T3N0 + nADT • PSA < 50	• 64 P + SV • 74 P + SV	• 60% • 71%	63 mo
Kuban et al. (83) IJROBP'08	• T1-3N0; no ADT	• 46 + 24 4-field • 46 + 32 4-field	• Low: 63%; Med: 65%; Hi:b 26% • Low: 88%; Med: 94%; Hi:b 63%	104 mo
Sathya JCO'05	• T2-3N0; no ADT	• 66 P + SV EBRT • 40 EBRT + 35 Ir-192	• 29% • 61%	?
Zeitman JAMA'05	• T1b-2b; no ADT • PSA < 15	• 50 ph + 20 pr P + SV • 50 ph + 29 pr P + SV	• Low: 84% Med: 79% • Low: 98% Med: 91%	66 mo

TARGET DELINEATION FOR PROSTATE INTENSITY-MODULATED RADIATION THERAPY

Low- and Intermediate-Risk Disease

- CTV1 = prostate and proximal seminal vesicles.
  - For low risk, no need to include seminal vesicles.
  - For intermediate risk, include 1 cm of the proximal seminal vesicles.
- PTV = CTV1 + 7 mm everywhere, but 5 mm posteriorly.
- Figure 29-2 shows CT-based target delineation for an intermediate-risk patient.

High-Risk Disease with Nodes at Risk

- CTV1 = prostate and proximal 2 cm of seminal vesicles.
  - CTV is expanded as needed for known extracapsular extension (as determined by digital rectal exam, MR, or CT imaging).

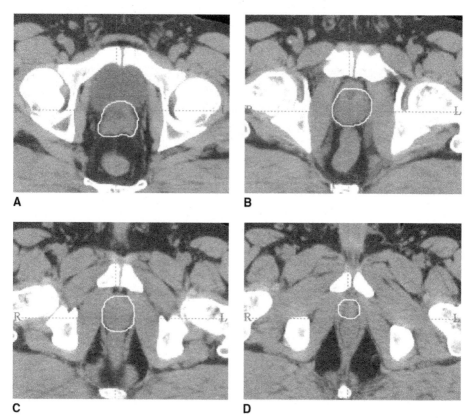

FIGURE 29-2. IMRT target delineation for a patient with intermediate-risk prostate cancer. The *white line* is the CTV1 or high-risk volume.

- CTV2 = CTV1 + elective pelvic nodes (if your institution does this).
  - Obturator nodes
  - Internal iliac nodes to the body of the sacrum
  - Medial external iliac nodes
  - Common iliac nodes to the sacral promontory below the L5-S1 interspace
  - Presacral nodes
  - Small published an excellent guide to contouring pelvic nodes (78).
    - The guide is for gynecologic cancers. But, it is applicable to prostate cancers.
- PTV = CTV1 + 7 mm everywhere, but 5 mm posteriorly.
- Planning parameters.
  - Radiation prescription is prescribed as a minimum dose to the respective PTVs.
  - CTV2 receives 45.0 to 50.4 Gy in 1.8 Gy per day fractions.
  - CTV1 receives 75.6 to 79.2 Gy in 1.8 Gy per day fractions.
- Figure 29-3 shows CT-based target delineation for a high-risk patient.

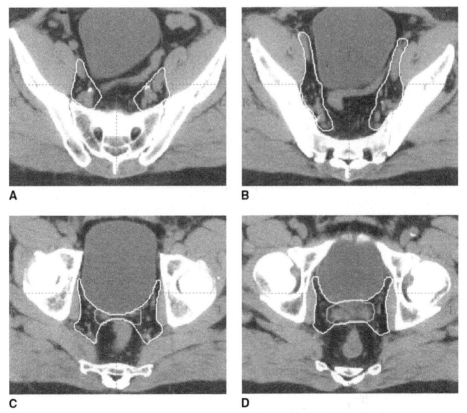

A B C D

FIGURE 29-3. IMRT target delineation for a patient with high-risk prostate cancer. The *outer white line* is CTV1 or intermediate-risk volume, whereas the *inner gray line* is the CTV2 or high-risk volume.

INTERSTITIAL IRRADIATION

- Brachytherapy classically used permanently implanted low–dose rate seeds.
  - Classic low–dose rate isotopes:
    - Iodine-125 (I-125) with 60 days half-life and 28-keV energy.
    - Palladium-103 (Pd-103) with 17 days half-life and 21-keV energy.
    - Isotopes considered equivalent in terms of disease control.
    - Anecdotally, iodine needs fewer seeds to build a dose cloud than palladium.
      - Iodine plans often need fewer seeds than palladium plans.
      - But iodine dose clouds can be harder to shape around organs at risk.
  - Increasingly, temporarily implanted high-dose rate seeds are being used (91–93).
    - Standard high-dose rate isotope is Iridium-192 (Ir-192) with 73.8-day half-life.
  - This section concerns low–dose rate brachytherapy unless otherwise noted.
- Brachytherapy contraindications:
  - TURP defect
  - T3+ disease
  - Large median lobe
  - Pubic arch interference
  - Poor baseline urinary function
    - International Prostate Symptom Score (or IPSS) greater than 20
    - (per American Brachytherapy Society or ABS)
    - American Urological Association Score (or AUA) greater than 15
    - (per the Radiation Therapy Oncology Group or RTOG)
  - Prostate volume greater than 60 cc (can attempt shrinking with 2 months of hormonal ablation)
  - Prostate volume less than 20 cc (stricture risk too great)
  - Unable to use ultrasound
  - Unable to safely tolerate anesthesia
- ABS recommends prostate brachy monotherapy if low risk (94,95).
  - I-125 monotherapy prescription: 145 Gy
  - Pd-103 monotherapy prescription: 125 Gy
- Patients with more risk factors benefit from combination therapy (95,96).
  - Combination therapy can give higher biologic equivalent dose (BED).
  - I-125 dual therapy prescription: 100 to 110 Gy after 45-Gy beam radiation.
  - Pd-103 dual therapy prescriptions: 90 to 100 Gy after 45-Gy beam radiation.
  - Beam radiation to CTV1 ± CTV2 as described, above, except to 45 Gy.
- For further dosimetry details, consider the following detailed guidelines:
  - American Association of Physicists in Medicine Task Group Report #64 (97)
  - American Association of Physicists in Medicine Report re: Pd-103 (98)
- Constraints for low–dose rate brachytherapy (these can vary by institution):
  - Dx% of organ y is the dose to x% of the volume of organ y.
    - Example 1:
      D90% of prostate = 100% means:
      "dose to 90% of the prostate is 100% of prescribed dose."

- Vx% of organ y is the v.
  - Example 2:
    V200% less than 20% of the prostate:
    "Less than 20% of the prostate gets 200% of the prescribed dose."
- Prostate:
  - D90% = 90% to 125% of prescription dose
    ○ This range optimizes biochemical control (99).
  - V100% greater than 95%
  - V150% less than 60% (to minimize chronic GU toxicity)
  - V200% less than 20% (to minimize acute GU toxicity)
- Urethra:
  - V125% less than 30%
  - V150% less than 5%
- Rectum:
  - V100% less than 1 cc

POSTOPERATIVE RADIATION THERAPY

- Terminology:
  - Postprostatectomy radiation is either adjuvant or salvage.
  - Adjuvant radiation is immediate radiation even if post-op PSA is undetectable.
  - Salvage radiation is delayed radiation after post-op PSA becomes detectable.
- No consensus exists for which patients benefit from adjuvant (versus salvage) radiation.
  - An EORTC trial suggested that patients with positive margins benefit (100,101).
    - pT3 or margin-positive men randomized to adjuvant 60 Gy or surveillance.
      ○ pT3a is extracapsular extension.
      ○ pT3b is seminal vesicle invasion.
    - 5-year biochemical progression-free survival was 74% versus 53%.
    - On subset analysis, only men with positive margins benefited.
    - A separate study reported these rates of positive margins after surgery (102):
      ○ 10% in pT1b patients
      ○ 18% in pT2a patients
      ○ 50% to 60% in pT2b patients
  - Other studies suggest men with pT3 disease do benefit from adjuvant radiation.
    - In a German trial, 5-year biochemical control was 72% versus 54% (103).
    - A SWOG trial found improved overall and distant metastatic-free survival (104).
  - Despite these trials, many surgeons often refer for salvage (versus adjuvant) radiation.
    - Why? Because no trial has *prospectively* and directly compared outcomes for immediate adjuvant radiation versus later salvage radiation. Thus, some surgeons feel that adjuvant radiation overtreats patients because not all pT3 or margin-positive men go on to fail biochemically and need salvage.
    - *But,* in a *retrospective* matched analysis, immediate adjuvant radiation had better 5-year biochemical control compared to delayed salvage radiation (105).

- o 5-year control from surgery date: 75% versus 66% for adjuvant versus salvage radiation
- o 5-year control from end of radiation: 73% versus 50%

Postprostatectomy Salvage Radiotherapy

- As noted above, there is no consensus on who benefits from adjuvant versus salvage radiation.
- Stephenson retrospectively identified factors that predicted salvage success (106,107).
  - This group published a nice multifactor nomogram.
    - The original report has a typo that miscalculates the salvage success rates.
    - The updated report corrects the typo (107).
  - A particularly important factor: preradiotherapy PSA level.
  - If preradiation PSA is ≤0.5 ng/mL, 6-year biochemical control is approximately 50%.
  - If preradiation PSA is greater than 1.5 ng/mL, 6-year biochemical control is approximately 20%.

TARGET DELINEATION FOR POSTPROSTATECTOMY INTENSITY-MODULATED RADIATION THERAPY

- CTV1—Prostate bed
  - RTOG Consensus Guidelines describe postprostatectomy CTV borders (108).
    - Inferiorly: the GU diaphragm
    - Laterally: the obturator muscles
    - Posteriorly: the anterior rectal wall
    - Superiorly: the level previously occupied by the seminal vesicles
    - Anteriorly: approximately 1 cm of the posterior-inferior bladder wall
    - Below the top of the pubic symphysis, the CTV encompasses the bladder neck, which has been pulled inferiorly to anastomose to the penile urethra.
    - Above the pubic symphysis, the CTV takes a "bow tie" shape as it encompasses the periprostatic and the obturator tissues as well as the thin strip of tissue between the bladder and the rectum.
- PTV1 = CTV1 + 8 mm everywhere but 6 mm posteriorly (with daily IGRT)
- CTV2—Elective pelvic nodal irradiation
  - This is controversial.
  - If included, the delineation is the same as for the intact prostate, described above.
  - Ramey et al. reported better biochemical control with elective nodal radiation (109).
    - 5-year PSA control of 62% versus 49% without elective nodal irradiation
    - 5-year PSA control of 55% versus 50% without hormonal ablation

Planning Parameters: Postoperative CTV1

- Target is prescribed 64.8 Gy for adjuvant or low-risk salvage disease.
- Patients with gross disease at recurrence are treated to a higher dose (66 to 70 Gy).
- Figure 29-4 shows CT-based target delineation for a patient being planned for postprostatectomy IMRT.

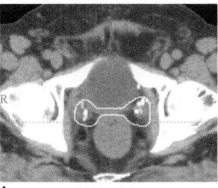
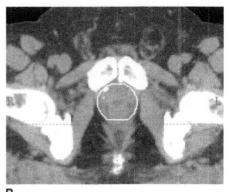

A   **B**

FIGURE 29-4. Target delineation for postprostatectomy IMRT. The *white line* is the CTV1 or high-risk volume.

Normal Tissue Complications: QUANTEC Results

- Radiation damage to the bladder was discussed in Chapter 31.
- Viswanathan et al. (110) gave particular note to 3DCRT and IMRT optimizations in prostate cancer treatment to constrain high dosages to the bladder.

SEQUELAE OF THERAPY

Radiation Therapy

- Dziuk has published an excellent pocket reference for the management of common acute radiation-related reactions (111).
- Acute gastrointestinal side effects during irradiation (in 3% to 5% of patients) (112,113):
  - Loose stool/diarrhea managed with:
    - Diphenoxylate/atropine sulfate (Lomotil)
    - Loperamide (Imodium)
    - Opium preparations such as paregoric
    - Emollients such as kaolin and pectin
  - Rectal discomfort or, less commonly, rectal bleeding:
    - Rule out hemorrhoids.
    - Small enemas with hydrocortisone (e.g., Proctofoam, Cortifoam).
    - Anti-inflammatory suppositories containing bismuth, benzyl benzoate, zinc oxide, or Peruvian balsam (e.g., Anusol, Medicone, Rowasa, Wyanoids) with or without cortisone.
    - Low-residue diet without grease/spices.
    - Increased/supplemental fiber (e.g., Metamucil, FiberCon).
    - In more severe cases, laser therapy or cauterization may be necessary.

- Acute genitourinary symptoms include dysuria, frequency, nocturia, and hematuria.
  - Phenazopyridine hydrochloride (Pyridium).
  - Flavoxate hydrochloride (Urispas) or hyoscyamine sulfate (Cystospaz).
  - Fluid intake should be at least 2,000 to 2,500 mL daily.
  - Rule out urinary tract infection first (especially in the first couple weeks of therapy).
- Acute skin erythema and desquamation may develop.
  - Proper skin hygiene
  - Topical petrolatum (Vaseline), Aquaphor, or lanolin
- Acute grade 5 (fatal) toxicities are vanishingly rare with radiotherapy (less than 0.2%) (114).
- Chronic leg, scrotal, or penile edema is generally rare (less than 1%) (115).
  - But, rates may approach 10% to 30% if pelvic nodes irradiated or dissected.
- Chronic GI toxicity (e.g., incontinence) is rare (1% to 2%).
- Chronic urinary cystitis is also rare (less than 5%), esp. if bladder dose is kept below 75 Gy.
- Chronic urinary incontinence or urethral stricture occurs in 1% to 3% of patients.
  - TURP before or during irradiation increases risk (approximately 2.0% versus 0.2%) (12,23).
  - 11% to 13% of men leaked more than a few drops of urine postradiation (116).
- Chronic erectile dysfunction is relatively common postradiotherapy (51,116).
  - Unlike surgery, few men have erectile dysfunction during or immediately after treatment (unless hormonally ablated). But, incidence can increase over time.
  - 77% of men reported full or partial erection before radiation therapy (116).
  - 22% of men reported full erection postradiation (116).
  - 41% of men reported partial erection postradiation (116).
  - Another series reported erectile bother in 14% to 50% of men postradiation (51).
  - Management for erectile dysfunction:
    - Psychotherapy with active participation of the sexual partner
    - Vacuum devices
    - Intrapenile/intraurethral injections of papaverine, phentolamine, or PgE$_1$
    - Oral tadalafil (Cialis), vardenafil (Levitra), and sildenafil citrate (Viagra)
    - Semirigid or inflatable penile implants
- Chronic lumbosacral plexopathy is rare but morbid (117).

Combined Surgery and Irradiation

- Combined surgery and radiation can be more morbid than surgery or radiation alone.
- Lower extremity and genital edema may occur in 10% to 20% of combined therapy patients.
  - 0% of men that got radiation only developed lower extremity edema (118).
  - 16% of men that got radiation + limited nodal dissection developed edema (118).
  - 66% of men that got radiation + extended dissection developed edema (118).
- Urinary stress incontinence may or may not be more frequent after combined therapy.
  - 6% of combined therapy patients reported urinary incontinence (119).
  - 8% of surgery-only patients reported urinary incontinence (119).

- Urethral stricture is observed in approximately 5% to 10% of patients (120).
- Sexual potency after nerve-sparing surgery alone is 30% to 40% (102).
  - No great data on erectile dysfunction rates in combined therapy patients.
  - 1-year potency was 44% versus 48% in the adjuvant radiation versus surgery-only arms (119).

References

1. Coakley FV, Hricak H. Radiologic anatomy of the prostate gland: a clinical approach. *Radiol Clin North Am* 2000;38(1):15–30.
2. Scales CD Jr, Moul JW, Curtis LH, et al. Prostate cancer in the Baby Boomer generation: results from CaPSURE. *Urology* 2007;70(6):1162–1167.
3. Eifler JB, et al. An updated prostate cancer staging nomogram (Partin tables) based on cases from 2006 to 2011. *BJU Int* 2013;111(1):22–29.
4. Diaz A, et al. Indications for and the significance of seminal vesicle irradiation during 3D conformal radiotherapy for localized prostate cancer. *Int J Radiat Oncol Biol Phys* 1994;30(2):323–329.
5. Nguyen PL, Chen MH, Hoffman KE, et al. Predicting the risk of pelvic node involvement among men with prostate cancer in the contemporary era. *Int J Radiat Oncol Biol Phys* 2009;74(1):104–109.
6. Roach M III. Equations for predicting the pathologic stage of men with localized prostate cancer using the preoperative prostate specific antigen. *J Urol* 1993;150:1923–1924.
7. Roach M III, et al. Pretreatment prostate-specific antigen and Gleason score predict the risk of extracapsular extension and the risk of failure following radiotherapy in patients with clinically localized prostate cancer. *Semin Urol Oncol* 2000;18(2):108–114.
8. Cagiannos I, et al. A preoperative nomogram identifying decreased risk of positive pelvic lymph nodes in patients with prostate cancer. *J Urol* 2003;170(5):1798–1803.
9. Weckermann D, et al. Reliability of preoperative diagnostics and location of lymph node metastases in presumed unilateral prostate cancer. *BJU Int* 2007;99(5):1036–1040.
10. McMahon CJ, Rofsky NM, Pedrosa I. Lymphatic metastases from pelvic tumors: anatomic classification, characterization, and staging. *Radiology* 2010;254(1):31–46.
11. Chung HT, Speight JL, Roach M III. Intermediate- and high-risk prostate cancer. In: Halperin EC, Perez CA, Brady LW, eds. *Principles and practice of radiation oncology*, 5th ed. Philadelphia, PA: Lippincott Williams & Wilkins, 2008:1483–1502.
12. Perez CA. Prostate. In: Perez CA, Brady LW, eds. *Principles and practice of radiation oncology*, 3rd ed. Philadelphia, PA: Lippincott–Raven, 1998:1583–1694.
13. Crawford ED, et al. Comorbidity and mortality results from a randomized prostate cancer screening trial. *J Clin Oncol* 2011;29(4):355–361.
14. Hugosson J, et al. Mortality results from the Goteborg randomised population-based prostate-cancer screening trial. *Lancet Oncol* 2010;11(8):725–732.
15. Schroder FH, et al. Prostate-cancer mortality at 11 years of follow-up. *N Engl J Med* 2012;366(11):981–990.
16. National Comprehensive Cancer Network (NCCN). Prostate Cancer (Version 2.2017). https://www.nccn.org/professionals/physician_gls/pdf/prostate_blocks.pdf. Accessed January 26, 2018.
17. Carlsson S, et al. Prostate cancer screening: facts, statistics, and interpretation in response to the US Preventive Services Task Force Review. *J Clin Oncol* 2012;30(21):2581–2584.
18. Shimbo M, et al. PSA doubling time as a predictive factor on repeat biopsy for detection of prostate cancer. *Jpn J Clin Oncol* 2009;39(11):727–731.
19. Thompson IM, et al. Prevalence of prostate cancer among men with a prostate-specific antigen level < or =4.0 ng per milliliter. *N Engl J Med* 2004;350(22):2239–2246.
20. Vickers AJ, Brewster SF. PSA velocity and doubling time in diagnosis and prognosis of prostate cancer. *Br J Med Surg Urol* 2012;5(4):162–168.

21. Emiliozzi P, Scarpone P, DePaula F, et al. The incidence of prostate cancer in men with prostate specific antigen greater than 4.0 ng/ml: a randomized study of 6 versus 12 core transperineal prostate biopsy. *J Urol* 2004;171(1):197–199.

22. Amin MB, Edge SB, Greene FL, et al. *AJCC cancer staging manual*, 8th ed. New York, NY: Springer Verlag, 2017.

23. Zelefsky MJ, Valicenti RK, Hunt M, et al. Low-risk prostate cancer. In: Halperin EC, Perez CA, Brady LW, eds. *Principles and practice of radiation oncology*, 5th ed. Philadelphia, PA: Lippincott Williams & Wilkins, 2008:1439–1482.

24. Chan TY, Partin AW, Walsh PC, et al. Prognostic significance of Gleason score 3 + 4 versus Gleason score 4 + 3 tumor at radical prostatectomy. *Urology* 2000;56(5):823–827.

25. Sakr WA, Tefilli MV, Grignon DJ, et al. Gleason score 7 prostate cancer: a heterogeneous entity? Correlation with pathologic parameters and disease-free survival. *Urology* 2000;56(5):730–734.

26. Zumsteg ZS, et al. A new risk classification system for therapeutic decision making with intermediate-risk prostate cancer patients undergoing dose-escalated external-beam radiation therapy. *Eur Urol* 2013;64(6):895–902.

27. Partin AW, Mangold LA, Lamm DM, et al. Contemporary update of prostate cancer staging nomograms (Partin Tables) for the new millennium. *Urology* 2001;58(6):843–848.

28. Partin AW, Yoo J, Carter HB, et al. The use of prostate specific antigen, clinical stage and Gleason score to predict pathological stage in men with localized prostate cancer. *J Urol* 1993;150(1):110–114.

29. Prestidge BR, Kaplan I, Cox RS, et al. Predictors of survival after a positive post-irradiation prostate biopsy. *Int J Radiat Oncol Biol Phys* 1994;28(1):17–22.

30. Hall MC, Navone NM, Troncoso P, et al. Frequency and characterization of p53 mutations in clinically localized prostate cancer. *Urology* 1995;45(3):470–475.

31. Albain KS, Unger JM, Crowley JJ, et al. Racial disparities in cancer survival among randomized clinical trials patients of the Southwest Oncology Group. *J Natl Cancer Inst* 2009;101(14):984–992.

32. Freedland SJ, Banez LL, Sun LL, et al. Obese men have higher-grade and larger tumors: an analysis of the duke prostate center database. *Prostate Cancer Prostatic Dis* 2009;12(3):259–263.

33. Thompson IM, et al. The influence of finasteride on the development of prostate cancer. *N Engl J Med* 2003;349(3):215–224.

34. Gleason DF, Mellinger GT. Prediction of prognosis for prostatic adenocarcinoma by combined histological grading and clinical staging. *J Urol* 1974;111(1):58–64.

35. Gleason DF. Histologic grade, clinical stage, and patient age in prostate cancer. *NCI Monogr* 1988(7):15–18.

36. Hattab EM, et al. Tertiary Gleason pattern 5 is a powerful predictor of biochemical relapse in patients with Gleason score 7 prostatic adenocarcinoma. *J Urol* 2006;175(5):1695–1699; discussion 1699.

37. Reese JH, Freiha FS, Gelb AB, et al. Transitional cell carcinoma of the prostate in patients undergoing radical cystoprostatectomy. *J Urol* 1992;147(1):92–95.

38. Sarris A, Dimopoulos M, Pugh W, et al. Primary lymphoma of the prostate: good outcome with doxorubicin-based combination chemotherapy. *J Urol* 1995;153(6):1852–1854.

39. Mostofi FK, Sesterhenn IA, Davis CJ Jr. A pathologist's view of prostatic carcinoma. *Cancer* 1993;71(3 Suppl):906–932.

40. Gunderson LL, Tepper JE, Bogart JA. *Clinical radiation oncology*, 4th ed. Philadelphia, PA: Elsevier Saunders, 2015.

41. Albertsen PC, Hanley JA, Fine J. 20-Year outcomes following conservative management of clinically localized prostate cancer. *JAMA* 2005;293(17):2095–2101.

42. Johansson JE, Holmberg L, Johansson S, et al. Fifteen-year survival in prostate cancer. A prospective, population-based study in Sweden. *JAMA* 1997;277(6):467–471.

43. Hamdy FC, et al. 10-Year outcomes after monitoring, surgery, or radiotherapy for localized prostate cancer. *N Engl J Med* 2016;375(15):1415–1424.

44. Grimm P, et al. Comparative analysis of prostate-specific antigen free survival outcomes for patients with low, intermediate and high risk prostate cancer treatment by radical therapy. Results from the Prostate Cancer Results Study Group. *BJU Int* 2012;109(Suppl 1):22–29.

45. Benaim EA, Pace CM, Roehrborn CG. Gleason score predicts androgen independent progression after androgen deprivation therapy. *Eur Urol* 2002;42(1):12–17.

46. Neri R. Antiandrogens: preclinical and clinical studies. *Urology* 1994;44:53–60.

47. Iversen P, Tyrrell CJ, Kaisary AV, et al. Casodex (bicalutamide) 150-mg monotherapy compared with castration in patients with previously untreated nonmetastatic prostate cancer: results from two multicenter randomized trials at a median follow-up of 4 years. *Urology* 1998;51(3):389–396.

48. Shearer RJ, Hendry WF, Sommerville IF, et al. Plasma testosterone: an accurate monitor of hormone treatment in prostatic cancer. *Br J Urol* 1973;45(6):668–677.

49. Geller J, Albert J, Yen SS. Treatment of advanced cancer of prostate with megestrol acetate. *Urology* 1978;12(5):537–541.

50. Worgul TJ, Santen RJ, Samojlik E, et al. Clinical and biochemical effect of aminoglutethimide in the treatment of advanced prostatic carcinoma. *J Urol* 1983;129(1):51–55.

51. Zinreich ES, Derogatis LR, Herpst J, et al. Pre and posttreatment evaluation of sexual function in patients with adenocarcinoma of the prostate. *Int J Radiat Oncol Biol Phys* 1990;19(3):729–732.

52. Rhee H, et al. Adverse effects of androgen-deprivation therapy in prostate cancer and their management. *BJU Int* 2015;115(Suppl 5):3–13.

53. McCloskey EV, et al. From relative risk to absolute fracture risk calculation: the FRAX algorithm. *Curr Osteoporos Rep* 2009;7(3):77–83.

54. Viani GA, Bernardes da Silva LG, Stefano EJ. Prevention of gynecomastia and breast pain caused by androgen deprivation therapy in prostate cancer: tamoxifen or radiotherapy? *Int J Radiat Oncol Biol Phys* 2012;83(4):e519–e524.

55. Zelefsky MJ, et al. Biochemical response to androgen deprivation therapy before external beam radiation therapy predicts long-term prostate cancer survival outcomes. *Int J Radiat Oncol Biol Phys* 2013;86(3):529–533.

56. Nanda A, et al. Hormonal therapy use for prostate cancer and mortality in men with coronary artery disease-induced congestive heart failure or myocardial infarction. *JAMA* 2009;302(8):866–873.

57. Jones CU, et al. Radiotherapy and short-term androgen deprivation for localized prostate cancer. *N Engl J Med* 2011;365(2):107–118.

58. D'Amico AV, Chen MH, Renshaw AA, et al. Androgen suppression and radiation vs. radiation alone for prostate cancer: a randomized trial. *JAMA* 2008;299(3):289–295.

59. Denham JW, et al. Short-term neoadjuvant androgen deprivation and radiotherapy for locally advanced prostate cancer: 10-year data from the TROG 96.01 randomised trial. *Lancet Oncol* 2011;12(5):451–459.

60. Pisansky TM, et al. Duration of androgen suppression before radiotherapy for localized prostate cancer: radiation therapy oncology group randomized clinical trial 9910. *J Clin Oncol* 2015;33(4):332–339.

61. Bolla M, de Reijke TM, Van Tienhoven G, et al. Duration of androgen suppression in the treatment of prostate cancer. *N Engl J Med* 2009;360(24):2516–2527.

62. Bolla M, et al. External irradiation with or without long-term androgen suppression for prostate cancer with high metastatic risk: 10-year results of an EORTC randomised study. *Lancet Oncol* 2010;11(11):1066–1073.

63. Zapatero A, et al. High-dose radiotherapy with short-term or long-term androgen deprivation in localised prostate cancer (DART01/05 GICOR): a randomised, controlled, phase 3 trial. *Lancet Oncol* 2015;16(3):320–327.

64. Nabid A, et al. Duration of androgen deprivation therapy in high risk prostate cancer: final results of a randomized phase III trial. *J Clin Oncol* 2017;35(15 Suppl):5008.

65. Carrie C, et al. Salvage radiotherapy with or without short-term hormone therapy for rising prostate-specific antigen concentration after radical prostatectomy (GETUG-AFU 16): a randomised, multicentre, open-label phase 3 trial. *Lancet Oncol* 2016;17(6):747–756.

66. Shipley WU, et al. Radiation with or without antiandrogen therapy in recurrent prostate cancer. *N Engl J Med* 2017;376(5):417–428.

67. Honger B, Schwegler N. Experience with prophylactic irradiation of the breast in prostatic carcinoma patients being treated with estrogen. *Helv Chir Acta* 1980;47:427–430.

68. McLeod DG, Iversen P. Gynecomastia in patients with prostate cancer: a review of treatment options. *Urology* 2000;56(5):713–720.

69. Hanks GE, Lee WR, Hanlon AL, et al. Conformal technique dose escalation for prostate cancer: biochemical evidence of improved cancer control with higher doses in patients with pretreatment prostate-specific antigen > or = 10 ng/mL. *Int J Radiat Oncol Biol Phys* 1996;35(5):861–868.

70. Leibel SA, Zelefsky MJ, Kutcher GJ, et al. Three-dimensional conformal radiation therapy in localized carcinoma of the prostate: interim report of a phase 1 dose-escalation study. *J Urol* 1994;152(5 Pt 2):1792–1798.

71. Zelefsky MJ, Kelly WK, Scher HI, et al. Results of a phase II study using estramustine phosphate and vinblastine in combination with high-dose three-dimensional conformal radiotherapy for patients with locally advanced prostate cancer. *J Clin Oncol* 2000;18(9):1936–1941.

72. Pommier P, Chabaud S, Lagrange JL, et al. Is there a role for pelvic irradiation in localized prostate adenocarcinoma? Preliminary results of GETUG-01. *J Clin Oncol* 2007;25(34):5366–5373.

73. Lawton CA, DeSilvio M, Roach M III, et al. An update of the phase III trial comparing whole pelvic to prostate only radiotherapy and neoadjuvant to adjuvant total androgen suppression: updated analysis of RTOG 94-13, with emphasis on unexpected hormone/radiation interactions. *Int J Radiat Oncol Biol Phys* 2007;69(3):646–655.

74. Roach M III, DeSilvio M, Lawton C, et al. Phase III trial comparing whole-pelvic versus prostate-only radiotherapy and neoadjuvant versus adjuvant combined androgen suppression: Radiation Therapy Oncology Group 9413. *J Clin Oncol* 2003;21(10):1904–1911.

75. Pilepich MV, Krall JM, Johnson RJ, et al. Extended field (periaortic) irradiation in carcinoma of the prostate—analysis of RTOG 75-06. *Int J Radiat Oncol Biol Phys* 1986;12(3):345–351.

76. Asbell SO, Krall JM, Pilepich MV, et al. Elective pelvic irradiation in stage A2, B carcinoma of the prostate: analysis of RTOG 77-06. *Int J Radiat Oncol Biol Phys* 1988;15(6):1307–1316.

77. Lawton CA, Michalski J, El-Naqa I, et al. RTOG GU Radiation oncology specialists reach consensus on pelvic lymph node volumes for high-risk prostate cancer. *Int J Radiat Oncol Biol Phys* 2009;74(2):383–387.

78. Small W Jr, et al. Consensus guidelines for delineation of clinical target volume for intensity-modulated pelvic radiotherapy in postoperative treatment of endometrial and cervical cancer. *Int J Radiat Oncol Biol Phys* 2008;71(2):428–434.

79. Wu CC, et al. Rectal balloon use in intensity modulated radiation therapy planning for posthysterectomy gynecological malignancies can limit rectal dose and toxicity as well as limit vaginal displacement. *Int J Radiat Oncol Biol Phys* 2016;96(2):E300–E301.

80. Padmanabhan R, Pinkawa M, Song DY. Hydrogel spacers in prostate radiotherapy: a promising approach to decrease rectal toxicity. *Future Oncol* 2017;13(29):2697–2708.

81. Dearnaley DP, Sydes MR, Graham JD, et al. Escalated-dose versus standard-dose conformal radiotherapy in prostate cancer: first results from the MRC RT01 randomised controlled trial. *Lancet Oncol* 2007;8(6):475–487.

82. Al-Mamgani A, van Putten WL, Heemsbergen WD, et al. Update of Dutch multicenter dose-escalation trial of radiotherapy for localized prostate cancer. *Int J Radiat Oncol Biol Phys* 2008;72(4):980–988.

83. Kuban DA, Tucker SL, Dong L, et al. Long-term results of the M.D. Anderson randomized dose-escalation trial for prostate cancer. *Int J Radiat Oncol Biol Phys* 2008;70(1):67–74.
84. Zelefsky MJ, Yamada Y, Fuks Z, et al. Long-term results of conformal radiotherapy for prostate cancer: impact of dose escalation on biochemical tumor control and distant metastases-free survival outcomes. *Int J Radiat Oncol Biol Phys* 2008;71(4):1028–1033.
85. Hegemann NS, et al. Hypofractionated radiotherapy for prostate cancer. *Radiat Oncol* 2014;9:275.
86. Pollack A, et al. Randomized trial of hypofractionated external-beam radiotherapy for prostate cancer. *J Clin Oncol* 2013;31(31):3860–3868.
87. King CR, et al. Stereotactic body radiotherapy for localized prostate cancer: pooled analysis from a multi-institutional consortium of prospective phase II trials. *Radiother Oncol* 2013;109(2):217–221.
88. Zietman AL, DeSilvio ML, Slater JD, et al. Comparison of conventional-dose vs. high-dose conformal radiation therapy in clinically localized adenocarcinoma of the prostate: a randomized controlled trial. *JAMA* 2005;294(10):1233–1239.
89. Kim S, et al. Late gastrointestinal toxicities following radiation therapy for prostate cancer. *Eur Urol* 2011;60(5):908–916.
90. Roach M III, Hanks G, Thames H Jr, et al. Defining biochemical failure following radiotherapy with or without hormonal therapy in men with clinically localized prostate cancer: recommendations of the RTOG-ASTRO Phoenix Consensus Conference. *Int J Radiat Oncol Biol Phys* 2006;65(4):965–974.
91. Blasko JC, Wallner K, Grimm PD, et al. Prostate specific antigen based disease control following ultrasound guided iodine-125 implantation for stage T1/T2 prostatic carcinoma. *J Urol* 1995;154(3):1096–1099.
92. Martinez A, Gonzalez J, Stromberg J, et al. Conformal prostate brachytherapy: initial experience of a phase I/II dose-escalating trial. *Int J Radiat Oncol Biol Phys* 1995;33(5):1019–1027.
93. Wallner K, Roy J, Harrison L. Dosimetry guidelines to minimize urethral and rectal morbidity following transperineal I-125 prostate brachytherapy. *Int J Radiat Oncol Biol Phys* 1995;32(2):465–471.
94. Nag S, Beyer D, Friedland J, et al. American Brachytherapy Society (ABS) recommendations for transperineal permanent brachytherapy of prostate cancer. *Int J Radiat Oncol Biol Phys* 1999;44(4):789–799.
95. Rivard MJ, et al. American Brachytherapy Society recommends no change for prostate permanent implant dose prescriptions using iodine-125 or palladium-103. *Brachytherapy* 2007;6(1):34–37.
96. Stone NN, Potters L, Davis BJ, et al. Multicenter analysis of effect of high biologic effective dose on biochemical failure and survival outcomes in patients with Gleason score 7–10 prostate cancer treated with permanent prostate brachytherapy. *Int J Radiat Oncol Biol Phys* 2009;73(2):341–346.
97. Yu Y, Anderson LL, Li Z, et al. Permanent prostate seed implant brachytherapy: report of the American Association of Physicists in Medicine Task Group No. 64. *Med Phys* 1999;26(10):2054–2076.
98. Williamson JF, Coursey BM, DeWerd LA, et al. Recommendations of the American Association of Physicists in Medicine on ^{103}Pd interstitial source calibration and dosimetry: implications for dose specification and prescription. *Med Phys* 2000;27(4):634–642.
99. Stock RG, Stone NN, Tabert A, et al. A dose-response study for I-125 prostate implants. *Int J Radiat Oncol Biol Phys* 1998;41(1):101–108.
100. Bolla M, van Poppel H, Collette L, et al. Postoperative radiotherapy after radical prostatectomy: a randomised controlled trial (EORTC trial 22911). *Lancet* 2005;366(9485):572–578.
101. Van der Kwast TH, Bolla M, Van Poppel H, et al. Identification of patients with prostate cancer who benefit from immediate postoperative radiotherapy: EORTC 22911. *J Clin Oncol* 2007;25(27):4178–4186.

102. Catalona WJ, Smith DS. 5-Year tumor recurrence rates after anatomical radical retropubic prostatectomy for prostate cancer. *J Urol* 1994;152(5 Pt 2):1837–1842.

103. Wiegel T, Bottke D, Steiner U, et al. Phase III postoperative adjuvant radiotherapy after radical prostatectomy compared with radical prostatectomy alone in pT3 prostate cancer with postoperative undetectable prostate-specific antigen: ARO 96-02/AUO AP 09/95. *J Clin Oncol* 2009;27(18):2924–2930.

104. Thompson IM, Tangen CM, Paradelo J, et al. Adjuvant radiotherapy for pathological T3N0M0 prostate cancer significantly reduces risk of metastases and improves survival: long-term followup of a randomized clinical trial. *J Urol* 2009;181(3):956–962.

105. Trabulsi EJ, Valicenti RK, Hanlon AL, et al. A multi-institutional matched-control analysis of adjuvant and salvage postoperative radiation therapy for pT3-4N0 prostate cancer. *Urology* 2008;72(6):1298–1302; discussion 1302–1294.

106. Stephenson AJ, Shariat SF, Zelefsky MJ, et al. Salvage radiotherapy for recurrent prostate cancer after radical prostatectomy. *JAMA* 2004;291(11):1325–1332.

107. Tendulkar RD, et al. Contemporary update of a multi-institutional predictive nomogram for salvage radiotherapy after radical prostatectomy. *J Clin Oncol* 2016: pii: JCO679647. [Epub ahead of print].

108. Michalski JM, Lawton C, El Naqa I, et al. Development of RTOG Consensus Guidelines for the definition of the clinical target volume for postoperative conformal radiation therapy for prostate cancer. *Int J Radiat Oncol Biol Phys* 2010;76(2):361–368.

109. Ramey SJ, et al. Multi-institutional evaluation of elective nodal irradiation and/or androgen deprivation therapy with postprostatectomy salvage radiotherapy for prostate cancer. *Eur Urol* 2018;74(1):99–106.

110. Viswanathan AN, Yorke ED, Marks LB, et al. Radiation dose-volume effects of the urinary bladder. *Int J Radiat Oncol Biol Phys* 2010;76(3 Suppl):S116–S122.

111. Dziuk TW. *Commonly prescribed medications in radiation oncology*, 9th ed. Austin, TX: Southwest Regional Cancer Center, 2007.

112. Perez CA, Michalski J, Brown KC, et al. Nonrandomized evaluation of pelvic lymph node irradiation in localized carcinoma of the prostate. *Int J Radiat Oncol Biol Phys* 1996;36(3):573–584.

113. Perez CA, Michalski JM, Purdy JA, et al. Three-dimensional conformal therapy or standard irradiation in localized carcinoma of prostate: preliminary results of a nonrandomized comparison. *Int J Radiat Oncol Biol Phys* 2000;47(3):629–637.

114. Lawton CA, Won M, Pilepich MV, et al. Long-term treatment sequelae following external beam irradiation for adenocarcinoma of the prostate: analysis of RTOG studies 7506 and 7706. *Int J Radiat Oncol Biol Phys* 1991;21(4):935–939.

115. Pilepich MV, Asbell SO, Krall JM, et al. Correlation of radiotherapeutic parameters and treatment related morbidity—analysis of RTOG Study 77-06. *Int J Radiat Oncol Biol Phys* 1987;13(7):1007–1012.

116. Jonler M, Ritter MA, Brinkmann R, et al. Sequelae of definitive radiation therapy for prostate cancer localized to the pelvis. *Urology* 1994;44(6):876–882.

117. Thomas JE, Cascino TL, Earle JD. Differential diagnosis between radiation and tumor plexopathy of the pelvis. *Neurology* 1985;35(1):1–7.

118. Pilepich MV, Pajak T, George FW, et al. Preliminary report on phase III RTOG studies of extended-field irradiation in carcinoma of the prostate. *Am J Clin Oncol* 1983;6(4):485–491.

119. Formenti SC, Lieskovsky G, Simoneau AR, et al. Impact of moderate dose of postoperative radiation on urinary continence and potency in patients with prostate cancer treated with nerve sparing prostatectomy. *J Urol* 1996;155(2):616–619.

120. Schild SE, Wong WW, Grado GL, et al. The result of radical retropubic prostatectomy and adjuvant therapy for pathologic stage C prostate cancer. *Int J Radiat Oncol Biol Phys* 1996;34(3):535–541.

CHAPTER 30

TESTIS

EPIDEMIOLOGY AND RISK FACTORS

- Testicular cancer is the most common malignancy in men aged 15 to 40 (1) with approximately 72,000 cases per year worldwide (2).
- In the United States, white males are four times more likely to present with testicular cancer than are African Americans (3). Other known risk factors include cryptorchidism, contralateral testicular cancer, and family history. There are no data supporting an association between vasectomy and testicular cancer (4).
- Seminomas and nonseminomatous germ cell tumors (NSGCTs) account for 95% of testicular cancer.
- The usual types of NSGCTs are embryonal carcinoma, teratoma (and mature, immature, and malignant), yolk sac tumors, and choriocarcinoma (caries worst prognosis). Many NSGCTs are mixed.
- Sex cord stromal tumors make up less than 5% of adult testicular cancers. The two main types are Leydig cell and Sertoli cell tumors.

NATURAL HISTORY

- Prior to the significant medical advances in the 1970s, testicular cancer accounted for approximately 11% of all cancer deaths in men aged 25 to 35 with long-term cure rates of approximately 25% (5). With the advent of cisplatin-based chemotherapy, improved staging, better surgical techniques, and the availability of serum tumor markers, the 5-year survival of men with testicular germ cell tumors is now greater than 95%.
- Germ cell neoplasia in situ is a premalignant condition that progresses to invasive malignancy in approximately 50% to 70% of patients (1,6). The incidence of carcinoma *in situ* of the contralateral testis in patients who have developed one testicular tumor is approximately 2.7% to 5.0%.
- Pure seminoma spreads in an orderly fashion, initially to the retroperitoneal lymph nodes, then the mediastinum and supraclavicular fossae. NSGCTs have a higher tendency to spread by hematogenous routes to involve lung parenchyma, bone, liver, or brain (7).

CLINICAL PRESENTATION

- The most common presentation is a lump in the testes although about 5% of patients will have extragonadal manifestations in the retroperitoneum or mediastinum, or metastatic disease.
- About 80% of seminomas are localized at presentation and infrequently spread beyond retroperitoneal lymph nodes.
- Leydig cell tumors can cause gynecomastia, impotence, and loss of libido when secreting estrogens. Androgen-secreting tumors can cause precocious puberty in young boys.

DIAGNOSTIC WORKUP

- The tests usually obtained are listed in Table 30-1. The contralateral testis should be carefully examined and a testicular ultrasound obtained.

Table 30-1
Diagnostic Workup for Tumors of the Testis
General
History (document cryptorchidism and previous inguinal or scrotal surgery) Physical examination
Laboratory Studies
Complete blood cell count Biochemistry profile (including lactate dehydrogenase) Serum assays Alpha-fetoprotein β-hCG LDH
Surgery
Radical inguinal orchiectomy
Diagnostic Radiology
Chest x-ray CT scan of chest for NSGCT CT scan of abdomen and pelvis Ultrasound of contralateral testis (baseline)
Special Studies
Semen analysis

- A testicular biopsy is typically not necessary. A biopsy can be considered in unusual situations such as the presence of metastatic disease in uncommon locations (e.g., bone) or a discrepancy in tumor markers raising questions about the diagnosis.
- If a testicular cancer is suspected, serum tumor markers should be assayed before and after orchiectomy.
- NSGCTs are associated with elevated β-human chorionic gonadotropin (β-hCG) and α-fetoprotein (AFP).
- β-hCG may be modestly elevated in 15% to 20% of patients with pure seminomas, but an elevation of AFP indicates nonseminomatous elements and these tumors are generally treated as NSGCTs.
- Computed tomography (CT) scans of the abdomen and pelvis and CXR should be performed to evaluate lymph nodes and metastatic disease. A CT scan of the chest is added for NSGCT. The use of FDG-PET scan as initial staging is not recommended because of the rate of false negatives; however, it is sometimes used to evaluate a residual mass after treatment of seminoma (1,8).
- Semen analysis and sperm banking should routinely be discussed with all patients undergoing treatment for testicular cancer.
- Pulmonary function tests should be performed for patients who receive bleomycin chemotherapy and a hearing evaluation for patients considered for cisplatin.

STAGING

- Testicular cancers are staged using the TNM system developed by the American Joint Committee on Cancer (AJCC) and the Union for International Cancer Control (UICC).
- Prognostic group is formed by combining the TNM stage with serum tumor markers for β-hCG, AFP, and LDH, as measured after orchiectomy.
- Several modifications to the staging of testicular cancer have been introduced in the 8th edition of the AJCC staging manual but not the 8th edition of the UICC. These include the following:
  - Intratubular germ cell neoplasia (carcinoma in situ) has been renamed germ cell neoplasia in situ (GCNIS).
  - For pure seminoma only, pT1 is divided into pT1a (less than 3 cm) and pT1b (greater than 3 cm).
  - Invasion of the epididymis is upstaged to pT2 from pT1.
  - Invasion of hilar soft tissue is new and staged as pT2. This is adipose and connective tissue beyond the rete testis.
  - Tumor adjacent to or surrounding the vas deferens is to be identified as spermatic cord invasion pT3.
  - Discontinuous involvement of the spermatic cord and soft tissues via LVI is considered metastatic and staged as pM1.
  - Spermatocytic seminoma has been renamed spermatocytic tumor by the 2016 WHO classification and is not part of the testicular cancer staging because of its excellent prognosis.

PROGNOSTIC FACTORS

- Extent of primary and lymph node disease is prognostic in both seminoma and NSGCT, as apparent in the staging and prognostic grouping of testicular cancers.
- In a pooled analysis of patients with stage I seminoma, tumor size greater than 4 cm and rete testes invasion were associated with an increased risk of relapse of up to 30% (9). However, only size, and not rete testis invasion, was found to be a significant predictor of relapse when validated on an independent data set (10).
- The most important risk factor for relapse in stage I NSGCTs is lymphovascular invasion. Other risk factors include the presence of a significant embryonal carcinoma component, slow decrease in serum tumor markers, and absence of yolk sac elements (11).
- The International Prognostic Factors Study Group has identified several risk factors for relapse in metastatic GCTs treated with chemotherapy. Risk factors include mediastinal NSGCTs, progression-free interval greater than 3 months, response to prior chemotherapy, elevated AFP and hCG at salvage, and metastases to the liver, bone, and brain (12).

GENERAL MANAGEMENT

- The initial management of a suspected malignant germ cell tumor of the testis begins with a radical inguinal orchiectomy.
- Subsequent management is based on the pathologic diagnosis and the extent of disease. The specimen should be reviewed by an experienced pathologist as the distinction between seminoma and nonseminoma is essential.
- Carcinoma in situ can be treated with radical orchiectomy, RT (20 Gy/10), or surveillance with regular ultrasounds. Surveillance is appropriate for fertile men wishing to father children, and should be discussed on a case-by-case basis.
- In rare cases, patients presenting with life-threatening metastatic disease can be treated with upfront chemotherapy and delayed orchiectomy.

STAGE I SEMINOMA

- For stage I seminoma, orchiectomy is usually curative.
- Active surveillance after orchiectomy is the preferred approach to minimize overtreatment and morbidity from adjuvant therapies. Even with relapse rates of approximately 15%, an active surveillance strategy ultimately confers an excellent prognosis with long-term survival approaching 100% (13,14).
- Patients unlikely to comply with follow-up and those who decline surveillance can be offered adjuvant RT to the paraaortic lymph nodes. Two randomized trials have demonstrated low rates of recurrence with 20 Gy versus 30 Gy, and PALN RT versus dog-leg RT (PALN and ipsilateral iliac LNs) (15,16) (Fig. 30-1).

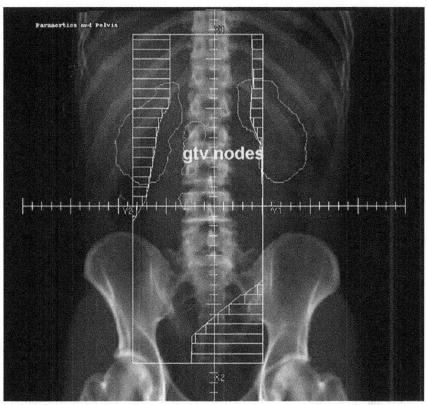

FIGURE 30-1. A modified dog-leg field, also showing contours of gross lymphadenopathy. (Courtesy of Dr. Padraig Warde, Princess Margaret Cancer Centre, Toronto, Canada.)

- An alternative to RT is adjuvant single-agent carboplatin with 1 to 2 cycles. A randomized trial of adjuvant RT versus carboplatin showed similar 5-year relapse rates of approximately 5% (17).
- The decision to use adjuvant RT or carboplatin in patients unsuitable for surveillance should include a discussion on the relative side effects of treatment including infertility, second malignancy, late cardiac disease (see Treatment-Related Toxicity section), as well as the availability of long-term outcomes.

STAGE II TO III SEMINOMA

- The treatment of stage II seminoma depends on the bulk of lymph node disease.
- For patients with relapsed stage I, stage IIA (LN size less than 2 cm), and stage IIB (LN size 2 to 5 cm), RT to the paraaortic and ipsilateral pelvic nodes achieves a relapse rate of 5% to 10% and an overall survival approaching 100% (18).

- For stage IIB disease, chemotherapy with 3 cycles of BEP or 4 cycles of EP is an alternative with similar oncologic outcomes but a different toxicity profile (19).
- Chemotherapy is preferred in patients with stage IIA to B seminoma with a horseshoe kidney, a history of inflammatory bowel disease, or prior RT.
- Patients with IIC disease are at risk of distant relapse. Stage IIC to III seminomas are treated with BEP or EP (especially in patients with decreased pulmonary or renal function), or PEI (cisplatin, etoposide, ifosfamide), according to their IGCCCG risk classification (20).
- Restaging examinations after 1 to 2 cycles of chemotherapy will occasionally reveal decreasing tumor markers but a growing mass. A diagnosis of growing teratoma should be entertained and resection of the mass considered immediately, or after the completion of chemotherapy.

SURVEILLANCE PROTOCOLS

- Surveillance protocols for stage I GCTs are directed at retroperitoneal and pelvic lymphadenopathy and thoracic/mediastinal spread. NSGCTs are more likely than are seminomas to experience thoracic recurrences and elevated tumor markers.
- The majority of patients with GCTs who relapse do so within the first 2 years; therefore, most protocols reduce the frequency of imaging after 2 to 3 years (21–23).
- Serum tumor markers are rarely elevated in the absence of radiologic disease in stage I seminoma, and their use for surveillance is not recommended (24,25).
- A reasonable surveillance protocol after orchiectomy for stage I seminoma is as follows:
  - Physical examination every 3 to 6 months in year 1, every 6 months in year 2 to 3, then annually in year 4 to 5.
  - CT scan of the abdomen and pelvis at 3, 6, and 12 months in year 1, every 6 months in years 2 to 3, then annually in years 4 to 5.
  - CXR annually in years 1 to 3 (or as clinically indicated).
- Active surveillance protocols for stage I NSGCT generally mandate regular CXRs for at least 5 years as well as serum tumor markers. We refer the reader to the National Comprehensive Cancer Network (NCCN) guidelines for examples of active surveillance protocols (NCCN.org).
- Low-dose CT scans have been shown to reduce radiation exposure with minimal loss of diagnostic quality and are recommended in some protocols (26).
- MRI surveillance is currently being compared with CT in the phase III randomized trial TE24—Trial of Imaging and Schedule in Seminoma Testis.

NONSEMINOMA

- After inguinal orchiectomy, the management of NSGCTs is based on stage and risk factors (see section on Prognostic Factors).
- RT is generally reserved for palliation.

- Stage IA and IB patients with no risk factors can be managed with on active surveillance protocols.
- High-risk patients are considered for adjuvant BEP chemotherapy for 1 cycle or RPLND as their risk of relapse approaches 40%.
- Stage IS with persistent elevation in tumor markers after orchiectomy are considered to have micrometastatic disease and treated with adjuvant chemotherapy.
- Patients with clinical stage IIA to C disease are considered for RPLND or chemotherapy (3 cycles of BEP or 4 cycles of EP) depending on the volume of disease. Patients with pathologic IIA-C after RPLND are considered for adjuvant chemotherapy.
- Patients with metastatic disease are treated with chemotherapy based on their risk stratification by the international Germ Cell Cancer Collaborative Group (iGCCCG).
- Residual lymphadenopathy greater than 1 cm usually mandates RPLND. Smaller residual lesions can be considered for observation.
- Patients with brain metastases at presentation have on average a 40% to 50% 3-year survival, significantly higher than those with brain relapse, possibly revealing a component of chemotherapy resistance (27). The optimal management for patients with brain metastases is not defined. Cisplatin-based chemotherapy is recommended in most patients, but the value of multimodality treatment with RT or surgery is controversial.

TREATMENT-RELATED TOXICITY

- Acute toxicity can be significant even with 20 Gy/10. In a randomized trial, patients treated with 20 Gy/10 had 18% grade 3 nausea/vomiting, 5% grade 3 to 4 fatigue, and almost 30% were unable to work at 4 weeks (16).
- Other acute toxicity includes leukopenia, dyspepsia, diarrhea, and decreased spermatogenesis.
- Late effects include peptic ulcers (6%), decreased spermatogenesis, and second malignancy (15,16).
- Careful shielding of the remaining testis can reduce the dose received by this testis to less than 1% of the prescription dose (28).
- In population-based studies, patients treated with subdiaphragmatic RT have a 1.4- to 2.6-fold lifetime increase in risk of second malignancies. Very long-term estimates are challenging, but patients may have an absolute risk increase of 10% or more, 40 years after treatment (29–31).
- Patients who received chemotherapy (BEP or PVB) similarly had a 2-fold increase in second malignancy risk, as well as a 1.7-fold increase in cardiovascular disease (32).
- Long-term toxicity data from patients treated with adjuvant single-agent carboplatin in stage I seminoma are not yet available. Relapses after adjuvant single-agent carboplatin usually occur in retroperitoneal LNs; therefore, patients will require ongoing cross-sectional surveillance of the abdomen (33) and those who relapse may ultimately undergo two courses of chemotherapy.

RADIATION THERAPY TECHNIQUES

Adjuvant RT for Stage I Seminoma

- Adjuvant RT can be delivered to PALN alone with doses in the range of 20 Gy/10 or 25 Gy/20.
- Patients are simulated supine with a clamshell shield to protect the contralateral testis.
- Field arrangement is AP-PA to limit dose to kidneys, liver, and bowel. IMRT may reduce high-dose areas to OARs but also increases kidney, liver, and bowel Dmean and D50% (34).
- Typical treatment fields are as follows:
  - Superiorly: top of T11 vertebral body. However, there are data supporting low rates of recurrence with the superior border at T12 (35,36).
  - Inferiorly: bottom of L5.
  - Laterally: approximately 9 to 11 cm wide encompassing the tips of transverse processes. For left-sided tumors, the ipsilateral renal hilum can be included.
- Modified dog-leg fields are also used, as this technique decreases the rate of pelvic relapses and precludes the need for ongoing CT surveillance.
- RT fields can also be informed by volumetric expansion on the aorta and IVC down to the bifurcation (see section on RT for Stage II Seminoma).

RT for Stage II Seminoma

- RT is typically delivered with modified dog-leg fields encompassing PALNs and ipsilateral iliac LNs.
- Typical dog-leg fields are as follows:
  - Superiorly: top of T11 or T12 (see above)
  - Inferiorly: below L4, the field extends diagonally to the top of acetabulum
  - Laterally: tips of transverse processes
- RT fields can also be informed by volumetric expansions on the IVC and aorta to approximate the location of PALNs. One approach is to add a 1.2-cm CTV on the IVC and 1.9-cm CTV on the aorta, followed by a 5-mm PTV for setup error and 7-mm PTV for penumbra to field edge. Appropriate shielding is used to reduce irradiated volume and to include the left kidney hilum (36).
- A cone-down boost of 10 Gy/5 or 16 Gy/8 can be added for gross nodes greater than 2 to 3 cm in size although data for this are limited. A 2-cm margin to field edge is typically used.

References

1. Winter C, Albers P. Testicular germ cell tumors: pathogenesis, diagnosis and treatment. *Nat Rev Endocrinol* 2011;7(1):43–53.
2. Global Burden of Disease Cancer Collaboration, et al. Global, regional, and national cancer incidence, mortality, years of life lost, years lived with disability, and disability-adjusted life-years for 32 cancer groups, 1990 to 2015: a systematic analysis for the global burden of disease study. *JAMA Oncol* 2017;3(4):524–548.

3. Gajendran VK, Nguyen M, Ellison LM. Testicular cancer patterns in African-American men. *Urology* 2005;66(3):602–605.

4. Moller H, Knudsen LB, Lynge E. Risk of testicular cancer after vasectomy: cohort study of over 73,000 men. *Br Med J* 1994;309(6950):295–299.

5. Einhorn LH. Treatment of testicular cancer: a new and improved model. *J Clin Oncol* 1990;8(11):1777–1781.

6. von der Maase H, et al. Carcinoma in situ of contralateral testis in patients with testicular germ cell cancer: study of 27 cases in 500 patients. *Br Med J (Clin Res Ed)* 1986;293(6559):1398–1401.

7. Morton G, Thomas G. Testis. In: Halperin EC, Perez CA, Brady LW, eds. *Principles and practice of radiation oncology*, 5th ed. Philadelphia, PA: Lippincott Williams & Wilkins, 2008.

8. De Santis M, et al. Predictive impact of 2-18fluoro-2-deoxy-D-glucose positron emission tomography for residual postchemotherapy masses in patients with bulky seminoma. *J Clin Oncol* 2001;19(17):3740–3744.

9. Warde P, et al. Prognostic factors for relapse in stage I seminoma managed by surveillance: a pooled analysis. *J Clin Oncol* 2002;20(22):4448–4452.

10. Chung P, et al. Evaluation of a prognostic model for risk of relapse in stage I seminoma surveillance. *Cancer Med* 2015;4(1):155–160.

11. Krege S, et al. European consensus conference on diagnosis and treatment of germ cell cancer: a report of the second meeting of the European Germ Cell Cancer Consensus group (EGCCCG): part I. *Eur Urol* 2008;53(3):478–496.

12. International Prognostic Factors Study Group, et al. Prognostic factors in patients with metastatic germ cell tumors who experienced treatment failure with cisplatin-based first-line chemotherapy. *J Clin Oncol* 2010;28(33):4906–4911.

13. Kollmannsberger C, et al. Patterns of relapse in patients with clinical stage I testicular cancer managed with active surveillance. *J Clin Oncol* 2015;33(1):51–57.

14. Chung P, Warde P. Stage I seminoma: adjuvant treatment is effective but is it necessary? *J Natl Cancer Inst* 2011;103(3):194–196.

15. Fossa SD, et al. Optimal planning target volume for stage I testicular seminoma: a Medical Research Council randomized trial. Medical Research Council Testicular Tumor Working Group. *J Clin Oncol* 1999;17(4):1146.

16. Jones WG, et al. Randomized trial of 30 versus 20 Gy in the adjuvant treatment of stage I testicular seminoma: a report on Medical Research Council Trial TE18, European Organisation for the Research and Treatment of Cancer Trial 30942 (ISRCTN18525328). *J Clin Oncol* 2005;23(6):1200–1208.

17. Oliver RT, et al. Randomized trial of carboplatin versus radiotherapy for stage I seminoma: mature results on relapse and contralateral testis cancer rates in MRC TE19/EORTC 30982 study (ISRCTN27163214). *J Clin Oncol* 2011;29(8):957–962.

18. Classen J, et al. Radiotherapy for stages IIA/B testicular seminoma: final report of a prospective multicenter clinical trial. *J Clin Oncol* 2003;21(6):1101–1106.

19. Garcia-del-Muro X, et al. Chemotherapy as an alternative to radiotherapy in the treatment of stage IIA and IIB testicular seminoma: a Spanish Germ Cell Cancer Group Study. *J Clin Oncol* 2008;26(33):5416–5421.

20. International Germ Cell Consensus Classification: a prognostic factor-based staging system for metastatic germ cell cancers. International Germ Cell Cancer Collaborative Group. *J Clin Oncol* 1997;15(2):594–603.

21. Mortensen MS, et al. A nationwide cohort study of stage I seminoma patients followed on a surveillance program. *Eur Urol* 2014;66(6):1172–1178.

22. Mortensen MS, et al. Late relapses in stage I testicular cancer patients on surveillance. *Eur Urol* 2016;70(2):365–371.

23. Nayan M, et al. Conditional risk of relapse in surveillance for clinical stage I testicular cancer. *Eur Urol* 2017;71(1):120–127.
24. Gilligan TD, et al. American Society of Clinical Oncology Clinical Practice Guideline on uses of serum tumor markers in adult males with germ cell tumors. *J Clin Oncol* 2010;28(20):3388–3404.
25. Vesprini D, et al. Utility of serum tumor markers during surveillance for stage I seminoma. *Cancer* 2012;118(21):5245–5250.
26. O'Malley ME, et al. Comparison of low dose with standard dose abdominal/pelvic multidetector CT in patients with stage 1 testicular cancer under surveillance. *Eur Radiol* 2010;20(7):1624–1630.
27. Feldman DR, et al. Brain metastases in patients with germ cell tumors: prognostic factors and treatment options—an analysis from the Global Germ Cell Cancer Group. *J Clin Oncol* 2016;34(4):345–351.
28. Lieng H, et al. Testicular seminoma: scattered radiation dose to the contralateral testis in the modern era. *Pract Radiat Oncol* 2018;8(2):e57–e62.
29. de Gonzalez AB, et al. Proportion of second cancers attributable to radiotherapy treatment in adults: a cohort study in the US SEER cancer registries. *Lancet Oncol* 2011;12(4):353–360.
30. Travis LB, et al. Second cancers among 40,576 testicular cancer patients: focus on long-term survivors. *J Natl Cancer Inst* 2005;97(18):1354–1365.
31. van den Belt-Dusebout AW, et al. Treatment-specific risks of second malignancies and cardiovascular disease in 5-year survivors of testicular cancer. *J Clin Oncol* 2007;25(28):4370–4378.
32. van den Belt-Dusebout AW, et al. Long-term risk of cardiovascular disease in 5-year survivors of testicular cancer. *J Clin Oncol* 2006;24(3):467–475.
33. Mead GM, et al. Randomized trials in 2466 patients with stage I seminoma: patterns of relapse and follow-up. *J Natl Cancer Inst* 2011;103(3):241–249.
34. Zilli T, et al. Bone marrow-sparing intensity-modulated radiation therapy for Stage I seminoma. *Acta Oncol* 2011;50(4):555–562.
35. Bruns F, et al. Adjuvant radiotherapy in stage I seminoma: is there a role for further reduction of treatment volume? *Acta Oncol* 2005;44(2):142–148.
36. Wilder RB, et al. Radiotherapy treatment planning for testicular seminoma. *Int J Radiat Oncol Biol Phys* 2012;83(4):e445–e452.

CHAPTER 31

URETHRA AND PENIS

FEMALE URETHRA

- Carcinoma of the urethra in women is rare; approximately 1,600 cases have been reported in the literature.

Anatomy

- The female urethra is approximately 4.0 cm long and extends from the urinary bladder through the urogenital diaphragm to the vestibule, where it forms the urethral meatus.
- The lymphatic drainage of the urethral meatus parallels that of the vulva to the superficial and deep inguinal and external iliac lymph nodes. The primary drainage of the entire urethra is mainly to the obturator and internal and external iliac nodes.

Clinical Presentation

- A tumor of the urethral meatus at an early stage may resemble a urethral caruncle or a prolapse of the mucosa through the urethral orifice. As the lesion progresses, it enlarges and eventually ulcerates.
- Advanced tumors (stages II and III) of the urethra have been associated with a 35% to 50% incidence of inguinal or pelvic lymph node involvement (1).

Diagnostic Workup

- A routine history and general physical examination should be performed in all patients.
- A detailed pelvic examination under anesthesia is necessary to fully evaluate the clinical extent of the disease. It can be performed at the time of urethroscopy and cystoscopy.
- Routine radiographic evaluation should include chest radiographs, an intravenous urogram, and a computed tomography (CT) scan of the abdomen and pelvis.

| **NEW!** | **SUMMARY OF CHANGES TO AJCC STAGING** |

PRIMARY TUMOR STAGING (T STAGE)

* Now includes prostatic urothelial carcinoma.
* Tis now refers to both Tis pu (carcinoma in situ of the prostatic urethra) and/or Tis pd (carcinoma in situ of the prostatic ducts and acini.)
* T1 prostatic urothelial cancers involve the subepithelial connective tissues of the prostatic urethra.
* T4 now includes urethral cancer extension to the bladder wall, consistent with bladder cancer staging where T4 disease extends to the prostate.

REGIONAL LYMPH NODE STAGING (N STAGE)

* N1 now refers to single regional lymph node metastasis in the inguinal region, true pelvis (viz, perivesical, obturator, internal or hypogastric, and external iliac) or pre-sacral nodes.
* N2 now refers to multiple nodal metastases in the same basins covered by N1.

See: Amin MB, Edge SB, Greene FL, et al, eds. *AJCC cancer staging manual*, 8th ed. New York: Springer, 2017.

Staging

* Urethral cancer staged according to the American Joint Committee on Cancer (AJCC) system.
* AJCC 8 was adopted in January 2018, replacing the AJCC 7 adopted in 2009 (2).

Prognostic Factors

* Tumor size and location are the most important factors in determining prognosis and survival.
* Eighty-one percent of patients with lesions less than 2 cm had 5-year progression-free survival, compared with 37% of those with lesions 2 to 4 cm and 7% of patients with lesions greater than 4 cm ($p = 0.0001$) (3).
* Bladder neck involvement, parametrial extension, and inguinal lymph node involvement are poor prognostic factors.

General Management

Anterior Urethral Cancer

* Open excision, electroexcision, fulguration, or laser coagulation can be used to treat tumors at the meatus or *in situ* involvement of the distal urethra (stage 0).
* For larger and more invasive lesions (stage I), interstitial irradiation or combined interstitial and external beam irradiation are alternatives to surgical resection of the distal third of the urethra.

- Anterior urethral lesions that recur after treatment by local excision or radiation therapy may require anterior exenteration and urinary diversion.
- If no inguinal adenopathy exists, node dissection is not recommended, but prophylactic groin irradiation is recommended for patients with invasive lesions (3).

Posterior Urethral Cancer

- Cancers of the posterior or entire urethra (stages II to IV) are usually associated with invasion of the bladder and a high incidence of inguinal and pelvic lymph node metastases.
- The best results have been achieved with preoperative irradiation with exenterative surgery and urinary diversion.
- A report on 97 patients with urethral carcinoma who were treated using radiotherapy (RT) either in the adjuvant or the definitive setting showed 5- and 10-year survival rates of 41% and 31%, respectively. Five-year local control was 64%. Forty-nine percent of those who achieved local control developed complications including urethral stenosis, fistula, necrosis, hemorrhage, or cystitis (4).

Radiation Therapy Techniques

- Interstitial implant is the usual method for treating meatal carcinomas. Radioactive needles forming a double-plane or a volume implant have been used. After radiographs are used to verify needle placement, a dose of 60 to 70 Gy with low-dose rate (LDR) brachytherapy can be given in 6 to 7 days (0.4 Gy per hour to the target volume) when an implant alone is used.
- Large tumors extending into the labia, vagina, entire urethra, or base of the bladder cannot be treated with an implant alone. A combination of external beam irradiation and implant is recommended (5). The external beam portal should flash the perineum to cover the entire urethra. The portal should be wide enough to cover the inguinal nodes (6) and extend cephalad to the L5-S1 interspace to include the pelvic nodes. A bolus, appropriate for the photon energy used, should be added to the groins when inguinal nodes are positive. The whole pelvis is treated to a dose of 50 Gy. A boost of 10 to 15 Gy is delivered to positive nodes through reduced anterior photon or en face electron fields (7).
- For advanced disease, the primary tumor is treated with a vaginal cylinder to bring the dose to the entire urethra to approximately 60 Gy. An interstitial implant is used to raise the total tumor dose to 70 to 80 Gy LDR brachytherapy. Intracavitary irradiation simultaneously with a vaginal cylinder and an interstitial implant should be used with caution because of the resultant high-dose rate at the vaginal mucosa interface of the intracavitary and interstitial implants (7).
- A limiting factor in the use of external beam irradiation is the tolerance of the perineal skin (confluent moist desquamation).
- Extensive disease combined with advanced age can be formidable obstacles to completing radiation therapy. Diligent personal hygiene and individualized care are necessary if patients are to complete the course of treatment (5).

Sequelae of Treatment

- Urethral strictures develop in some patients, necessitating dilatation or urinary diversion.
- Incontinence, cystitis, and vaginal stenosis may also develop.
- Severe complications are fistula formation, bowel obstruction, and occasionally operative mortality.
- With advanced neoplasms, fistula formation may be unavoidable because of tumor erosion of the organ and subsequent tumor necrosis.

PENIS AND MALE URETHRA

Anatomy

- The basic structural components of the penis include two corpora cavernosa and the corpus spongiosum. Distally, the corpus spongiosum expands into the glans penis, which is covered by a skin fold (prepuce).
- The male urethra, composed of a mucous membrane and the submucosa, extends from the bladder neck to the external urethral meatus.
- The posterior urethra is subdivided into the membranous urethra (portion passing through urogenital diaphragm) and the prostatic urethra, which passes through the prostate (Fig. 31-1). The anterior urethra passes through the corpus spongiosum and is subdivided into the fossa navicularis, a widening within the glans; the penile urethra, which passes through the pendulous part of the penis; and the bulbous urethra, the dilated proximal portion of the anterior urethra.
- The lymphatic channels of the prepuce and the skin of the shaft drain into the superficial inguinal nodes located above the fascia lata. The rich anastomotic network of the lymphatics within the penis and at its base means that, for practical purposes, lymphatic drainage may be considered bilateral.
- The so-called sentinel nodes, located above and medial to the junction of the epigastric and saphenous veins, have been identified as the primary drainage sites in carcinoma of the penis (Fig. 31-2). This group of nodes is of obvious importance in assessment of tumor extent because, if they are not involved in the tumor, a complete nodal dissection may not be necessary.
- The lymphatics of the fossa navicularis and the penile urethra follow those of the penis to the superficial and deep inguinal lymph nodes.
- The lymphatics of the bulbomembranous and prostatic urethra may follow three routes: Some pass under the pubic symphysis to the external iliac nodes, some go to the obturator and internal iliac nodes, and others end in the presacral lymph nodes.
- The pelvic (iliac) lymph nodes are rarely affected in the absence of inguinal lymph node involvement (8).

Natural History

- Most carcinomas of the penis start within the preputial area, arising in the glans, coronal sulcus, or the prepuce (9).

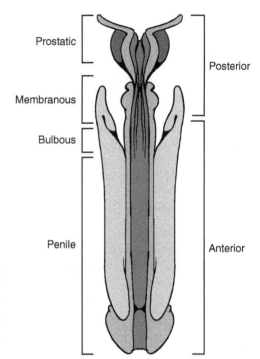

Prostatic

Membranous

Bulbous

Penile

Posterior

Anterior

FIGURE 31-1. Anatomic subdivisions of the male urethra. (Reprinted with permission from Mansur DB, Chao KS. Penis and male urethra. In: Halperin EC, Perez CA, Brady LW, eds. *Principles and practice of radiation oncology*, 5th ed. Philadelphia, PA: Lippincott Williams & Wilkins, 2008:1519–1531. © Wolters Kluwer.)

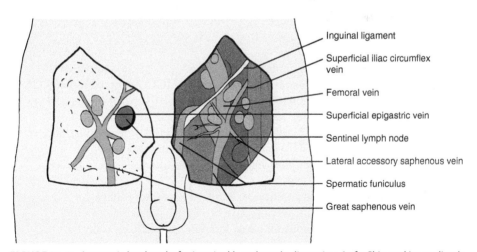

Inguinal ligament

Superficial iliac circumflex vein

Femoral vein

Superficial epigastric vein

Sentinel lymph node

Lateral accessory saphenous vein

Spermatic funiculus

Great saphenous vein

FIGURE 31-2. Anatomic landmarks for inguinal lymph node dissection. **Left:** Skin and immediately surrounding adipose tissue are removed to expose sentinel lymph node. Deep fatty stratum remains. Other lymph nodes and great saphenous vein and tributaries are indicated by dashed lines. **Right:** Sentinel lymph node and superficial and deep fascia are removed to expose other superficial and deep lymph nodes. (Reprinted with permission from Cabanas RM. An approach for the treatment of penile carcinoma. *Cancer* 1977;39:456–466.)

- The inguinal lymph nodes are the most common site of metastatic spread. In patients with clinically nonpalpable inguinal nodes, between 20% and 40% have micrometastasis.
- Pathologic evidence of nodal metastases is reported in approximately 35% of all patients and in approximately 50% of those with palpable lymph nodes.
- Urethral cancers tend to spread by direct extension to adjacent structures. Invasion into the vascular space of the corpus spongiosum in the periurethral tissues is common. Malignancies beginning in the bulbomembranous urethra often invade the deep structures of the perineum, including the urogenital diaphragm, prostate, and adjacent skin. In most prostatic urethral tumors, the bulk of the prostate gland is involved at the time of diagnosis.

Clinical Presentation

- Carcinoma of the penis may present as either an infiltrative-ulcerative or an exophytic papillary lesion.
- Patients with urethral carcinoma may present with obstructive symptoms, tenderness, dysuria, urethral discharge, and occasionally, initial hematuria.

Diagnostic Workup

- Urethroscopy and cystoscopy are essential to the diagnostic workup.
- Inguinal lymph nodes should be thoroughly evaluated. Chest x-ray films and intravenous pyelogram are routinely obtained.
- CT is useful in the identification of enlarged pelvic and periaortic lymph nodes in patients with involved inguinal lymph nodes.

Staging Systems

- Penile cancer staged according to the AJCC system.
- AJCC 8 was adopted in January 2018, replacing the AJCC 7 adopted in 2009 (2).
- Major changes in the AJCC 8 system include (2):
  - Histologic grading (G grade)
    - The three-tiered World Health Organization (WHO)/International Society of Urological Pathology (ISUP) grading system was adopted.
    - The presence of any amount of anaplastic cells constitutes grade 3 disease.
  - Primary tumor staging (T stage)
    - Ta broadened to include noninvasive localized squamous carcinoma.
    - T1a and T1b now also include negative or positive perineural invasion.
    - T1 now includes definitions for glans, foreskin, and shaft invasion.
    - T2 now includes corpus spongiosum invasion.
    - T3 now includes corpora cavernosum invasion.
  - Regional lymph node staging (N stage)
    - pN1a now includes ≤2 unilateral inguinal metastases without extranodal extension.
    - pN2 now includes ≥3 unilateral inguinal metastases or any bilateral metastases.

- Obsolete staging systems include:
  - The Jackson (10) penile carcinoma staging system, and
  - The Ray (11) urethral staging system.

Pathologic Classification

- Most malignant penile tumors are well-differentiated squamous cell carcinomas.
- Approximately 80% of urethral carcinomas in men can be classified as squamous cell carcinomas, usually well or moderately differentiated (12).
- Transitional cell carcinoma, adenocarcinoma, and undifferentiated or mixed carcinomas represent approximately 15%, 5%, and 1%, respectively.

Prognostic Factors

- Extent of the primary lesion and status of the lymph nodes are the principal prognostic factors in carcinoma of the penis.
- Tumor-free regional nodes imply excellent (85% to 90%) long-term survival or even cure.
- Patients with involvement of the inguinal nodes fare considerably worse and only 40% to 50% survive long term (13,14). Pelvic lymph node involvement implies the worst prognosis; less than 20% of these patients survive (13,15,16). Distal urethral cancer generally has a prognosis similar to that of carcinoma of the penis.
- Lesions of the bulbomembranous urethra are usually quite extensive and are associated with a dismal prognosis.
- Tumors of the prostatic urethra show prognostic features similar to those in bladder carcinoma.

General Management

Carcinoma of the Penis

- Surgical intervention at the primary site for carcinoma of the penis ranges from local excision or chemosurgery (17) (in a small group of highly selected cases, particularly those with small lesions of the prepuce) to partial or total penectomy.
- The ideal surgical procedure eliminates the disease and preserves sexual and urinary function, although this is not always possible depending on the extent of disease. Radical surgery, especially total penectomy, may be psychologically devastating to the patient.
- Lesions confined to the prepuce may be treated with wide circumcision.
- Lesions on the glans penis traditionally have been treated by partial penectomy; however, brachytherapy is an alternative.
- Circumcision is associated with a 40% local recurrence rate.
- Partial penectomy is the procedure of choice if surgical margins of 2 cm can be achieved.

- It is possible for some patients to remain sexually active after partial penectomy. Jensen (18) reported that 45% of patients with 4 to 6 cm and 25% of patients with 2 to 4 cm of penile stump could have sexual intercourse.
- The 2018 update of the NCCN Guidelines for Penile Carcinoma are worthwhile reading.

Radiation therapy

- The primary advantage of radiation therapy is preservation of the phallus. This is particularly important to young, sexually active men with a small, invasive lesion localized to the glans.
- Modalities to deliver radiation to the penis include megavoltage external beam irradiation, ^{192}Ir mold plesiotherapy, and interstitial implant using ^{192}Ir wires (17,19–22).
- Grabstald and Kelley (23) reported 90% local tumor control in ten patients with stage I lesions treated with external beam irradiation (51 to 52 Gy in 6 weeks).
- De Crevoisier et al. (24) reported 80% of 10-year local tumor control in 144 patients with squamous cell carcinoma of the penis, confined to the glans, treated with interstitial LDR brachytherapy.
- Crook et al. (25) reported 5-year actuarial cause-specific survival of 90% and 5-year actuarial penile preservation rate of 86.5% for 49 patients with T1-T4 squamous cell carcinoma of the penis treated with penile brachytherapy.
- A series of clinical trials at the M. D. Anderson Cancer Center, Houston, Texas, demonstrated 80% local control and retention of the phallus in early-stage disease (26).
- Duncan and Jackson (27) reported 90% local control for stage I lesions treated with a megavoltage treatment unit delivering 50 to 57 Gy over 3 weeks.
- Ozsahin et al. (28) reported that local tumor control is superior with surgery in patients with penile cancer, but no difference in survival was noted between surgery and definitive RT.
- Irradiation of the involved regional lymph nodes in patients with carcinoma of the penis results in permanent control and cure in a substantial proportion of patients. In the classic series of Staubitz et al. (29), 5 of 13 patients (38%) with proven involvement of regional lymph nodes who received nodal irradiation survived 5 years.
- Inguinal lymph node irradiation for nonpalpable nodes is an integral component of successful treatment; control has been achieved in 95% of cases. Without irradiation to the inguinal lymph nodes, as many as 20% of patients can be expected to develop positive nodes later.

Chemoirradiation

- Because most lesions are squamous cell carcinoma, one would expect platinum-based agents to be effective when performing chemoirradiation.
- Doxorubicin, bleomycin sulfate, and methotrexate may be useful in the management of advanced-stage lesions, and perhaps in early-stage disease as well.

Carcinoma of the Male Urethra

- The primary therapy for carcinoma of the male urethra is surgical excision.
- In lesions of the distal urethra, results with either penectomy or radiation therapy are similar to those for carcinoma of the penis; 5-year survival rates also are comparable (50% to 60%).

Radiation Therapy Techniques

Carcinoma of the Penis

- Circumcision, if indicated, must be performed before irradiation is initiated. The purpose of this procedure is to minimize radiation-associated morbidity (swelling, skin irritation, moist desquamation, and secondary infection).
- External beam therapy has become prevalent in the treatment of primary lesions in carcinoma of the penis; plastic molds or interstitial implants are still occasionally used (9).

External Irradiation

- External beam therapy requires specially designed accessories (including bolus) to achieve homogeneous dose distribution to the entire penis.
- Frequently, a plastic box with a central circular opening that can be fitted over the penis is used. The space between the skin and the box must be filled with tissue-equivalent material (Fig. 31-3). This box can be treated with parallel-opposed megavoltage beams.
- An ingenious alternative to the box technique is the use of a water-filled container to envelop the penis while the patient is in a prone position (30).
- In many series, fraction size ranges from 2.5 to 3.5 Gy (total dose of 50 to 55 Gy), although a smaller daily fraction size (1.8 to 2.0 Gy) and a higher total dose are preferable.
- A total of 60 to 65 Gy, with the last 5 to 10 Gy delivered to a reduced portal, should result in a reduced incidence of late fibrosis.
- Regional lymphatics may be treated with external beam megavoltage irradiation. Both groins should be irradiated. The fields should include inguinal and pelvic (external iliac and hypogastric) lymph nodes (Fig. 31-4).
- Depending on the extent of nodal disease and the proximity of detectable tumor to the skin surface, or the presence of skin invasion, application of a bolus to the inguinal area should be considered.
- If clinical and radiographic evaluations show no gross enlargement of the pelvic lymph nodes, dose to these nodes may be limited to 50 Gy. In patients with palpable lymph nodes, doses of approximately 70 to 75 Gy over 7 to 8 weeks (1.8 to 2.0 Gy per day) with reducing fields (after 50 Gy) are advised.

Brachytherapy

- For brachytherapy, a mold is usually built in the form of a box or a cylinder, with a central opening and channels for placement of radioactive sources (needles or wires) in the periphery of the device. The cylinder and sources should be long enough to prevent underdosage at the tip of the penis.

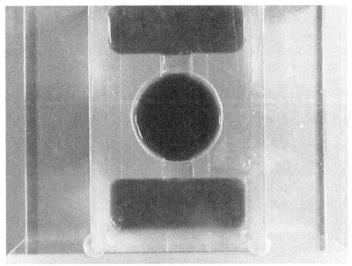

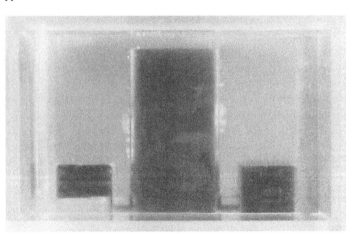

FIGURE 31-3. A: View from above of plastic box with central cylinder for external irradiation of the penis. Patient is treated in the prone position. The penis is placed in the central cylinder, and water is used to fill the surrounding volume in the box. Depth dose is calculated at the central point of the box. **B:** Lateral view. (Reprinted with permission from Mansur DB, Chao KS. Penis and male urethra. In: Halperin EC, Perez CA, Brady LW, eds. *Principles and practice of radiation oncology*, 5th ed. Philadelphia, PA: Lippincott Williams & Wilkins, 2008:1519–1531. © Wolters Kluwer.)

- A dose of 60 to 65 Gy at the surface and approximately 50 Gy at the center of the organ is delivered over 6 to 7 days.
- The mold can be applied either continuously (in which case an indwelling catheter should be in place) or intermittently. Intermittent application requires precise time record keeping.
- Alternatively, single- or double-plane implants can be used to deliver 60 to 70 Gy in 5 to 7 days (21).

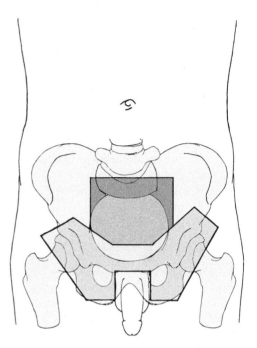

FIGURE 31-4. Portals encompassing inguinal and pelvic lymph nodes. (Reprinted with permission from Mansur DB, Chao KS. Penis and male urethra. In: Halperin EC, Perez CA, Brady LW, eds. *Principles and practice of radiation oncology*, 5th ed. Philadelphia, PA: Lippincott Williams & Wilkins, 2008:1519–1531. © Wolters Kluwer.)

Carcinoma of the Male Urethra

- Radiation therapy for carcinoma of the anterior (distal) urethra is similar to that for carcinoma of the penis.
- Lesions of the bulbomembranous urethra can be treated with a set of parallel-opposed fields covering the groins and pelvis, followed by perineal and inguinal boost.
- Lesions of the prostatic urethra can be treated with techniques and doses similar to those used for carcinoma of the prostate.

Chemotherapy

- Experience with the use of chemotherapy in carcinoma of the penis is even more limited than with other modalities.
- Tumor regression occasionally has been observed with antineoplastic agents such as bleomycin sulfate, 5-fluorouracil, or methotrexate. In some instances, however, chemotherapy has been combined with irradiation or surgery, making assessment of the response more difficult (31).
- Response to cisplatin has been reported in a few patients. Ahmed et al. (32) treated 12 patients with penile cancer with intravenous cisplatin (70 to 120 mg per m^2) every 3 weeks and noted three responses, with a duration of 2 to 8 months. Gagliano et al. (33) observed no complete response and only four partial responses (15.4%) in 26 patients with stage III or IV epidermal carcinoma of the penis who received cisplatin (50 mg per m^2) intravenously on day 1 and then every 28 days; response duration was 1 to 3 months.

Normal Tissue Complications—QUANTEC Results

Recommendations from the QUANTEC review for penile bulb given by Roach et al. (34) include the following: According to the data available, it is prudent to keep the mean dose to 95% of the penile bulb volume to less than 50 Gy. It may also be prudent to limit the $D_{70\%}$ and $D_{90\%}$ to 70 and 50 Gy, respectively, but coverage of the planning target volume should not be compromised. It is acknowledged that the penile bulb may not be the critical component of the erectile apparatus, but it seems to be a surrogate for yet-to-be-determined structure(s) critical for erectile function for at least some techniques. Readers are also referred to Chapters 31 and 28 for discussion on dose limits to the bladder and rectum, respectively.

A schematic picture of the penile anatomy, as well as CT and MRI scans (35), are given in Figure 31-5.

Sequelae of Treatment

• Irradiation of the penis produces a brisk erythema, dry or moist desquamation, and swelling of the subcutaneous tissue of the shaft in virtually all patients. Although quite uncomfortable, these are reversible reactions that subside within a few weeks, with conservative treatment.

• Telangiectasia is a common late consequence of radiation therapy and is usually asymptomatic.

• In the reported series, meatal-urethral strictures occur with a frequency of 0% to 40% (19,36–39). This incidence compares favorably with the incidence of urethral stricture following penectomy. Most strictures following radiation therapy are at the meatus.

• Ulceration, necrosis of the glans, and necrosis of the skin of the shaft are rare complications.

• Lymphedema of the legs has been reported after inguinal and pelvic irradiation, but the role of irradiation in the development of this complication is controversial. Many patients with this symptom have active disease in the lymphatics that may be responsible for lymphatic blockage.

• Of all male genitourinary cancers, penile cancer poses the greatest threat to sexual function. It also carries the risk of castration, which can be psychologically devastating. Despite recent advances in treatment, however, sexual function is not likely to be adequately preserved in some patients. These patients and their partners need information about physical impairments after surgical intervention and should be taught adjustment skills before treatment is started. Referral to a trained sexual consultant or therapist for help is indicated.

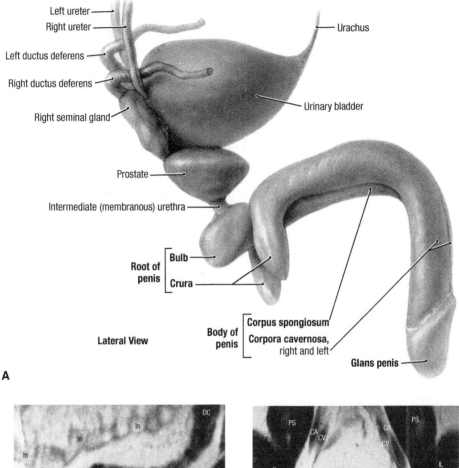

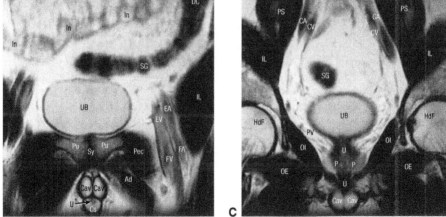

FIGURE 31-5. **A:** Major tissues of male urogential system. **B** and **C:** Coronal MRI of sections of male pelvis. (Reprinted with permission from Agur AMR, Dalley AF, eds. *Grant's Atlas of anatomy*, 12th ed. Philadelphia, PA: Lippincott Williams & Wilkins, 2009:266, 278. © Wolters Kluwer.)

References

1. Eng TY. Femle urethra. In: Halperin EC, Perez CA, Brady LW, eds. *Principles and practice of radiation oncology*, 5th ed. Philadelphia, PA: Lippincott Williams & Wilkins, 2008:1682–1691.

2. Amin MA, Greene FL, Edge S, et al. *AJCC cancer staging manual*, 8th ed. New York, NY: Springer, 2017.

3. Grigsby PW. Female urethra. In: Perez CA, Brady LW, eds. *Principles and practice of radiation oncology*, 3rd ed. Philadelphia, PA: Lippincott–Raven, 1998:1473–1581.

4. Garden AS, Zagars GK, Delclos L. Primary carcinoma of the female urethra. Results of radiation therapy. *Cancer* 1993;71(10):3102–3108.

5. Klein FA, Ali MM, Kersh R. Carcinoma of the female urethra: combined iridium Ir 192 interstitial and external beam radiotherapy. *South Med J* 1987;80(9):1129–1132.

6. Foens CS, Hussey DH, Staples JJ, et al. A comparison of the roles of surgery and radiation therapy in the management of carcinoma of the female urethra. *Int J Radiat Oncol Biol Phys* 1991;21(4):961–968.

7. Grigsby PW, Corn BW. Localized urethral tumors in women: indications for conservative versus exenterative therapies. *J Urol* 1992;147(6):1516–1520.

8. Crawford ED, Dawkins CA. Cancer of the penis. In: Skinner DG, Lieskovsky G, eds. *Diagnosis and management of genitourinary cancer*. Philadelphia, PA: WB Saunders, 1988:549–563.

9. Mansur DB, Chao KSC. Penis and male urethra. In: Halperin EC, Perez CA, Brady LW, eds. *Principles and practice of radiation oncology*, 5th ed. Philadelphia, PA: Lippincott Williams & Wilkins, 2008:1519–1531.

10. Jackson SM. The treatment of carcinoma of the penis. *Br J Surg* 1966;53(1):33–35.

11. Ray B, Canto AR, Whitmore WF Jr. Experience with primary carcinoma of the male urethra. *J Urol* 1977;117(5):591–594.

12. Narayana AS, Olney LE, Loening SA, et al. Carcinoma of the penis: analysis of 219 cases. *Cancer* 1982;49(10):2185–2191.

13. de Kernion JB, Tynberg P, Persky L, et al. Proceedings: carcinoma of the penis. *Cancer* 1973;32(5):1256–1262.

14. Skinner DG, Leadbetter WF, Kelley SB. The surgical management of squamous cell carcinoma of the penis. *J Urol* 1972;107(2):273–277.

15. Cabanas RM. An approach for the treatment of penile carcinoma. *Cancer* 1977;39(2):456–466.

16. Hardner GJ, Bhanalaph T, Murphy GP, et al. Carcinoma of the penis: analysis of therapy in 100 consecutive cases. *J Urol* 1972;108(3):428–430.

17. Rosemberg SK. Carbon dioxide laser treatment of external genital lesions. *Urology* 1985;25(6):555–558.

18. Jensen MO. Cancer of the penis in Denmark 1942 to 1962 (511 cases). *Dan Med Bull* 1977;24(2):66–72.

19. Haile K, Delclos L. The place of radiation therapy in the treatment of carcinoma of the distal end of the penis. *Cancer* 1980;45(7 suppl):1980–1984.

20. Mazeron JJ, Langlois D, Lobo PA, et al. Interstitial radiation therapy for carcinoma of the penis using iridium 192 wires: the Henri Mondor experience (1970-1979). *Int J Radiat Oncol Biol Phys* 1984;10(10):1891–1895.

21. Pierquin B, Chassagne D, Chahbazian C, et al. *Brachytherapy*. St. Louis, MO: Warren Green, 1978.

22. Pointon R. External beam therapy. *Proc R Soc Med* 1975;68:779–781.

23. Grabstald H, Kelley CD. Radiation therapy of penile cancer: six to ten-year follow-up. *Urology* 1980;15(6):575–576.

24. de Crevoisier R, Slimane K, Sanfilippo N, et al. Long-term results of brachytherapy for carcinoma of the penis confined to the glans (N- or NX). *Int J Radiat Oncol Biol Phys* 2009;74(4):1150–1156.
25. Crook JM, Jezioranski J, Grimard L, et al. Penile brachytherapy: results for 49 patients. *Int J Radiat Oncol Biol Phys* 2005;62(2):460–467.
26. Haddad F. Letter to the editor. *J Urol* 1989;141:959.
27. Duncan W, Jackson SM. The treatment of early cancer of the penis with megavoltage x-rays. *Clin Radiol* 1972;23(2):246–248.
28. Ozsahin M, Jichlinski P, Weber DC, et al. Treatment of penile carcinoma: to cut or not to cut?. *Int J Radiat Oncol Biol Phys* 2006;66(3):674–679.
29. Staubitz WJ, Lent MH, Oberkircher OJ. Carcinoma of the penis. *Cancer* 1955;8(2):371–378.
30. Sagerman RH, Yu WS, Chung CT, et al. External-beam irradiation of carcinoma of the penis. *Radiology* 1984;152(1):183–185.
31. Yagoda A, Mukherji B, Young C, et al. Bleomycin, an antitumor antibiotic. Clinical experience in 274 patients. *Ann Intern Med* 1972;77(6):861–870.
32. Ahmed T, Sklaroff R, Yagoda A. Sequential trials of methotrexate, cisplatin and bleomycin for penile cancer. *J Urol* 1984;132(3):465–468.
33. Gagliano RG, Blumenstein BA, Crawford ED, et al. cis-Diamminedichloroplatinum in the treatment of advanced epidermoid carcinoma of the penis: a Southwest Oncology Group Study. *J Urol* 1989;141(1):66–67.
34. Roach M III, Nam J, Gagliardi G, et al. Radiation dose-volume effects and the penile bulb. *Int J Radiat Oncol Biol Phys* 2010;76(3 suppl):S130–S134.
35. Wallner KE, Merrick GS, Benson ML, et al. Penile bulb imaging. *Int J Radiat Oncol Biol Phys* 2002;53(4):928–933.
36. Ekstrom T, Edsmyr F. Cancer of the penis; a clinical study of 229 cases. *Acta Chir Scand* 1958;115(1-2):25–45.
37. Kelley CD, Arthur K, Rogoff E, et al. Radiation therapy of penile cancer. *Urology* 1974;4(5):571–573.
38. Mandler JI, Pool TL. Primary carcinoma of the male urethra. *J Urol* 1966;96(1):67–72.
39. Newaishy GA, Deeley TJ. Radiotherapy in the treatment of carcinoma of the penis. *Br J Radiol* 1968;41(487):519–522.

CHAPTER 32

UTERINE CERVIX

EPIDEMIOLOGY

- The incidence of cervical cancer in 2017 in the United States is estimated to be 12,820, whereas the number of deaths from cervical cancer is estimated to be 4,120 (1).
- Worldwide, cervical cancer is the fourth most common malignancy and the fourth leading cause of cancer death among women, with an estimated 527,624 new cases and 265,672 deaths in 2012 (2).
- Ninety percent of cervical cancer deaths occur in developing countries because of high rates of human papillomavirus (HPV) infection and lack of access to preventative testing and vaccination (2).
- Incidence of cervical cancer in the United States has declined by approximately 65% over the past four decades because of the implementation of screening programs (2).
- Cervical cancer is most commonly diagnosed in the fifth decade of life in the United States (2).
- Risk factors for cervical cancer include: HPV infection with high-risk strains, early onset of sexual activity, history of sexually transmitted diseases, high number of lifetime sexual partners, tobacco exposure, prolonged oral conceptive use, chronic immunosuppression (HIV, systemic lupus erythematosus, and history of organ transplant), micronutrient deficiency, and human leukocyte antigen (HLA) type (3).

ANATOMY

- The uterus is located in the midline of the true pelvis anterior to the rectum and posterior to the bladder. It is attached to surrounding structures by the broad ligament, round ligament, and uterosacral ligaments.
- The cardinal ligaments, also known as the transverse cervical ligaments, arise at the upper lateral margins of the cervix and insert into the pelvic diaphragm.
- The uterus is divided into the uterine corpus and the uterine cervix, which meet at the isthmus of the uterus (Fig. 32-1A) (4).

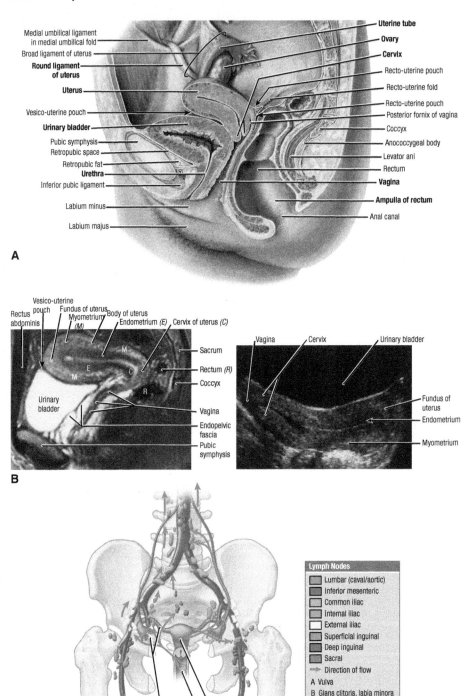

FIGURE 32-1. Pelvic anatomy. **A:** Female pelvic anatomy, median section. **B:** Female reproductive anatomy. **C:** Lymphatic drainage of the pelvis and perineum. (Reprinted with permission from Agur AMR, Dalley AF, eds. *Grant's atlas of anatomy*, 14th ed. Philadelphia, PA: Wolters Kluwer, 2017: 387.)

- The uterus has two orifices, the internal orifice (os), which connects the uterine corpus to the uterine cervix, and the external os, which connects the uterine cervix to the vaginal vault.
- The uterine cervix is divided into the ectocervix and the endocervix. The endocervix (supravaginal component) extends from the internal os to the external os and surrounds the cervical canal. The ectocervix (vaginal component) surrounds the external os and protrudes into the vagina (Fig. 32-1B).
- The ectocervix is lined by nonkeratinizing stratified squamous epithelium, whereas the endocervix is lined by simple columnar mucin-secreting epithelium.
- The ectocervix and endocervix epithelia meet at the squamocolumnar junction known as the transformation zone, where cervical remodeling and metaplasia of columnar to squamous epithelium takes place.
- The arterial supply of the uterine cervix is the uterine artery, which originates from the internal iliac artery.
- Venous drainage occurs via a plexus within the broad ligament that drains to the uterine veins.
- Regional draining lymph node (LN) basins include the paracervical, parametrial, obturator, internal iliac, external iliac, common iliac, and sacral LNs (Fig. 32-1C).

NATURAL HISTORY AND PATTERNS OF SPREAD

- The vast majority of squamous cell carcinomas of the cervix originate within the squamocolumnar junction at the transformation zone. Adenocarcinomas more commonly arise higher in the endocervix.
- Mildly dysplastic cells (LSIL/CIN1) can progress over 10 to 20 years to moderate/severe dysplasia (HSIL/CIN 2 to 3) and carcinoma *in situ* (CIS). Invasive carcinoma occurs once cells have broken through the basement membrane and invaded into the cervical stroma.
- In historical longitudinal analyses of patients diagnosed with CIN2/3 or CIS who were not treated, approximately 40% and 80%, respectively, experienced progression to invasive cervical cancer (5,6).
- The tumor can progress exophytically onto the ectocervix or infiltrate into the endocervix. Local spread can occur to the adjacent vaginal fornices, myometrium of the lower uterine segment and corpus, parametrial tissues, vagina, and pelvic walls. In advanced cases, there can be direct invasion into the bladder, rectum, or both.
- Regional lymphatic or hematogenous spread frequently occurs to the internal iliac, external iliac, presacral, common iliac, and/or paraaortic LN chains.
- Lymphatic vessels drain along three principal routes:
  - Laterally within the broad ligament to the regional and external iliac nodes.
  - Posterolaterally within the transverse cervical ligament to the internal iliac nodes.
  - Posteriorly within the uterosacral ligament to the sacral and common iliac nodes.
  - The external iliac and internal iliac nodes then drain to the common iliac and paraaortic LNs.
- Distant metastatic spread occurs most frequently to the lungs, mediastinal and supraclavicular LN basins, bones, and liver.

CLINICAL PRESENTATION

- The most common presenting symptoms of cervical cancer are abnormal vaginal bleeding, postcoital spotting, and abnormal vaginal discharge.
- Postcoital spotting is an early manifestation that may progress to limited metrorrhagia (intermenstrual bleeding) or menorrhagia (prominent menstrual bleeding).
- If chronic or severe bleeding occurs, the patient may experience fatigue or other symptoms of acute or chronic anemia.
- Pelvic pain may be caused by tumor necrosis or associated pelvic inflammatory disease.
- Pain in the lumbosacral region suggests paraaortic LN involvement with extension into the lumbosacral roots or hydronephrosis.
- Urinary and rectal symptoms (hematuria and rectal bleeding) may occur in patients with advanced stage disease.

SCREENING AND DIAGNOSTIC WORKUP

Human Papillomavirus

- The greatest risk factor for the development of cervical cancer is persistent infection with a high-risk HPV subtype. HPV is detectable in greater than 90% of cervical cancers and its precursor lesions (7).
- There are 19 known high-risk HPV subtypes. Over 70% of cases of cervical cancer are caused by the HPV-16 and HPV-18 subtypes, of which HPV-18 is considered to be more aggressive and more commonly associated with LN involvement and distant metastatic spread (8,9).
  - Other high-risk subtypes include HPV-31, -33, -35, -39, -45, -51, -52, -56, and -58.
- There are 5 known low-risk HPV subtypes. Of these, HPV-6 and HPV-11 are the most common and are associated with genital warts.
  - Other low-risk subtypes include HPV-42, -43, and -44.
- The interaction of viral E6 and E7 proteins with cell cycle–regulating proteins p53 and RB leads to the disruption of normal growth regulatory mechanisms. The E6 oncoprotein binds and inactivates p53, thereby facilitating ubiquitination-mediated degradation. The E7 oncoprotein inactivates RB-mediated inhibition of transcription factor E2F, leading to constitutive activation of E2F and subsequent increased transcription and unregulated progression through the cell cycle.
- There are currently three HPV vaccines licensed in the United States and internationally. The first HPV vaccine was approved in 2006 and covered the HPV-6, -11, -16, and -18 subtypes (10). In 2014, a nonavalent vaccine covering the HPV-6, -11, -16, -18, -31, -33, -45, -52, and -58 subtypes was approved by the U.S. Food and Drug Administration (FDA) (11). These vaccines demonstrated 100% efficacy against HPV subtype–related CIN3 (10).
- The American Cancer Society (ACS) currently recommends vaccination of males and females between the ages of 9 and 26 to protect against HPV infections and potentially prevent a total of 28,500 cases of cervical cancer annually (12).

- Approximately 8% of cervical cancers do not have HPV transcripts. HPV-independent cervical cancer is more common in older women, and these patients have decreased survival compared to their HPV-positive counterparts. HPV-independent cervical cancer may have a distinct gene expression profile including TP53, PI3K, and WNT mutations (13).

Papanicolaou Smear and Screening Guidelines

- Screening for CIS or early invasive carcinomas can be performed using the cytologic Papanicolaou (Pap) smear and HPV testing prior to development of symptoms.
- For average-risk asymptomatic adults, the 2017 ACS recommendations state that cervical cancer screening should begin at age 21 (Table 32-1) (14).
- American Society for Colposcopy and Cervical Pathology (ASCPP) guidelines recommend further workup for patients with abnormal screening tests (15).

Table 32-1

Guidelines for Cervical Cancer Screening for Average-Risk Asymptomatic Adults

Cervical Cancer Screening		
Population	Test	Frequency
Ages 21–29	Pap smear	Every 3 y
Ages 30–65	Pap smear and HPV test	Every 5 y
	Pap smear	Every 3 y
Ages ≥65	Testing not indicated, unless: • History of CIN2 disease in previous 20 y • ≤3 consecutive negative Pap smears and ≤ 2 consecutive negative Pap smears and HPV tests within the last 5 y	
Treatment for Abnormal Screening Tests		
Results	Treatment	Progression[a]
Pap negative, HPV positive	• Undergo repeat cotesting or HPV genotyping in 12 mo. • If results persistent, refer for colposcopy.	
ASCUS	• Reflex HPV cotesting. • If HPV positive, refer colposcopy.	<1%
AGUS	• Colposcopy and endocervical curettage. • Endometrial sampling if over 40 years old.	
LSIL	• Colposcopy followed by repeat cytology in 12 mo.	5%
HSIL/ASC-H	• Colposcopy with excision/ablation of the transformation zone or diagnostic excisional procedure. • Repeat cotesting annually for 2 y.	22%

[a]Progression to invasive cervical cancer if untreated.
AGUS, atypical glandular cells of undetermined significance; ASC-H, atypical squamous cells: cannot exclude high-grade squamous epithelial lesions; ASCUS, atypical squamous cells of undetermined significance; HSIL, high-grade squamous epithelial lesions; LSIL, low-grade squamous intraepithelial lesions.

Physical Exam, Blood Work, and Biopsy (Table 32-2)

- After a general physical examination with special attention to the abdomen, liver, left supraclavicular node (Virchow), left axillary node (Irish), and umbilicus (Sister Mary Joseph), a careful pelvic examination should be performed including bimanual palpation of the pelvis.
- For abnormal Pap smears with lesions that are not clinically visible, colposcopy with biopsy should be performed with endocervical curettage as appropriate. Endometrial sampling should be performed for patients older than 35 years or with symptoms concerning for endometrial neoplasia.

Table 32-2

Diagnostic Workup for Carcinoma of the Uterine Cervix

General
History
Physical examination, including bimanual pelvic and rectal examinations

Diagnostic Procedures
Cytologic smear (Papanicolaou), if not bleeding
Colposcopy and biopsy
Conization, if colposcopy negative
Cystoscopy and rectosigmoidoscopy (stages IIB, III, and IVA)

Staging Studies
FIGO staging:
Physical exam
Colposcopy and cervical biopsy with endocervical curettage ± endometrial sampling
Cold knife conization or loop electrosurgical excision procedure (LEEP)[a]
Punch biopsy (for gross lesions)
Exam under anesthesia
Chest x-ray
Cystoscopy/rectosigmoidoscopy under anesthesia[b]
Skeletal x-ray[c]
Lymphangiogram[c]
Commonly performed if available, but not part of FIGO staging:
Computed tomography[d]
Magnetic resonance imaging
Positron emission tomography

Laboratory Studies
Complete blood cell count (CBC) plus differential
Complete metabolic profile with liver function panel
Urinalysis
HIV testing may be considered

[a]If cervical biopsy is insufficient, conization (preferred) or LEEP can be performed.
[b]If suspected bladder or rectal extension.
[c]Optional studies that may be used for FIGO staging.
[d]Hydronephrosis noted on CT imaging can be used for FIGO staging.

- Conization should be performed if the cervical biopsy is inadequate to define invasion, further assessment of microinvasive carcinoma is required, or when an endocervical tumor is suspected. Cold knife conization is preferred, whereas loop electrosurgical excision procedure (LEEP) may be appropriate if adequate margins and a nonfragmented specimen can be obtained without electrosurgical artifact.
- When a gross lesion of the cervix is present, multiple punch biopsies should be obtained from the margin of any suspicious area, all four quadrants of the cervix, and any suspicious areas in the vagina.
- For invasive carcinoma, patients should have complete peripheral blood evaluation, complete metabolic profile with liver function panel, and urinalysis. HIV testing may be considered.
- Cystoscopy or rectosigmoidoscopy should be performed in patients with suspected bladder or rectal extension.

Imaging

- National Comprehensive Cancer Network (NCCN) recommendations (16)
  - For stage I disease, a chest radiograph (CXR) can be considered. If an abnormality is noted, computed tomography (CT) scan without contrast can be performed.
  - For women interested in fertility-sparing treatment, pelvic magnetic resonance imaging (MRI) scan or transvaginal ultrasound should be performed to assess local disease extent and proximity of disease to the internal os.
  - If disease is found incidentally following total hysterectomy, pelvic MRI may be performed to evaluate for pelvic residual disease, and whole-body positron emission tomography (PET)/CT or CT scan of the chest, abdomen, and pelvis may be performed to evaluate for metastatic disease.
  - For patients with stage IB disease or above, imaging of the urinary tract is required via CT, MRI, or intravenous pyelogram.
  - Imaging studies such as PET/CT and/or MRI are recommended for patients with stage IB2 disease or above for evaluation of nodal or extrapelvic disease.
  - For patients with stage II to IV, whole-body PET/CT or CT scan of the chest, abdomen, and pelvis should be performed.
  - PET/CT is the most sensitive imaging modality for nodal staging, whereas MRI is the most sensitive for detecting parametrial or vaginal involvement.
  - PET/CT and MRI posttreatment have been shown to be predictive of locoregional control and disease-free survival (DFS) (17,18).

STAGING

- Cervical cancer is clinically staged using the International Federation of Gynecology and Obstetrics (FIGO) schema, which enables consistent staging with low-resource countries (19).
- The gynecologic oncologist and radiation oncologist should jointly stage each tumor with bimanual pelvic and rectal examination.

- Surgical staging can be reported using the American Joint Committee on Cancer (AJCC) Tumor-Node-Metastases (TNM) staging schema (20).
- Diagnostic studies:
  - Studies that can be used in FIGO staging include: physical exam, exam under anesthesia, colposcopy, hysteroscopy, cystoscopy, rectosigmoidoscopy, intravenous pyelogram, chest x-ray, and skeletal x-ray.
  - CT, MRI, PET, lymphangiogram, and ultrasound scans, although commonly performed in the United States and used to inform prognosis and treatment decisions, should not be used for FIGO staging. Findings from laparoscopy and/or laparotomy should also not be included in the FIGO stage (21).
  - Hydronephrosis noted on imaging may be used in FIGO staging.
- Staging should ideally be done prior to institution of therapy, but is occasionally postponed until the time of radical hysterectomy or first intracavitary brachytherapy insertion.
- General description of FIGO staging:
  - For lesions that are not clinically visible (stage IA), tumor stage reflects extent of historical spread and depth of invasion of the cervical stroma.
  - Clinically visible lesions confined to the cervix are staged based on size (stage IB1 to IB2).
  - Lesions not confined to the cervix are staged based on extension to involve the parametrial tissues (stage IIB), lower third of the vagina (stage IIIA), pelvic side wall (stage IIIB), or the bladder or rectum (stage IVA).
  - Disease causing hydronephrosis or damage to the kidney is considered stage IIIB.
  - Nodal disease is not incorporated by FIGO staging but is considered to be AJCC stage IIIB.
- Should a disagreement arise regarding clinical staging, the earlier stage should be selected.
- Suspected invasion of the bladder or rectum should be confirmed by biopsy.

Surgical Staging

- For patients with stage IA1 disease without lymphovascular space invasion (LVSI), conservative treatment with conization may be sufficient. Those with evidence of LVSI are recommended to undergo conization with sentinel lymph node (SLN) mapping or pelvic lymphadenectomy.
- Radical hysterectomy with bilateral pelvic lymph node dissection (LND) or SLN mapping is recommended for patients with stage IA2 to IIA1 cancer.

NEW! SUMMARY OF CHANGES TO AJCC STAGING

- N0(i+) is defined as isolated tumor cells in regional LNs smaller than 0.2 mm.

See: Amin MB, Edge SB, Greene FL, et al., eds. *AJCC cancer staging manual*, 8th ed. New York, NY: Springer, 2017.

- Meta-analyses have shown sensitivity of detection by SLN mapping to be 89% to 90% and may reduce the need for pelvic LND (22,23).
- Current NCCN guidelines recommend consideration of SLN mapping for patients with tumors less than 2 cm followed by side-specific nodal dissection in cases of failed mapping or for removal of suspicious or enlarged nodes (16).
- Surgical staging via intraperitoneal or laparoscopic LND may be considered for patients with advanced disease for evaluation of nodal stations before or after chemoradiation (24,25).
- 2016 American Society of Clinical Oncology (ASCO) consensus guidelines recommend paraaortic LN sampling in place of paraaortic LND for patients who meet Sedlis criteria.
- A combined retrospective analysis of Gynecologic Oncology Group (GOG) trials suggested improved prognosis for patients following surgical evaluation of paraaortic LNs compared to radiographic staging alone (26). A randomized controlled trial evaluating PET/CT versus laparoscopic extraperitoneal staging for the evaluation of paraaortic LN involvement is currently ongoing (27).

PATHOLOGIC CLASSIFICATION

- Approximately 80% of cervical cancers are of squamous cell histology, whereas 10% to 20% are adenocarcinomas. Adenocarcinomas are likely to have a higher rate of LN involvement.
- Less common histologies can include: adenosquamous, endometrioid, adenoid cystic, clear cell, glassy cell, small cell, verrucous, or basaloid carcinomas. Primary sarcomas or lymphomas of the cervix have also been reported.
- Adenosquamous carcinoma is relatively rare (2% to 5%) and consists of intermingled epithelial cell cores and glandular structures.
- Adenoid cystic carcinoma is rare (less than 1%) and has a similar appearance to its counterparts in the salivary gland or bronchial tree.
- Glassy cell carcinoma is considered a poorly differentiated adenosquamous tumor with a distinctive histologic appearance. Survival is poor after surgery or irradiation.
- Small cell carcinoma arises from endocervical argyrophil cells. One-third to one-half stain positively for neuroendocrine markers such as chromogranin, serotonin, or somatostatin. Lymphatic and vascular invasion are substantially more common in small cell carcinoma.
- Verrucous carcinoma is a variant of a very well-differentiated squamous cell carcinoma that has a tendency to recur locally, but not to metastasize.
- Basaloid carcinoma (or adenoid basal carcinoma) is extremely rare and is characterized by nests or cords of small basaloid cells.
- Primary sarcomas of the cervix (leiomyosarcoma, rhabdomyosarcoma, stromal sarcoma, and carcinosarcoma) have been described occasionally.
- Malignant primary or secondary lymphomas are sporadically reported. They behave and should be treated as other lymphomas.

PROGNOSTIC FACTORS

Risk of Lymph Node Involvement (Table 32-3)

- Kim et al. (28) constructed a nomogram predicting preoperative risk of LN metastasis from 493 patients with stage IA2 to IIA cervical cancer using age, tumor size, and LN involvement on PET scan.
- In a retrospective analysis of 665 patients with stage IA to IIA cervical cancer who underwent hysterectomy and pelvic LND, younger age, deep stromal invasion, and LVSI were each associated with increased risk of pelvic LN metastasis (29).
- Presence of pelvic LN metastases, primary tumor size greater than 2 cm, and metastasis of the common iliac nodes have been shown to be associated with paraaortic LN involvement (30,31).

Recurrence and Survival

- Overall, LN involvement is the most significant negative prognostic factor for the risk of recurrence and survival for patients without widely metastatic disease, followed by clinical stage, tumor size, and performance status (32–34). Other prognostic factors include LVSI, depth of stromal invasion, histology, and tobacco use.
- Rose et al. generated prognostic nomograms for 2-year progression-free survival (PFS), 5-year overall survival (OS), and risk of pelvic recurrence based on a number of clinicopathologic variables using 2,042 patients with locally advanced cervical cancer limited to the pelvis who were enrolled in Gynecologic Oncology Group clinical trials (33).

Table 32-3
Risk of Lymph Node Involvement and Overall Survival by Stage

FIGO Stage	Pelvic LN	Paraaortic LN	5-Year OS
IA1	0%–5%	<2%	95%
IA2	0%–5%	<2%	93%
IB1	15%	<5%	87%
IB2	30%	10%	70%
IIA	35%–40%	15%	60%
IIB	35%–40%	15%	60%
IIIA	50%–60%	25%–30%	35%–40%
IIIB	50%–60%	25%–30%	35%–40%
IVA	50%–60%	25%–30%	25%–30%
IVB	70%	60%	20%

Percentages derived from National Cancer Database (NCDB) 2004–2014.
LN, lymph node; OS, overall survival.

- Kidd et al. created prognostic nomograms for recurrence-free survival (RFS), disease-specific survival (DSS), and OS using 234 patients with stage IB1 to IVA cervical cancer treated with definitive radiotherapy or concurrent chemoradiotherapy who underwent PET/CT scan at diagnosis. SUV_{max} of the cervical tumor, tumor volume as defined on PET scan, and highest level of LN involvement were utilized to produce a combined prognostic model with more accurate prediction of disease prognosis than models that included FIGO stage, histology, and age (35).
- Kang et al. developed a model for prediction of 5-year distant recurrence for patients with locally advanced cervical cancer using pelvic and paraaortic nodal positivity on PET/CT, nonsquamous cell histology, and pretreatment serum squamous cell carcinoma antigen (36).
- Surrogate markers of tumor hypoxia such as low hemoglobin (Hb) levels have been associated with decreased survival and increased risk of recurrence (37–39). A more recent retrospective cohort analysis, however, revealed no association of Hb with risk of recurrence. Furthermore, a phase II clinical trial evaluating use of recombinant human erythropoietin (rhEPO) in women with stage IIB to IVA cervical cancer with Hb levels between 8.0 and 12.5 demonstrated decreased PFS and OS as well as an increased incidence of deep venous thrombosis compared to historical rates in women who did not receive rhEPO (40,41).

GENERAL MANAGEMENT

- Treatment should involve close collaboration between the gynecologic oncologist and the radiation oncologist, with an integrated team approach vigorously pursued.
- Because of the increased morbidity associated with trimodality therapy, surgical resection is generally reserved for patients with small tumors confined to the cervix and who have a low probability of requiring postoperative radiation or chemoradiation.
- Preinvasive disease is generally treated with excision (conization/LEEP), ablation, total abdominal hysterectomy (TAH), or radical trachelectomy.
- For patients with early-stage disease (IA1 to IB1), treatment options include TAH or definitive radiation (42,43).
- Surgery may be preferred for early-stage patients considered to be at very low risk of needing adjuvant treatment because of shorter treatment time and improved long-term toxicity profile.
  - Patients who undergo hysterectomy should receive adjuvant radiation if found to have at least two of the following three criteria: LVSI, greater than 4 cm disease, or greater than ⅓ invasion into the stroma (Sedlis criteria) (44).
  - If found to have close or positive margins, positive LNs, or microscopic parametrial invasion, adjuvant chemoradiation with or without brachytherapy should be given (Peters criteria) (45–47).
- For stage IB1/IIA1, radical hysterectomy with pelvic LND or definitive external beam radiation therapy (EBRT) with or without concurrent cisplatin-based chemotherapy followed by high-dose rate (HDR) brachytherapy is recommended. Surgery is

generally reserved in this setting for women with smaller lesions or those requesting fertility preservation.

- For stage IB2/IIA2 and above, definitive EBRT with concurrent cisplatin-based chemotherapy followed by HDR brachytherapy is recommended (48,49).
- For patients treated with concurrent chemoradiation followed by brachytherapy, all treatment should be completed within 8 weeks as overall treatment time greater than this has been shown to be associated with decreased survival (50–52). More recent studies, however, have not demonstrated a significant association between overall treatment time and outcomes (53–56).
- Treatment for recurrent or progressive disease is limited and highly dependent on factors including history of prior radiation, centrality of disease within the pelvis, and performance status. Overall, outcomes following local recurrence or disease progression are poor.
- For metastatic disease, treatment with cisplatin/paclitaxel or carboplatin/paclitaxel with or without bevacizumab and individualized recommendations for EBRT is appropriate (57,58).
- Smoking cessation should be counseled in all patients with cervical cancer who are current smokers.

TREATMENT RECOMMENDATIONS BY STAGE (TABLE 32-4)

Carcinoma *In Situ*

- The preferred treatment option for patients with CIS is TAH.
- Fertility-sparing treatment may be offered with therapeutic conization, LEEP, cryotherapy, or radical trachelectomy. For lesions within the endocervical canal, conization should always be performed.
- Definitive radiation can be considered for patients with medical contraindications to surgery or with multifocal CIS.

Stage IA1

- Treatment recommendations for women with stage IA1 disease are based on several factors, including desire for fertility preservation, surgical eligibility, and pathologic findings on cone biopsy. As incidence of LN metastasis for patients with stage IA1 disease is minimal (less than 1%), evaluation of nodal basins is not needed unless there are positive margins or evidence of LVSI.
- For fertility-sparing treatment, specimens from cone biopsy should be evaluated to ensure no foci of invasion beyond 3 mm, LVSI, or dysplasia at the margin.
  - Negative margins, no evidence of LVSI: observation.
  - Positive margins: repeat cone biopsy or radical trachelectomy.
  - Evidence of LVSI: conization or radical trachelectomy with SLN mapping/pelvic LND with or without paraaortic LN sampling, as appropriate.

Table 32-4

Treatment Recommendations by Stage

FIGO Stage	Management
IA1	Negative margins without LVSI: • TAH. • Pelvic EBRT (45 Gy) + HDR brachytherapy (6 Gy × 4 fractions) to >75 EQD$_2$ (Gy). Positive margins or LVSI: • MRH with SLN mapping/pelvic LND. • Pelvic EBRT (45 Gy) + brachytherapy (6 Gy × 4 fractions) to >75 EQD$_2$ (Gy).
IA2	• MRH with SLN mapping/pelvic LND. • Pelvic EBRT (45 Gy) + brachytherapy (6 Gy × 4 fractions) to >75 EQD$_2$ (Gy).
IB1/IIA1	Low risk of needing adjuvant radiation: • MRH with SLN mapping/pelvic LND ± paraaortic sampling.[a] Higher suspicion of adverse features requiring adjuvant radiation: • Chemoradiation[b] + brachytherapy (5.5 Gy × 5 fractions) to 80–85 EQD$_2$ (Gy).
IB2/IIA2	• Chemoradiation + brachytherapy (5.5–6 Gy × 5 fractions) to 80–85 EQD$_2$ (Gy).
IIB-IVA	Without evidence of lymph node involvement: • Chemoradiation ± parametrial boost + brachytherapy (5.5–6 Gy × 5 fractions) to 85–90 EQD$_2$ (Gy). With evidence of lymph node involvement: • Chemoradiation + boost to LN basins ± boost to the parametrium + brachytherapy to 85–90 EQD$_2$ (Gy).
IVB	• Systemic chemotherapy with or without bevacizumab. • EBRT or HDR brachytherapy individualized to the patient may be given for palliative purpose.

EBRT (45 Gy) to the pelvis with concurrent cisplatin-based chemotherapy followed by HDR brachytherapy.
[a]Paraaortic LND may be performed for patients with larger tumors and suspected pelvic node involvement.
[b]Chemoradiation refers to cisplatin-based chemotherapy with concurrent pelvic EBRT to 45 Gy. If concurrent chemotherapy is given with EBRT, 5.5 Gy × 5 Fx should be given for cases with <4 cm residual disease, whereas 6 Gy × 5 Fx should be given for cases with >4 cm residual disease.
EBRT, external beam radiation therapy; EQD$_2$, total equieffective dose in 2-Gy fractions; Gy, gray; LND, lymphadenectomy; LVSI, lymphovascular space invasion; MRH, modified radical hysterectomy; SLN, sentinel lymph node; TAH, total abdominal hysterectomy.

Stage IA2

• Treatment recommendations for women with stage IA2 disease are based on factors including desire for fertility preservation and surgical eligibility.
• Fertility-sparing treatment includes radical trachelectomy and SLN mapping/pelvic LND.

Stages IB and IIA

• Treatment recommendations for women with stage IB and IIA disease include surgery, radiation, or concurrent chemoradiation, depending on tumor size and extent of disease.

- Surgery is considered for select patients with stage IB1/IIA1, whereas concurrent chemoradiation is preferred for patients with stage IB2/IIA2 or evidence of nodal disease (43,46).
- Definitive chemoradiation is preferred over surgical management for tumors above stage IB2 and those that are suspected of needing adjuvant radiation because of increased toxicity with trimodality management (59,60). Adjuvant hysterectomy following chemotherapy or chemoradiation is no longer typically performed because of a lack of evidence supporting survival benefit while increasing morbidity but may be considered for patients with residual disease or uterine anatomy that is unable to be adequately covered by brachytherapy (16,59,61).
- Fertility-sparing surgery may be considered for select patients with IB1 tumors, with consideration of MRI and PET/CT to rule out more extensive local as well as extrapelvic disease.
  - Radical vaginal trachelectomy (less than 2 cm) or abdominal trachelectomy (2 to 4 cm) as well as sentinel LN mapping/pelvic LND with or without paraaortic LN sampling.

Stage IIB to IVB

- Patients eligible for definitive therapy (stage IIB to IVA) should be treated with definitive chemoradiation.
- Patients with very advanced disease (stage IIIB to IVB) for whom definitive therapy is not reasonable should be offered palliative treatment options including palliative radiation, surgery, or chemotherapy, as appropriate.

Recurrent Disease

- Treatment for recurrent disease is dependent on history of previous radiation and distribution of recurrent disease.
  - No prior radiation:
    - Consider surgical resection.
    - EBRT with or without concurrent chemotherapy with or without brachytherapy.
  - Prior radiation with central disease:
    - Size less than 2 cm: radical hysterectomy or definitive brachytherapy.
    - Size greater than 2 cm: pelvic exenteration with or without intraoperative radiation.
  - Prior radiation with noncentral disease:
    - EBRT with or without chemotherapy.
    - Resection with intraoperative radiation or adjuvant EBRT.
    - Consider clinical trial, chemotherapy alone, or palliative care.
- At the time of a second recurrence, palliative treatment options should be discussed, including appropriate clinical trials, chemotherapy, or symptom-directed care.

Small Cell Carcinoma of the Cervix

- Gynecologic Cancer InterGroup (GCIG) consensus review (62).
  - Stage IA to IIA, less than 4 cm: radical hysterectomy and LND followed by chemotherapy using etoposide and cisplatin with or without radiation therapy.
  - Stage IA to IIA, greater than 4 cm: neoadjuvant chemotherapy followed by radical hysterectomy and LND and chemotherapy with etoposide and cisplatin with or without radiation.
  - Stage IIB to IV or nonsurgical candidate: definitive concurrent chemoradiation.
- Radical hysterectomy should be offered only to patients with low probability of requiring adjuvant radiation because of increased toxicity associated with trimodality therapy.
- Etoposide with cisplatin is the most common chemotherapy regimen for small cell carcinoma, although a multidrug regimen consisting of vincristine, adriamycin, and cyclophosphamide alternating with cisplatin and etoposide has also been used (62,63).
- Women with small cell carcinoma of the cervix should not be treated with radical trachelectomy because of the aggressive nature of the disease.
- There is conflicting evidence regarding the benefit of adjuvant chemotherapy for patients with small cell carcinoma of the cervix. Although some studies demonstrated a survival benefit following treatment with adjuvant chemotherapy, others did not (63–65). Future studies with greater homogeneity of the patient population and type of systemic therapy may be of benefit.
- The benefit of radiation either following surgery or with concurrent chemotherapy remains unclear (66–68).

Invasive Cancer Incidentally Diagnosed Following Simple Hysterectomy

- Occasionally, invasive carcinoma is identified on pathologic review of specimens following simple hysterectomy. Treatment recommendations depend on stage, presence of LVSI, and evidence of nodal involvement on imaging.
- NCCN recommendations (16)
  - Stage IA1 disease without evidence of LVSI: surveillance may be offered.
  - Stage IA1 disease with LVSI or greater than stage IA1 disease:
    - Negative surgical margins, no evidence of nodal involvement on imaging:
      - Observation or pelvic EBRT with or without vaginal brachytherapy can be performed, particularly in cases with large primary tumors, deep stromal invasion, or LVSI. Alternatively, a complete parametrectomy, upper vaginectomy, and pelvic LND with or without paraaortic LN sampling can be performed.
    - Positive surgical margins, parametrium, nodal disease, or gross residual disease:
      - Pelvic EBRT with concurrent cisplatin is recommended with consideration of brachytherapy for positive vaginal margins.
      - If imaging is positive for nodal disease, surgical debulking of grossly enlarged LNs (greater than 5 cm) can be performed followed by EBRT with concurrent cisplatin-based chemotherapy with or without brachytherapy.

Chemotherapy Regimens

- Weekly cisplatin or cisplatin plus 5-fluorouracil (5-FU) every 3 to 4 weeks is recommended as concurrent chemotherapy regimens with EBRT (60).
- Consolidation of chemotherapy regimens following concurrent chemoradiation is currently under investigation as part of the OUTBACK (GOG 0274) trial (69–71). A phase III clinical trial comparing concurrent chemoradiation with gemcitabine and cisplatin followed by adjuvant chemotherapy with concurrent chemoradiation with cisplatin alone without adjuvant chemotherapy demonstrated increased survival outcomes with manageable toxicity.
- For stage IV or recurrent disease, cisplatin or carboplatin plus paclitaxel with or without bevacizumab may be considered (72–74).

RADIATION THERAPY

Introduction

- Radiation therapy is a critical component of the standard of care for treatment of cervical cancer, either following hysterectomy for disease with high-risk features or as definitive treatment with concurrent chemoradiation for locally advanced disease.

External Beam Radiation Therapy

- EBRT is utilized to treat the primary tumor, cervix, uterus, local tumor extension, and regional pelvic LNs.

Simulation and Image Fusion

- Prior to simulation, a radiopaque marker may be inserted at the vaginal apex.
- Patients should be immobilized during simulation and treatment to achieve consistent placement of the upper body, trunk, and proximal legs.
- A CT (or MRI) simulation scan with slice thickness no greater than 3 mm should be obtained for treatment planning. Intravenous contrast should be used for vessel delineation. Scans should be performed with both a full and empty bladder to account for potential variability of internal organ motion within the pelvis.
- Relevant imaging studies, including the empty bladder scan, T2-weighted MR scan, and FDG-PET scan, ideally taken in the treatment position, should be fused to the simulation scan.
- The treatment planning CT will be utilized for delineation of the gross tumor volume (GTV), clinical target volume (CTV), internal target volume (ITV), and planning target volume (PTV).

Volume Delineation

- Consensus guidelines for CTV delineation for both definitive and postoperative radiation therapy utilizing intensity-modulated radiation therapy (IMRT) have been published and should be referenced during volume delineation (Table 32-5) (75,76).

Table 32-5

Volume Definitions

	3D Image–Based Treatment Planning
GTV	• Gross disease including extension to the parametria, uterosacral ligaments, and vagina.
CTV1	• GTV + cervix and entire uterus.
CTV2	• Parametria, ovaries, and vaginal tissues. • Minimal or no involvement of the vagina: include upper ½ of the vagina. • Extensive involvement of the vagina: include entire vagina.
CTV3	• Internal iliac, external iliac, common iliac nodal chains and adjacent soft tissues, contoured superiorly to 7 mm below the L4/L5 intervertebral space at the bifurcation of the aorta superiorly and inferiorly to the level of the femoral heads. • Common iliac node involvement: paraaortic nodes should be contoured superiorly to 7 mm below the L1/L2 intervertebral space. • Paraaortic node involvement: paraaortic nodes should be contoured superiorly to 7 mm below the T11/T12 intervertebral space. • The presacral nodal basin should be contoured inferiorly to the level of S3 with 1–2 cm anterior extension from the sacral segments.
ITV	• CTV2 plus vagina and paravaginal tissues on both empty and full bladder scans. • The ITV should include the anterior ⅓–½ of the rectum as well as 1–2 cm of the posterior aspect of the bladder. • The inferior border of the ITV should be at least 1 cm below the obturator foramen and include the proximal 3 cm of the vagina, approximately at the level of the upper ⅓ of the symphysis. • The lateral margin of the ITV should be at the obturator muscle.
PTV	• The PTV should include a 1.5 cm expansion of CTV1 (cervix, uterus), a 1.0 cm of the ITV (parametrium, vaginal tissues), and a 7 mm expansion of CTV3 (lymph nodes).
	GEC-ESTRO Definitions (Brachytherapy)
GTV	• Macroscopic tumor extension at the time of brachytherapy.
HR CTV	• MRI-based: cervix + tumor extension. • CT-based: width of cervix + parametrial extension + suspected GRD.[a]
IR CTV	• Expansion of the HR CTV by 5–15 mm depending on tumor size, location, potential tumor spread, tumor regression, and treatment strategy.

continued

Table 32-5	
Volume Definitions *(continued)*	
	ICRU/GOG Definitions (Brachytherapy)
Point A	• 2 cm superior to the cervical os and 2 cm lateral to the tandem. ABS guidelines currently recommend using the top of the ovoids on 3D imaging. • Corresponds to the paracervical triangle where the uterine vessels cross the ureter.
Point B	• 2 cm superior to the cervical os and 5 cm lateral to the patient midline. • Represents the parametrium and obturator nodes.
Bladder Point	• Posterior surface of a Foley balloon filled with 7 cc of contrast and water.
Rectum Point	• 5 mm posterior to the vaginal wall between the ovoids at the most distal extent of the last tandem source.
Vaginal Surface Point	• Lateral edge of the ovoids on AP films and center of ovoids on lateral films.

[a]If accurate delineation of the cervix is suboptimal, a height of ~3 cm should be contoured. The superior border of the cervix should be at least 1 cm above the uterine vessels or the point at which the uterus begins to enlarge. CTV, clinical target volume; GRD, gross residual disease; GTV, gross tumor volume; HR CTV, high risk; IR, intermediate risk; ITV, internal target volume; PTV, planning target volume.

• Contour delineation should be performed on the full bladder treatment planning scan.
• The GTV is defined as all known gross disease as derived from clinical information, physical exam, CT simulation, MR imaging, and PET scan. No GTV should be delineated for patients receiving radiation following hysterectomy.
• The CTV is defined as the anatomical area considered to be at high risk for microscopic disease and should include the proximal pelvic structures and nodal CTV.
• The ITV is defined as the volume of the vagina and paravaginal tissues present in both the empty and full bladder scans and is utilized to account for internal organ motion.
• The PTV is an expansion from the CTV and ITV to account for interfraction variability of the treatment setup.
• Nodal groups to be covered within the CTV include involved nodes as well as appropriate regional draining basins.
• Normal pelvic structures including the rectum, bladder, sigmoid colon, bowel, and proximal femurs should be delineated as described by the RTOG consensus guidelines (77).

Target Volumes

• The RTOG consensus atlas and current clinical trial protocols should be referenced during volume delineation (http://www.rtog.org) (78,79).
• Given the risk of recurrence within the uterine fundus or corpus, the entire uterus should be included in the CTV (80,81).

- The boundaries of the parametria are as described (75):
  - Anterior: posterior wall of the bladder or of the external iliac vessel.
  - Posterior: uterosacral ligaments and mesorectal fascia.
  - Lateral: medial edge of the internal obturator muscle or ischial ramus bilaterally.
  - Superior: top of the fallopian tube or broad ligament.
  - Inferior: urogenital diaphragm.
- Nodal contours should include the vessel and perinodal tissue, excluding bowel, bone, and muscle. The superior border of the nodal CTV should be approximately 7 mm below the appropriate intervertebral space to account for PTV expansion.
- The obturator nodes should be contoured to include the upper ⅓ of the obturator fossa.

Radiation Treatment Fields

- Traditional pelvic portals
  - Anteroposterior/posteroanterior (AP/PA):
    - Superior: level of L4-L5.
    - Lateral: 1 to 2 cm lateral to the widest true pelvic diameter.
    - Inferior border: at least 4 cm beyond the vaginal cuff below the obturator foramen.
    - Margins of at least 1 cm should be assured beyond the common iliac nodes. The obturator foramina should not be blocked.
  - Lateral:
    - Superior/inferior: identical to AP/PA.
    - Anterior: a line drawn through the symphysis pubis and at least 1 cm anterior to the common iliac nodes at L4-L5.
    - Posterior border: include S3-S4.
    - Anterior small bowel should be shielded, assuring a 1-cm margin from the common and external iliac nodes. The sacrum may be split to assure adequate margin for presacral nodes. The most posterior aspect of the rectum may be blocked.
- Parametrial boost fields
  - AP/PA:
    - Superior: 1 cm superior to the bottom of the sacroiliac joint.
    - Lateral/inferior: identical to pelvic AP/PA fields.
    - Customized midline shielding with a 4- to 5-cm central block should be used to block central high-dose region.
- Paraaortic fields
  - AP/PA:
    - Superior: T11/12 (paraaortic involvement) or L1/L2 (common iliac involvement).
    - Inferior: extending from pelvic field border.
    - Lateral: just outside the transverse processes.
    - The kidneys and bowels should be blocked.
  - Lateral:
    - Superior/inferior: identical to AP/PA fields.
    - Anterior: at least 2 cm anterior to the vertebral body and/or 1 cm anterior to the paraaortic nodal contours.
    - Posterior: at least 1 cm posterior to the paraaortic nodal contours and/or 1 to 1.5 cm into the vertebral body.

Normal Pelvic Structures

- Organs at risk (OARs) should be contoured on the full bladder treatment planning scan (77).
- The anus and rectum should be contoured from the anal verge to the level of the sigmoid flexure as it moves into the anterior pelvis. Full rectal sparing should be avoided because of the high interfraction variability of rectal filling and the concentration of high-risk clinical volume within the adjacent soft tissues, including the presacral nodes, uterosacral ligaments, and internal iliac nodes.
- The sigmoid colon should be contoured from the superior aspect of the anorectum to the connecting point with the ascending colon.
- The bowel should be contoured from the most inferior bowel loop to 2 cm above the PTV. It should include all loops of small and large bowel to the edge of the peritoneum to account for motion.
- The full bladder should be contoured in its entirety.
- The proximal femurs should be contoured from the lowest level of the ischial tuberosities to the top of the ball of the femur including the trochanters.
- The kidneys may be contoured bilaterally, assuring two thirds of each kidney to be outside of the treatment field.
- The spinal cord should be contoured.

Technique

- 3D conformal radiotherapy (3DCRT) using image-guided planning to the whole pelvis typically employs AP/PA and opposed lateral photon fields. Although effective at controlling disease, WPRT results in significant dose delivery to OARs including the rectum, bladder, femoral heads, and occasionally small bowel. This can lead to increased rates of acute and late gastrointestinal and genitourinary toxicity, while also potentially restricting the dose that may safely be delivered to the CTV because of dose constraints.
- IMRT utilizes photon beams of varying intensity across each beam to achieve highly conformal tumor volume coverage while sparing normal tissues. The treatment plan is produced by an automated process called inverse planning to achieve a series of dose-volume constraints and dose limits. IMRT is able to achieve greater conformality of the dose distribution to the target volume, thereby reducing off-target dose to the OARs (82).
- Use of IMRT for whole pelvic radiation has been demonstrated to effectively deliver highly conformal dose to the high-risk clinical volume, including the pelvic LN chains, while achieving significant reduction of dose to normal pelvic organs and spinal cord as compared to treatment plans using 3DCRT (83). Furthermore, IMRT has been shown to improve dose conformity and homogeneity while achieving superior coverage of the target volume as compared with 3DCRT (Fig. 32-2) (84).
- Boosts to the parametria and/or LNs are generally performed sequentially following brachytherapy, but can also be delivered using a simultaneous integrated boost (SIB) technique.

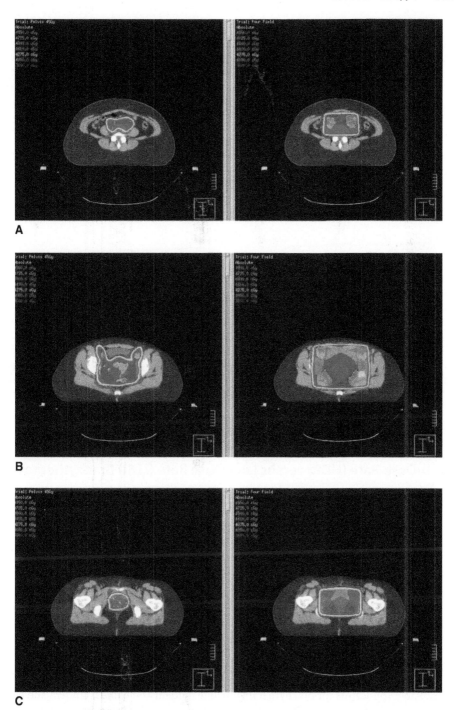

FIGURE 32-2. Representative four-field and intensity-modulated radiotherapy (IMRT) treatment plans for intact cervical cancer patient. **A:** Near level of aortic bifurcation. **B:** At superior aspect of femoral heads. **C:** At level of obturator foramen.

- Among patients treated with whole pelvic radiotherapy, use of IMRT technique has been shown to significantly decrease the rate of acute and chronic gastrointestinal toxicity, hematologic toxicity, and grade 1 to 3 toxicity overall as compared to 3DCRT (39,85–89). A randomized trial comparing 3DCRT versus IMRT with concurrent cisplatin in patients with stage IIB to IIIB squamous cell carcinoma of the cervix demonstrated that IMRT achieved equivalent coverage of the target volume, reduced dose to the OARs, and decreased incidence of acute and chronic gastrointestinal toxicities as compared to 3DCRT treatment plans (90).
- With increased conformality, however, comes increased need for precision in volume delineation. Appropriate margins for creation of the ITV to account for bladder and rectal motion are critical to account for intrafraction and interfraction variability. Image-guided radiation therapy techniques such as cone beam CT and heightened quality assurance protocols are commonly employed to assure accurate dose delivery.

Brachytherapy

- Brachytherapy allows for dose escalation to the cervix and high-risk clinical volume while avoiding delivery of excessive dose to normal pelvic structures.
- Use of brachytherapy in combination with EBRT to the whole pelvis has been shown to be critical in achieving tumor control and increasing survival outcomes (91,92).
- Alternate forms of dose escalation (i.e., stereotactic body radiation therapy [SBRT], protons, IMRT) are not currently recommended as an alternative to brachytherapy for dose escalation.
- Brachytherapy should be started following the initiation of EBRT, ideally prior to stenosis development within the vaginal canal, but following evidence of response to treatment in order to achieve a smaller brachytherapy dose field.

High-Dose Rate (HDR) versus Low-Dose Rate (LDR) Brachytherapy

- LDR brachytherapy delivers iridium-192 (Ir-192) or cesium-37 (Cs-37) via a manually loaded or remote afterloader at a rate of 0.4 to 2 Gy/h over a course of 72 hours while the patient is admitted to the hospital. HDR brachytherapy delivers Ir-192 using a remote afterloader at a rate of greater than 12 Gy/h, typically on an outpatient basis.
- A meta-analysis of retrospective and prospective trials demonstrated statistically equivalent tumor control, survival outcomes, as well as toxicity between LDR and HDR (91,93).
- Use of LDR is declining in favor of HDR because of its increased flexibility of dose distribution, greater reproducibility, decreased exposure to medical personal and ability to the performed on an outpatient basis (94,95).

Applicator Selection and Intraoperative Procedure

- Available applicators for brachytherapy include tandem and ovoids, tandem and ring, tandem and cylinder, tandem and ovoid/ring with guides for interstitial catheters, and interstitial templates.

- Tandem and ovoids are appropriate for patients with a barrel-shaped cervix. The largest ovoid that fits well into the fornices should be used. A cervical flange, when available, can be used to prevent perforation and assure tandem depth.
- Tandem and ring is appropriate for patients with shallow vaginal fornices. It produces a narrower dose distribution than ovoids and can achieve a higher vaginal dose.
- Tandem and cylinder is indicated for patients with upper vaginal stenosis causing inability to place ovoids or ring or for patients with superficial disease involving the lower vagina that is less than 5 mm thick. Tandem and cylinder is associated with higher dose to the bladder and rectum as well as lower dose to the parametrial tissues.
- Tandem and ring/ovoids with short interstitial needles may be appropriate for patients with large, bulky tumors in order to cover the entire cervix while minimizing dose to OARs.
- Interstitial brachytherapy is appropriate for large lesions, suboptimally fitting applicators, gross residual disease involving the sidewall, or lower vaginal involvement greater than 5 mm thick.
- Patients who have not undergone hysterectomy should be treated with a tandem with or without interstitial catheters to adequately dose the superior cervix and uterus.
- The patient should have an absolute neutrophil count of at least 500 mm (3) on the day of applicator placement.
- For HDR cases using tandem and ovoid/ring/cylinder, a Smit sleeve may be placed under general or spinal anesthesia. For subsequent fractions, intravenous conscious sedation, a paracervical block, or oral analgesia may be used. Alternatively, general or spinal anesthesia can be used for each HDR fraction.
- Interstitial needles should be placed under general or spinal anesthesia. Fiducial markers may be placed to help identify location and extent of residual disease.
- Epidural catheter placement is an option for patients who will remain hospitalized for postoperative pain management.
- For LDR cases, each applicator placement should be performed under general, spinal, or epidural anesthesia.
- For tandem and ovoid/ring applicators, anterior and posterior packing or balloons should be used to displace the bladder and rectum from the radiation source.
- Criteria for an adequate implant is based on radiographic criteria (96):
  - The tandem should split the ovoids/ring on AP and lateral images.
  - Ovoids should be symmetrical and not displaced inferiorly from the flange on lateral images. The tandem should be one half to one third of the distance between the symphysis and the sacral promontory.
  - The superior tip of the tandem should be located below the sacral promontory within the pelvis.
  - No packing should be visible superior to the ovoids.
- An analysis of RTOG 0116 and RTOG 0128 demonstrated that improper ovoid positioning was associated with decreased rates of locoregional control and DFS. Inappropriate packing was also associated with decreased DFS (97).

CT Versus MR Imaging for Volume Delineation

- The use of 3D imaging for treatment planning is critical for accurate volume delineation because of the rapid fall-off of dose. Furthermore, 3D imaging allows for better soft tissue delineation of gynecologic tissues as well as OARs compared to 2D imaging.
- In a recent meta-analysis, patients treated with image-based brachytherapy were shown to demonstrate significant improvement in pelvic control and DFS compared to patients treated with ICRU point A specification (98).
- MRI is considered to be the most accurate imaging modality for identifying normal pelvic tissues as well as residual disease.
- In a recent meta-analysis of 13 studies comparing CT- versus MR-based imaging for treatment planning, CT imaging was found to overestimate the width and underestimate the height of the cervix leading to insufficient dose delivered to the HR-CTV (99,100).
- The Groupe Européen Curietherapie-European Society of Therapeutic Radiation Oncology (GEC-ESTRO) has published consensus guidelines for the delineation of clinical target volumes for CT- and MR image–based brachytherapy (101). In a comparison of CT- versus MR-contoured volumes by experts in the field of gynecologic radiation oncology, the mean tumor volume was found to be smaller on MR plans. This difference occurred particularly in cases that involved parametrial extension. The greatest difference between volume delineation using CT- versus MR-based planning occurred in cases with parametrial extension.
- In a comparison of women with locally advanced cervical cancer treated with MR-guided versus CT-guided interstitial brachytherapy, local control and OS rates were significantly increased for patients who underwent MR-guided brachytherapy while toxicity was equivalent (102).
- Tumor volume and rate of regression as determined by sequential MRIs before and during primary therapy have been shown to be predictive of local recurrence and cancer-specific survival (103,104).

Nomenclature for Treatment Volumes and Dose Prescriptions

- In 2005, the ABS and GEC-ESTRO agreed to adopt the GEC-ESTRO guidelines for 3D image–based treatment planning for cervical cancer in the United States (Table 32-5) (105–107).
- The International Commission on Radiation Units and Measurements (ICRU) Report No. 38 defines the dose and volume specifications for reporting intracavitary therapy in gynecologic procedures (108).

Dosimetry

- Cumulative dose prescriptions must be integrated to include dose delivered by EBRT and brachytherapy to assure appropriate target volume coverage (Table 32-6) while meeting constraints for OARs (Table 32-7).
- External radiation using EBRT or IMRT is typically prescribed to a dose of 45 to 50.4 Gy. Brachytherapy dose is dependent on stage, amount of residual

Table 32-6

Dose Prescription Recommendations

Tumor Stage	External Irradiation		HDR Brachytherapy	Total Dose (EQD$_2$)
	EBRT/IMRT	Boost[a]	Fractionation[b,c]	
IA1/IA2, (N0)	45 Gy		6 Gy × 4 Fx	>75 Gy
IB1/IIA1, (N0)	45 Gy		5.5 Gy × 5 Fx	80–85 Gy
IB2/IIA2, (N0)	45 Gy		5.5–6 Gy × 5 Fx[d]	80–85 Gy
IIB-IVA, (N0)	45 –50 Gy	Parametrial boost: total 60–65 Gy	5.5–6 Gy × 5 Fx[d]	85–90 Gy
IA1-IVA, (N1)	45 –50 Gy	Parametrial boost: total 60–65 Gy Gross LN: total 65–70 Gy	5.5–6 Gy × 5 Fx[d]	75–90 Gy

[a]Total dose represents dose from EBRT, any dose from brachytherapy, and additional EBRT boost. Typically, boost doses to achieve these total doses range from 5.4 to 9 Gy for the parametrial boost and 5.4 to 25 Gy for the nodal boost.
[b]Interstitial brachytherapy: fractionation schemes can include 3.5 Gy × 9 Fx, 4.25 Gy × 7 Fx, and 5 Gy × 5 Fx.
[c]Low-dose rate (LDR): 35–45 Gy with a dose rate of 0.4–0.6 Gy/h.
[d]If concurrent chemotherapy is given with EBRT, 5.5 Gy × 5 Fx should be given for cases with <4 cm residual disease, whereas 6 Gy × 5 Fx should be given for cases with >4 cm residual disease.
EBRT, external beam radiation therapy; EQD$_2$, equivalent dose in 2 Gy fractions; Fx, fractions; Gy, gray; HDR, high-dose rate; IMRT, intensity-modulated radiation therapy; LN, lymph node.

disease following EBRT, utilization of concurrent chemotherapy, and technique (Table 32-6).

- Typically, a lower dose per fraction (5.5 Gy) can be used for patients who are receiving concurrent chemotherapy or who have residual disease following EBRT less than 4 cm, whereas a higher dose per fraction (6 Gy) is recommended for patients who are not receiving chemotherapy or who have residual disease following EBRT greater than 4 cm.
- LDR brachytherapy is typically prescribed to a dose of 35 to 45 Gy at a rate of 0.4 to 0.6 Gy/h.
- Fractionation schemes for interstitial brachytherapy can include 3.5 Gy × 9 fractions (Fx), 4.25 Gy × 7 Fx, or 5 Gy × 5 Fx.
- The parametrial boost generally ranges from 5.4 to 9 Gy to achieve a cumulative dose of 60 to 65 Gy.
- The boost to gross LNs generally ranges from 5.4 to 25 Gy using sequential or SIB technique to achieve a total dose of 65 to 70 Gy.
- It is recommended to report dose to point A in addition to DVH parameters (i.e., D$_{90\%}$ to HR-CTV; EQD$_2$) for 3D planning.
- D$_{90\%}$ for HR CTV ≤ 87 Gy has been shown to be associated with an increased risk of local recurrence (4% versus 20%) (109).

Table 32-7

Dose Constraints

Structure	Constraint
HR CTV	$D_{90\%} > 95\%–100\%$ $EQD_2 \geq 80$ Gy, if <4 cm residual disease $EQD_2 = 85–90$ Gy, if >4 cm residual disease
IR CTV	$EQD_2 \geq 60$ Gy
Rectum	Maximum dose < 115% $D_{2cc} < 70–75$ Gy ICRU point < 70 Gy
Sigmoid	$D_{2cc} < 70–75$ Gy
Bowel	Maximum dose < 115% $D_{2cc} < 65$ Gy
Bladder	Maximum dose < 115% $D_{2cc} < 90$ Gy ICRU point < 75 Gy
Femoral heads	Maximum dose < 115%
Spinal cord	Maximum dose < 45 Gy
Bone marrow	$V_{10} < 90\%$ $V_{20} < 75\%$
Vaginal surface	Point dose < 140%–160% of point A (HDR) Total dose < 100–120 Gy (LDR)

D_x, dose (D, Gy) receiving greater than specified percentage or volume of dose (X); D_{2cc}, maximum point dose to volume of 2 cc; Gy: gray; HDR, high-dose rate; HR, high risk; IR, intermediate risk; LDR, low-dose rate; V_x, volume (V, cc, or %) receiving greater than specified dose in Gy (x).

SEQUELAE OF RADIATION THERAPY

- Acute side effects of pelvic irradiation can include fatigue, enteritis (diarrhea, abdominal cramping), proctitis (rectal discomfort or bleeding), cystourethritis (dysuria, frequency), dermatitis (erythema, desquamation within the perineum or intergluteal folds), and vaginitis.
- Late side effects of pelvic irradiation include intestinal, rectal, or vaginal ulcers, rectal or ureteral strictures, hematuria, bladder contracture, necrosis or perforation of the uterus, and vaginal dryness, stenosis, fistulas, or ulcers.
- Late irradiation sequelae are closely related to the total dose, dose per fraction, volume treated, and tissue type.
- Image-guided brachytherapy treatment planning is associated with a significant decrease in grade 3 to 4 toxicity (2.6% versus 22.7%) (110). In the RetroEMBRACE study, the 5-year grade 3 to 5 rates of bladder, gastrointestinal, and vaginal toxicity following image-guided brachytherapy were 5%, 7%, and 5%, respectively (111).

- An analysis from the EMBRACE study demonstrated significant associations between the D2cc, D0.1cc, and dose-point parameters with the probability of rectal toxicity. D2cc ≥ 65 Gy was associated with significantly increased risk of proctitis, whereas D2cc ≥ 75 Gy was associated with a significantly increased risk of fistula at 3 years (112).
- The actuarial probability of grade 3 vaginal morbidity in the EMBRACE study was found to be 3.6%, whereas mild and moderate vaginal symptoms were 89% (grade 1) and 29% (grade ≥ 2), respectively (113).
- D2cc ≥ 95 Gy was associated with significantly increased rates of grade 2 to 4 bladder toxicity (114).
- An analysis of 73 women ≥70 years old treated with concurrent chemoradiation followed by HDR brachytherapy demonstrated that rates of grade 3 to 4 acute hematologic, gastrointestinal, and urinary toxicity were 31.5%, 19.1%, and 12.3%, respectively, whereas rates of grade 3 to 4 chronic gastrointestinal and genitourinary toxicities were 4.1% and 2.7%, respectively (115).
- A retrospective analysis of the EMBRACE study reported an overall incidence of pelvic insufficiency fractures to be 20% (116). The majority of fractures were located in the sacrum (77%). Age over 50 years, the sacrum D50%, and the dose and volume associated with radiation of the elective CTV were associated with incidence of fractures. Risk of fracture decreased from 45% to 22% when the sacrum EQD$_2$ was decreased from 40 to 35 Gy.
- Use of a vaginal dilator one to two times per week starting 2 to 4 weeks after radiotherapy has been shown to significantly decrease the incidence of vaginal stenosis (117).

CARCINOMA OF THE CERVIX AND PREGNANCY

- The concurrent presence of CIS or invasive carcinoma of the uterine cervix and pregnancy, although rare, poses a therapeutic dilemma.
- Cervical cancer is the most common gynecologic malignancy diagnosed during pregnancy (118). Approximately 1% to 3% of women diagnosed with cervical cancer will be pregnant or peripartum at the time of diagnosis (119).
- According to a retrospective review of women at Brigham and Women's Hospital and Massachusetts General Hospital diagnosed with cervical cancer while pregnant, the majority were found to be stage IB1, and the mean gestational age at diagnosis was 17.4 weeks (120).
- A pregnant woman diagnosed with cervical cancer must decide whether to delay treatment until fetal maturity or to proceed with treatment.
- For patients with stage IB1 disease or greater, a chest x-ray and MRI are recommended for complete staging.
- Laparoscopic lymphadenectomy for the evaluation of LN status can safely be performed between the 13th and 22nd weeks of pregnancy without adverse fetal outcomes and is recommended for women with stage IA2 disease or greater (121,122).

Management

- Currently, there are no guidelines for management of cervical cancer in pregnant women within the United States; consensus guidelines are available, however, from the European Society for Gynecological Oncology (122).
- Factors influencing treatment recommendations will include gestational age, stage of disease at diagnosis, and patient preferences.
- Women at a gestational age of greater than 22 to 25 weeks diagnosed with stage IA and IB1 tumors less than 2 cm can delay treatment until delivery. If progression of disease is observed, early delivery or neoadjuvant chemotherapy should be recommended.
- Women who elect to delay treatment should undergo delivery by cesarean section and may undergo concurrent radical hysterectomy and pelvic node dissection.
- If possible, elective surgery should be postponed until the second trimester because of the increased risk of miscarriage associated with surgery in the first trimester.
- If at a gestational age earlier than 22 weeks, women with stage IA1 disease may be managed by conization. Women with stage IA2 and IB1 tumors may be considered for simple trachelectomy or large conization.
- Several case reports have described conization or radical trachelectomy with preservation of pregnancy for women with early-stage cervical cancer (123–126). Other reports, however, have described an approximately 32% risk of pregnancy loss following radical trachelectomy. Large conization is associated with a 19.1% risk of pregnancy loss, which may be improved with cerclage.
- Neoadjuvant chemotherapy may be considered until fetal maturity is reached for women with a stage IB1 tumor larger than 2 cm with negative pelvic LNs or for women with stage IB2 or greater disease.
- Preferred neoadjuvant chemotherapy regimens are platinum-based, preferably with paclitaxel (127).
- Women found to have positive LNs should be counseled to undergo termination of the pregnancy and receive stage-appropriate treatment.
- For women who elect to terminate the pregnancy and pursue definitive radiation therapy with or without concurrent chemotherapy, whole pelvic radiotherapy should be recommended. A spontaneous abortion will generally occur followed by involution of the uterus. Following completion of radiation, careful evacuation of the uterus and intracavitary insertion may be performed under general anesthesia.

Outcomes in Pregnant Patients

- The risk of recurrence in pregnant patients with early-stage cervical cancer who delay treatment is reported to be approximately 5%.
- In a retrospective analysis of 76 women with stage IB1 cervical cancer who delayed treatment, there was a reported 95% survival rate at a median follow-up of 37.5 months (128). There were no reported recurrences in patients with biopsy-proven negative involvement of LNs.
- In a retrospective analysis of pregnant versus nonpregnant women diagnosed with cervical cancer, there was a trend toward decreased survival among pregnant women

(89.3% versus 98.1%, p = 0.09). Of the patients who died, however, none had delayed cancer treatment. Of the 28 pregnant women evaluated in this analysis, 21 did not terminate the pregnancy and delivered at a mean gestational age of 36.1 weeks with a mean birthweight of 2,820 g (120).

- Of the 47 women who received neoadjuvant chemotherapy in order to achieve fetal maturity, 67.4% of neonates were safely delivered with a median weight of 2,213 g. Complete or partial response was achieved in 73.4% of patients, whereas 3.3% experienced progression of disease (127).
- Higher recurrence rates and worse OS have been reported for pregnant women with cervical cancer who undergo vaginal delivery as compared to cesarean delivery (129).
- Radical hysterectomy at the time of cesarean delivery has been demonstrated to be associated with increased blood loss compared to radical hysterectomy postpartum (130).

CARCINOMA OF THE CERVICAL STUMP

- Carcinoma of the cervical stump may occur following subtotal hysterectomy.
- The natural history of carcinoma of the cervical stump is similar to that of the cervix in the intact uterus. The diagnostic workup, clinical staging, and basic principles of therapy are also the same.
- Surgical management may be more difficult because of the history of prior surgeries and presence of pelvic adhesions.
- The lack of a uterine cavity can make insertion of a tandem more difficult.
- Occasionally, transvaginal irradiation may be used to boost the dose delivered to central disease located on the cervical stump.
- If bulky disease is present in the cervix, parametrium, or vagina, additional interstitial therapy should be recommended.
- Because of the close proximity of the intracavitary source to the bladder, rectum, and small intestine in patients posthysterectomy, the rate of complications may be more frequent than that seen in cases with an intact uterus.

SEMINAL RANDOMIZED CLINICAL TRIALS

Summary

- For patients with early-stage disease (stage IB to IIA), survival and recurrence outcomes are equivalent between hysterectomy (with adjuvant radiation as needed) and definitive radiation (42,43).
- Adjuvant pelvic EBRT following hysterectomy increases PFS and decreases risk of locoregional recurrence (LRR) in patients who have two or more of the following criteria: (a) greater than ⅓ stromal invasion, (b) LVSI, and (c) tumor size greater than 4 cm (Sedlis criteria) (44,131). These patients are considered "intermediate risk."
- Adjuvant pelvic EBRT with concurrent chemotherapy with or without vaginal brachytherapy following hysterectomy and pelvic LND increases OS in patients with

at least one of the following criteria: (a) positive pelvic nodes, (b) positive surgical margins, and (c) positive parametrium (Peters criteria) (46,132). These patients are considered "high risk."
- Neoadjuvant chemotherapy and/or radiation prior to hysterectomy are not associated with a recurrence or survival benefit (133,134).
- For patients with stage IB2 disease and above, concurrent chemoradiation with cisplatin is associated with decreased LRR and increased PFS and OS compared to radiation alone (135,136).
- Neoadjuvant chemotherapy with or without radiation prior to hysterectomy is inferior to concurrent chemoradiation (59).
- For metastatic or recurrent disease, outcomes are equivalent between cisplatin/paclitaxel and carboplatin/paclitaxel (57). The addition of bevacizumab to cisplatin/paclitaxel is associated with increased OS (47).

Definitive Radiation Therapy Versus Surgery for Early-Stage Cervical Cancer

- Landoni et al.: Radical hysterectomy versus definitive radiation therapy in stage IB to IIA cervical cancer (42,43).
  - *Patients*: 343 women with clinical stage IB or IIA cervical cancer.
  - *Methods*: Phase III randomized trial (1986–1991) comparing radical hysterectomy plus pelvic LND versus EBRT followed by LDR brachytherapy (median total dose of 76 Gy to point A). Paraaortic nodes were included in the radiation treatment field in cases of nodal involvement to 45 Gy. Women who underwent surgery received adjuvant radiation (50.4 Gy/28 fractions) if found to have surgical stage greater than pT2a, less than 3 mm of uninvolved cervical stroma, or LN involvement.
  - *Findings*: At 20-year follow-up, there was not a significant difference in OS (72% [surgery] versus 77%) or local recurrence (28% versus 28%) between treatment groups. Significant risk factors for survival on multivariate analysis included histology, tumor size, and LN status. Morbidity was significantly increased in the surgical arm. Women with adenocarcinoma trended toward increased survival with surgery (71% versus 47%, $p = 0.09$). A large number of patients (64%) required adjuvant radiation following surgery. Grade 2 to 3 morbidity was significantly higher in the surgery arm (28% versus 12%).
  - *Conclusion*: Hysterectomy and definitive radiation have equivalent survival and recurrence outcomes for women with early-stage cervical cancer. Morbidity is increased following surgery and approximately two thirds of patients required adjuvant radiation.

Adjuvant Therapy after Radical Hysterectomy

- GOG 92: Adjuvant radiation versus observation in stage IB cervical cancer with poor prognostic features (44,131).
  - *Patients*: 277 women with stage IB cervical cancer who underwent radical hysterectomy and found to have negative nodes but at least two of the following risk factors: LVSI, greater than 4-cm primary tumor, and greater than ⅓ stromal invasion.

- *Methods*: Phase III randomized trial (1988–1995) comparing observation versus pelvic EBRT (46 to 50.4 Gy in 28 fractions).
- *Findings*: At 12-year follow-up, radiation was associated with a significant reduction in local recurrence (13.9% versus 20.7%), distant recurrence (2.9% versus 8.6%), and a significant increase in PFS (78.1% versus 65.0%). There was a trend toward increased OS in the EBRT treatment group (28.6% versus 19.7%, $p = 0.07$). Risk of local recurrence was most significantly decreased in adenocarcinomas and adenosquamous carcinomas when treated with adjuvant radiation (44% versus 8.8%).
- *Conclusion*: Adjuvant radiation decreases risk of local or distant recurrence and increases OS benefit in patients with at least two risk factors (Sedlis criteria).
- GOG 109 (SWOG 87-97): Adjuvant concurrent chemoradiation versus radiation in high-risk stage IA2 to IIA cervical cancer (46).
  - *Patients*: 268 women with stage IA2 to IIA cervical cancer who underwent radical hysterectomy and pelvic LND and found to have positive pelvic LNs, positive margins, or microscopic involvement of the parametrium.
  - *Methods*: Phase III randomized trial (1991–1996) comparing concurrent chemoradiation (cisplatin and 5-FU) versus radiation alone (49.3 Gy in 29 fractions).
  - *Findings*: At 4-year follow-up, concurrent chemoradiation was associated with a significant increase in PFS (80% versus 63%) and OS (81% versus 71%). Rates of grade 3 and 4 hematologic and gastrointestinal toxicity were increased with concurrent chemoradiation. Chemoradiation did not increase survival for women with tumors less than 2 cm and only one positive node compared to radiation alone.
  - *Conclusion*: Concurrent chemoradiation increases PFS and OS in patients with positive pelvic nodes, margins, or involvement of the parametrium (Peters criteria).

Definitive Concurrent Chemoradiation Versus Radiotherapy Alone

- RTOG 90-01: Definitive concurrent chemoradiation versus extended field radiation therapy (EFRT) (135).
  - *Patients*: 228 women with stage IIB to IVA cancer or stage IB to IIA cancer either greater than 5 cm or with positive pelvic LN involvement.
  - *Methods*: Phase III randomized trial (1990–1997) comparing EFRT (with coverage of the paraaortic LN chain to L1/L2) without chemotherapy versus definitive concurrent chemoradiation with cisplatin and 5-FU. Radiation in both arms included brachytherapy prescribed to a dose of 85 Gy at point A.
  - *Findings*: At 8-year follow-up, concurrent chemoradiation was associated with significantly increased OS (67% versus 41%) and DFS (61% versus 36%), and significantly decreased locoregional failure (18% versus 35%) and distant metastasis (20% versus 35%). The greatest benefit from concurrent therapy was seen in patients with stage IB to IIB disease. There was no noted difference in late treatment-related side effects.
  - *Conclusions*: Definitive concurrent chemoradiation is associated with significantly decreased risk of local and regional recurrence as well as significantly increased DFS and OS.

- Meta-analysis (Green et al.) of trials evaluating concurrent chemoradiation versus radiation (136).
  - *Patients*: 3,656 women with stage IB to IVA cervical cancer.
  - *Methods*: Meta-analysis of 19 randomized clinical trials comparing concurrent chemoradiation versus radiotherapy. Patients were not excluded if they underwent surgery or received adjuvant chemotherapy.
  - *Findings*: Concurrent chemoradiation was significantly associated with increased OS (52% versus 40%), PFS (63% versus 47%), local recurrence, and distant recurrence. Survival benefit was greatest in trials that enrolled a high proportion of stage I and II patients. Grade 3 to 4 hematologic (5.6% versus 3.8%) or gastrointestinal (9% versus 4%) toxicity was increased with concurrent chemoradiation. Patients who were most likely to benefit from chemoradiation had involved pelvic LNs, large cervical lesions, or stage IB to IIB disease.
  - *Conclusion*: Definitive concurrent chemoradiation is associated with significantly decreased risk of LRR as well as increased OS and PFS.

Chemotherapy Regimens

- GOG 120: Cisplatin-based regimens versus hydroxyurea chemotherapy with concurrent radiation (60,137).
  - *Patients*: 526 patients with stage IIB to IVA cervical cancer without evidence of nodal involvement.
  - *Methods*: Phase III randomized trial (1992–1997) comparing cisplatin versus cisplatin/5-FU/hydroxyurea versus hydroxyurea with concurrent EBRT (40.8 to 51 Gy/24 to 30 fractions) followed by 30 to 40 Gy intracavitary brachytherapy to a total dose to point A of approximately 81 Gy.
  - *Findings*: At 10-year follow-up, patients receiving cisplatin-based regimens had significantly increased PFS (46% versus 26%) and OS (53% versus 34%), as well as decreased risk of LRR (22% versus 34%).
  - *Conclusion*: The greatest benefit from concurrent chemoradiation is seen with cisplatin-based regimens. Cisplatin-based regimens are also better tolerated than those involving hydroxyurea.
- GOG 240: Benefit of bevacizumab in combination chemotherapy in metastatic or recurrent disease (47).
  - *Patients*: 452 patients with stage IVB, recurrent, or persistent cervical cancer.
  - *Methods*: Phase III randomized trial (2009–2012) comparing cisplatin/paclitaxel and topotecan/paclitaxel with or without bevacizumab.
  - *Findings*: In a pooled analysis, patients who received bevacizumab had increased OS (17.0 versus 13.3 months). Topotecan/paclitaxel was noninferior to cisplatin/paclitaxel. Bevacizumab was associated with increased toxicity, but quality of life was not statistically different.
  - *Conclusion*: The addition of bevacizumab to paclitaxel and either cisplatin or topotecan is associated with improved outcomes in metastatic or recurrent disease.

- Meta-analysis (Lorusso et al.) of trials evaluating cisplatin/paclitaxel versus carboplatin/paclitaxel in metastatic or recurrent disease (57).
  - *Patients*: 1,181 women with stage IVB, recurrent, or persistent cervical cancer.
  - *Methods*: Meta-analysis of 17 randomized clinical trials comparing cisplatin/paclitaxel and carboplatin/paclitaxel.
  - *Findings*: There was no significant difference in the risk of recurrence (48.5% [cisplatin/paclitaxel] versus 49.3%) or median OS (12.9 versus 10.0 months).
  - *Conclusion*: Carboplatin/paclitaxel and cisplatin/paclitaxel are largely equivalent regimens in metastatic or recurrent disease.

Clinical Trials

- Awaiting data maturity
  - OUTBACK (GOG 0274) [NCT01414608]: A phase III trial of adjuvant chemotherapy as primary treatment for locally advanced cervical cancer compared to chemoradiation alone: the OUTBACK trial.
  - GOG 0179 [NCT00003945]: Randomized phase III study of cisplatin versus cisplatin plus topotecan versus MVAC in stage IVB, recurrent, or persistent squamous cell carcinoma of the cervix.
  - MD Anderson Cancer Center [NCT01365156]: A phase III randomized study of pretherapeutic paraaortic lymphadenectomy in women with locally advanced cervical cancer dispositioned to definitive chemoradiotherapy.
  - TIME-C (RTOG 1203) [NCT01672892]: A randomized phase III study of standard versus IMRT pelvic radiation for postoperative treatment of endometrial and cervical cancer.

References

1. Siegel RL, Miller KD, Jemal A. Cancer Statistics, 2017. *CA Cancer J Clin* 2017;67(1):7–30.
2. Torre LA, Bray F, Siegel RL, et al. Global cancer statistics, 2012. *CA Cancer J Clin* 2015;65(2):87–108.
3. International Collaboration of Epidemiological Studies of Cervical Cancer. Comparison of risk factors for invasive squamous cell carcinoma and adenocarcinoma of the cervix: collaborative reanalysis of individual data on 8,097 women with squamous cell carcinoma and 1,374 women with adenocarcinoma from 12 epidemiological studies. *Int J Cancer* 2007;120(4):885–891.
4. Agur A, Dalley A. *Grant's atlas of anatomy*, 14th ed. Philadelphia, PA: Wolters Kluwer, 2016.
5. Kottmeier HL. The development and treatment of epitheliomas. *Rev Fr Gynecol Obstet* 1961;56:821–826.
6. Petersen O, Wiklund E. Further studies on the spontaneous course of cervical precancerous conditions. *Acta Radiol Suppl* 1959;188:210–215.
7. National Institutes of Health Consensus Development Conference statement on cervical cancer. April 1–3, 1996. *Gynecol Oncol* 1997;66(3):351–361.
8. Munoz N, Bosch FX, de Sanjose S, et al. Epidemiologic classification of human papillomavirus types associated with cervical cancer. *N Engl J Med* 2003;348(6):518–527.
9. Clifford GM, Smith JS, Aguado T, et al. Comparison of HPV type distribution in high-grade cervical lesions and cervical cancer: a meta-analysis. *Br J Cancer* 2003;89(1):101–105.
10. FUTURE II Study Group. Quadrivalent vaccine against human papillomavirus to prevent high-grade cervical lesions. *N Engl J Med* 2007;356(19):1915–1927.

11. Petrosky E, Bocchini JA Jr, Hariri S, et al. Use of 9-valent human papillomavirus (HPV) vaccine: updated HPV vaccination recommendations of the advisory committee on immunization practices. *MMWR Morb Mortal Wkly Rep* 2015;64(11):300–304.

12. Saslow D, Andrews KS, Manassaram-Baptiste D, et al. Human papillomavirus vaccination guideline update: American Cancer Society guideline endorsement. *CA Cancer J Clin* 2016;66(5):375–385.

13. Banister CE, Liu C, Pirisi L, et al. Identification and characterization of HPV-independent cervical cancers. *Oncotarget.* 2017;8(8):13375-13386.

14. Smith RA, Andrews KS, Brooks D, et al. Cancer screening in the United States, 2017: a review of current American Cancer Society guidelines and current issues in cancer screening. *CA Cancer J Clin* 2017;67(2):100–121.

15. Massad LS, Einstein MH, Huh WK, et al. 2012 Updated consensus guidelines for the management of abnormal cervical cancer screening tests and cancer precursors. *J Low Genit Tract Dis* 2013;17(5 Suppl 1):S1–S27.

16. National Cancer Center Network. Cervical Cancer (Version 1.2017). http://www.nccn.org/professionals/physician_gls/pdf/cervical.pdf. Accessed August 27, 2017.

17. Herrera FG, Breuneval T, Prior JO, et al. [(18)F]FDG-PET/CT metabolic parameters as useful prognostic factors in cervical cancer patients treated with chemo-radiotherapy. *Radiat Oncol* 2016;11:43.

18. Kim JY, Byun SJ, Kim YS, et al. Disease courses in patients with residual tumor following concurrent chemoradiotherapy for locally advanced cervical cancer. *Gynecol Oncol* 2017;144(1):34–39.

19. FIGO staging for carcinoma of the vulva, cervix, and corpus uteri. *Int J Gynaecol Obstet* 2014;125(2):97–98.

20. Edge S, Byrd D, Compton C, et al. *AJCC cancer staging manual,* 7th ed. France: Springer, 2010.

21. Sharma DN, Thulkar S, Goyal S, et al. Revisiting the role of computerized tomographic scan and cystoscopy for detecting bladder invasion in the revised FIGO staging system for carcinoma of the uterine cervix. *Int J Gynecol Cancer* 2010;20(3):368–372.

22. Lecuru F, Mathevet P, Querleu D, et al. Bilateral negative sentinel nodes accurately predict absence of lymph node metastasis in early cervical cancer: results of the SENTICOL study. *J Clin Oncol* 2011;29(13):1686–1691.

23. Wu Y, Li Z, Wu H, et al. Sentinel lymph node biopsy in cervical cancer: a meta-analysis. *Mol Clin Oncol* 2013;1(6):1025–1030.

24. Kohler C, Mustea A, Marnitz S, et al. Perioperative morbidity and rate of upstaging after laparoscopic staging for patients with locally advanced cervical cancer: results of a prospective randomized trial. *Am J Obstet Gynecol* 2015;213(4):503.e501–507.e501.

25. Marnitz S, Martus P, Kohler C, et al. Role of Surgical Versus Clinical Staging in Chemoradiated FIGO Stage IIB-IVA Cervical Cancer Patients-Acute Toxicity and Treatment Quality of the Uterus-11 Multicenter Phase III Intergroup Trial of the German Radiation Oncology Group and the Gynecologic Cancer Group. *Int J Radiat Oncol Biol Phys* 2016;94(2):243–253.

26. Gold MA, Tian C, Whitney CW, et al. Surgical versus radiographic determination of paraaortic lymph node metastases before chemoradiation for locally advanced cervical carcinoma: a Gynecologic Oncology Group Study. *Cancer* 2008;112(9):1954–1963.

27. Frumovitz M, Querleu D, Gil-Moreno A, et al. Lymphadenectomy in locally advanced cervical cancer study (LiLACS): phase III clinical trial comparing surgical with radiologic staging in patients with stages IB2-IVA cervical cancer. *J Minim Invasive Gynecol* 2014;21(1):3–8.

28. Kim DY, Shim SH, Kim SO, et al. Preoperative nomogram for the identification of lymph node metastasis in early cervical cancer. *Br J Cancer* 2014;110(1):34–41.

29. Li X, Yin Y, Sheng X, et al. Distribution pattern of lymph node metastases and its implication in individualized radiotherapeutic clinical target volume delineation of regional lymph nodes in patients with stage IA to IIA cervical cancer. *Radiat Oncol* 2015;10:40.

30. Huang H, Liu J, Li Y, et al. Metastasis to deep obturator and para-aortic lymph nodes in 649 patients with cervical carcinoma. *Eur J Surg Oncol* 2011;37(11):978–983.

31. Shim SH, Kim DY, Lee SJ, et al. Prediction model for para-aortic lymph node metastasis in patients with locally advanced cervical cancer. *Gynecol Oncol* 2017;144(1):40–45.

32. Stehman FB, Bundy BN, DiSaia PJ, et al. Carcinoma of the cervix treated with radiation therapy. I. A multi-variate analysis of prognostic variables in the Gynecologic Oncology Group. *Cancer* 1991;67(11):2776–2785.

33. Rose PG, Java J, Whitney CW, et al. Nomograms predicting progression-free survival, overall survival, and pelvic recurrence in locally advanced cervical cancer developed from an analysis of identifiable prognostic factors in patients from NRG Oncology/Gynecologic Oncology Group randomized trials of chemoradiotherapy. *J Clin Oncol* 2015;33(19):2136–2142.

34. Kidd EA, Siegel BA, Dehdashti F, et al. Lymph node staging by positron emission tomography in cervical cancer: relationship to prognosis. *J Clin Oncol* 2010;28(12):2108–2113.

35. Kidd EA, El Naqa I, Siegel BA, et al. FDG-PET-based prognostic nomograms for locally advanced cervical cancer. *Gynecol Oncol* 2012;127(1):136–140.

36. Kang S, Nam BH, Park JY, et al. Risk assessment tool for distant recurrence after platinum-based concurrent chemoradiation in patients with locally advanced cervical cancer: a Korean gynecologic oncology group study. *J Clin Oncol* 2012;30(19):2369–2374.

37. Grogan M, Thomas GM, Melamed I, et al. The importance of hemoglobin levels during radiotherapy for carcinoma of the cervix. *Cancer* 1999;86(8):1528–1536.

38. Girinski T, Pejovic-Lenfant MH, Bourhis J, et al. Prognostic value of hemoglobin concentrations and blood transfusions in advanced carcinoma of the cervix treated by radiation therapy: results of a retrospective study of 386 patients. *Int J Radiat Oncol Biol Phys* 1989;16(1):37–42.

39. Brixey CJ, Roeske JC, Lujan AE, et al. Impact of intensity-modulated radiotherapy on acute hematologic toxicity in women with gynecologic malignancies. *Int J Radiat Oncol Biol Phys* 2002; 54(5):1388–1396.

40. Mountzios G, Aravantinos G, Alexopoulou Z, et al. Lessons from the past: long-term safety and survival outcomes of a prematurely terminated randomized controlled trial on prophylactic vs. hemoglobin-based administration of erythropoiesis-stimulating agents in patients with chemotherapy-induced anemia. *Mol Clin Oncol* 2016;4(2):211–220.

41. Lavey RS, Liu PY, Greer BE, et al. Recombinant human erythropoietin as an adjunct to radiation therapy and cisplatin for stage IIB-IVA carcinoma of the cervix: a Southwest Oncology Group study. *Gynecol Oncol* 2004;95(1):145–151.

42. Landoni F, Colombo A, Milani R, et al. Randomized study between radical surgery and radiotherapy for the treatment of stage IB-IIA cervical cancer: 20-year update. *J Gynecol Oncol* 2017; 28(3):e34.

43. Landoni F, Maneo A, Colombo A, et al. Randomised study of radical surgery versus radiotherapy for stage Ib-IIa cervical cancer. *Lancet* 1997;350(9077):535–540.

44. Rotman M, Sedlis A, Piedmonte MR, et al. A phase III randomized trial of postoperative pelvic irradiation in Stage IB cervical carcinoma with poor prognostic features: follow-up of a gynecologic oncology group study. *Int J Radiat Oncol Biol Phys* 2006;65(1):169–176.

45. Monk BJ, Wang J, Im S, et al. Rethinking the use of radiation and chemotherapy after radical hysterectomy: a clinical-pathologic analysis of a Gynecologic Oncology Group/Southwest Oncology Group/Radiation Therapy Oncology Group trial. *Gynecol Oncol* 2005;96(3):721–728.

46. Peters WA III, Liu PY, Barrett RJ II, et al. Concurrent chemotherapy and pelvic radiation therapy compared with pelvic radiation therapy alone as adjuvant therapy after radical surgery in high-risk early-stage cancer of the cervix. *J Clin Oncol* 2000;18(8):1606–1613.

47. Tewari KS, Sill MW, Long HJ III, et al. Improved survival with bevacizumab in advanced cervical cancer. *N Engl J Med* 2014;370(8):734–743.

48. Stehman FB, Ali S, Keys HM, et al. Radiation therapy with or without weekly cisplatin for bulky stage 1B cervical carcinoma: follow-up of a Gynecologic Oncology Group trial. *Am J Obstet Gynecol* 2007;197(5):503.e501–503.e506.

49. Chemoradiotherapy for Cervical Cancer Meta-Analysis Collaboration. Reducing uncertainties about the effects of chemoradiotherapy for cervical cancer: a systematic review and meta-analysis of individual patient data from 18 randomized trials. *J Clin Oncol* 2008;26(35):5802–5812.

50. Girinsky T, Rey A, Roche B, et al. Overall treatment time in advanced cervical carcinomas: a critical parameter in treatment outcome. *Int J Radiat Oncol Biol Phys* 1993;27(5):1051–1056.

51. Perez CA, Grigsby PW, Castro-Vita H, et al. Carcinoma of the uterine cervix. I. Impact of prolongation of overall treatment time and timing of brachytherapy on outcome of radiation therapy. *Int J Radiat Oncol Biol Phys* 1995;32(5):1275–1288.

52. Chen SW, Liang JA, Yang SN, et al. The adverse effect of treatment prolongation in cervical cancer by high-dose-rate intracavitary brachytherapy. *Radiother Oncol* 2003;67(1):69–76.

53. Tergas AI, Neugut AI, Chen L, et al. Radiation duration in women with cervical cancer treated with primary chemoradiation: a population-based analysis. *Cancer Invest* 2016;34(3):137–147.

54. Huang EY, Lin H, Wang CJ, et al. Impact of treatment time-related factors on prognoses and radiation proctitis after definitive chemoradiotherapy for cervical cancer. *Cancer Med* 2016; 5(9):2205–2212.

55. Pathy S, Kumar L, Pandey RM, et al. Impact of treatment time on chemoradiotherapy in locally advanced cervical carcinoma. *Asian Pac J Cancer Prev* 2015;16(12):5075–5079.

56. Erridge SC, Kerr GR, Downing D, et al. The effect of overall treatment time on the survival and toxicity of radical radiotherapy for cervical carcinoma. *Radiother Oncol* 2002;63(1):59–66.

57. Lorusso D, Petrelli F, Coinu A, et al. A systematic review comparing cisplatin and carboplatin plus paclitaxel-based chemotherapy for recurrent or metastatic cervical cancer. *Gynecol Oncol* 2014; 133(1):117–123.

58. Monk BJ, Sill MW, McMeekin DS, et al. Phase III trial of four cisplatin-containing doublet combinations in stage IVB, recurrent, or persistent cervical carcinoma: a Gynecologic Oncology Group study. *J Clin Oncol* 2009;27(28):4649–4655.

59. Keys HM, Bundy BN, Stehman FB, et al. Cisplatin, radiation, and adjuvant hysterectomy compared with radiation and adjuvant hysterectomy for bulky stage IB cervical carcinoma. *N Engl J Med* 1999;340(15):1154–1161.

60. Rose PG, Bundy BN, Watkins EB, et al. Concurrent cisplatin-based radiotherapy and chemotherapy for locally advanced cervical cancer. *N Engl J Med* 1999;340(15):1144–1153.

61. Kokka F, Bryant A, Brockbank E, et al. Hysterectomy with radiotherapy or chemotherapy or both for women with locally advanced cervical cancer. *Cochrane Database Syst Rev* 2015;(4):CD010260.

62. Satoh T, Takei Y, Treilleux I, et al. Gynecologic Cancer InterGroup (GCIG) consensus review for small cell carcinoma of the cervix. *Int J Gynecol Cancer* 2014;24(9 Suppl 3):S102–S108.

63. Tokunaga H, Nagase S, Yoshinaga K, et al. Small cell carcinoma of the uterine cervix: clinical outcome of concurrent chemoradiotherapy with a multidrug regimen. *Tohoku J Exp Med* 2013; 229(1):75–81.

64. Huang L, Liao LM, Liu AW, et al. Analysis of the impact of platinum-based combination chemotherapy in small cell cervical carcinoma: a multicenter retrospective study in Chinese patients. *BMC Cancer* 2014;14:140.

65. Kuji S, Hirashima Y, Nakayama H, et al. Diagnosis, clinicopathologic features, treatment, and prognosis of small cell carcinoma of the uterine cervix; Kansai Clinical Oncology Group/ Intergroup study in Japan. *Gynecol Oncol* 2013;129(3):522–527.

66. Viswanathan AN, Deavers MT, Jhingran A, et al. Small cell neuroendocrine carcinoma of the cervix: outcome and patterns of recurrence. *Gynecol Oncol* 2004;93(1):27–33.

67. Hoskins PJ, Swenerton KD, Pike JA, et al. Small-cell carcinoma of the cervix: fourteen years of experience at a single institution using a combined-modality regimen of involved-field irradiation and platinum-based combination chemotherapy. *J Clin Oncol* 2003;21(18):3495–3501.

68. Chen TC, Huang HJ, Wang TY, et al. Primary surgery versus primary radiation therapy for FIGO stages I-II small cell carcinoma of the uterine cervix: a retrospective Taiwanese Gynecologic Oncology Group study. *Gynecol Oncol* 2015;137(3):468–473.

69. Duenas-Gonzalez A, Zarba JJ, Patel F, et al. Phase III, open-label, randomized study comparing concurrent gemcitabine plus cisplatin and radiation followed by adjuvant gemcitabine and cisplatin versus concurrent cisplatin and radiation in patients with stage IIB to IVA carcinoma of the cervix. *J Clin Oncol* 2011;29(13):1678–1685.

70. Mabuchi S, Isohashi F, Okazawa M, et al. Chemoradiotherapy followed by consolidation chemotherapy involving paclitaxel and carboplatin and in FIGO stage IIIB/IVA cervical cancer patients. *J Gynecol Oncol* 2017;28(1):e15.

71. Zhao H, Li L, Su H, et al. Concurrent paclitaxel/cisplatin chemoradiotherapy with or without consolidation chemotherapy in high-risk early-stage cervical cancer patients following radical hysterectomy: preliminary results of a phase III randomized study. *Oncotarget* 2016;7(43):70969–70978.

72. Perren TJ, Swart AM, Pfisterer J, et al. A phase 3 trial of bevacizumab in ovarian cancer. *N Engl J Med* 2011;365(26):2484–2496.

73. Tewari KS, Sill MW, Monk BJ, et al. Prospective Validation of Pooled Prognostic Factors in Women with Advanced Cervical Cancer Treated with Chemotherapy with/without Bevacizumab: NRG Oncology/GOG Study. *Clin Cancer Res* 2015;21(24):5480–5487.

74. Chuang LT, Temin S, Camacho R, et al. Management and care of women with invasive cervical cancer: American Society of Clinical Oncology Resource-Stratified Clinical Practice Guideline. *J Glob Oncol* 2016;2(5):311–340.

75. Lim K, Small W Jr, Portelance L, et al. Consensus guidelines for delineation of clinical target volume for intensity-modulated pelvic radiotherapy for the definitive treatment of cervix cancer. *Int J Radiat Oncol Biol Phys* 2011;79(2):348–355.

76. Small W Jr, Mell LK, Anderson P, et al. Consensus guidelines for delineation of clinical target volume for intensity-modulated pelvic radiotherapy in postoperative treatment of endometrial and cervical cancer. *Int J Radiat Oncol Biol Phys* 2008;71(2):428–434.

77. Gay HA, Barthold HJ, O'Meara E, et al. Pelvic normal tissue contouring guidelines for radiation therapy: a Radiation Therapy Oncology Group consensus panel atlas. *Int J Radiat Oncol Biol Phys* 2012;83(3):e353–e362.

78. Small W, Mundt A. Guidelines for the delineation of the CTV in postoperative pelvic RT. RTOG Foundation Contouring Atlases https://www.rtog.org/CoreLab/ContouringAtlases/GYN.aspx. Accessed September 4, 2017.

79. RTOG 0724/GOG-0724: Chemotherapy and Pelvic Radiation Therapy with or without Additional Chemotherapy in Treating Patients with High-Risk Early-Stage Cervical Cancer after Radical Hysterectomy [NCT00980954]. Radiation Therapy Oncology Group, 2010.

80. Bali A, Weekes A, Van Trappen P, et al. Central pelvic recurrence 7 years after radical vaginal trachelectomy. *Gynecol Oncol* 2005;96(3):854–856.

81. Diaz JP, Sonoda Y, Leitao MM, et al. Oncologic outcome of fertility-sparing radical trachelectomy versus radical hysterectomy for stage IB1 cervical carcinoma. *Gynecol Oncol* 2008;111(2):255–260.

82. Webb S. The physical basis of IMRT and inverse planning. *Br J Radiol* 2003;76(910):678–689.

83. Heron DE, Gerszten K, Selvaraj RN, et al. Conventional 3D conformal versus intensity-modulated radiotherapy for the adjuvant treatment of gynecologic malignancies: a comparative dosimetric study of dose-volume histograms. *Gynecol Oncol* 2003;91(1):39–45.

84. Lukovic J, Patil N, D'Souza D, et al. Intensity-modulated radiation therapy versus 3D conformal radiotherapy for postoperative gynecologic cancer: are they covering the same planning target volume? *Cureus* 2016;8(1):e467.

85. Mundt AJ, Mell LK, Roeske JC. Preliminary analysis of chronic gastrointestinal toxicity in gynecology patients treated with intensity-modulated whole pelvic radiation therapy. *Int J Radiat Oncol Biol Phys* 2003;56(5):1354–1360.

86. Mundt AJ, Lujan AE, Rotmensch J, et al. Intensity-modulated whole pelvic radiotherapy in women with gynecologic malignancies. *Int J Radiat Oncol Biol Phys* 2002;52(5):1330–1337.

87. Beriwal S, Jain SK, Heron DE, et al. Clinical outcome with adjuvant treatment of endometrial carcinoma using intensity-modulated radiation therapy. *Gynecol Oncol* 2006;102(2):195–199.

88. Lujan AE, Mundt AJ, Yamada SD, et al. Intensity-modulated radiotherapy as a means of reducing dose to bone marrow in gynecologic patients receiving whole pelvic radiotherapy. *Int J Radiat Oncol Biol Phys* 2003;57(2):516–521.

89. Yang B, Zhu L, Cheng H, et al. Dosimetric comparison of intensity modulated radiotherapy and three-dimensional conformal radiotherapy in patients with gynecologic malignancies: a systematic review and meta-analysis. *Radiat Oncol* 2012;7:197.

90. Gandhi AK, Sharma DN, Rath GK, et al. Early clinical outcomes and toxicity of intensity modulated versus conventional pelvic radiation therapy for locally advanced cervix carcinoma: a prospective randomized study. *Int J Radiat Oncol Biol Phys* 2013;87(3):542–548.

91. Patankar SS, Tergas AI, Deutsch I, et al. High versus low-dose rate brachytherapy for cervical cancer. *Gynecol Oncol* 2015;136(3):534–541.

92. Han K, Milosevic M, Fyles A, et al. Trends in the utilization of brachytherapy in cervical cancer in the United States. *Int J Radiat Oncol Biol Phys* 2013;87(1):111–119.

93. Liu R, Wang X, Tian JH, et al. High dose rate versus low dose rate intracavity brachytherapy for locally advanced uterine cervix cancer. *Cochrane Database Syst Rev* 2014;(10):CD007563.

94. Eifel PJ, Ho A, Khalid N, et al. Patterns of radiation therapy practice for patients treated for intact cervical cancer in 2005 to 2007: a quality research in radiation oncology study. *Int J Radiat Oncol Biol Phys* 2014;89(2):249–256.

95. Grover S, Harkenrider MM, Cho LP, et al. Image guided cervical brachytherapy: 2014 survey of the American Brachytherapy Society. *Int J Radiat Oncol Biol Phys* 2016;94(3):598–604.

96. Viswanathan AN, Thomadsen B. American Brachytherapy Society consensus guidelines for locally advanced carcinoma of the cervix. Part I: general principles. *Brachytherapy* 2012;11(1):33–46.

97. Viswanathan AN, Moughan J, Small W Jr, et al. The quality of cervical cancer brachytherapy implantation and the impact on local recurrence and disease-free survival in radiation therapy oncology group prospective trials 0116 and 0128. *Int J Gynecol Cancer* 2012;22(1):123–131.

98. Mayadev J, Viswanathan A, Liu Y, et al. American Brachytherapy Task Group Report: a pooled analysis of clinical outcomes for high-dose-rate brachytherapy for cervical cancer. *Brachytherapy* 2017;16(1):22–43.

99. Wang F, Tang Q, Lv G, et al. Comparison of computed tomography and magnetic resonance imaging in cervical cancer brachytherapy: a systematic review. *Brachytherapy* 2017;16(2):353–365.

100. Viswanathan AN, Dimopoulos J, Kirisits C, et al. Computed tomography versus magnetic resonance imaging-based contouring in cervical cancer brachytherapy: results of a prospective trial and preliminary guidelines for standardized contours. *Int J Radiat Oncol Biol Phys* 2007;68(2):491–498.

101. Viswanathan AN, Erickson B, Gaffney DK, et al. Comparison and consensus guidelines for delineation of clinical target volume for CT- and MR-based brachytherapy in locally advanced cervical cancer. *Int J Radiat Oncol Biol Phys* 2014;90(2):320–328.

102. Kamran SC, Manuel MM, Cho LP, et al. Comparison of outcomes for MR-guided versus CT-guided high-dose-rate interstitial brachytherapy in women with locally advanced carcinoma of the cervix. *Gynecol Oncol* 2017;145(2):284–290.

103. Mongula JE, Slangen BF, Lambregts DM, et al. Consecutive magnetic resonance imaging during brachytherapy for cervical carcinoma: predictive value of volume measurements with respect to persistent disease and prognosis. *Radiat Oncol* 2015;10:252.

104. Wang JZ, Mayr NA, Zhang D, et al. Sequential magnetic resonance imaging of cervical cancer: the predictive value of absolute tumor volume and regression ratio measured before, during, and after radiation therapy. *Cancer* 2010;116(21):5093–5101.

105. Haie-Meder C, Potter R, Van Limbergen E, et al. Recommendations from Gynaecological (GYN) GEC-ESTRO Working Group (I): concepts and terms in 3D image based 3D treatment planning in cervix cancer brachytherapy with emphasis on MRI assessment of GTV and CTV. *Radiother Oncol* 2005;74(3):235–245.

106. Potter R, Haie-Meder C, Van Limbergen E, et al. Recommendations from gynaecological (GYN) GEC ESTRO working group (II): concepts and terms in 3D image-based treatment planning in cervix cancer brachytherapy-3D dose volume parameters and aspects of 3D image-based anatomy, radiation physics, radiobiology. *Radiother Oncol* 2006;78(1):67–77.

107. Viswanathan AN, Erickson BA. Three-dimensional imaging in gynecologic brachytherapy: a survey of the American Brachytherapy Society. *Int J Radiat Oncol Biol Phys* 2010;76(1):104–109.

108. International Commission on Radiation Units and Measurements. *Dose and volume specification for reporting intracavitary therapy in gynecology. ICRU Report 38.* Bethesda, MD: Author, 1985.

109. Dimopoulos JC, Lang S, Kirisits C, et al. Dose-volume histogram parameters and local tumor control in magnetic resonance image-guided cervical cancer brachytherapy. *Int J Radiat Oncol Biol Phys* 2009;75(1):56–63.

110. Charra-Brunaud C, Harter V, Delannes M, et al. Impact of 3D image-based PDR brachytherapy on outcome of patients treated for cervix carcinoma in France: results of the French STIC prospective study. *Radiother Oncol* 2012;103(3):305–313.

111. Sturdza A, Potter R, Fokdal LU, et al. Image guided brachytherapy in locally advanced cervical cancer: improved pelvic control and survival in RetroEMBRACE, a multicenter cohort study. *Radiother Oncol* 2016;120(3):428–433.

112. Mazeron R, Fokdal LU, Kirchheiner K, et al. Dose-volume effect relationships for late rectal morbidity in patients treated with chemoradiation and MRI-guided adaptive brachytherapy for locally advanced cervical cancer: results from the prospective multicenter EMBRACE study. *Radiother Oncol* 2016;120(3):412–419.

113. Kirchheiner K, Nout RA, Tanderup K, et al. Manifestation pattern of early-late vaginal morbidity after definitive radiation (chemo)therapy and image-guided adaptive brachytherapy for locally advanced cervical cancer: an analysis from the EMBRACE study. *Int J Radiat Oncol Biol Phys* 2014;89(1):88–95.

114. Kim Y, Kim YJ, Kim JY, et al. Toxicities and dose-volume histogram parameters of MRI-based brachytherapy for cervical cancer. *Brachytherapy* 2017;16(1):116–125.

115. Wang W, Hou X, Yan J, et al. Outcome and toxicity of radical radiotherapy or concurrent chemoradiotherapy for elderly cervical cancer women. *BMC Cancer* 2017;17(1):510.

116. Ramlov A, Pedersen EM, Rohl L, et al. Risk factors for pelvic insufficiency fractures in locally advanced cervical cancer following intensity modulated radiation therapy. *Int J Radiat Oncol Biol Phys* 2017;97(5):1032–1039.

117. Wolfson AH, Varia MA, Moore D, et al. ACR Appropriateness Criteria(R) role of adjuvant therapy in the management of early stage cervical cancer. *Gynecol Oncol* 2012;125(1):256–262.

118. Hunter MI, Tewari K, Monk BJ. Cervical neoplasia in pregnancy. Part 2: current treatment of invasive disease. *Am J Obstet Gynecol* 2008;199(1):10–18.

119. Nguyen C, Montz FJ, Bristow RE. Management of stage I cervical cancer in pregnancy. *Obstet Gynecol Surv* 2000;55(10):633–643.

120. Bigelow CA, Horowitz NS, Goodman A, et al. Management and outcome of cervical cancer diagnosed in pregnancy. *Am J Obstet Gynecol* 2017;216(3):276.e271–276.e276.

121. Vercellino GF, Koehler C, Erdemoglu E, et al. Laparoscopic pelvic lymphadenectomy in 32 pregnant patients with cervical cancer: rationale, description of the technique, and outcome. *Int J Gynecol Cancer* 2014;24(2):364–371.

122. Amant F, Halaska MJ, Fumagalli M, et al. Gynecologic cancers in pregnancy: guidelines of a second international consensus meeting. *Int J Gynecol Cancer* 2014;24(3):394–403.

123. Abu-Rustum NR, Tal MN, DeLair D, et al. Radical abdominal trachelectomy for stage IB1 cervical cancer at 15-week gestation. *Gynecol Oncol* 2010;116(1):151–152.

124. Sopracordevole F, Rossi D, Di Giuseppe J, et al. Conservative treatment of stage IA1 adenocarcinoma of the uterine cervix during pregnancy: case report and review of the literature. *Case Rep Obstet Gynecol* 2014;2014:296253.

125. van de Nieuwenhof HP, van Ham MA, Lotgering FK, et al. First case of vaginal radical trachelectomy in a pregnant patient. *Int J Gynecol Cancer* 2008;18(6):1381–1385.

126. Yahata T, Numata M, Kashima K, et al. Conservative treatment of stage IA1 adenocarcinoma of the cervix during pregnancy. *Gynecol Oncol* 2008;109(1):49–52.

127. Zagouri F, Sergentanis TN, Chrysikos D, et al. Platinum derivatives during pregnancy in cervical cancer: a systematic review and meta-analysis. *Obstet Gynecol* 2013;121(2 Pt 1):337–343.

128. Morice P, Uzan C, Gouy S, et al. Gynaecological cancers in pregnancy. *Lancet* 2012;379(9815):558–569.

129. Sood AK, Sorosky JI, Mayr N, et al. Cervical cancer diagnosed shortly after pregnancy: prognostic variables and delivery routes. *Obstet Gynecol* 2000;95(6 Pt 1):832–838.

130. Leath CA III, Bevis KS, Numnum TM, et al Comparison of operative risks associated with radical hysterectomy in pregnant and nonpregnant women. *J Reprod Med* 2013;58(7–8):279–284.

131. Sedlis A, Bundy BN, Rotman MZ, et al. A randomized trial of pelvic radiation therapy versus no further therapy in selected patients with stage IB carcinoma of the cervix after radical hysterectomy and pelvic lymphadenectomy: a Gynecologic Oncology Group Study. *Gynecol Oncol* 1999;73(2):177–183.

132. Trifiletti DM, Swisher-McClure S, Showalter TN, et al. Postoperative chemoradiation therapy in high-risk cervical cancer: re-evaluating the findings of Gynecologic Oncology Group Study 109 in a large, population-based cohort. *Int J Radiat Oncol Biol Phys* 2015;93(5):1032–1044.

133. Eddy GL, Bundy BN, Creasman WT, et al. Treatment of ("bulky") stage IB cervical cancer with or without neoadjuvant vincristine and cisplatin prior to radical hysterectomy and pelvic/paraaortic lymphadenectomy: a phase III trial of the gynecologic oncology group. *Gynecol Oncol* 2007;106(2):362–369.

134. Keys HM, Bundy BN, Stehman FB, et al. Radiation therapy with and without extrafascial hysterectomy for bulky stage IB cervical carcinoma: a randomized trial of the Gynecologic Oncology Group. *Gynecol Oncol* 2003;89(3):343–353.

135. Eifel PJ, Winter K, Morris M, et al. Pelvic irradiation with concurrent chemotherapy versus pelvic and para-aortic irradiation for high-risk cervical cancer: an update of radiation therapy oncology group trial (RTOG) 90-01. *J Clin Oncol* 2004;22(5):872–880.

136. Green JA, Kirwan JM, Tierney JF, et al. Survival and recurrence after concomitant chemotherapy and radiotherapy for cancer of the uterine cervix: a systematic review and meta-analysis. *Lancet* 2001;358(9284):781–786.

137. Kunos C, Tian C, Waggoner S, et al. Retrospective analysis of concomitant Cisplatin during radiation in patients aged 55 years or older for treatment of advanced cervical cancer: a gynecologic oncology group study. *Int J Gynecol Cancer* 2009;19(7):1258–1263.

CHAPTER 33

ENDOMETRIUM

ANATOMY

- The uterus is a pear-shaped hollow muscular organ that is divided into three parts: the fundus, body, and cervix (Fig. 33-1).
- The three layers of the uterine wall are the endometrium, myometrium, and serosa.
- The endometrium is the lining inside the uterine cavity and is composed of columnar cells.
- The myometrium is the muscular layer of the uterus and is composed of smooth muscle fibers.
- The serosa is the peritoneum covering the uterus and forms the broad ligaments laterally.
- Blood supply to the uterus comes from the ovarian and uterine arteries.
- The primary lymphatic drainage of the cervix and lower uterine segment is to the pelvic lymph nodes, including internal and external iliac, obturator, presacral and parametrial lymph nodes.
- Additional lymphatic drainage of the fundus includes direct drainage to the paraaortic (PA) nodes.

EPIDEMIOLOGY

- Uterine corpus cancers are the most common gynecologic malignancy in the United States.
- The incidence peaks in the 50- to 70-year-old age group.
- Uterine corpus cancer is the fourth most common cancer in females, after breast, lung, and colorectal (1).
- Uterine corpus cancer is the sixth leading cause of death in females, after lung, breast, colorectal, pancreas, and ovarian (1).
- The American Cancer Society estimated that the number of new cases in 2017 was 61,380 (1).
- The American Cancer Society estimated that the number of deaths was 10,920 (1).

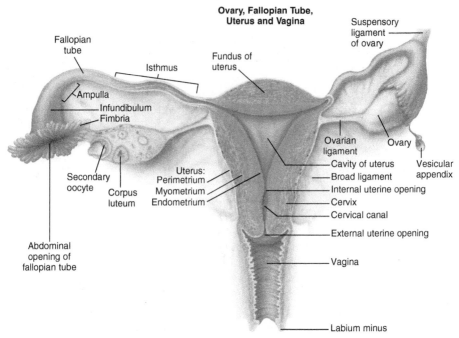

FIGURE 33-1. Female reproductive system. (Reprinted with permission from Agur AMR, Dalley AF, eds. *Grant's atlas of anatomy*, 14th ed. Philadelphia, PA: Wolters Kluwer, 2017: Chapter 5.)

- The overall 5-year survival for all stage uterine corpus cancers is 82% (1).
- The 5-year survival for local uterine corpus cancer is 95%, regional uterine corpus cancer is 69%, and distant uterine corpus cancer is 17% (1).
- The following are risk factors for developing carcinoma of the endometrium:
  - Unopposed estrogen exposure (exogenous or endogenous, which includes obesity, functional ovarian tumors, polycystic ovarian syndrome, late menopause, nulliparity)
  - Tamoxifen use
  - Older age
  - Lynch syndrome
  - Diabetes mellitus

NATURAL HISTORY

- Most endometrial carcinomas are confined to the uterus at the time of diagnosis.
- Tumors arising from the endometrium commonly spread into the myometrium and to contiguous areas, including direct extension into the cervix, vagina, parametrial tissue, bladder, or rectum.
- The risk of pelvic and paraaortic lymph node metastases increases as tumor grade and depth of myometrial invasion increase (Table 33-1).

Table 33-1

Risk of Lymph Node Involvement Depends on Grade and Depth of Invasion

Depth of Invasion	Grade 1 (n = 180)		Grade 2 (n = 288)		Grade 3 (n = 153)	
	Aortic Node (%)	Pelvic Node (%)	Aortic Node (%)	Pelvic Node (%)	Aortic Node (%)	Pelvic Node (%)
Endometrium only (n = 86)	0 (0)	0 (0)	1 (3)	1 (3)	0 (0)	0 (0)
Superficial (n = 281)	1 (1)	3 (3)	5 (4)	7 (5)	2 (4)	5 (9)
Middle (n = 115)	1 (5)	0 (0)	0 (0)	6 (9)	0 (0)	1 (4)
Deep (n = 139)	1 (6)	2 (11)	8 (14)	11 (19)	15 (23)	22 (34)

Data from Prat J. FIGO Committee on Gynecologic Oncology. Staging classification for cancer of the ovary, fallopian tube, and peritoneum. *Int J Gynaecol Obstet* 2014; 124(1):1–5.

- Peritoneal seeding of endometrial cancer may occur because an endometrial lesion may penetrate the uterine wall or seed transtubally. This is most common with papillary serous or clear cell histologies.
- Hematogenous metastases are infrequent at presentation but are seen in end-stage patients.

CLINICAL PRESENTATION

- Vaginal bleeding or discharge is the most common presenting symptom and occurs in about 75% of cases.
- Back pain or pressure symptoms may occur as a result of an enlarged uterus on the bowel or bladder.
- More advanced tumors may present with symptoms associated with invasion of nearby structures (rectal bleeding, constipation) or extensive lymph node involvement (lower extremity edema), or peritoneal seeding (ascites).

DIAGNOSTIC WORKUP

- Currently, there is no screening method for detecting endometrial carcinoma.
- Diagnosis is dependent on endometrial biopsy or aspiration curettage, which is indicated in postmenopausal women with vaginal bleeding or perimenopausal women with abnormal bleeding.
- Fractional dilation and curettage and cervical biopsy are indicated when there is a high degree of suspicion of cancer, and diagnosis cannot be made by endometrial biopsy or aspiration curettage.

Table 33-2
Diagnostic Workup for Endometrial Cancer
All Stages
History Physical examination, including pelvic examination Endometrial biopsy or aspiration curettage Fractional dilatation and curettage (if biopsy or aspiration does not reveal cancer) Chest radiograph Cervical biopsy Urinary imaging study in all patients before surgery (intravenous pyelogram, ultrasound, CT) Complete blood cell count, urinalysis, blood chemistry including LFTs Consideration of genetic testing/counseling for patients (<50 y) with a significant family history of endometrial and/or colorectal cancer
Advanced Disease or If Symptoms Warrant
Transvaginal ultrasound Cystoscopy Sigmoidoscopy CT scan or MRI with contrast unless contraindicated Intravenous pyelogram Barium enema

- The recommended diagnostic workup by the National Comprehensive Cancer Network and the Society of Gynecologic Oncology is summarized in Table 33-2.
- Computed tomography (CT) of the pelvis and abdomen is recommended for all patients with high-grade tumors or with stage II or higher disease to detect possible nodal or extrauterine spread of cancer.
- Magnetic resonance imaging (MRI) is not helpful in detecting nodal or peritoneal spread; however, it is useful in demonstrating the depth of myometrial invasion, with an accuracy of approximately 80% (2,3).
- Ultrasound measurement of endometrial thickness in premenopausal women has no diagnostic value and is not recommended. Endometrial thickness of 5 mm or less on ultrasonography in postmenopausal women had a sensitivity of 90% and a specificity of 54% for the detection of endometrial cancer (4).
- The tumor marker CA-125 is elevated in 59% of patients with advanced or recurrent endometrial carcinoma; however, the marker is not specific (5).

STAGING SYSTEM

- Endometrial cancer is most commonly surgically staged according to the guidelines of the International Federation of Gynecology and Obstetrics.
- For inoperable patients, the International Federation of Gynecology and Obstetrics clinical staging system, which is based on bimanual pelvic examination under anesthesia and on the diagnostic procedures previously discussed, is recommended.

- For definition of regional lymph node (N), distinctions have been made to include isolated tumor cells in regional LNs, N0(i+), as well as micrometastasis, including regional lymph node metastasis greater than 0.2 mm but not greater than 2.0 mm, N1mi (pelvic LN), or N2mi (paraaortic LN).

See: Amin MB, Edge SB, Greene FL, et al., eds. *AJCC cancer staging manual*, 8th ed. New York, NY: Springer, 2017.

PATHOLOGIC CLASSIFICATION

- Endometrioid adenocarcinoma is the most common form of carcinoma of the endometrium, accounting for 75% to 80% of cases.
- Endometrioid adenocarcinoma is divided into four subtypes: papillary, secretory, ciliated cells, and adenocarcinoma with squamous differentiation. The ciliated subtype is associated with prior estrogen use and carries an excellent prognosis.
- Serous, clear cell, and pure squamous cell carcinomas are the most aggressive cancers arising from the endometrium.
- About 5% of cases are uterine sarcomas, which have a higher rate of lymph node involvement (carcinosarcoma and endometrial stromal sarcoma) and distant metastases (carcinosarcoma, leimyosarcoma, and endometrial stromal sarcoma).

PROGNOSTIC FACTORS

- The most significant prognostic factor is the clinical or pathologic stage.
- Tumor grade and depth of invasion into the myometrium are important prognostic indicators as both factors have an impact on the incidence of lymph node involvement and on prognosis (6–8) (Table 33-1). Deep myometrial invasion is more common with higher-grade tumors.
- Lymphovascular space involvement (LVSI) significantly increases the risk of tumor recurrence after surgery, especially distant relapse (9–11).

GENERAL MANAGEMENT

Operable FIGO Stage I Endometrial Carcinoma

- Total hysterectomy and bilateral salpingo-oophorectomy (TH/BSO) is the standard surgical procedure for the initial treatment of endometrial carcinoma.
- Peritoneal cytology does not affect staging, but FIGO and AJCC recommend that it is obtained and reported.
- Pelvic lymph node dissection is an important part of surgical staging for selected uterine-confined endometrial cancer. External iliac, internal iliac, obturator, and common iliac nodes are frequently removed for staging purposes.

- Although the therapeutic benefit of lymphadenectomy has not been shown in randomized trials (12,13), retrospective analyses have shown benefits to pelvic lymph node dissection (14) and paraaortic lymph node dissection in intermediate- and high-risk patients (15).
- Adjuvant therapy determinations are made on the basis of pathologic findings and risk stratification. Adverse risk factors include grade, depth of invasion, LVSI, and age. A summary of risk groups for endometrial cancer is listed in Table 33-3.

Operable FIGO Stage II Endometrial Carcinoma

- Patients with stage II endometrial carcinoma have cervical stromal invasion, and 5-year survival for this patient population is about 70%.
- The incidence of pelvic lymph node involvement varies from 20% to 50% in patients with cervical stromal involvement and therefore strongly argues for treatment of nodal areas and parametrial tissues with external pelvic irradiation.
- In patients with stage II, grade 3 disease, national guidelines support consideration of adjuvant chemotherapy.

Adjuvant Radiation Therapy in Early-Stage Disease

- Radiation therapy (RT) is tailored to histopathologic factors found in the uterine specimen in addition to nodal status and presence of nodal information.
- Clinical practice guidelines, endorsed by ASTRO (American Society of Radiation Oncology) and SGO (Society of Gynecologic Oncology), for adjuvant radiation in the treatment of endometrial cancer have been published and are outlined below (16).

Table 33-3	
Risk Groups in Endometrial Cancer	
Low Risk	Stage IA (<50% MI), grade 1
Intermediate Risk	Stage IA (<50% MI), grade 2
Low-intermediate risk	Stage IA (<50% MI), grade 3
High-intermediate risk	Stage IB (>50% MI), grade 1 or 2
PORTEC definition	Risk factors: age > 60 y, grade 3, deep invasion (>50%)
	2 or more risk factors
	Risk factors: grade 2 or 3, outer 1/3rd myometrial involvement, +LVSI
GOG 99 definition	Any age with 3 risk factors
	Age ≥ 50 y and 2 risk factors
	Age ≥ 70 y and 1 risk factor
High Risk	Stage IB (>50% MI), grade 3
	Stage II (cervical stroma), any grade
	Papillary serous or clear cell carcinoma histology, any stage
	Stage III–IV

Omission of Adjuvant Radiation Therapy

- No adjuvant RT is reasonable for patients with endometrioid histology and:
  - No residual disease in surgical pathology (positive biopsy only)
  - Stage IA, grade 1 or 2 disease, especially when no other high-risk features are present, including age greater than 60 years and/or LVSI
- Omission of adjuvant radiation may be considered in patients with endometrioid histology and:
  - Grade 3 disease without myometrial invasion
  - Stage IA, grade 1 or 2, with age greater than 60 years and/or LVSI

Vaginal Cuff Radiation

- Vaginal cuff brachytherapy (VCB) is as effective as external beam radiation therapy (EBRT) in terms of vaginal recurrence but has slightly higher rates of pelvic recurrence with lower toxicity.
- VCB alone is recommended for patients with endometrioid histology and:
  - Stage IB, grade 1 or 2 disease
  - Stage IA, grade 3 disease

Pelvic External Beam Radiation Therapy

- Pelvic EBRT decreased pelvic recurrence rates but does not improve overall survival (OS) in early-stage patients.
- Pelvic EBRT is recommended for patients with:
  - Stage IB, grade 3 disease
  - Stage II (cervical stromal involvement)
  - Serous or clear cell histology, stage IB or greater
- Pelvic EBRT may benefit patients with:
  - Stage IB, grade 1 or 2, with other risk factors including age greater than 60 years and/or LVSI
  - Serous or clear cell histology, stage IA

Advanced Stage FIGO Stage III to IV

- Treatment for patients with advanced endometrial cancer includes pelvic EBRT, extended field RT, and chemotherapy.
- Historically, whole abdominal irradiation (WAI) was used for stage II/IV endometrial cancer patients. Adjuvant chemotherapy alone was adopted into practice after the results from GOG 122 demonstrated superior progression-free survival (PFS) and OS for stage III/IV endometrial cancer patients treated with doxorubicin and cisplatin versus WAI (17).
- Several randomized trials have examined combined modality adjuvant treatment (sequential or concurrent chemotherapy and pelvic or extended RT) in high-risk patients with mixed results.

Radiation Therapy

- Adjuvant chemotherapy alone for advanced disease is often employed; however, it must be acknowledged that patients with cervical, adnexal, and/or deep myometrial disease will remain at significant increased risk (20% to 40%) to have pelvic failure if RT is not used (17,18).
- RTOG 97-08 was a phase II trial that enrolled 46 patients to examine postoperative chemoradiation (45 Gy to pelvis with cisplatin plus vaginal brachytherapy) followed by adjuvant chemotherapy (cisplatin + Taxol) for high-risk endometrial adenocarcinoma (stage IC grade 2 to 3, stage II or III). At a median follow-up of 4 years, locoregional control was excellent at 2% (19).
- Retrospective evidence also supports the use of pelvic EBRT in advanced stage patients with excellent locoregional control and improved survival in stage IIIC (20,21).

Hormonal Therapy

- Although endometrial adenocarcinoma cells possess steroid receptors, multiple randomized trials failed to show a statistically significant improvement in overall or disease-free survival with the use of adjuvant progestational therapy (12,22).

Chemotherapy

- Results from GOG 122 demonstrated superior PFS and OS for stage III/IV endometrial cancer patients treated with doxorubicin and cisplatin versus WAI (17).
- Since GOG 122, several additional randomized trials have examined combined modality adjuvant treatment (sequential or concurrent chemotherapy with pelvic or extended RT) in high-risk patients with mixed results. These studies include a multi-institutional randomized study from Italy (Maggi et al., 2006), GOG 38, RTOG 9708, NSGO EC-9501/EORTC-55991, and MaNGO ILIADE-III.
- A combined analysis of NSGO EC-9501/EORTC-55991 and MaNGO ILIADE-III showed that the addition of chemotherapy improved cancer-specific survival (CSS) (HR 0.55, CI 0.35 to 0.88; $p = 0.01$) and had a trend toward improving OS (HR 0.69, CI 0.46 to 1.03; $p = 0.07$) (23).
- Several new combined modality trials are underway testing chemotherapy versus combined chemotherapy and RT (GOG 258) and pelvic radiotherapy with or without concurrent and adjuvant chemotherapy (PORTEC-3).
- The optimal sequencing of chemotherapy and RT for patients with advanced stage disease remains to be defined.

Medically Inoperable Patients

- For patients with severe medical comorbidities that render them medically inoperable, definitive or curative intent RT can be offered.
- Intrauterine brachytherapy alone may be given to patients at low risk for extrauterine spread (24).
- The decision to give EBRT to the pelvis is based on the risk of extrauterine disease. It is usually used in grade 3 disease, larger uterine volume, or cervical involvement (25).

- Treatment with intrauterine brachytherapy with or without EBRT, several studies have shown substantial local control and DSS rates. For patients with clinical stage I disease, 5-year uterine control rates of 70% to 90% and disease-free survival rates of 50% to 80% have been reported (26,27).

Recurrent Endometrial Carcinoma

- Early diagnosis is crucial for successful treatment of recurrent endometrial carcinoma (28).
- Approximately 70% of all relapses occur within the first 2 years after completion of initial therapy; frequent follow-up examinations are highly recommended.
- The rates of pelvic recurrence in patients with early-stage disease after surgery alone range between 5% and 15%, and 70% to 75% are isolated vaginal recurrences (9,29).
- The reported salvage rate with radical irradiation is 65% to 80% in patients with isolated vaginal relapses (as high as 80% to 90% in patients with lesions confined to the vaginal mucosa) compared with 25% to 60% salvage rate in patients with pelvic and/or regional recurrences (30,31).
- Isolated vaginal recurrences are rare, particularly in patients who have received adequate initial RT. Vaginal recurrences usually coexist with more extensive pelvic disease.
- Patients with disseminated tumors are treated with progestational agents, which may be given alone or combined with chemotherapy, depending on the status of estrogen or progesterone receptors.
- RT is indicated for palliation of bleeding or pain.

RADIATION THERAPY TECHNIQUES

External Beam Radiation Treatment

- CT simulation is helpful for accurate identification of blood vessels and surrounding critical structures for using three-dimensional conformal RT or intensity-modulated radiation therapy (IMRT) techniques.
- Patient should be simulated in the supine or prone position, with a comfortably filled bladder (or two scans: full bladder and empty bladder, to create an integrated target volume [ITV]), and scanned with CT with intravenous contrast performed with less than or equal to 3-mm slice thickness (32). If there is vaginal involvement, a radiopaque marker should be placed at the most caudal extent of disease (32).
- For pelvic radiation, the clinical target volume (CTV) encompasses the parametrial tissues, proximal half of the vagina (upper 3 cm and the lateral paravaginal soft tissue), and the pelvic lymph node regions, including the internal and external iliac and common iliac lymph nodes. For patients with cervical stromal invasion, it is recommended to include the presacral lymph node region in the CTV. If the distal one third of the vagina is involved, the inguinal nodes should be included in the CTV (32,33).
- A four-field box technique has been traditionally used, and the borders are as follows: superior = L4/5 (or level of bifurcation of the aorta), inferior = lower half of the vagina

or obturator foramen, lateral = 1.5 cm lateral to pelvic brim, posterior = split sacrum to S3, and anterior = pubic symphysis).

- IMRT is an attractive treatment for pelvic radiotherapy in endometrial cancer because of the reduction in the volume of small bowel within the field and consequently the decreased risk of bowel side effects, but long-term outcome data are limited, and current trials are investigating the benefits in this patient population (34).
- Extended field radiation is used to treat the pelvis and paraaortic lymph node regions in high-risk patients. Patients are usually treated in the supine position with CT-based planning for 3D conformal or IMRT to spare the kidneys and bowel. The superior field is at the T12-L1 junction but may be individualized based on patient anatomy and the clinical scenario.
- Doses for pelvic and paraaortic treatment are 45 to 50.4 Gy in 1.8-Gy fractions with a boost to lymph nodes that are grossly involved (5 Gy or higher depending on volume of disease and normal tissue constraints).
- Weekly imaging should be performed with megavoltage portal, kilovoltage imaging, or cone beam CT to verify treatment setup. Daily imaging should be performed if using IMRT, particularly if small margins are being used.

Brachytherapy

- Vaginal cuff irradiation is delivered with colpostats or vaginal cylinders. The dose with low-dose rate (LDR) brachytherapy is 100 cGy/h or 60 to 70 Gy to the vaginal mucosa in one or two insertions. With high-dose rate (HDR) brachytherapy, a common prescription utilized is 7 Gy per fraction at 0.5 cm depth; 3 fractions are delivered 1 to 2 weeks apart. However, this fractionation may be associated with increased vaginal toxicities, and an extended fractionation schedule (i.e., 4 to 6 fractions) to reduce vaginal morbidity could be considered depending on the patient (35). Table 33-4 summarizes common dose and fractionation schedules for vaginal brachytherapy in endometrial cancer (36).
- The American Brachytherapy Society (ABS) recommends treating the proximal 3 to 5 cm of the vagina. In rare circumstances when the histology is serous or clear cell, grade 3 disease, or extensive LVI is present, consideration could be given to treat the

Table 33-4	
Standard Vaginal Brachytherapy Dose and Fractionation Regimens	
Vaginal Brachytherapy (monotherapy)	7 Gy × 3 fractions to 0.5 cm depth 6 Gy × 5 fractions to the surface 4 Gy × 6 fractions to the surface
Vaginal Brachytherapy (boost with EBRT)	45 Gy EBRT + 6 Gy × 3 fractions to the vaginal mucosa 50.4 Gy EBRT + 6 Gy × 2 fractions to the vaginal mucosa

Data from Small W Jr, et al. American Brachytherapy Society consensus guidelines for adjuvant vaginal cuff brachytherapy after hysterectomy. *Brachytherapy* 2012;11(1):58–67.

entire length of the vagina (36). If there is tumor extension into the vagina, the entire length of the organ should be treated.
- When treating with a vaginal cylinder, it is critical to select the largest diameter cylinder that will comfortably fit the patient so that the vaginal mucosa is in contact with the applicator surface for an effective dose distribution.
- The prescription dose should be delivered to the surface or to a depth of 0.5 cm.

Medically Inoperable

- Patients with clinical stage IA, with well- or moderately differentiated tumors, without evidence of myometrial infiltration or lymph node metastasis from CT or MRI scans, can be treated with intracavitary brachytherapy (ICB) alone.
- When using LDR intracavitary brachytherapy, one or two applications are performed to deliver a dose of 70 to 75 Gy to point A.
- HDR applicators for definitive treatment of endometrial cancer include tandem and ovoids, tandem and ring, or tandem and cylinder.
- Dose-fractionation schedules for definitive treatment with HDR brachytherapy alone in medically inoperable patients with superficial invasion include 8.5 Gy × 4 fractions, 7.3 Gy × 5 fractions, 6.4 Gy × 6 fractions, 6 Gy × 6 fractions, and 5 Gy × 9 to 10 fractions (24).
- Patients with stage IB disease, poorly differentiated or deeply invasive tumors, as well as patients with inoperable stage II disease, should be treated with a combination of EBRT (45 to 50 Gy) and ICB (24).
- Patients with inoperable stage III disease could be potentially treated for the pelvis only, followed by ICB in the absence of nodal pelvic or retroperitoneal metastasis, or with extended field RT and ICB in those patients with nodal disease, followed by chemotherapy or enrollment in a clinical trial.

Recurrent Endometrial Carcinoma

- For patients with recurrent cancer in the pelvis who have not received previous irradiation, external beam irradiation to the whole pelvis (45 to 50 Gy in 5 to 6 weeks) is recommended followed by a boost. The 5-year OS with combination EBRT and brachytherapy ranges from 35% to 75% (37).
- The amount of vagina to include in treatment volumes for EBRT is highly practitioner dependent. For recurrences in the upper half of the vagina, some experts would treat a 3- to 4-cm margin on the most distal extent of disease, and others recommend treating the whole vagina. For recurrences in the lower half of the vagina, there is consensus to treat the entire vagina (37).
- Vaginal recurrences can receive boost irradiation with intracavitary or interstitial RT to bring the total tumor dose to 75 to 80 Gy (37). The volume of disease to be included for brachytherapy should depend on initial volume, extent, and response of disease.
- The choice of intracavitary device depends on tumor bulk and location. If the thickness of tumor is greater than 0.5 cm, interstitial brachytherapy should be offered.

- An additional boost to the tumor bulk can be delivered with external beam irradiation when the tumor involves the central pelvis or the pelvic side wall or when brachytherapy cannot be performed.
- Palliative RT commonly employs a short course of treatment, and in endometrial cancer, this can be delivered in 3- to 4-Gy fractions to a total dose of 20 or 30 Gy. Shorter courses have been utilized (38) based on clinical symptoms and overall health status of the patient.
- There is no consensus on the addition of concurrent or adjuvant chemotherapy, but both could be considered.

SEQUELAE OF TREATMENT

- The mortality rate for patients who undergo a total abdominal hysterectomy and BSO is less than 1%; however, concomitant medical problems (obesity, hypertension, and heart disease) increase the risk for complications (e.g., infection, wound dehiscence, fistula formation, and bleeding).
- Acute complications resulting from pelvic irradiation include fatigue, diarrhea, and cystitis.
- Desquamation of vulvar skin from irradiation of the vagina is not uncommon.
- Anorexia and vomiting may occur if the paraaortic lymph node region is irradiated.
- Late complications such as chronic cystitis, bowel obstruction, and fistula formation are generally seen in fewer than 10% of patients.
- Although vaginal stenosis occurs, it is successfully managed with routine use of a vaginal dilator and vaginal estrogen applications.

RANDOMIZED STUDIES FOR ADJUVANT RADIATION

- Several landmark prospective trials (PORTEC-1, GOG 99, ASTEC/EN.5, and PORTEC-2) have shown that the use of adjuvant RT in the intermediate- and high-intermediate-risk groups decreases locoregional recurrence but does not impact OS.
- Aalders et al. (6) randomized 500 patients with stage I endometrial cancer after TAH/BSO without lymph node sampling to IVB (LDR 60 Gy) versus IVB + WPRT (40 Gy). Addition of WPRT decreased pelvic and vaginal recurrences from 7% to 2%. On subset analysis, high-grade disease ICG3 showed a larger improvement with WPRT from 20% to 5%.
- In GOG 99 (9), 392 patients with IB, IC, and occult II endometrial cancer were randomized after TAH/BSO with selective pelvic and paraaortic lymph node sampling to WPRT versus observation. WPRT reduced the local recurrence rate from 12% to 3%. Subset analysis defined the "high-intermediate-risk" subgroup as those patients with grade 2 and 3 tumors, presence of LVSI, and deep myometrial involvement. Patients younger than 50 years with all three risk factors, or older than 50 but younger than 70 with two factors, or those older than 70 with any one of the risk factors, were most

likely to benefit from EBRT. The 4-year cumulative locoregional recurrence rates were 13% in the RT arm and 27% in the observation arm.

- In the PORTEC trial (39), 714 patients with IB grade 2 and 3 and IC grade 1 and 2 endometrial cancer were randomized after TAH/BSO with sampling of suspicious lymph nodes to observation versus WPRT (46 Gy). WPRT decreased pelvic and vaginal recurrences from 14% to 4%, with 75% of failures occurring in the vaginal vault. A subset analysis defined a group of patients at intermediate to high risk (greater than 15%) of recurrence when at least two of the three following major risk factors present: age 60 or greater, deep (outer, 50%) myometrial invasion if grades 1 and 2, or superficially invasive grade 3 histology. Adjuvant pelvic RT given to this intermediate- to high-risk group lessened local relapse from 21.7% to 7.5% (40).

- PORTEC-2 (41) is the first randomized trial comparing the efficacy of vaginal brachytherapy (VBT) and EBRT to determine which treatment provides optimal local control with best quality of life. 427 patients with stage I or IIA disease after TAHB/BSO (surgical lymphadenectomy was excluded) were randomized to pelvic EBRT (46 Gy in 23 fractions) or VBT (21 Gy HDR in 3 fractions or 30 Gy LDR). Eligible patients had a high-intermediate-risk EC: age more than 60 and stage IC grades 1 and 2 or stage IB grade 3; any age and stage IIA grades 1 and 2 or 3 with less than 50% invasion. At a median follow-up of 45 months, 5-year rates of vaginal recurrence were 1.8% in the VBT arm and 1.6% after EBRT ($p = 0.74$). Five-year rates of LRR were 5.1% in the VBT arm and 2.1% in the EBRT arm ($p = 0.17$). There were no significant differences in 5-year OS (84.8% versus 79.6% $p = 0.57$). Rates of acute GI toxicity were significantly lower in the VBT group, 12.6% versus 53.8%. Given the equivalent recurrence and survival outcomes between VBT alone and EBRT, VBT should be the treatment of choice for patients with high-intermediate-risk endometrial carcinoma to reduce toxicity.

- ASTEC/EN.5 (42) included 905 patients with intermediate- or high-risk disease and randomized to observation or EBRT after hysterectomy and BSO. Patients in these trials could have lymphadenectomy, and VBT was allowed in either arm for stage I or IIA patients, resulting in 52% receiving VBT in the observation arm and 54% receiving VBT in the EBRT group. The 5-year LRR rate was decreased in the EBRT group (3.2% versus 6.1%), but there was no difference in OS between groups.

- In a 2012 Cochrane review (43) on the role of adjuvant RT in early-stage disease, analysis demonstrated that EBRT reduced locoregional recurrence but with significant acute and late toxicities and reduced quality of life. This included results from eight clinical trials, including ASTEC/EN.5, GOG 99, PORTEC-1, PORTEC-2, and trials by Aalders et al., Soderini et al. in 2003, and Sorbe et al. in 2009 and 2011.

- GOG 249 is a randomized phase III trial with the primary objective of determining if VCB and chemotherapy could increase recurrence-free survival compared to pelvic EBRT in patients with high-intermediate-risk stage I endometrioid histology, stage II, or stage I/II serous or clear cell histology. A total of 601 patients were enrolled, and the recurrence-free survival was 82% for both treatment arms at a median follow-up of 53 months (44).

- GOG 258 is a randomized phase III trial in patients with stage III/IVA uterine cancer or stage I/II with serous or clear cell histology and positive cytology, testing whether treatment with concurrent cisplatin and EBRT followed by carboplatin and paclitaxel reduces the rate of recurrence compared to chemotherapy with carboplatin and paclitaxel alone. With a median follow-up of 47 months, concurrent chemoradiation reduced vaginal (HR 0.36, 95% CI 0.16 to 0.82), pelvic, and paraaortic recurrences (HR 0.43, 95% CI 0.28 to 0.66) compared to chemotherapy alone, but there was no difference in recurrence-free survival (HR 0.9, 95% CI 0.74 to 1.10) (45).

- PORTEC-3 investigated the benefit of adjuvant chemotherapy during and after radiation versus pelvic radiation alone in patients with high-risk endometrial cancer (FIGO stage I grade 3 with deep myometrial invasion and/or LVSI, stage II or III, or serous/clear cell histology). OS and failure-free survival were co-primary end points. Adjuvant chemotherapy given during and after pelvic radiotherapy for treatment of HREC compared with RT alone did not significantly improve 5-year FFS (0.77 [0.58 to 1.03, p = 0.078]) and OS (HR 0.79 [95% CI 0.57 to 1.12, p = 0.183]). Stage III demonstrated greater FFS benefit with concurrent chemoradiation and adjuvant chemotherapy compared to chemotherapy alone (5-year FFS 69.3% versus 58.0%, p = 0.032) (46).

RANDOMIZED STUDIES FOR LYMPHADENECTOMY

- The ASTEC surgical study group (47) investigated whether pelvic lymphadenectomy could improve survival of women with endometrial cancer. One thousand four hundred and eight women with histologically proven endometrial carcinoma, which was thought preoperatively to be confined to the corpus, were randomized to standard surgery (hysterectomy and BSO, peritoneal washings, and palpation of paraaortic nodes; n = 704) or standard surgery plus lymphadenectomy (n = 704). No evidence of benefit in terms of overall or recurrence-free survival for pelvic lymphadenectomy was found in women with early endometrial cancer.
- Benedetti Panici et al. (13) randomized 514 women with FIGO stage I endometrial carcinoma to undergo TAH/BSO with or without lymphadenectomy. Both early and late postoperative complications occurred statistically significantly more frequently in the patients with lymphadenectomy. The 5-year disease-free and OS rates in an intention-to-treat analysis were similar between arms (81.0% and 85.9% in the lymphadenectomy arm and 81.7% and 90.0% in the no-lymphadenectomy arm, respectively).

RANDOMIZED STUDIES FOR CHEMOTHERAPY

- GOG 122 randomized 396 patients with III/IV disease treated with surgery with maximal residual disease less than 2 cm to WAI (30 Gy + 15 Gy pelvic boost + 15 Gy paraaortic boost if pelvic lymph node + or no sampling) or chemotherapy (cisplatin + doxorubicin). Chemotherapy improved disease-free survival from 38% to 50% and 5-year OS from 42% to 55% (17).
- A multi-institutional study from Italy (Maggi et al., 2006) randomized 345 patients with high-risk endometrial cancer treated with surgery (stage IC or II grade 3 with

greater than 50% invasion or stage III) to pelvic radiotherapy (45 to 50 Gy) or five cycles of CDDP, Adriamycin, and Cytoxan. With a median follow-up of 95.5 months, there was no difference in 5-year DFS or OS. Radiotherapy reduced locoregional recurrence rate (7% versus 11%), and chemotherapy reduced distant failures (16% versus 21%) (48).

- GOG 34 randomized patients, from November 1977 to July 1986, between RT alone and RT with Adriamycin. Chemotherapy in addition to radiation did not improve outcome when compared to radiation alone (3 years OS 68% versus 75%) (49).
- RTOG 9708 (Greven et al., 2006) was a phase II trial examining the use of concurrent chemotherapy (cisplatin) with pelvic RT (45 Gy) and VCB followed by four cycles of chemotherapy (cisplatin + paclitaxel). Patients with stage I to III surgical staged endometrial cancer were included if they had grade 2 to 3 disease, greater than 50% invasion, cervical stroma involvement, extrauterine disease (pelvic only), and positive cytology washings. The 4-year locoregional relapse rate was 4%, and the distant failure rate was 19%, translating to an 81% DFS and 85% OS (19). These promising data led to the development of a phase III trial, RTOG 9901, but it closed for lack of accrual.
- NSGO EC-9501/EORTC-55991 enrolled 382 patients from 1996 to 2007 who were surgical stage I, II, IIIA, or IIIC with high risk for micrometastatic disease or serous, clear cell, or anaplastic carcinoma regardless of other risk factors. Patients were randomized to pelvic radiotherapy (greater than or equal to 44 Gy) with optional VCB or pelvic radiotherapy with chemotherapy either before or after radiotherapy. The primary end point of progression-free survival showed an advantage for chemotherapy and radiation (HR 0.64, 95% CI 0.41 to 0.99; $p = 0.04$) (23).
- MaNGO ILIADE-III was a multicenter study, which included endometrioid histology, stage IIB, IIIA to IIIC disease (stage IIIA with positive cytology alone without other risk factors was not included). Patients were randomized to receive RT alone (45 Gy pelvic with or without paraaortic fields or vaginal brachytherapy) or chemotherapy (doxorubicin + cisplatin) followed by RT within 4 weeks. There was no significant difference in PFS, OS, or CSS (23).
- A combined analysis of NSGO EC-9501/EORTC-55991 and MaNGO ILIADE-III showed that the addition of chemotherapy improved cancer-specific survival (CSS) (HR 0.55, CI 0.35 to 0.88; $p = 0.01$) and had a trend toward improving OS (HR 0.69, CI 0.46 to 1.03; $p = 0.07$) (23).

References

1. American Cancer Society. *Cancer Facts & Figures 2017*. Atlanta: American Cancer Society, 2017.
2. Gordon AN, et al. Preoperative assessment of myometrial invasion of endometrial adenocarcinoma by sonography (US) and magnetic resonance imaging (MRI). *Gynecol Oncol* 1989;34(2):175–179.
3. Ortashi O, et al. Evaluation of the sensitivity, specificity, positive and negative predictive values of preoperative magnetic resonance imaging for staging endometrial cancer. A prospective study of 100 cases at the Dorset Cancer Centre. *Eur J Obstet Gynecol Reprod Biol* 2008;137(2):232–235.
4. Timmermans A, et al. Endometrial thickness measurement for detecting endometrial cancer in women with postmenopausal bleeding: a systematic review and meta-analysis. *Obstet Gynecol* 2010;116(1):160–167.

5. Schwartz PE, et al. Circulating tumor markers in the monitoring of gynecologic malignancies. *Cancer* 1987;60(3):353–361.

6. Aalders J, et al. Postoperative external irradiation and prognostic parameters in stage I endometrial carcinoma: clinical and histopathologic study of 540 patients. *Obstet Gynecol* 1980;56(4):419–427.

7. Grigsby PW, et al. Clinical stage I endometrial cancer: prognostic factors for local control and distant metastasis and implications of the new FIGO surgical staging system. *Int J Radiat Oncol Biol Phys* 1992;22(5):905–911.

8. Morrow CP, et al. Relationship between surgical-pathologic risk factors and outcome in clinical stage I and II carcinoma of the endometrium: a Gynecologic Oncology Group study. *Gynecol Oncol* 1991;40(1):55–65.

9. Keys HM, et al. A phase III trial of surgery with or without adjunctive external pelvic radiation therapy in intermediate risk endometrial adenocarcinoma: a Gynecologic Oncology Group study. *Gynecol Oncol* 2004;92(3):744–751.

10. Creutzberg CL, et al. Outcome of high-risk stage IC, grade 3, compared with stage I endometrial carcinoma patients: the Postoperative Radiation Therapy in Endometrial Carcinoma Trial. *J Clin Oncol* 2004;22(7):1234–1241.

11. Briet JM, et al. Lymphvascular space involvement: an independent prognostic factor in endometrial cancer. *Gynecol Oncol* 2005;96(3):799–804.

12. Martin-Hirsch P, Jarvis G, Kitchener H. Progestagens for endometrial cancer. *Cochrane Database Syst Rev* 2000;2:CD001040.

13. Benedetti Panici P, et al. Systematic pelvic lymphadenectomy vs. no lymphadenectomy in early-stage endometrial carcinoma: randomized clinical trial. *J Natl Cancer Inst* 2008;100(23):1707–1716.

14. Kilgore LC, et al. Adenocarcinoma of the endometrium: survival comparisons of patients with and without pelvic node sampling. *Gynecol Oncol* 1995;56(1):29–33.

15. Todo Y, et al. Survival effect of para-aortic lymphadenectomy in endometrial cancer (SEPAL study): a retrospective cohort analysis. *Lancet* 2010;375(9721):1165–1172.

16. Klopp A, et al. The role of postoperative radiation therapy for endometrial cancer: executive summary of an American Society for Radiation Oncology evidence-based guideline. *Pract Radiat Oncol* 2014;4(3):137–144.

17. Randall ME, et al. Randomized phase III trial of whole-abdominal irradiation versus doxorubicin and cisplatin chemotherapy in advanced endometrial carcinoma: a Gynecologic Oncology Group Study. *J Clin Oncol* 2006;24(1):36–44.

18. Mundt AJ, et al. Significant pelvic recurrence in high-risk pathologic stage I–IV endometrial carcinoma patients after adjuvant chemotherapy alone: implications for adjuvant radiation therapy. *Int J Radiat Oncol Biol Phys* 2001;50(5):1145–1153.

19. Greven K, et al. Final analysis of RTOG 9708: adjuvant postoperative irradiation combined with cisplatin/paclitaxel chemotherapy following surgery for patients with high-risk endometrial cancer. *Gynecol Oncol* 2006;103(1):155–159.

20. Shaikh T, et al. The role of adjuvant radiation in lymph node positive endometrial adenocarcinoma. *Gynecol Oncol* 2016;141(3):434–439.

21. Wong AT, et al. Utilization of adjuvant therapies and their impact on survival for women with stage IIIC endometrial adenocarcinoma. *Gynecol Oncol* 2016;142(3):514–519.

22. von Minckwitz G, et al. Adjuvant endocrine treatment with medroxyprogesterone acetate or tamoxifen in stage I and II endometrial cancer—a multicentre, open, controlled, prospectively randomised trial. *Eur J Cancer* 2002;38(17):2265–2271.

23. Hogberg T, et al. Sequential adjuvant chemotherapy and radiotherapy in endometrial cancer—results from two randomised studies. *Eur J Cancer* 2010;46(13):2422–2431.

24. Schwarz JK, et al. Consensus statement for brachytherapy for the treatment of medically inoperable endometrial cancer. *Brachytherapy* 2015;14(5):587–599.

25. Gunderson L, Tepper J. Chapter 57. Endometrial cancer. In: Gunderson LL, Tepper JE, eds. *Clinical radiation oncology*, 3rd ed. Philadelphia, PA: Elsevier, 2012.

26. Grigsby PW, et al. Medically inoperable stage I adenocarcinoma of the endometrium treated with radiotherapy alone. *Int J Radiat Oncol Biol Phys* 1987;13(4):483–488.

27. Knocke TH, et al. Primary treatment of endometrial carcinoma with high-dose-rate brachytherapy: results of 12 years of experience with 280 patients. *Int J Radiat Oncol Biol Phys* 1997;37(2):359–365.

28. Hoekstra CJ, Koper PC, van Putten WL. Recurrent endometrial adenocarcinoma after surgery alone: prognostic factors and treatment. *Radiother Oncol* 1993;27(2):164–166.

29. Creutzberg CL, et al. Survival after relapse in patients with endometrial cancer: results from a randomized trial. *Gynecol Oncol* 2003;89(2):201–209.

30. Nag S, et al. Interstitial brachytherapy for salvage treatment of vaginal recurrences in previously unirradiated endometrial cancer patients. *Int J Radiat Oncol Biol Phys* 2002;54(4):1153–1159.

31. Petignat P, et al. Salvage treatment with high-dose-rate brachytherapy for isolated vaginal endometrial cancer recurrence. *Gynecol Oncol* 2006;101(3):445–449.

32. Pravati AJ, Simpson D, Yashar CM, et al. Uterine cancer. In: Lee NY, Riaz N, Lu JJ, eds. *Target volume delineation for conformal and intensity-modulated radiation therapy*. Switzerland: Springer, 2015.

33. Small W Jr, et al. Consensus guidelines for delineation of clinical target volume for intensity-modulated pelvic radiotherapy in postoperative treatment of endometrial and cervical cancer. *Int J Radiat Oncol Biol Phys* 2008;71(2):428–434.

34. Jhingran A, et al. A phase II study of intensity modulated radiation therapy to the pelvis for postoperative patients with endometrial carcinoma: radiation therapy oncology group trial 0418. *Int J Radiat Oncol Biol Phys* 2012;84(1):e23–e28.

35. Sorbe B, Straumits A, Karlsson L. Intravaginal high-dose-rate brachytherapy for stage I endometrial cancer: a randomized study of two dose-per-fraction levels. *Int J Radiat Oncol Biol Phys* 2005;62(5):1385–1389.

36. Small W Jr, et al. American Brachytherapy Society consensus guidelines for adjuvant vaginal cuff brachytherapy after hysterectomy. *Brachytherapy* 2012;11(1):58–67.

37. Kamrava M, et al. American Brachytherapy Society recurrent carcinoma of the endometrium task force patterns of care and review of the literature. *Brachytherapy* 2017;16(6):1129–1143.

38. Spanos W Jr, et al. Phase II study of multiple daily fractionations in the palliation of advanced pelvic malignancies: preliminary report of RTOG 8502. *Int J Radiat Oncol Biol Phys* 1989;17(3):659–661.

39. Creutzberg CL, et al. Surgery and postoperative radiotherapy versus surgery alone for patients with stage-1 endometrial carcinoma: multicentre randomised trial. PORTEC Study Group. Post Operative Radiation Therapy in Endometrial Carcinoma. *Lancet* 2000;355(9213):1404–1411.

40. Scholten AN, et al. Postoperative radiotherapy for Stage 1 endometrial carcinoma: long-term outcome of the randomized PORTEC trial with central pathology review. *Int J Radiat Oncol Biol Phys* 2005;63(3):834–838.

41. Nout RA, et al. Vaginal brachytherapy versus pelvic external beam radiotherapy for patients with endometrial cancer of high-intermediate risk (PORTEC-2): an open-label, non-inferiority, randomised trial. *Lancet* 2010;375(9717):816–823.

42. Group AES, et al. Adjuvant external beam radiotherapy in the treatment of endometrial cancer (MRC ASTEC and NCIC CTG EN.5 randomised trials): pooled trial results, systematic review, and meta-analysis. *Lancet* 2009;373(9658):137–146.

43. Kong A, et al. Adjuvant radiotherapy for stage I endometrial cancer. *Cochrane Database Syst Rev* 2012;(4):CD003916.

44. Randall M. A phase 3 trial of pelvic radiation therapy versus vaginal cuff brachytherapy followed by paclitaxel/carboplatin chemotherapy in patients with high-risk, early-stage endometrial cancer: a Gynecology Oncology Group Study. *Int J Radiat Oncol Biol Phys* 2017;99(2 Suppl):S1–S272, e1–e759.

45. Matei D. A randomized phase III trial of cisplatin and tumor volume directed irradiation followed by carboplatin and paclitaxel vs. carboplatin and paclitaxel for optimally debulked, advanced endometrial carcinoma. *J Clin Oncol* 2017;35(15 Suppl):5505.

46. de Boer SM. Final results of the international randomized PORTEC-3 trial of adjuvant chemotherapy and radiation therapy (RT) versus RT alone for women with high-risk endometrial cancer. *J Clin Oncol* 2017;35(15 Suppl):5502–5502.

47. ASTEC Study Group, et al. Efficacy of systematic pelvic lymphadenectomy in endometrial cancer (MRC ASTEC trial): a randomised study. *Lancet* 2009;373(9658):125–36.

48. Maggi R, et al. Adjuvant chemotherapy vs radiotherapy in high-risk endometrial carcinoma: results of a randomised trial. *Br J Cancer* 2006;95(3):266–271.

49. Morrow CP, et al. Doxorubicin as an adjuvant following surgery and radiation therapy in patients with high-risk endometrial carcinoma, stage I and occult stage II: a Gynecologic Oncology Group Study. *Gynecol Oncol* 1990;36(2):166–171.

CHAPTER 34

OVARY AND FALLOPIAN TUBE

INTRODUCTION

- There are projected to be 22,400 estimated new cases of carcinoma of the ovary, fallopian tube, or primary peritoneum in the United States in 2017, with an estimated death toll of 14,080 (1).
- Ovarian cancer is the second most common gynecologic malignancy and the leading cause of death from gynecologic cancer. Overall, it is the fifth leading cause of cancer death among women (1).
- The highest age-adjusted incidence rates are observed in Europe and North America, whereas they are lowest in Asia and Africa (2).
- Carcinoma of the fallopian tube and primary peritoneum are now diagnosed, staged, and managed similarly to carcinoma of the ovary. Unless noted below, the information regarding ovarian carcinoma relates also to carcinoma of the fallopian tube and primary peritoneum.

EPIDEMIOLOGY

- Carcinoma of the ovary is a disease of older women, with a peak incidence in the sixth or seventh decades of life (1). Although rarely diagnosed prior to menarche, when identified they are predominantly of ovarian germ cell histology at this early age.
- Family history of ovarian cancer, particularly of a first-degree relative, is one of the most significant risk factors for development of ovarian cancer. Known genetic syndromes constitute approximately 36% of ovarian cancers (3,4).
- Hereditary breast and ovarian cancer (HBOC) syndrome is caused by germ-line mutations in *BRCA1* or *BRCA2* genes and is associated with a 39% to 46% and 10% to 27% risk of ovarian cancer, respectively, by the age of 70 (3).
- Hereditary nonpolyposis colorectal cancer (HNPCC), or Lynch's syndrome, confers an increased risk of ovarian cancer, endometrial cancer, and colorectal cancer (3).
- Peutz-Jeghers syndrome is associated with an increased risk of ovarian sex cord–stromal tumors, as well as cervical and breast cancers (3).

- The Cancer Genome Atlas (TCGA) study demonstrated that of 316 primary specimens of *de novo* high-grade serous carcinoma, 96% demonstrated mutations of the *TP53* gene, whereas 17% demonstrated germ-line mutations in either the *BRCA1* or *BRCA2* genes. (5,6) Mutations in other genes involved in DNA repair such as *CHEK2, PALB2, RAD50, BARD1,* and *BRIP1* have also been identified.
- Hormonal and reproductive factors have been strongly implicated in the pathogenesis of ovarian cancer, particularly for the endometrioid and clear cell subtypes, and are potentially related to the number of uninterrupted ovulatory cycles in a woman's life. Nulliparity is associated with a 30% to 60% increased risk of ovarian cancer compared to women who have borne children, whereas each additional pregnancy is associated with an approximately 15% further decrease in risk. Younger age at first full-term pregnancy, breast-feeding, and use of oral contraceptives are also considered to be protective, particularly for endometrioid and clear cell subtypes (7,8).
- Other reported risk factors include use of hormone replacement therapy, increased levels of C-reactive protein, and history of depression, while women who undergo hysterectomy or tubal ligation have been shown to be at a reduced risk (9–12).
- Smoking has been associated with an increased risk of the mucinous subtype of ovarian cancer, but a decreased risk of the endometrioid and clear cell subtypes (13). An elevated body mass index has been linked to an increased risk of endometrioid ovarian cancers (14).

ANATOMY

- The paired ovaries are light gray and approximately the size and shape of large almonds (Fig. 34-1A and B).
- The fallopian tubes are hollow, muscular viscera positioned horizontally within the superior part of the broad ligament. Each fallopian tube extends from the ipsilateral ovary to the superoposterior aspect of the uterine fundus. Each tube is lined with ciliated columnar epithelium with secretory cells.
- During the reproductive years, each ovary weighs 3 to 6 g and measures approximately 1.5 × 2.5 × 4.0 cm.
- The mesovarium ligament, ovarian ligament, and infundibular pelvic ligament (suspensory ligament of the ovary) determine the anatomic mobility of the ovary.
- The mesovarium ligament contains the arterial anastomotic branches of the ovarian and uterine arteries.
- The ovarian ligament is a narrow, short, fibrous band that extends over the lower pole of the ovary to the uterus.
- The suspensory ligament attaches the ovary to the lateral pelvic walls and contains the ovarian artery, veins, and accompanying nerves.
- Regional lymphatic nodes of the ovaries include the internal iliac, obturator, sacral, external iliac, common iliac, paraaortic, and inguinal nodes.
- The arterial supply to the ovary is from the ovarian and uterine arteries, which are derived from the aorta and internal iliac arteries, respectively.

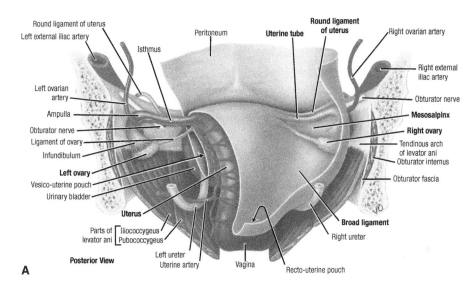

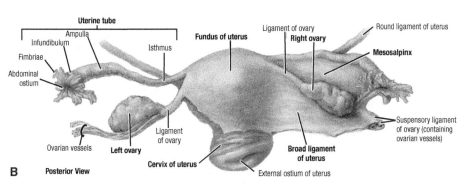

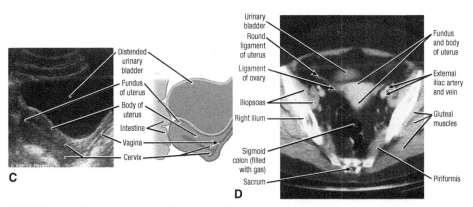

FIGURE 34-1. Pelvic anatomy. **A:** Female pelvic anatomy, paramedian section. **B:** Female reproductive anatomy. **C:** Longitudinal ultrasound image of the uterus and uterine adnexa. **D:** Transverse (axial) CT of the uterus and uterus adnexa. (Reprinted with permission from Agur AMR, Dalley AF, eds. *Grant's atlas of anatomy*, 14th ed. Philadelphia, PA: Wolters Kluwer, 2017: Chapter 5. © Wolters Kluwer.)

NATURAL HISTORY

- Ovarian tumors arise from one of three cell types: epithelial cells, stromal cells, and germ cells. Approximately 90% of tumors are epithelial, whereas 5% to 6% are sex cord–stromal tumors, and 2% to 3% are germ cell tumors (15). In 2014, the World Health Organization (WHO) and the International Federation of Gynecology and Obstetrics (FIGO) adopted a unified classification of the common epithelial, germ cell, sex cord, and stromal ovarian tumors (16).

- Historically, epithelial ovarian carcinoma was believed to originate from the malignant transformation of the ovarian surface epithelium that is entrapped in ovarian inclusion cysts during ovulation. More recently, however, emerging evidence has suggested that a large percentage of epithelial ovarian cancers may originate from the epithelium of the fallopian tube fimbria that then spread to the ovary or peritoneal cavity (17). A third site of origin may include mesothelium-lined surfaces within the peritoneal cavity.

- Sex cord–stromal tumors arise from the ovarian stroma, which consists of granulosa cells, theca cells, and fibroblasts, whereas germ cell tumors most commonly arise from the primitive streak.

- Dissemination can occur through transcoelomic, lymphatic, hematogenous, or direct spread. Exfoliation of tumor cells from the ovarian surface can lead to tumor implantation of the omentum and peritoneal surfaces.

- All peritoneal surfaces are at risk for tumor implantation and nodule growth. The peritoneal surfaces of the diaphragm, liver, and spleen are frequently coated by tumor in advanced disease.

- The Surveillance, Epidemiology and End Results (SEER) database between 2007 and 2013 reported that 15% of newly diagnosed cases were localized, 20% had spread to regional lymph nodes, and 60% had metastasized to distant sites (18).

- The most frequently involved nodal regions are the pelvic and paraaortic lymph nodes, which are involved in approximately 10% to 20% of patients with clinically localized disease and up to 80% of those with advanced disease (19,20).

- Hematogenous metastases most frequently spread to the liver, lung, and pleura, and less frequently to the bones, kidneys, bladder, skin, adrenal glands, and spleen.

- Despite optimal treatment, up to 25% of patients experience disease recurrence less than 6 months following completion of primary chemotherapy and 60% will eventually experience relapse (21).

PATHOLOGIC CLASSIFICATION

- The main histologic subtypes of epithelial ovarian cancer are high-grade serous (70%), endometrioid (10%), mucinous (10% to 15%), clear cell (5%), low-grade serous (less than 5%), and transitional cell (1% to 2%).

- Borderline tumors, also known as tumors of low malignant potential, do not demonstrate stromal invasion, and have excellent prognosis (22).

- High-grade serous epithelial ovarian tumors are thought to arise from atypical lesions within the fimbriae of the epithelium of the fallopian tube that then shed into the ovary, whereas low-grade serous epithelial ovarian tumors may be derived from transplanted tubal epithelium (23,24).
- Endometrioid and clear cell epithelial ovarian tumors may arise from endometriotic cysts, whereas mucinous tumors may arise from transitional cell nests at the tubal-mesothelial junction (25,26).
- Transitional cell tumors are considered to be a subset of epithelial tumors that resemble transitional cells of the urinary tract and demonstrate increased sensitivity to chemotherapy and favorable outcomes (27,28).
- Bilateral tumors may be identified in up to 30% of patients with serous tumors, 15% of patients with endometrioid tumors, and 5% to 10% of patients with mucinous tumors.
- Low-grade serous, endometrioid, clear cell, mucinous, and borderline ovarian carcinomas are considered to be type I tumors, whereas high-grade serous ovarian carcinomas are considered to be type II tumors.
- Type I tumors frequently demonstrate mutations encoding the B-raf and KRAS proteins, whereas type II tumors more commonly have mutations in the TP53 proteins.

SCREENING

- The location of the ovaries, nonspecific symptoms related to disease presentation, as well as the relatively low incidence of disease renders early diagnosis of ovarian cancer challenging, particularly for early-stage disease or in younger women.
- Routine screening is not currently recommended by any professional society because of a lack of demonstrated mortality benefit with currently available screening tests, including serum levels of cancer antigen 125 (CA-125), human epididymis (HE4), or transvaginal ultrasonography (TVUS).

CA-125

- CA-125 is an ovarian tumor-associated antigen that is elevated in approximately 80% of women with ovarian cancer (29). CA-125 demonstrates greater sensitivity for the detection of serous subtypes, whereas levels are lower in cases of mucinous subtypes (30).
- CA-125 is considered at this time to be inadequate for use as a screening test either alone or in conjunction with TVUS. The Prostate, Lung, Colorectal and Ovarian (PLCO) Cancer Screening Randomized Controlled Trial of 72,816 women revealed no significant reduction in mortality among women screened with CA-125 and TVUS (31). Combined screening tests such as the OVA1 and OvaSure, which include other potential biomarkers of ovarian cancer in addition to CA-125, are also not recommended as screening tests of ovarian cancer (32).
- The UK Collaborative Trial of Ovarian Cancer Screening (UKCTOCS) evaluated multimodality screening of postmenopausal women with TVUS and CA-125 versus

TVUS alone or no screening. Primary analysis revealed a nonsignificant 10% reduction in mortality with multimodality screening. However, when women who were previously diagnosed with ovarian cancer were excluded, the use of multimodality screening was associated with a 20% reduction in mortality that was statistically significant (33).

- Preoperative elevation of CA-125 and HE4 in conjunction with a symptom index has been demonstrated to have an 83% positive predictive value and an 89% negative predictive value for the prediction of localized ovarian cancer in women with pelvic masses (34).
- Preoperative level and relative decrease of CA-125 following resection has been shown to be prognostic for residual tumor burden, tumor recurrence, progression-free survival (PFS), and overall survival (OS) (35–37).
- If levels are elevated at diagnosis, routine surveillance of CA-125 is recommended following definitive treatment (38). Following evidence of biochemical recurrence, median time to clinical recurrence is 2 to 6 months (39).

CLINICAL PRESENTATION

- Common symptoms at presentation include abdominal or pelvic pain, abdominal distention, and gastrointestinal symptoms such as constipation, bloating, and early satiety.
- In early-stage disease, symptoms are rare and the diagnosis is usually made incidentally by palpation of an asymptomatic adnexal mass on routine examination.
- Most adnexal masses are not malignant and in premenopausal women, invasive cancer represents fewer than 5% of adnexal neoplasms. An adnexal mass in a postmenopausal woman has a higher likelihood of malignancy and surgical exploration is usually indicated.
- Unfortunately, most women are diagnosed after the disease has spread beyond the pelvis and present with abdominal pain or discomfort with increased abdominal girth related to ascites or large intra-abdominal masses.
- The majority of women with ovarian cancer are diagnosed with stage III to IV disease (40).

DIAGNOSTIC WORKUP

- The diagnostic workup and preoperative evaluation of a patient suspected of having an ovarian malignancy should include a full history and physical assessment, including bimanual pelvic examination.
- TVUS is a sensitive imaging study, especially when combined with color flow Doppler, and is generally utilized for initial evaluation of an adnexal mass. A complex mass seen on TVUS with multiple irregular septa, irregular borders, or solid and cystic elements is concerning for malignancy.
- Computed tomography (CT) scan, magnetic resonance imaging (MRI) scan with contrast, or positron emission tomography (PET)/CT scan can be performed to help determine malignant characteristics of an ovarian mass as well as to evaluate for upper abdominal or retroperitoneal disease.

- Routine laboratory studies should include a complete blood cell count, blood urea nitrogen, creatinine, and liver enzymes.
- Serum tumor markers can be assessed as clinically indicated. CA-125 is associated with serous epithelial tumors, whereas human chorionic gonadotropin (β-hCG), alpha-fetoprotein (AFP), and lactate dehydrogenase (LDH) are the most useful markers for germ cell tumors. Yolk sac tumors commonly demonstrate elevated levels of AFP, whereas choriocarcinomas and embryonal carcinomas demonstrate elevated levels of β-hCG, and dysgerminomas frequently demonstrate elevated levels of LDH. Immature teratomas oftentimes have normal serum levels but may show elevated levels of AFP.
- Diagnosis of an ovarian or fallopian tube cancer is made based on pathologic analysis of a surgical specimen. Fine needle aspiration (FNA) should not be performed in patients with suspected early-stage disease because of concern of seeding of disease into the peritoneum.

STAGING SYSTEMS

- The FIGO staging classification is the most widely used system (Table 34-1) (41).
- FIGO staging requires a thorough surgical exploration as outlined by the Gynecologic Oncology Group (GOG).
- Approximately 30% of patients presumed to have early-stage disease are upstaged following surgical staging.
- Patients who did not undergo complete surgical staging at the time of the initial surgical procedure should have a second-look laparotomy (42).

Table 34-1		
Staging Classification for Cancer of the Ovary, Fallopian Tube, and Peritoneum		
FIGO[a,b]	TNM	Definition
—	TX	Primary tumor cannot be assessed
—	T0	No evidence of primary tumor
I	**T1**	**Tumor limited to ovaries or fallopian tube(s)**
IA	T1a	Tumor limited to one ovary or fallopian tube; no tumor on ovarian or fallopian tube surface; no malignant cells in the ascites or peritoneal washings
IB	T1b	Tumor limited to both ovaries (capsules intact) or fallopian tubes; no tumor on ovarian or fallopian tube surface; no malignant cells in the ascites or peritoneal washings

continued

Table 34-1		
Staging Classification for Cancer of the Ovary, Fallopian Tube, and Peritoneum *(continued)*		
FIGO*a,b*	TNM	Definition
IC	T1c	Tumor limited to one or both ovaries or fallopian tubes, with any of the following:
IC1	T1c1	Surgical spill
IC2	T1c2	Capsule ruptured before surgery or tumor on ovarian or fallopian tube surface
IC3	T1c3	Malignant cells in the ascites or peritoneal washings.
II	**T2**	**Tumor involves one or both ovaries with pelvic extension and/or implants**
IIA	T2a	Extension and/or implants on uterus and/or fallopian tubes and/or ovaries.
IIB	T2b	Extension to other pelvic intraperitoneal tissues.
III	**T3**	**Tumor involves one or both ovaries or fallopian tubes, or primary peritoneal cancer, with cytologically or histologically confirmed spread to the peritoneum outside the pelvis and/or metastasis to the retroperitoneal lymph nodes.**
IIIA1	T1-2 N1	Positive retroperitoneal lymph nodes only (cytologically or histologically proven)
IIIA1(i)	T1-2 N1	Metastasis of retroperitoneal lymph nodes up to and including 10mm in greatest dimension
IIIA1(ii)	T1-2 N1	Metastasis of retroperitoneal lymph nodes greater than 10mm in greatest dimension
IIIA2	T3a N0-1	Microscopic extrapelvic (above the pelvic brim) peritoneal involvement with or without positive retroperitoneal lymph nodes.
IIIB	T3b N0-1	Macroscopic peritoneal metastasis beyond the pelvis 2 cm or less in greatest dimension with or without positive retroperitoneal lymph nodes.
IIIC	T3c N0-1	Macroscopic peritoneal metastasis beyond the pelvis 2 cm or greater in greatest dimension with or without positive retroperitoneal lymph nodes, or extension of tumor to capsule of liver and spleen without parenchymal involvement.
IV	Tx Nx M1	Distant metastasis excluding peritoneal metastases
IVA		Pleural effusion with positive cytology
IVB		Parenchymal metastases and metastases to extra-abdominal organs (including inguinal lymph nodes and lymph nodes outside of the abdominal cavity).

*a*Data from Prat J; FIGO Committee on Gynecologic Oncology. Staging classification for cancer of the ovary, fallopian tube, and peritoneum. *Int J Gynaecol Obstet* 2014;124(1):1–5.
*b*FIGO no longer includes stage 0 (Tis).

PROGNOSTIC FACTORS

Lymph Node Involvement

* Increased risk of lymph node involvement is associated with serous and high-grade histology, presence of ascites or positive cytologic washings, and tumor bilaterality (19,43,44).
* Nomograms for risk of pelvic and paraaortic lymph node involvement in patients with stage I to II ovarian cancer have been created based on stage, histology, and bilaterality (19).
* Tumors of high-grade serous, endometrioid, and undifferentiated subtypes are more likely to demonstrate lymph node involvement compared to tumors of low-grade serous or clear cell subtypes (19).

Survival

* An analysis of the SEER database for patients diagnosed between 2007 and 2013 reported a 5-year relative survival rate of 92.5% for patients with localized disease, 73.0% for patients with disease spread to the regional lymph nodes, and 28.9% for disease that had spread to distant sites (18).
* A nomogram for survival rates among women with epithelial ovarian cancer utilized age, time of surgery, residual disease, histology, FIGO Stage, WHO performance status, presence of ascites, and *BRCA* status (45).
* An analysis of over 1,500 patients with stage I epithelial ovarian cancer demonstrated that grade was the most important prognostic factor for PFS, followed by capsule rupture, stage, and age (46).
* Several meta-analyses of retrospective studies and prospective trials have demonstrated that among patients with advanced ovarian cancer the volume of postoperative residual disease is the most important prognostic factor for PFS and OS (21,47).
* In a retrospective analysis of patients with FIGO stage I to IV epithelial ovarian cancer enrolled in one of twelve prospective randomized GOG protocols, clear cell histology was associated with longer PFS times among patients with early-stage disease, whereas serous histology was associated with longer OS times among patients with advanced stage disease (48).
* In a prospective case-control study, longer disease-free interval following clinical remission was associated with longer PFS. Among patients who had been free of disease for 5 years, 97.7% remained disease free for a subsequent 3 years (49).

GENERAL MANAGEMENT

* Ovarian cancer is generally treated via primary cytoreduction followed by systemic chemotherapy (Table 34-2).
* Surgical management for a newly diagnosed ovarian mass with disease confined to the pelvis generally consists of staging laparotomy with total abdominal hysterectomy

Table 34-2

General Treatment Strategy for Serous Epithelial Ovarian Cancer Following Surgical Staging

FIGO Stage	Grade	Management
IA–IB	Grade 1	Observation
	Grade 2	Observation 3–6 cycles IV carboplatin/paclitaxel
	Grade 3	3–6 cycles IV carboplatin/paclitaxel
IC–II	Grade 1	Observation 3–6 cycles IV carboplatin/paclitaxel Hormone therapy
IC	Grade 2–3	3–6 cycles IV carboplatin/paclitaxel
II	Grade 2–3	Optimally debulked: 6 cycles IP/IV carboplatin/paclitaxel Not optimally debulked: 6 cycles IV carboplatin/paclitaxel
III	Grades 1–3	Optimally debulked: 6 cycles IP/IV carboplatin/paclitaxel Not optimally debulked: 6 cycles IV carboplatin/paclitaxel
IV	Grades 1–3	6 cycles IV carboplatin/paclitaxel

(TAH), bilateral salpingo-oophorectomy (BSO), omentectomy, dissection of the paraaortic and pelvic lymph nodes, peritoneal lavage, and peritoneal biopsies.

- Fertility-sparing surgical staging consisting of unilateral salpingo-oophorectomy (USO) may be considered for carefully selected patients with early-stage and low-risk disease.
- Adjuvant systemic intravenous (IV) chemotherapy with or without intraperitoneal (IP) chemotherapy is indicated for patients with epithelial and germ cell tumors that are stage IC disease or above as well as patients with Stage IA to B Grade 3 disease and may be considered for patients with stage IA to B Grade 2 disease. There is no evidence that adjuvant chemotherapy improves outcomes for patients with sex cord or stromal tumors.
- The chemotherapeutic regimen of choice is generally carboplatin and paclitaxel for women with epithelial tumors, whereas germ cell tumors are treated with bleomycin, etoposide, and a platinum-based regimen.
- Neoadjuvant chemotherapy followed by interval cytoreduction may be performed for patients considered to be poor surgical candidates or with a low likelihood of achieving optimal debulking with primary cytoreduction.
- Secondary cytoreduction, chemotherapy, and palliative radiotherapy may be considered for patients who experience relapsed disease.
- Following initial therapy, patients should be followed closely for clinical signs of recurrent disease, such as pelvic pain, weight loss, or bloating, with imaging studies ordered as clinically indicated (50).
- Monitoring of serum CA-125 levels may be considered for patients who demonstrated elevated CA-125 levels at diagnosis (50). Treatment based upon biochemical

relapse alone, however, has not been shown to be associated with longer survival as compared to treatment following clinical evidence of recurrence (51). Hormonal therapies may be considered for patients with increasing serum CA-125 levels without clinical evidence of recurrence (52).

Surgery

- Surgery is the initial treatment strategy for most cases of newly diagnosed ovarian cancer in order to achieve pathologic diagnosis, surgical staging, and cytoreduction.
- Cytoreductive surgery is a critical component of surgical management in patients with ovarian cancer. There are three types of cytoreductive surgery: primary cytoreduction is performed prior to adjuvant therapy; interval cytoreduction is performed following suboptimal debulking and/or induction chemotherapy; and secondary cytoreduction is performed in a patient with recurrent disease who has completed primary treatment.
- Complete debulking is defined as resection of all gross residual disease. Optimal debulking is defined as macroscopic disease up to 1 cm in diameter following primary surgery. Suboptimal debulking is defined as macroscopic disease greater than 1 cm in size following primary surgery. Maximal cytoreduction of disease has been shown to be associated with longer median survival times independent of adjuvant therapy (53).
- Comprehensive staging laparotomy including a TAH and BSO should be performed by a gynecologic oncologist. The extent of initial disease, whether a complete or incomplete resection was achieved, and a description of the size and number of any residual lesions following debulking should be described in the operative report (54).

General Surgical Approach

- For most patients, an open laparotomy with a vertical midline abdominal incision is performed. TAH and BSO should be performed with the goal of keeping an encapsulated mass intact during removal. A minimally invasive surgical approach may be considered for women with early-stage disease. Conversion to an open procedure should be performed should optimal debulking not be feasible using a minimally invasive approach (38).
- A meta-analysis of randomized clinical trials demonstrated no statistically significant difference in risk of locoregional recurrence or death between patients treated with laparotomy versus laparoscopy (55).
- Upon entering the abdomen, aspiration of ascites or peritoneal lavage of the pelvis, paracolic gutters, and infradiaphragmatic area should be performed for cytologic analysis.
- All peritoneal surfaces, including the undersurface of both diaphragms as well as the serosa and mesentery of the entire gastrointestinal tract should be visualized and palpated for evidence of metastatic disease. Any peritoneal surface or adhesion suspicious for metastatic involvement should be excised or biopsied. If no lesions are visualized, random peritoneal biopsies should be performed.
- Careful inspection and biopsy or removal of the omentum should be performed.

- Bilateral pelvic and paraaortic lymph node sampling or dissection should be performed in all patients. Any suspicious or enlarged nodes and all remaining gross disease within the abdominal cavity should be resected.
- For patients with disease involving the upper abdomen, maximum cytoreduction of disease should be performed and may include partial or total resection of involved organs including the diaphragm, colon, appendix, bladder, gallbladder, liver, stomach, and pancreas.
- Women diagnosed with primary invasive mucinous tumors should undergo appendectomy, as well as careful evaluation of the upper and lower gastrointestinal tract to rule out an occult primary.

Lymph Node Evaluation

- Lymphadenectomy is highly recommended, particularly for patients with extrapelvic tumor nodules that are ≤2 cm in maximal dimension.
- Pelvic lymph node dissection consists of removal of the lymph nodes overlying and anterolateral or anteromedial to the bilateral common iliac vessels, external iliac vessels, and hypogastric vessels, as well as within the obturator fossa.
- Paraaortic lymph node dissection is performed by stripping the nodal tissue from the vena cava and aorta to at least the level of the inferior mesenteric artery.
- Systematic pelvic and paraaortic lymphadenectomy among patients with presumed clinical early-stage epithelial ovarian carcinoma is associated with a higher rate of identification of involved lymph nodes and subsequent upstaging compared to resection of macroscopic lymph nodes alone and can inform clinical management decisions regarding adjuvant chemotherapy.
- Lymphadenectomy has been shown in a randomized trial to be associated with longer PFS (56,57). An exploratory analysis of three randomized trials demonstrated that lymphadenectomy was associated with significantly longer OS times (58).

Advanced Stage

- The Society of Gynecologic Oncology (SGO) and American Society of Clinical Oncology (ASCO) 2016 Clinical Practice Guideline recommends primary cytoreductive surgery for women with suspected stage IIIC or IV disease thought to have a high likelihood of achieving cytoreduction to less than 1 cm with acceptable morbidity.
- Women determined to have high perioperative morbidity risk or a low likelihood of achieving cytoreduction to less than 1 cm should receive neoadjuvant chemotherapy followed by possible interval cytoreduction.
- In two randomized clinical trials of women with stage III to IV disease (EORTC 55971 and the CHORUS trial), neoadjuvant chemotherapy followed by interval cytoreductive surgery was found to be noninferior to primary cytoreductive surgery with respect to PFS and OS (59,60). Secondary analyses suggested that primary cytoreductive surgery was associated with longer survival among women with stage IIIC cancer and smaller burden of metastatic disease, whereas women with stage IV cancer and greater burden of metastatic disease had longer survival with neoadjuvant chemotherapy followed by interval debulking surgery (61).

- A meta-analysis of three randomized clinical trials found no statistically significant benefit of interval cytoreduction following primary cytoreduction and adjuvant chemotherapy compared to primary cytoreduction and adjuvant chemotherapy alone (62).
- Ultraradical surgery to achieve debulking of large-volume involvement of the upper abdomen can be associated with significant morbidity and complications. Tumor burden, patient age greater than 70 years, significant comorbidity, and poor performance status are all factors that should be considered to determine if optimal debulking without significant postoperative complication is likely to be achieved (63,64).

Recurrent Disease

- For patients clinically suspected of recurrent ovarian cancer, secondary cytoreduction can be considered for select patients with the goal of achieving complete tumor debulking.
- A meta-analysis of retrospective studies demonstrated that patients with recurrent disease who underwent secondary cytoreduction and achieved complete debulking experienced longer overall post-recurrence survival as compared to those for whom complete debulking was not achieved (65).
- Given the potential morbidity associated with surgery and the limited benefit for patients who achieve suboptimal debulking, patient factors that should be considered in determining eligibility for secondary cytoreduction include (1) a disease-free interval of at least 6 to 12 months; (2) sensitivity to platinum chemotherapy; (3) oligometastatic or localized disease without evidence of ascites or carcinomatosis; and (4) good performance status (66).

Risk-Reducing Salpingo-Oophorectomy

- Risk-reducing salpingo-oophorectomy (RRSO) is recommended for women determined to be at high risk for hereditary breast and ovarian cancer syndromes.
- During this procedure, pelvic washings and BSO should be performed with removal of 2 cm of the proximal ovarian vasculature and infundibular pelvic ligaments as well as all surrounding peritoneum. The fallopian tubes from the fimbriae to the insertion point into the uterus should be removed. Both the ovaries and fallopian tubes should be carefully sectioned and examined for evidence of disease.
- Concurrent hysterectomy or salpingectomy alone without oophorectomy is controversial.
- Minimally invasive techniques may be considered for patients undergoing RRSO.

SYSTEMIC THERAPY FOR EPITHELIAL OVARIAN CARCINOMA

- Following cytoreduction, systemic platinum-based chemotherapy is the standard of care for all but the lowest risk patients (stage IA to IB, Grade 1) with epithelial ovarian cancer.

- Recommended adjuvant or neoadjuvant IV and IV/IP chemotherapy regimens for patients with stage II to IV epithelial ovarian, fallopian tube, or primary peritoneal cancer generally consist of carboplatin and paclitaxel with or without bevacizumab for 6 cycles. Reduced dose chemotherapy regimens for 18 cycles can be used for patients with poor performance status.
- If used upfront, bevacizumab may also be considered as a maintenance regimen for a total of 22 cycles (38).
- Docetaxel with carboplatin may be an appropriate regimen for patients at high risk for peripheral neuropathy.
- 6 cycles of chemotherapy are recommended for patients with advanced stage disease, whereas 3 to 6 cycles may be considered for patients with early-stage disease.
- Maintenance chemotherapy with pazopanib or paclitaxel may be considered for women who achieve complete remission following initial therapy.

Early-Stage Disease

- A meta-analysis of four randomized clinical trials evaluating adjuvant chemotherapy for patients with FIGO stage I to IIA epithelial ovarian cancer demonstrated that women with high-risk early-stage disease who received cisplatin-based chemotherapy following primary cytoreduction had significantly increased 10-year OS and PFS compared to women who were observed (67). Subgroup analyses were unable to conclude whether women with low-risk early-stage disease would derive a substantial benefit from adjuvant chemotherapy.
- Currently, NCCN guidelines recommend observation for patients with stage IA or IB Grade 1 disease given their high rates of OS with surgical resection alone (38).
- Hormone therapy may be considered for patients with Grade 1 disease.

Advanced-Stage Disease

1. Women with stage II to IV disease should be offered adjuvant IV chemotherapy generally consisting of 6 cycles of carboplatin and paclitaxel. Patients who achieve optimal debulking may be offered combination IP and IV chemotherapy consisting of six cycles of IV/IP paclitaxel with IP cisplatin.
   - In GOG-172, a Phase III clinical trial of patients with stage III ovarian or primary peritoneal cancer with residual disease less than 1 cm following cytoreductive surgery, women were randomized to receive either IP administration of cisplatin with IV/IP paclitaxel or IV chemotherapy alone. The IV/IP chemotherapy regimen was associated with a 16-month increase in median OS and a 21.6% decrease in risk of death (68).
   - More recently, patients with stage III ovarian cancer who underwent primary cytoreduction with no residual disease followed by IP/IV chemotherapy demonstrated a median OS of 110 months (69). Each additional cycle of IP chemotherapy has been shown to lengthen median OS (70).
   - Dose-dense chemotherapy regimens have demonstrated conflicting results. In the randomized clinical trial JGOG 3016, patients treated with dose-dense chemotherapy with weekly paclitaxel and carboplatin demonstrated significantly

longer PFS and OS times compared to patients treated with conventional treatment regimens (71). A recent study, however, did not show longer PFS with dose-dense treatment with carboplatin and paclitaxel (72).

- Results from GOG-178 demonstrated that among women who achieved a complete clinical response following initial therapy, 12 months of maintenance paclitaxel was associated with significantly longer PFS compared to no maintenance therapy (73). Results from GOG-175, however, demonstrated that maintenance weekly paclitaxel for 6 months was not associated with a longer recurrence-free interval (74).
- Treatment with upfront bevacizumab with carboplatin and paclitaxel followed by maintenance bevacizumab has been shown in two randomized clinical trials to be associated with a 2- to 4-month increase in PFS and may confer a particular survival benefit among women with ascites or with a poor prognosis (75,76).
- Post-remission treatment with 12 monthly cycles of pazopanib was demonstrated in a randomized clinical trial to be associated with increased PFS and may therefore be considered for patients with stage II to IV epithelial ovarian cancer, fallopian tube cancer, or primary peritoneal cancer who achieve complete clinical remission following initial therapy (77).
- For patients undergoing neoadjuvant chemotherapy, a minimum of 6 cycles is recommended, including 3 cycles of adjuvant chemotherapy following interval cytoreduction. Bevacizumab should be used with caution as it can affect healing following surgery.
- Patients with poor performance status, older age, significant comorbidities, or stage IV disease may not be able to tolerate certain regimens and may require weekly dosing of a combined chemotherapy regimen or single-agent platinum-based chemotherapy alone (78).

RECURRENT DISEASE

- Chemotherapy regimens for patients with recurrent disease are based on platinum-sensitivity, histology, number of previous lines of systemic treatment, and *BRCA* status.
- For patients with platinum-sensitive recurrent disease, combination platinum-based regimens with or without bevacizumab are recommended. The OCEANS trial demonstrated that patients with platinum-sensitive disease had significantly longer PFS, but not OS, when treated with bevacizumab with chemotherapy compared to chemotherapy alone (79).
- In GOG-213, women with recurrent ovarian, primary peritoneal, or fallopian tube cancer who had achieved a complete clinical response to primary platinum-based chemotherapy and were disease-free for at least 6 months were randomized to chemotherapy with or without induction and maintenance therapy with bevacizumab. Women with platinum-sensitive recurrent disease in the bevacizumab arm experienced longer median OS (80).
- For patients with platinum-resistant recurrent disease, sequential single-agent regimens or combination regimens with bevacizumab are generally recommended. In the

AURELIA trial, patients with platinum-resistant disease had modestly longer PFS and objective response rates when treated with bevacizumab in addition to chemotherapy compared to chemotherapy alone (81).

* Olaparib and rucaparib may be considered for women with known *BRCA* mutations who have progressed following at least two lines of chemotherapy.
* Patients who have experienced progression of disease following two consecutive chemotherapy regimens without experiencing clinical benefit have a poor prognosis and may derive little minimal benefit from further systemic therapy (82).

MANAGEMENT OF LESS COMMON OVARIAN HISTOLOGIES

* Histopathologies other than serous epithelial carcinoma include borderline epithelial tumors, carcinosarcoma (malignant mixed mullerian tumor), clear cell carcinoma, mucinous carcinoma, transitional cell carcinoma, malignant sex cord–stromal tumors, and malignant germ cell tumors.
* Diagnostic workup is the same as for serous epithelial carcinoma, whereas additional tumor markers including inhibin, β-hCG, AFP, and CEA may be obtained for patients suspected of having a germ cell or sex cord–stromal tumor.
* As with serous epithelial carcinoma, patients with less common histopathologies should undergo primary cytoreduction and complete surgical staging. These tumors more commonly present at early stages, and patients may be candidates for fertility-sparing surgery, if desired.
* Prospective studies regarding less common histopathologies are limited.

Borderline Epithelial Tumors

* Patients without evidence of invasive implants following surgical staging may be observed. Patients with invasive implants should be treated as low-grade serous epithelial carcinoma.
* Patients with high-grade disease should be treated as serous epithelial carcinoma.

Carcinosarcoma

* Carcinosarcomas are rare and are associated with a poor prognosis. Following surgical staging, all patients with carcinosarcoma should undergo chemotherapy as per the recommendations for serous epithelial carcinoma (83).
* Alternative chemotherapy regimens for carcinosarcoma include platinum- or taxane-based chemotherapy with ifosfamide.

Clear Cell Carcinoma

* Clear cell carcinoma is considered a high-grade tumor (84). Advanced stage disease is associated with a poor prognosis (85).

- Tumors of clear cell histology are more likely to be confined to the pelvis and demonstrate increased chemoresistance compared to their histologic counterparts (48,86).
- Systematic lymphadenectomy has been shown to be associated with increased OS for patients with clear cell tumors, and is recommended for all patients (85).
- Patients with stage IA to IC clear cell carcinoma should receive 3 to 6 cycles of IV carboplatin and taxane chemotherapy (87). A recent multicenter retrospective study suggested that recurrence and survival was equivalent among patients with stage IA to II disease who received 3 as compared to 6 cycles of platinum-based chemotherapy (88).
- Patients with stage II to IV disease should be managed as serous epithelial ovarian carcinoma.

Mucinous Carcinoma of the Ovary

- Mucinous tumors are associated with younger age at diagnosis and larger size tumors. Patients diagnosed with mucinous tumors have a favorable prognosis (89).
- In addition to surgical staging generally including an appendectomy, patients with mucinous carcinoma should undergo comprehensive gastrointestinal evaluation and testing for carcinoembryonic antigen (CEA).
- Patients with stage IA to IB disease may be considered for fertility-sparing surgery and may be observed following primary cytoreduction.
- Women with stage IC disease may be observed or offered chemotherapy, whereas all patients with stage II to IV disease should be offered chemotherapy.
- Recommended chemotherapy regimens include standard platinum-/taxane-based chemotherapy. Alternative regimens include 5-fluorouracil (5-FU) with leucovorin or capecitabine with oxaliplatin.

Malignant Sex Cord–Stromal Tumors

- Malignant sex cord–stromal tumors include granulosa cell and Sertoli-Leydig cell tumors and generally present with early stage disease. Generally, these tumors are considered to be indolent and are associated with a good prognosis.
- Patients with stage IA to IC disease may be offered fertility-sparing surgery with complete staging with or without lymphadenectomy (90).
- Following surgical staging, patients with low-risk stage I disease may be observed. Intermediate-risk or high-risk patients may be observed or offered platinum-based chemotherapy (91).
- Patients with stage II to IV disease should be offered platinum-based chemotherapy or radiation therapy for limited disease.
- Recommended chemotherapy regimens for malignant sex cord–stromal tumors include platinum- and taxane-based and bleomycin, etoposide, cisplatin (BEP) regimens.

Malignant Germ Cell Tumors

- Germ cell tumor types include dysgerminomas, immature teratomas, embryonal tumors, and endodermal sinus tumors.

- Germ cell tumors primarily occur in young women with a median age of 16 to 20, and are associated with a good prognosis following surgical treatment (92).
- Patients with stage I dysgerminoma or stage I, grade 1 immature teratoma may be observed following surgical staging. All other patients (embryonal tumors, endodermal sinus tumors, stage II to IV dysgerminoma, and other teratomas) may be offered adjuvant chemotherapy with 3 to 4 cycles of BEP chemotherapy (93).
- Patients should be assessed for residual tumor following primary cytoreduction by imaging studies and measurement of serum tumor markers. If there is evidence of residual disease, chemotherapy may be considered.

RADIATION THERAPY

- Historically, whole abdominal radiotherapy (WAR) was a standard component of treatment for ovarian cancer following surgical resection, with the rationale of sterilizing micrometastatic IP disease. With the introduction of effective chemotherapeutic regimens and the toxicity associated with WAR, however, the use of radiation as an adjuvant therapy fell out of favor.
- Older techniques such as two-dimensional external beam radiation therapy (EBRT) or wide-field irradiation were associated with high levels of acute- and long-term toxicity, and efficacy was limited because of the dose constraints of normal bowel structures.
- The introduction of newer techniques for the planning and delivery of radiotherapy such as three-dimensional conformal radiation therapy (3D-CRT), intensity-modulated radiation therapy (IMRT) with image guidance radiation therapy (IGRT), and stereotactic body radiation therapy (SBRT) has led to renewed interest regarding the potential role of adjuvant or salvage radiotherapy for certain subgroups of patients.

Colloidal Intraperitoneal Phosphorus-32

- Colloidal IP phosphorus-32 (^{32}P) was investigated as both an adjuvant and consolidation therapy in several clinical trials that enrolled through the early 1990s.
- Use of IP ^{32}P was consistently associated with increased toxicity without lengthening time to recurrence or death either compared to chemotherapy alone or following chemotherapy as a consolidative treatment (94–96).

Adjuvant Radiotherapy

- Early studies suggested that treatment of early-stage patients with WAR following primary cytoreduction lengthened survival as compared to observation alone or pelvic radiation plus chlorambucil (97,98).
- Subsequent trials, however, demonstrated that women with early-stage ovarian cancer treated with adjuvant WAR had either decreased or equivalent survival compared to women treated with adjuvant chemotherapy either alone or with pelvic radiotherapy (99–102).

- More recently, the multicenter OVAR-IMRT trial evaluated the tolerability of consolidative IMRT to the whole abdomen among 20 patients who achieved complete remission following chemotherapy. This technique achieved excellent coverage of the treatment volume with effective sparing of organs at risk and was well-tolerated with acceptable levels of acute toxicity (103).
- Long-term follow-up results of 16 patients treated with IMRT to the whole abdomen demonstrated median recurrence-free survival (RFS) of 27.6 months and median OS of 42.1 months. The most frequent site of initial failure following IMRT was within the peritoneal cavity (104).

Consolidative Radiotherapy

- Trials evaluating WAR as a consolidation therapy following primary cytoreduction, adjuvant chemotherapy, and second-look surgery compared to either observation or further chemotherapy alone have demonstrated inconsistent results.
- Several studies demonstrated equivalent treatment outcomes between both treatment arms, but increased toxicity following WAR (105–107). The West Midlands Ovarian Cancer Group Trial II showed survival was not significantly increased with WAR as compared to chlorambucil chemotherapy alone following primary cytoreduction, chemotherapy, and second-look surgery (107).
- A prospective trial conducted in Austria demonstrated longer RFS and OS among women treated with WAR as compared to observation alone, with the greatest benefit seen among women with stage III disease (108).
- Similarly, a Swedish prospective trial demonstrated that WAR is associated with longer PFS and OS among women who achieve pathologic complete response following induction cytoreduction and chemotherapy, but not among women with either microscopic or macroscopic residual disease (109).

Salvage Radiotherapy

- The use of radiotherapy for the treatment of ovarian cancer in the modern era has been primarily in the setting of disease progression or for palliative intent (110). To date, there are no currently published randomized trials evaluating outcomes following radiotherapy as compared to chemotherapy in this setting.
- A number of retrospective studies have provided initial support for involved field radiation therapy (IFRT) among women with locoregionally recurrent ovarian cancer (111–115).
- An analysis of 102 patients with epithelial ovarian cancer treated at the MD Anderson Cancer Center with definitive IFRT to localized lymph nodes or pelvic masses demonstrated an in-field control rate of 71% at 5 years (112).
- A smaller analysis compared women with locoregional recurrence of disease who received tumor-directed radiotherapy with an unmatched cohort of similar patients, who received further chemotherapy. The cohort of patients who received radiotherapy experienced longer median OS compared to the cohort of patients who received chemotherapy. The 10-year rate of locoregional recurrence-free survival (LRFS) for patients treated with radiotherapy was 60% (111).

- Among patients who experience disease recurrence, lymph node involvement, sensitivity to platinum agents, and complete resection following secondary cytoreductive surgery have been shown to be associated with longer PFS in multivariable analyses (113,116).
- SBRT has more recently been evaluated as a potential technique for the treatment of locally recurrent or oligometastatic disease. Several small institutional cohort analyses have provided initial evidence that SBRT may be a safe and effective treatment modality with minimal toxicity and high rates of local control for patients with limited recurrent disease (117–119). Disease progression outside of the treatment field, however, remained high.
- A small phase I study evaluating the safety of sequential carboplatin and gemcitabine followed the next day with SBRT demonstrated acceptable rates of toxicity (120).

Clear Cell Carcinoma

- Because of the enhanced chemoresistance of clear cell tumors, but high likelihood of remaining confined to the pelvis, there has been a particular interest in exploring the potential benefit of radiotherapy for this population of patients.
- A small prospective study of 28 women with stage I to III ovarian clear cell carcinoma treated with adjuvant platinum-based chemotherapy versus adjuvant WAR alone following primary cytoreduction demonstrated significantly increased OS and disease-free survival (DFS) within the radiotherapy arm (121).
- Two retrospective analyses have additionally suggested a potential role for adjuvant or consolidative radiotherapy among subsets of patients with clear cell carcinoma. One retrospective analysis of patients who underwent primary cytoreduction followed by adjuvant carboplatin and paclitaxel chemotherapy with or without consolidation WAR demonstrated that receipt of radiotherapy was associated with longer DFS among women with nonruptured stage IC and II disease (122).
- A large retrospective Canadian study subsequently demonstrated significantly longer DFS and OS among patients with stage I and II ovarian carcinomas of clear cell, endometrioid, and mucinous histologies who received adjuvant radiotherapy, but not among patients with stage III disease or serous histology (123).
- A retrospective analysis of patients who received IMRT to an involved site of recurrence revealed a particular benefit of radiotherapy among patients with clear cell carcinoma. These patients showed significantly increased 5 years PFS (75% versus 20%) and OS (88% versus 37%) compared to patients with tumors of other subtypes (112).

Palliative Radiotherapy

- Palliative radiotherapy can be effectively utilized in patients with symptomatic localized or metastatic disease.
- In a recent prospective cohort of patients with symptomatic locoregionally recurrent or residual disease, palliative radiotherapy effectively controlled abdominal pain, vaginal bleeding, and vaginal discharge, particularly among patients with limited disease bulk (124).

- A separate retrospective analysis of patients with symptomatic recurrence of disease demonstrated significant improvement in pain, bleeding, and obstruction following receipt of palliative radiation (125).

RADIATION THERAPY TECHNIQUES

Whole Abdomen Radiation Therapy

Three-Dimensional Conformal Radiation Therapy

- CT-guided treatment planning should be performed with the patient appropriately immobilized in a supine position with her arms above her head. Four-dimensional treatment planning with coverage of the diaphragm at terminal respiration is preferred.
- If using 3D-CRT, an open field is utilized to treat the entire peritoneal cavity and diaphragm. The superior border of the field should be placed 2 cm above the domes of the diaphragm during quiet respiration. The inferior border should be placed at the inferior aspect of the obturator foramen. Lateral borders should extend 2 cm beyond the lateral peritoneum.
- The general dose recommendation for WAR is 22.5 Gy in 18 daily fractions. There has been no demonstrated benefit to additional dose beyond 22.5 Gy (126). The liver should be shielded above doses of 25 Gy, whereas the dose to the kidney should be limited to 18 Gy.
- Anterioposterior/posteroanterior (AP/PA) technique is commonly used, using posterior blocks to shield the liver and kidneys. The femoral heads and bony pelvis should also be blocked.
- Following WAR, a boost to the pelvis to achieve a total pelvic dose of 45 to 50.4 Gy is commonly performed. For the boost, the patient should undergo repeat treatment planning in the prone position with consideration of abdominal compression. The bladder should be full. Further boost to residual or paraaortic nodal disease may also be considered.
- Studies evaluating the tolerability of WAR using standard 3D-CRT demonstrated that up to one-third of patients required treatment breaks during therapy, even then up to 15% of patients were unable to complete therapy because of myelosuppression.

Intensity-Modulated Radiation Therapy

- IMRT utilizes inverse planning with multiple nonuniform static or dynamic beams to achieve conformal dose delivery to the planning target volume (PTV) while minimizing dose to organs at risk (Fig. 34-2).
- The OVAR-IMRT Phase 1/2 clinical trial utilized IMRT to deliver WAR to women with stage III ovarian cancer following primary cytoreduction with less than 1 cm residual disease followed by adjuvant chemotherapy with carboplatin and docetaxel. Static beams or helical tomotherapy were utilized to deliver 30 Gy in 20 fractions to the PTV (103,127). The clinical target volume (CTV) included the entire peritoneal

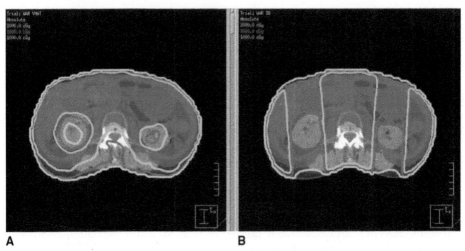

FIGURE 34-2. Representative treatment plans for whole abdomen radiation therapy (WAR). **A:** Intensity modulated radiation therapy (IMRT). **B:** Three-dimensional conformal radiation therapy (3D-CRT).

cavity including the diaphragm, Douglas cavity, and both pelvic and paraaortic nodal basins. The PTV was defined as a 1.5-cm axial and 2.5-cm superior-inferior expansion from the CTV with exclusion of the kidneys and all but the 1-cm outer border of the liver. Other organs at risk included the lungs, pelvic bones, vertebral bodies, heart, and spinal cord, and were limited to the Tolerance Dose 5/5 for each organ.

- Results from the Phase 1 component demonstrated excellent coverage of the PTV with acceptable sparing of critical structures (128). Preliminary results regarding treatment tolerability, acute toxicity, and quality of life from the Phase 2 component demonstrated a tolerability rate of 95%. No patient experienced a grade 3 or higher acute gastrointestinal toxicity while mean global health status returned to baseline 6 weeks following WAR (103).

Involved Field Radiation Therapy

- Definitive or salvage radiation therapy to sites of disease recurrence has been described in several single-institution analyses. In these studies, patients treated using either IMRT or 3D-CRT to a median dose ranging between 45 and 60 Gy achieved high levels of local control (111,112). A review of previously published studies recommends use of IMRT to achieve adequate dose delivery while minimizing toxicity (110).

Stereotactic Body Radiation Therapy

- SBRT utilizes high doses per fraction to deliver highly conformal radiation therapy over 3 to 5 fractions.
- Patients should be immobilized using a vacuum-type body mold and undergo CT-based treatment planning with co-registration of PET or MRI images in the treatment position. IV contrast or four-dimensional scans should be performed as

NEW!   SUMMARY OF CHANGES TO AJCC STAGING

TNM STAGE

- Malignant tumors arising in the ovary, fallopian tube, and primary peritoneum now share the same staging system as of the FIGO Committee's consensus recommendations published in 2014, as listed in Table 34-1. The following describes changes incorporated in the AJCC 8th edition as compared to the FIGO Staging (130).
- N0(i+) now denotes isolated tumor cells in regional lymph node(s) less than or equal to 0.2 mm.
- N1 has been subdivided into N1a and N1b to differentiate between the size of nodal metastasis.
- N1a: Metastasis up to and including 10 mm in greatest dimension.
- N1b: Metastasis greater than 10 mm in greatest dimension.
- M1 has been subdivided into M1a and M1b to differentiate between malignant pleural effusion and involvement of extrapelvic organs.
- M1a: Pleural effusion with positive cytology.
- M1b: Liver or splenic parenchymal metastases and metastases to extra-abdominal organs including inguinal lymph nodes, or transmural involvement of the intestine.

From: Amin MB, Edge SB, Greene FL, et al., eds. *AJCC cancer staging manual*, 8th ed. New York, NY: Springer, 2017.

needed. The known disease burden should be delineated as the CTV/ITV, and the PTV should include a 3–5-mm margin expansion from the CTV. Although fractionation schemes can vary, published treatment regimens using 8 Gy × 3 fractions or 6 Gy × 5 fractions have achieved excellent local control rates (117,120,129).

SEQUELAE OF RADIATION THERAPY

- Historically, WAR using 3D-CRT was associated with significant toxicity, with a large number of patients unable to complete treatment as prescribed. Acute toxicity included diarrhea, nausea, fatigue, and hematologic effects. Long-term toxicities included radiation pneumonitis, liver damage, and bowel toxicity. Small bowel obstruction occurred among 10% to 15% of patients.
- With IMRT, WAR has been shown in preliminary analyses to be reasonably well-tolerated with minimal acute or long-term toxicity.

References

1. Siegel RL, Miller KD, Jemal A. Cancer statistics, 2017. *CA Cancer J Clin* 2017;67(1):7–30.
2. Ferlay J, Soerjomataram I, Ervik M, et al. GLOBOCAN 2012 v1.0, Cancer Incidence and Mortality Worldwide: IARC CancerBase No. 11 [Internet], 2013; http://globocan.iarc.fr/, accessed on February 10, 2017.

3. Lancaster JM, Powell CB, Chen LM, et al. Society of Gynecologic Oncology statement on risk assessment for inherited gynecologic cancer predispositions. *Gynecol Oncol* 2015;136(1):3–7.

4. Bahcall OG. iCOGS collection provides a collaborative model. Foreword. *Nat Genet* 2013;45(4):343.

5. Dong A, Lu Y, Lu B. Genomic/epigenomic alterations in ovarian carcinoma: translational insight into clinical practice. *J Cancer* 2016;7(11):1441–1451.

6. Vang R, Levine DA, Soslow RA, et al. Molecular alterations of TP53 are a defining feature of ovarian high-grade serous carcinoma: a rereview of cases lacking TP53 mutations in the cancer genome atlas ovarian study. *Int J Gynecol Pathol* 2016;35(1):48–55.

7. Modan B, Hartge P, Hirsh-Yechezkel G, et al. Parity, oral contraceptives, and the risk of ovarian cancer among carriers and noncarriers of a BRCA1 or BRCA2 mutation. *N Engl J Med* 2001;345(4):235–240.

8. Wentzensen N, Poole EM, Trabert B, et al. Ovarian cancer risk factors by histologic subtype: an analysis from the Ovarian Cancer Cohort Consortium. *J Clin Oncol* 2016;34(24): 2888–2898.

9. Reid BM, Permuth JB, Sellers TA. Epidemiology of ovarian cancer: a review. *Cancer Biol Med* 2017;14(1):9–32.

10. Walker JL, Powell CB, Chen LM, et al. Society of Gynecologic Oncology recommendations for the prevention of ovarian cancer. *Cancer* 2015;121(13):2108–2120.

11. Beral V, Bull D, Green J, et al. Ovarian cancer and hormone replacement therapy in the Million Women Study. *Lancet* 2007;369(9574):1703–1710.

12. Zeng F, Wei H, Yeoh E, et al. Inflammatory markers of CRP, IL6, TNFalpha, and soluble TNFR2 and the risk of ovarian cancer: a meta-analysis of prospective studies. *Cancer Epidemiol Biomarkers Prev* 2016;25(8):1231–1239.

13. Beral V, Gaitskell K, Hermon C, et al. Ovarian cancer and smoking: individual participant meta-analysis including 28,114 women with ovarian cancer from 51 epidemiological studies. *Lancet Oncol* 2012;13(9):946–956.

14. Gates MA, Rosner BA, Hecht JL, et al. Risk factors for epithelial ovarian cancer by histologic subtype. *Am J Epidemiol* 2010;171(1):45–53.

15. Chen VW, Ruiz B, Killeen JL, et al. Pathology and classification of ovarian tumors. *Cancer* 2003;97(10 Suppl):2631–2642.

16. Kurman RJ, Carcangiu ML, Harrington CS, et al. *WHO classification of tumors of female reproductive organs*, 4th ed. Vol 6. Lyon, France: IARC Publications, 2014.

17. Levanon K, Crum C, Drapkin R. New insights into the pathogenesis of serous ovarian cancer and its clinical impact. *J Clin Oncol* 2008;26(32):5284–5293.

18. SEER 18 2007–2013, All Races, Females by SEER Summary Stage 2000. Surveillance, Epidemiology, and End Results (SEER) Program (http://www.seer.cancer.gov/) Research Data (1973–2014), National Cancer Institute, DCCPS, Surveillance Research Program, released April 2017, based on the November 2016 submission. Accessed November, 2017.

19. Bogani G, Tagliabue E, Ditto A, et al. Assessing the risk of pelvic and para-aortic nodal involvement in apparent early-stage ovarian cancer: a predictors- and nomogram-based analyses. *Gynecol Oncol* 2017;147(1):61–65.

20. Bachmann C, Bachmann R, Kraemer B, et al. Prevalence and distribution pattern of nodal metastases in advanced ovarian cancer. *Mol Clin Oncol* 2016;5(4):483–487.

21. du Bois A, Reuss A, Pujade-Lauraine E, et al. Role of surgical outcome as prognostic factor in advanced epithelial ovarian cancer: a combined exploratory analysis of 3 prospectively randomized phase 3 multicenter trials: by the Arbeitsgemeinschaft Gynaekologische Onkologie Studiengruppe Ovarialkarzinom (AGO-OVAR) and the Groupe d'Investigateurs Nationaux Pour les Etudes des Cancers de l'Ovaire (GINECO). *Cancer* 2009;115(6):1234–1244.

22. Barnhill D, Heller P, Brzozowski P, et al. Epithelial ovarian carcinoma of low malignant potential. *Obstet Gynecol* 1985;65(1):53–59.

23. Labidi-Galy SI, Papp E, Hallberg D, et al. High grade serous ovarian carcinomas originate in the fallopian tube. *Nat Commun* 2017;8(1):1093.

24. Li J, Abushahin N, Pang S, et al. Tubal origin of 'ovarian' low-grade serous carcinoma. *Mod Pathol* 2011;24(11):1488–1499.

25. Seidman JD, Khedmati F. Exploring the histogenesis of ovarian mucinous and transitional cell (Brenner) neoplasms and their relationship with Walthard cell nests: a study of 120 tumors. *Arch Pathol Lab Med* 2008;132(11):1753–1760.

26. Veras E, Mao TL, Ayhan A, et al. Cystic and adenofibromatous clear cell carcinomas of the ovary: distinctive tumors that differ in their pathogenesis and behavior: a clinicopathologic analysis of 122 cases. *Am J Surg Pathol* 2009;33(6):844–853.

27. Ingin RJ, Andola SK, Zubair AA. Transitional cell carcinoma of the ovary: case series and review of literature. *J Clin Diagn Res* 2014;8(8):Fd07–Fd08.

28. Guseh SH, Rauh-Hain JA, Tambouret RH, et al. Transitional cell carcinoma of the ovary: a case-control study. *Gynecol Oncol* 2014;132(3):649–653.

29. Shimizu Y, Fujiwara H, Akagaki E, et al. Significance of CA 125 antigen levels in patients with ovarian cancer. *Gan To Kagaku Ryoho* 1986;13(1):46–52.

30. Duffy MJ, Bonfrer JM, Kulpa J, et al. CA125 in ovarian cancer: European Group on Tumor Markers guidelines for clinical use. *Int J Gynecol Cancer* 2005;15(5):679–691.

31. Buys SS, Partridge E, Black A, et al. Effect of screening on ovarian cancer mortality: the Prostate, Lung, Colorectal and Ovarian (PLCO) Cancer Screening Randomized Controlled Trial. *JAMA* 2011;305(22):2295–2303.

32. Committee Opinion No. 477: the role of the obstetrician-gynecologist in the early detection of epithelial ovarian cancer. *Obstet Gynecol* 2011;117(3):742–746.

33. Jacobs IJ, Menon U, Ryan A, et al. Ovarian cancer screening and mortality in the UK Collaborative Trial of Ovarian Cancer Screening (UKCTOCS): a randomised controlled trial. *Lancet* 2016;387(10022):945–956.

34. Goff BA, Agnew K, Neradilek MB, et al. Combining a symptom index, CA125 and HE4 (triple screen) to detect ovarian cancer in women with a pelvic mass. *Gynecol Oncol* 2017;147(2):291–295.

35. Muallem MZ, Parashkevova A, Almuheimid J, et al. Preoperative CA-125 values as a predictive factor for the postoperative outcome in primary serous ovarian cancer. *Anticancer Res* 2017;37(6):3157–3161.

36. Juretzka MM, Barakat RR, Chi DS, et al. CA125 level as a predictor of progression-free survival and overall survival in ovarian cancer patients with surgically defined disease status prior to the initiation of intraperitoneal consolidation therapy. *Gynecol Oncol* 2007;104(1):176–180.

37. van Altena AM, Kolwijck E, Spanjer MJ, et al. CA125 nadir concentration is an independent predictor of tumor recurrence in patients with ovarian cancer: a population-based study. *Gynecol Oncol* 2010;119(2):265–269.

38. National Cancer Center Network. Ovarian cancer including fallopian tube cancer and primary peritoneal cancer (Version 3.2017). http://www.nccn.org/professionals/physician_gls/pdf/cervical.pdf. Accessed August 27, 2017.

39. Verheijen RH, Cibula D, Zola P, et al. Cancer antigen 125: lost to follow-up?: a European society of gynaecological oncology consensus statement. *Int J Gynecol Cancer* 2012;22(1):170–174.

40. Heintz AP, Odicino F, Maisonneuve P, et al. Carcinoma of the ovary. FIGO 26th Annual Report on the results of treatment in gynecological cancer. *Int J Gynaecol Obstet* 2006;95(Suppl 1):S161–S192.

41. Prat J. Staging classification for cancer of the ovary, fallopian tube, and peritoneum. *Int J Gynaecol Obstet* 2014;124(1):1–5.

42. Young RC, Decker DG, Wharton JT, et al. Staging laparotomy in early ovarian cancer. *JAMA* 1983;250(22):3072–3076.

43. Zhou J, Sun JY, Wu SG, et al. Risk factors for lymph node metastasis in ovarian cancer: implications for systematic lymphadenectomy. *Int J Surg* 2016;29:123–127.

44. Powless CA, Aletti GD, Bakkum-Gamez JN, et al. Risk factors for lymph node metastasis in apparent early-stage epithelial ovarian cancer: implications for surgical staging. *Gynecol Oncol* 2011;122(3):536–540.

45. Rutten MJ, Boldingh JH, Schuit E, et al. Development and internal validation of a prognostic model for survival after debulking surgery for epithelial ovarian cancer. *Gynecol Oncol* 2014;135(1):13–18.

46. Vergote I, De Brabanter J, Fyles A, et al. Prognostic importance of degree of differentiation and cyst rupture in stage I invasive epithelial ovarian carcinoma. *Lancet* 2001;357(9251): 176–182.

47. Elattar A, Bryant A, Winter-Roach BA, et al. Optimal primary surgical treatment for advanced epithelial ovarian cancer. *Cochrane Database Syst Rev* 2011;(8):Cd007565.

48. Oliver KE, Brady WE, Birrer M, et al. An evaluation of progression free survival and overall survival of ovarian cancer patients with clear cell carcinoma versus serous carcinoma treated with platinum therapy: an NRG Oncology/Gynecologic Oncology Group experience. *Gynecol Oncol* 2017;147(2):243–249.

49. Kurta ML, Edwards RP, Moysich KB, et al. Prognosis and conditional disease-free survival among patients with ovarian cancer. *J Clin Oncol* 2014;32(36):4102–4112.

50. Salani R, Backes FJ, Fung MF, et al. Posttreatment surveillance and diagnosis of recurrence in women with gynecologic malignancies: Society of Gynecologic Oncologists recommendations. *Am J Obstet Gynecol* 2011;204(6):466–478.

51. Miller RE, Rustin GJ. How to follow-up patients with epithelial ovarian cancer. *Curr Opin Oncol* 2010;22(5):498–502.

52. Markman M, Webster K, Zanotti K, et al. Use of tamoxifen in asymptomatic patients with recurrent small-volume ovarian cancer. *Gynecol Oncol* 2004;93(2):390–393.

53. Bristow RE, Tomacruz RS, Armstrong DK, et al. Survival effect of maximal cytoreductive surgery for advanced ovarian carcinoma during the platinum era: a meta-analysis. *J Clin Oncol* 2002;20(5):1248–1259.

54. Cliby WA, Powell MA, Al-Hammadi N, et al. Ovarian cancer in the United States: contemporary patterns of care associated with improved survival. *Gynecol Oncol* 2015;136(1):11–17.

55. Galaal K, Bryant A, Fisher AD, et al. Laparoscopy versus laparotomy for the management of early stage endometrial cancer. *Cochrane Database Syst Rev* 2012;(9):Cd006655.

56. Maggioni A, Benedetti Panici P, Dell'Anna T, et al. Randomised study of systematic lymphadenectomy in patients with epithelial ovarian cancer macroscopically confined to the pelvis. *Br J Cancer* 2006;95(6):699–704.

57. Panici PB, Maggioni A, Hacker N, et al. Systematic aortic and pelvic lymphadenectomy versus resection of bulky nodes only in optimally debulked advanced ovarian cancer: a randomized clinical trial. *J Natl Cancer Inst* 2005;97(8):560–566.

58. du Bois A, Reuss A, Harter P, et al. Potential role of lymphadenectomy in advanced ovarian cancer: a combined exploratory analysis of three prospectively randomized phase III multicenter trials. *J Clin Oncol* 2010;28(10):1733–1739.

59. Kehoe S, Hook J, Nankivell M, et al. Primary chemotherapy versus primary surgery for newly diagnosed advanced ovarian cancer (CHORUS): an open-label, randomised, controlled, non-inferiority trial. *Lancet* 2015;386(9990):249–257.

60. Vergote I, Trope CG, Amant F, et al. Neoadjuvant chemotherapy or primary surgery in stage IIIC or IV ovarian cancer. *N Engl J Med* 2010;363(10):943–953.

61. van Meurs HS, Tajik P, Hof MH, et al. Which patients benefit most from primary surgery or neoadjuvant chemotherapy in stage IIIC or IV ovarian cancer? An exploratory analysis of the European Organisation for Research and Treatment of Cancer 55971 randomised trial. *Eur J Cancer* 2013;49(15):3191–3201.

62. Tangjitgamol S, Manusirivithaya S, Laopaiboon M, et al. Interval debulking surgery for advanced epithelial ovarian cancer. *Cochrane Database Syst Rev* 2016;(1):Cd006014.

63. Aletti GD, Eisenhauer EL, Santillan A, et al. Identification of patient groups at highest risk from traditional approach to ovarian cancer treatment. *Gynecol Oncol* 2011;120(1):23–28.

64. Wright JD, Lewin SN, Deutsch I, et al. Defining the limits of radical cytoreductive surgery for ovarian cancer. *Gynecol Oncol* 2011;123(3):467–473.

65. Bristow RE, Puri I, Chi DS. Cytoreductive surgery for recurrent ovarian cancer: a meta-analysis. *Gynecol Oncol* 2009;112(1):265–274.

66. Diaz-Montes TP, Bristow RE. Secondary cytoreduction for patients with recurrent ovarian cancer. *Curr Oncol Rep* 2005;7(6):451–458.

67. Lawrie TA, Winter-Roach BA, Heus P, et al. Adjuvant (post-surgery) chemotherapy for early stage epithelial ovarian cancer. *Cochrane Database Syst Rev* 2015;(12):Cd004706.

68. Armstrong DK, Bundy B, Wenzel L, et al. Intraperitoneal cisplatin and paclitaxel in ovarian cancer. *N Engl J Med* 2006;354(1):34–43.

69. Landrum LM, Java J, Mathews CA, et al. Prognostic factors for stage III epithelial ovarian cancer treated with intraperitoneal chemotherapy: a Gynecologic Oncology Group study. *Gynecol Oncol* 2013;130(1):12–18.

70. Tewari D, Java JJ, Salani R, et al. Long-term survival advantage and prognostic factors associated with intraperitoneal chemotherapy treatment in advanced ovarian cancer: a gynecologic oncology group study. *J Clin Oncol* 2015;33(13):1460–1466.

71. Katsumata N, Yasuda M, Isonishi S, et al. Long-term results of dose-dense paclitaxel and carboplatin versus conventional paclitaxel and carboplatin for treatment of advanced epithelial ovarian, fallopian tube, or primary peritoneal cancer (JGOG 3016): a randomised, controlled, open-label trial. *Lancet Oncol* 2013;14(10):1020–1026.

72. Chan JK, Brady MF, Penson RT, et al. Weekly vs. every-3-week paclitaxel and carboplatin for ovarian cancer. *N Engl J Med* 2016;374(8):738–748.

73. Markman M, Liu PY, Moon J, et al. Impact on survival of 12 versus 3 monthly cycles of paclitaxel (175 mg/m^2) administered to patients with advanced ovarian cancer who attained a complete response to primary platinum-paclitaxel: follow-up of a Southwest Oncology Group and Gynecologic Oncology Group phase 3 trial. *Gynecol Oncol* 2009;114(2):195–198.

74. Mannel RS, Brady MF, Kohn EC, et al. A randomized phase III trial of IV carboplatin and paclitaxel × 3 courses followed by observation versus weekly maintenance low-dose paclitaxel in patients with early-stage ovarian carcinoma: a Gynecologic Oncology Group Study. *Gynecol Oncol* 2011;122(1):89–94.

75. Ferriss JS, Java JJ, Bookman MA, et al. Ascites predicts treatment benefit of bevacizumab in front-line therapy of advanced epithelial ovarian, fallopian tube and peritoneal cancers: an NRG Oncology/GOG study. *Gynecol Oncol* 2015;139(1):17–22.

76. Oza AM, Cook AD, Pfisterer J, et al. Standard chemotherapy with or without bevacizumab for women with newly diagnosed ovarian cancer (ICON7): overall survival results of a phase 3 randomised trial. *Lancet Oncol* 2015;16(8):928–936.

77. du Bois A, Floquet A, Kim JW, et al. Incorporation of pazopanib in maintenance therapy of ovarian cancer. *J Clin Oncol* 2014;32(30):3374–3382.

78. Pignata S, Scambia G, Katsaros D, et al. Carboplatin plus paclitaxel once a week versus every 3 weeks in patients with advanced ovarian cancer (MITO-7): a randomised, multicentre, open-label, phase 3 trial. *Lancet Oncol* 2014;15(4):396–405.

79. Aghajanian C, Blank SV, Goff BA, et al. OCEANS: a randomized, double-blind, placebo-controlled phase III trial of chemotherapy with or without bevacizumab in patients with platinum-sensitive recurrent epithelial ovarian, primary peritoneal, or fallopian tube cancer. *J Clin Oncol* 2012;30(17):2039–2045.

80. Coleman RL, Brady MF, Herzog TJ, et al. Bevacizumab and paclitaxel-carboplatin chemotherapy and secondary cytoreduction in recurrent, platinum-sensitive ovarian cancer (NRG Oncology/Gynecologic Oncology Group study GOG-0213): a multicentre, open-label, randomised, phase 3 trial. *Lancet Oncol* 2017;18(6):779–791.

81. Pujade-Lauraine E, Hilpert F, Weber B, et al. Bevacizumab combined with chemotherapy for platinum-resistant recurrent ovarian cancer: the AURELIA open-label randomized phase III trial. *J Clin Oncol* 2014;32(13):1302–1308.

82. Griffiths RW, Zee YK, Evans S, et al. Outcomes after multiple lines of chemotherapy for platinum-resistant epithelial cancers of the ovary, peritoneum, and fallopian tube. *Int J Gynecol Cancer* 2011;21(1):58–65.

83. Berton-Rigaud D, Devouassoux-Shisheboran M, Ledermann JA, et al. Gynecologic Cancer InterGroup (GCIG) consensus review for uterine and ovarian carcinosarcoma. *Int J Gynecol Cancer* 2014;24(9 Suppl 3):S55–S60.

84. Kobel M, Kalloger SE, Huntsman DG, et al. Differences in tumor type in low-stage versus high-stage ovarian carcinomas. *Int J Gynecol Pathol* 2010;29(3):203–211.

85. Magazzino F, Katsaros D, Ottaiano A, et al. Surgical and medical treatment of clear cell ovarian cancer: results from the multicenter Italian Trials in Ovarian Cancer (MITO) 9 retrospective study. *Int J Gynecol Cancer* 2011;21(6):1063–1070.

86. Pectasides D, Fountzilas G, Aravantinos G, et al. Advanced stage clear-cell epithelial ovarian cancer: the Hellenic Cooperative Oncology Group experience. *Gynecol Oncol* 2006;102(2):285–291.

87. Okamoto A, Glasspool RM, Mabuchi S, et al. Gynecologic Cancer InterGroup (GCIG) consensus review for clear cell carcinoma of the ovary. *Int J Gynecol Cancer* 2014;24(9 Suppl 3):S20–S25.

88. Prendergast EN, Holzapfel M, Mueller JJ, et al. Three versus six cycles of adjuvant platinum-based chemotherapy in early stage clear cell ovarian carcinoma—a multi-institutional cohort. *Gynecol Oncol* 2017;144(2):274–278.

89. Massad LS, Gao F, Hagemann I, et al. Clinical outcomes among women with mucinous adenocarcinoma of the ovary. *Gynecol Obstet Invest* 2016;81(5):411–415.

90. Ray-Coquard I, Brown J, Harter P, et al. Gynecologic Cancer InterGroup (GCIG) consensus review for ovarian sex cord stromal tumors. *Int J Gynecol Cancer* 2014;24(9 Suppl 3):S42–S47.

91. Park JY, Jin KL, Kim DY, et al. Surgical staging and adjuvant chemotherapy in the management of patients with adult granulosa cell tumors of the ovary. *Gynecol Oncol* 2012;125(1):80–86.

92. Mangili G, Sigismondi C, Gadducci A, et al. Outcome and risk factors for recurrence in malignant ovarian germ cell tumors: a MITO-9 retrospective study. *Int J Gynecol Cancer* 2011;21(8):1414–1421.

93. Kang H, Kim TJ, Kim WY, et al. Outcome and reproductive function after cumulative high-dose combination chemotherapy with bleomycin, etoposide and cisplatin (BEP) for patients with ovarian endodermal sinus tumor. *Gynecol Oncol* 2008;111(1):106–110.

94. Varia MA, Stehman FB, Bundy BN, et al. Intraperitoneal radioactive phosphorus (32P) versus observation after negative second-look laparotomy for stage III ovarian carcinoma: a randomized trial of the Gynecologic Oncology Group. *J Clin Oncol* 2003;21(15):2849–2855.

95. Young RC, Brady MF, Nieberg RK, et al. Adjuvant treatment for early ovarian cancer: a randomized phase III trial of intraperitoneal 32P or intravenous cyclophosphamide and cisplatin—a gynecologic oncology group study. *J Clin Oncol* 2003;21(23):4350–4355.

96. Bolis G, Colombo N, Pecorelli S, et al. Adjuvant treatment for early epithelial ovarian cancer: results of two randomised clinical trials comparing cisplatin to no further treatment or chromic phosphate (32P). G.I.C.O.G.: Gruppo Interregionale Collaborativo in Ginecologia Oncologica. *Ann Oncol* 1995;6(9):887–893.

97. Dembo AJ. Radiation therapy in the management of ovarian cancer. *Clin Obstet Gynaecol* 1983;10(2):261–278.

98. Smith JP, Rutledge FN, Delclos L. Postoperative treatment of early cancer of the ovary: a random trial between postoperative irradiation and chemotherapy. *Natl Cancer Inst Monogr* 1975;42:149–153.

99. Chiara S, Conte P, Franzone P, et al. High-risk early-stage ovarian cancer. Randomized clinical trial comparing cisplatin plus cyclophosphamide versus whole abdominal radiotherapy. *Am J Clin Oncol* 1994;17(1):72–76.

100. Klaassen D, Shelley W, Starreveld A, et al. Early stage ovarian cancer: a randomized clinical trial comparing whole abdominal radiotherapy, melphalan, and intraperitoneal chromic phosphate: a National Cancer Institute of Canada Clinical Trials Group report. *J Clin Oncol* 1988;6(8):1254–1263.

101. Sell A, Bertelsen K, Andersen JE, et al. Randomized study of whole-abdomen irradiation versus pelvic irradiation plus cyclophosphamide in treatment of early ovarian cancer. *Gynecol Oncol* 1990;37(3):367–373.

102. Redman CW, Mould J, Warwick J, et al. The West Midlands epithelial ovarian cancer adjuvant therapy trial. *Clin Oncol (R Coll Radiol)* 1993;5(1):1–5.

103. Arians N, Kieser M, Benner L, et al. Adjuvant intensity modulated whole-abdominal radiation therapy for high-risk patients with ovarian cancer (International Federation of Gynecology and Obstetrics Stage III): first results of a prospective phase 2 study. *Int J Radiat Oncol Biol Phys* 2017;99(4):912–920.

104. Rochet N, Lindel K, Katayama S, et al. Intensity-modulated whole abdomen irradiation following adjuvant carboplatin/taxane chemotherapy for FIGO stage III ovarian cancer: four-year outcomes. *Strahlenther Onkol* 2015;191(7):582–589.

105. Hoskins PJ, Swenerton KD, Wong F, et al. Platinum plus cyclophosphamide plus radiotherapy is superior to platinum alone in 'high-risk' epithelial ovarian cancer (residual negative and either stage I or II, grade 3, or stage III, any grade). *Int J Gynecol Cancer* 1995;5(2):134–142.

106. Lambert HE, Rustin GJ, Gregory WM, et al. A randomized trial comparing single-agent carboplatin with carboplatin followed by radiotherapy for advanced ovarian cancer: a North Thames Ovary Group study. *J Clin Oncol* 1993;11(3):440–448.

107. Lawton F, Luesley D, Blackledge G, et al. A randomized trial comparing whole abdominal radiotherapy with chemotherapy following cisplatinum cytoreduction in epithelial ovarian cancer. West Midlands Ovarian Cancer Group Trial II. *Clin Oncol (R Coll Radiol)* 1990;2(1):4–9.

108. Pickel H, Lahousen M, Petru E, et al. Consolidation radiotherapy after carboplatin-based chemotherapy in radically operated advanced ovarian cancer. *Gynecol Oncol* 1999;72(2):215–219.

109. Sorbe B. Consolidation treatment of advanced (FIGO stage III) ovarian carcinoma in complete surgical remission after induction chemotherapy: a randomized, controlled, clinical trial comparing whole abdominal radiotherapy, chemotherapy, and no further treatment. *Int J Gynecol Cancer* 2003;13(3):278–286.

110. De Felice F, Marchetti C, Di Mino A, et al. Recurrent ovarian cancer: the role of radiation therapy. *Int J Gynecol Cancer* 2017;27(4):690–695.

111. Albuquerque K, Patel M, Liotta M, et al. Long-term benefit of tumor volume-directed involved field radiation therapy in the management of recurrent ovarian cancer. *Int J Gynecol Cancer* 2016;26(4):655–660.

112. Brown AP, Jhingran A, Klopp AH, et al. Involved-field radiation therapy for locoregionally recurrent ovarian cancer. *Gynecol Oncol* 2013;130(2):300–305.

113. Lee SW, Park SM, Kim YM, et al. Radiation therapy is a treatment to be considered for recurrent epithelial ovarian cancer after chemotherapy. *Tumori* 2011;97(5):590–595.

114. Macrie BD, Strauss JB, Helenowski IB, et al. Patterns of recurrence and role of pelvic radiotherapy in ovarian clear cell adenocarcinoma. *Int J Gynecol Cancer* 2014;24(9):1597–1602.

115. Yahara K, Ohguri T, Imada H, et al. Epithelial ovarian cancer: definitive radiotherapy for limited recurrence after complete remission had been achieved with aggressive front-line therapy. *J Radiat Res* 2013;54(2):322–329.

116. Chundury A, Apicelli A, DeWees T, et al. Intensity modulated radiation therapy for recurrent ovarian cancer refractory to chemotherapy. *Gynecol Oncol* 2016;141(1):134–139.

117. Kunos CA, Brindle J, Waggoner S, et al. Phase II clinical trial of robotic stereotactic body radiosurgery for metastatic gynecologic malignancies. *Front Oncol* 2012;2:181.

118. Kunos CA, Spelic M. Role of stereotactic radiosurgery in gynecologic cancer. *Curr Opin Oncol* 2013;25(5):532–538.

119. Mesko S, Sandler K, Cohen J, et al. Clinical outcomes for stereotactic ablative radiotherapy in oligometastatic and oligoprogressive gynecological malignancies. *Int J Gynecol Cancer* 2017;27(2):403–408.

120. Kunos CA, Sherertz TM, Mislmani M, et al. Phase I trial of carboplatin and gemcitabine chemotherapy and stereotactic ablative radiosurgery for the palliative treatment of persistent or recurrent gynecologic cancer. *Front Oncol* 2015;5:126.

121. Nagai Y, Inamine M, Hirakawa M, et al. Postoperative whole abdominal radiotherapy in clear cell adenocarcinoma of the ovary. *Gynecol Oncol* 2007;107(3):469–473.

122. Hoskins PJ, Le N, Gilks B, et al. Low-stage ovarian clear cell carcinoma: population-based outcomes in British Columbia, Canada, with evidence for a survival benefit as a result of irradiation. *J Clin Oncol* 2012;30(14):1656–1662.

123. Swenerton KD, Santos JL, Gilks CB, et al. Histotype predicts the curative potential of radiotherapy: the example of ovarian cancers. *Ann Oncol* 2011;22(2):341–347.

124. Bansal A, Rai B, Kumar S, et al. Fractionated palliative pelvic radiotherapy as an effective modality in the management of recurrent/refractory epithelial ovarian cancers: an institutional experience. *J Obstet Gynaecol India* 2017;67(2):126–132.

125. Jiang G, Balboni T, Taylor A, et al. Palliative radiation therapy for recurrent ovarian cancer: efficacy and predictors of clinical response. *Int J Gynecol Cancer* 2018;28(1):43–50.

126. Fyles AW, Thomas GM, Pintilie M, et al. A randomized study of two doses of abdominopelvic radiation therapy for patients with optimally debulked Stage I, II, and III ovarian cancer. *Int J Radiat Oncol Biol Phys* 1998;41(3):543–549.

127. Rochet N, Kieser M, Sterzing F, et al. Phase II study evaluating consolidation whole abdominal intensity-modulated radiotherapy (IMRT) in patients with advanced ovarian cancer stage FIGO III—the OVAR-IMRT-02 study. *BMC Cancer* 2011;11:41.

128. Rochet N, Sterzing F, Jensen AD, et al. Intensity-modulated whole abdominal radiotherapy after surgery and carboplatin/taxane chemotherapy for advanced ovarian cancer: phase I study. *Int J Radiat Oncol Biol Phys* 2010;76(5):1382–1389.

129. Deodato F, Macchia G, Grimaldi L, et al. Stereotactic radiotherapy in recurrent gynecological cancer: a case series. *Oncol Rep* 2009;22(2):415–419.

130. Edge SB, Compton CC. The American Joint Committee on Cancer: the 7th edition of the AJCC cancer staging manual and the future of TNM. *Ann Surg Oncol* 2010;17(6):1471–1474.

CHAPTER 35

VAGINA

ANATOMY

- The vagina is a distensible, fibromuscular tube, approximately 7.5 cm in length, that extends from the vulva externally to the uterine cervix internally. It is located posterior to the bladder and anterior to the rectum.
- Histologically, the vaginal wall consists of three layers—an inner mucosa composed of nonkeratinized stratified squamous epithelium with an underlying lamina propria, a middle layer of circular smooth muscle, and an outer adventitia composed of loose connective tissue.
- The upper posterior wall is separated from the rectum by a reflection of peritoneum called the pouch of Douglas. The vaginal lumen surrounding the uterine cervix is divided into four fornices—the anterior, posterior, right lateral, and left lateral fornices.
- The primary blood supply to the vagina is supplied by the vaginal arteries, which are branches of the internal iliac arteries. Lymphatic drainage is generally to the external iliac and paraaortic nodes for the upper third of the vagina, the common and internal iliac nodes for the middle third, and the inguinal and femoral nodes for the lower third.

EPIDEMIOLOGY AND NATURAL HISTORY

- Primary cancer of the vagina is a rare entity that comprises about 3% of all female genital tract malignancies. The most common histology is squamous cell carcinoma (SCC).
- Approximately 80% of vaginal cancers are metastatic, primarily from the cervix or endometrium.
- Mean age of diagnosis is 60 years.
- Human papillomavirus (HPV) DNA is detected in 64% to 91% of invasive primary vaginal cancers. HPV serotype 16 is the most common, detected in 55.4% of invasive cancers (1).

- Risk factors for vaginal cancer include multiple lifetime sexual partners, early age at first intercourse, smoking, and vaginal intraepithelial neoplasia (VAIN) (2).
- VAIN is the presence of squamous cell dysplasia without invasion. The estimated lifetime risk of malignant transformation of VAIN to invasive vaginal carcinoma is estimated to be 9% to 10% (3).
- The posterior wall of the upper one third of the vagina is the most common site of primary vaginal carcinoma. In one review, tumors occurred in the upper, middle, and lower third in 50%, 20%, and 30% of cases, respectively (4).
- Vaginal tumors may invade locally and disseminate by several routes: direct extension to other pelvic soft structures, lymphatic spread to pelvic and paraaortic lymph nodes, and hematogenous dissemination to other organs including the lungs, liver, and bone.
- Lymphatic drainage generally mirrors that of the cervix for upper third vaginal tumors and that of the vulva for lower third tumors. Given the complex lymphatic drainage of the vagina, however, any nodal group is at risk of involvement regardless of location of the primary lesion.
- Approximately 13% of patients present with distant metastatic disease (5).

CLINICAL PRESENTATION

- Abnormal vaginal bleeding is the most common clinical presentation of vaginal cancer. Bleeding may be associated with a malodorous discharge. A vaginal mass may be noted by the patient.
- Local extension of disease may lead to urinary symptoms (dysuria and hematuria), gastrointestinal (tenesmus and hematochezia) symptoms, and/or pain.
- Up to 20% of women are asymptomatic at the time of diagnosis. These cancers may be detected as incidentally on pelvic exam or as result of screening for cervical cancer.
- A vaginal lesion involving the external os of the cervix should be considered and treated as cervical cancer; similarly, a tumor involving both the vulva and vagina should be treated as vulvar cancer.

DIAGNOSTIC WORKUP

- Key elements of the diagnostic evaluation are the history, pelvic examination, vaginal cytology, and vaginal biopsy (Table 35-1).
- A complete history should assess for prior history of cervical or vulvar neoplasia, which could exclude a diagnosis of vaginal cancer.
- A complete pelvic exam including speculum examination and palpation are essential. The anterior and posterior blades of the speculum must be rotated such that the anterior and posterior walls of the vagina can be thoroughly inspected. A rectovaginal exam is performed to assess for extravaginal spread of disease.
- The inguinal region should be palpated to assess for lymph node involvement.
- A vaginal cytology specimen should be obtained during pelvic exam, and any abnormal lesions should be biopsied. Colposcopy of the vagina and cervix with acetic acid followed by Lugol iodine stain may help visualize lesions and aid directed biopsies.

Table 35-1

Diagnostic Workup for Vaginal Tumors

General
  History—assess for prior history of cervical or vulvar neoplasia
  Physical, including careful pelvic, rectovaginal, and bimanual examination
Special studies
  Exfoliative cytology
  Colposcopy and directed biopsies
  Biopsies and examination under anesthesia to determine extent
  Cystoscopy
  Proctosigmoidoscopy (as indicated)
Radiographic studies
  Imaging studies recommended by FIGO
    Chest radiographs
    Intravenous pyelogram
  Complementary imaging studies
    Computed tomography scans of abdomen/pelvis
    MRI pelvis
    PET/CT scan
Laboratory studies
  Complete blood cell count
  Blood chemistry
  Urinalysis

Reprinted with permission from Halperin EC, Brady LW, Perez CA, Wazer DE. In Halperin EC, Perez CA, Brady LW. *Principles and practice of radiation oncology*, 6th ed. Philadelphia, Lippincott Williams & Wilkins, 2013:1490. © Wolters Kluwer.

- Exam under anesthesia may be necessary for women unable to tolerate office examination.
- Cystoscopy and proctoscopy are recommended if significant extravaginal spread of disease is suspected.
- Although chest and skeletal radiography are the only imaging studies recommended for staging workup by International Federation of Gynecology and Obstetrics (FIGO), computed tomography (CT), magnetic resonance imaging (MRI), and positron emission tomography/CT (PET/CT) imaging are commonly used to aid in staging and treatment planning.

STAGING

- Vaginal cancer is staged using the FIGO or American Joint Committee on Cancer (AJCC) staging systems.
- FIGO uses a clinical staging system that is based upon findings from physical exam, cystoscopy, proctoscopy, and chest and skeletal radiography. The results of a biopsy or fine needle aspiration (FNA) of lymph nodes may be included in clinical staging.

- In cases treated with a definitive surgical procedure, the pathology findings should not change the clinical staging, but they should be recorded as pathologic staging using the AJCC system.
- Per FIGO, cases with clinical involvement of the cervix or the vulva should be classified as primary cervical or vulvar cancers, respectively.

NEW! **SUMMARY OF CHANGES TO AJCC STAGING**

- In AJCC 8th edition, notable changes compared to AJCC 7th edition include subdivision of T1 and T2 stages into "a" and "b" substages based on tumor size, with "a" representing tumor sizes less than or equal to 2 cm and the "b" representing tumor sizes greater than 2 cm; in addition, there is now a N0(i+) nodal stage, which represents isolated tumor cells in regional lymph node(s) no greater than 2 mm. Overall stage I and II groups are divided into "A" and "B" subgroups corresponding to T1 and T2 "a" and "b" substage divisions.

PATHOLOGY

Squamous Cell Carcinoma

- SCC accounts for approximately 90% of vaginal cancers.
- Grossly, it appears as an ulcerating lesion, a fungating mass, or an annular, constricting mass.
- Though vaginal cancer is associated with HPV infection, vaginal epithelium is more stable than cervical epithelium, which undergoes constant metaplasia, and thus is less susceptible to oncogenic viruses.
- Verrucous carcinoma is an uncommon variant of vaginal SCC that is well-differentiated and has low malignant potential. It typically presents as a large, warty, cauliflower-like mass that is locally aggressive but rarely metastasizes.

Adenocarcinoma

- Adenocarcinoma comprises about 5% of primary vaginal tumors overall, though it represents nearly all primary vaginal cancers in women younger than 20 years old, particularly in those with a history of *in utero* exposure to diethylstilbestrol (DES).
- Clear cell carcinoma is the most common variant of adenocarcinoma associated with DES exposure and has a good overall prognosis. Adenocarcinoma that occurs in non–DES-exposed women has poorer outcomes.

Melanoma

- Melanoma arising on the vaginal mucosa is rare and is thought to originate from mucosal melanocytes. It is seen primarily in older Caucasian women.

- Tumors often appear as discolored masses or ulcerations, though lesions may be non-pigmented. Vaginal melanomas are aggressive tumors with high rates of local failure and distant metastases that predispose to a poor overall prognosis.

Sarcoma

- Leiomyosarcomas, endometrial stromal sarcomas, malignant mixed müllerian tumors, and rhabdomyosarcomas are the common types of primary vaginal sarcomas.
- Leiomyosarcomas comprise 70% of vaginal sarcomas in adults, whereas rhabdomyosarcomas comprise 90% of cases occurring in children under the age of 5.
- Embryonal rhabdomyosarcoma (sarcoma botryoides) is a highly malignant tumor that occurs in the vagina during infancy and early childhood. It presents as soft nodules that fill and protrude from the vagina, resembling grapes, and is therefore also known as sarcoma botryoides.

Others

- Primary vaginal neuroendocrine small cell carcinoma is a rare, aggressive entity that may occur either in pure form or associated with squamous or glandular elements.
- Primary vaginal lymphomas are most commonly diffuse large B-cell types. They present as a submucosal mass with an intact vaginal mucosa.

GENERAL MANAGEMENT

- There are no randomized trials that define optimal treatment strategy for primary vaginal squamous cell cancer. Treatment strategies are extrapolated from management of cervical and anal cancers.
- In addition to tumor characteristics such as location, size, and clinical stage, treatment decisions should also take into account psychosexual issues including the patient's desire to maintain a functional vagina.
- Radiation therapy is the treatment of choice for most patients with vaginal cancer. Primary surgery is appropriate in well-selected patients with early stage when curative resection can be achieved without exenteration or functionally morbid surgery (Fig. 35-1).
- The role of chemotherapy is unclear; it is often used concurrently with radiation therapy in the treatment of advanced disease.

Vaginal Intraepithelial Neoplasia

- VAIN may be multifocal in the vagina in up to 60% of patients (6) making diagnosis and treatment of lesions challenging.
- Treatments with surgical excision, laser vaporization, and intravaginal topical 5-FU have been used as first-line therapies and proven variably effective (7).

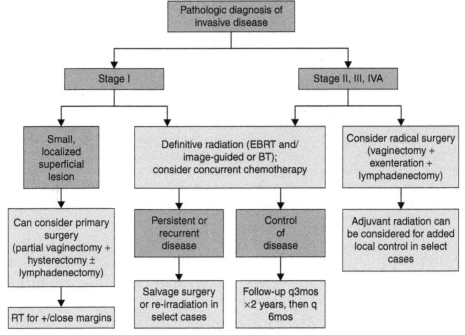

FIGURE 35-1. Proposed treatment algorithm for invasive squamous cell cancer of the vagina. (Reprinted with permission from Kang J, Viswanathan AN. Vaginal cancer. In: Halperin EC, Perez CA, Brady LW, eds. *Principles and practice of radiation oncology*, 6th ed. Philadelphia, Lippincott Williams & Wilkins, 2013:1490. © Wolters Kluwer.)

- Intracavitary brachytherapy alone may be employed for select cases of high-grade VAIN, but this approach should not be selected as first-line therapy given long-term risks of radiation therapy. Control of VAIN using intracavitary brachytherapy approaches 100% (8).

Stage I

- Patients with small, superficial tumors may be adequately treated with brachytherapy alone with reported long-term control rates between 67% and 100% (9). There may be an increased risk of local failure if the extent of submucosal disease is underestimated.
- External beam radiation therapy (EBRT) is often used in conjunction with a brachytherapy boost depending on the extent of disease. A total radiation dose of at least 70 to 75 Gy is recommended with 45 to 50 Gy delivered with EBRT and the additional dose delivered with brachytherapy.
- Surgical resection is a feasible approach for patients with limited early-stage disease in whom a potentially curative resection can be achieved without extensive functional morbidity.
- Surgery frequently entails a radical hysterectomy, vulvovaginectomy in addition to pelvic and/or inguinal lymph node dissection to achieve negative margins.
- Disease-specific survival rates for stage I disease treated with definitive radiation range from 75% to 95% (10).

Stage II

- Combination of whole pelvis EBRT with or without a parametrial boost followed by brachytherapy is the primary treatment for stage II vaginal cancer.
- Inguinal lymph nodes are included in radiation fields if tumor involves the distal vaginal canal.
- Extensive or deeply infiltrating tumors may not be suited for brachytherapy; in such cases, treatment with conformal EBRT may yield superior outcomes than suboptimal brachytherapy.
- Studies demonstrate improved outcomes when the tumor volume receives a minimum of 75 to 80 Gy using combined EBRT and brachytherapy (11).
- Neoadjuvant chemotherapy followed by radical surgery may be an alternative approach to radiation therapy. A small prospective study of 11 patients with stage II disease showed that treatment with three 3-week cycles of cisplatin and paclitaxel followed by surgery yielded a clinical response in 91% of patients and a pathologic complete response rate in 27% (10).

Stage III to IVA

- Radiation therapy is first-line therapy for patients with advanced vaginal cancers.
- Surgical treatment typically requires a pelvic exenteration, an extensive procedure that may be associated with a high degree of morbidity.
- Concurrent cisplatin-based chemotherapy is frequently administered with radiation therapy in patients with advanced disease, extrapolating from data showing improved outcomes with combination treatment in cervical cancer.
- Data to support a combined chemoradiation approach are largely limited to small retrospective series, which demonstrate improved outcomes without significant increase in long-term toxicity.
- One single-institution series of 71 patients treated with definitive RT with or without concurrent chemoradiation showed that the addition of chemotherapy resulted in improvement in 3-year disease-free survival (43% versus 73%) and 3-year overall survival (56% versus 79%) (12).
- Radiation therapy alone is a reasonable option for patients who are not candidates for concurrent chemotherapy and radiation.

OTHER HISTOLOGIES

Clear Cell Adenocarcinoma

- The optimal management of clear cell adenocarcinoma is unclear. These cases are often treated with a similar approach as SCCs.
- These tumors may be more amenable to surgical resection, as they tend to present at earlier stages than SCCs. However, given the young age of many patients, there is an emphasis on preservation of ovarian and vaginal function.

Melanoma

- Given the rarity of primary vaginal melanoma, optimal treatment approaches are not known.
- A general treatment approach consists of wide local excision followed by adjuvant radiation therapy and systemic therapy. Limited retrospective evidence suggests that radiation therapy may improve local control following resection (13).
- Regardless of primary treatment, outcomes have been poor given the high propensity for local and distant failure.
- Immunotherapy is often added to overall management to reduce risk of distant metastases.

Sarcoma

- Most adult vaginal sarcomas are diagnosed at an advanced stage with poor overall outcomes.
- Treatment approaches are extrapolated from high-grade sarcomas in other regions of the body and consist of surgery followed by adjuvant radiation to reduce the risk of recurrence.
- Systemic therapy with doxorubicin is standard for treatment of leiomyosarcoma.

Outcomes

- A review of the National Cancer Database, which evaluated 4,885 women with vagina cancer between 1985 and 1994, found 5-year survival rates of 73% for stage I, 58% for stage II, and 36% for stages III and IV (14).
- Rates of locoregional recurrence follow definitive therapy range from 10% to 20% for stage I disease, 30% to 40% for stage II disease, and may approach 60% to 70% for stage III to IV disease (9).
- Local recurrence is the most common pattern of failure with most failures occurring within the first 3 years with a median time to recurrence of 6 to 12 months (15).

RADIATION THERAPY TECHNIQUES

External Beam Radiation Therapy

- Definitive treatment of primary vaginal cancer with radiation involves EBRT, brachytherapy, or more typically a combination of the two.
- With advances in conformal radiation therapy delivery, dose to tumor can be escalated, whereas dose to surrounding normal structures is minimized.
- CT-based three-dimensional treatment planning has become standard practice. This allows for more accurate delineation of target structures and organs-at-risk.

Simulation

- Patients are simulated in the supine position with a neutral head position and arms crossed. A frog leg position can be considered if planning to treat inguinal lymph nodes or in order to minimize inguinal skin folds.
- Full and empty bladder CT scans should be performed particularly if intensity-modulated radiation therapy (IMRT) is being considered (see below).
- A Vac-Lok bag may be used for immobilization.
- The distal extent of the vaginal tumor may be marked with a radiopaque marker at the time of simulation.
- If available, an MRI or PET/CT simulation may be performed to aid in treatment planning.
- IV and oral contrast may be used to help with delineation of tumor, lymph nodes, and bowel.

Two-Dimensional (2D) Treatment Planning

- 2D EBRT is commonly delivered with either a two-field (opposed anterior and posterior fields) or four-field (anterior, posterior, lateral fields) approach.
- Fields are generally designed to ensure coverage of the vagina, common iliac, external iliac, hypogastric, and obturator lymph nodes.
- Field borders for a standard treatment field consist of the following:
  - The superior border is located at the L5/S1 interspace; if there are positive pelvic lymph nodes, it should be raised to the L4/L5 interspace in order to cover the common iliac nodes.
  - The inferior border lies at the vaginal introitus or 4 cm distal to the most caudal aspect of the vaginal tumor, whichever is lower.
  - Lateral borders are 1.5 to 2 cm lateral to the pelvic brim; they should be extended to include the inguinal lymph nodes, if warranted.
  - Lateral fields, when utilized, should extend anteriorly to the pubic symphysis and posteriorly to the S2-S3 interspace.

Three-Dimensional (3D) Treatment Planning

- Most centers currently use CT-based simulation for treatment planning. When available, an MRI and/or a PET/CT simulation may also be performed. MRI and PET imaging is fused with the treatment planning CT to enable more accurate delineation of target volumes.
- Gross tumor volume (GTV) is defined as the extent of gross disease noted on exam and imaging.
- Clinical target volume (CTV) generally includes the GTV as well as the entire length of the vagina, parametrial tissue, and bilateral pelvic lymph nodes. The CTV is expanded by 1 cm to obtain the planning target volume (PTV). If a full and empty bladder CT scans are performed, an internal target volume (ITV) should be generated

based on CTVs delineated on the two data sets. If there is a large amount of gas in the rectum, consideration should be made to either resimulate the patient with an empty rectum or extend the CTV several centimeters into the rectum.

- Standard EBRT dose to the pelvis is 45 to 50.4 Gy in 1.8 Gy fractions. An additional boost of up to 15 Gy may be delivered to the parametrium. Following EBRT, a brachytherapy boost may be delivered to escalate dose to the primary tumor to 75 to 80 Gy (low-dose rate [LDR] equiv) total dose.

Intensity-Modulated Radiation Therapy

- The use of IMRT in the treatment of vaginal cancers is becoming more common, as it offers highly conformal treatment with increased sparing of normal structures (Fig. 35-2).
- IMRT is more sensitive to day-to-day shifts in tumor position that may result from normal tissue changes such as bladder and rectal filling or tumor regression during treatment.

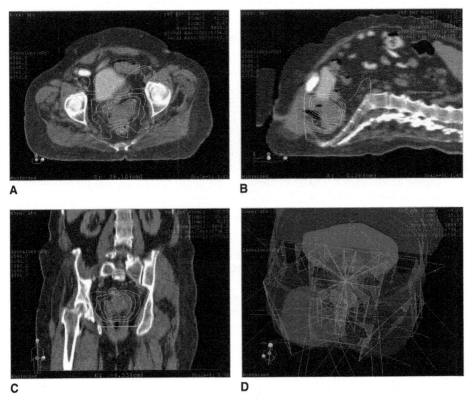

FIGURE 35-2. A: Axial dose distribution intensity-modulated radiation therapy (IMRT) plan for vaginal cancer. **B:** Sagittal dose distribution IMRT plan for vaginal cancer. **C:** Coronal dose distribution IMRT plan for vaginal cancer. **D:** Beam arrangement IMRT plan for vaginal cancer. (Reprinted with permission from Halperin EC, Perez CA, Brady LW, eds. *Principles and practice of radiation oncology*, 5th ed. Philadelphia: Lippincott Williams & Wilkins, 2008. © Wolters Kluwer.)

- Patients may be simulated with both full and empty bladder, which allows for the creation of an internal target volume (ITV) that accounts for potential day-to-day shifts in tumor position.
- IMRT may allow for dose escalation to gross disease in cases where extensive or diffusely infiltrative disease is inaccessible to brachytherapy.

Brachytherapy

- Patients are reevaluated following EBRT to assess their suitability for brachytherapy.
- Brachytherapy can be delivered via intracavitary or interstitial approaches, using low-dose rate or high-dose rate techniques.
- Superficial residual disease that is less than 5 mm in thickness may be treated with intracavitary brachytherapy, whereas thicker lesions require interstitial brachytherapy.
- Brachytherapy is typically used after EBRT to safely boost the cumulative dose to the primary tumor up to 80 Gy (LDR equiv dose) while minimizing dose to normal pelvic structures.

Intracavitary Brachytherapy

- Intracavitary brachytherapy is most commonly performed using a vaginal cylinder loaded with cesium-137 (low-dose rate) or iridium-192 (high-dose rate) sources.
- An applicator with the largest diameter that can be comfortably accommodated by the patient should be used to improve ratio of mucosa to tumor dose.
- Compared to low-dose rate brachytherapy, high-dose rate brachytherapy delivers treatment over a span of minutes and has the potential advantages of limiting dose to caregivers, as well as optimized dose distribution through the use of varying dwell times.
- A variety of high-dose rate (HDR) treatment regimens may be used, ranging from one to six insertions with doses of 3 to 8 Gy per fraction. There is no consensus on the optimal dose fractionation schedule to use.
- Dose is typically prescribed 0.5 cm from the surface of the applicator.

Interstitial Brachytherapy

- Candidates for interstitial brachytherapy include patients with lesions thicker than 5 mm, distal vaginal extension of tumor, or those with a vagina that is unable to accommodate standard intracavitary applicators (Fig. 35-3).
- Clinical examination and imaging following EBRT allows for determination of extent of residual tumor and aids in planning for interstitial brachytherapy.
- Insertion of brachytherapy catheters is typically performed under anesthesia in the operating room with image guidance using a transrectal ultrasound or with direct laparoscopic visualization.
- Catheters may be inserted with guidance from a perineal template or in a "free-hand" manner with the goal of covering the residual disease with a 1- to 2-cm margin.

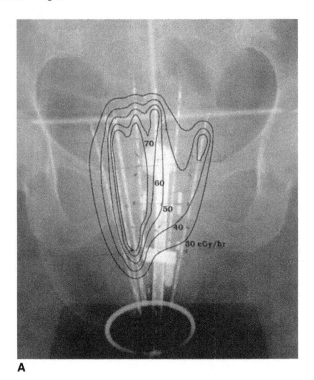

A

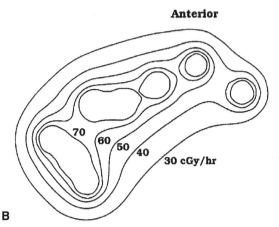

B

FIGURE 35-3. Interstitial implant of a squamous carcinoma involving the anterior and right lateral wall of the vagina. Needles were placed transperineally while the position of the needles was monitored by fingers in the vagina and rectum. A plastic cylinder in the vagina displaced uninvolved tissues from the needles, which were loaded with iridium-192 sources. Needles were placed, and sources were selected to deliver a somewhat higher dose to the thickest portion of the tumor on the right lateral wall of the vagina. Isodose contours represent the dose rates (in centigray per hour [cGy/h]) delivered to the tissue's coronal plane at the approximate center of the implant **(A)** and in a transverse plane through the center of the implant **(B)**. (Reprinted with permission from DeVita VT, Lawrence TS, Rosenberg SA. *DeVita, Hellman, and Rosenberg's cancer principles & practice of oncology*, 9th ed. Philadelphia. PA: Wolters Kluwer Health, 2011.)

- The use of 3D imaging for subsequent treatment planning has become more common; this allows for determination of depth and location of inserted needles.
- Although LDR or HDR techniques may be used, the HDR technique has the advantage of limiting exposure to caregivers and the ability to optimize dose distribution using 3D treatment planning.
- Different HDR brachytherapy fractionation regimens may be used ranging from 3 to 5 fractions of 4.5 to 6.5 Gy per fraction to 9 to 10 fractions of 2 to 3 Gy per fraction.
- During treatment planning, a high-risk CTV (HR-CTV) is defined as any residual disease and the entire circumference of the adjacent vagina at the level of the residual tumor. An intermediate-risk CTV (IR-CTV) is defined as the region of initial tumor extension and the remaining vagina.
- The rectum, sigmoid, bladder, and small bowel are the organs at risk of interest while treating with interstitial brachytherapy. The maximum dose that 2 cc (D2cc) of the rectum and sigmoid receives should be less than 70 to 75 Gy, whereas that of the bladder should be less than 90 Gy (16).

SEQUELAE OF TREATMENT

- Pathologic changes in the vaginal mucosa after radiation treatment include mucosal atrophy and fibrosis of the underlying connective tissues.
- These changes may manifest clinically as vaginal stenosis and shortening in the months following radiation therapy. Reviews of patients treated with cervical cancer reveal that the 10-year incidence of severe vaginal shortening, defined as greater than 50% of length, may be 5% (17).
- Other complications include formation of rectovaginal and vesicovaginal fistulas as well as rectal ulceration, proctitis, and rectal strictures.
- Patient-related factors associated with increased risk of side effects include older patient age, invasion of primary tumor into bladder and/or rectum, and a history of smoking. Treatment-related factors include surface vaginal dose greater than 70 Gy (18), dose fractionation scheme, and history of prior surgery.

References

1. Bosch FX, et al. Comprehensive control of human papillomavirus infections and related diseases. *Vaccine* 2013;31:I1–I31.
2. Daling JR, Madeleine MM, Schwartz SM, et al. A population-based study of squamous cell vaginal cancer: HPV and cofactors. *Gynecol Oncol* 2002;84(2):263.
3. Aho M, Vesterinen E, Meyer B, et al. Natural history of vaginal intraepithelial neoplasia. *Cancer* 1991;68(1):195.
4. Hiniker SM, Roux A, Murphy JD, et al. Primary squamous cell carcinoma of the vagina: prognostic factors, treatment patterns, and outcomes. *Gynecol Oncol* 2013;131(2):380–385.
5. Hacker NF, Eifel PJ. Vaginal cancer. In: Berek JS, Hacker NF, eds. *Berek and Hacker's gynecologic oncology*, 6th ed. Philadelphia, PA: Lippincott Williams & Wilkins, 2015:608.
6. Dodge JA, et al. Clinical features and risk of recurrence among patients with vaginal intraepithelial neoplasia. *Gynecol Oncol* 2001;83:363–369.

7. Petrilli ES, et al. Vaginal intraepithelial neoplasia: biologic aspects and treatment with topical 5-fluorouracil and the carbon dioxide laser. *Am J Obstet Gynecol* 1980;138:321–328.
8. Graham K, et al. 20-Year retrospective review of medium dose rate intracavitary brachytherapy in VAIN3. *Gynecol Oncol* 2007;106:105–111.
9. Frank SJ, et al. Definitive radiation therapy for squamous cell carcinoma of the vagina. *Int J Radiat Oncol Biol Phys* 2005;62(1):138–147.
10. Perez CA, et al. Factors affecting long-term outcome of irradiation in carcinoma of the vagina. *Int J Radiat Oncol Biol Phys* 1999;44(1):37–45.
11. Puthawala A, et al. Integrated external and interstitial radiation therapy for primary carcinoma of the vagina. *Obstet Gynecol* 1983;62(3):367–372.
12. Samant R, Lau B, E C, et al. Primary vaginal cancer treated with concurrent chemoradiation using Cis-platinum. *Int J Radiat Oncol Biol Phys* 2007;69:746.
13. Buchanan DJ, Schlaerth J, Kurosaki T. Primary vaginal melanoma: thirteen-year disease-free survival after wide local excision and review of recent literature. *Am J Obstet Gynecol* 1998; 178(6):1177–1184.
14. Creasman WT, Phillips JL, Menck HR. The National Cancer Data Base report on cancer of the vagina. *Cancer* 1998;83(5):1033–1040.
15. Tabata T, et al. Treatment failure in vaginal cancer. *Gynecol Oncol* 2002;84(2):309–314.
16. Viswanathan AN, et al. The American Brachytherapy Society Treatment Recommendations for Locally Advanced Carcinoma of the Cervix. Part II: High Dose-Rate Brachytherapy. *Brachytherapy* 2012;11(1):47–52.
17. Eifel PJ, et al. Time course and incidence of late complications in patients treated with radiation therapy for FIGO stage IB carcinoma of the uterine cervix. *Int J Radiat Oncol Biol Phys* 1995;32(5):1289–1300.
18. Lian J, et al. Twenty-year review of radiotherapy for vaginal cancer: an institutional experience. *Gynecol Oncol* 2008;111(2):298–306.

CHAPTER 36

VULVA

INTRODUCTION

- Vulvar cancer is the fourth most common gynecologic cancer and constitutes 5% of malignancies of the female genital tract (1,2).
- In the United States, an estimated 5,950 new cases and 1,110 deaths from vulvar cancer occurred in 2016 (3).
- Vulvar cancer occurs with a bimodal age distribution.
- Younger patients more frequently smoke and are at higher risk of human papillomavirus (HPV) infection, and their invasive cancers are more commonly associated with vulvar intraepithelial neoplasia (VIN) (4).
- More commonly, patients are older with disease associated with lichen sclerosus and squamous hyperplasia (5).

ANATOMY

- The vulva is composed of the mons pubis, clitoris, labia majora and minora, vaginal vestibule, perineal body, posterior fourchette, and their supporting subcutaneous tissues.
- The Bartholin glands, two small mucus-secreting glands, are located within the subcutaneous tissues of the posterior labia majora. Malignancies arising from these structures are grouped with vulvar cancers.

NATURAL HISTORY

- The most common sites of vulvar malignancies are the labia majora and minora (70%), clitoris (10% to 15%), and perineum and fourchette (4% to 5%) (6).
- Less common sites include the vestibule, Bartholin's gland, and clitoral prepuce, accounting for less than 1% of vulvar cancers.
- Approximately 5% of vulvar cancers are multifocal and 20% present synchronously with cervical cancer (7).

- Multifocal disease and concurrent cervical tumors are more common in HPV-positive tumors.
- Patients with HPV-positive tumors have decreased risk of recurrence and death from vulvar cancer compared to HPV-negative tumors (5,8).
- All vulvar cancers spread by direct extension to adjacent structures including the vagina, urethra, perineum, anus, and ischial rami.
- Lymphatic drainage of the perineum, clitoris, and anterior labia minora is often bilateral, whereas lymphatic flow from well-lateralized sites in the vulva is predominantly to the ipsilateral groin (Fig. 36-1).
- Lymphatics of the labia drain into the superficial inguinal and superficial femoral nodes, which penetrate the cribriform fascia and reach the deep femoral nodes.
- From the deep femoral nodes, lymph drains under the inguinal ligaments into the external and common iliac lymph nodes (pelvic lymphatics).
- Lymphatics of the fourchette, perineum, prepuce, and glans clitoris follow the lymphatics of the labia.
- Metastases to the femoral lymph nodes without involvement of the superficial inguinal lymph nodes have been reported, especially from carcinomas of the clitoris and Bartholin's gland.
- The overall incidence of inguinal lymph node metastases in surgically staged patients is 6% to 50%, depending on depth of tumor invasion (9,10).

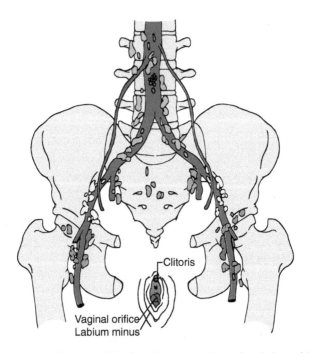

FIGURE 36-1. Lymphatic drainage of the female pelvis in the vulva. (Adapted from Agur AMR, Dalley AF, eds. *Grant's atlas of anatomy*, 14th ed. Philadelphia, PA: Lippincott Williams & Wilkins, 2017: 407. © Wolters Kluwer.)

- In nonmidline lesions, only 8% of patients on GOG 36 had a positive contralateral node, and only 2.5% of patients without a positive ipsilateral node had a positive contralateral node (11).
- Lymphadenectomy will detect metastatic involvement to pelvic nodes in approximately 5% of all cases.
- In those with metastases to inguinal nodes, approximately 15% to 20% have positive pelvic nodes (9).
- Metastases to pelvic nodes may occur without involvement of the superficial inguinal lymph nodes, especially from carcinomas of midline structures such as clitoris and Bartholin's gland (12,13).
- Hematogenous spread is uncommon in the absence of prior inguinofemoral lymph node involvement.
- The most common sites of metastatic disease are liver, lungs, and bones.

CLINICAL PRESENTATION

- Up to 20% of patients are asymptomatic.
- Patients most commonly present with a vulvar mass or ulcer often associated with a variable history of pruritus or vulvar pain.
- Extensive lesions may be associated with dysuria, difficulty with defecation, bleeding, or discharge.
- Advanced inguinal node involvement is rare and may present with ulcerating masses in the groins or lower extremity edema secondary to obstruction.

DIAGNOSTIC WORKUP

- A complete history and physical examination including assessment of the vulva, anus, and perineum is required for diagnosis.
- A pelvic examination including Papanicolaou smear of the cervix and vagina and bimanual pelvic examination is mandatory for detection of synchronous disease.
- Exam under anesthesia, cystoscopy, or proctoscopy may be needed for advanced disease.
- Consider chest imaging with plain chest radiography.
- Consider pelvic magnetic resonance imaging (MRI) to aid in surgical and/or radiation treatment planning (14).
- Consider whole-body positron emission tomography/computed tomography (PET/CT) or chest/abdominal/pelvic CT for T2 or larger tumors if metastasis is suspected (15–17).
- A punch biopsy is most commonly performed for pathologic confirmation at the primary site.
- Biopsy enlarged or fludeoxyglucose (FDG)-avid lymph nodes with image-guided needle aspiration or local excision.
- Appropriate patients should receive smoking cessation counseling and HPV testing.
- Diagnostic workup is outlined in Figure 36-2.

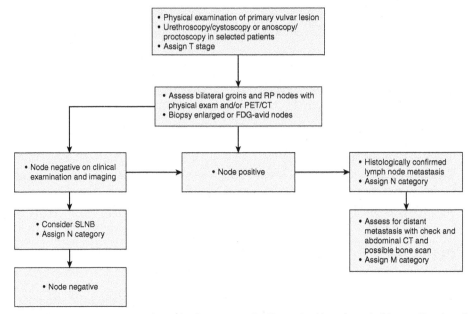

FIGURE 36-2. Diagnostic workup of vulvar cancer. SLNB, sentinel lymph node biopsy. (Reprinted with permission from Russell AH, Van der Zee AGJ. Vulvar and vaginal carcinoma. In: Gunderson LL, Tepper JE, eds. *Clinical radiation oncology*, 3rd ed. Philadelphia, PA: Elsevier, 2012:1276.)

STAGING

- The International Federation of Gynecology and Obstetrics (FIGO) adopted a modified surgical staging system for vulvar cancer in 1989, in which tumor assessment is based on physical exam with endoscopy in bulky disease, and nodal status is determined by surgical evaluation of the groins (18,19).
- The FIGO system was updated in 2009. Major changes include combination of former stage I and II as well as classification based on number and size of involved lymph nodes (20).
- The American Joint Committee on Cancer Staging was released in 2016.
- For details of the current staging system, please refer to the AJCC staging system, 8th edition (21).

PATHOLOGIC CLASSIFICATION

- Between 2% and 5% of VIN 3 lesions will progress to invasive carcinoma (22).
- Over 90% of vulvar carcinoma is squamous cell carcinoma (22). There are two subtypes:
  - Keratinizing, differentiated, or simplex is more common, present in 65% to 80% of cases. It is unrelated to HPV infection but is associated with vulvar dystrophies including lichen sclerosis and chronic venereal granulomatous disease.
  - Classic, warty, or Bowenoid type is associated most commonly with HPV 16, 18, or 33 and occurs in 20% to 35% of cases (23).

- Verrucous cancer is a distinct variant of squamous cell carcinoma that exhibits hyperkeratosis microscopically and is cauliflower-like in appearance. These are a discrete clinicopathologic subset of vulvar cancer and are treated with surgical excision (24,25).
- Melanomas are the second most common malignancy of the vulva although they account for less than 10% of primary vulvar tumors (18).
- Sarcomas including leiomyosarcoma, rhabdomyosarcoma, liposarcoma, angiosarcoma, neurofibrosarcoma, epithelioid sarcoma, and undifferentiated/unclassified soft tissue sarcomas constitute 1% to 2% of vulvar malignancies (26,27).
- Vulvar Paget's disease is the same pathologically as diseases in the breast and accounts for less than 1% of all vulvar malignancies (28).
- Less common vulvar tumors also include basal cell carcinoma, Merkel cell tumors, carcinoid, transitional cell carcinomas, and adenoid cystic carcinoma.
- Adenocarcinomas may originate from periurethral Skene's glands but most commonly arises in Bartholin's gland.
- Bartholin's gland carcinoma is most commonly adenoid cystic (10%) and constitutes only 0.1% of all vulvar malignancies (29).
- Bartholin's gland carcinoma may be squamous cell when it originates near the orifice of the duct or papillary if it arises from transitional epithelium of the duct.

PROGNOSTIC FACTORS

- Lymph node metastasis is considered the most important prognostic factor and determinant of treatment in vulvar cancer (30).
- Patients with negative lymph nodes have a 5-year overall survival from 83% to 100%, whereas those with involved lymph nodes have an average 5-year overall survival of 38% to 61% (31).
- Lymph node involvement correlates well with FIGO clinical stage. Regional nodes are reported in 8.9% to 15%, 25.3% to 40%, 31.1% to 80%, and 62.5% to 100% of patients with clinical stage I, II, III, and IV diseases, respectively (32).
- Predictors of groin node metastases include tumor size, depth of invasion, histologic subtype, and degree of lymphovascular invasion (11,33).
- Invasion of 1, 2, or 3 mm has been shown to correspond to 2.6%, 7%, and 17% incidence of lymph node involvement, respectively (11,33).
- Extracapsular extension is an independent risk factor in patients with positive lymph nodes (34,35).
- Predictors of local recurrence after primary surgery include stage, width of surgical margin, depth of invasion, tumor thickness, growth pattern, and presence of vascular space invasion.
- Multiple studies have shown an association between risk of vulvar recurrence and surgical margins. When pathologic margins are ≤8 mm, local recurrence may be up to 30%. A minimal clinical space of 1 cm of uninvolved normal, unfixed tissue is recommended (36).

GENERAL MANAGEMENT

Stage I and II Tumors

- Historically, all patients were staged and treated with en bloc radical vulvectomy and bilateral inguinofemoral lymphadenectomy (37).
- In current practice, radical local excision (also known as radical partial vulvectomy, radical hemivulvectomy, or modified radical vulvectomy) is typically used when feasible.
- En bloc lymphadenectomy is now more commonly replaced by a triple incision procedure including a vulvectomy incision and two separate incisions in the groin for inguinal lymphadenectomy (38).
- Radical wide excision is possible in the case of T1 lesions with no extension to adjacent perineal structures. This operation is as effective as radical vulvectomy in preventing local recurrence (36,39,40).
- A tumor-free margin greater than or equal to 1 cm is required because of the increased risk of local recurrence with smaller margins (36).
- For patients with tumor at or close to surgical margins, re-excision or radiation therapy is indicated to reduce the risk of local recurrence (41,42).
- For patients with T1 tumors with less than or equal to 1 mm depth of invasion, inguinofemoral lymph node evaluation is not required because of the low risk of lymph node metastases (27,43–45).
- For patients with T1 or smaller T2 tumors with greater than 1 mm invasion, primary treatment is dependent on tumor location.
- Patients with lateralized lesions located greater than or equal to 2 cm from vulvar midline should undergo radical local resection or modified radical vulvectomy and ipsilateral groin node evaluation (44,46).
- Patients with midline vulvar lesions should undergo radical local resection or modified radical vulvectomy and bilateral groin node evaluation with sentinel lymph node biopsy or inguinofemoral lymph node dissection (43,44).
- Sentinel lymph node biopsy (SLNB) has been shown to have a sensitivity of 91.7%, with false negative predictive value of 3.7% on GOG 173 (47).
- GROINSS-V enrolled women with T1/T2 tumors less than 4 cm and demonstrated a 2.5% groin failure and 90% disease-specific survival with no additional therapy after negative SLNB and inguinofemoral lymphadenectomy for positive sentinel lymph node or no sentinel lymph node detected (48,49).
- A higher risk of groin recurrence was observed with increasing tumor size (less than 1 cm 0%, 1 to 2 cm 3.3%, and greater than 2 cm 14.3%) in a prospective study of women with stage I or II vulvar cancer undergoing SLNB (50).
- Eligibility criteria for SLNB are still evolving, and most offer SLNB to patients with vulvar cancer who meet GROINSS-V criteria with tumor diameter less than 4 cm, as well as greater than 1 mm depth of invasion, no palpable groin lymph nodes, unifocal disease, and sufficient surgical expertise.

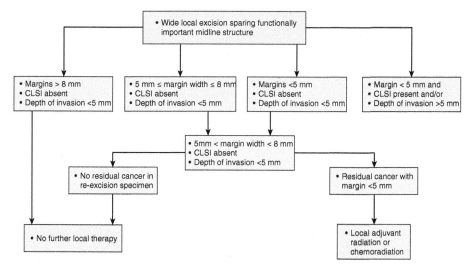

FIGURE 36-3. Algorithm illustrating various therapeutic options for patients with favorable and unfavorable operable carcinoma of the vulva. CLSI, capillary–lymphatic space invasion. (Reprinted with permission from Russell AH, Van der Zee AGJ. Vulvar and vaginal cancer. In: Gunderson LL, Tepper JE, eds. *Clinical radiation oncology*, 3rd ed. Philadelphia, PA: Elsevier, 2012:1276.)

- Groin evaluation can be performed by SLNB or ipsilateral inguinofemoral lymph node dissection if a SLNB is not possible or no sentinel lymph node is detected.
- Therapeutic options for early stage vulvar cancers are indicated in Figure 36-3.

Stage III and IV Tumors

- Historically, locally advanced cancers were treated with radical surgeries with significant postoperative complications and poor quality of life.
- There has been a shift to multimodality treatment to improve organ preservation and reduce surgical morbidity.
- Preoperative radiation alone was shown in early studies to decrease tumor size, and chemotherapy was added in later studies as a radiosensitizer (51,52).
- GOG 101 demonstrated a pathologic complete clinical response rate of 48%, pathologic complete response in 31%, and negative margin resection in 85% in patients with T3/T4 or N2/N3 tumors after 47.6 Gy in 1.7 Gy fractions in a split course with concurrent cisplatin/5FU (53,54).
- GOG 205 treated patients with T3/T4 disease to 57.6 Gy with weekly cisplatin. Patients with pathologic complete response were observed, and those with residual disease underwent surgery. Complete clinical response was observed in 64% and pathologic complete response in 50% (53).
- High pathologic complete response rates from chemoradiation therapy have led many to believe that surgery can be avoided in locally advanced tumors who achieve a clinical complete response.
- Therapeutic options for patients with locally advanced or inoperable tumors are given in Figure 36-4.

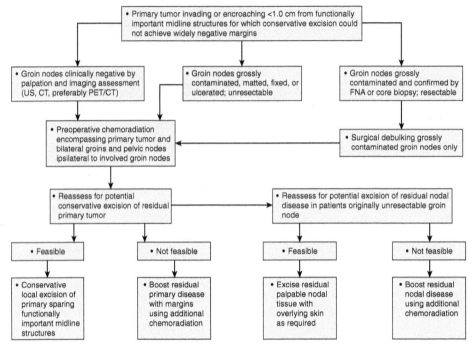

FIGURE 36-4. Algorithm illustrating therapeutic options for patients with locally advanced carcinoma of the vulva. FNA, fine needle aspiration. (Reprinted with permission from Russell AH, Van der Zee AGJ. Vulvar and vaginal cancer. In: Gunderson LL, Tepper JE, eds. *Clinical radiation oncology*, 3rd ed. Philadelphia, PA: Elsevier, 2012:1276.)

Adjuvant Therapy

- Postoperative radiation therapy to the inguinal and pelvic nodes is indicated for patients with involvement of two or more nodes or extranodal extension based on results of GOG 37, which demonstrated improved progression-free and overall survival in patients treated with postoperative radiation therapy (33,55).
- Postoperative radiation therapy may be considered for patients with 1 or more positive nodes with macroscopic metastases (greater than 2 mm) based on results of the AGO CaRE-1 study, demonstrating 3-year progression-free survival and overall survival of 35% and 56% in node-positive compared to 75% and 90% in node-negative patients (56).
- Inclusion of residual vulva and tumor bed when groins and pelvic nodes require irradiation is controversial.
- Adjuvant radiation therapy to the vulva is indicated for positive margins and extracapsular extension (ECE) (57).
- Relative indications for adjuvant radiation to the vulva include close margins if re-resection is not possible, lymphovascular space invasion, and 1 or more lymph nodes (57).
- For bulky nodal disease, the addition of concurrent chemotherapy should be considered.

RADIATION THERAPY TECHNIQUES

- In general, radiation will encompass the vulva, inguinofemoral lymph nodes, and pelvic nodes up to the bifurcation of the external and internal iliac vessels depending on the indications for treatment, while minimizing dose to organs at risk.
- Historically, a wide range of approaches have been used. In an attempt to standardize radiation use and techniques, an international survey with consequent recommendations has been reported.

Patient Positioning and Simulation

- Instruct patients to take a Fleet enema the day prior to simulation.
- Patients are generally positioned in the supine position with lower extremities abducted (Fig. 36-5).
- Immobilization in a vacuum-evacuated device to ensure reproducibility in setup.
- Radiopaque wire is used to identify areas of gross disease the postoperative tumor bed.
- A marker on the anus, urethra, and clitoris and wiring of any scars will aid in planning.
- Bolus of 0.5 to 1 cm thickness for the vulvar region at the time of treatment planning for daily treatments should be considered depending on the clinical situation and skin dose. Bolus in the inguinal region should be considered for gross extension to the skin. Thermoluminescent dosimeters (TLDs) should be used at the beginning of treatment to evaluate skin dose.
- Image using a CT or PET/CT simulation using 3- to 5-mm slice thickness with oral and IV contrast, typically from L2 through mid thigh.
- Patients should be treated with full bladder and empty rectum.
- Setup daily using kV and cone beam CT (CBCT) imaging.

Radiation Therapy Doses

- Doses range from 59.4 to 64.8 Gy in 1.8-Gy fractions for unresectable disease or definitive treatment of medically inoperable patients. For larger tumors, a boost may be given to 70 Gy (57,58).
- Patients with advanced lesions involving surrounding structures should receive preoperative radiation. Doses range from 45 to 57.5 Gy in 1.8-Gy fractions (57,58).
- For adjuvant therapy, irradiation alone to doses of 45 to 54 Gy is recommended, partially depending on margin status (57,58).
- Clinically uninvolved lymph nodes without lymph node dissection may be treated electively to 45 to 50 Gy in 1.8- to 2.0-Gy daily fractions in the appropriate clinical setting (57,58).
- Involved nodes should be boosted to 60 to 65 Gy (57,58).

Radiation Therapy Targets

- In patients undergoing primary radiotherapy with lesions less than 2 cm in diameter, the probability of pelvic nodal involvement is low and irradiation of inguinofemoral nodes alone may be appropriate if imaging is otherwise negative.

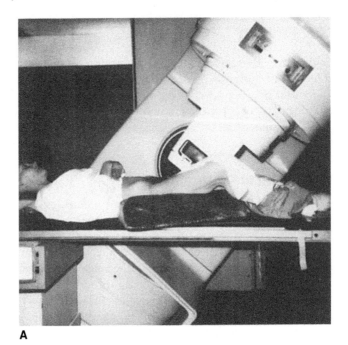

A

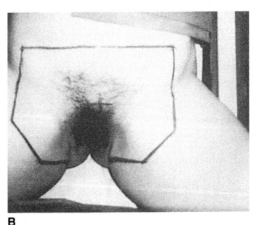

B

FIGURE 36-5. A: Supine frog-leg position for irradiation of vulva and inguinal pelvic lymph nodes. **B:** Example of portal used for irradiation of vulva and inguinofemoral lymph nodes with patient in treatment position. (Reprinted with permission from Pao WM, Perez CA, Kuske RR, et al. Radiation therapy and conservation surgery for primary and recurrent carcinoma of the vulva: report of 40 patients and a review of the literature. *Int J Radiat Oncol Biol Phys* 1988;14:1123–1132. © Elsevier.)

- When an inguinal lymph node dissection is performed and only superficial node involvement is detected, postoperative irradiation is given only to the inguinofemoral nodes.
- Patients with metastatic deep inguinofemoral nodes may benefit from postoperative irradiation including pelvic lymphatics.

Radiation Therapy Techniques

3D Treatment Planning

- Either anteroposterior beam or differentially loaded parallel-opposed anteroposterior-posteroanterior or electron beam can be used.
- If only vulva and inguinofemoral lymph nodes are treated, 4- to 6-MV x-rays through an anterior portal or higher energy x-rays through a posterior portal may be sufficient (Fig. 36-6A).
- The superior field border should be no lower than the sacroiliac joints or higher than the L4/L5 junction unless pelvic nodes are involved. The super border should be raised 5 cm above the most cephalad positive nodes if pelvic lymph nodes are involved (Fig. 36-6B).
- The lateral border will be a vertical line from the anteroinferior iliac spine.
- To adequately cover the inguinal nodes, inferolateral inguinal node border is placed parallel to the inguinal crease and inferior enough to encompass the inguinofemoral node bed and intertrochanteric line of the femur, 1.5 to 2 cm distal to the saphenofemoral junction.
- The inferior vulvar border should be at least 2 cm below the distal most part of the vulva.
- Gross tumor in the vulva or nodes may be boosted with en face electrons. The energy for the vulva is typically 6 to 9 MeV, using a 1.0- to 1.5-cm bolus (Fig. 36-7).
- Electron-beam energy to irradiate lymph nodes depends on the depth, which must be determined by CT scanning.
- Partial-transmission blocks may be used to reduce dose to femoral heads (59,60).
- A midline block should only be used if there are no risk factors at the primary site in postoperative cases.

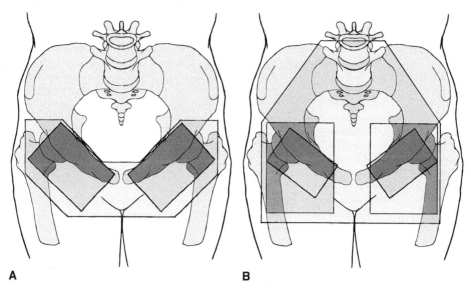

A　　　　　　　　　　　　　　**B**

FIGURE 36-6. **A:** Portal for elective irradiation of regional lymphatics in patients with no clinical evidence of lymph node involvement. **B:** Portal for irradiation of pelvic and inguinofemoral lymph nodes and vulvar area. (Adapted with permission from Perez CA, Grigsby PW, Chao KSC, et al. Vulva. In: Perez CA, Brady LW, eds. *Principles and practice of radiation oncology*, 3rd ed. Philadelphia, PA: Lippincott-Raven, 1998:1915–1942. © Wolters Kluwer.)

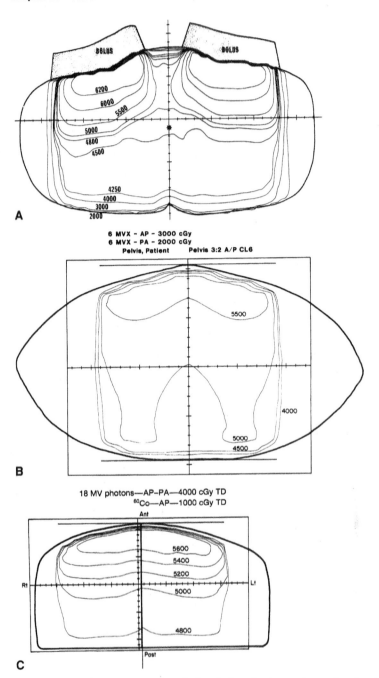

FIGURE 36-7. Representative treatment plans for irradiation of vulvar region and regional lymphatics. **A:** Parallel-opposed 18-MV photon beams, preferentially loaded anteriorly (2,700 cGy anteriorly; 1,800 cGy posteriorly); bolus is added over the inguinal areas to improve dose distribution in subcutaneous tissues in that area. A 1,500-cGy boost using 16-MeV electrons (without bolus) is added to the groin. **B** and **C:** Alternate setups with different beam energies and loading.

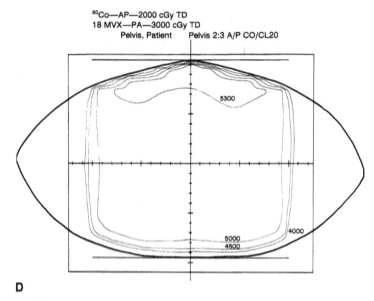

⁶⁰Co—AP—2000 cGy TD
18 MVX—PA—3000 cGy TD
Pelvis, Patient   Pelvis 2:3 A/P CO/CL20

D

FIGURE 36-7. *(Continued)* **D:** Another alternative setup with different beam energy and loading. (Reprinted with permission from Perez CA, Brady LW, Halperin EC, et al., eds. *Principles and practice of radiation oncology*, 4th ed. Philadelphia, PA: Lippincott Williams & Wilkins, 2004. © Wolters Kluwer.)

- Blocks should not be placed lateral to the medial obturator foramen in postoperative cases to avoid undertreating the inguinal nodes.

IMRT Treatment Planning

- The vulvar and nodal targets should be contoured on the planning CT.
- The gross vulvar disease should be contoured as a gross target volume (GTV) including any visible and/or palpable extension into the vagina (Fig. 36-8).
- The vulvar clinical target volume (CTV) is the GTV or tumor bed including adjacent skin, mucosa, and subcutaneous tissue of the vulva excluding bony tissue.
- The inguinofemoral nodal CTV extends laterally from the inguinofemoral vessels to the medial border of the sartorius and rectus femoris muscles, posteriorly to the anterior vastus medialis muscle, and medially to the pectineus muscle. Anteriorly, the volume should extend to the anterior border of the sartorius muscle. The caudal extent of the inguinofemoral nodal basin is the top of the lesser trochanter of the femur (61).
- The pelvic nodal CTV is the vasculature of the bilateral external iliac, obturator, and internal iliac nodal regions with a minimum of 7 mm of symmetric expansion excluding bone and muscle (61).
- The groin CTV should not extend outside the skin and should be trimmed by 3 mm without skin involvement. With skin involvement, the CTV should extend to the skin with bolus material applied during treatment. In thin patients with ECE, bolus should also be considered.
- Planning treatment volume (PTV) expansion is then 7 to 10 mm.

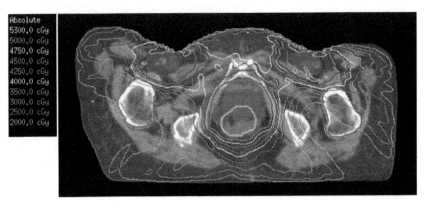

FIGURE 36-8. Representative initial treatment volume for irradiation of stage IVA, T3N0M0, vulvar cancer located at the left vulvar introitus extending into the distal vagina using IMRT. The primary GTV (*purple colorwash*), primary CTV (*red colorwash*), and elective nodal CTV (*blue colorwash*) encompassed by a PTV (*blue outline*) were treated to 4,500 cGy.

- Intensity-modulated radiation therapy (IMRT) target volumes for definitive therapy are listed in Table 36-1.
- IMRT target volumes for postoperative therapy are listed in Table 36-2.

Table 36-1

Carcinoma of the Vulva: Intensity-Modulated Radiation Therapy (IMRT) Treatment Targets

Definitive IMRT: Primary Vulvar Region

GTV
  Use clinical exam, MRI if available
CTV
  Entire vulva
Special considerations:
  If GTV extends beyond vulva, this region + 1 cm = CTV
  If GTV invades muscle, include a rim of muscle in CTV
  If GTV involves vagina, include GTV + 3-cm vaginal tissue in CTV
  If GTV involves vaginal with uncertainty on full extent or LVSI, include entire vaginal length
  If GTV involves anus, anal canal, or bladder, GTV + 2 cm anorectum or bladder is included in CTV
  If GTV is periurethral, GTV + 2 cm urethra included in CT

Definitive IMRT Target Volumes: Lymph Nodes

LN for primary vulvar involving vulva only; vulva and distal vagina; periurethral, or periclitoral
  Bilateral inguinofemoral
  Bilateral obturator
  Bilateral internal and external iliacs
LN for proximal half posterior vaginal wall
  Consider including presacral LN from S1-S3
LN for primary vulvar lesions involving anus or anal canal
  Bilateral inguinofemoral
  Bilateral obturator
  Bilateral internal and external iliacs
  Perirectal (including mesorectum) and presacral LN

Table 36-2

Carcinoma of the Vulva: Intensity-Modulated Radiation Therapy (IMRT) Treatment Targets

Postoperative IMRT

Primary site
  Negative margins
    CTV should cover the entire operative bed
  Positive margins
    2-cm margins on areas of close or positive margins
Positive groin
  Bilateral inguinofemoral nodes
  Bilateral obturator nodes
  Bilateral internal and external iliacs to L5/S1 interspace

TREATMENT FOR RECURRENT LESIONS

- Given the rarity of primary vulvar cancer, data for treating recurrences are scarce and no clear standard of care exists.
- Isolated local recurrences can often be treated with radical local excision (62,63).
- Additional postoperative therapy is indicated by margin and nodal status.
- Nonsurgical therapy for recurrence includes external beam radiation therapy with or without brachytherapy and/or concurrent chemotherapy (58).
- Pelvic exenteration can be considered for select cases with a central recurrence (64,65).
- For patients with nodal recurrence or distant metastases, chemotherapy, palliative/best supportive care, or clinical trial enrollment is recommended (58).
- If recurrence is limited to the groin and no prior radiation was given, consideration of resection of positive nodes followed by EBRT with or without chemotherapy may be considered (58).

SEQUELAE OF TREATMENT

- Radical vulvectomy with *en bloc* resection of inguinal and/or pelvic lymph nodes was associated with a high morbidity rate including an approximately 50% risk of wound infections and major problems for the patient concerning relationship, sexual function, body image, and self-assurance (37,66).
- More modern procedures show markedly lower rates of wound-healing disorders (38).
- Complications are more common after complete lymphadenectomy as compared to sentinel lymph node biopsy. In GROINNS-V, authors found 11.7%, 1.9%, and 45% of wound break down, lymphedema, and cellulitis after SLNB as compared to 34.0%, 25.2%, and 21.3% after complete lymphadenectomy (48).
- Reported incidence of wound infection varies from 5.7% to 50% (9,67).
- Incidence of wound dehiscence and necrosis varies from 30% to 50% (9).
- Operative mortality varies from 3% to 6%.

- All patients treated with radiation therapy are anticipated to have some degree of desquamation. This may range from patchy, moist desquamation to confluent, most desquamation over the entire treatment volume. In general, this reaction heals 2 to 3 weeks after completion of therapy.
- Necrosis and fracture of the femoral head/neck may be observed. Grigsby et al. reported 5% actuarial 5-year incidence of fractures in patients receiving doses of 50 Gy or higher using 2D techniques (68).
- Updated Society of Gynecologic Oncology recommendations for post-treatment surveillance are based on the patient's risk for recurrence and personal preferences (69).
- History and physical exam is recommended every 3 to 6 months for the first 2 years, every 6 to 12 months for another 3 to 5 years, and then annually.
- Patients with high-risk disease may be assessed more frequently.
- Annual cervical/vaginal cytology should be considered as clinically indicated.
- Imaging is recommended as indicated by suspicious examination findings or symptoms of recurrence.

RANDOMIZED STUDIES

- GOG 37 randomized patients treated with radical vulvectomy and bilateral lymph node dissection with positive inguinal nodes to either pelvic lymph node dissection or radiotherapy to the pelvis and groins from 45 to 50 Gy. At 2 years, radiotherapy resulted in improved overall survival (68% versus 54%) and lower incidence of groin recurrences (5.1% versus 23.6%). The greatest survival benefit was observed in patients with ECE or two or more positive nodes (70).
- A 6-year update of GOG 37 did not show a statistically significant survival benefit in patients overall. However, the survival benefit persisted in patients with ECE or 2 or more positive lymph nodes. Cancer-related death and groin failure rate were significantly improved with radiation (55).
- GOG 88 randomized patients with clinically negative inguinal lymph nodes after radical vulvectomy to either inguinal lymph node dissection or radiotherapy to the groin. The study was closed early due to higher rates of groin recurrences in the radiotherapy arm, 19% versus 0%, and decreased overall survival, 63% versus 88% (71). However, the study did not use CT-based treatment planning. Radiation was prescribed to a depth of 3 cm from the anterior skin. With appropriate nodal coverage, radiotherapy to the groin did not produce statistically significant differences in local control (91% versus 100%) or cause-specific survival (63% versus 88%) (71,72).

References

1. Siegel RL, Miller KD, Jemal A. Cancer statistics, 2016. *CA Cancer J Clin* 2016;66:7–30.
2. Hunter DJS. Carcinoma of the vulva: a review of 361 patients. *Gynecol Oncol* 1975;3:117–123.
3. *Cancer facts & figures 2016.* Atlanta, GA: American Cancer Society, 2016.
4. Crum CP, McLachlin CM, Tate JE, et al. Pathobiology of vulvar squamous neoplasia. *Curr Opin Obstet Gynecol* 1997;9:63–69.
5. Monk BJ, Burger RA, Lin F, et al. Prognostic significance of human papillomavirus DNA in vulvar carcinoma. *Obstet Gynecol* 1995;85:709–715.

6. Petereit D, Mehta M, Buchler D, et al. *Lymphatic system of the female genitalia: the morphological basis of oncologic diagnosis and therapy.* Philadelphia, PA: WB Saunders, 1971.

7. Collins CG, Lee F, Roman-Lopez J. Invasive carcinoma of the vulva with lymph node metastasis. *Am J Obstet Gynecol* 1971;109:446.

8. Lee L, Howitt B, Vatalano P, et al. Prognostic importance of human papillomavirus (HPV) and p16 positivity in squamous cell carcinoma of the vulva treated with radiotherapy. *Gynecol Oncol* 2016;142:293–298.

9. Boutselis J. Radical vulvectomy for invasive squamous cell carcinoma of the vulva. *Obstet Gynecol* 1972;39:827–836.

10. Wang CJ, Chin YY, Leung SW, et al. Topographic distribution of inguinal lymph nodes metastasis: Significance in determination of treatment margin for elective inguinal lymph nodes irradiation of low pelvic tumors. *Int J Radiat Oncol Biol Phys* 1996;35:133–136.

11. Homesley HD, Bundy BN, Sedlis A, et al. Prognostic factors for groin node metastasis in squamous cell carcinoma of the vulva (a Gynecologic Oncology Group study). *Gynecol Oncol* 1993;49:279–283.

12. Chu J, Tamimi H, Figge D. Femoral node metastases with negative superficial inguinal nodes in early vulvar cancer. *Am J Obstet Gynecol* 1981;140:337–339.

13. Burke T, Levenback C, Coleman RL, et al. Surgical therapy of T1 and T2 vulvar carcinoma. Further experience with radical wide excision and selective inguinal lymphadenectomy. *Gynecol Oncol* 1995;57:215–220.

14. Kataoka MY, Sala E, Baldwin P, et al. The accuracy of magnetic resonance imaging in staging of vulvar cancer: A retrospective multi-centre study. *Gynecol Oncol* 2010;117:82–87.

15. Cohn DE, Dehdashti F, Gibb RK, et al. Prospective evaluation of positron emission tomography for the detection of groin node metastases from vulvar cancer. *Gynecol Oncol* 2002;85:179–184.

16. Kamran MW, O'Toole F, Meghen K, et al. Whole-body [18F]fluoro-2-deoxyglucose positron emission tomography scan as combined PET-CT staging prior to planned radical vulvectomy and inguinofemoral lymphadenectomy for squamous vulvar cancer: a correlation with groin node metastasis. *Eur J Gynaecol Oncol* 2014;35:230–235.

17. Robertson NL, Hricak H, Sonoda Y, et al. The impact of FDG-PET/CT in the management of patients with vulvar and vaginal cancer. *Gynecol Oncol* 2016;140:420–424.

18. Creasman W. New gynecologic cancer staging. *Obstet Gynecol* 1990;75:287–288.

19. Shepherd J. Revised FIGO staging for gynecologic cancer. *Br J Obstet Gynaecol* 1989;96:889–892.

20. Pecorelli S, Zigliani L, Odicino F. Revised FIGO staging for carcinoma of the cervix. *Int J Gynecol Obstet* 2009;105:107–108.

21. Amin MB, Edge SB, Greene FL, et al., eds. *AJCC cancer staging manual*, 8th ed. New York, NY: Springer, 2017.

22. Sideri M, Jones RW, Wilkinson EJ, et al. Squamous vulvar intraepithelial neoplasia: 2004 modified terminology, ISSVD Vulvar Oncology Subcommittee. *J Reprod Med* 2005;50:807–810.

23. Medeiros F, Nascimento AF, Crum CP. Early vulvar squamous neoplasia: advances in classification, diagnosis, and differential diagnosis. *Adv Anat Pathol* 2005;12:20–26.

24. Partridge E, Murad T, Shingleton H, et al. Verrucous lesions of the female genitalia II. Verrucous carcinoma. *Am J Obstet Gynecol* 1980;137:419–424.

25. Japaze H, Van Dinh T, Woodruff JD. Verrucous carcinoma of the vulva: study of 24 cases. *Obstet Gynecol* 1982;60:462–466.

26. Ulutin HC, Zellars RC, Frassica D. Soft tissue sarcoma of the vulva: a clinical study. *Int J Gynecol Cancer* 2003;13:528–531.

27. Homesley HD. Management of vulvar cancer. *Cancer* 1995;76:2159–2170.

28. Parker LP, Parker JR, Bodurka-Bevers D, et al. Paget's disease of the vulva: pathology, pattern of involvement, and prognosis. *Gynecol Oncol* 2000;77:183–189.

29. Leuchter RS, Hacker NF, Voet RL, et al. Primary carcinoma of the Bartholin gland: a report of 14 cases and review of the literature. *Obstet Gynecol* 1982;60:361–368.

30. Figge D, Tamimi H, Greer B. Lymphatic spread in carcinoma of the vulva. *Obstet Gynecol* 1985;152:387–394.

31. Beller U, Maissoneuve P, Benedet J. Carcinoma of the vulva. *Int J Gynecol Obstet* 2003;83(suppl 1): 7–26.

32. Donaldson E, Powell D, Hanson M, et al. Prognostic parameters in invasive vulvar cancer. *Gynecol Oncol* 1981;11:184–190.

33. Sedlis A, Homesley H, Bundy BN, et al. Positive groin lymph nodes in superficial squamous cell vulvar cancer. A gynecologic oncology group study. *Am J Obstet Gynecol* 1987;156:1159–1164.

34. Origoni M, Sideri M, Garsia S, et al. Prognostic value of pathological patterns of lymph node positivity in squamous cell carcinoma of the vulva Stage III and IVA FIGO. *Gynecol Oncol* 1992;45:313–316.

35. van der Velden K, Ansink A. Primary groin irradiation vs primary groin surgery for early vulvar cancer. *Cochrane Database Syst Rev* 2001;CD002224.

36. Heaps JM, Fu YS, Montz FJ, et al. Surgical-pathologic variables predictive of local recurrence in squamous cell carcinoma of the vulva. *Gynecol Oncol* 1990;38:309–314.

37. Way S. The anatomy of the lymphatic drainage of the vulva and its influence on the radical operation for carcinoma. *Ann R Coll Surg Engl* 1948;3:187–209.

38. Hacker NF, Leuchter RS, Berek JS, et al. Radical vulvectomy and bilateral inguinal lymphadenectomy through separate groin incisions. *Obstet Gynecol* 1981;58:574–579.

39. Tantipalakorn C, Robertson G, Marsden DE, et al. Outcome and patterns of recurrence for International Federation of Gynecology and Obstetrics (FIGO) stages I and II squamous cell vulvar cancer. *Obstet Gynecol* 2009;113:895–901.

40. De Hullu JA, Oonk MHM, Ansink AC, et al. Pitfalls in the sentinel lymph node procedure in vulvar cancer. *Gynecol Oncol* 2004;94:10–15.

41. Rouzier R, Haddad B, Dubernard G, et al. Inguinofemoral dissection for carcinoma of the vulva: Effect of modifications of extent and technique on morbidity and survival. *J Am Coll Surg* 2003;196:442–450.

42. Gonzalez Bosquet J, Magrina JF, Magtibay PM, et al. Patterns of inguinal groin metastases in squamous cell carcinoma of the vulva. *Gynecol Oncol* 2007;105:742–746.

43. Hacker NF, Van der Velden J: Conservative management of early vulvar cancer. *Cancer* 1993;71:1673–1677.

44. Benedet JL, Bender H, Jones H III, et al. Staging classifications and clinical practice guidelines of gynaecologic cancers. *Int J Gynecol Obstet* 2000;70:207–312.

45. Magrina JF, Gonzalez-Bosquet J, Weaver AL, et al. Squamous cell carcinoma of the vulva stage IA: long-term results. *Gynecol Oncol* 2000;76:24–27.

46. Hacker NF, Berek JS, Lagasse LD, et al. Management of regional lymph nodes and their prognostic influence in vulvar cancer. *Obstet Gynecol* 1983;61:408–412.

47. Levenback CF, Ali S, Coleman RL, et al. Lymphatic mapping and sentinel lymph node biopsy in women with squamous cell carcinoma of the vulva: a gynecologic oncology group study. *J Clin Oncol* 2012;30:3786–3791.

48. Van der Zee AGJ, Oonk MH, De Hullu JA, et al. Sentinel node dissection is safe in the treatment of early-stage vulvar cancer. *J Clin Oncol* 2008;26:884–889.

49. te Grootenhuis N, van der Zee A, van Doorn H, et al. Sentinel nodes in vulvar cancer: long-term follow-up of the GROningen INternational Study on Sentinel nodes in Vulvar cancer (GROINSS-V) I. *Gynecol Oncol* 2016;140:8–14.

50. Robison K, Roque D, McCourt C, et al. Long-term follow-up of vulvar cancer patients evaluated with sentinel lymph node biopsy alone. *Gynecol Oncol* 2014;133:416–420.

51. Boronow RC, Hickman BT, Reagan MT, et al. Combined therapy as an alternative to exenteration for locally advanced vulvovaginal cancer. II. Results, complications, and dosimetric and surgical considerations. *Am J Clin Oncol* 1987;10:171–181.

52. Thomas G, Dembo A, DePetrillo A, et al. Concurrent radiation and chemotherapy in vulvar carcinoma. *Gynecol Oncol* 1989;34:263–267.
53. Moore DH, Thomas GM, Montana GS, et al. Preoperative chemoradiation for advanced vulvar cancer: a phase II study of the Gynecologic Oncology Group. *Int J Radiat Oncol Biol Phys* 1998;42:79–85.
54. Montana GS, Thomas GM, Moore DH, et al. Preoperative chemo-radiation for carcinoma of the vulva with N2/N3 nodes: a gynecologic oncology group study. *Int J Radiat Oncol Biol Phys* 2000;48:1007–1013.
55. Kunos C, Simpkins F, Gibbons H, et al. Radiation therapy compared with pelvic node resection for node-positive vulvar cancer: a randomized controlled trial. *Obstet Gynecol* 2009;114:537–546.
56. Mahner S, Jueckstock J, Hilpert F, et al. Adjuvant therapy in lymph node-positive vulvar cancer: the AGO-CaRE-1 study. *J Natl Cancer Inst* 2015;107. doi: 10.1093/jnci/dju426.
57. Russell A, Van Der Zee AGJ. Vulvar and vaginal carcinoma. In: Gundreson L, Tepper J, eds. *Clinical radiation oncology*. Philadelphia, PA: Elsevier Ltd., 2012:1241–1276.
58. NCCN Guidelines Version 1.2017 Vulvar Cancer (Squamous Cell Carcinoma), 2017.
59. King GC, Sonnik DA, Kalend AM, et al. Transmission block technique for the treatment of the pelvis and perineum including the inguinal lymph nodes: dosimetric considerations. *Med Dosim* 1993;18:7–12.
60. Kalnicki S, Zide A, Maleki N, et al. Transmission block to simplify combined pelvic and inguinal radiation therapy. *Radiology* 1987;164:578–580.
61. Kim CH, Olson AC, Kim H, et al. Contouring inguinal and femoral nodes; how much margin is needed around the vessels? *Pract Radiat Oncol* 2012;2:274–278.
62. Maggino T, Landoni F, Sartori E, et al. Patterns of recurrence in patients with squamous cell carcinoma of the vulva. A multicenter CTF Study. *Cancer* 2000;89:116–122.
63. Piura B, Masotina A, Murdoch J, et al. Recurrent squamous cell carcinoma of the vulva: a study of 73 cases. *Gynecol Oncol* 1993;48:189–195.
64. Forner DM, Lampe B. Exenteration as a primary treatment for locally advanced cervical cancer: long-term results and prognostic factors. *Am J Obstet Gynecol* 2011;205(2):148.e1–148.e8. doi: 10.1016/j.ajog.2011.03.057.
65. Miller B, Morris M, Levenback C. Pelvic exenteration for primary and recurrent vulvar cancer. *Gynecol Oncol* 1995;58:202–205.
66. Günther V, Malchow B, Schubert M, et al. Impact of radical operative treatment on the quality of life in women with vulvar cancer—a retrospective study. *Eur J Surg Oncol* 2014;40:875–882.
67. Iversen T, Aalders JG, Christensen A, et al. Squamous cell carcinoma of the vulva: A review of 424 patients, 1956–1974. *Gynecol Oncol* 1980;9:271–279.
68. Grigsby PW, Roberts HL, Perez CA. Femoral neck fracture following groin irradiation. *Int J Radiat Oncol Biol Phys* 1995;32:63–67.
69. Salani R, Backes FJ, Fung Kee Fung M, et al. Posttreatment surveillance and diagnosis of recurrence in women with gynecologic malignancies: Society of Gynecologic Oncologists recommendations. *Am J Obstet Gynecol* 2011;204:466–478.
70. Homesley HD, Bundy BN, Sedlis A, et al. Radiation therapy versus pelvic node resection for carcinoma of the vulva with positive groin nodes. *Obstet Gynecol* 1986;68:733–740.
71. Stehman FB, Bundy BN, Thomas G, et al. V GOG 88 N0, RT [v] LND: Groin dissection versus groin radiation in carcinoma of the vulva: a Gynecologic Oncology Group study. *Int J Radiat Oncol Biol Phys* 1992;24:389–396.
72. Petereit DG, Mehta MP, Buchler DA, et al. Inguinofemoral radiation of N0,N1 vulvar cancer may be equivalent to lymphadenectomy if proper radiation technique is used. *Int J Radiat Oncol Biol Phys* 1993;27:963–967.

CHAPTER 37

HODGKIN LYMPHOMA

NATURAL HISTORY AND CLINICAL PRESENTATION

- Hodgkin lymphoma (HL) has a bimodal age distribution. The first peak is from ages 25 to 30 years, and the second peak is from ages 75 to 80 years (1).
- Many studies have shown an association of Hodgkin lymphoma with the Epstein-Barr virus (2–6).
- HL nearly always begins in the lymph nodes.
- More than 80% of patients with HL present with cervical lymph node involvement, and more than 50% have mediastinal disease.
- Patients with HL generally present with painless lymphadenopathy.
- Some patients may note systemic symptoms such as unexplained fevers, drenching night sweats, and weight loss (B symptoms). Other symptoms include generalized pruritus, neurologic symptoms, and alcohol-induced pain in tissues involved by HL.
- The theory of contiguity of spread and the development of treatment programs, including presumptive treatment of uninvolved sites, were important conceptual advances in the treatment of HL (7).
- Nearly all patients with hepatic or bone marrow involvement by HL have extensive involvement of the spleen (8).
- HL rarely involves Waldeyer's ring, Peyer's patches, the upper aerodigestive tract, central nervous system, or skin.
- One third of patients present with B symptoms: fever, night sweats, or 10% weight loss within the past 6 months. Fevers may present in a classic waxing and waning Pel-Ebstein pattern (5% to 10%). Night sweats may be drenching, requiring a change of bedclothes.
- HL may be diagnosed during pregnancy, and many women become pregnant after successful treatment.
- Historically, children had a better prognosis than did adults; however, advances in treatment have lead to equivalent outcomes in the adult population.

DIAGNOSTIC WORKUP

- Diagnostic and staging procedures commonly used for HL are listed in Table 37-1.
- The erythrocyte sedimentation rate (ESR) is a prognostic factor for patients with stage I to II disease; anemia, lymphopenia, and hypoalbuminemia are adverse prognostic factors for patients with stage III to IV disease (9,10).
- Computed tomography (CT) scan is less sensitive, specific, and accurate (65%, 92%, and 87%, respectively) for detection of disease in the retroperitoneal nodes than is classic bipedal lymphangiography, although the latter technique has largely fallen out of favor (11).

Table 37-1
Diagnostic and Staging Procedures for Hodgkin Lymphoma
History
Systemic B symptoms: unexplained fever, night sweats, weight loss >10% of body weight in the last 6 months Other symptoms: alcohol intolerance, pruritus, respiratory problems, energy loss
Physical Examination
Palpable nodes (note number, size, location, shape, consistency, mobility) Palpable viscera
Laboratory Studies

Standard
   Complete blood cell count
   Platelet count
   Liver and renal function tests
   Blood chemistry profile
   Erythrocyte sedimentation rate
Optional
   Serum copper
   β_2-microglobulin

Radiologic Studies
Chest radiograph: posteroanterior and lateral Computed tomography (CT) of thorax, abdomen, and pelvis CT of neck if indicated FDG-PET scan (current preferred imaging)
Special Tests

Standard
   Pathologic specimen (excisional biopsy of affected lymph node)
   Cytologic examination of effusions, if present
   Bone marrow, needle biopsy (if subdiaphragmatic disease or B symptoms)
Optional
   Percutaneous liver biopsy (if abnormal LFTs but normal CT)

- The criterion for enlarged lymph nodes on CT scan is typically a short axis diameter that exceeds 1 cm (12).
- The criterion for bulky mediastinal lymphadenopathy is when the maximum width of the mediastinal mass divided by the maximum transthoracic diameter (near the level of the diaphragm) on a standing posteroanterior chest radiograph exceeds 1/3. Other definitions include a mass greater than 10 cm, and a ratio of mediastinal mass to the chest diameter at T5-6 exceeding 0.35 (used by the European Organization for the Treatment of Cancer [EORTC]).
- Gallium imaging has been replaced by 2-fluoro-2-deoxy-D-glucose positron emission tomography (FDG-PET). FDG-PET is routinely used as part of the initial staging in HL, and is more sensitive than is CT or gallium imaging (13,14).
- Magnetic resonance imaging (15) is an alternative to CT, and is useful in the staging of women who are pregnant (16).
- The incidence of bone marrow involvement in HL is only 5%. Therefore, a bone marrow biopsy is performed only in those patients who present with stage III to IV disease, bulky adenopathy, or B symptoms.
- Low-risk populations for subdiaphragmatic extension are (a) patients with clinical disease limited to intrathoracic sites (yield approximately 0%); (b) women with stage I disease (yield approximately 6%); (c) men with stage I disease and lymphocyte predominance or interfollicular histology (yield approximately 4%); and (d) women with stage II disease and with three or fewer sites of clinical involvement and who are younger than 27 years of age (yield approximately 9%) (17). In the past, these criteria have been used to define patients not requiring staging laparotomy; however, FDG-PET scanning has supplanted the need for laparotomy in contemporary patients.

STAGING SYSTEM

- The Ann Arbor staging system for HL has been in use since 1971 (18). The lymphoid regions defined in this system are shown in Figure 37-1.
- Because staging laparotomy has been discontinued, instead of clinical and pathologic stage, the generic term stage is now employed.
- Inadequacies of the Ann Arbor system include failure to consider bulk of disease and lack of a more precise definition of the E lesion (19).
- The descriptor "X" is employed to designate bulky mediastinal adenopathy in Cotswolds modification of the Ann Arbor system (20).

PATHOLOGIC CLASSIFICATION

- The neoplastic cell of HL is the Reed-Sternberg cell. It is typically binucleate, with a prominent, centrally located nucleolus in each nucleus. It also has a well-demarcated nuclear membrane and eosinophilic cytoplasm with a perinuclear halo.
- Reed-Sternberg cells are derived from monoclonal B cells, and are CD15 and CD30 positive.

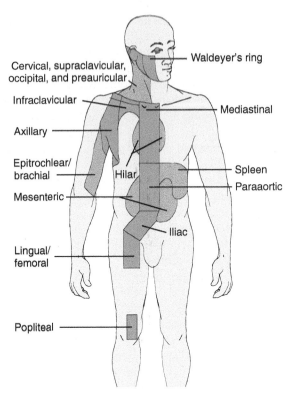

FIGURE 37-1. Lymphoid regions as defined in the Ann Arbor staging system. Note that the cervical, supraclavicular, occipital, and preauricular nodes are included in a single region. The mediastinum and pulmonary hila make up three regions. (Reprinted from Hoppe RT. The non-Hodgkin's lymphomas: pathology, staging, and treatment. *Curr Probl Cancer* 1987;11:379, with permission.)

- They usually account for less than 1% of the cells in a HL-infiltrated lymph node. The majority of the cells in involved nodes are nonmalignant lymphoid cells, plasma cells, eosinophils, and other benign cells.
- The World Health Organization (WHO) modification of the Lukes and Butler system has five histologic subtypes (21). These include the four subtypes of classical HL: nodular sclerosis, lymphocyte rich, mixed cellularity, and lymphocyte depleted. The fifth subtype is nodular lymphocyte predominance HL.
- Nodular lymphocyte predominance HL (nLPHL) is predominantly composed of normal-appearing lymphocytes and has few abnormal cells. Unlike the subtypes of classical HL, the abnormal cells in nLPHL are strongly positive for CD20 and CD45 and negative for CD15 and CD30. The abnormal cells are called "L and H cells" or "popcorn cells." Patients frequently present with a solitary peripheral node and early-stage disease. Systemic symptoms are uncommon (less than 10%). Some patients may have a late relapse, but it has the best overall survival of any HL histologic subtype.
- Lymphocyte-predominant HL (LPHL) is often diagnosed in young people. Patients frequently present with early-stage disease, and systemic symptoms are uncommon. The natural history is the most favorable of the classical HL histologic subtypes.

NEW! **SUMMARY OF CHANGES TO STAGING**

HODGKIN AND NON-HODGKIN LYMPHOMAS

The current staging system is the Lugano classification, which is adapted from the Ann Arbor staging system with Cotswolds modifications for Hodgkin lymphoma. The Lugano classification incorporated the stage groupings from the previous system while adding criteria for involvement of a given site using FDG-PET/CT and other imaging. The Lugano recommendations also put forth a system for definitions of response assessment following treatment as well as preferences for classification of Hodgkin lymphoma (e.g., the designation of the longest measurable diameter of lymph nodes rather than the traditional "X" designation).

See: Amin MB, Edge SB, Greene FL, et al., eds. *AJCC cancer staging manual*, 8th ed. New York: Springer, 2017; Lister TA, Crowther D, et al. Report of a committee convened to discuss the evaluation and staging of patients with Hodgkin's disease: Cotswolds meeting. *J Clin Oncol* 1989;7(11):1630–1636; Cheson BD, Fisher RI, Barrington SF, et al. Recommendations for initial evaluation, staging, and response assessment of Hodgkin and non-Hodgkin lymphoma: the Lugano classification. *J Clin Oncol* 2014;32(27):3059–3068.

- Nodular sclerosing HL (NSHL) is the most common histologic subtype. The mediastinum is often clinically involved. One third of these patients have B symptoms. The natural history of NSHL is less favorable than that of LPHL.
- Mixed cellularity HL (MCHL) patients more commonly present with advanced disease (e.g., subdiaphragmatic involvement). Its natural history is less favorable than that of NSHL.
- Lymphocyte-depleted HL (LDHL) tends to occur in older patients and is more likely to be associated with advanced disease and B symptoms. It has the worst prognosis of all histologic subtypes of HL.

PROGNOSTIC FACTORS

- Men have a slightly worse outcome than do women (22).
- After the extent of disease has been determined, histologic subtype seems to have little additional impact on prognosis.
- Ann Arbor stage is the most important prognostic factor influencing therapy.
- Bulky disease, especially in the mediastinum, is reported to be associated with greater risk of relapse after single-modality therapy.
- The International Prognostic Score was created from a large study that evaluated prognostic factors for 5,141 patients with advanced HL. There were seven factors identified that had a significant impact on prognosis: age, gender, albumin, white cell count, lymphocyte count, hemoglobin, and Ann Arbor stage. If patients have three or more adverse risk factors, they are considered to be in an unfavorable prognostic group for advanced HL (9).

GENERAL MANAGEMENT

Radiation Therapy

- Irradiation is the most effective single agent for the treatment of patients with HL. Actuarial relapse-free survival at 5 years for all stages ranges from 94% for LPHL, 74% for NSHL, and 75% for mixed-cellularity HL to 45% for lymphocyte-depleted HL (23).
- However, irradiation as a monotherapy has largely been abandoned in favor on multidrug chemotherapeutic approaches, often in a combined modality setting incorporating involved-field radiotherapy (IFRT). This is due to the late toxicities associated with radiation therapy given as monotherapy for Hodgkin lymphoma.

Chemotherapy

- The first successful drug combination for treating HL was mechlorethamine hydrochloride (nitrogen mustard), vincristine sulfate (Oncovin), procarbazine hydrochloride, and prednisone (MOPP) (24).
- After the development of doxorubicin (Adriamycin), many trials utilized this drug in novel combinations. Adriamycin, bleomycin, vinblastine, and dacarbazine (AVBD) is now the "gold standard" based on a randomized trial comparing MOPP, ABVD, and MOPP/ABVD (25,26).
- Other drug combinations that are used are MOPP-ABV hybrid, MOPP/ABVD combination, and newer regimens such as Stanford V and BEACOPP (27–30).
- Ongoing trials are seeking to determine if drugs in the common regimens can be safely left out. In the future, biologic agents may be a part of the standard up-front treatment for Hodgkin lymphoma.

Combined-Modality Therapy

- Typically, treatment is initiated with chemotherapy, which has the advantage of treating all disease sites at the outset (particularly important in stage III and IV). Another advantage of initial chemotherapy treatment is a reduction in the size of bulky disease to facilitate subsequent radiotherapy with minimization of normal tissue irradiation (especially in the mediastinum).
- Combined-modality therapy programs generally use a reduced number of cycles of chemotherapy and/or "safer" drugs, as well as reduced irradiation fields and/or doses.
- The radiation dose used in combined-modality studies in adults ranges from 20 to 36 Gy (29,31).
- Is chemotherapy alone a reasonable option in early-stage Hodgkin lymphoma? Two trials with MOPP gave contradictory results (32,33). The decision not to treat with radiotherapy in these trials was not linked to tumor response. Subsequent numerous studies using more modern chemotherapy regimens indicate that combined modality therapy offers improved relapse-free survival/event-free survival compared with chemotherapy alone. The EORTC-GELA H9-F trial randomized early-stage favorable HL patients to no IFRT, 20 Gy IFRT, or 36 Gy IFRT after achieving a complete

response to six cycles of epirubicin, bleomycin, vinblastine, and prednisone (EBVP) chemotherapy; the 4-year event-free survival was inferior in the no IFRT arm (70%) versus the 20 Gy (84%) and 36 Gy (87%) arms, and the results were recently published, which suggest that omission of radiotherapy may be detrimental to patients (34). The EORTC H10 trial addresses a similar issue with demonstration of increased relapse rate with chemotherapy alone; however, it is unclear if this impacts overall survival (35).

RADIATION THERAPY TECHNIQUES

- The principal objective of radiation therapy in HL is to treat involved and contiguous lymphatic chains to a dose associated with a high likelihood of tumor eradication using IFRT.
- In the rare circumstance when radiation alone is used in the modern era, the Patterns of Care Study recommendation for a tumoricidal dose of radiation is 35 to 44 Gy fractionated at a rate of 7.5 to 10.0 Gy per week (36). In this setting, generally extended fields of irradiation are used (e.g., subtotal nodal irradiation) rather than IFRT. Indeed, a key component in curative irradiation monotherapy programs is the use of "prophylactic" treatment to clinically uninvolved areas. A study by the German Hodgkin's Disease Study Group indicates that 30 Gy is an adequate dose for such prophylactic treatment (37).
- Most commonly, combined modality therapy is used in the modern management of HL, for which the range of irradiation doses is 20 to 30 Gy for nonbulky and 20 to 36 Gy for bulky disease (38).
- Evenly weighted opposed-field treatments are generally used; all fields are treated daily with fractions of 1.5 to 1.8 Gy.
- The beam energy used is typically in the 6 to 15 MV range. If an energy greater than 6 MV is used for the supraclavicular and inguinofemoral lymph nodes, bolus should generally be added.
- As combined modality treatment has become more prevalent, "classic" radiation fields (e.g., total lymphoid irradiation, subtotal lymphoid irradiation, full mantle, inverted-Y) are being used less often in favor of more tailored IFRT.
- Recently, the use of involved site radiation therapy (ISRT) is becoming the new standard treatment for consolidative radiotherapy in patients with Hodgkin lymphoma (39).
- The use of 3D-conformal, intensity-modulated radiation therapy (IMRT), breath hold, and other techniques to minimize toxicity are being more widely used.

Mantle

- The full mantle is rarely treated in contemporary management; however, involved fields are portions of the classic treatment field. A description of one setup for a classic mantle field is given in Table 37-2. An example of typical mantle field blocking is shown in Figure 37-2.

Table 37-2
Classic Mantle Setup

Patient Supine with Head Fully Extended

Superior margin: bisects the mandible and passes about 1–2 cm above the mastoid

Lateral margin: flash axillae (humeral head blocks)

Inferior margin:
   Axillae—inferior tips of scapulae
   Mediastinum—encompass inferior extent of mediastinal disease with 5 cm margin (around T10-11 interspace)

Lung blocks: 1–1.5-cm margin around mediastinal contours and hilar nodes; superior point no higher than the inferior tip of the head of the clavicle; taper laterally parallel to the projection of the posterior ribs (to treat high axillary/infraclavicular nodes)

- In addition to lung blocks, blocks can be placed over the occipital region and spinal cord posteriorly, the larynx anteriorly, and the humeral heads both anteriorly and posteriorly.
- Spinal cord shielding may not be necessary with compensated fields if the prescribed tumor dose is only 36 Gy, but should be used when the prescribed dose is more than 40 Gy.
- For significant mediastinal disease with subcarinal extension or pericardial involvement, the entire cardiac silhouette is irradiated to 15 Gy, with a block placed over the apex of the heart thereafter.
- After a dose of 30 Gy has been delivered, a block is placed in the subcarinal region (approximately 5 cm below the carina), shielding additional pericardium and myocardium.

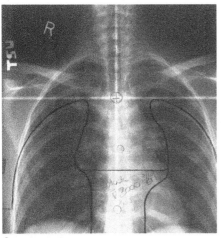 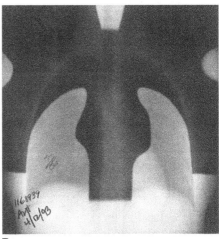

A   **B**

FIGURE 37-2. Anterior mantle setup **(A)** and anterior mantle portal films **(B)** for a patient with a small mediastinal mass. (Reprinted from Hoppe RT. Hodgkin's disease. In: Leibel S, Phillips T, eds. *Textbook of radiation oncology.* Philadelphia, PA: WB Saunders, 1998, with permission.)

- Bolus can be used if disease extends to the anterior chest wall.
- If the pulmonary hilar lymph nodes are involved and a patient is being treated with irradiation alone, a 37% transmission lung block can be used to deliver 15.0 to 16.5 Gy to the lung (40).
- Given issues of potentially excessive pulmonary irradiation with bulky mediastinal disease, the postchemotherapy width of disease (plus about 1.5 to 2 cm margin) is often used as the target volume. However, superior and inferior field margins should encompass the initial (prechemotherapy) extent of disease.

Preauricular Field

- The preauricular field can be treated with opposed lateral or unilateral photons or, preferably, with a unilateral 6- to 9-MeV electron field to spare the contralateral parotid.
- In some cases, the primary site of enlarged nodes may include bulky high cervical nodes, which extend very near the upper border of the typical mantle field. In this setting, large, opposed lateral Waldeyer fields can be used to encompass the upper cervical and adjacent nodes (Fig. 37-3).

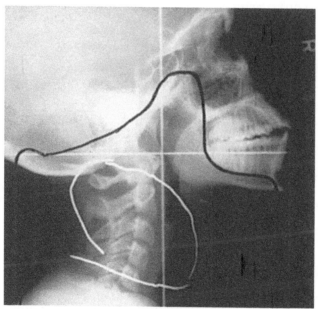

FIGURE 37-3. Large Waldeyer field. This field is appropriate to use when there is a primary component of large cervical adenopathy, as outlined by a lead wire in this setup film. This field should include the submandibular, preauricular, occipital, and high cervical nodes. The inferior border of the field is matched to the mantle low in the neck, below the cervical adenopathy. In most cases, regression of disease after the first 25 to 30 Gy permits switching to a standard mantle with a high superior border matched to a small preauricular field. (Reprinted from Hoppe RT. Hodgkin's disease. In: Perez CA, Brady LW, eds. *Principles and practice of radiation oncology*, 3rd ed. Philadelphia, PA: Lippincott-Raven, 1998:1963–1986, with permission.)

Subdiaphragmatic Fields

- The classic subdiaphragmatic irradiation field for HL is the "inverted Y," which includes the paraaortic (retroperitoneal) and pelvic lymph nodes (Fig. 37-4).
- For paraaortic nodes only, the inferior border of the subdiaphragmatic field is drawn at the L4-5 interspace (paraaortic/splenic pedicle field) or below the bifurcation of the aorta to include the common iliac nodes (spade field).
- The width of the paraaortic field generally coincides with the width of the transverse processes but with adequate margin on the patient's lymphomatous disease. However, for bulky paraaortic adenoapthy, one option is to design the width of the field based on the postchemotherapy extent of disease plus 1.5 to 2 cm margin.
- If the spleen is intact, the entire spleen, not just the splenic hilar region, is included in the field. Respiratory motion has to be considered when planning the splenic field; therefore, generous superior/inferior margins, respiratory gating, and/or 4D CT have to be utilized.
- Sequential treatment to a mantle field and inverted-Y field is referred to as total lymphoid irradiation. When the subdiaphragmatic field does not include the pelvis, the term subtotal lymphoid irradiation is used.
- Low-dose hepatic irradiation may be used for involvement if irradiation alone is being used as primary treatment, or in combined-modality programs when the liver is involved. A 50% transmission block delivers 20 to 22 Gy to the liver during the same period in which the paraaortic nodes would receive 40 to 44 Gy.

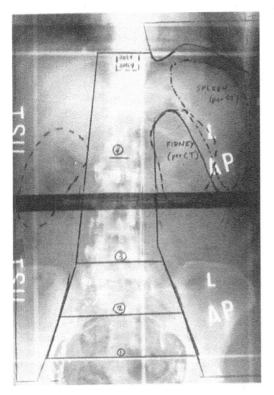

FIGURE 37-4. Subdiaphragmatic irradiation in the absence of a staging laparotomy. The splenic and renal volumes are reconstructed according to computed tomography data. Inferior borders 1 and 2 correspond to reasonable lower margins of the field for men and women, respectively, when the common iliac nodes are to be included in the treatment field. Border 3 defines the inferior limit of a paraaortic field. Line 4 indicates the inferior position for placement of a posterior cord block, if necessary, to limit the cord dose to 40 Gy. (Reprinted from Hoppe RT. The lymphomas. In: Khan F, Potish R, eds. *Treatment planning in radiation oncology*. Baltimore, MD: Williams & Wilkins, 1997:418, with permission.)

- In women, the ovaries normally overlie the iliac lymph nodes. To avoid radiation-induced amenorrhea, an oophoropexy must be performed. The surgeon marks the ovaries with radiopaque sutures or clips and places them medially and as low as possible behind the uterine body. A double-thickness (10 half-value layer) midline block is then used; its location is guided by the position of the opacified nodes and transposed ovaries. When the ovaries are at least 2 cm from the edge of this block, the dose is decreased to 8% of that delivered to the iliac nodes (41) (Fig. 37-5).
- In men, use of a double-thickness midline block and specially constructed testicular shield can reduce testicular dose from 10% to from 0.75% to 3.00% (17,23).

3D Treatment Planning

- Planning with 3D simulation allows the use of more tailored treatment fields to limit late effects (42).
- The gross tumor volume (GTV) is defined as palpable nodes, nodes enlarged on CT, or nodes avid on PET.
- The clinical target volume (CTV) is the GTV plus the entire involved lymph node region (Fig. 37-1), and possibly the inclusion of adjacent uninvolved nodal regions (extended CTV).

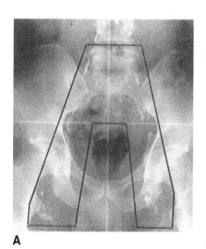 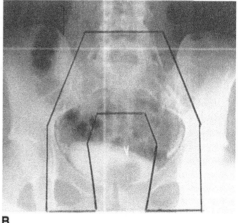

A **B**

FIGURE 37-5. Typical setup films for pelvic irradiation. Note that the opacified nodes from the lymphangiogram permit maximum tailoring of the field to minimize amount of bone marrow being irradiated. (In the modern era of computed tomography–based treatment planning, similar customized planning can be achieved by contouring of the iliac vessels.) The field is matched superiorly to the paraaortic/splenic pedicle field, or the two fields can be treated together (inverted Y). When the pelvic nodes are involved, the midline pelvic block is deleted. **A:** Male pelvic field. A narrow midline block protects rectum, anus, and genitalia. A testicular shield is used during therapy. **B:** Female pelvic field. A wide, double-thickness (10 half-value layer) midline block protects rectum, anus, and ovaries. The ovaries have been transposed to the midline and are marked by wire sutures (in this case, surgical clips). Every attempt should be made to ensure that the ovaries are no closer than 2 cm from the edge of the block. (Reprinted from Hoppe RT. Hodgkin's disease. In: Perez CA, Brady LW, eds. *Principles and practice of radiation oncology*, 3rd ed. Philadelphia, PA: Lippincott–Raven, 1998:1963–1986, with permission.)

- The PTV includes the CTV (or extended CTV) plus a 1 to 1.5 cm margin.
- Modern treatment involves the use of ISRT following guidelines from the International Lymphoma Radiation Oncology Group (ILROG). Rather than having the CTV cover the entire lymph node region, current practice is to treat more limited volumes.

Favorable Prognosis Stage I to IIA Disease (Supradiaphragmatic)

- Patients are considered favorable if they have no B symptoms or bulky mediastinal disease. In addition, risk stratification paradigms from Europe and Canada classify patients with an elevated ESR (greater than 50), extralymphatic extension, multiple sites of disease (e.g., greater than 2 to 3), unfavorable histology (mixed cellularity or lymphocyte depleted), and age greater than 50 as unfavorable. Each clinical trial group has slight variations in the differentiation of early favorable and early unfavorable disease.
- The current management for these early-stage favorable patients is combined modality therapy with an expected freedom from progression of 90% to 95%. Trials using abbreviated chemotherapy along with involved-field radiation therapy (IFRT) include the Milan trial of Adriamycin, bleomycin, vinblastine, and dacarbazine (ABVD) for four cycles plus 36 Gy IFRT (43); the British trial of vinblastine, Adriamycin, prednisone, etoposide, cyclophosphamide, and bleomycin (VAPEC-B) for 4 weeks, followed by 30 to 40 Gy IFRT (44); and the Stanford University trial of 8 weeks of Stanford V chemotherapy followed by 30 Gy IFRT (45).
- The optimal duration of chemotherapy and dose of irradiation are being tested in several trials. The GHSG HD10 trial randomized favorable patients to two versus four cycles of ABVD and 20 versus 30 Gy IFRT and long-term outcomes support the use of 2 cycles of ABVD followed by 20 Gy RT for favorable patients (a subset of "favorable" Hodgkin patients).
- Radiation alone was historically the treatment of choice for this group, but has fallen out of favor secondary to concerns over late effects due to the large fields and relatively high doses of irradiation delivered. Results from large trials have shown 10-year survival rate of 90% and freedom from progression of 80% with radiation alone (46).
- Trials that have attempted to eliminate radiation therapy have been inconclusive. The NCCTG HD-6/ECOG JHD06 trial arms included ABVD alone, subtotal lymphoid irradiation alone for favorable patients, and ABVD for two cycles and subtotal lymphoid irradiation for unfavorable patients. The freedom from progression in the two radiation arms of the trial was higher compared to ABVD alone (93% versus 87%; $p = 0.006$); however, neither of the radiation therapy arms on this trial are considered appropriate in modern management (47).
- In the EORTC-GELA H9-F trial, favorable prognosis HL patients were treated with EBVP chemotherapy; if they had a complete response to chemotherapy, they were randomized to no further therapy, IFRT 20 Gy, or IFRT 36 Gy. The 4-year event-free survival in the EBVP-alone arm was unacceptably low at 70%; therefore, that arm of the study was closed early (48).

Favorable Prognosis Stage I to IIA Disease (Subdiaphragmatic)

* Less than 10% of patients with stage I or II HL present with involvement limited to subdiaphragmatic sites.
* The treatment (combined modality therapy) and outcomes are approximately the same as for supradiaphragmatic disease (49,50).

Limited Presentations of Stage I to IIA Nodular Lymphocyte Predominance HL

* Unlike patients with classical HL, patients with limited presentations of nodular lymphocyte predominance HL (nLPHL) may achieve long-term disease-free survival after treatment with involved or slightly extended field irradiation alone (51–54).
* The usual dose is 30 to 36 Gy, and there is no apparent added benefit to chemotherapy.

Unfavorable Prognosis Stage I to II (Supradiaphragmatic) Classical HL

* Unfavorable prognosis stage I to II patients usually have either B symptoms or a large mediastinal mass.
* The patients with bulky disease are best treated with combined modality therapy. The expected freedom from progression is 80% to 90% (46,55).
* The recommended radiation dose is 30 to 36 Gy. Doses at the higher end of this spectrum are usually recommended for incomplete response to chemotherapy, residual PET-FDG positivity after chemotherapy, or abbreviated chemotherapy course (29,43,56).
* Treatment may be to the area of initial bulk (e.g., mediastinum) or all initially involved sites. When treatment is limited to the mediastinum, it is reasonable to include the adjacent bilateral supraclavicular areas.
* The German HD11 trial for patients with intermediate prognosis HL randomized patients to BEACOPP versus ABVD and to 20 versus 30 Gy of radiation.
* Approximately 15% to 20% of patients with stage I or II disease have B symptoms.
* Patients who have B symptoms are sometimes managed similar to stage III or IV disease. However, because these patients have limited anatomic disease, one can make an argument to include consolidative involved-field radiation in the treatment of these patients as a component of a combined modality regimen.

Stage III or IV Disease

* The appropriate chemotherapy for advanced stage HL was determined by a major landmark trial by the Cancer and Leukemia Group B. In this study, patients with stage IIIA2, IIIB, or IV HL were randomly assigned to treatment with either MOPP (6 to 8 cycles), MOPP/ABVD (12 months), or ABVD (6 to 8 cycles). Both the

ABVD-containing regimens were equivalent and superior to MOPP alone. The patients in the ABVD chemotherapy group had a complete response rate of 82%, a 5-year failure-free survival of 61%, and a 5-year survival rate of 73% (26).

- There are several studies that have assessed whether there is any benefit to combined modality therapy (including radiotherapy) over chemotherapy alone. A number of studies found that combined modality therapy was superior (57,58). The rationale for a combined modality approach is that when patients relapse, they typically do so at the initial site of disease (59). However, these early trials were either poorly designed, used outdated chemotherapy, or had inadequate accruals.

- A more relevant trial to address this question was the EORTC-GPMC (Groupe Pierre-et-Marie Curie) H34 (20884) trial. Patients received six to eight cycles of nitrogen mustard, vincristine, procarbazine, prednisone, Adriamycin, bleomycin, and vinblastine (MOPP-ABV) chemotherapy; if they had a complete response, they were randomized 24 Gy IFRT versus no further therapy. There were no differences between the groups in freedom from failure or overall survival (60). However, those patients who had only a partial response to chemotherapy all received 30 Gy IFRT, and the freedom from treatment failure and survival for this group were similar to those of patients who had a complete response to chemotherapy (61). This study suggests merit to adding IFRT after chemotherapy for those patients that achieve only a partial response to chemotherapy.

- Therefore, the general recommendation is to reserve IFRT for those patients who achieve a partial response, and to forego IFRT if there is a complete response to a full course of chemotherapy. Some institutions treat initial sites of bulky disease in advanced stage patients with consolidative radiotherapy.

- However, if an abbreviated chemotherapy regimen is used, such as the Stanford V program, then IFRT is an essential component of treatment.

- The Stanford V is composed of 12 weeks of chemotherapy (versus 6 to 8 cycles of ABVD), with reduced doses of doxorubicin (50% less) and bleomycin (25% less). Typically, 36-Gy radiation therapy is delivered to initially bulky (greater than 5 cm) lymph node sites and macroscopic splenic disease. Radiation is delivered 1 to 3 weeks after completion of chemotherapy. Using this approach, the 12-year freedom from progression is 83% and the 12-year survival is 95%, with minimal late complications of treatment (62,63).

- The Stanford V chemotherapy regimen without the standard associated radiation protocol results in significantly inferior results (64,65).

- The Eastern Cooperative Oncology Group (ECOG) 2496 intergroup trial demonstrates comparable results with ABVD and Stanford V chemotherapy programs (66).

Pediatric and Elderly Management

- Excellent outcome is reported for programs that combine chemotherapy (with non-leukemogenic ABVD regimen) and low-dose (20 to 25 Gy) involved-field irradiation in the management of pediatric and elderly populations. The 5-year survival rates are approximately 90% and relapse-free survival rates are at least 80% for children treated with these regimens (67,68).

- To reduce growth effects, limitation of radiation doses to 15 to 25 Gy is warranted unless bulky disease has not responded to chemotherapy.
- For pediatric patients, enrollment on a clinical trial, if available, should be strongly considered.
- For people older than 65 to 70 years of age, treatment should be tailored to respect their quality of life without threatening their "normal" survival. Although late effects of treatment are the major problem in childhood, it is immediate intolerance that is problematic in the elderly.
- Chemotherapy regimens that are better tolerated by older adults include PAVe (procarbazine, Alkeran, and vinblastine), ChlVPP (chlorambucil, vinblastine, procarbazine and prednisolone), and VBM (vinblastine, bleomycin, and methotrexate) (45,58,69).

Hodgkin Lymphoma during Pregnancy and in Human Immunodeficiency Virus–Infected Patients

- Staging may be hampered if HL is diagnosed during pregnancy because CT scan is contraindicated. With a photon beam of 25 MV, the maximum dose received by the uterus and the fetus is approximately 5.5 cGy from a mantle field; the dose is much greater (10.0 to 13.6 cGy) with cobalt (70). Therefore, during the first 3 months, the major question is whether the pregnancy is to be maintained or not. The answer depends on the clinical aggressiveness of the HL.
- If there is limited disease (e.g., stage IA), an involved-field irradiation field (e.g., neck) could potentially allow staging to be postponed until delivery.
- During the final 3 months of gestation, fetal development is advanced enough to allow an induced premature delivery or to wait a few weeks until childbirth. A multidisciplinary discussion and coordination of care with the oncology team, a pediatrician and obstetrician allows for optimal management.
- Some chemotherapeutic agents do not cross the placenta (e.g., vincristine sulfate or vinblastine sulfate), and may be useful if treatment is necessary.
- HL is clinically different among human immunodeficiency virus–positive patients. In most cases, the mediastinum is not involved but gut, pleura, meningeal, or Waldeyer ring involvement are common. Patients tend to present at stage III and IVB disease with bone marrow involvement.
- The pathologic pattern is different, with a high frequency of mixed cellularity type, and the response to chemotherapy is not as good as in human immunodeficiency virus–negative patients. Three major prognostic factors are no acquired immunodeficiency syndrome before HL diagnosis, CD4 counts more than 250 to 300, and response to HL treatment (70).

Treatment for Relapse

- Individualized treatment plans are made for each patient considering site(s) of initial disease, initial treatment and response, patient performance status, and relapse site(s).

- For initial stage I to II disease, if the patient was treated initially with radiation alone, he or she should generally receive chemotherapy as the primary salvage treatment (71–73). Salvage chemotherapy has a long-term freedom from relapse greater than 60%. The benefit of adding radiation to salvage chemotherapy is not well defined, but it is often given after completion of chemotherapy (72). Typically, 15 to 25 Gy is delivered to sites that have been previously irradiated and 30 to 36 Gy to those areas that have never received any radiation.
- There is no consensus for the management of patients who have initial stage I to II disease treated with chemotherapy alone (46). Because many of these patients may have limited relapse at their initial sites of disease, radiation is often considered as an option in the treatment algorithm. The effectiveness of radiation has been shown in some patients with initially advanced disease who have limited relapse (74).
- Stage III to IV patients who relapse after achieving a complete response to chemotherapy or combined-modality therapy are typically salvaged with high-dose chemotherapy and autologous stem cell transplant. The long-term progression-free survival is approximately 50% (75). Factors associated with a favorable prognosis are a longer duration of response to primary therapy and absence of extranodal disease (76,77).
- The management of relapse or refractory Hodgkin lymphoma involves specialty care. Consideration of stem cell transplant should be undertaken with appropriate specialists.
- The discovery of new agents for patients with relapsed or refractory Hodgkin lymphoma is a subject of current investigation. Currently, biologic therapy and immunotherapy are active areas of research.

Stem Cell Transplant

- Total body irradiation (TBI) is a part of some protocols for stem cell transplant. However, studies that have used regimens with or without fractionated TBI have reported similar results (78).
- Radiation doses that are often used in TBI programs (12 to 15 Gy) have been shown to eradicate disease in only about 20% of sites (79).
- Therefore, locoregional radiation is typically given instead of TBI. Some studies have given local radiation pretransplant, but most have delivered it posttransplant.
- The time from transplant to radiation varies from 1 to 4 months, and usual doses are 18 to 40 Gy depending on the bulk of disease and response to therapy (80).
- The areas of treatment include sites of initial bulky relapse, areas of residual disease after high-dose chemotherapy, or in some protocols all involved sites at the time of relapse.
- In several studies, significantly improved freedom from relapse was seen with the addition of radiation to a high-dose chemotherapy transplant regimen (81–83).

FOLLOW-UP

- Follow-up visits should be approximately every 2 to 4 months during the first 2 years, every 4 to 6 months during the 3rd and 4th years, and annually thereafter.

- All initially abnormal studies (CT, PET, etc.) should be repeated after treatment is finished to document the extent of response to therapy.
- A good history and physical examination, chest radiograph, complete blood count, alkaline phosphatase level, serum thyroxine (T4), and thyroid-stimulating hormone (TSH) level should be done at every visit. After 2 years, the chest radiograph can be performed annually (15). If any other serum markers were abnormal at presentation (e.g., ESR, serum albumin), these should also be obtained at every visit (84).
- A challenging problem in follow-up evaluation is the interpretation of residual mediastinal abnormality on chest radiograph or chest CT scan (85,86). The use of FDG-PET has been helpful in this circumstance (87–89).
- Generally, any suspicion of relapse should be documented by biopsy, as reactive hyperplasia is common in nonirradiated lymph nodes adjacent to previously treated radiation portals. In addition to reactive hyperplasia, other benign processes, such as a progressive transformation of germinal centers or the rebound growth of the thymus in young patients, may be FDG-avid on PET scanning and therefore confused with relapsed Hodgkin lymphoma (90).

SEQUELAE OF TREATMENT

- Radiation pneumonitis develops in less than 5% of patients within 6 to 12 weeks after completion of mantle irradiation. The risk is related to the volume of lung irradiated, total dose, and fraction size. Symptomatic management is generally sufficient; however, a small number of patients require treatment with corticosteroids.
- Radiation pericarditis after well-executed mantle therapy is seen in less than 5% of patients and can be managed with conservative medical treatment.
- Subclinical hypothyroidism develops in approximately one half of patients with HL (91), manifested by an elevation of the sensitive TSH even with a normal thyroxine (T4) level. Thyroid replacement therapy with levothyroxine is recommended, with an initial dose of 0.1 mg/d.
- Herpes zoster occurs during treatment for HL, or within the first 1 to 2 years after treatment, in 10% to 15% of patients (92).
- Lhermitte's sign develops in approximately 10% to 15% of patients after mantle therapy; it generally resolves spontaneously after 2 to 6 months.
- Postsplenectomy sepsis can be caused by *Streptococcus pneumoniae*, meningococcus, and *Haemophilus* strains. This risk can be minimized by prior immunization against these organisms.
- In men, pelvic irradiation may be followed by azoospermia if no special precautions are taken to shield the testes. MOPP or MOPP-like chemotherapy that includes alkylating agents and procarbazine causes sterility in most men. However, the ABVD and Stanford V regimens seem to spare male fertility (93).
- Even with a proper oophoropexy and well-planned pelvic irradiation, the scattered dose of radiation may be sufficient to affect ovarian function and cause menopausal symptoms in women older than 30 years; younger women may not be affected. In contrast to MOPP, the ABVD and Stanford V combinations appear to spare female fertility (93).

- The most important long-term hazards are secondary malignancies and cardiovascular disease. Secondary malignancies include leukemia, lymphoma, and solid tumors. Overall, the relative risk for developing a second malignancy after treatment for HL is 1.3 to 2.9, and the absolute risk is 44.5 to 47.2 (i.e., 44.5 to 47.2 excess cases) per 10,000 patients per year (9,94,95).

- Long-term cardiovascular sequelae include coronary artery disease, pericarditis, pancarditis, and valvular disease (96). The relative risk of death from cardiac disease is 3.1.

- As radiation therapy field's volumes and treatment doses are being reduced with advanced radiotherapy techniques, the long-term side effects of treatment will likely be lower in the future.

References

1. Medeiros LJ, Greiner TC. Hodgkin's disease. *Cancer* 1995;75(1 suppl):357–369.
2. Deconinck E, Foussard C, Milpied N, et al. High-dose therapy followed by autologous purged stem-cell transplantation and doxorubicin-based chemotherapy in patients with advanced follicular lymphoma: a randomized multicenter study by GOELAMS. *Blood* 2005;105(10):3817–3823.
3. Glaser SL, Lin RJ, Stewart SL, et al. Epstein-Barr virus-associated Hodgkin's disease: epidemiologic characteristics in international data. *Int J Cancer* 1997;70(4):375–382.
4. Hjalgrim H, Askling J, Sorensen P, et al. Risk of Hodgkin's disease and other cancers after infectious mononucleosis. *J Natl Cancer Inst* 2000;92(18):1522–1528.
5. Mueller N, Evans A, Harris NL, et al. Hodgkin's disease and Epstein-Barr virus. Altered antibody pattern before diagnosis. *N Engl J Med* 1989;320(11):689–695.
6. Weiss LM, Movahed LA, Warnke RA, et al. Detection of Epstein-Barr viral genomes in Reed-Sternberg cells of Hodgkin's disease. *N Engl J Med* 1989;320(8):502–506.
7. Kaplan HS. The radical radiotherapy of regionally localized Hodgkin's disease. *Radiology* 1962;78:553–561.
8. Hoppe RT, Cox RS, Rosenberg SA, et al. Prognostic factors in pathologic stage III Hodgkin's disease. *Cancer Treat Rep* 1982;66(4):743–749.
9. Hasenclever D, Diehl V. A prognostic score for advanced Hodgkin's disease. International Prognostic Factors Project on Advanced Hodgkin's Disease. *N Engl J Med* 1998;339(21):1506–1514.
10. Henry-Amar M, Friedman S, Hayat M, et al. Erythrocyte sedimentation rate predicts early relapse and survival in early-stage Hodgkin disease. The EORTC Lymphoma Cooperative Group. *Ann Intern Med* 1991;114(5):361–365.
11. Castellino RA, Hoppe RT, Blank N, et al. Computed tomography, lymphography, and staging laparotomy: correlations in initial staging of Hodgkin disease. *AJR Am J Roentgenol* 1984;143(1):37–41.
12. Cheson BD, Pfistner B, Juweid ME, et al. Revised response criteria for malignant lymphoma. *J Clin Oncol* 2007;25(5):579–586.
13. Huic D, Dodig D. Fluorine-18-fluorodeoxyglucose positron emission tomography metabolic imaging in patients with lymphoma. *Croat Med J* 2002;43(5):541–545.
14. Partridge S, Timothy A, O'Doherty MJ, et al. 2-Fluorine-18-fluoro-2-deoxy-D glucose positron emission tomography in the pretreatment staging of Hodgkin's disease: influence on patient management in a single institution. *Ann Oncol* 2000;11(10):1273–1279.
15. Dryver ET, Jernstrom H, Tompkins K, et al. Follow-up of patients with Hodgkin's disease following curative treatment: the routine CT scan is of little value. *Br J Cancer* 2003;89(3):482–486.
16. Castellino RA. Diagnostic imaging evaluation of Hodgkin's disease and non-Hodgkin's lymphoma. *Cancer* 1991;67(4 suppl):1177–1180.

17. Hoppe R. Hodgkin Lymphoma. In: Halperin E, Perez C, Brady L, eds. *Principles and practice of radiation oncology.* Philadelphia, PA: Lippincott Williams & Wilkins, 2008:1721–1738.

18. Carbone PP, Kaplan HS, Musshoff K, et al. Report of the Committee on Hodgkin's Disease Staging Classification. *Cancer Res* 1971;31(11):1860–1861.

19. Connors JM, Klimo P. Is it an E lesion or stage IV? An unsettled issue in Hodgkin's disease staging. *J Clin Oncol* 1984;2(12):1421–1423.

20. Lister TA, Crowther D, Sutcliffe SB, et al. Report of a committee convened to discuss the evaluation and staging of patients with Hodgkin's disease: Cotswolds meeting. *J Clin Oncol* 1989;7(11):1630–1636.

21. Swerdlow SH, Campo E, Pileri SA, et al. The 2016 revision of the World Health Organization classification of lymphoid neoplasms. *Blood* 2016;127(20):2375–2390. doi: 10.1182/blood-2016-01-643569.

22. Ries L, Hankey BF, Miller BA, et al., eds. *Cancer statistics review 1973–88. (NIH publication no. 91-2789.).* Bethesda, MD: National Cancer Institute, 1991.

23. Hoppe R. Hodgkin's disease. In: Perez CA Brady L, eds. *Principles and practice of radiation oncology,* 3rd ed. Philadelphia, PA: Lippincott–Raven, 1998:1963–1986.

24. De Vita VT Jr, Hubbard SM, Longo DL. The chemotherapy of lymphomas: looking back, moving forward--the Richard and Hinda Rosenthal Foundation award lecture. *Cancer Res* 1987;47(22):5810–5824.

25. Bonadonna G. Chemotherapy strategies to improve the control of Hodgkin's disease: the Richard and Hinda Rosenthal Foundation Award Lecture. *Cancer Res* 1982;42(11):4309–4320.

26. Canellos GP, Anderson JR, Propert KJ, et al. Chemotherapy of advanced Hodgkin's disease with MOPP, ABVD, or MOPP alternating with ABVD. *N Engl J Med* 1992;327(21):1478–1484.

27. Bonadonna G, Valagussa P, Santoro A. Alternating non-cross-resistant combination chemotherapy or MOPP in stage IV Hodgkin's disease. A report of 8-year results. *Ann Intern Med* 1986;104(6):739–746.

28. Engel C, Loeffler M, Schmitz S, et al. Acute hematologic toxicity and practicability of dose-intensified BEACOPP chemotherapy for advanced stage Hodgkin's disease. German Hodgkin's Lymphoma Study Group (GHSG). *Ann Oncol* 2000;11(9):1105–1114.

29. Horning SJ, Williams J, Bartlett NL, et al. Assessment of the stanford V regimen and consolidative radiotherapy for bulky and advanced Hodgkin's disease: Eastern Cooperative Oncology Group pilot study E1492. *J Clin Oncol* 2000;18(5):972–980.

30. Klimo P, Connors JM. MOPP/ABV hybrid program: combination chemotherapy based on early introduction of seven effective drugs for advanced Hodgkin's disease. *J Clin Oncol* 1985;3(9):1174–1182.

31. Fabian CJ, Mansfield CM, Dahlberg S, et al. Low-dose involved field radiation after chemotherapy in advanced Hodgkin disease. A Southwest Oncology Group randomized study. *Ann Intern Med* 1994;120(11):903–912.

32. Biti GP, Cimino G, Cartoni C, et al. Extended-field radiotherapy is superior to MOPP chemotherapy for the treatment of pathologic stage I-IIA Hodgkin's disease: eight-year update of an Italian prospective randomized study. *J Clin Oncol* 1992;10(3):378–382.

33. Longo DL, Glatstein E, Duffey PL, et al. Radiation therapy versus combination chemotherapy in the treatment of early-stage Hodgkin's disease: seven-year results of a prospective randomized trial. *J Clin Oncol* 1991;9(6):906–917.

34. Thomas J, et al. Comparison of 36 Gy, 20 Gy, or No Radiation Therapy After 6 Cycles of EBVP Chemotherapy and Complete Remission in Early-Stage Hodgkin Lymphoma Without Risk Factors: Results of the EORT-GELA H9-F Intergroup Randomized Trial. *Int J Radiat Oncol Biol Phys* 2018;100(5):1133–1145.

35. Raemakers JM, et al. Omitting radiotherapy in early positron emission tomography-negative stage I/II Hodgkin lymphoma is associated with an increased risk of early relapse: Clinical results of the preplanned interim analysis of the randomized EORTC/LYSA/FIL H10 trial. *J Clin Oncol* 2014;32(12):1188–1194.

36. Hoppe RT, Hanlon AL, Hanks GE, et al. Progress in the treatment of Hodgkin's disease in the United States, 1973 versus 1983. The Patterns of Care Study. *Cancer* 1994;74(12):3198–3203.

37. Duhmke E, Diehl V, Loeffler M, et al. Randomized trial with early-stage Hodgkin's disease testing 30 Gy vs. 40 Gy extended field radiotherapy alone. *Int J Radiat Oncol Biol Phys* 1996;36(2):305–310.

38. Hoppe RT, Advani RH, Bierman PJ, et al. Hodgkin disease/lymphoma. Clinical practice guidelines in oncology. *J Natl Compr Canc Netw* 2006;4(3):210–230.

39. Specht L, et al. Modern radiation therapy for Hodgkin lymphoma: field and dose guidelines from the international lymphoma radiation oncology group (ILROG). *Int J Radiat Oncol Biol Phys* 2014;89(4):854–862.

40. Palos B, Kaplan HS, Karzmark CJ. The use of thin lung shields to deliver limited whole-lung irradiation during mantle-field treatment of Hodgkin's disease. *Radiology* 1971;101(2):441–442.

41. Le Floch O, Donaldson SS, Kaplan HS. Pregnancy following oophoropexy and total nodal irradiation in women with Hodgkin's disease. *Cancer* 1976;38(6):2263–2268.

42. Girinsky T, van der Maazen R, Specht L, et al. Involved-node radiotherapy (INRT) in patients with early Hodgkin lymphoma: concepts and guidelines. *Radiother Oncol* 2006;79(3):270–277.

43. Bonadonna G, Bonfante V, Viviani S, et al. ABVD plus subtotal nodal versus involved-field radiotherapy in early-stage Hodgkin's disease: long-term results. *J Clin Oncol* 2004;22(14):2835–2841.

44. Moody AM, Pratt J, Hudson GV, et al. British National Lymphoma Investigation: pilot studies of neoadjuvant chemotherapy in clinical stage Ia and IIa Hodgkin's disease. *Clin Oncol (R Coll Radiol)* 2001;13(4):262–268.

45. Horning SJ, Ang PT, Hoppe RT, et al. The Stanford experience with combined procarbazine, Alkeran and vinblastine (PAVe) and radiotherapy for locally extensive and advanced stage Hodgkin's disease. *Ann Oncol* 1992;3(9):747–754.

46. Hoppe RT, Coleman CN, Cox RS, et al. The management of stage I--II Hodgkin's disease with irradiation alone or combined modality therapy: the Stanford experience. *Blood* 1982;59(3):455–465.

47. Meyer RM, Gospodarowicz MK, Connors JM, et al. Randomized comparison of ABVD chemotherapy with a strategy that includes radiation therapy in patients with limited-stage Hodgkin's lymphoma: National Cancer Institute of Canada Clinical Trials Group and the Eastern Cooperative Oncology Group. *J Clin Oncol* 2005;23(21):4634–4642.

48. Thomas J, Fermé C, Noordijk EM, et al. Comparison of 36 Gy, 20 Gy, or no radiation therapy after 6 cycles of EBVP chemotherapy and complete remission in early-stage Hodgkin lymphoma without risk factors: results of the EORT-GELA H9-F Intergroup Randomized Trial. *Int J Radiat Oncol Biol Phys* 2018;100(5):1133–1145. doi: 10.1016/j.ijrobp.2017.10.015.

49. Darabi K, Sieber M, Chaitowitz M, et al. Infradiaphragmatic versus supradiaphragmatic Hodgkin lymphoma: a retrospective review of 1,114 patients. *Leuk Lymphoma* 2005;46(12):1715–1720.

50. Vassilakopoulos TP, Angelopoulou MK, Siakantaris MP, et al. Pure infradiaphragmatic Hodgkin's lymphoma. Clinical features, prognostic factor and comparison with supradiaphragmatic disease. *Haematologica* 2006;91(1):32–39.

51. Bodis S, Kraus MD, Pinkus G, et al. Clinical presentation and outcome in lymphocyte-predominant Hodgkin's disease. *J Clin Oncol* 1997;15(9):3060–3066.

52. Nogova L, Reineke T, Eich HT, et al. Extended field radiotherapy, combined modality treatment or involved field radiotherapy for patients with stage IA lymphocyte-predominant Hodgkin's lymphoma: a retrospective analysis from the German Hodgkin Study Group (GHSG). *Ann Oncol* 2005;16(10):1683–1687.

53. Sutcliffe SB, Gospodarowicz MK, Bergsagel DE, et al. Prognostic groups for management of localized Hodgkin's disease. *J Clin Oncol* 1985;3(3):393–401.

54. Wirth A, Yuen K, Barton M, et al. Long-term outcome after radiotherapy alone for lympho-cyte-predominant Hodgkin lymphoma: a retrospective multicenter study of the Australasian Radiation Oncology Lymphoma Group. *Cancer* 2005;104(6):1221–1229.

55. Hoppe RT. Hodgkin's disease: complications of therapy and excess mortality. *Ann Oncol* 1997;8(suppl 1):115–118.

56. Behar RA, Horning SJ, Hoppe RT. Hodgkin's disease with bulky mediastinal involvement: effec-tive management with combined modality therapy. *Int J Radiat Oncol Biol Phys* 1993;25(5): 771–776.

57. Salloum E, Doria R, Farber LR, et al. Combined modality therapy in previously untreated patients with advanced Hodgkin's disease: a 24-year follow-up study. *Cancer J Sci Am* 1995;1(4):267–273.

58. Yahalom J, Ryu J, Straus DJ, et al. Impact of adjuvant radiation on the patterns and rate of relapse in advanced-stage Hodgkin's disease treated with alternating chemotherapy combinations. *J Clin Oncol* 1991;9(12):2193–2201.

59. Young RC, Canellos GP, Chabner BA, et al. Patterns of relapse in advanced Hodgkin's disease treated with combination chemotherapy. *Cancer* 1978;42(2 suppl):1001–1007.

60. Aleman BM, Raemaekers JM, Tirelli U, et al., Involved-field radiotherapy for advanced Hodgkin's lymphoma. *N Engl J Med* 2003;348(24):2396–2406.

61. Aleman BM, Raemaekers JM, Tomisic R, et al. Involved-field radiotherapy for patients in partial remission after chemotherapy for advanced Hodgkin's lymphoma. *Int J Radiat Oncol Biol Phys* 2007;67(1):19–30.

62. Horning S, Hoppe R, Advani R, et al. Efficacy and late effects of Stanford V chemotherapy and radiotherapy in untreated Hodgkin's disease: Mature data in early and advanced stage patients. *Blood* 2004;104:92a(abst).

63. Horning SJ, Hoppe RT, Breslin S, et al. Stanford V and radiotherapy for locally extensive and advanced Hodgkin's disease: mature results of a prospective clinical trial. *J Clin Oncol* 2002;20(3):630–637.

64. Federico M, Levis S, Luminari S, et al. ABVD vs Stanford V (SV) vs MOPP-EBV-CAD (MEC) in advanced Hodgkin lymphoma. Final results of the IIL HD9601 randomized trial. *J Clin Oncol* 2004;22:559s(abst).

65. Gobbi PG, Levis A, Chisesi T, et al. ABVD versus modified stanford V versus MOPPEBVCAD with optional and limited radiotherapy in intermediate- and advanced-stage Hodgkin's lym-phoma: final results of a multicenter randomized trial by the Intergruppo Italiano Linfomi. *J Clin Oncol* 2005;23(36):9198–9207.

66. Gordon LI, Hong F, Fisher RI, et al. Randomized phase III trial of ABVD versus Stanford V with or without radiation therapy in locally extensive and advanced-stage Hodgkin lymphoma: an intergroup study coordinated by the Eastern Cooperative Oncology Group (E2496). *J Clin Oncol* 2013;31(6):684–691. doi: 10.1200/JCO.2012.43.4803.

67. Donaldson SS, Hudson MM, Lamborn KR, et al. VAMP and low-dose, involved-field radiation for children and adolescents with favorable, early-stage Hodgkin's disease: results of a prospective clinical trial. *J Clin Oncol* 2002;20(14):3081–3087.

68. Hudson MM, Krasin M, Link MP, et al. Risk-adapted, combined-modality therapy with VAMP/ COP and response-based, involved-field radiation for unfavorable pediatric Hodgkin's disease. *J Clin Oncol* 2004;22(22):4541–4550.

69. Horning SJ, Hoppe RT, Mason J, et al. Stanford-Kaiser Permanente G1 study for clinical stage I to IIA Hodgkin's disease: subtotal lymphoid irradiation versus vinblastine, methotrexate, and bleomycin chemotherapy and regional irradiation. *J Clin Oncol* 1997;15(5):1736–1744.

70. Eghbali H, Soubeyran P, Tchen N, et al. Current treatment of Hodgkin's disease. *Crit Rev Oncol Hematol* 2000;35(1):49–73.

71. Ng AK, Li S, Neuberg D, et al. Comparison of MOPP versus ABVD as salvage therapy in patients who relapse after radiation therapy alone for Hodgkin's disease. *Ann Oncol* 2004;15(2):270–275.

72. Roach M III, Brophy N, Cox R, et al. Prognostic factors for patients relapsing after radiotherapy for early-stage Hodgkin's disease. *J Clin Oncol* 1990;8(4):623–629.

73. Specht L, Horwich A, Ashley S. Salvage of relapse of patients with Hodgkin's disease in clinical stages I or II who were staged with laparotomy and initially treated with radiotherapy alone. A report from the international database on Hodgkin's disease. *Int J Radiat Oncol Biol Phys* 1994;30(4):805–811.

74. Roach M III, Kapp DS, Rosenberg SA, et al. Radiotherapy with curative intent: an option in selected patients relapsing after chemotherapy for advanced Hodgkin's disease. *J Clin Oncol* 1987;5(4):550–555.

75. Lavoie JC, Connors JM, Phillips GL, et al. High-dose chemotherapy and autologous stem cell transplantation for primary refractory or relapsed Hodgkin lymphoma: long-term outcome in the first 100 patients treated in Vancouver. *Blood* 2005;106(4):1473–1478.

76. Brice P, Bouabdallah R, Moreau P, et al. Prognostic factors for survival after high-dose therapy and autologous stem cell transplantation for patients with relapsing Hodgkin's disease: analysis of 280 patients from the French registry. Societe Francaise de Greffe de Moelle. *Bone Marrow Transplant* 1997;20(1):21–26.

77. Sweetenham JW, Taghipour G, Milligan D, et al. High-dose therapy and autologous stem cell rescue for patients with Hodgkin's disease in first relapse after chemotherapy: results from the EBMT. Lymphoma Working Party of the European Group for Blood and Marrow Transplantation. *Bone Marrow Transplant* 1997;20(9):745–752.

78. Nademanee A, O'Donnell MR, Snyder DS, et al. High-dose chemotherapy with or without total body irradiation followed by autologous bone marrow and/or peripheral blood stem cell transplantation for patients with relapsed and refractory Hodgkin's disease: results in 85 patients with analysis of prognostic factors. *Blood* 1995;85(5):1381–1390.

79. Kaplan HS. Evidence for a tumoricidal dose level in the radiotherapy of Hodgkin's disease. *Cancer Res* 1966;26(6):1221–1224.

80. Ferme C, Mounier N, Divine M, et al. Intensive salvage therapy with high-dose chemotherapy for patients with advanced Hodgkin's disease in relapse or failure after initial chemotherapy: results of the Groupe d'Etudes des Lymphomes de l'Adulte H89 Trial. *J Clin Oncol* 2002;20(2):467–475.

81. Lancet JE, Rapoport AP, Brasacchio R, et al. Autotransplantation for relapsed or refractory Hodgkin's disease: long-term follow-up and analysis of prognostic factors. *Bone Marrow Transplant* 1998;22(3):265–271.

82. Nachman JB, Sposto R, Herzog P, et al. Randomized comparison of low-dose involved-field radiotherapy and no radiotherapy for children with Hodgkin's disease who achieve a complete response to chemotherapy. *J Clin Oncol* 2002;20(18):3765–3771.

83. Poen JC, Hoppe RT, Horning SJ. High-dose therapy and autologous bone marrow transplantation for relapsed/refractory Hodgkin's disease: the impact of involved field radiotherapy on patterns of failure and survival. *Int J Radiat Oncol Biol Phys* 1996;36(1):3–12.

84. Torrey MJ, Poen JC, Hoppe RT. Detection of relapse in early-stage Hodgkin's disease: role of routine follow-up studies. *J Clin Oncol* 1997;15(3):1123–1130.

85. Jochelson M, Mauch P, Balikian J, et al. The significance of the residual mediastinal mass in treated Hodgkin's disease. *J Clin Oncol* 1985;3(5):637–640.

86. Thomas F, Cosset JM, Cherel P, et al. Thoracic CT-scanning follow-up of residual mediastinal masses after treatment of Hodgkin's disease. *Radiother Oncol* 1988;11(2):119–122.

87. de Wit M, Bohuslavizki KH, Buchert R, et al. 18FDG-PET following treatment as valid predictor for disease-free survival in Hodgkin's lymphoma. *Ann Oncol* 2001;12(1):29–37.

88. Hutchings M, Mikhaeel NG, Fields PA, et al. Prognostic value of interim FDG-PET after two or three cycles of chemotherapy in Hodgkin lymphoma. *Ann Oncol* 2005;16(7):1160–1168.

89. Naumann R, Vaic A, Beuthien-Baumann B, et al. Prognostic value of positron emission tomography in the evaluation of post-treatment residual mass in patients with Hodgkin's disease and non-Hodgkin's lymphoma. *Br J Haematol* 2001;115(4):793–800.

90. Hansmann ML, Fellbaum C, Hui PK, et al. Progressive transformation of germinal centers with and without association to Hodgkin's disease. *Am J Clin Pathol* 1990;93(2):219–226.

91. Hancock SL, Cox RS, McDougall IR. Thyroid diseases after treatment of Hodgkin's disease. *N Engl J Med* 1991;325(9):599–605.

92. Guinee VF, Guido JJ, Pfalzgraf KA, et al. The incidence of herpes zoster in patients with Hodgkin's disease. An analysis of prognostic factors. *Cancer* 1985;56(3):642–648.

93. Viviani S, Santoro A, Ragni G, et al. Gonadal toxicity after combination chemotherapy for Hodgkin's disease. Comparative results of MOPP vs ABVD. *Eur J Cancer Clin Oncol* 1985;21(5):601–605.

94. Dores GM, Metayer C, Curtis RE, et al. Second malignant neoplasms among long-term survivors of Hodgkin's disease: a population-based evaluation over 25 years. *J Clin Oncol* 2002;20(16):3484–3494.

95. Swerdlow AJ, Barber JA, Hudson GV, et al. Risk of second malignancy after Hodgkin's disease in a collaborative British cohort: the relation to age at treatment. *J Clin Oncol* 2000;18(3):498–509.

96. Hancock SL, Tucker MA, Hoppe RT. Factors affecting late mortality from heart disease after treatment of Hodgkin's disease. *JAMA* 1993;270(16):1949–1955.

CHAPTER 38

NON-HODGKIN LYMPHOMAS

- The estimated number of new cases of non-Hodgkin lymphoma (NHL) in the United States in 2006 was 59,000, and the number of deaths was 19,000 (1). The highest incidence rate of NHL in the world is in the United States, and the lowest is in Asia (2,3). There has been an alarming increase in the incidence of NHL over the last four decades, with a doubling from 1970 to 1990. However, in the last decade, the rate of increase has started to plateau (4). [See SEER Cancer Statistics Review, 1975 to 2003 (5). Available at: http://seercancergov/csr/1975_2003/2005. Accessed November 2005.]
- The postulated reasons for the increase are multifactorial. They include an aging population, HIV/AIDS, occupational exposure, infectious agents, and advances in diagnostic techniques (6). The exact cause has yet to be determined.

ETIOLOGY

- There has been a significant increase in the incidence of NHL in immunocompromised patients, particularly AIDS patients and organ transplantation patients on prolonged immunosuppression (7,8).
- Epstein-Barr virus (EBV) infection is associated with Burkitt's lymphoma, post-transplantation lymphoproliferative disorders, HIV/AIDS-associated primary CNS lymphoma, T/NK cell lymphomas, and lymphomas associated with congenital deficiency (9).
- Other NHL associations with infectious agents include human T-cell lymphotropic virus type 1 (HTLV-1) with T/NK cell lymphomas and *Helicobacter pylori* with gastric mucosa-associated lymphoid tissue (MALT) lymphomas (10).
- NHL has been linked to many occupational and environmental exposures, including radiation exposure (11).

NATURAL HISTORY

- The principal cellular component of lymphoma is the lymphocyte, and tumors may arise in any area of lymphoid aggregation, such as the lymph nodes, spleen, Waldeyer's ring, bone marrow, gastrointestinal (GI) tract, and other tissues in which lymphoid cells may be circulating. NHL may be found in nonlymphoid organs.
- The median age at diagnosis is 65 years (12).
- Approximately two-thirds of NHLs have a nodal presentation and one-third are extranodal (versus for Hodgkin lymphoma [HL], extranodal disease is rare) (13).
- Systemic B symptoms are present in 20% to 30% of patients, and lymph nodes can undergo spontaneous regression and subsequent regrowth.
- The most commonly involved nodal sites are the neck (70%), groin (60%), and axilla (50%) (14). Typically, 2/3 of patients with an initially localized presentation are found to have more advanced disease upon completion of a full staging workup (15).
- Nodal presentations are often follicular B-cell histology. Patients with this histology tend to run an indolent course; many patients present with advanced disease, but the median survival is typically relatively long.
- The case for lymphatic contiguity is much weaker for NHL than for HL.
- Epitrochlear and brachial nodes are sometimes involved, especially in patients with follicular lymphoma (FL).
- The most commonly involved extranodal site in the United States is the GI tract, and the patient often presents with epigastric discomfort, abdominal pain, and/or bleeding.
- Waldeyer's ring, although rarely involved in patients with HL, is not an uncommon extranodal site involved in patients with NHL. This can present as a sore throat or dysphagia.
- If nodal and extranodal disease presentations have the same histology, stage, and other prognostic variables, they are often treated in a similar manner and have approximately equivalent outcomes (16).

DIAGNOSTIC WORKUP

- Routine staging investigations include a full physical examination with careful evaluation of all lymph node-bearing areas, liver, and spleen; complete blood cell count; erythrocyte sedimentation rate; liver function tests; lactate dehydrogenase (LDH); imaging tests; and a bone marrow biopsy. A pregnancy test is necessary for premenopausal women. Assessment for HIV and hepatitis viral infections is standard.
- The minimum imaging investigations include chest x-ray and computed tomography (CT) scanning of the chest, abdomen, and pelvis (17). CT scans of the head and neck are done when clinically indicated.
- CT scans are useful for identifying mesenteric lymph node involvement.
- CT scan of the chest reveals abnormalities in 7% to 30% of patients with initially normal chest x-rays and additional abnormalities in 25% of patients with abnormal chest x-rays (18,19).

- The use of PET and PET/CT imaging has significantly increased. Studies have reported that the sensitivity of PET exceeds 90%, which is significantly better than that of conventional CT at 60% to 70% (20,21).
- PET scanning (typically, PET/CT) is now considered a standard part of the initial staging evaluation for patients with NHL.
- Patients with positive functional imaging (FDG-avidity on PET) after completion of therapy have a poor prognosis associated with an early relapse. Conversely, those patients with only abnormalities on CT that are PET negative generally have the same prognosis as those patients with an absence of any abnormalities seen on PET or CT (22–24).

STAGING SYSTEM

- The Ann Arbor staging was slightly altered in the Cotswolds modification by adding the subscript "X" to designate bulky disease. Also, the criteria for liver and spleen involvement were changed to any focal defects seen in the organ with greater than two imaging modalities. Abnormal liver function tests do not play a role in staging.
- In the Ann Arbor classification, Waldeyer's ring, thymus, spleen, appendix, and Peyer's patches of the small intestine are considered lymphatic tissues; involvement of these areas does not constitute an "E" lesion, which was defined originally as extralymphatic involvement. Because of the unique pathologic and clinical characteristics of primary lymphomas affecting these organs, many clinicians consider these as separate entities.

NEW!   SUMMARY OF CHANGES TO STAGING

NON-HODGKIN LYMPHOMAS

The current staging system is the Lugano classification, which is adapted from the Ann Arbor staging system with Cotswolds modifications for non-Hodgkin lymphoma. The Lugano classification incorporated the stage groupings from the previous system while adding criteria for involvement of a given site using FDG-PET/CT and other imagings. The Lugano recommendations also put forth a system for definitions of response assessment following treatment and preferences for classification of non-Hodgkin lymphoma (e.g., the designation of the longest measurable diameter of lymph nodes rather than the traditional "X" designation).

See: Amin MB, Edge SB, Greene FL, et al., eds. *AJCC cancer staging manual*, 8th ed. New York, NY: Springer; 2017; and Cheson BD, Fisher RI, Barrington SF, et al. Recommendations for initial evaluation, staging, and response assessment of Hodgkin and non-Hodgkin lymphoma: the Lugano classification. *J Clin Oncol* 2014;32(27):3059–3068.

PATHOLOGIC CLASSIFICATION

- The Working Formulation was developed to facilitate translation between various classifications and promote the uniformity of reporting applied to B-cell (but not T-cell) lymphomas (Table 38-1).
- In 1994, a group of European and American pathologists published the Revised European American Lymphoma (REAL) classification and described malignant lymphomas as series of distinct disease entities (25).
- The REAL classification recognizes three major categories of lymphoid malignancies: B-cell, T-cell, and HL, with emphasis on cytology rather than architecture and the recognition of a wide spectrum of morphologic grades and clinical aggressiveness.
- The REAL classification has been subsequently modified, mainly through the inclusion of myeloid neoplasms, to form the World Health Organization (WHO) classification or the REAL/WHO classification (26).
- The WHO classification divides NHL into B- and T-cell neoplasms with 31 unique lymphomas detailed (Table 38-2) (27).
- The most common pathologic types, in order of decreasing frequency, are diffuse large B-cell lymphoma (DLBCL), FL, marginal zone lymphoma (MZL), mantle cell lymphoma (MCL), peripheral T-cell lymphoma (PTCL), and small lymphocytic lymphoma B-cell/chronic lymphocytic leukemia (SLLB-CLL) (28).

Table 38-1

Pathologic Classification of Non-Hodgkin Lymphoma: Working Formulation of Non-Hodgkin Lymphomas for Clinical Usage

Low Grade

Malignant lymphoma, small lymphocytic
Malignant lymphoma, follicular, predominantly small cleaved cell
Malignant lymphoma, follicular, mixed small cleaved and large cell

Intermediate Grade

Malignant lymphoma, follicular, predominantly large cell
Malignant lymphoma, diffuse small cleaved cell
Malignant lymphoma, diffuse, mixed small and large cell
Malignant lymphoma, diffuse large cell

High Grade

Malignant lymphoma, large cell immunoblastic
Malignant lymphoma, lymphoblastic
Malignant lymphoma, small noncleaved cell

Miscellaneous

Composite
Mycosis fungoides
Histiocytic
Extramedullary plasmacytoma
Unclassifiable

Table 38-2

World Health Organization Classification of Lymphoid Neoplasms

B-cell neoplasms
  Precursor B-cell neoplasm
  Precursor B-lymphocytic leukemia/lymphoma (precursor B-cell acute lymphoblastic leukemia)
Mature (peripheral) B-cell neoplasms[a]
  B-cell chronic lymphocytic leukemia/small lymphocytic lymphoma
  B-cell prolymphocytic leukemia
  Lymphoplasmacytic lymphoma
  Splenic marginal zone B-cell lymphoma (±villous lymphocytes)
  Hairy cell leukemia
  Plasma cell myeloma/plasmacytoma
  Extranodal marginal zone B-cell lymphoma of mucosa-associated lymphoid tissue type
  Nodal marginal zone B-cell lymphoma (±monocytoid B cells)
  Follicular lymphoma
  Mantle cell lymphoma
  Diffuse large B-cell lymphoma
  Mediastinal large B-cell lymphoma
  Primary effusion lymphoma
  Burkitt's lymphoma/Burkitt cell leukemia
T-cell neoplasms
Precursor T-cell neoplasm
Precursor T-lymphoblastic lymphoma/leukemia (precursor T-cell auto lymphoblastic leukemia)
Mature (peripheral) T-cell neoplasms[a]
  T-cell prolymphocytic leukemia
  T-cell granular lymphocytic leukemia
  Aggressive NK cell leukemia
  Adult T-cell lymphoma/leukemia (human T-cell leukemia virus type 1 positive)
  Extranodal NK/T-cell lymphoma, nasal type
  Enteropathy-type T-cell lymphoma
  Hepatosplenic gamma-delta T-cell lymphoma
  Subcutaneous panniculitislike T-cell lymphoma
  Mycosis fungoides/Sezary's syndrome
  Anaplastic large-cell lymphoma, T-/null cell, primary cutaneous type
  Peripheral T-cell lymphoma, not otherwise characterized
  Angioimmunoblastic T-cell lymphoma
  Anaplastic large cell lymphoma, T-/null cell, primary systemic type
Hodgkin lymphoma
  Nodular lymphocyte-predominant Hodgkin lymphoma
  Classic Hodgkin lymphoma
    Nodular sclerosis Hodgkin lymphoma
    Lymphocyte-rich Hodgkin lymphoma
    Mixed cellularity Hodgkin lymphoma
    Lymphocyte-depleted Hodgkin lymphoma

[a]B-cell and T-/NK cell neoplasms are grouped according to major clinical presentations (predominantly disseminated/leukemic, primary extranodal, predominantly nodal).
NK, natural killer.
Source: Jaffe ES, Harris NL, Stein H, Vardiman JW, eds. *Pathology and genetics of tumours of haematoporetic and lymphoid tissue. World Health Organization Classification of tumours.* Lyon, France: IARC Press, 2001.

- Cytogenetic abnormalities can be identified in 85% of NHL specimens.
- *MYC* translocation and overexpression are characteristics of Burkitt's lymphoma.
- The t(14;18) translocation is observed in 90% of FLs.
- A *BCL-2* oncogene identified on the chromosome 18 side of the breakpoint is essential for apoptosis.
- Trisomy 12 and *BCL-3* translocation t(14;19) are characteristics of CLL.
- The most common types of NHL seen in North America are follicular small cleaved cell lymphoma (20% to 30%) and diffuse large cell lymphoma (30% to 40%). The former is a low-grade lymphoma; the latter is intermediate-grade lymphoma (25).
- MALT lymphomas are usually low-grade B-cell tumors. Typically, a characteristic lymphoepithelial lesion infiltrating the glandular epithelium of the mucosa is identified. MALT lymphomas arise in the stomach, thyroid, thymus, salivary glands, breast, and bladder. They show a tendency toward localized disease and toward cure with local therapy.
- MCL occurs in older adults and presents with generalized disease with spleen, bone marrow, and GI tract involvement. It is generally not curable; median survival is 3 to 5 years, and there is little information on response to irradiation in stage I and II disease.
- PTCLs are a heterogeneous group of T-cell neoplasms, more common in Asia, that usually affect adults and are commonly generalized at presentation. In Asia, PTCL typically occurs in the head and neck, while presentation in the skin is more common in the United States and Europe. An aggressive clinical course is typical. Although potentially curable, some are resistant to existing chemotherapeutic regimens. A subtype of PTCL is intestinal T-cell lymphoma, previously called malignant histiocytosis of the intestine; it usually involves the jejunum and is associated with a history of gluten-sensitive enteropathy in approximately 50% of cases (enteropathy-associated T-cell lymphoma).
- Angiocentric lymphoma, which includes disorders previously known as lethal midline granuloma, nasal T-cell lymphoma, and lymphomatoid granulomatosis, is characterized by an angiocentric and angioinvasive infiltrate.
- Anaplastic large cell (CD30+) lymphoma is a distinct entity with a predilection for skin involvement and generalized disease.

PROGNOSTIC FACTORS

- Ten-year cause-specific survivals for patients with stage I, II, III, and IV FLs are 68%, 56%, 42%, and 18%, respectively (29).
- Although stage is an important prognostic factor, many other factors influence the outcome in patients with NHL.
- The International Prognostic Index (IPI) is based on patient age (≤60 years versus greater than 60 years), serum LDH (normal versus elevated), performance status (ECOG 0 or 1 versus 2 to 4), stage (I to II versus III to IV), and number of involved extranodal sites (≤ 1 versus greater than 1); the IPI score provides a relatively simple, clinically based method to predict prognosis in NHL

Table 38-3

International Prognostic Index for Non-Hodgkin Lymphomas

Risk Factors	Unfavorable Feature	Risk Group	Unfavorable Factors (n)	5-Year Survival (%)
Age	>60 y	Low	0 or 1	73
Lactate dehydrogenase	>1X normal	Low-intermediate	2	51
Performance status	ECOG 2–4	High-intermediate	3	43
Stage	III–IV Ann Arbor	High	4 or 5	26
Extranodal involvement	>1 site	—	—	—

ECOG, Eastern Cooperative Oncology Group.
Reprinted with permission from Gospodarowicz MK, Wasserman TH. Non-Hodgkin's lymphomas. In: Perez CA, Brady LW, eds. *Principles and practice of radiation oncology*, 3rd ed. Philadelphia, PA: Lippincott–Raven, 1998:1987–2011. © Wolters Kluwer.

(Table 38-3). Five-year survival rates for patients treated with doxorubicin-based chemotherapy, with or without radiation therapy, were 73% for the low-risk group (0 or 1 adverse factor), 51% for the low-intermediate group (2 adverse factors), 43% for the high-intermediate group (3 adverse factors), and 26% for the high-risk group (4 or 5 adverse factors) (30). Of note, patients with involvement of bone marrow, liver, spleen, central nervous system, lung, or GI tract had a higher risk of relapse (31).

- The IPI was developed mainly for DLBCL, but it has been modified for PTCL (32–34) and FL (Table 38-4) (35).
- Elevated serum LDH is an adverse prognostic factor, which is thought to be a reflection of a patient's tumor burden (30).
- Serum calcium elevation is an adverse factor in patients with T-cell lymphoma in Japan.

Table 38-4

Follicular Lymphoma International Prognostic Index

Adverse Factors	Risk Group	10-Year Survival (%)
Age > 60 y	Low (none to 1 factor)	70.7
Nodal sites > 4	Intermediate (2 factors)	50.9
Ann Arbor stage III–IV	High (>3 factors)	35.5
Elevated serum lactate dehydrogenase		
Hgb < 12.0 g/dL		

Adapted with permission from Prosnitz LR, Ng A. Non-Hodgkin's lymphoma. In: Halperin EC, Perez CA, Brady LW, eds. *Principles and practice of radiation oncology*, 5th ed. Philadelphia, PA: Lippincott Williams & Wilkins, 2008:1739–1765. © Wolters Kluwer.

- An abnormal level of cerebrospinal fluid protein is a prognostic factor in patients with primary brain lymphoma.
- Male gender is an independent adverse prognostic factor in patients with low-grade NHL.
- The presence of B symptoms is generally correlated with advanced disease, large tumor bulk, and elevated LDH levels, indicators of high tumor burden.
- Tumor bulk or burden is one of the most important prognostic factors in NHL. In patients with stage IA and IIA intermediate- and high-grade NHL treated with radiation therapy alone, 39% of those with tumor bulk less than 5 cm relapsed, while 62% of those with tumor bulk greater than 5 cm relapsed (36).
- Bulk greater than 10 cm is one the most important factors in patients with stage III and IV disease treated with chemotherapy.
- Other indicators of high tumor burden associated with poor outcome include presence of a large mediastinal mass (greater than one-third of chest diameter), presence of a palpable abdominal mass, and a combination of paraaortic and pelvic node involvement in stage III and IV disease (37).
- The number of sites of involvement is an independent prognostic factor for disease-free and overall survival in patients treated with chemotherapy or combined-modality therapy (CMT).
- Almost 50% of patients with stage I and II NHL have disease in extranodal sites (38). The GI tract is an adverse site of extranodal presentation due to the impact of locally advanced, bulky, and unresectable disease.
- High proliferative activity, as determined by Ki-67 expression in more than 60% of malignant cells, was a predictor of poor survival, independent of age, stage, B symptoms, bulk, and LDH level (39).

GENERAL MANAGEMENT

- The main modalities used to treat NHL are radiation therapy and chemotherapy, with surgery limited to secure the diagnosis or manage selected extranodal sites.
- The initial decision in curative situations is between the use of local treatment alone versus a local and systemic approach. The choice is based on recognition of the potential for local control, inherent risk of occult distant disease, and availability of curative chemotherapy. NHL represents a diverse set of lymphoproliferative malignancies and recognition of the differences in biology and behavior affects the selection of appropriate curative and palliative treatments.

RADIATION THERAPY

- Involved-field, extended-field, and total lymphoid irradiation are common terms used to describe the extent of radiation therapy. In recent years, the use of involved site and involved nodal radiation is more commonly used in the treatment of NHL.

- Involved-field irradiation is most commonly used in localized lymphomas and implies treatment to the involved nodal regions (not just involved nodes) with adequate margins or to the extranodal site and its immediate lymph node drainage area.
- Extended-field radiation therapy is a treatment plan including radiation therapy to the next-echelon lymph nodes.
- Doses of 40 to 50 Gy have been used to treat intermediate-grade lymphomas, especially the diffuse large cell type. When high doses are used for diffuse lymphomas, local recurrence rates vary from 15% to 20%. However, when radiation is delivered as a component of a combined-modality program with chemotherapy, typical irradiation doses are 30 to 40 Gy.
- Data from Princess Margaret Hospital reveal that for MZL, especially MALT of the stomach, local control rates of 95% are achieved with about 30 Gy (40,41). Similarly, a local control rate of 100% was achieved with 30 Gy in a smaller series from Memorial Sloan-Kettering Cancer Center (42).
- Most patients with intermediate-grade lymphomas are treated with CMT with rituximab, cyclophosphamide, doxorubicin, vincristine sulfate, and prednisone (R-CHOP) chemotherapy, followed by involved-field irradiation. Data suggest that the radiation dose can be limited to 30 to 36 Gy in patients who respond to chemotherapy (43).
- The usual pattern of failure after CMT for DLBCL is distant, with few patients failing locally (44). However, more local failure is seen if chemotherapy is used as the sole treatment modality (45). When patients are treated with CMT, nodal failures adjacent to areas of original disease are rarely seen. This forms the basis for using primarily involved-field radiation therapy (IFRT) when treating with CMT.
- The decision whether to treat the pre- or postchemotherapy volume is dependent on the site of the tumor and the radiotolerance of the surrounding normal structures. In certain situations, the entire organ is treated (e.g., DLBCL of stomach) regardless of chemotherapy response.
- For head and neck sites such as tonsil, base of tongue, or nasopharynx, 3D conformal radiation therapy (3DCRT) or intensity modulated radiation therapy (IMRT) plan is generally recommended. Again, the irradiation of Waldeyer's ring is not generally recommended unless there is involvement of this lymph node group.
- Those patients presenting with a large mediastinal mass typically have their postchemotherapy tumor volume treated in the lateral dimensions, while superiorly and inferiorly the field margins may be more generous and generally are based on prechemotherapy extent of disease.
- If radiation therapy is to be delivered on both sides of the diaphragm, an appropriate gap must be calculated between the fields at the surface of the skin on both the anteroposterior (AP) and posteroanterior portals to account for the normal divergence of the beam from each of the two fields. The objective of this calculation is to have the 50% isodose lines of the superior and inferior fields match exactly at the midplane.
- Unlike in HL, mesenteric lymph nodes are often involved in NHL. In addition, the GI tract is a common site for primary extranodal lymphoma. Therefore, in NHL, the whole-abdominal cavity is rarely, but occasionally, treated. If doses over 20 Gy are used, posterior renal shielding is recommended to limit the dose to the anterior surface of both kidneys to 20 Gy.

- To treat abdominal disease, whole-abdomen irradiation based on an isocentric setup is planned (46). The upper abdominal field is set up on a four-field basis on a simulator. Initial treatment consists of simple anterior and posterior fields from the dome of the diaphragm to approximately the level of the iliac crests (assuming that the inferior margin does not cut across known tumor). When massive tumor occurs at this level, the entire abdominal contents, from diaphragm to the floor of the pelvis, are treated in one large field. When possible, lead blocks are placed over the lateral portions of each ileum to attempt to protect iliac bone marrow.

- With large fields, the dose should not exceed 1.5 Gy per day. A tumor dose of approximately 15 Gy over 2 to 3 weeks is administered to these large anterior and posterior fields.

- Throughout the initial portion of treatment, the right lobe of the liver is protected by an anterior lead block to minimize the dose that the liver receives; this will be compensated in the second portion of treatment to the abdominal field. The second portion of the abdominal treatment continues to treat the upper abdominal field by lateral fields.

- For massive abdominal disease, a pelvic (iliofemoral) portion of the irradiation field may continue by opposing AP techniques. The upper abdominal field receives opposing cross-table lateral fields with the patient in the supine position and with blocks to protect both kidneys. The kidneys are localized with CT scans or an infusion of contrast material in the treatment position on a simulator. The posterior margin of the lateral portal is placed anterior to the kidneys but posterior to the periaortic nodes. The anterior margin of the lateral portal should extend to the anterior abdominal wall. By use of these two opposing lateral fields, with carefully positioned kidney blocks, the upper abdomen (including the liver) receives another 15 Gy over approximately 2 weeks, which brings the dose to the nodes to approximately 30 Gy over approximately 4 to 5 weeks.

- When kidney location prevents the use of lateral field technique, AP irradiation techniques are required, and the use of 5-cm-thick lead kidney blocks is necessary posteriorly to keep the total renal dose under 25 Gy.

- The final portion of the upper abdominal technique is a wide paraaortic field using anterior and posterior fields. The lateral width of the upper portion of this wide paraaortic field extends from the margin of one kidney to the margin of the opposite kidney. The total dose delivered to the central abdomen is 45 Gy over approximately 6 to 7 weeks.

- Caution should be used when blood cell counts are low or when prior chemotherapy has been used; pelvic therapy can be deferred until the upper abdominal irradiation is completed.

- In patients with advanced follicular lymphocytic lymphoma or follicular mixed lymphoma, total body irradiation (TBI) may be used for palliation (47). Fractionation can be delivered in several ways, but typically a dose of approximately 1.5 Gy midplane over 5 weeks is administered, often at the rate of 30 cGy per week in 2 or 3 fractions per week (10 to 15 cGy per fraction) (25). TBI is tolerated well symptomatically.

- More modern treatment involves the use of involved site or involved nodal radiation, particularly in patients treated with CMT where radiation treatment is delivered after initial chemotherapy. Guidelines published by the International Lymphoma Radiation Oncology Group (ILROG) can be used to guide treatment (48,49).

CHEMOTHERAPY AND COMBINED-MODALITY THERAPY

- Malignant lymphomas are very responsive to chemotherapy; however, the specific type of NHL often determines whether a given lymphoma is curable.
- The only variant in the WHO classification that has consistent curability is DLBCL and sometimes PTCL or anaplastic large T/null cell lymphoma (ALCL).
- The indolent lymphomas (e.g., FL) are generally not curable with chemotherapy.
- A wide variety of chemotherapy combinations have been used, but the most common is CHOP (cyclophosphamide, doxorubicin, vincristine, prednisone) (50). When used for DLBCL, this combination has a 50% to 60% complete response (CR) rate and a cure rate of 30% to 40% (51).
- The efficacy of CHOP is significantly improved with the addition of rituximab (an anti-CD20 antibody) such that R-CHOP is now the standard of care.
- R-CHOP is also the most commonly used regimen for FL, although its superiority over other regimens for this histology has yet to be proven in large phase III trials (52).
- The choice of chemotherapy regimen is based on histology, irrespective of the site of disease.
- In most instances when chemotherapy and irradiation are combined, chemotherapy is given first to allow assessment of response and reduction of disease bulk.

MANAGEMENT BY HISTOLOGIC TYPE, SITE, AND STAGE

Diffuse Large B-Cell Lymphomas: Stage I/II

- In the pre-chemotherapy era, DLBCL was treated with irradiation alone. Typically, doses of 30 to 60 Gy were used with 10-year failure-free survival (FFS) in the range of 30% to 60%, with stage II FFS approximately 25% and stage I 50% to 60% (53,54).
- This radiation-only approach has been superceded by a CMT approach of using chemotherapy than radiation. The most efficacious chemotherapy is generally CHOP/R-CHOP, and IFRT typically is used after chemotherapy. This approach has yielded a substantial improvement in FFS over radiation alone, with FFS of approximately 70% to 85% with CMT (37,55).
- There are two major randomized trials which have led to CMT being a commonly accepted treatment approach for early-stage DLBCL.
- The Southwest Oncology Group (SWOG) 8735 trial enrolled 401 patients comparing 8 cycles of CHOP with 3 cycles of CHOP followed by IFRT. Radiation doses were 40 to 55 Gy. The 5-year results showed the CMT arm to be superior with FFS and OS of 77% and 82% (versus 64% and 72% with chemotherapy alone). Toxicity was also found to be worse in the chemotherapy-alone arm (44). With longer follow-up, however, disease outcome differences between the arms no longer persisted.
- The Eastern Cooperative Oncology Group (ECOG) E1484 trial of 352 patients compared 8 cycles of CHOP with or without IFRT. Those with a complete response to chemotherapy received either 30 Gy of radiation or observation, whereas those with a partial response received 40 Gy. There was a statistically significantly improved

6-year disease-free survival of 73% for the CMT group versus 56% for chemotherapy alone. Also, there was a trend towards improved overall survival (82% versus 71%), although this was not significant (56).

- One has to keep in mind that neither of these two studies incorporated rituximab.
- A recent French study demonstrated that for stage I/II intermediate-grade lymphoma, a more aggressive chemotherapy regimen of ACVBP was superior to CMT incorporating IFRT (57).

Diffuse Large B-Cell Lymphomas: Stage III/IV

- The standard therapy is R-CHOP combination chemotherapy. Traditionally, radiation has not been used in consolidation following treatment. However, institutions will consolidate initial sites of bulky disease and/or patients with residual FDG-PET-avid disease following chemotherapy.
- Many combinations of chemotherapy have been tried, but CHOP appears to have equal or better efficacy than other regimens with less toxicity (50).
- A review that analyzed 35 randomized trials incorporating 22,000 patients demonstrated that for aggressive advanced-stage NHL, CHOP was curative in 1/3 of patients (58).
- Several trials have shown the value of adding rituximab to CHOP. For example, the GELA LNH98-5 study of 399 patients who were greater than 60 years old compared CHOP with R-CHOP. The 5-year progression-free survival and OS improved from 30% to 54% and 45% to 58%, respectively, with the addition of rituximab (51).
- Another European trial by the MInT group compared R-CHOP-like to CHOP-like chemotherapy alone in 824 patients aged 18 to 60 years with DLBCL. Radiation was also given to selected patients with bulky and extranodal disease. The 3-year OS rates were 93% and 84% for R-CHOP-like and CHOP-like, respectively (59).
- Some studies have attempted to use high-dose chemotherapy and autologous stem cell transplant to improve the results of R-CHOP regimens but with mixed results.
- There is an increasing interest in using radiation in CMT for patients with advanced DLBCL. The rationale is that studies have found that when relapses occur, they are usually at the sites of initial disease, particularly bulky disease (60,61). Several centers have explored this therapeutic approach with good results to date; however, it needs to be validated in large phase III trials (62–64).

Follicular Lymphoma: Stages I and II

- Stage I and II FL patients treated with irradiation alone have excellent survival. The overall survival rate at 5 years is 80% to 100% (65).
- For these patients, no clear evidence shows benefit to extended-field irradiation.
- Large phase III studies of CMT including DLBCL and FL have not shown any benefit to CMT over radiation alone for FL. The caveat is that there were few FL patients in these studies. Additionally, CMT studies including rituximab have not been reported (66–69).

- Low-grade lymphomas are more responsive to radiation therapy: doses of 20 to 35 Gy delivered in 10 to 20 fractions over 2 to 4 weeks result in local control rates of over 95%. Many centers use a dose of approximately 24 to 30 Gy. Large clinical trials have supported the use of 24 Gy in most cases. Additionally, so-called boom boom regimens of 4 to 8 Gy delivered in two fractions can be used for palliation. In the up-front setting, this approach may have increased failure rates, but no difference in survival compared to 24 Gy.

Follicular Lymphoma: Stages III and IV

- For stage III low-grade lymphomas, excellent 5- and 10-year survival can be expected with conservative management in asymptomatic patients with treatment deferred until symptoms develop (70).
- Median survival can be from 6 to 11 years with or without therapy.
- In one non-randomized study, 10-year OS was 73% in selected patients observed without therapy. There was also about a 25% spontaneous regression rate. Transformation to a higher-grade lymphoma was seen at the same rate for patients treated versus not treated at the outset. Similar findings were confirmed in a randomized trial by Groupe d'Etude des Lymphomes Folliculaires (GELF) (71,72).
- Once a patient develops symptoms, treatment may include small-field, low-dose irradiation for symptom relief. Alternatively, a single oral alkylating agent (e.g., chlorambucil or cyclophosphamide) may be used. Oftentimes, the decision of treatment can be based on whether symptoms are localized (e.g., painful lymph nodes) or generalized (e.g., B symptoms)
- Intensive chemotherapy appears to be associated with not only a high probability of response but also a continuous risk of relapse.
- Many novel agents are being investigated to alter the natural history of advanced FL.
- Rituximab has a response rate of 50% and 70% for treatment of relapse and first-line therapy, respectively. A variety of chemotherapy combinations have been tried with rituximab, but the optimal therapy is unclear. In the United States, the most commonly used regimen is R-CHOP (52,73,74).
- There are two radioimmunotherapy agents that have also been thoroughly investigated for use in FL. The first is Y-90 ibritumomab (Zevalin), a pure beta emitter, and the second is I-131 tositumomab (Bexxar), a combination of gamma and beta emitter. Both agents have response rates of 60% to 80% in relapsed FL patients. The agents have yielded good response when combined with chemotherapy, but combinations have to be done cautiously due to myelotoxicity (75–77).
- Interferon given with combination chemotherapy has been shown to be efficacious, but it is generally not given secondary to its adverse side effect profile (78).
- Several studies have looked at using either autologous or allogeneic transplantation for FL in first remission after induction chemotherapy or in relapsed FL. These studies have shown no benefit in the setting of relapsed FL but have shown some benefit in FFS for first remission. However, the OS results have yet to mature for these trials (79–81).
- Radiation therapy has been investigated by several groups as consolidative treatment after chemotherapy for stage III/IV FL. A trial of 118 patients entailed randomization

to CVP chemotherapy with or without IFRT (35 to 45 Gy) to initially involved sites. The 7-year relapse-free survival rates were 33% and 66% in the groups treated with chemotherapy alone and CMT including IFRT, respectively (82). Further studies are needed to confirm these findings.

- There is an aggressive subset of FL, and that group is FL grade 3 in the WHO classification. It comprises 15% of all cases of FL and is generally managed similar to DLBCL with a CMT approach. The dose of radiation typically used is 30 to 36 Gy. Prognosis is intermediate between that for low-grade FL and DLBCL (83–85).

Marginal Zone Lymphomas

- MZL (MALT) lymphomas are usually extranodal, with the stomach constituting the most common location.
- MALT lymphomas outside of the GI tract behave similar to those in the GI tract; however, there is no association with *H. pylori.*
- MALTomas are very responsive to radiation, and they have a local control and OS rate of 97% and 96%, respectively. Doses of approximately 24 to 30 Gy are used (40,41).
- Chemotherapy is palliative, and it is reserved for patients with symptomatic generalized disease.
- Patients with asymptomatic generalized disease are usually observed, similar to FL.
- Those patients with nodal and splenic MZL usually have generalized disease and are managed similar to advanced FL.

Peripheral T-Cell Lymphomas

- A nodal PTCL is very similar to DLBCL in its presentation and treatment, except it generally has a worse prognosis (86,87).
- The treatment usually consists of 3 to 6 cycles of CHOP and IFRT, and there is no role for rituximab as its use is restricted to histologies of B-cell origin. However, there are minimal data on the role of radiation in advanced PTCL.
- The ALCL variant of PTCL has a much better prognosis. ALCL patients respond fairly well to CHOP, especially if they are positive for the anaplastic lymphoma kinase (ALK) gene (88).

Small Lymphocytic Lymphoma

- SLL is treated with the same approach as B-CLL. It is responsive to combination chemotherapy such as CHOP or a single agent such as chlorambucil; similar to FL and MZL, either approach produces equivalent results. Rituximab is also a major part of the treatment regimen (89,90).
- Radiation may be considered in those rare circumstances of localized disease (i.e., stage I or II). Typically, a dose of 30 Gy with generous fields is employed.

Mantle Cell Lymphoma

- MCL has a very poor prognosis (10-year OS of 8%), and although many chemotherapy regimens have been, there is no standard therapy (91–93).
- High-dose chemotherapy with stem cell transplantation has also been explored with some benefit in FFS but not OS. Therefore, enrollment on a clinical trial is recommended for treating MCL patients (94).
- Although localized MCL is exceedingly rare, in this setting radiation alone may have a role (95).

PRIMARY EXTRANODAL LYMPHOMAS

- Approximately 35% to 40% of all patients with NHL have extranodal lymphomas. The most common sites involved, in decreasing order, are the GI tract, the head and neck region (including Waldeyer's ring and other head and neck sites, but excluding brain), and skin.

Gastrointestinal Lymphoma

- The stomach is the most common site of involvement (50% to 80%). Other GI sites include the small and large intestine, primarily ileum, followed by colon and rectum.
- Approximately 90% to 95% of stomach lymphomas are MALT or DLBCL, and the two entities are about equivalent in their frequency of occurrence.
- Historically, surgery was the mainstay of therapy, and resection was usually followed by adjuvant chemotherapy and irradiation.
- In a report from the Princess Margaret Hospital, a primarily surgical approach led to FFS of 81% and CSS of 88% (96).
- However, subsequently many investigators have explored using a combination of chemotherapy and radiotherapy instead of surgery. There are now numerous studies showing equivalent outcomes using a chemoradiation approach compared with surgery (97–99).

DLBCL Gastric Lymphoma

- DLBCL gastric lymphoma is typically treated with chemotherapy alone or CMT. Chemotherapy commonly consists of R-CHOP.
- Radiation doses are 30 to 36 Gy after chemotherapy (100).
- The local control with this regimen is 90%, and the FFS and OS for patients with stage I and II disease are 70% to 80% (96,101,102).
- The radiation portal typically encompasses the entire stomach, celiac axis nodes, and other involved areas with a margin of several centimeters. Appropriate technique should be utilized to minimize the dose to the kidneys. A common field arrangement is parallel-opposed anterior and posterior fields. However, a more complex plan with 3D conformal radiotherapy or IMRT may be necessary to minimize kidney dose.

MALT Gastric Lymphoma

- *Helicobacter pylori* infection is seen in over 90% of patients with MALT gastric lymphoma (11).
- Recommended antibiotic therapy includes metronidazole (400 mg t.i.d.), ampicillin (500 mg t.i.d.), and omeprazole (Prilosec) (20 mg b.i.d.) or tinidazole, clarithromycin (Biaxin), and omeprazole (25). The expected rate of eradication of *H. pylori* is 75% to 90%.
- Antibiotic therapy has a complete response (CR) rate of approximately 75%. Two-thirds of these patients with a CR will remain in remission at 5 years. Therefore, the 5-year FFS is about 50%, and the 5-year OS is 90%.
- The t(11:18) translocation is a predictor of antibiotic resistance.
- For treatment with radiation therapy, the CR rate exceeds 95% and the relapse rate is less than 10% with a dose of 30 Gy.
- General recommendations are for initial therapy with antibiotics and close follow-up. Radiation, with techniques similar to those used for gastric DLBCL, is generally utilized after a patient has failed antibiotics.
- There is no general role for adjuvant chemotherapy, although rituximab has been used in patients who are not suitable candidates for radiation.

Intestinal Lymphoma

- The majority are DLBCL.
- Similar to gastric lymphoma, the presenting symptoms are usually abdominal pain, anorexia, and weight loss. However, in contrast to gastric lymphoma, ileus or perforation is much more common (up to 40% of patients) (98).
- Typically, diagnosis and treatment are achieved with surgery.
- For DLBCL, resection is typically followed by treatment with anthracycline-based chemotherapy.
- Some authors recommend whole-abdominal radiation, with a dose of 20 to 25 Gy in 1 to 1.25 Gy fractions, if surgical resection is incomplete (96).
- Overall long-term survival is approximately 50%.
- Waldeyer's ring lymphoma (tonsil, base of tongue, nasopharynx)
- Traditionally, involved-field irradiation (primary tumor plus draining neck nodes) and moderate doses have been used for Waldeyer's ring lymphoma with survival rates of 50% to 60% for stage IE lesions and 25% to 50% for IIE lesions (103).
- CMT using doxorubicin-based chemotherapy and irradiation to the primary tumor and neck nodes result in local control rates of over 80% and overall survival rates of 60% to 75%.

Salivary Gland Lymphoma

- Lymphoma of the salivary gland occurs commonly in patients with Sjögren's syndrome. Myoepithelial sialadenitis, considered part of the spectrum of MALT lymphoma, is also characteristic of Sjögren's syndrome.
- Radiation therapy offers excellent local control for limited-stage salivary gland lymphomas.

Thyroid Lymphoma

- With locoregional, moderate-dose irradiation, local control is achieved in over 75% of patients with thyroid lymphoma.
- Linkage between the GI tract and Waldeyer's ring progression agrees with the categorization of thyroid lymphoma within the MALT system.

Orbital Lymphoma

- Symptoms of orbital lymphoma include ptosis, blurred vision, chemosis, and epiphora.
- Tumors of the retrobulbar region present with swelling and proptosis, with disturbance of ocular movement.
- Delineation of local disease extent is as important as staging evaluation to rule out generalized lymphoma.
- Bilateral lesions do not have the unfavorable prognosis of generalized lymphoma, and in some series, the incidence of distant relapse is similar for unilateral (30%) and bilateral (25%) cases (25).
- Orbital lesions are easily controlled with low-to-moderate radiation doses.
- Treatment with an anterior orthovoltage x-ray field or electron beam provides satisfactory therapy for anterior lesions limited to the eyelid or bulbar conjunctiva, with the advantage of sparing orbital structures compared with the use of a photon beam.
- If an anterior orthovoltage field is used, a small, lead eye shield suspended in the beam to shield the lens can result in a lens dose of less than 5% to 10% (104).
- For unilateral retrobulbar tumors, a two-field technique can be used (4- to 6-MV photons), with a corneal shield placed in the anterior and lateral fields, angled posteriorly, to spare the lens in both eyes (105).
- An alternative arrangement uses an isocentric technique with two oblique (wedged) fields with a shield potentially inserted in each, with the patient looking at the shield for each treatment field.
- Radiation therapy (20 to 30 Gy in 10 to 20 daily fractions) results in a local control rate of over 95% for patients with low-grade orbital and conjunctival lymphomas.
- Fewer data are available for intermediate- and high-grade lymphomas, but dose-control data for lymphoma suggest that for patients with small bulk tumors, a dose of 35 Gy provides excellent local control (106). For patients with larger intermediate- and high-grade tumors, short-duration doxorubicin-based chemotherapy followed by radiation therapy is recommended (106).

Breast Lymphoma

- High-grade breast lymphomas in young women, which are commonly bilateral, tend to be associated with pregnancy and lactation and may disseminate rapidly to the central nervous system.
- Breast preservation is possible in most cases.
- Radiation therapy to the whole breast (45 to 50 Gy) and to the ipsilateral axillary lymph nodes (40 to 45 Gy) results in excellent local control (75% to 78%).

- The current treatment recommendation in all patients with intermediate- and high-grade lymphomas is CMT. Patients with low-grade lymphomas may be successfully treated with irradiation alone.
- Central nervous system prophylaxis should be given to all patients with high-grade histology, especially those with bulky or bilateral disease.

Testicular Lymphoma

- Lymphoma accounts for 25% to 50% of primary testicular tumors in men older than 50 years of age and is the most common testicular tumor in patients over 60 years (107).
- The incidence of bilateral involvement is as high as 18% to 20%.
- Essentially, all primary lymphomas of the testis are intermediate or high grade, with diffuse large cell lymphoma being most common.
- Historically, postorchiectomy therapy involved radiation therapy to the paraaortic and ipsilateral pelvic lymph nodes, with cure rates of 40% to 50% for stage I and 20% to 30% for stage II disease.
- Doxorubicin-based chemotherapy improves survival to 93% at 4 years for patients with localized testicular lymphoma (108). The role of radiation therapy is less clear. However, low-dose irradiation (approximately 25 to 36 Gy) to the contralateral testis minimizes the risk of failure at this site, carries little morbidity, and is generally recommended for all patients with primary testicular lymphoma.
- Central nervous system prophylaxis with intrathecal methotrexate is an essential part of treatment.

Bone Lymphoma

- Long bones are the most common presentation site of bone lymphoma.
- Patients with primary bone lymphoma should be treated with anthracycline-based chemotherapy and subsequent radiation therapy to the whole bone to a minimum dose of 35 Gy; however, some clinicians question the need to treat the entire bone.
- With current CMT, overall survival and relapse-free rates exceed 70% at 5 years.
- Magnetic resonance imaging is important in revealing extension of disease beyond that visualized by CT or radionuclide imaging.

Primary Central Nervous System Lymphoma

- Primary central nervous system lymphoma (PCNSL) accounts for approximately 10% of all extranodal lymphomas.
- Two-thirds of patients with PCNSL present with cerebral disease (usually in the periventricular region), with only a subset having meningeal, spinal cord, or ocular disease.
- Pathologies are mostly of diffuse histology, predominantly B-cell tumors.
- Most patients present with a solitary brain lesion; however, the leptomeninges are involved in approximately 30% of cases and the eye in 20%. Therefore, a lumbar puncture and full ophthalmologic examination are warranted as part of the initial workup.

- Surgery only plays a role in diagnosis, typically via stereotactic biopsy. Occasionally, surgical decompression and shunt placement are necessary for elevated intracranial pressure.
- Corticosteroids reduce intracranial pressure and also have antitumor activity. However, steroids should be withheld until after a biopsy such that tumor regression does not lead to difficulties in establishing the diagnosis (109).
- Radiation therapy improves median survival, but only to approximately 15 months.
- Irradiation fields are usually to the whole brain, with extension to the upper cervical spinal cord and typically to the posterior orbits.
- Patients in a North Central Cancer Group and Eastern Cooperative Oncology Group trial were given CHOP for two cycles followed by radiation therapy to the whole brain, including C-2 extension, to 50.4 Gy. Unfortunately, the results of this study did not show any improvement over use of irradiation alone (110).
- Methotrexate in high doses penetrates the blood-brain barrier, and therefore, it has been tried with whole brain radiation therapy (WBRT) with demonstrated efficacy.
- RTOG 93-10 treated patients with combination chemotherapy (including high-dose methotrexate) and WBRT. The results were much improved over historical controls, with 5-year OS of 32% and PFS of 25%. A similar therapeutic approach has been utilized at Memorial Sloan-Kettering Cancer Center (111).
- There is a significant risk of treatment-related neurotoxicity, including leukoencephalopathy and dementia, with the combination of high-dose methotrexate and WBRT. Such neurotoxicity is more common in patients greater than 60 years (109,112). Accordingly, it is reasonable to defer WBRT to the salvage setting for older patients with a complete response to high-dose methotrexate-based chemotherapy.

Cutaneous Lymphoma

- Primary lymphomas of the skin are divided into three categories: low-grade, small lymphocytic type T-cell lymphoma (mycosis fungoides/Sézary syndrome) (65%); T-cell lymphoma of larger cells (pleomorphic, immunoblastic, and anaplastic) (10%); and cutaneous B-cell lymphoma (25%) (113).
- Infection with *Borrelia burgdorferi* has been implicated in the development of cutaneous B-cell lymphoma.
- Total body electron irradiation is the preferred treatment modality, with very high local control rates (85% to 100%) and favorable survival (113).
- Both irradiation and chemotherapy produce an initial response, but rapid extracutaneous dissemination occurs in large cell T-cell lymphoma.

References

1. Jemal A, Siegel R, Ward E, et al. Cancer statistics, 2006. *CA Cancer J Clin* 2006;56(2):106–130.
2. Anderson JR, Armitage JO, Weisenburger DD. Epidemiology of the non-Hodgkin's lymphomas: distributions of the major subtypes differ by geographic locations. Non-Hodgkin's Lymphoma Classification Project. *Ann Oncol* 1998;9(7):717–720.
3. Seow A, Lee J, Sng I, et al. Non-Hodgkin's lymphoma in an Asian population: 1968–1992 time trends and ethnic differences in Singapore. *Cancer* 1996;77(9):1899–1904.

4. Newton R, Ferlay J, Beral V, et al. The epidemiology of non-Hodgkin's lymphoma: comparison of nodal and extra-nodal sites. *Int J Cancer* 1997;72(6):923–930.

5. Ries L, Harkins D, Krapcho M, et al., eds. *SEER cancer statistics review, 1975–2003*. Bethesda, MD: National Cancer Institute, 2005.

6. Fisher SG, Fisher RI. The epidemiology of non-Hodgkin's lymphoma. *Oncogene* 2004;23(38):6524–6534.

7. Behler CM, Kaplan LD. Advances in the management of HIV-related non-Hodgkin lymphoma. *Curr Opin Oncol* 2006;18(5):437–443.

8. Gottschalk S, Rooney CM, Heslop HE. Post-transplant lymphoproliferative disorders. *Annu Rev Med* 2005;56:29–44.

9. Gandhi MK, Tellam JT, Khanna R. Epstein-Barr virus-associated Hodgkin's lymphoma. *Br J Haematol* 2004;125(3):267–281.

10. Ratner L. Human T cell lymphotropic virus-associated leukemia/lymphoma. *Curr Opin Oncol* 2005;17(5):469–473.

11. Wotherspoon AC, Ortiz-Hidalgo C, Falzon MR, et al. *Helicobacter pylori*-associated gastritis and primary B-cell gastric lymphoma. *Lancet* 1991;338(8776):1175–1176.

12. Glass AG, Karnell LH, Menck HR. The National Cancer Data Base report on non-Hodgkin's lymphoma. *Cancer* 1997;80(12):2311–2320.

13. d'Amore F, Christensen BE, Brincker H, et al. Clinicopathological features and prognostic factors in extranodal non-Hodgkin lymphomas. Danish LYFO Study Group. *Eur J Cancer* 1991;27(10):1201–1208.

14. Straus DJ, Filippa DA, Lieberman PH, et al. The non-Hodgkin's lymphomas. I. A retrospective clinical and pathologic analysis of 499 cases diagnosed between 1958 and 1969. *Cancer* 1983;51(1):101–109.

15. Chabner BA, Fisher RI, Young RC, et al. Staging of non-Hodgkin's lymphoma. *Semin Oncol* 1980;7(3):285–291.

16. Sutcliffe S, Gospodarowicz M. Primary extranodal lymphomas. In: Canellos G, Lister T, Sklar J, eds. *The lymphomas*. Philadelphia, PA: W.B. Saunders Company, 1998:449–479.

17. Sandrasegaran K, Robinson PJ, Selby P. Staging of lymphoma in adults. *Clin Radiol* 1994;49(3):149–161.

18. Castellino RA, Hilton S, O'Brien JP, et al. Non-Hodgkin lymphoma: contribution of chest CT in the initial staging evaluation. *Radiology* 1996;199(1):129–132.

19. Khoury MB, Godwin JD, Halvorsen R, et al. Role of chest CT in non-Hodgkin lymphoma. *Radiology* 1986;158(3):659–662.

20. Juweid ME, Wiseman GA, Vose JM, et al. Response assessment of aggressive non-Hodgkin's lymphoma by integrated International Workshop Criteria and fluorine-18-fluorodeoxyglucose positron emission tomography. *J Clin Oncol* 2005;23(21):4652–4661.

21. Schoder H, Meta J, Yap C, et al. Effect of whole-body (18)F-FDG PET imaging on clinical staging and management of patients with malignant lymphoma. *J Nucl Med* 2001;42(8):1139–1143.

22. Juweid ME, Cheson BD. Role of positron emission tomography in lymphoma. *J Clin Oncol* 2005;23(21):4577–4580.

23. Lavely WC, Delbeke D, Greer JP, et al. FDG PET in the follow-up management of patients with newly diagnosed Hodgkin and non-Hodgkin lymphoma after first-line chemotherapy. *Int J Radiat Oncol Biol Phys* 2003;57(2):307–315.

24. Spaepen K, Stroobants S, Dupont P, et al. Prognostic value of pretransplantation positron emission tomography using fluorine 18-fluorodeoxyglucose in patients with aggressive lymphoma treated with high-dose chemotherapy and stem cell transplantation. *Blood* 2003;102(1):53–59.

25. Gospodarowicz M, Wasserman T. Non-Hodgkin's lymphomas. In: Perez C, Brady L, eds. *Principles and practice of radiation oncology*, 3rd ed. Philadelphia, PA: Lippincott–Raven, 1998:1987–2011.

26. Prosnitz L, Ng A. Non-Hodgkin's lymphoma. In: Halperin E, Perez C, Brady L, eds. *Principles and practice of radiation oncology.* Philadelphia, PA: Lippincott Williams & Wilkins, 2008: 1739–1765.

27. Jaffe E, Harris N, Stein H, et al., eds. *Pathology and genetics of tumours of hematoporetic and lymphoid tissue. World Health Organization classification of tumours.* Lyon, France: IARC Press, 2001.

28. Armitage JO, Weisenburger DD. New approach to classifying non-Hodgkin's lymphomas: clinical features of the major histologic subtypes. Non-Hodgkin's Lymphoma Classification Project. *J Clin Oncol* 1998;16(8):2780–2795.

29. Gospodarowicz MK, Bush RS, Brown TC, et al. Prognostic factors in nodular lymphomas: a multivariate analysis based on the Princess Margaret Hospital experience. *Int J Radiat Oncol Biol Phys* 1984;10(4):489–497.

30. International N-HsLPFP. A predictive model for aggressive non-Hodgkin's lymphoma. The International Non-Hodgkin's Lymphoma Prognostic Factors Project. *N Engl J Med* 1993;329(14):987–994.

31. Couderc B, Dujols JP, Mokhtari F, et al. The management of adult aggressive non-Hodgkin's lymphomas. *Crit Rev Oncol Hematol* 2000;35(1):33–48.

32. Gallamini A, Stelitano C, Calvi R, et al. Peripheral T-cell lymphoma unspecified (PTCL-U): a new prognostic model from a retrospective multicentric clinical study. *Blood* 2004;103(7): 2474–2479.

33. Sonnen R, Schmidt WP, Muller-Hermelink HK, et al. The International Prognostic Index determines the outcome of patients with nodal mature T-cell lymphomas. *Br J Haematol* 2005;129(3):366–372.

34. Went P, Agostinelli C, Gallamini A, et al. Marker expression in peripheral T-cell lymphoma: a proposed clinical-pathologic prognostic score. *J Clin Oncol* 2006;24(16):2472–2479.

35. Solal-Celigny P, Roy P, Colombat P, et al. Follicular lymphoma international prognostic index. *Blood* 2004;104(5):1258–1265.

36. Sutcliffe SB, Gospodarowicz MK, Bush RS, et al. Role of radiation therapy in localized non-Hodgkin's lymphoma. *Radiother Oncol* 1985;4(3):211–223.

37. Prestidge BR, Horning SJ, Hoppe RT. Combined modality therapy for stage I-II large cell lymphoma. *Int J Radiat Oncol Biol Phys* 1988;15(3):633–639.

38. Bush R, Gospodarowicz M. The place of radiation therapy in the management of patients with localized non-Hodgkin's lymphoma. In: Rosenberg S, Kaplan H, eds. *Malignant lymphomas: etiology, immunology, pathology, treatment. Bristol Myers Cancer Symposia.* New York, NY: Academic Press, 1982.

39. Grogan TM, Lippman SM, Spier CM, et al. Independent prognostic significance of a nuclear proliferation antigen in diffuse large cell lymphomas as determined by the monoclonal antibody Ki-67. *Blood* 1988;71(4):1157–1160.

40. Tsang RW, Gospodarowicz MK, Pintilie M, et al. Stage I and II MALT lymphoma: results of treatment with radiotherapy. *Int J Radiat Oncol Biol Phys* 2001;50(5):1258–1264.

41. Tsang RW, Gospodarowicz MK, Pintilie M, et al. Localized mucosa-associated lymphoid tissue lymphoma treated with radiation therapy has excellent clinical outcome. *J Clin Oncol* 2003;21(22):4157–4164.

42. Schechter NR, Portlock CS, Yahalom J. Treatment of mucosa-associated lymphoid tissue lymphoma of the stomach with radiation alone. *J Clin Oncol* 1998;16(5):1916–1921.

43. Connors JM, Klimo P, Fairey RN, et al. Brief chemotherapy and involved field radiation therapy for limited-stage, histologically aggressive lymphoma. *Ann Intern Med* 1987;107(1):25–30.

44. Miller TP, Dahlberg S, Cassady JR, et al. Chemotherapy alone compared with chemotherapy plus radiotherapy for localized intermediate- and high-grade non-Hodgkin's lymphoma. *N Engl J Med* 1998;339(1):21–26.

45. Miller TP, Jones SE. Initial chemotherapy for clinically localized lymphomas of unfavorable histology. *Blood* 1983;62(2):413–418.

46. Valicenti RK, Wasserman TH, Monyak DJ, et al. Non-Hodgkin lymphoma: whole-abdomen irradiation as an adjuvant to chemotherapy. *Radiology* 1994;192(2):571–576.

47. Carabell SC, Chaffey JT, Rosenthal DS, et al. Results of total body irradiation in the treatment of advanced non-Hodgkin's lymphomas. *Cancer* 1979;43(3):994–1000.

48. Yahalom J, Illidge T, Specht L, et al.; International Lymphoma Radiation Oncology Group. Modern radiation therapy for extranodal lymphomas: field and dose guidelines from the International Lymphoma Radiation Oncology Group. *Int J Radiat Oncol Biol Phys* 2015;92(1):11–31. doi: 10.1016/j.ijrobp.2015.01.009.

49. Illidge T, Specht L, Yahalom J, et al.; International Lymphoma Radiation Oncology Group. Modern radiation therapy for nodal non-Hodgkin lymphoma-target definition and dose guidelines from the International Lymphoma Radiation Oncology Group. *Int J Radiat Oncol Biol Phys* 2014;89(1):49–58. doi: 10.1016/j.ijrobp.2014.01.006.

50. Fisher RI, Gaynor ER, Dahlberg S, et al. Comparison of a standard regimen (CHOP) with three intensive chemotherapy regimens for advanced non-Hodgkin's lymphoma. *N Engl J Med* 1993;328(14):1002–1006.

51. Feugier P, Van Hoof A, Sebban C, et al. Long-term results of the R-CHOP study in the treatment of elderly patients with diffuse large B-cell lymphoma: a study by the Groupe d'Etude des Lymphomes de l'Adulte. *J Clin Oncol* 2005;23(18):4117–4126.

52. Czuczman MS, Weaver R, Alkuzweny B, et al. Prolonged clinical and molecular remission in patients with low-grade or follicular non-Hodgkin's lymphoma treated with rituximab plus CHOP chemotherapy: 9-year follow-up. *J Clin Oncol* 2004;22(23):4711–4716.

53. Kaminski MS, Coleman CN, Colby TV, et al. Factors predicting survival in adults with stage I and II large-cell lymphoma treated with primary radiation therapy. *Ann Intern Med* 1986;104(6):747–756.

54. Vaughan Hudson B, Vaughan Hudson G, MacLennan KA, et al. Clinical stage 1 non-Hodgkin's lymphoma: long-term follow-up of patients treated by the British National Lymphoma Investigation with radiotherapy alone as initial therapy. *Br J Cancer* 1994;69(6):1088–1093.

55. Shenkier TN, Voss N, Fairey R, et al. Brief chemotherapy and involved-region irradiation for limited-stage diffuse large-cell lymphoma: an 18-year experience from the British Columbia Cancer Agency. *J Clin Oncol* 2002;20(1):197–204.

56. Horning SJ, Weller E, Kim K, et al. Chemotherapy with or without radiotherapy in limited-stage diffuse aggressive non-Hodgkin's lymphoma: Eastern Cooperative Oncology Group study 1484. *J Clin Oncol* 2004;22(15):3032–3038.

57. Reyes F, Lepage E, Ganem G, et al. ACVBP versus CHOP plus radiotherapy for localized aggressive lymphoma. *N Engl J Med* 2005;352(12):1197–1205.

58. Kimby E, Brandt L, Nygren P, et al. A systematic overview of chemotherapy effects in aggressive non-Hodgkin's lymphoma. *Acta Oncol* 2001;40(2–3):198–212.

59. Pfreundschuh M, Trumper L, Osterborg A, et al. CHOP-like chemotherapy plus rituximab versus CHOP-like chemotherapy alone in young patients with good-prognosis diffuse large-B-cell lymphoma: a randomised controlled trial by the MabThera International Trial (MInT) Group. *Lancet Oncol* 2006;7(5):379–391.

60. Hallahan DE, Farah R, Vokes EE, et al. The patterns of failure in patients with pathological stage I and II diffuse histocytic lymphoma treated with radiation therapy alone. *Int J Radiat Oncol Biol Phys* 1989;17(4):767–771.

61. Shipp MA, Klatt MM, Yeap B, et al. Patterns of relapse in large-cell lymphoma patients with bulk disease: implications for the use of adjuvant radiation therapy. *J Clin Oncol* 1989;7(5):613–618.

62. Aviles A, Delgado S, Nambo MJ, et al. Adjuvant radiotherapy to sites of previous bulky disease in patients stage IV diffuse large cell lymphoma. *Int J Radiat Oncol Biol Phys* 1994;30(4):799–803.

63. Ferreri AJ, Dell'Oro S, Reni M, et al. Consolidation radiotherapy to bulky or semibulky lesions in the management of stage III-IV diffuse large B cell lymphomas. *Oncology* 2000;58(3):219–226.

64. Schlembach PJ, Wilder RB, Tucker SL, et al. Impact of involved field radiotherapy after CHOP-based chemotherapy on stage III-IV, intermediate grade and large-cell immunoblastic lymphomas. *Int J Radiat Oncol Biol Phys* 2000;48(4):1107–1110.

65. Chen MG, Prosnitz LR, Gonzalez-Serva A, et al. Results of radiotherapy in control of stage I and II non-Hodgkin's lymphoma. *Cancer* 1979;43(4):1245–1254.

66. Kelsey SM, Newland AC, Hudson GV, et al. A British National Lymphoma Investigation randomised trial of single agent chlorambucil plus radiotherapy versus radiotherapy alone in low grade, localised non-Hodgkin's lymphoma. *Med Oncol* 1994;11(1):19–25.

67. Monfardini S, Banfi A, Bonadonna G, et al. Improved five year survival after combined radiotherapy-chemotherapy for stage I-II non-Hodgkin's lymphoma. *Int J Radiat Oncol Biol Phys* 1980;6(2):125–134.

68. Nissen NI, Ersboll J, Hansen HS, et al. A randomized study of radiotherapy versus radiotherapy plus chemotherapy in stage I-II non-Hodgkin's lymphomas. *Cancer* 1983;52(1):1–7.

69. Yahalom J, Varsos G, Fuks Z, et al. Adjuvant cyclophosphamide, doxorubicin, vincristine, and prednisone chemotherapy after radiation therapy in stage I low-grade and intermediate-grade non-Hodgkin lymphoma. Results of a prospective randomized study. *Cancer* 1993;71(7):2342–2350.

70. Rosenberg SA. Karnofsky memorial lecture. The low-grade non-Hodgkin's lymphomas: challenges and opportunities. *J Clin Oncol* 1985;3(3):299–310.

71. Brice P, Bastion Y, Lepage E, et al. Comparison in low-tumor-burden follicular lymphomas between an initial no-treatment policy, prednimustine, or interferon alfa: a randomized study from the Groupe d'Etude des Lymphomes Folliculaires. Groupe d'Etude des Lymphomes de l'Adulte. *J Clin Oncol* 1997;15(3):1110–1117.

72. Horning SJ, Rosenberg SA. The natural history of initially untreated low-grade non-Hodgkin's lymphomas. *N Engl J Med* 1984;311(23):1471–1475.

73. Ghielmini M, Schmitz SF, Cogliatti SB, et al. Prolonged treatment with rituximab in patients with follicular lymphoma significantly increases event-free survival and response duration compared with the standard weekly x 4 schedule. *Blood* 2004;103(12):4416–4423.

74. Zinzani PL, Pulsoni A, Perrotti A, et al. Fludarabine plus mitoxantrone with and without rituximab versus CHOP with and without rituximab as front-line treatment for patients with follicular lymphoma. *J Clin Oncol* 2004;22(13):2654–2661.

75. Davies AJ, Rohatiner AZ, Howell S, et al. Tositumomab and iodine I 131 tositumomab for recurrent indolent and transformed B-cell non-Hodgkin's lymphoma. *J Clin Oncol* 2004;22(8):1469–1479.

76. Horning SJ, Younes A, Jain V, et al. Efficacy and safety of tositumomab and iodine-131 tositumomab (Bexxar) in B-cell lymphoma, progressive after rituximab. *J Clin Oncol* 2005;23(4):712–719.

77. Press OW, Unger JM, Braziel RM, et al. Phase II trial of CHOP chemotherapy followed by tositumomab/iodine I-131 tositumomab for previously untreated follicular non-Hodgkin's lymphoma: five-year follow-up of Southwest Oncology Group Protocol S9911. *J Clin Oncol* 2006;24(25):4143–4149.

78. Rohatiner AZ, Gregory WM, Peterson B, et al. Meta-analysis to evaluate the role of interferon in follicular lymphoma. *J Clin Oncol* 2005;23(10):2215–2223.

79. Deconinck E, Foussard C, Milpied N, et al. High-dose therapy followed by autologous purged stem-cell transplantation and doxorubicin-based chemotherapy in patients with advanced follicular lymphoma: a randomized multicenter study by GOELAMS. *Blood* 2005;105(10):3817–3823.

80. Hunault-Berger M, Ifrah N, Solal-Celigny P. Intensive therapies in follicular non-Hodgkin lymphomas. *Blood* 2002;100(4):1141–1152.

81. Lenz G, Dreyling M, Schiegnitz E, et al. Myeloablative radiochemotherapy followed by autologous stem cell transplantation in first remission prolongs progression-free survival in follicular lymphoma: results of a prospective, randomized trial of the German Low-Grade Lymphoma Study Group. *Blood* 2004;104(9):2667–2674.

82. Aviles A, Diaz-Maqueo JC, Sanchez E, et al. Long-term results in patients with low-grade nodular non-Hodgkin's lymphoma. A randomized trial comparing chemotherapy plus radiotherapy with chemotherapy alone. *Acta Oncol* 1991;30(3):329–333.

83. Hans CP, Weisenburger DD, Vose JM, et al. A significant diffuse component predicts for inferior survival in grade 3 follicular lymphoma, but cytologic subtypes do not predict survival. *Blood* 2003;101(6):2363–2367.

84. Rodriguez J, McLaughlin P, Hagemeister FB, et al. Follicular large cell lymphoma: an aggressive lymphoma that often presents with favorable prognostic features. *Blood* 1999;93(7):2202–2207.

85. Wendum D, Sebban C, Gaulard P, et al. Follicular large-cell lymphoma treated with intensive chemotherapy: an analysis of 89 cases included in the LNH87 trial and comparison with the outcome of diffuse large B-cell lymphoma. Groupe d'Etude des Lymphomes de l'Adulte. *J Clin Oncol* 1997;15(4):1654–1663.

86. Arrowsmith ER, Macon WR, Kinney MC, et al. Peripheral T-cell lymphomas: clinical features and prognostic factors of 92 cases defined by the revised European American lymphoma classification. *Leuk Lymphoma* 2003;44(2):241–249.

87. Lopez-Guillermo A, Cid J, Salar A, et al. Peripheral T-cell lymphomas: initial features, natural history, and prognostic factors in a series of 174 patients diagnosed according to the R.E.A.L. Classification. *Ann Oncol* 1998;9(8):849–855.

88. Falini B, Pileri S, Zinzani PL, et al. ALK+ lymphoma: clinico-pathological findings and outcome. *Blood* 1999;93(8):2697–2706.

89. Coiffier B, Thieblemont C, Felman P, et al. Indolent nonfollicular lymphomas: characteristics, treatment, and outcome. *Semin Hematol* 1999;36(2):198–208.

90. Dana BW, Dahlberg S, Nathwani BN, et al. Long-term follow-up of patients with low-grade malignant lymphomas treated with doxorubicin-based chemotherapy or chemoimmunotherapy. *J Clin Oncol* 1993;11(4):644–651.

91. Fisher RI. Mantle-cell lymphoma: classification and therapeutic implications. *Ann Oncol* 1996;7(suppl 6):S35–S39.

92. Ghielmini M, Schmitz SF, Cogliatti S, et al. Effect of single-agent rituximab given at the standard schedule or as prolonged treatment in patients with mantle cell lymphoma: a study of the Swiss Group for Clinical Cancer Research (SAKK). *J Clin Oncol* 2005;23(4):705–711.

93. Lenz G, Dreyling M, Hoster E, et al. Immunochemotherapy with rituximab and cyclophosphamide, doxorubicin, vincristine, and prednisone significantly improves response and time to treatment failure, but not long-term outcome in patients with previously untreated mantle cell lymphoma: results of a prospective randomized trial of the German Low Grade Lymphoma Study Group (GLSG). *J Clin Oncol* 2005;23(9):1984–1992.

94. Dreyling M, Lenz G, Hoster E, et al. Early consolidation by myeloablative radiochemotherapy followed by autologous stem cell transplantation in first remission significantly prolongs progression-free survival in mantle-cell lymphoma: results of a prospective randomized trial of the European MCL Network. *Blood* 2005;105(7):2677–2684.

95. Rosenbluth BD, Yahalom J. Highly effective local control and palliation of mantle cell lymphoma with involved-field radiation therapy (IFRT). *Int J Radiat Oncol Biol Phys* 2006;65(4):1185–1191.

96. Crump M, Gospodarowicz M, Shepherd FA. Lymphoma of the gastrointestinal tract. *Semin Oncol* 1999;26(3):324–337.

97. Ferreri AJ, Cordio S, Ponzoni M, et al. Non-surgical treatment with primary chemotherapy, with or without radiation therapy, of stage I-II high-grade gastric lymphoma. *Leuk Lymphoma* 1999;33(5–6):531–541.

98. Koch P, del Valle F, Berdel WE, et al. Primary gastrointestinal non-Hodgkin's lymphoma: I. Anatomic and histologic distribution, clinical features, and survival data of 371 patients registered in the German Multicenter Study GIT NHL 01/92. *J Clin Oncol* 2001;19(18):3861–3873.

99. Koch P, Probst A, Berdel WE, et al. Treatment results in localized primary gastric lymphoma: data of patients registered within the German multicenter study (GIT NHL 02/96). *J Clin Oncol* 2005;23(28):7050–7059.

100. Gospodarowicz MK, Sutcliffe SB, Clark RM, et al. Outcome analysis of localized gastrointestinal lymphoma treated with surgery and postoperative irradiation. *Int J Radiat Oncol Biol Phys* 1990;19(6):1351–1355.

101. Amer MH, el-Akkad S. Gastrointestinal lymphoma in adults: clinical features and management of 300 cases. *Gastroenterology* 1994;106(4):846–858.

102. Ibrahim EM, Ezzat AA, Raja MA, et al. Primary gastric non-Hodgkin's lymphoma: clinical features, management, and prognosis of 185 patients with diffuse large B-cell lymphoma. *Ann Oncol* 1999;10(12):1441–1449.

103. Conley SF, Staszak C, Clamon GH, et al. Non-Hodgkin's lymphoma of the head and neck: the University of Iowa experience. *Laryngoscope* 1987;97(3 Pt 1):291–300.

104. Dunbar SF, Linggood RM, Doppke KP, et al. Conjunctival lymphoma: results and treatment with a single anterior electron field. A lens sparing approach. *Int J Radiat Oncol Biol Phys* 1990;19(2):249–257.

105. Bessell EM, Henk JM, Wright JE, et al. Orbital and conjunctival lymphoma treatment and prognosis. *Radiother Oncol* 1988;13(4):237–244.

106. Chao CK, Lin HS, Devineni VR, et al. Radiation therapy for primary orbital lymphoma. *Int J Radiat Oncol Biol Phys* 1995;31(4):929–934.

107. Doll DC, Weiss RB. Malignant lymphoma of the testis. *Am J Med* 1986;81(3):515–524.

108. Connors JM, Klimo P, Voss N, et al. Testicular lymphoma: improved outcome with early brief chemotherapy. *J Clin Oncol* 1988;6(5):776–781.

109. DeAngelis LM. Primary CNS lymphoma: treatment with combined chemotherapy and radiotherapy. *J Neurooncol* 1999;43(3):249–257.

110. O'Neill BP, O'Fallon JR, Earle JD, et al. Primary central nervous system non-Hodgkin's lymphoma: survival advantages with combined initial therapy? *Int J Radiat Oncol Biol Phys* 1995;33(3):663–673.

111. Gavrilovic IT, Hormigo A, Yahalom J, et al. Long-term follow-up of high-dose methotrexate-based therapy with and without whole brain irradiation for newly diagnosed primary CNS lymphoma. *J Clin Oncol* 2006;24(28):4570–4574.

112. Blay JY, Conroy T, Chevreau C, et al. High-dose methotrexate for the treatment of primary cerebral lymphomas: analysis of survival and late neurologic toxicity in a retrospective series. *J Clin Oncol* 1998;16(3):864–871.

113. Rijlaarsdam J, Willemze R. Primary cutaneous B-cell lymphomas. *Leuk Lymphoma* 1994;14:213–218.

CHAPTER 39

MULTIPLE MYELOMA AND PLASMACYTOMAS

EPIDEMIOLOGY

- The incidence of plasma cell tumors is approximately the same as that for Hodgkin's disease and chronic lymphocytic leukemia (2 to 5 per 100,000).

NATURAL HISTORY

- Plasma cell neoplasms are associated with proliferation and accumulation of CD38/CD138-positive immunoglobulin-secreting cells derived from B-cell lymphocytes.

CLINICAL PRESENTATION

- Common presenting complaints include bone pain (68%), infection (12%), bleeding (7%), and easy fatigability (1).
- Peripheral blood examination usually reveals normocytic anemia.
- Thrombocytopenia, granulocytopenia, or both are present in one third of patients.
- Hyperglobulinemia can lead to hyperviscosity syndromes and coagulopathies.
- Hypercalcemia is present in 50% of patients. Skeletal radiographs demonstrate one of three common patterns: diffuse osteoporosis, well-demarcated lytic lesions, or localized cystic osteolytic lesions.
- Plasma cell tumors secrete a measurable paraprotein "M protein" in 95% to 99% of cases. Free light chain levels are informative in patients who lack measurable M protein. Solitary plasmacytomas secrete a measurable M protein 20% to 60% of the time.
- Immunoglobulin G is found in 50% to 60% of cases and immunoglobulin A in 20% to 25%.

Solitary Plasmacytoma

- Solitary plasmacytomas are localized lesions of the bone (80%) or soft tissue (20%).
- Solitary plasmacytomas account for 2% to 10% of all plasma cell tumors (1,2) and occur with a frequency of 0.34 per 100,000 person years (3).
- Solitary plasmacytomas are more common in African Americans than Whites with a ratio of 1.3:1.
- Solitary plasmacytomas of the bone most frequently involve the vertebral bodies or pelvic bones. Most patients presenting with a solitary plasmacytoma of the bone are considered to have precursor to myeloma (Fig. 39-1).
- A second type of localized presentation occurs in soft tissue (extramedullary plasmacytoma). It arises most frequently (80%) in the upper aerodigestive tract (e.g., nasal cavity, nasopharynx, paranasal sinuses, larynx, tonsils) but is also found in the lung, lymph nodes, spleen, and gastrointestinal tract.
- Survival is significantly better with solitary extramedullary plasmacytoma than with myeloma. Numerous (4) reports support a 40% survival rate at 10 years for osseous plasmacytoma versus 70% for extramedullary.

DIAGNOSTIC WORKUP

Multiple Myeloma

- A complete blood count with differential and peripheral blood smear microscopy should be obtained. Blood chemistries obtained include calcium, creatinine, total protein, albumin, lactate dehydrogenase, and C-reactive protein.

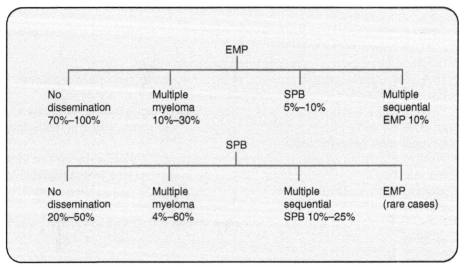

FIGURE 39-1. Evolution of extramedullary plasmacytoma (EMP) and solitary plasmacytoma of the bone (SPB). (Reprinted with permission from Wassermann TH. Multiple myeloma and plasmacytomas. In: Perez CA, Brady LW, eds. *Principles and practice of radiation oncology*, 3rd ed. Philadelphia, PA: Lippincott–Raven, 1998. © Wolters Kluwer.)

- Serum and urine protein electrophoresis, immunoglobulin, and free light chain quantification, along with 24-hour urinary protein excretion, are an essential part of the workup.
- β_2-Microglobulin is a low molecular mass protein that is a function of both myeloma cell mass and renal function. Therefore, the serum level ($\geq$5.5 mg/mL or <3.5 mg/dL) has been useful in staging and prediction of survival (5).
- A bone marrow biopsy must show that at least 10% of cells are plasma cells. Flow cytometry will show a monoclonal population of CD38+/CD138+ cells. Molecular studies of translocations by FISH and conventional cytogenetics are important in assigning risk group (6).
- A complete radiographic skeletal survey is more sensitive than bone scan with Technetium-99m in detecting bony lesions, as the bone lesions from myeloma are a purely lytic phenomenon (7).
- Localized areas of disease should be evaluated by computed tomography (CT) or magnetic resonance imaging (MRI). MRI is essential to assess the extent of myeloma-tous disease in certain disease sites, particularly in the spine where it can also detail the presence of spinal cord or nerve root compression.
- Imaging with 18F-fluorodeoxyglucose positron-emission tomography (FDG-PET) has also shown to be of benefit in assessing the functional definition of lesions seen with other modalities.
- Significant advances in diagnostic imaging have likely resulted in a "stage migration" phenomenon (8).
- Studies have shown that some patients with presumed osseous solitary plasmacytoma will be upstaged following the detection of multiple vertebral lesions or bone marrow disease by MRI and/or FDG-PET (9,10).
- A diagnosis of multiple myeloma requires a specified combination of at least one major and one minor criteria, from the following (11).

Major Criteria

- Biopsy-proven boney or extramedullary plasmacytoma
- Bone marrow plasmacytosis with greater than 10% plasma cells

Minor Criteria (CRAB and SLiM Features)

- Hypercalcemia: serum calcium greater than 1 mg/dL higher than the upper limit of normal or greater than 11 mg/dL.
- Renal dysfunction with creatinine clearance less than 40 mL per minute or serum creatinine greater than 2 mg/dL attributed to myeloma.
- Anemia: hemoglobin value of greater than 20 g/L below the lowest limit of normal.
- Bone disease ($\geq$1 lytic lesion on skeletal radiography, CT, or PET-CT). If the bone marrow has less than 10% clonal plasma cells, more than one bone lesion is required to distinguish from solitary plasmacytoma with minimal marrow involvement.
- Greater than 60% (Sixty) or greater clonal plasma cells found in bone marrow biopsy.
- Light chain involved/uninvolved ratio greater than 100.
- 1 or more focal lesion ($\geq$5 mm each) detected by MRI studies.

- Staging is performed using the International Myeloma Working Group Revised International Staging System, which incorporates chromosomal abnormalities detected by interphase FISH and LDH measurements (12). Older staging systems include the original International Staging System (ISS) (5) and the Durie and Salmon Staging System (15).

International Staging System for Multiple Myeloma

- ISS stage I: Serum beta 2 microglobulin less than 3.5 mg/L and serum albumin ≥3.5 g/dL
- ISS stage II: Not ISS stage I or III
- ISS stage III: Serum beta 2 microglobulin ≥5.5 mg/L

Revised International Staging System for Multiple Myeloma

- Revised International Staging System (R-ISS) stage I: ISS stage I *and* no high-risk chromosomal abnormalities *and* normal LDH.
- R-ISS stage II: Not ISS stage I and III.
- R-ISS stage III: ISS stage III *and* either high-risk chromosomal abnormalities by FISH or elevated LDH.
- High-risk chromosomal abnormalities are defined as del(17p) p53, t(4;14) MMSET, and t(14;16) MAF.

Plasmacytoma

- The workup of a suspected solitary plasmacytoma should be nearly identical to multiple myeloma. Priority should be given to biopsy of the lesion confirming monoclonal plasmacytes.
- A bone marrow biopsy must show less than 10% of cells are plasma cells, and none of the minor criteria (CRAB and SLiM) in multiple myeloma diagnosis (see above) should be met.
- No end-organ damage should be present.
- A trace amount of serum or urine M protein may sometimes be present. Low is defined as IgG less than 3.5 g/dL, IgA less than 2.0 g/dL, and urine monoclonal kappa or lambda less than 1.0 g/24 hours.
- About 30% to 50% of patients with apparent solitary plasmacytoma will have multiple asymptomatic lesions detected in the spine on MRI (13,14).

PROGNOSTIC FACTORS

- There has been a shift toward molecular definition of risk in multiple myeloma away from simply using clinical markers (6,11,15).
- High-risk patients are those with ISS stage II/III disease, or del17p13 (TP53 deletion), by FISH, those with high-risk gene expression profiling signature, or those with t(4:14) involving the FGFR3/MMSET oncogene. These patients have median OS of 2 years and comprise 20% of patients.

- Other high-risk features include t(14:16) involving the c-MAF oncogene locus (5%) and t(14;20) involving the MAFB transcription factor amplification of 1q21 by FISH, or deletion of 13, or evidence of hypodiploidy by cytogenetics.
- Standard-risk patients are those who lack any high- or low-risk abnormalities. They have median overall survival of 7 years.
- Low-risk patients are ISS stage I/II and have no cytogenetic abnormality and are aging less than 55. These have median overall survival approaching 10 years and comprise approximately 20% of patients.
- In a Southwest Oncology Group review of prognostic parameters in 482 patients with myeloma, factors associated with a shortened survival or remission duration were old age, severe anemia, hypercalcemia, blood urea nitrogen greater than 40 mg/dL, markedly elevated M protein, hypoalbuminemia, and high tumor cell burden (16).
- The most easily measurable, quantifiable, and strongest prognostic factors are the serum β_2-microglobulin (greater than 3.5 mg/L) and low serum albumin levels (17).

GENERAL MANAGEMENT

Solitary Plasmacytoma

- Radiation is the primary therapy for osseous solitary plasmacytoma. Surgery is only considered in the case of structural instability or cord compression with rapid neurologic decline (18).
- Even for those patients treated with surgery, postoperative radiation is still indicated secondary to a high likelihood for residual microscopic disease leading to an increased rate of local recurrence (19).
- The local control rate with radiation is 80% to 95%; however, survival with radiation alone is only 50% at 10 years. The reason for the discrepancy is the high rate of progression to multiple myeloma seen with osseous plasmacytomas, generally from 50% to 80% at a median of 2 to 3 years (20,21).
- If all the diagnostic criteria for solitary plasmacytoma are still met, the appropriate management is to give local radiation to the presenting site without systemic therapy (22).
- These patients have a 20% to 80% risk of progression to myeloma within 3 years, and chemotherapy can be started at the time of symptomatic progression. This risk is greater in osseous solitary tumors than extramedullary tumors.
- The use of adjuvant melphalan and prednisone, though shown to have some benefit, is not routinely recommended because of concerns with the effects of long-term alkylating agent use (23).
- A low-level M protein at presentation is very common and is not associated with an increased progression rate to multiple myeloma. However, if it persists postradiation, there is a high rate of subsequent systemic failure (24,25).
- Solitary extramedullary plasmacytomas may be cured by surgery alone if they are small. For larger lesions, inoperable tumors, or residual disease, local radiation should be utilized.

- The progression to myeloma for extramedullary plasmacytomas is much lower than for osseous plasmacytomas, approximately only 10% to 40%. Therefore, many patients are cured of their disease with local radiation alone (4,26,27).
- Although the 10-year survival rates vary, the two largest series report 10-year survival rates of 72% (19) and 78% (26).

Multiple Myeloma

- The initial management of myeloma involves induction therapy comprising of a proteasome inhibitor and immunomodulating agent. Those patients who are transplant eligible go on to receive autologous stem cell transplant (28).
- An important step in the management of symptomatic multiple myeloma is to determine whether the patient is eligible for autologous stem cell transplantation (ASCT). There are significant data from multiple trials showing that ASCT increases complete response, disease-free survival, and overall survival (29,30). Therefore, ASCT has become the standard of care for eligible patients.
- For patients who are transplant ineligible, chemotherapy is usually given until the M protein has reached a plateau followed by maintenance therapy in select patients. The use of lenalidomide maintenance therapy in patients who are transplant ineligible is under debate because of the long-term toxicity associated with treatment (31,32).
- The management of myeloma requires treating the disease as well as the complications from the disease process. Erythropoietic agents and bisphosphonates, along with interventional techniques such as vertebroplasty and kyphoplasty, are all being used more commonly. In particular, bisphosphonate therapy should be considered in all patients in frontline therapy even without the presence of lytic lesions.
- It is necessary to select those patients that will undergo ASCT up front, so that subsequent stem cell harvest is not compromised by induction therapy (33). The initial treatment approach to multiple myeloma is shown in Figure 39-2.

Autologous Stem Cell Transplantation

- Various regimens can be used for induction in ASCT. These include regimens such as bortezomib, lenalidomide, and dexamethasone or carfilzomib, lenalidomide, and dexamethasone. Older high-dose steroid-based and melphalan-based therapies without the inclusion of novel agents are less favored because of comparable or inferior response rates while incurring damage to hematopoietic stem cells (28,34–37).
- Melphalan-based regimens should be avoided as it decreases ASCT harvest yield. It is still a commonly used agent for the conditioning regimen especially in resource-poor environments.
- The mortality rates associated with ASCT are less than 2%, and the transplant is usually an outpatient procedure.
- Double (tandem) transplantation is a planned second ASCT after the patient has recovered from the first. A randomized trial of tandem versus single ASCT has shown increased overall survival with tandem transplant. However, on subsequent analysis,

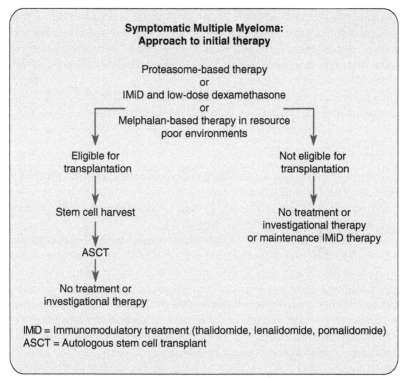

FIGURE 39-2. An approach to initial therapy with symptomatic multiple myeloma. (Adapted from Hodgson DC, Mikhael J, Tsang RW. Plasma cell myeloma and plasmacytoma. In: Halperin EC, Perez CA, Brady LW, eds. *Principles and practice of radiation oncology*, 5th ed. Philadelphia, PA: Lippincott Williams & Wilkins, 2008:1795. © Wolters Kluwer.)

this benefit was confined to those who did not achieve a 90% reduction in their burden of disease after the first ASCT (38). A second randomized trial of patients who received bortezomib-based induction randomized to either single or double transplants showed CR and nCR rates favoring the group randomized to tandem autologous transplant. The largest benefit was seen those who failed to achieve a CR following induction. Currently, tandem transplant is generally reserved for those patients with a suboptimal response to initial ASCT although future upfront use in high-risk patients is under consideration (39).

- Allogeneic stem cell transplant is a potentially curative treatment for myeloma. However, it can only be seriously considered in a small population of patients because of limitations such as age, lack of donors, graft versus host disease, and high treatment-related mortality (40).

Chemotherapy

- The goal of myeloma therapy is not cure, but instead, it is sequential therapy with various agents to prolong disease control and turn the disease into a chronic illness.

- For patients who are not candidates for transplant, induction with a three-drug regimen including a proteasome inhibitor, dexamethasone, and third immunomodulatory or cytotoxic agent is now the mainstay of therapy. Older nonproteasome-based induction regimens have been shown to be largely inferior in a meta-analysis of several phase III trials (41).
- Multiple prospective trials have demonstrated the superiority of adding a third agent to bortezomib and dexamethasone in induction therapy (42–44).

Novel Biologic Agents

- As the armamentarium for myeloma has grown, so has the median survival for patients to over 7 years in standard-risk patients.
- Relapse after ASCT is at a median of 4 years, so new therapies generally have to be added in an effort to prolong disease control.
- Options for therapy after relapse include novel combination of agents such as bortezomib, carfilzomib, and lenalidomide, second ASCT, or investigational targeted therapies. Lenalidomide, a derivative of thalidomide, is an immunomodulatory drug whose efficacy was demonstrated in a randomized trial that compared lenalidomide and dexamethasone with dexamethasone alone in induction therapy for newly diagnosed myeloma. The trial was stopped prematurely because of a significant benefit in favor of the combination arm (45). Lenalidomide with low-dose prednisone is now a mainstay for maintenance therapy for selected low-risk patients, transplant ineligible patients, and after ASCT given evidence from two randomized trials evaluating lenalidomide maintenance versus placebo following ASCT have shown increased PFS advantage of nearly 2 years (31,46).
- Daratumumab is an anti-CD38 human IgG-kappa monoclonal antibody, which has shown significant activity as monotherapy in the relapsed refractory setting (47).

Radiation Therapy

- Indications for radiation therapy include (a) primary treatment in localized presentations (solitary plasmacytomas of the bone and extramedullary plasmacytomas), (b) palliation of pain not controlled by chemotherapy from bone lesions of symptomatic myeloma, (c) prevention of pathologic fractures in weight-bearing bones, and (d) relief of spinal cord compression or nerve root compression.
- Local field external beam radiation with generous margins is the most common radiation technique used to treat myeloma.

TOTAL BODY AND HEMIBODY IRRADIATION

- Some centers incorporate total body irradiation (TBI) into their high-dose chemotherapy conditioning regimen as preparation for transplant. Data from several trials have shown no definitive benefit to the addition of TBI, but most have shown increased toxicity (48–50).

- Hemibody irradiation may be used to palliate diffuse bone pain, although it is rarely done today. The rationale is that the bone marrow in the unirradiated half of the body serves as a reserve for stem cells and it will slowly repopulate the irradiated portion (51–53).
- Pain relief with hemibody irradiation occurs in 80% to 90% of patients, often within 24 to 48 hours, which is more rapid than the pain relief following local irradiation.
- Doses are often 5 to 8 Gy in a single fraction.
- The sequential hemibody radiation technique has been tested as a systemic treatment in a large randomized trial. In a Southwest Oncology Group (SWOG) trial, patients initially treated with chemotherapy who were complete responders were randomized to either sequential hemibody radiation (7.5 Gy in five fractions to the upper hemibody, followed 6 weeks later by lower hemibody treatment) or further chemotherapy. Survival was found to be significantly worse in the radiation arm (54).

Radioimmunotherapy

- Radioimmunotherapy is being tested as an alternative to TBI for conditioning regimens. It is still in the early phases of study, and larger studies are needed to determine what its role may be (55–58).

RADIATION THERAPY TECHNIQUES

Solitary Plasmacytomas

- A common practice is to include one vertebral body above and one vertebral body below the grossly involved vertebra(e). This is based on data from relapse patterns after radiation to solid tumor spinal metastases. As such, it may not be directly applicable to solitary plasmacytoma.
- Radiation portals covering the entire bone, even for long bone lesions, have been recommended by some authors. However, covering the entire long bone is probably not necessary. A study found no marginal recurrences among 30 patients with solitary plasmacytoma treated with radiation to the tumor plus a margin (59).
- Plasmacytomas frequently extend into the adjacent soft tissues, requiring diligent evaluation for the true tumor extent.
- MRI is particularly helpful in defining boney and soft tissue extension.
- For osseous plasmacytoma, prophylactic nodal irradiation is not needed as the regional nodal failure rate after involved-field radiation is quite low (0% to 4%) (60).
- However, for extramedullary plasmacytomas, the necessity of prophylactic nodal radiation is controversial (27,61). For extramedullary plasmacytoma of Waldeyer's ring, first echelon cervical nodes should be included in the treatment fields. More generally for any extramedullary plasmacytoma of the head and neck, the elective nodes that would be covered if it were a squamous cell cancer should also be covered for the plasmacytoma.

- Treatment portals usually consist of parallel-opposed fields and include the gross tumor plus a 2- to 3-cm margin. However, more complex treatment plans including 3DCRT and IMRT are often needed for tumors located in areas such as the head and neck region and can be used for other sites as this represents curative, definitive treatment to doses of 45 to 50 Gy.
- Exact dose to be used is controversial. Several reports have shown good local control in greater than 85% of tumors that are less than 5 cm in size with 35 to 40 Gy. However, tumors greater than 5 cm, usually extramedullary plasmacytomas, require doses of 45 to 50 Gy (19,59,60).

Multiple Myeloma

- The role of radiation in myeloma is primarily for palliation or pain relief. A palliative dose of 20 to 30 Gy is recommended based on the extent of disease and whether or not there is cord compression (62,63).
- A multicenter study compared 30 Gy in 10 fractions, 10 Gy in 5 fractions, and 8 Gy in 1 fraction for patients who had cord compression. It found that the protracted course of 30 Gy in 10 fractions was associated with an improved neurologic recovery (64). Single fractions of 8 and 30 Gy in 10 fractions have similar analgesic efficacy in myeloma (65).
- Concurrent chemotherapy given with radiation appears not to have an impact on pain relief (63).
- Concurrent radiotherapy with novel proteasome agents has been shown to be safe without increased acute adverse events (66).
- It is important to use skin tattoos for reproducing patient setup and to assess the location of the field for future retreatment in cases in which 3D records are not available.
- It is mandatory to keep fields in the pelvis, and in other areas involving abundant bone marrow activity, as small as possible to maximize marrow function for future chemotherapy.
- In patients with large lytic lesions in weight-bearing bones such as the femur, orthopedic stabilization procedures should be considered. Whether irradiation is delivered before or after bone fixation is probably not of critical importance, although many institutions prefer delivering postoperative irradiation.

ACKNOWLEDGMENT

This is dedicated to the clinical and research team who worked in the Myeloma Group, Metabolism Branch of the National Cancer Institute during the years of 2012–2014—for their hard work, creativity, and pursuit of a cure for patients with multiple myeloma.

References

1. Wassermann T. Multiple myeloma and plasmacytomas. In: Perez C, Brady L, eds. *Principles and practice of radiation oncology*, 3rd ed. Philadelphia, PA: Lippincott–Raven, 1998:2013–2023.
2. Hodgson D, Mikhael J, Tsang R. Plasma cell myeloma and plasmacytoma. In: Halperin E, Perez C, Brady L, eds. *Principles and practice of radiation oncology*. Philadelphia, PA: Lippincott Williams & Wilkins, 2013:1606–1607.

3. Jawad MU, Scully SP. Skeletal plasmacytoma: progression of disease and impact of local treatment; an analysis of SEER database. *J Hematol Oncol* 2009;2:41.

4. Wiltshaw E. The natural history of extramedullary plasmacytoma and its relation to solitary myeloma of bone and myelomatosis. *Medicine* 1976;55(3):217–238.

5. Greipp PR, et al. International staging system for multiple myeloma. *J Clin Oncol* 2005;23(15): 3412–3420.

6. Avet-Loiseau H, et al. Combining fluorescent in situ hybridization data with ISS staging improves risk assessment in myeloma: an International Myeloma Working Group collaborative project. *Leukemia* 2013;27(3):711–717.

7. Durie BG, et al. Myeloma management guidelines: a consensus report from the Scientific Advisors of the International Myeloma Foundation. *Hematol J* 2003;4(6):379–398.

8. Feinstein AR, Sosin DM, Wells CK. The Will Rogers phenomenon. Stage migration and new diagnostic techniques as a source of misleading statistics for survival in cancer. *N Engl J Med* 1985;312(25):1604–1608.

9. Liebross RH, et al. Solitary bone plasmacytoma: outcome and prognostic factors following radiotherapy. *Int J Radiat Oncol Biol Phys* 1998;41(5):1063–1067.

10. Schirrmeister H, et al. Positron emission tomography (PET) for staging of solitary plasmacytoma. *Cancer Biother Radiopharm* 2003;18(5):841–845.

11. Rajkumar SV, et al. International Myeloma Working Group updated criteria for the diagnosis of multiple myeloma. *Lancet Oncol* 2014;15(12):e538–e548.

12. Palumbo A, et al. Revised International Staging System for multiple myeloma: a report from International Myeloma Working Group. *J Clin Oncol* 2015;33(26):2863–2869.

13. Mariette X, et al. Prognostic value of vertebral lesions detected by magnetic resonance imaging in patients with stage I multiple myeloma. *Br J Haematol* 1999;104(4):723–729.

14. Moulopoulos LA, et al. Magnetic resonance imaging in the staging of solitary plasmacytoma of bone. *J Clin Oncol* 1993;11(7):1311–1315.

15. Chng WJ, et al. IMWG consensus on risk stratification in multiple myeloma. *Leukemia* 2014;28(2):269–277.

16. Alexanian R, et al. Prognostic factors in multiple myeloma. *Cancer* 1975;36(4):1192–1201.

17. Bataille R, et al. Prognostic factors and staging in multiple myeloma: a reappraisal. *J Clin Oncol* 1986;4(1):80–87.

18. Sundaresan N, et al. Indications and results of combined anterior-posterior approaches for spine tumor surgery. *J Neurosurg* 1996;85(3):438–446.

19. Ozsahin M, et al. Outcomes and patterns of failure in solitary plasmacytoma: a multicenter rare cancer network study of 258 patients. *Int J Radiat Oncol Biol Phys* 2006;64(1):210–217.

20. Wilder RB, et al. Persistence of myeloma protein for more than one year after radiotherapy is an adverse prognostic factor in solitary plasmacytoma of bone. *Cancer* 2002;94(5):1532–1537.

21. Frassica DA, et al. Solitary plasmacytoma of bone: Mayo Clinic experience. *Int J Radiat Oncol Biol Phys* 1989;16(1):43–48.

22. Soutar R, et al. Guidelines on the diagnosis and management of solitary plasmacytoma of bone and solitary extramedullary plasmacytoma. *Br J Haematol* 2004;124(6):717–726.

23. Aviles A, et al. Improved outcome in solitary bone plasmacytoma with combined therapy. *Hematol Oncol* 1996;14(3):111–117.

24. Galieni P, et al. Solitary plasmacytoma of bone and extramedullary plasmacytoma: two different entities? *Ann Oncol* 1995;6(7):687–691.

25. Dimopoulos MA, et al. Curability of solitary bone plasmacytoma. *J Clin Oncol* 1992;10(4): 587–590.

26. Galieni P, et al. Clinical outcome of extramedullary plasmacytoma. *Haematologica* 2000; 85(1):47–51.

27. Strojan P, et al. Extramedullary plasmacytoma: clinical and histopathologic study. *Int J Radiat Oncol Biol Phys* 2002;53(3):692–701.

28. Cavo M, et al. International Myeloma Working Group consensus approach to the treatment of multiple myeloma patients who are candidates for autologous stem cell transplantation. *Blood* 2011;117(23):6063–6073.

29. Attal M, et al. A prospective, randomized trial of autologous bone marrow transplantation and chemotherapy in multiple myeloma. Intergroupe Francais du Myelome. *N Engl J Med* 1996;335(2): 91–97.

30. Kumar A, et al. Management of multiple myeloma: a systematic review and critical appraisal of published studies. *Lancet Oncol* 2003;4(5):293–304.

31. McCarthy PL, et al. Lenalidomide after stem-cell transplantation for multiple myeloma. *N Engl J Med* 2012;366(19):1770–1781.

32. Palumbo A, et al. Second primary malignancies with lenalidomide therapy for newly diagnosed myeloma: a meta-analysis of individual patient data. *Lancet Oncol* 2014;15(3):333–342.

33. Goldschmidt H, et al. Factors influencing collection of peripheral blood progenitor cells following high-dose cyclophosphamide and granulocyte colony-stimulating factor in patients with multiple myeloma. *Br J Haematol* 1997;98(3):736–744.

34. Alexanian R, et al. Primary dexamethasone treatment of multiple myeloma. *Blood* 1992;80(4): 887–890.

35. Samson D, et al. Infusion of vincristine and doxorubicin with oral dexamethasone as first-line therapy for multiple myeloma. *Lancet* 1989;2(8668):882–885.

36. Rajkumar SV, et al. Combination therapy with thalidomide plus dexamethasone for newly diagnosed myeloma. *J Clin Oncol* 2002;20(21):4319–4323.

37. Moreau P, Hulin C, Facon T. Frontline therapy for patients with multiple myeloma not eligible for stem cell transplantation. *Hematol Oncol Clin North Am* 2014;28(5):829–838.

38. Attal M, et al. Single versus double autologous stem-cell transplantation for multiple myeloma. *N Engl J Med* 2003;349(26):2495–2502.

39. Cavo M, et al. Prospective, randomized study of single compared with double autologous stem-cell transplantation for multiple myeloma: Bologna 96 clinical study. *J Clin Oncol* 2007;25(17): 2434–2441.

40. Tricot G, et al. Graft-versus-myeloma effect: proof of principle. *Blood* 1996;87(3):1196–1198.

41. Sonneveld P, et al. Bortezomib-based versus nonbortezomib-based induction treatment before autologous stem-cell transplantation in patients with previously untreated multiple myeloma: a meta-analysis of phase III randomized, controlled trials. *J Clin Oncol* 2013;31(26):3279–3287.

42. Cavo M, et al. Bortezomib with thalidomide plus dexamethasone compared with thalidomide plus dexamethasone as induction therapy before, and consolidation therapy after, double autologous stem-cell transplantation in newly diagnosed multiple myeloma: a randomised phase 3 study. *Lancet* 2010;376(9758):2075–2085.

43. Rosinol L, et al. Superiority of bortezomib, thalidomide, and dexamethasone (VTD) as induction pretransplantation therapy in multiple myeloma: a randomized phase 3 PETHEMA/GEM study. *Blood* 2012;120(8):1589–1596.

44. Cavo M, et al. Bortezomib-thalidomide-dexamethasone is superior to thalidomide-dexamethasone as consolidation therapy after autologous hematopoietic stem cell transplantation in patients with newly diagnosed multiple myeloma. *Blood* 2012;120(1):9–19.

45. Dimopoulos MA, et al. Long-term follow-up on overall survival from the MM-009 and MM-010 phase III trials of lenalidomide plus dexamethasone in patients with relapsed or refractory multiple myeloma. *Leukemia* 2009;23(11):2147–2152.

46. Attal M, et al. Lenalidomide maintenance after stem-cell transplantation for multiple myeloma. *N Engl J Med* 2012;366(19):1782–1791.

47. Lonial S, et al. Daratumumab monotherapy in patients with treatment-refractory multiple myeloma (SIRIUS): an open-label, randomised, phase 2 trial. *Lancet* 2016;387(10027):1551–1560.

48. Moreau P, et al. Comparison of 200 mg/m(2) melphalan and 8 Gy total body irradiation plus 140 mg/m(2) melphalan as conditioning regimens for peripheral blood stem cell transplantation in patients with newly diagnosed multiple myeloma: final analysis of the Intergroupe Francophone du Myelome 9502 randomized trial. *Blood* 2002;99(3):731–735.

49. Lahuerta JJ, et al. Myeloablative treatments for multiple myeloma: update of a comparative study of different regimens used in patients from the Spanish registry for transplantation in multiple myeloma. *Leuk Lymphoma* 2002;43(1):67–74.

50. Abraham R, et al. Intensification of the stem cell transplant induction regimen results in increased treatment-related mortality without improved outcome in multiple myeloma. *Bone Marrow Transplant* 1999;24(12):1291–1297.

51. Bosch A, Frias Z. Radiotherapy in the treatment of multiple myeloma. *Int J Radiat Oncol Biol Phys* 1988;15(6):1363–1369.

52. McSweeney EN, et al. Double hemibody irradiation (DHBI) in the management of relapsed and primary chemoresistant multiple myeloma. *Clin Oncol (R Coll Radiol)* 1993;5(6):378–383.

53. Tobias JS, et al. Hemibody irradiation in multiple myeloma. *Radiother Oncol* 1985;3(1):11–16.

54. Salmon SE, et al. Chemotherapy is superior to sequential hemibody irradiation for remission consolidation in multiple myeloma: a Southwest Oncology Group study. *J Clin Oncol* 1990;8(9):1575–1584.

55. Dispenzieri A, et al. A phase I study of 153Sm-EDTMP with fixed high-dose melphalan as a peripheral blood stem cell conditioning regimen in patients with multiple myeloma. *Leukemia* 2005;19(1):118–125.

56. Hogan WJ, et al. Successful treatment of POEMS syndrome with autologous hematopoietic progenitor cell transplantation. *Bone Marrow Transplant* 2001;28(3):305–309.

57. Giralt S, et al. 166Ho-DOTMP plus melphalan followed by peripheral blood stem cell transplantation in patients with multiple myeloma: results of two phase 1/2 trials. *Blood* 2003;102(7):2684–2691.

58. Kennedy GA, et al. Outcome of myeloablative allogeneic stem cell transplantation in multiple myeloma with a 153Sm-EDTMP-based preparative regimen. *Leukemia* 2005;19(5):879–880.

59. Jyothirmayi R, et al. Radiotherapy in the treatment of solitary plasmacytoma. *Br J Radiol* 1997;70(833):511–516.

60. Tsang RW, et al. Solitary plasmacytoma treated with radiotherapy: impact of tumor size on outcome. *Int J Radiat Oncol Biol Phys* 2001;50(1):113–120.

61. Hu K, Yahalom J. Radiotherapy in the management of plasma cell tumors. *Oncology (Williston Park)* 2000;14(1):101–108, 111; discussion 111–112, 115.

62. Mill WB, Griffith R. The role of radiation therapy in the management of plasma cell tumors. *Cancer* 1980;45(4):647–652.

63. Leigh BR, et al. Radiation therapy for the palliation of multiple myeloma. *Int J Radiat Oncol Biol Phys* 1993;25(5):801–804.

64. Rades D, et al. Short-course radiotherapy is not optimal for spinal cord compression due to myeloma. *Int J Radiat Oncol Biol Phys* 2006;64(5):1452–1457.

65. Rudzianskiene M, et al. Single vs. multiple fraction regimens for palliative radiotherapy treatment of multiple myeloma: a prospective randomised study. *Strahlenther Onkol* 2017;193(9):742–749.

66. Shin SM, et al. Feasibility and efficacy of local radiotherapy with concurrent novel agents in patients with multiple myeloma. *Clin Lymphoma Myeloma Leuk* 2014;14(6):480–484.

CHAPTER 40

PRIMARY BONE TUMORS, INCLUDING EWING'S SARCOMA

- Primary bone neoplasms are rare (0.2% of all cancer diagnoses, per SEER database) with about 3,260 new cases and 1,550 deaths in 2017 in the United States (1). The majority of bone lesions identified clinically or radiographically are metastatic lesions.
- The most common primary bone tumors (in order of decreasing prevalence and excluding multiple myeloma) are osteosarcoma, chondrosarcoma, and Ewing's sarcoma. Other histologies include fibrosarcoma, undifferentiated pleomorphic sarcoma (previously known as malignant fibrous histiocytoma), myxofibrosarcoma, giant cell tumor, aneurysmal bone cyst, adamantinoma, angiosarcoma, and chordoma.
- Osteosarcoma is the most common malignant bone tumor in children and adolescents. It has a bimodal distribution with the second peak of incidence occurring in adults older than 65 years of age.
  - Osteosarcoma is associated with Li-Fraumeni syndrome (germ-line TP53 mutation), retinoblastoma, bone dysplasia (e.g., Paget's disease), or prior chemotherapy or radiation.
- Ewing's sarcoma is a tumor of neuroectodermal origin and is the second most common malignant pediatric bone tumor (after osteosarcoma), affecting mostly young white adolescents.

ANATOMY

- Osteosarcomas occur in areas of rapid bone growth in the metaphyseal region of tubular long bones in 85% of cases, particularly in the distal femur or proximal tibia. Osteosarcomas of flat bones are rare and are usually associated with Paget's disease (2).
- Chondrosarcomas may occur in any bone but occur most commonly in the pelvis, proximal femur, and shoulder. Skull base chondrosarcomas usually arise from the sphenooccipital junction or the clivus.
- Similar to osteosarcomas, fibrosarcomas, undifferentiated pleomorphic sarcomas, and malignant giant cell tumors often occur in the femur or tibia, mostly in the metaphyseal or epiphyseal region.
- Chordomas are malignant tumors arising from embryonic notochord remnants. Fifty percent originate in the sacrococcygeal region, 35% in the base of the skull, and 15% in the remaining spine.

- Aneurysmal bone cysts can occur in any bone, but most frequently occur in lower extremity long bones and vertebrae.
- Ewing's sarcoma mostly occurs in the lower extremities (45%), followed by the pelvis (25%), chest wall (20%), and upper extremities (10%).

CLINICAL PRESENTATION AND NATURAL HISTORY

- Osteosarcomas (and chondrosarcomas) usually present with local swelling and pain of the involved area. Joint effusion and pathologic fracture at presentation are uncommon.
- Metastases from osteosarcoma are present in 15% to 20% of patients at diagnosis and in 80% at 18 months if treated without chemotherapy. The primary mode of spread is hematogenous, and the most common metastatic site is the lungs, followed by bones (3). Five-year overall survival (OS) for osteosarcoma is typically 60% to 75%, but only 20% if metastatic at presentation. Low-grade osteosarcomas rarely metastasize and are curable with surgical resection alone.
- Only a third of chondrosarcomas are high-grade. They may be more locally aggressive but follow a more indolent course than osteosarcomas.
- Distant metastasis is less common with chondrosarcoma than with osteosarcoma, but similar to osteosarcomas, the most common site of distant metastasis is the lungs. Chondrosarcomas may dedifferentiate to aggressive fibrosarcomas or osteosarcomas (4).
- Chondrosarcomas in the pediatric population are aggressive and behave like classic osteosarcomas (5). Five-year OS for chondrosarcoma is 50% to 70%.
- The histologic grade of fibrosarcomas (low, intermediate, and high or anaplastic) determines how they behave. High-grade fibrosarcomas are locally aggressive and behave like osteosarcomas, resulting in a 5-year survival rate of 27% (6). Periosteal and low-grade fibrosarcomas are less aggressive, with 5- and 10-year survival rates of 50%.
- Pathologic fractures are more common with fibrosarcomas and undifferentiated pleomorphic sarcomas than with other types of bone tumors.
- Chordomas are slow-growing, locally aggressive malignant tumors, which usually present late in the disease or with very large primary lesions (7). They have a 10% to 25% incidence of metastases (much lower distant metastasis rate at diagnosis of approximately 5%).
- The clinical symptoms of chordoma are dependent on location or presentation. Pain and abnormal gait may be related to cord compression or nerve root compression, which predominate in paraspinal and sacrococcygeal lesions. Other presenting symptoms include dysphagia, dysphonia, diplopia, headache, or cranial nerve deficits for H&N chordomas and GI symptoms for sacral chordomas.
- Undifferentiated pleomorphic sarcoma of bone is very aggressive locally and has a high rate of lung metastases, with most recurrences appearing within 21 months of diagnosis (8).

- Malignant transformation of benign giant cell tumors must be strongly suspected if recurrence is discovered more than 5 years after treatment. Malignant degeneration after surgery is usually of lower histologic grade than after radiation therapy.
- Ewing's sarcoma usually presents with localized pain and swelling of the affected bone, and some present with systemic symptoms. Twenty-five percent of the patients present with overt metastasis, usually to the lungs (50%). Even with localized disease, 25% of patients have micrometastases.

DIAGNOSTIC WORKUP

- Table 40-1 outlines the suggested diagnostic workup for malignant bone tumors.
- Standard imaging techniques include plain x-ray films ("sunburst" appearance, osteoid formation under the periosteum, and Codman's triangle are seen with osteosarcomas versus "onion skinning" and Codman's triangle in Ewing's sarcoma), computed tomography (CT), and magnetic resonance (MR) imaging of the affected bone and surrounding soft tissues. MRI is indispensable to evaluate involvement of nerves, vessels, and joint space. Whole-body radionuclide bone and chest CT scans (with IV contrast) are included to evaluate for lung and bone metastases (6,9). Positron emission tomography (PET)/CT is less sensitive than bone scan and chest CT.

Table 40-1

Diagnostic Workup for Bone Tumors

General
History
Physical examination

Special Studies
Open biopsy, avoiding incision over area not to be irradiated
Bone marrow aspiration and biopsy (for Ewing's sarcoma)

Radiologic Studies
Standard
Plain radiography of bone and chest
Computed tomography of affected bone, surrounding soft tissue, and lungs
Radionuclide bone scan
Magnetic resonance imaging of affected bone and surrounding soft tissue
Optional
Angiography, PET/CT

Laboratory Studies
Complete blood cell count on admission
Blood chemistry profile
Urinalysis
Erythrocyte sedimentation rate, alkaline phosphatase

- Site-specific CT and MR imaging are important in evaluating chordomas because of the presence of soft tissue component. Other radiologic features of chordoma include irregular bone destruction, with or without areas of calcification.
- The typical presentation of undifferentiated pleomorphic sarcoma (with or without a pathologic fracture) is a predominantly metaphyseal radiolucent lesion, frequently with epiphyseal extension.
- It is not possible to absolutely differentiate a benign from a malignant giant cell tumor by radiographic examination (6,9,10).
- Aneurysmal bone cysts are usually well-defined, expansile metaphyseal or diaphyseal lesions characterized by a blowout appearance with internal septa and ridges (9).

STAGING SYSTEMS

- There is no universally accepted staging system for primary bone sarcomas.
- The Musculoskeletal Tumor Society (MSTS) or Enneking staging system classifies tumors according to grade, local extent, and presence or absence of distant metastases (11) (Table 40-2).

NEW!   SUMMARY OF CHANGES TO AJCC STAGING

- Grading no longer has a G4, undifferentiated designation.
- T stage groupings differ based on site:
  - For tumors of the appendicular skeleton, trunk, skull, and facial bones, the T staging is unchanged, with less than or equal to 8 cm (T1), greater than 8 cm (T2), and discontinuous tumors (T3).
  - For primary spine tumors, T stage is based on number of segments and extension, with 1 to 2 adjacent segments (T1), 3 adjacent segments (T2), greater than or equal to 4 segments or nonadjacent segments (T3), and extension into the spinal canal (T4a) or great vessels (T4b).
  - For pelvic tumors, T stage is based on size and extension, with tumor in 1 segment without extraosseous extension (T1, less than or equal to 8 cm T1a, and greater than 8 cm T1b), 2 segments without or 1 segment with extraosseous extension (T2, less than or equal to 8 cm T2a, and greater than 8 cm T2b), 2 segments with extraosseous extension (T3, less than or equal to 8 cm T3a, and greater than 8 cm T3b), and 3 segments or crossing the sacroiliac joint (T4, involving sacroiliac joint and medial to sacral neuroforamen T4a, encasing external iliacs or tumor thrombus in major vessels T4b).
- M stage is unchanged, with M1a denoting lung-only metastases, and M1b denoting metastases to other distant sites.
- Overall staging changes are limited; effectively, all grade 2 disease moved into high-grade categories.

See Amin MB, Edge SB, Greene FL, et al., eds. *AJCC cancer staging manual*, 8th ed. New York, NY: Springer, 2017.

Table 40-2
Enneking Staging System for Bone Sarcomas

Grade (G)

G1, low grade	Parosteal osteosarcoma
	Endosteal osteosarcoma
	Secondary chondrosarcoma
	Fibrosarcoma, low grade
	Atypical undifferentiated pleomorphic sarcoma
	Giant cell tumor
	Adamantinoma
G2, high grade	Classic osteosarcoma
	Radiation-induced sarcoma
	Paget's sarcoma
	Primary chondrosarcoma
	Fibrosarcoma, high grade
	Undifferentiated pleomorphic sarcoma
	Giant cell sarcoma

Local Extent (T)

T1, intracompartmental	Intraosseous
	Paraosseous
T2, extracompartmental	Soft tissue extension
	Extrafascial or deep fascial extension

Metastases (M)

M0	No distant metastases
M1	Distant metastases exist

Staging Grouping

IA	G1	T1	M0
IB	G1	T2	M0
IIA	G2	T1	M0
IIB	G2	T2	M0
III	G1 or G2	T1 or T2	M1

Reprinted with permission from Enneking WF, Spanier SS, Goodman MA. A system for staging musculoskeletal sarcoma. *Clin Orthop* 1980;153:106.

PATHOLOGIC CLASSIFICATION

- Malignant osteoid (immature bone) production is a histologic hallmark of osteosarcomas. Classic or conventional osteosarcoma makes up about 80% of all osteosarcomas, arises from intramedullary bone, and is usually poorly differentiated. Juxtacortical osteosarcomas are less common and are usually low- or intermediate-grade.
- "Skip" bone metastasis may be seen with osteosarcomas. These consist of an additional, smaller focus of osteosarcoma in the same bone or a second bone lesion on the opposing side of a joint space, with no gross or microscopic continuity or pulmonary metastases.

- Conventional chondrosarcoma is the most common histologic subtype. They are classified according to grade (grade 1 [well differentiated] to 3 [poorly differentiated]) or as atypical cartilaginous tumor (grade 1) or malignant tumors (grade 2 or 3).
- Fibrosarcomas are rare malignant tumors characterized by the predominance of fibroblasts without osteoid or cartilage formation.
- Conventional chordomas (with characteristic physaliphorous cells) are the most common histologic subtypes. Chondroid and dedifferentiated chordomas are much less common.
- Undifferentiated pleomorphic sarcoma of bone is formed of a mixture of spindle-shaped fibroblasts, mononuclear cells with histiocytic morphology, and anaplastic giant cells. Like fibrosarcomas, there is no osteoid or cartilage formation. The extent of local spread on pathologic examination is almost always greater than is visible by routine radiography (6).
- Only 15% of giant cell tumors are malignant. These tumors have nonneoplastic multinucleated giant cells (osteoclastic origin) and neoplastic giant cell tumor stromal cells (osteoblastic origin). Grade is not a reliable prognosticator in giant cell tumors (also known as osteoclastomas).
- Ewing's sarcomas are characterized by small round blue cells of the bone marrow and characteristic gene fusions, most commonly t(11;22) EWS-FLI1 (85%), less commonly t(21:22) EWS-ERG (10%). All Ewing's sarcomas are automatically grade 4.

PROGNOSTIC FACTORS

- The most important prognostic factors in osteosarcoma are resectability and metastasis at presentation. Radiation-induced osteosarcoma has a worse prognosis.
- Prognostic factors in chondrosarcoma include histologic grade, size, cell type, location, stage at presentation, patient age, degree of local aggressiveness, and presence or absence of pain at presentation (12). Metastases developed in 0% of patients with grade 1 chondrosarcoma, 10% with grade 2, and 73% with grade 3 (13).
- The metastatic rate for low-grade fibrosarcoma is 5% to 15%. The rate of distant metastasis for high-grade fibrosarcoma is equal to that of osteosarcoma (5). The overall 5-, 10-, and 20-year survival rates are 34%, 28%, and 25%, respectively (12).
- The most important prognostic indicators for chordoma are site of origin and local extension of tumor (14,15).
- Although undifferentiated pleomorphic sarcoma is very aggressive with a poor prognosis (5), it is less aggressive than fibrosarcomas and osteosarcomas (16). Survival rates of 58% and 43% at 5 and 10 years, respectively, have been reported (6).
- For Ewing's sarcoma, pelvic/axial site, older age (greater than 15), size greater than 8 cm, and abnormal labs (especially erythrocyte sedimentation rate [ESR] and lactate dehydrogenase [LDH]) are associated with poor prognosis. Presence of metastatic disease is the worst prognostic factor. Tumor volumes of greater than 100 or greater than 200 mL have also been correlated with worse outcomes.

GENERAL MANAGEMENT

Osteosarcoma

- Initial management includes a small incision for biopsy and meticulous closure to promote healing; optimally, the biopsy will be performed by or under the direction of the operating surgeon and included in the management plan.
- The best treatment for osteosarcoma is a limb-sparing strategy, which includes neoadjuvant chemotherapy and surgical resection +/– adjuvant chemotherapy (17,18).
  - Patients treated with less radical (limb-salvage) surgery have the same survival characteristics as those treated with more aggressive procedures.
  - Soft tissue problems (e.g., wound necrosis), which are the most frequent complications in limb-salvage surgery, have decreased with the aggressive use of rotational and free flaps at the time of surgery.
- Rosen et al. (19) reported a response rate of 77% with doxorubicin, vincristine, high-dose methotrexate, and cyclophosphamide.
- A randomized trial by the European Organization for Research and Treatment of Cancer (EORTC) showed that a short-term, aggressive, preoperative chemotherapy regimen in operable osteosarcoma gives the same results (in terms of toxicity, percentage of necrosis, and outcome) as longer and more complex multiagent chemotherapy regimens (20).
- Postoperative adjuvant chemotherapy was shown to improve 6 year event-free survival (EFS, 11% versus 61%, $p < 0.001$) by the Multi-Institutional Osteosarcoma Study (21) and disease-free and overall survival in another randomized trial (22).
- One retrospective study showed that, in patients with nonmetastatic extremity osteosarcoma who refused surgery, fractionated external beam radiation therapy (EBRT) to 60 Gy showed excellent overall survival, local control, metastases-free survival, and limb function at 5 years only in patients with good response to induction chemotherapy (23).
- Combined radiation therapy and chemotherapy are recommended for extrapulmonary metastases and small primary lesions in patients with metastatic disease (19).
- A retrospective series suggested that EBRT can help improve local control in patients with close or positive surgical margins. Doses greater than 55 Gy are possibly associated with better control (24).
- For patients with pelvic osteosarcomas, chemotherapy and surgery are mainstay treatments, but radiotherapy improves overall survival in patients who cannot get surgery or when the margin is intralesional (25).
- Unresectable osteosarcomas of the trunk showed favorable response with excellent local control and functional status with carbon-ion radiotherapy (26).
- Resection of pulmonary metastases may improve patient survival (27). Pulmonary irradiation, either alone or with chemotherapy, has been investigated but has not been demonstrated to have significant benefit (28,29).

Chondrosarcoma

- The treatment of choice for chondrosarcoma is surgery.
- The 5-year survival rate for patients with chondrosarcoma is 6% with biopsy alone; average survival without therapy is 1.8 years (30).
- The standard surgical procedure is wide total excision with possible amputation, including the biopsy tract and avoiding tumor exposure during the operation. Maximal safe surgical resection is usually recommended for skull base chondrosarcoma.
- Radiation therapy has been advocated for inoperable lesions, close/positive margins, and for palliation (10,31,32). Skull base chondrosarcoma usually requires adjuvant radiation therapy because of the difficulty of obtaining negative margins.
- A retrospective study reported 98% 10-year local control in 200 patients with skull base chondrosarcoma treated with postoperative combined proton/photon radiotherapy (median dose 72 cobalt GyE [CGyE]) (33). Combined surgery and postoperative photon and/or proton irradiation for extracranial chondrosarcomas resulted in 5-year local control and overall survival of 57% and 68%, respectively.
- Unresectable non–skull base chondrosarcomas showed favorable response with excellent local control and functional status with carbon-ion radiotherapy (34).
- The role of chemotherapy is not well defined for chondrosarcomas; for mesenchymal subtypes, Ewing's sarcoma regimens are recommended, and for dedifferentiated chondrosarcoma, osteosarcoma management paradigms may be followed.

Undifferentiated Pleomorphic Sarcoma of Bone

- Primary treatment traditionally has been aggressive surgery involving radical resection, amputation, or disarticulation.
- Radiation therapy responses have occurred predominantly with histiocytic rather than fibrocytic histologies (12).
- Reagan et al. (35) reported postoperative tumor control in 75% of patients with undifferentiated pleomorphic sarcoma of bone who were treated with a combination of photons and electrons (median dose of 60 Gy in 43 days).
- Hirano et al. (36) reported encouraging results with intraoperative radiation therapy delivery of 15 to 30 Gy.

Giant Cell Tumor

- Cassady et al. (10) recommended surgery as the primary therapy for giant cell tumors, reserving irradiation for when specifically warranted.
- Radiation therapy is used for inoperable lesions, incomplete resections, and local recurrences after surgery. It is also used in cases in which significant functional disability will occur if surgery is performed.

Aneurysmal Bone Cyst

- Surgery with curettage and bone grafting or cryosurgery, if possible, is the preferred treatment.
- Nobler et al. (37) showed a decrease in local recurrence from 32% to 8% with 20 to 30 Gy of postoperative irradiation.
- Radiation therapy alone has excellent outcomes when surgery is not possible (38).

Chordoma

- A combination of surgery and postoperative irradiation is considered standard treatment for resectable chordomas. There is a high risk of seeding along biopsy tracts, which should be marked and surgically removed if a biopsy is performed.
- Radical surgery and radiation therapy often are limited with chordomas because of the proximity of neural structures, especially at the base of the skull and the spine, often resulting in local recurrence. In general, local control is worse for chordomas than for chondrosarcomas.
- Radiation therapy as a single modality is the standard procedure for definitive treatment when surgery is not indicated.
- Combined photon/proton radiotherapy or proton therapy alone has been associated with excellent local control rates for chordomas either treated definitively or following maximal safe surgical resection (39–41).
- Unresectable sacral chordomas treated with carbon-ion radiotherapy achieved 77% and 81% 5-year local control and overall survival, respectively, while maintaining 97% ambulation in surviving patients. Grade 3 and 4 toxicities were limited (42).
- The role of chemotherapy is not well defined for chordomas; tyrosine kinase inhibitors may be utilized, as well as mTOR inhibitors.

Ewing's Sarcoma

- Treatment overview: Induction chemotherapy (vincristine, doxorubicin, cyclophosphamide [VDC] alternating with ifosfamide and etoposide [IE]) for 12 weeks followed by local therapy, and further adjuvant chemotherapy for a total of 48 weeks (43–45).
- Both surgery and irradiation are acceptable local therapy options, depending on tumor location and resectability.
- Surgery is recommended when complete resection is possible. Postoperative radiation is recommended for positive margins and tumor spillage and with poor response to chemotherapy.
- Whole-lung irradiation is recommended for lung metastases (46). Alternatively, resection is accepted with limited number of metastases (fewer than 5).

RADIATION THERAPY TECHNIQUES

- Whenever possible, radiation therapy should be performed as part of a multidisciplinary management plan, with treatment volumes discussed with the surgical team and coordinated with systemic therapy where indicated.
- Definitive radiation therapy requires meticulous planning and patient immobilization; axial contrast-enhanced CT and MRI imaging should be obtained in the treatment position and registered or fused to treatment planning imaging to optimally delineate the target lesion.
- In the postoperative setting, identifying both the preoperative and postoperative extent of disease/postoperative cavity will be necessary to define target volumes.
  - In general, all gross disease (GTV) prior to systemic therapy (if administered) and surgery should be treated with a clinical target volume (CTV) expansion of at least 1 cm, as well as a planning target volume (PTV) expansion defined by the treating institution (generally 0.5 to 1 cm) to doses of 45 to 50.4 Gy in conventional 1.8 to 2 Gy fractions. Additional radiation therapy to a reduced/cone-down field can be administered with definitive intent or to residual/postchemotherapy disease, with lower doses for chemotherapy-sensitive tumors such as Ewing's sarcoma and higher doses for chemotherapy- and/or radiation therapy-insensitive tumors such as chordoma, chondrosarcoma, and osteosarcoma.
- Preoperative radiation therapy can also be utilized for patients where positive margins are expected and can be given concurrently with chemotherapy; this is generally given in doses of 36 to 50.4 Gy in conventional 1.8 to 2 Gy fractions, generally with a 1- to 2-cm CTV margin on the preoperative extent of disease with a 0.5- to 1-cm PTV expansion. A postoperative boost can still be considered following resection based on final pathologic features.
- Use of blocking with customized Lipowitz metal block (cerrobend) shielding or multileaf collimation, or advanced techniques such as intensity-modulated radiation therapy (IMRT) or particle beam therapy, is necessary to reduce doses to nearby organs at risk (OARs), and for extremity lesions, to spare of a strip of skin (1.5 to 2.0 cm, if possible) on one side to limit distal extremity edema and constrictive fibrosis.
- For lesions in the base of the skull and/or cervical spine, immobilization with a five-point mask is required to reduce motion uncertainty and facilitate patient setup for treatment. For extremities, immobilization of all joints above and below the lesion is necessary to maintain reproducible setup. For example, for a lesion in the tibia, the patient should be immobilized at the hip, knee, and ankle; for a lesion in the humerus, the patient should be immobilized at the hand/wrist, elbow, and shoulder.
- Use of particle beam irradiation has been extensively explored because bone tumors are not considered to be very sensitive to radiation therapy at conventionally fractionated doses and are frequently located in areas in which a sharp dose gradient is essential to prevent severe side effects (e.g., lesions of the base of the skull and mobile spine). Several retrospective studies have shown increased local tumor control when particle beams were used (47).
  - In a phase II study using high-dose mixed photon/proton radiation therapy in the preoperative and postoperative management of spine sarcomas, patients received

50.4 CGyE to the operative bed and margin, a boost to 70.2 CGyE to microscopic residual, and up to 77.4 CGyE to GTV in 1.8 CGyE fractions. In this setting, the spinal cord was constrained to 63 CGyE to the cord surface and 54 CGyE to the cord center (48). In long-term follow-up, no myelopathy was noted, and 8-year actuarial local control was 85% for primary tumors (49).

- For lesions in close proximity to or abutting the dura, delivery of an adequate dose to optimally control the tumor following resection may not be possible because of the radiation tolerance of the spinal cord and/or cauda equina. If there is concern for residual microscopic disease at the dural surface, intraoperative radiation therapy may be considered (either electron beam or brachytherapy plaque) to supplement dose delivery, and has not been associated with increased risk of adverse effect (50–52).
- Hypofractionated radiation delivery techniques (stereotactic body radiation therapy or stereotactic ablative radiosurgery) have been explored for primary bone tumors, which may potentially yield improved local control over conventionally fractionated treatments in these relatively radiation-insensitive histologies, but may carry risk of increased long-term effects on muscle, connective, bone, and nerve tissue. Long-term follow-up will be necessary (53,54).

Osteosarcoma

- Although radiation therapy is usually not incorporated into the primary management of osteosarcoma, numerous radiation therapy approaches have been investigated for osteosarcoma when it is deemed unresectable, or when resection has been attempted with significant residual disease.
  - A multicenter trial using combined intra-arterial chemotherapy and irradiation (up to 46 Gy in 2- to 3-Gy fractions) reported a local tumor control rate of 98.5% in 66 patients, 60 of whom underwent limb-sparing surgery (55). Similar results were reported by Temple et al. (56).
  - An 81% local tumor control rate was reported in 21 patients treated palliatively with hypofractionated accelerated irradiation with or without chemotherapy, whereas a 92% local tumor control rate was noted in 13 patients treated with combined modalities for cure (57).
  - Similar impressive local tumor control rates have been achieved with 50 to 60 Gy of intraoperative radiation therapy, with or without preoperative chemotherapy (58).
- In general, postoperative treatment to 45 to 55.8 Gy in 1.8 Gy fractions to the operative bed with a 1- to 2-cm CTV expansion and 0.5- to 1-cm PTV expansion, followed by a boost of 9 to 20 Gy for microscopic to gross residual disease may be used for R1/R2 resection; for unresectable disease, total doses of 70 Gy may be required.

Chondrosarcoma

- Incorporation of radiation therapy in the primary management of chondrosarcoma is generally done postoperatively, or definitively in the setting of unresectable disease.
- Margins and doses are similar to those used in osteosarcoma; doses in excess of 70 Gy are required for unresectable lesions and lesions resected with gross residual tumor.

- Particle beams have been extensively used to treat chondrosarcoma, to allow dose escalation near critical structures such as the spinal cord.

Undifferentiated Pleomorphic Sarcoma of Bone

- Incorporation of radiation therapy in the primary management of undifferentiated pleomorphic sarcoma of bone is generally done postoperatively, or definitively in the setting of unresectable disease. Margins and doses are as noted above; there is an increasing role for the incorporation of chemotherapy in the treatment of undifferentiated pleomorphic sarcoma.

Giant Cell Tumor

- An 80% local tumor control rate was reported in patients with giant cell tumors who were treated with 45 to 55 Gy (59); similar control rates have been reported by other researchers.
- All GTV should be treated with an in-bone CTV expansion of at least 1 cm, as well as a PTV expansion defined by the treating institution (generally 0.5 to 1 cm) to doses of 45 to 50.4 Gy in conventional 1.8 to 2 Gy fractions. If an extraosseous component is present, this will also need an approximately 1 cm CTV expansion.

Chordoma

- Surgery is the mainstay of treatment for chordoma. However, because surgical excision is usually incomplete because of tumor location (base of skull or spine), radiation therapy also plays a significant role in treating this disease.
- Doses of 50 to 60 Gy have been reported to provide significant tumor control (60–62); however, optimal control does seem to require escalated doses of 70 Gy or more. For microscopic residual disease, a final CTV dose of at least 70 Gy is recommended; for gross residual or unresectable disease, a final CTV dose of 78 Gy should be attempted.
- Particle beams have been extensively used to treat chordoma, to allow dose escalation near critical structures such as the spinal cord.

Ewing's Sarcoma

- Patients who undergo complete surgical excision of involved bone/soft tissue disease with adequate surgical margins (defined in AEWS0031 as 2 mm on fascia, periosteum, and intramuscular septae; 5 mm on fat or muscle; and 10 mm on bone) do not require additional radiation therapy.
- For GTV (definitive or postoperative with gross residual), doses of 55.8 Gy are recommended (typically 45 Gy to prechemo, preop volume followed by a cone down to 55.8 Gy to the postchemo, postop residual). For postoperative cases with only microscopic disease, 50.4 Gy is enough. "Pushing border" techniques should be used when contouring preop, prechemo volumes near the bowel/lungs (see Fig. 40-1).

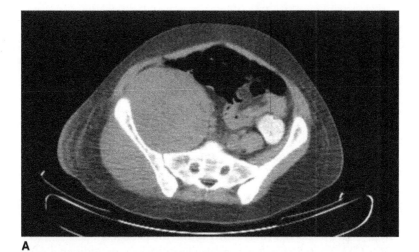

FIGURE 40-1. "Pushing border" example for Ewing's sarcoma. **A:** An axial CT image showing the prechemotherapy extent of the disease arising from and involving the right iliac bone. The soft tissue extent of the tumor extends into and displaces the bowel medially. Following initial chemotherapy, there was significant response in the tumor. **B:** A planning CT image shows the prechemotherapy GTV extent of the disease in *blue* and the postchemotherapy GTV in *red*. For planning purposes, the postchemotherapy volume may be reduced to allow for "pushing borders" resulting from the bowel falling into the area previously occupied by the tumor, as well as anatomic boundaries such as the anterior abdominal wall. The resulting modified postchemo GTV in *green* may be used for further planning.

- When planning treatment for Ewing's sarcoma, the following volumes are used:
  - Initial volumes:
    - GTV1: All pretreatment clinical and radiographic disease. This volume may be edited based on the altered appearance of the tumor on the treatment planning scan, where tumor regression would allow lung, intestine, bladder, or other tissues to fall into the space previously occupied by the tumor.
    - CTV1: GTV1 + 1.5 cm, constrained within the patient.
    - PTV1: CTV1 + 0.5 to 1.0 cm, generally treated to 45 Gy in 25 fractions; if pathologically involved lymph nodes are present, the involved basin will receive 50.4 Gy in 28 fractions to PTV1.
  - Boost volumes:
    - GTV2: All pretreatment bony involvement and postchemotherapy soft tissue disease, or residual primary disease after preoperative radiation and surgery, or unresected lymph nodes.
    - CTV2: GTV2 + 1.0 cm, constrained within the patient.
    - PTV2: CTV2 + 0.5 to 1.0 cm, generally treated to an additional 10.8 Gy in 6 fractions; if the area previously received 50.4 Gy in 28 fractions (see note for PTV1 above if pathologically involved lymph nodes are present), boost is reduced to 5.4 Gy in 3 fractions.
  - Special cases:
    - If GTV2 is only defined for unresected lymph nodes; if resected, only treat initial volumes.
    - If pleura is involved, patients require irradiation of ipsilateral hemithorax in the initial volume. The initial volume receives 15 Gy in 10 fractions for patients less than or equal to 10 years of age, or 12 Gy in 8 fractions if less than 6 years of age. Residual disease then receives additional boost radiation.
    - For extraosseous tumors with complete chemotherapy response, boost to PTV2 will be only 5.4 Gy in 3 fractions.
    - For vertebral body primaries, there is no boost.
    - Radiation may be given preoperatively to 45 Gy in 25 fractions to PTV1. If completely resected with adequate margins, no boost is required; if residual disease is present, this requires a boost to 10.8 Gy in 6 fractions as with PTV2 above.
- For localized bone disease, there is no difference in local control between whole bone versus involved field irradiation (63); since INT-0091, the involved field approach is standard.
- Whole-lung radiation dose is 15 Gy in 10 fractions, with coverage of the entire pulmonary and pleural space. The field generally extends from 1 cm above first rib (apex) to the inferior diaphragmatic attachments, with appropriate kidney blocks.

SEQUELAE OF TREATMENT

- The effects of radiation therapy on bone are directly related to the dose and treatment volume and inversely related to age at time of treatment.
- Clinically evident growth abnormalities are evident 6 months and 1 year after treatment in infants and in older children, respectively. Premature epiphyseal closure can occur with doses greater than 20 Gy.

- Scoliosis after vertebral irradiation is limited and is frequently compensated for by pelvic tilt.
- Irradiated bone is more prone to infection, fracture, and osteoradionecrosis because of radiation-induced small vessel changes.
- Irradiation can also cause lymphedema, joint fibrosis, limitation in range of motion, and secondary cancers (especially leukemia or sarcoma).

FOLLOW-UP/SURVEILLANCE

- If needed, refer to physical therapy as soon as possible. Functional assessments should be performed at each follow-up visit.
- Follow-up with primary/local site and chest imaging every 3 months for the post-treatment years 1 and 2, every 4 months for posttreatment year 3, every 6 months for posttreatment years 4 and 5, and then annually thereafter.
  - PET/CT or bone imaging may be performed as well, especially for Ewing's sarcoma; pediatric patients are generally followed more frequently for the first year, every 2 months.
- Indefinite (life-long) follow-up is recommended because of the risk of late recurrence and potential late effects from surgery, radiation therapy, and chemotherapy.

References

1. Siegel RL, Miller KD, Jemal A. Cancer Statistics, 2017. *CA Cancer J Clin* 2017;67(1):7–30.
2. Mirabello L, Troisi RJ, Savage SA. Osteosarcoma incidence and survival rates from 1973 to 2004: data from the Surveillance, Epidemiology, and End Results Program. *Cancer* 2009;115(7):1531–1543.
3. Mialou V, et al. Metastatic osteosarcoma at diagnosis: prognostic factors and long-term outcome—the French pediatric experience. *Cancer* 2005;104(5):1100–1109.
4. Cortes EP, Holland JF, Glidewell O. Osteogenic sarcoma studies by the Cancer and Leukemia Group B. *Natl Cancer Inst Monogr* 1981;(56):207–209.
5. Schajowicz F. *Tumors and tumorlike lesions of bones and joints.* New York, NY: Springer-Verlag, 1981.
6. Dahlin D, Unni K. *Bone tumor: general aspects and data on 8542 cases.* Springfield, IL: Charles C Thomas Publisher, 1986.
7. Saunders WM, et al. Early results of ion beam radiation therapy for sacral chordoma. A Northern California Oncology Group Study. *J Neurosurg* 1986;64(2):243–247.
8. Dunham WK, Wilborn WH. Malignant fibrous histiocytoma of bone. Report of two cases and review of the literature. *J Bone Joint Surg Am* 1979;61(6A):939–942.
9. Edeiken J. *Roentgen diagnosis of diseases of bone*, 3rd ed. Baltimore, MD: Williams & Wilkins, 1981.
10. Cassady J. Radiation therapy in less common primary bone tumors. In: Jaffe N, ed. *Solid tumors in childhood.* Boca Raton, FL: CRC Press, 1983:205.
11. Enneking WF, Spanier SS, Goodman MA. A system for the surgical staging of musculoskeletal sarcoma. *Clin Orthop Relat Res* 1980;(153):106–120.
12. Huvos AG, et al. Mesenchymal chondrosarcoma. A clinicopathologic analysis of 35 patients with emphasis on treatment. *Cancer* 1983;51(7):1230–1237.
13. Simon MA, Kirchner PT. Scintigraphic evaluation of primary bone tumors. Comparison of technetium-99m phosphonate and gallium citrate imaging. *J Bone Joint Surg Am* 1980;62(5):758–764.

14. Bjornsson J, et al. Chordoma of the mobile spine. A clinicopathologic analysis of 40 patients. *Cancer* 1993;71(3):735–740.

15. Coffin CM, et al. Chordoma in childhood and adolescence. A clinicopathologic analysis of 12 cases. *Arch Pathol Lab Med* 1993;117(9):927–933.

16. McCarthy EF, Matsuno T, Dorfman HD. Malignant fibrous histiocytoma of bone: a study of 35 cases. *Hum Pathol* 1979;10(1):57–70.

17. Simon MA. Limb salvage for osteosarcoma. *J Bone Joint Surg Am* 1988;70(2):307–310.

18. Taylor WF, et al. Trends and variability in survival among patients with osteosarcoma: a 7-year update. *Mayo Clin Proc* 1985;60(2):91–104.

19. Rosen G, et al. Combination chemotherapy and radiation therapy in the treatment of metastatic osteogenic sarcoma. *Cancer* 1975;35(3):622–630.

20. Bramwell VH, et al. A comparison of two short intensive adjuvant chemotherapy regimens in operable osteosarcoma of limbs in children and young adults: the first study of the European Osteosarcoma Intergroup. *J Clin Oncol* 1992;10(10):1579–1591.

21. Link MP, et al. Adjuvant chemotherapy of high-grade osteosarcoma of the extremity. Updated results of the Multi-Institutional Osteosarcoma Study. *Clin Orthop Relat Res* 1991;(270):8–14.

22. Eilber F, et al. Adjuvant chemotherapy for osteosarcoma: a randomized prospective trial. *J Clin Oncol* 1987;5(1):21–26.

23. Machak GN, et al. Neoadjuvant chemotherapy and local radiotherapy for high-grade osteosarcoma of the extremities. *Mayo Clin Proc* 2003;78(2):147–155.

24. DeLaney TF, et al. Radiotherapy for local control of osteosarcoma. *Int J Radiat Oncol Biol Phys* 2005;61(2):492–498.

25. Ozaki T, et al. Osteosarcoma of the pelvis: experience of the Cooperative Osteosarcoma Study Group. *J Clin Oncol* 2003;21(2):334–341.

26. Matsunobu A, et al. Impact of carbon ion radiotherapy for unresectable osteosarcoma of the trunk. *Cancer* 2012;118(18):4555–4563.

27. Harting MT, et al. Long-term survival after aggressive resection of pulmonary metastases among children and adolescents with osteosarcoma. *J Pediatr Surg* 2006;41(1):194–199.

28. Breur K, et al. Prophylactic irradiation of the lungs to prevent development of pulmonary metastases in patients with osteosarcoma of the limbs. *Natl Cancer Inst Monogr* 1981;(56):233–236.

29. Burgers JM, et al. Osteosarcoma of the limbs. Report of the EORTC-SIOP 03 trial 20781 investigating the value of adjuvant treatment with chemotherapy and/or prophylactic lung irradiation. *Cancer* 1988;61(5):1024–1031.

30. Huvos AG, et al. Telangiectatic osteogenic sarcoma: a clinicopathologic study of 124 patients. *Cancer* 1982;49(8):1679–1689.

31. Harwood AR, Krajbich JI, Fornasier VL. Radiotherapy of chondrosarcoma of bone. *Cancer* 1980;45(11):2769–2777.

32. Suit HD, et al. Definitive radiation therapy for chordoma and chondrosarcoma of base of skull and cervical spine. *J Neurosurg* 1982;56(3):377–385.

33. Rosenberg AE, et al. Chondrosarcoma of the base of the skull: a clinicopathologic study of 200 cases with emphasis on its distinction from chordoma. *Am J Surg Pathol* 1999;23(11):1370–1378.

34. Maruyama K, et al. Carbon ion radiation therapy for chondrosarcoma. *IJROBP*, 2012;84(3):S139.

35. Reagan MT, et al. Radiation therapy in the treatment of malignant fibrous histiocytoma. *Int J Radiat Oncol Biol Phys* 1981;7(3):311–315.

36. Hirano T, et al. Curative local control of malignant tumors in the acetabulum by intraoperative radiotherapy. *Arch Orthop Trauma Surg* 1994;113(4):215–217.

37. Nobler MP, Higinbotham NL, Phillips RF. The cure of aneurysmal bone cyst. Irradiation superior to surgery in an analysis of 33 cases. *Radiology* 1968;90(6):1185–1192.

38. Zhu S, Hitchcock KE, Mendenhall WM. Radiation therapy for aneurysmal bone cysts. *Am J Clin Oncol* 2017;40(6):621–624.
39. Habrand JL, et al. Proton therapy in pediatric skull base and cervical canal low-grade bone malignancies. *Int J Radiat Oncol Biol Phys* 2008;71(3):672–675.
40. Noel G, et al. Chordomas of the base of the skull and upper cervical spine. One hundred patients irradiated by a 3D conformal technique combining photon and proton beams. *Acta Oncol* 2005;44(7):700–708.
41. Hug EB, et al. Proton radiotherapy in management of pediatric base of skull tumors. *Int J Radiat Oncol Biol Phys* 2002;52(4):1017–1024.
42. Imai R, Kamada T, Araki N. Carbon ion radiation therapy for unresectable sacral chordoma: an analysis of 188 cases. *Int J Radiat Oncol Biol Phys* 2016;95(1):322–327.
43. Grier HE, et al. Addition of ifosfamide and etoposide to standard chemotherapy for Ewing's sarcoma and primitive neuroectodermal tumor of bone. *N Engl J Med* 2003;348(8):694–701.
44. Burgert EO Jr, et al. Multimodal therapy for the management of nonpelvic, localized Ewing's sarcoma of bone: intergroup study IESS-II. *J Clin Oncol* 1990;8(9):1514–1524.
45. Nesbit ME Jr, et al. Multimodal therapy for the management of primary, nonmetastatic Ewing's sarcoma of bone: a long-term follow-up of the First Intergroup study. *J Clin Oncol* 1990;8(10):1664–1674.
46. Paulussen M, et al. Primary metastatic (stage IV) Ewing tumor: survival analysis of 171 patients from the EICESS studies. European Intergroup Cooperative Ewing Sarcoma Studies. *Ann Oncol* 1998;9(3):275–281.
47. Brady L, Montemaggi P, Horowitz S, et al. Bone with special section of Ewing's sarcoma. In: Perez C, Brady L, eds. *Principles and practice of radiation oncology*, 3rd ed. Philadelphia, PA: Lippincott–Raven, 1998:2025–2049.
48. DeLaney TF, et al. Phase II study of high-dose photon/proton radiotherapy in the management of spine sarcomas. *Int J Radiat Oncol Biol Phys* 2009;74(3):732–739.
49. DeLaney TF, et al. Long-term results of Phase II study of high dose photon/proton radiotherapy in the management of spine chordomas, chondrosarcomas, and other sarcomas. *J Surg Oncol* 2014;110(2):115–122.
50. DeLaney TF, et al. Intraoperative dural irradiation by customized 192iridium and 90yttrium brachytherapy plaques. *Int J Radiat Oncol Biol Phys* 2003;57(1):239–245.
51. Folkert MR, et al. Local recurrence outcomes using the (3)(2)P intraoperative brachytherapy plaque in the management of malignant lesions of the spine involving the dura. *Brachytherapy* 2015;14(2):202–208.
52. Kondo T, et al. Intraoperative radiotherapy combined with posterior decompression and stabilization for non-ambulant paralytic patients due to spinal metastasis. *Spine (Phila Pa 1976)* 2008;33(17):1898–1904.
53. Chang UK, Lee DH, Kim MS. Stereotactic radiosurgery for primary malignant spinal tumors. *Neurol Res* 2014;36(6):597–606.
54. Jiang B, et al. CyberKnife radiosurgery for the management of skull base and spinal chondrosarcomas. *J Neurooncol* 2013;114(2):209–218.
55. Wanebo HJ, et al. Preoperative regional therapy for extremity sarcoma. A tricenter update. *Cancer* 1995;75(9):2299–2306.
56. Temple WJ, et al. Limb salvage surgery for widely infiltrating bony sarcomas. *Can J Surg* 1994;37(6):479–482.
57. Lombardi F, et al. Hypofractionated accelerated radiotherapy in osteogenic sarcoma. *Int J Radiat Oncol Biol Phys* 1992;24(4):761–765.

58. Yamamuro T, Kotoura Y. Intraoperative radiation therapy for osteosarcoma. In: Humphrey GB, ed. *Osteosarcoma in adolescents and young adults.* Boston, MA: Kluwer Academic Publishers, 1993:177.

59. Chen ZX, et al. Radiation therapy of giant cell tumor of bone: analysis of 35 patients. *Int J Radiat Oncol Biol Phys* 1986;12(3):329–334.

60. Amendola BE, et al. Chordoma: role of radiation therapy. *Radiology* 1986;158(3):839–843.

61. Fuller DB, Bloom JG. Radiotherapy for chordoma. *Int J Radiat Oncol Biol Phys* 1988;15(2): 331–339.

62. Keisch ME, Garcia DM, Shibuya RB. Retrospective long-term follow-up analysis in 21 patients with chordomas of various sites treated at a single institution. *J Neurosurg* 1991;75(3):374–377.

63. Donaldson SS, et al. A multidisciplinary study investigating radiotherapy in Ewing's sarcoma: end results of POG #8346. Pediatric Oncology Group. *Int J Radiat Oncol Biol Phys* 1998;42(1): 125–135.

CHAPTER 41

SOFT TISSUE SARCOMA

RETROPERITONEAL SOFT TISSUE SARCOMA

Anatomy

- The retroperitoneum is the region of the trunk delineated by specific anatomic boundaries:
  - It is covered anteriorly by the parietal peritoneum.
  - Superiorly (cephalad), it is bounded by the 12th rib and the diaphragm.
  - The pelvic diaphragm with the fascia of the levator ani and coccygeus muscles forms the inferior (caudad) boundary.
  - Posteriorly, it is bounded by the fascia of the abdominal wall muscles (Fig. 41-1).
- Because of the rigidity of the posterior, cephalad, and caudal boundaries, the most common route of expansion and invasion for retroperitoneal tumors is anteriorly into the abdominal cavity.

Natural History

- The histology of a retroperitoneal tumor tends to predict the mode of invasion.
  - Benign soft tissue tumors and well-differentiated sarcomas (e.g., myxoid liposarcomas) tend to grow in an expansile manner.
  - High-grade sarcomas often invade and surround the aorta and its main tributaries, and the vena cava. Small round cell tumors (neuroblastoma and rhabdomyosarcoma) can invade the intervertebral foramina in a dumbbell shape.
- The incidence of adjacent organ involvement is 60% to 70% (1,2).

Clinical Presentation

- Patients present with complaints of abdominal pain and/or a mass in 60% to 80% of cases.
- Fifty percent of patients present with weight loss and loss of appetite at diagnosis.

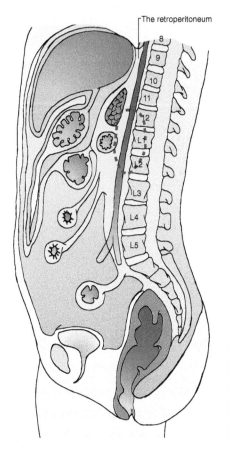

The retroperitoneum

FIGURE 41-1. Sagittal view of the trunk, showing the retroperitoneal space (*shaded area*). The kidney is outlined by the *dashed line*. (Reprinted with permission from Buchsbaum JC, Douglas JG, Dasgupta B, et al. Retroperitoneal cancer. In: Halperin EC, Perez CA, Brady LW, eds. *Principles and practice of radiation oncology*, 6th ed. Philadelphia, PA: Lippincott Williams & Wilkins, 2013:1517. © Wolters Kluwer.)

- Patients with sarcomas tend to seek medical treatment only when the tumors are large, because these tumors are usually asymptomatic or associated with vague abdominal symptoms. Patients with a germ cell tumor or lymphoma tend to become more acutely ill because of more rapid growth and other factors.
- Several retroperitoneal tumors are associated with paraneoplastic syndromes. Germ cell tumors can cause precocious puberty in children, and neuroblastoma can produce opsoclonic myoclonus. Retroperitoneal liposarcoma or lipoma can produce intermittent hypoglycemia due to pancreatic involvement/compromise. Extraadrenal retroperitoneal paraganglioma can produce signs of excessive catecholamine.
- The liver is the most common location of metastasis for retroperitoneal sarcomas.

Diagnostic Workup

- Evaluation should focus on three factors: physiologic status of the patient, extent of tumor involvement, and histologic characteristics.
- In addition to thorough history and physical examination, complete blood cell count and blood studies are required to assess the baseline bone marrow, hepatic, and renal status.

- Computed tomography (CT) has changed the detection and staging of retroperitoneal neoplasms because it can delineate tumor size and extent with more than 90% accuracy (3).
- CT guidance has allowed us to obtain histologic and cytologic specimens by needle biopsy, thus enabling a diagnosis without a laparotomy (4,5). Imaging should always precede biopsy.
- Magnetic resonance imaging (MRI) can also be used to study retroperitoneal tumors. Chang et al. (6) from the National Cancer Institute (NCI) showed that MRI was significantly better than CT at delineating tumors from muscle in sarcomas using T2-weighted spin echo and inversion recovery sequences in a study of 20 patients.

Staging System

- In the AJCC 7 staging system, staging of retroperitoneal tumors depended on histology. All retroperitoneal sarcomas are considered to be "deep" tumors.
- Staging of extremity soft tissue sarcomas (STS) has changed significantly and is reflected in the eighth edition of the *AJCC Cancer Staging Manual*. The changes are summarized in the box below.

Pathologic Classification

- Retroperitoneal neoplasms are extremely diverse because of the embryologic origin of the region in which the mesoderm, urogenital ridge, and neural crest develop (Table 41-1).
- Mesenchymal neoplasms predominate in adults. Lipoma and liposarcoma, the most common histopathologic subtypes, constitute 25% to 50% of cases in most studies and can recur if not excised with a wide margin (7–12).
- The most common retroperitoneal malignancy in children is rhabdomyosarcoma, followed by lymphoma.

NEW!   **SUMMARY OF CHANGES TO AJCC STAGING**

- AJCC 8 T staging and grading are the same as those for extremity soft tissue sarcoma.
- The primary difference between extremity and retroperitoneal staging in the AJCC 8 system is in overall stage grouping. Overall stage I soft tissues sarcomas are nonmetastatic, low grade, and without nodal spread; stage II are nonmetastatic grade 2 or 3 T1 lesions without nodal spread; stage III are nonmetastatic T2-4 grade 2 or 3 lesions with or without nodal spread; and stage IV are metastatic lesions of any grade with or without nodal spread.

See Amin MB, Edge SB, Greene FL, et al., eds. *AJCC cancer staging manual*, 8th ed. New York, NY: Springer, 2017.

Table 41-1			
Relative Incidence of Retroperitoneal Tumors			
Benign Tumors (*n* = 198)	%	Malignant Tumors (*n* = 1,080)	%
Lipoma	18	Lymphoma	27
Pheochromocytoma	12	Liposarcoma	18
Ganglioneuroma	9	Fibrosarcoma	11
Leiomyoma	6	Leiomyosarcoma	8
Teratoma	6	Neuroblastoma	8
Neurilemoma	4	Unclassified sarcoma	6
Neurofibroma	4	Rhabdomyosarcoma	4
Fibroma	3	Mesodermal sarcoma	2
Paraganglioma	2	Neurofibrosarcoma	1
Lymphangioma	2	Myxosarcoma	1
Myxoma	2	Malignant fibrous histiocytoma	1
Adenoma	2	Hemangiosarcoma	1
Hemangioma	1	Schwannoma	1
Cyst	29	Carcinoma	3
		Teratocarcinoma	1
		Unclassified tumor	4
		Metastatic tumor	3

- Primary germ cell tumors of the retroperitoneum theoretically arise from the embryonic urogenital ridge. Before a definite diagnosis can be made, a thorough examination of the genitalia is necessary. A physical and ultrasonographic examination of the testes is adequate in most patients. In six small series, 6 of 18 patients (33%) underwent biopsy or autopsy that showed a malignant tumor in the testes (13).

Prognostic Factors

- Preoperatively, the major prognostic factors are histology, invasiveness, and resectability of retroperitoneal tumors.
- A validated postoperative nomogram for 7-year disease-free survival and overall survival has been created for patients with primary retroperitoneal sarcomas as a collaborative project between the National Cancer Institute in Italy, MD Anderson Cancer Center, and the University of California at Los Angeles (14). This nomogram takes into account patient age, tumor size, histology, unifocality versus multifocality, and completeness of resection.

General Management

- The management of retroperitoneal sarcoma is complex and optimally performed at a specialized center, with experienced multidisciplinary management (15).
- Whenever possible, biopsy should be obtained prior to radical resection of tumor, unless there is a consensus that no preoperative therapy will be recommended or needed, or if the imaging is pathognomonic (15).
  - Optimal biopsy is performed using ultrasound- or CT-based percutaneous biopsy, by obtaining multiple cores. FDG-avid or solid, well-perfused areas of tumor should be sampled.
- In the past, surgical resection was the only means of curing most patients with retroperitoneal tumors (16,17); this is still true in STS.
  - Nonresectability criteria include involvement of the aorta, vena cava, iliac, or superior mesenteric vessels, as well as spinal cord or nerve plexus, peritoneal seeding, and distant metastases (1). Wist et al. (12) showed that 45% of patients survived for 5 years after complete excision, whereas only 8% survived after partial excision or biopsy.
- Radiation therapy is often required for many malignant retroperitoneal tumors because of their infiltrative nature into retroperitoneal soft tissues.
- A strong rationale exists for using preoperative irradiation to decrease the likelihood of tumor seeding; this facilitates complete tumor resection and minimizes the risk of complications.
- The primary treatment paradigms for retroperitoneal sarcomas are as follows:
  - Surgical resection +/– intraoperative radiation therapy (IORT) (12 to 15 Gy) followed by postop RT (45 to 50 Gy).
  - Preop RT +/– chemo followed by surgery +/– IORT.
- For resectable gastrointestinal stromal tumors (GIST), surgery is the primary treatment modality followed by observation or imatinib. Unresectable or R1/R2-resected GISTs are usually treated with imatinib followed by surgery, if possible.
- For operable desmoid tumors, surgery is the primary treatment modality followed by postop RT to 50 Gy for positive margins. Inoperable desmoids are treated with definitive RT to 56 to 60 Gy.
- Intraoperative Radiation Therapy (IORT) is a standard technique used to improve local control of retroperitoneal sarcomas. In a study conducted by the NCI, one of the only randomized studies performed for retroperitoneal sarcoma, 35 patients with resectable retroperitoneal sarcomas were randomized to determine whether an intraoperative irradiation (20 Gy IORT) boost was better than conventional irradiation alone after complete surgical resection. Both arms received postop XRT (35 to 40 Gy in the IORT group and 50 to 55 Gy in the other). Survival was not affected, although the locoregional control rate (80%) was higher in the IORT arm than in the conventional arm (35%) at 5 years. The incidence of enteritis was significantly decreased from 60% in the conventional arm to 7% with IORT, but radiation-related neuropathy was more frequent with IORT (18).
- Carbon-ion radiotherapy for unresectable retroperitoneal sarcomas yielded 50% and 69% for overall survival and local control at 5 years, respectively, with an excellent safety profile (19).

Chemotherapy

- The use of neoadjuvant or adjuvant chemotherapy has not been clearly defined in the management of retroperitoneal sarcoma, but may be most relevant in the setting of unresectable or borderline resectable high-grade lesions, and in retroperitoneal sarcoma histologies with known sensitivity to chemotherapy, including synovial sarcoma and leiomyosarcoma.
- The role of chemotherapy in childhood rhabdomyosarcoma is well established. Vincristine sulfate, doxorubicin, actinomycin D (dactinomycin), and cyclophosphamide are the most commonly used agents.
- Germ cell tumors are responsive to etoposide, cisplatin, bleomycin, and vincristine.
- Disease-free survival for patients with germ cell tumors who have complete responses is 75% to 90%, compared with less than 5% in patients who do not completely respond. If disease is present after retroperitoneal dissection, a radiation dose of 40 to 45 Gy can be delivered (20,21).
- In both germ cell tumor and rhabdomyosarcoma, chemotherapy is often the initial treatment, followed by surgery and irradiation.
- In one prospective randomized NCI study, 108 patients were accrued after removal of the primary tumor (22). Among patients assigned to chemotherapy, survival was better in those with extremity tumors. Patients with head and neck or trunk lesions (including retroperitoneal sarcomas) did not benefit; the 5-year survival rate was approximately 40% in both arms.

Radiation Therapy Techniques

- Whenever possible, radiation therapy should be performed as part of a multidisciplinary management plan, with treatment volumes discussed with the surgical team and coordinated with systemic therapy where indicated.
- In the treatment of retroperitoneal STS with radiation therapy, preoperative irradiation with possible intraoperative or postoperative boost is considered the optimal sequencing (13). This usually requires an initial procedure (either needle biopsy, if adequate tissue can be obtained, or a small operative procedure) to obtain tissue for histology.
  - Preoperative irradiation is preferred for three reasons: (a) the extent of local disease is usually easily defined by CT scan or MRI; (b) radiation therapy morbidity usually is less with preoperative irradiation than with postoperative therapy, because the large primary tumor mass acts to push normal tissues (such as the bowel) out of the irradiation field, and facilitates boost dose delivery to unresectable structures such as the major vessels and spinal column; and (c) preoperative irradiation may shrink the tumor, which may allow for complete resection.
- When preoperative irradiation fields are designed, planning based on axial contrast-enhanced CT and/or MRI imaging is of great value. Contrast studies of the stomach or small bowel can be useful also to differentiate critical structures.

- At times, the tumor is well outlined by air-filled bowel seen on a simple radiograph; this can help confirm the location determined by CT scan.
- When retroperitoneal tumors are irradiated, careful attention must be paid to the location and radiation tolerance of kidneys, liver, small bowel, and stomach (23).
  - It is common for at least one kidney to be entirely within the irradiation field (or to be resected at the time of definitive resection of the retroperitoneal sarcoma). In this situation, the function of the other kidney should be documented with a differential renal scan or using CT with IV contrast (15), and the total renal function should be determined to ensure adequate residual renal function (24). The contralateral kidney should receive no more than 18 Gy to 15% of the kidney volume; if both kidneys remain intact, the mean kidney dose should be kept to less than 15 Gy, with less than 15% of either kidney receiving 18 Gy (25).
  - The mean dose to the liver after surgery should be less than 26 Gy. If substantial portions of the liver are treated with high doses, the dose to the remainder of the liver should be decreased to allow for hepatic regeneration.
  - Small bowel constraints are often difficult to meet, especially in the postoperative setting, but optimally a V15 Gy less than 120 cc and V55 Gy of less than 20 cc if contouring individual loops of bowel, or a V15 Gy less than 830 cc and V45 Gy of 195 cc if contouring the entire bowel potential space as a constraint volume are desired (25,26).
  - The stomach and duodenum should be constrained such that the entire structure does not receive more than 45 Gy, with a V50 less than 50% and a maximum dose of 56 Gy (25).
- Radiation therapy fields must be individualized for the exact location of the tumor in each patient. CT simulation techniques and three-dimensional treatment planning are required.
- Anteroposterior-posteroanterior fields or moderately oblique fields will often produce reasonable distribution; lateral fields should be used sparingly, as they often result in much larger volumes of irradiation to normal tissue especially the liver in the upper abdomen.
  - Advanced techniques such as intensity-modulated radiation therapy (IMRT) or charged particle therapy usually improve target coverage while reducing dose to organs at risk, and are generally preferred for optimal management.
- In most cases, high-energy photons (≥10 MV) should be used.
- Traditionally, margins of 3 cm or more around gross tumors in the retroperitoneum were needed, but applying these large margins is no longer consistent with best practices. Generally, experienced institutions will expand the GTV by 0.5 to 1.5 cm to the CTV, and then apply a 0.5- to 1-cm PTV expansion, with or without adjustment for respiratory motion. Margin expansion into visceral structures should be minimized, with emphasis on expansion into unresectable retroperitoneal structures (paraspinal tissues, major vessels), where the risk of local recurrence is greatest (Fig. 41-2).

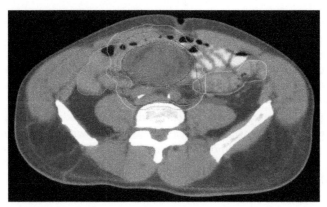

FIGURE 41-2. Preoperative treatment of retroperitoneal sarcoma. A 59-year-old male presented with a large abdominopelvic myxoid sarcoma, confirmed on ultrasound-guided biopsy prior to any therapy. A preoperative CT of the abdomen and pelvis had shown a large mass arising in the superior midline pelvis, 13 × 9.6 × 9.6 cm. In the planning image, the GTV (*red*) is expanded by 1.5 cm to the CTV (*blue*); this is limited to only 0.5 cm of overlap with small (*orange*) and large (*cyan*) bowel, but is more generous around the unresectable large vessels. An additional expansion of 0.5 cm off the CTV results in the PTV (*green*), using image guidance. The patient underwent treatment using arc IMRT techniques to 50 Gy in 25 fractions using 10-MV photons; he subsequently underwent curative resection.

- Treatment guidelines have been published by Baldini et al. (25):
- Motion assessment and internal margin expansion are recommended for all upper abdominal tumors; the incorporation of motion is used to generate an ITV from the sum of the GTV in key respiratory phases, or through a maximum intensity projection (MIP).
  - The ITV is expanded by 1.5 cm to create the clinical target volume (CTV); the CTV is edited according to surrounding tissue by removing the retroperitoneal component, bone, kidney, and liver; allowing up to 0.5 cm overlap with the bowel and air cavity; and under the skin by 0.3 to 0.5 cm. Of note, if the tumor extends to the inguinal canal, an inferior expansion of 3 cm is recommended because of concern for tumor extension.
  - The CTV is then expanded to the PTV by 0.5 cm if image guidance is used, or by 0.9 to 1.2 cm if image-guided radiation therapy (IGRT) is not used.
  - Recommended dose fractionation is 50.4 Gy in 1.8 Gy fractions or 50 Gy in 2 Gy fractions, preferably with IMRT or 3DCRT.
- The portion of tumor protruding into the peritoneal cavity usually does not produce significant risk of local recurrence; the primary concern is invasion of unresectable structures such as major vessels, nerve structures, axial skeleton, posterior abdominal wall, pelvic sidewall, and presacral tissues.
- Following preoperative radiation therapy, surgery is generally performed in 4 to 6 weeks. At the time of resection, the radiation oncologist should be present to evaluate the need for further radiation therapy.

- If the surgical margins are close to or positive for critical structures, additional intraoperative or postoperative therapy may be considered. Supplemental radiation therapy may be given with external beam therapy following surgery, via an interstitial brachytherapy implant placed in the tumor bed, or at the time of surgery with IORT (using either electron beam or brachytherapy-based applicators); of these approaches, only IORT is recommended because of the risk of excessive radiation dose to nearby critical structures with external beam or closed interstitial approaches.
  - For IORT, 10 to 15 Gy are generally given in a single fraction for microscopic residual disease; 15 Gy or higher can be given for gross residual disease.
  - For postoperative external beam boost, recommended doses are 16 to 20 Gy for microscopic residual disease, and 20 to 26 Gy for gross residual disease in 1.8 to 2 Gy per fraction, if needed.
  - For interstitial brachytherapy boost, high dose rate brachytherapy to 15 to 16 Gy for microscopic residual disease, or 18 to 24 Gy for gross residual disease in 3 to 4 Gy per fraction delivered BID are recommended.
  - If at all possible, repeat resection is recommended for positive margins or gross residual disease.
- Although postoperative radiation therapy is suboptimal, it may be considered based on concern for local recurrence, especially if positive margins or gross residual disease are present and repeat resection is not possible. If surgical clips have been placed, they can be used to define the extent of tumor. If not, the information must be transferred from the preoperative imaging studies to the simulation film to determine the extent of the irradiation field. Generally, the fields should be of the same extent as for preoperative therapy, remembering that the retroperitoneum is the site at highest risk for local failure. Normal tissue tolerances need to be respected as for preoperative therapy, but the total dose often is limited to 50 Gy because of the tolerance of the small intestine and stomach (11,27,28).

Sequelae of Treatment

- The acute sequelae of irradiation treatment are nausea and vomiting, as well as gastrointestinal disturbances such as gassiness, bloating, and diarrhea.
- The long-term major sequelae of surgery and irradiation are small bowel enteropathy, which is linked to the number of laparotomies the patient has had as well as irradiation dose and volume (29), and small bowel obstruction.

Follow-Up/Surveillance

- Follow-up with primary/local site and chest imaging every 3 months for posttreatment years 1 and 2, every 4 months for posttreatment year 3, every 6 months for posttreatment years 4 and 5, and annually thereafter.
- Indefinite (life-long) follow-up is recommended because of the risk of late recurrence and potential late effects from surgery, radiation therapy, and chemotherapy.

SOFT TISSUE SARCOMAS (EXCLUDING RETROPERITONEUM)

- Sarcomas constitute a relatively rare group of malignancies arising from the mesoderm or connective tissues of the body. The mesenchymal soft tissues constitute approximately 50% of body weight.
- STS are the most common type of sarcomas.
- Median age range is 40 to 60 years with a slight male prevalence among the 12,390 cases expected in 2017, according to the American Cancer Society.
- STS can occur within any organ or anatomic location within the musculoskeletal system.
- Other sarcomas (pediatric and bone) are discussed in different chapters of this book.

Anatomy

- Because STS initially remain confined to the muscle compartment of origin, knowledge of the anatomic location of these muscle groups is important to the radiation oncologist to permit appropriate positioning of the limb. This, in turn, ensures that the compartment at risk is encompassed, that the tumor receives adequate coverage during radiation therapy (RT), and that compartments that are not involved are avoided.
- The thigh is the most common subsite of origin (25) and is divided into three compartments; anterior, posterior, and medial (or adductor). The muscle compartments of the lower leg and upper extremity are defined in a similar fashion, and tumors tend to stay within one compartment.
- Most common sites in decreasing prevalence: lower extremity, trunk, upper extremity, retroperitoneum, then head and neck.

Clinical Presentation and Risk Factors

- In general, the tumor presents as a painless lump lasting a few weeks or months, and growing initially by direct spread along the longitudinal axis of the muscle compartment without traversing, or violating the major fascial planes or bone. Sudden increase in size at presentation or afterward is usually due to hematoma formation.
- Invasion proceeds to adjacent muscle, skin, nerves, and bone.
- Tumors of the trunk, head, and neck may invade adjacent structures earlier.
- Lymph node metastases are uncommon (less than 5% overall), but are an ominous sign when they occur. Some histologies such as angiosarcomas, synovial cell sarcomas, clear cell sarcomas, rhabdomyosarcomas, and epithelioid sarcomas have a higher rate of nodal involvement (15% to 20%) (26).
- Skin involvement is seen in approximately 10% of patients.

- Hematogenous metastasis is the most common pattern of metastatic spread and occurs more frequently in high-grade tumors and large tumors. The lung is the most common site of metastatic disease.
- Risk factors: NF-1 (MPNST), Rb (leiomyosarcoma), Gardner syndrome (desmoid), Li-Fraumeni (STS), chronic lymphedema (Stewart-Treves syndrome/lymphangiosarcoma), viral infection (HHV-8 for Kaposi's sarcoma), prior radiation (RR of 3 for secondary sarcomas in children receiving XRT), chemical exposure (vinyl chloride, herbicide exposure, arsenic exposure).

Pathologic Classification

- Over 100 types of STS have been classified by the World Health Organization.
- The most common soft tissue sarcoma is pleomorphic undifferentiated sarcoma (previously known as malignant fibrous histiocytoma), which occurs in 30% of cases. Other sarcomas include (from most to least common) liposarcoma, leiomyosarcoma, synovial sarcoma, MPNST, fibrosarcoma, myxoid liposarcoma, rhabdomyosarcoma, and other rare histologies.

Diagnostic Workup

- A detailed family history and specific questioning with regard to prior therapeutic irradiation are critical.
- The physical examination must detail the size and characteristics of the mass, and, for limb lesions, the proximity to joints.
- Evidence of neurovascular compromise and fixation to bone should be evaluated with magnetic resonance imaging or computed tomography with contrast, keeping in mind the potential for limb-sparing surgical procedures. Imaging should precede biopsy.
- Careful lymph node examination should be performed.
- Biopsy should be performed in the same center as surgery, preferably by the same surgeon. Incisional or core needle biopsies are preferred over excisional biopsy, which may lead to field contamination.
- The diagnostic workup for patients with STS is shown in Table 41-2.

Staging System

- Staging of extremity STS has changed significantly in the eighth edition of the *AJCC Cancer Staging Manual*. The box below summarizes the changes made in the eighth edition.
- Along with stage, the histologic grade of the tumor, primary tumor site, superficial or deep compartment involvement, regional lymph node involvement, and distant metastases should be described.

Table 41-2

Diagnostic Workup for Patients with Soft Tissue Sarcomas

Multidisciplinary Team Management
Routine studies
    History and physical examination
    Complete blood cell count and chemistry profile
    Plain radiograph of involved area
    CT or MRI of involved site
    Chest radiograph or chest CT scan
    Incisional or core needle biopsy
Complementary studies
    FDG-PET
    Bone scan
    Arteriography or magnetic resonance angiogram
    Lymphangiogram
    Ultrasound

NEW! SUMMARY OF CHANGES TO AJCC STAGING

- T stage is no longer simply less than or equal to 5 cm (T1), and greater than 5 cm (T2) with distinction of superficial (a) or deep (b) location; T staging is now less than or equal to 5 cm (T1), greater than 5 but less than or equal to 10 cm (T2), greater than 10 but less than or equal to 15 cm (T3), and greater than 15 cm (T4). Of note, there is no difference in overall stage for T3 versus T4 disease.

- Grade has been incorporated and defined directly in the AJCC 8 staging system, incorporating a differentiation score, mitotic count score, and necrosis score, which contributes to overall stage.

- Soft tissue sarcomas of the head and neck have their own staging system and different T staging, with less than or equal to 2 cm (T1), greater than 2 but less than or equal to 4 cm (T2), greater than 4 cm without invasion (T3), and tumors of any size invading adjoining structures (T4); denoted T4a if invading orbit, skull base, dura, central compartment viscera, facial skeleton, or pterygoid muscles, and T4b if invading brain parenchyma or prevertebral muscles, encasing the carotid arteries, or exhibiting perineural spread.

- Overall stage I soft tissues sarcomas are nonmetastatic, low grade, and without nodal spread; stage II are nonmetastatic grade 2 or 3 T1 lesions without nodal spread; stage III are nonmetastatic T2-4 grade 2 or 3 lesions without nodal spread; and stage IV are node positive or metastatic lesions of any grade.

See Amin MB, Edge SB, Greene FL, et al., eds. *AJCC cancer staging manual*, 8th ed. New York, NY: Springer, 2017.

Prognostic Factors

- Tumor grade is the most important factor in overall and disease-free survival, and has been incorporated into the AJCC 8 staging system.
- In an analysis of prospectively collected data from a population of 1,041 adult patients with localized extremity soft tissue sarcomas at Memorial Sloan-Kettering Cancer Center (MSKCC), significant independent adverse prognostic factors for local recurrence included age greater than 50 years, recurrent disease, positive surgical margins, and the histologic subtypes fibrosarcoma and MPNST. For distant metastasis, tumor size, high grade, deep location, recurrent disease, leiomyosarcoma, and nonliposarcoma histology were independent adverse prognostic factors (27).
- Other nomograms have been established for outcomes in sarcoma. The sarcoma-specific death at 12 years nomogram (28) and the local recurrence after limb-sparing surgery without RT nomogram (29) were developed at MSKCC and are useful tools for patient counseling and prognostication. Additionally, a validated international nomogram based on age, tumor size, grade, and histology can be used to predict 5- and 10-year overall survival, and 5- and 10-year rates of distant metastasis.

General Management

- The management of extremity sarcoma is complex and optimally performed at a specialized center, with experienced multidisciplinary management.
- Surgical approaches to soft tissue sarcomas can be grouped into different categories, based on the surgical plane of dissection:
  - An intralesional procedure is performed for biopsy, but presents the problem of seeding along the wound; biopsy should be performed either by percutaneous image-guided biopsy or by the managing surgical/orthopedic oncologist planning to perform definitive surgery.
  - A marginal procedure removes the tumor within the confines of the pseudocapsule, but with a significant likelihood of subclinical disease being left behind. Local recurrence rate is approximately 80%. With more extensive excision, residual tumor has been reported in 45% to 49% of specimens (30).
  - In wide local excision, the tumor is removed with a margin of normal tissue (usually 2 cm) from within the same muscle compartment. Local recurrence of 30% to 60% with this operation reflects the wide variability of the surgical procedures used.
  - A radical excision removes the entire tumor and the structures of origin en bloc. The local recurrence rate is approximately 10% to 20%, although this procedure is frequently associated with substantial functional compromise.
  - Amputation, which is not recommended for extremity sarcomas in most cases and is used in only approximately 5% of patients, may fall within any category, depending on the location within the extremity and the margins of tissue obtained around the tumor.
- The efficacy of radiation therapy is greatly influenced by the quality of the surgical procedure.

- If there is doubt concerning the amount of residual tumor or adequacy of the excision, reexcision should be considered; this is because positive margins greatly increase the risk of local recurrence, even when postoperative irradiation is given.
- Surgical scars are at risk for subclinical disease and should be oriented longitudinally in the extremity. Circumferential irradiation of scars oriented other than in a longitudinal fashion is hazardous because of the impact on lymphatics draining the extremity.
- Surgical clips should be used to mark the tumor bed and the tumor volume to aid in patient positioning for treatment planning.
- Complete resection and adjuvant RT (+/– concurrent chemotherapy) can replace limb amputation (31,32), and is the current standard of care. The rationale for combining RT and surgery is to avoid the functional and cosmetic deficits of radical resection and the late consequences of high doses of radiation alone to large volumes of normal tissues.
- Local recurrences of low-grade lesions often can be reexcised with organ conservation, unlike intermediate- and high-grade sarcomas, which require more aggressive management.
- Radiation therapy is not indicated for initial treatment of small, low-grade (stage I) sarcomas, except for those where recurrence would be particularly debilitating, and should be reserved for tumors with positive margins, deep lesions that are difficult to follow, questionable margins, and location in which local recurrence would require amputation.
- The current standard of care for stage II or III soft tissue sarcomas is limb-preserving surgery and preoperative, intraoperative, or postoperative radiation therapy, with or without chemotherapy. Neoadjuvant or adjuvant chemotherapy is generally reserved for large-size tumors or high-grade lesions because of the increased risk of distant metastases.
- For stage IV disease with controlled primary, surgical resection should be attempted in selected patients with limited metastases to improve survival.
- Carbon ion radiotherapy for nonsurgical extremity STS yielded 5-year local control and overall survival of 76% and 56%, respectively (33).

Radiation Therapy Techniques

- Adjuvant brachytherapy improves local control after complete limb-sparing resection of soft tissue sarcomas; an early study by Rosenberg et al. demonstrated that limb-sparing surgery with adjuvant brachytherapy did not compromise survival relative to amputation (31). This improvement in local control was later observed to be limited to patients with high-grade histopathology (34).
- For patients with high-grade tumors and positive surgical margins, external beam RT and/or brachytherapy yielded a higher local regional control rate than the group that did not receive radiation therapy, 74% versus 56% at 5 years, respectively (35).
- Radiation therapy in moderate doses (60 to 65 Gy in 6 to 7 weeks, generally at 1.8 Gy per fraction delivered daily) is effective in eradicating microscopic extension of the excised gross lesion (36).
- IMRT has been shown to have improved local control over brachytherapy (37) and conventional EBRT (38).

- When designing a radiation therapy treatment plan, it is important to keep the following issues in mind:
  - Immobilization at all proximal and distal joints to the lesion, and also comfortable, reproducible positioning are critical. When using 2D or 3D techniques, treating inner thigh lesions in the frog-leg position may be beneficial (Fig. 41-3); when using IMRT techniques with or without conformal arcs, the affected limb should be straight, if possible. Moving the contralateral limb further away from the affected limb may offer increased flexibility in beam angles. Occasionally, treatment of posterior lesions in the prone position may be beneficial, but comfort should be assessed as it may affect reproducibility.
  - Beam energies of 4- to 6-MV photons (or higher) are necessary to ensure homogeneity of radiation dose delivery.
  - Three-dimensional treatment planning is important to ensure coverage of the target area while sparing normal tissues. A combination of photons and electrons may enhance optimization of the dose in the treated volume, although electrons are rarely if ever needed if IMRT techniques are used.

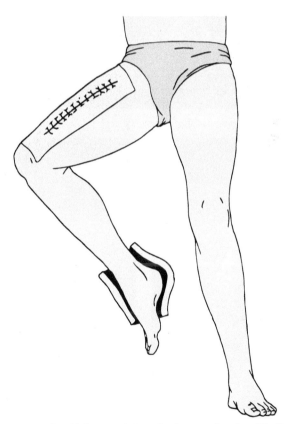

FIGURE 41-3. To treat anterior thigh musculature, the leg may be placed in the frog-leg position. This separates the anterior thigh from the posterior and medial compartments.

- Bolus may be used for skin or superficial subcutaneous tissue involvement by tumor; in this setting, one should bolus scar or drain sites until 50 Gy unless using tangential beams. Note that no extra effort is needed to increase dose to skin that is planned for excision.
- A 1-cm strip of skin (minimum) should be preserved, particularly in the extremities, to reduce the risk of lymphedema.
- MRI-based imaging should be used to define preoperative extent of tumor. Include T2 edema in the CTV with 3 to 4 cm longitudinal and 1 to 1.5 cm circumferential expansion; smaller longitudinal margins may be considered for small, low-grade MRI-defined lesions. Elective nodal coverage is not recommended (Fig. 41-4).

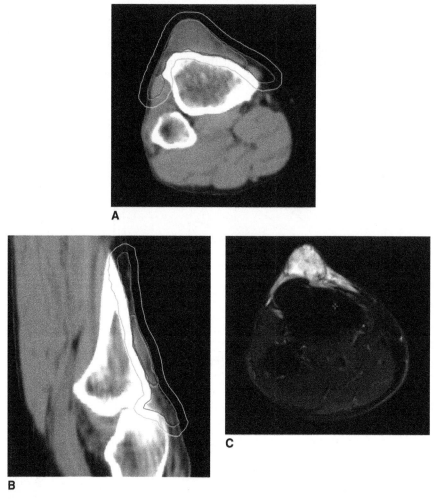

FIGURE 41-4. Extremity sarcoma preoperative treatment. Axial **(A)** and sagittal **(B)** planning images of a patient with a pretibial grade 2 pleomorphic undifferentiated sarcoma, with **(C)** planning MRI axial T2 image. The GTV (*red*) includes the MRI-defined tumor, the CTV (*blue*) is an expansion of approximately 1.5 cm radially and 3 cm sup-inf and excluding bone, and the PTV (*green*) is a 0.5 cm uniform expansion off the CTV.

- A 0.5-cm CTV to PTV expansion is sufficient when using IGRT; otherwise, a margin of 1 cm is recommended.
  - Surgery should be performed 4 to 6 weeks after preoperative RT; if given postoperatively, RT may start as early as 2 to 3 weeks after surgery and should start no later than 8 weeks after surgery.
- IGRT has been shown to reduce late toxicities in patients with extremity STS treated with preoperative RT without compromising local control (RTOG 0630) (39). In these cases, GTV was defined using T1 contrast-enhanced MRI images. For intermediate- to high-grade tumors ≥8 cm, GTV was expanded by 3 cm longitudinally to create the CTV. For low-grade tumors or those less than 8 cm, GTV was expanded by 2 cm longitudinally to create the CTV. The GTV to CTV radial margin was 1.5 cm for intermediate- to high-grade tumors ≥8 cm; and 1 cm for low-grade tumors or those less than 8 cm. CTV is further expanded to cover suspicious edema in any direction as needed and is constrained by anatomic barriers. The CTV was expanded by 5 mm to create the PTV.
- Guidelines for preoperative and postoperative external beam radiotherapy for extremity STS are summarized in Table 41-3 (40).
- Radiation doses should be reduced when chemotherapy is given; 2 or 3 days should elapse before and after administration of doxorubicin (Adriamycin) before radiation therapy is begun.

Table 41-3

Treatment Guidelines for Extremity Soft Tissue Sarcomas

	Preoperative	Postoperative
Dose	50–50.4 Gy Consider postoperative boost for close or positive margins identified following definitive resection 1.8–2.0 Gy/fraction	45–50.4 Gy to PTV_1 followed by boost of 10–16 Gy to PTV_2 (total dose 60–66 Gy) 1.8–2.0 Gy/fraction
Target delineation	CTV = GTV plus 3–4 cm in the longitudinal direction and 1–1.5 cm radially, including peritumoral edema but not expanded beyond bone surface, joints, or fasciae. PTV = CTV plus 0.5–1 cm depending on setup reproducibility and image guidance.	CTV_1 = tumor bed plus 3–4 cm in the longitudinal direction and 1.5 cm radially, including peritumoral edema, surgical clips, scar, and drain site but not expanded beyond bone surface, joints, or fasciae. PTV_1 = CTV_1 plus 0.5–1 cm depending on setup reproducibility and image guidance. CTV_2 = tumor bed plus 1–2 cm in the longitudinal direction and 1–1.5 cm radially, including peritumoral edema but not expanded beyond bone surface, joints, or fasciae. PTV_2 = CTV_2 plus 0.5–1 cm depending on setup reproducibility and image guidance.

Preoperative External Beam Radiation Therapy

- Preoperative radiation therapy has the potential advantages of rendering an unresectable tumor resectable, allowing limb-salvage surgery, reducing the risk of seeding at the time of surgery, and irradiating smaller volumes.
  - Preoperative radiation therapy has fewer late treatment side effects, such as fibrosis, edema, and joint stiffness, than postoperative treatment (41).
- In 110 patients with locally advanced disease treated with preoperative radiation therapy, the local failure rate was 10% and the local control rate 83% at 5 years (42). Suit et al. (43) reported a local failure rate of 10% with 181 patients treated in a similar fashion.
- In the event of positive margins noted following definitive resection, observation or additional postoperative boost radiation therapy can be considered; generally, 16 to 18 Gy in 1.8- to 2-Gy fractions for microscopic residual disease, and 20 to 26 Gy in 1.8- to 2-Gy fractions for gross residual disease. Whenever possible, repeated resection should be considered for microscopic or gross residual disease.
- Preoperative hypofractionated radiotherapy using 25 Gy in 5 consecutive fractions of 5 Gy per fraction followed by immediate surgery (and boost for R1 resection) for extremity and trunk STS showed favorable results and acceptable toxicity (44).

Postoperative External Beam Radiation Therapy

- Various studies show local failure rates of 10% to 22% for postoperative irradiation (30,32,43,45).
- Reduced survival in patients with stage IIB and IIIB disease is attributed to distant metastases. However, preoperative irradiation results for these patients are better than postoperative results, perhaps because there is less seeding at the time of surgery.
- A randomized trial of preoperative versus postoperative radiotherapy in soft tissue sarcomas of the limb was conducted by the NCI Canada (46). Radiation doses were 50 Gy preop (plus boost if close or positive margins) versus 66 Gy postop. Five-year results revealed no differences in local control, recurrence-free survival, or overall survival between the two arms. While preoperative RT was associated with a significantly increased rate of wound complications compared to postoperative RT (35% versus 17%), postoperative RT was associated with worse long-term functional impact due to fibrosis, edema, or joint stiffness (41).

Brachytherapy

- Although brachytherapy is used less frequently than external beam approaches, indications exist for treatment of extremity sarcomas, offering an abbreviated course of therapy compared to external beam approaches.
- Consensus recommendations for therapy have been published by the American Brachytherapy Society (ABS) (47,48).

- Treatment is delivered after placing multiple catheters into the operative bed at the time of the surgery. Catheters are placed 1 to 1.5 cm apart, generally with a single-plan implant. The treatment region should extend at least 2 cm longitudinally past the extent of the tumor bed, and at least 1 cm laterally. Treatment is delivered more than 5 days postoperatively to reduce the risk of complications, but can be delivered earlier with staged reconstruction. Treatment depth is 0.5 to 1 cm from the applicators.
- Brachytherapy alone may be recommended in the setting of high-grade lesions less than 10 cm in size with negative margins on resection, treated to 30 to 50 Gy in 2 to 4 Gy fractions delivered twice daily. For larger lesions or lesions with close/positive margins, external beam radiation therapy is generally added.

Intraoperative Radiation Therapy

- IORT with electron beam radiation therapy or high dose rate brachytherapy may be given at the time of surgery to improve local control (48–50).
- This may be used as a supplement to preoperative radiation therapy, or followed by postoperative radiation therapy as indicated.
  - For IORT, doses of 10 to 15 Gy are generally given in a single fraction for microscopic residual disease; doses of 15 Gy or higher can be given for gross residual disease.

Chemotherapy

- Numerous clinical trials have investigated the value of chemotherapy for patients with soft tissue sarcomas, but the data are difficult to interpret because of the heterogeneity of the tumors studied, the relatively small number of patients in each trial, and the variety of drugs and dosage schedules investigated (51).
- Recent data clearly indicate that multidrug chemotherapy regimens, combined with radiation therapy, may significantly improve local control and ultimate outcome.
- The most common regimens include cyclophosphamide, vincristine, doxorubicin, and dacarbazine, or a combination of doxorubicin and ifosfamide.
- A meta-analysis by Pervaiz et al. showed that adjuvant chemotherapy improves local control and reduces risk of distant metastases. The addition of ifosfamide to doxorubicin improved overall survival as well (52).
- In the United States, patients with stages II and III (high-grade) tumors currently are offered multiagent chemotherapy.
- In general, certain sarcomas are considered sensitive to single-agent or combination regimens; these include synovial sarcoma, leiomyosarcoma, myxoid liposarcomas, pleomorphic sarcoma, and angiosarcoma (53). Resistant sarcomas include alveolar soft part sarcoma, clear cell sarcoma, well-differentiated liposarcoma, and malignant solitary fibrous tumor (54).
- Use of immunotherapy, biologic agents, and novel combinations of radiation and systemic treatment are areas of active investigation.

Sequelae of Treatment

- Short-term sequelae of radiation therapy usually are limited to moist desquamation in the high-dose volume, particularly if the beams are tangential to the skin. The risk is increased in patients with more than 50% of the diameter of the extremity included in the field, as well as in those receiving concurrent doxorubicin (51). Notably, recall reactions are described with doxorubicin.
- Patients undergoing treatment for truncal tumors may experience nausea or thrombocytopenia.
- Major wound complications (requiring subsequent invasive procedure) occur in approximately 10% of patients after surgical resection, with or without postoperative irradiation. This rate may be somewhat higher in patients treated with preoperative irradiation or brachytherapy within 5 days after surgical resection (51,55).
- Long-term sequelae after conservative surgery and irradiation for extremity lesions may significantly limit the function of the preserved limb. These sequelae include decreased range of motion and muscle strength, contracture of the joint, edema, pain, and bone fracture. Complications can be reduced by sparing a strip of normal tissue and uninvolved muscle to allow lymphatic drainage from the extremity.
- Multiple dose constraints are used to reduce the risk of bone fracture: V40 Gy less than 64% and max point dose less than 59 Gy (56), or avoiding circumferential bone coverage with the 50-Gy isodose line (57). Other factors that increase the risk of fracture include periosteal stripping during surgery and perioperative chemotherapy (57–59). A nomogram has been created to predict the risk of femoral fracture after combined modality treatment of STS of the thigh (58).
- Physical therapy is essential in minimizing disabilities. Mobility of the extremity should be stressed, and patients should be placed on an exercise and range-of-motion program early in the course of therapy.
- High-dose radiation does not appear to compromise the viability of skin grafts used to repair defects after sarcoma surgery, assuming adequate time is allotted for healing (at least 3 weeks) (51,55).
- Fertility can be preserved in men undergoing irradiation for lower-extremity sarcomas by using a gonadal shield to decrease testicular dose.
- IMRT can permit enhanced target volume coverage in soft tissue sarcomas while maximally sparing normal tissues with the goal of decreased morbidity (60) as well as potentially improved local control (38).
- Secondary malignancy risk is a major consideration especially in the pediatric or adolescent population.

Follow-Up/Surveillance

- If needed, refer patients to physical therapy as soon as possible. Functional assessments should be performed at each follow-up visit.
- Follow up with primary/local site and chest imaging should occur every 3 months for the posttreatment years 1 and 2, every 4 months for posttreatment year 3, every 6 months for posttreatment years 4 and 5, and then annually thereafter.
- Indefinite (lifelong) follow-up is recommended because of the risk of late recurrence and potential late effects from surgery, radiation therapy, and chemotherapy.

References

1. Cody HS III, et al. The continuing challenge of retroperitoneal sarcomas. *Cancer* 1981;47(9):2147–2152.
2. Pack GT, Tabah EJ. Primary retroperitoneal tumors: a study of 120 cases. *Int Abstr Surg* 1954;99(4):313–341.
3. Stephens DH, et al. Diagnosis and evaluation of retroperitoneal tumors by computed tomography. *AJR Am J Roentgenol* 1977;129(3):395–402.
4. Husband JE, Golding SJ. The role of computed tomography-guided needle biopsy in an oncology service. *Clin Radiol* 1983;34(3):255–260.
5. Zornoza J, et al. Fine needle aspiration biopsy of retroperitoneal lymph nodes and abdominal masses: an updated report. *Radiology* 1977;125(1):87–88.
6. Chang AE, et al. Magnetic resonance imaging versus computed tomography in the evaluation of soft tissue tumors of the extremities. *Ann Surg* 1987;205(4):340–348.
7. Harrison LB, Gutierrez E, Fischer JJ. Retroperitoneal sarcomas: the Yale experience and a review of the literature. *J Surg Oncol* 1986;32(3):159–164.
8. Kinne DW, et al. Treatment of primary and recurrent retroperitoneal liposarcoma. Twenty-five-year experience at Memorial Hospital. *Cancer* 1973;31(1):53–64.
9. McGrath PC, et al. Improved survival following complete excision of retroperitoneal sarcomas. *Ann Surg* 1984;200(2):200–204.
10. Storm FK, et al. Retroperitoneal sarcomas: a reappraisal of treatment. *J Surg Oncol* 1981;17(1):1–7.
11. Tepper JE, et al. Radiation therapy of retroperitoneal soft tissue sarcomas. *Int J Radiat Oncol Biol Phys* 1984;10(6):825–830.
12. Wist E, et al. Primary retroperitoneal sarcomas. A review of 36 cases. *Acta Radiol Oncol* 1985;24(4):305–310.
13. Wasserman T, Tepper J. Retroperitoneum. In: Perez C, Brady L, eds. *Principles and practice of radiation oncology*, 3rd ed. Philadelphia, PA: Lippincott–Raven, 1998:1943–1956.
14. Raut CP, et al. External validation of a multi-institutional retroperitoneal sarcoma nomogram. *Cancer* 2016;122(9):1417–1424.
15. Trans-Atlantic RPSWG. Management of primary retroperitoneal sarcoma (RPS) in the adult: a consensus approach from the Trans-Atlantic RPS Working Group. *Ann Surg Oncol* 2015;22(1):256–263.
16. Donnelly B. Primary retroperitoneal tumors. *Surg Gynecol Obstet* 1946;83:705.
17. Moore SV, Aldrete JS. Primary retroperitoneal sarcomas: the role of surgical treatment. *Am J Surg* 1981;142(3):358–361.
18. Sindelar WF, et al. Intraoperative radiotherapy in retroperitoneal sarcomas. Final results of a prospective, randomized, clinical trial. *Arch Surg* 1993;128(4):402–410.
19. Serizawa I, et al. Carbon ion radiotherapy for unresectable retroperitoneal sarcomas. *Int J Radiat Oncol Biol Phys* 2009;75(4):1105–1110.
20. Hussey DH, Luk KH, Johnson DE. The role of radiation therapy in the treatment of germinal cell tumors of the testis other than pure seminoma. *Radiology* 1977;123(1):175–180.
21. Lack EE, Travis WD, Welch KJ. Retroperitoneal germ cell tumors in childhood. A clinical and pathologic study of 11 cases. *Cancer* 1985;56(3):602–608.
22. Rosenberg SA. Prospective randomized trials demonstrating the efficacy of adjuvant chemotherapy in adult patients with soft tissue sarcomas. *Cancer Treat Rep* 1984;68(9):1067–1078.
23. Goffinet DR, et al. Abdominal irradiation in non-Hodgkin's lymphomas. *Cancer* 1976;37(6):2797–2805.
24. Dubovsky EV, Russell CD. Quantitation of renal function with glomerular and tubular agents. *Semin Nucl Med* 1982;12(4):308–329.

25. Baldini EH, et al. Treatment guidelines for preoperative radiation therapy for retroperitoneal sarcoma: preliminary consensus of an International Expert Panel. *Int J Radiat Oncol Biol Phys* 2015;92(3):602–612.

26. Kavanagh BD, et al. Radiation dose-volume effects in the stomach and small bowel. *Int J Radiat Oncol Biol Phys* 2010;76(3 Suppl):S101–S107.

27. Sindelar WF, et al. Experimental and clinical studies with intraoperative radiotherapy. *Surg Gynecol Obstet* 1983;157(3):205–219.

28. Whittington R, et al. Radiotherapy of unresectable pancreatic carcinoma: a six year experience with 104 patients. *Int J Radiat Oncol Biol Phys* 1981;7(12):1639–1644.

29. Potish RA. Importance of predisposing factors in the development of enteric damage. *Am J Clin Oncol* 1982;5(2):189–194.

30. Arrowsmith ER, et al. Peripheral T-cell lymphomas: clinical features and prognostic factors of 92 cases defined by the revised European American lymphoma classification. *Leuk Lymphoma* 2003;44(2):241–249.

31. Brennan MF, et al. Lessons learned from the study of 10,000 patients with soft tissue sarcoma. *Ann Surg* 2014;260(3):416–421; discussion 421–422.

32. Ariel IM. Incidence of metastases to lymph nodes from soft-tissue sarcomas. *Semin Surg Oncol* 1988;4(1):27–29.

33. Pisters PW, et al. Analysis of prognostic factors in 1,041 patients with localized soft tissue sarcomas of the extremities. *J Clin Oncol* 1996;14(5):1679–1689.

34. Kattan MW, Leung DH, Brennan MF. Postoperative nomogram for 12-year sarcoma-specific death. *J Clin Oncol* 2002;20(3):791–796.

35. Cahlon O, et al. A postoperative nomogram for local recurrence risk in extremity soft tissue sarcomas after limb-sparing surgery without adjuvant radiation. *Ann Surg* 2012;255(2):343–347.

36. Lindberg RD, et al. Conservative surgery and postoperative radiotherapy in 300 adults with soft-tissue sarcomas. *Cancer* 1981;47(10):2391–2397.

37. Rosenberg SA, et al. The treatment of soft-tissue sarcomas of the extremities: prospective randomized evaluations of (1) limb-sparing surgery plus radiation therapy compared with amputation and (2) the role of adjuvant chemotherapy. *Ann Surg* 1982;196(3):305–315.

38. Yang JC, et al. Randomized prospective study of the benefit of adjuvant radiation therapy in the treatment of soft tissue sarcomas of the extremity. *J Clin Oncol* 1998;16(1):197–203.

39. Sugahara S, et al. Carbon ion radiotherapy for localized primary sarcoma of the extremities: results of a phase I/II trial. *Radiother Oncol* 2012;105(2):226–231.

40. Pisters PW, et al. Long-term results of a prospective randomized trial of adjuvant brachytherapy in soft tissue sarcoma. *J Clin Oncol* 1996;14(3):859–868.

41. Alektiar KM, et al. Adjuvant radiotherapy for margin-positive high-grade soft tissue sarcoma of the extremity. *Int J Radiat Oncol Biol Phys* 2000;48(4):1051–1058.

42. Mundt AJ, et al. Conservative surgery and adjuvant radiation therapy in the management of adult soft tissue sarcoma of the extremities: clinical and radiobiological results. *Int J Radiat Oncol Biol Phys* 1995;32(4):977–985.

43. Alektiar KM, Brennan MF, Singer S. Local control comparison of adjuvant brachytherapy to intensity-modulated radiotherapy in primary high-grade sarcoma of the extremity. *Cancer* 2011;117(14):3229–3234.

44. Folkert MR, et al. Comparison of local recurrence with conventional and intensity-modulated radiation therapy for primary soft-tissue sarcomas of the extremity. *J Clin Oncol* 2014;32(29):3236–3241.

45. Wang D, et al. Significant reduction of late toxicities in patients with extremity sarcoma treated with image-guided radiation therapy to a reduced target volume: results of Radiation Therapy Oncology Group RTOG-0630 Trial. *J Clin Oncol* 2015;33(20):2231–2238.

46. Haas RL, et al. Radiotherapy for management of extremity soft tissue sarcomas: why, when, and where? *Int J Radiat Oncol Biol Phys* 2012;84(3):572–580.

47. Davis AM, et al. Late radiation morbidity following randomization to preoperative versus post-operative radiotherapy in extremity soft tissue sarcoma. *Radiother Oncol* 2005;75(1):48–53.

48. Barkley HT Jr, et al. Treatment of soft tissue sarcomas by preoperative irradiation and conservative surgical resection. *Int J Radiat Oncol Biol Phys* 1988;14(4):693–699.

49. Suit H, Rosenberg A, Harmon D, et al. Soft tissue sarcomas. In: Halnan K, Sikora K, eds. *Treatment of cancer*, 2nd ed. London, UK: Chapman and Hall, 1990:657–677.

50. Kosela-Paterczyk H, et al. Preoperative hypofractionated radiotherapy in the treatment of localized soft tissue sarcomas. *Eur J Surg Oncol* 2014;40(12):1641–1647.

51. Potter DA, et al. High-grade soft tissue sarcomas of the extremities. *Cancer* 1986;58(1):190–205.

52. O'Sullivan B, et al. Preoperative versus postoperative radiotherapy in soft-tissue sarcoma of the limbs: a randomised trial. *Lancet* 2002;359(9325):2235–2241.

53. Holloway CL, et al. American Brachytherapy Society (ABS) consensus statement for sarcoma brachytherapy. *Brachytherapy* 2013;12(3):179–190.

54. Naghavi AO, et al. American Brachytherapy Society consensus statement for soft tissue sarcoma brachytherapy. *Brachytherapy* 2017;16(3):466–489.

55. Calvo FA, et al. Limb-sparing management with surgical resection, external-beam and intraoperative electron-beam radiation therapy boost for patients with primary soft tissue sarcoma of the extremity: a multicentric pooled analysis of long-term outcomes. *Strahlenther Onkol* 2014;190(10):891–898.

56. Roeder F, et al. Excellent local control with IOERT and postoperative EBRT in high grade extremity sarcoma: results from a subgroup analysis of a prospective trial. *BMC Cancer* 2014;14:350.

57. McGinn C, Lawrence T. Soft tissue sarcomas (excluding retroperitoneum). In: Perez C, Brady L, eds. *Principles and practice of radiation oncology*, 3rd ed. Philadelphia, PA: Lippincott–Raven, 1998:2051–2072.

58. Pervaiz N, et al. A systematic meta-analysis of randomized controlled trials of adjuvant chemotherapy for localized resectable soft-tissue sarcoma. *Cancer* 2008;113(3):573–581.

59. D'Adamo DR. Appraising the current role of chemotherapy for the treatment of sarcoma. *Semin Oncol* 2011;38(Suppl 3):S19–S29.

60. Noujaim J, et al. Histology-driven therapy: the importance of diagnostic accuracy in guiding systemic therapy of soft tissue tumors. *Int J Surg Pathol* 2016;24(1):5–15.

61. Ray M, McGinn C. Soft tissue sarcomas (excluding retroperitoneum). In: Halperin E, Perez C, Brady L, eds. *Principles and practice of radiation oncology*. Philadelphia, PA: Lippincott Williams & Wilkins, 2008:1808–1821.

62. Dickie CI, et al. Bone fractures following external beam radiotherapy and limb-preservation surgery for lower extremity soft tissue sarcoma: relationship to irradiated bone length, volume, tumor location and dose. *Int J Radiat Oncol Biol Phys* 2009;75(4):1119–1124.

63. Bishop AJ, et al. Treatment-related fractures after combined modality therapy for soft tissue sarcomas of the proximal lower extremity: can the risk be mitigated? *Pract Radiat Oncol* 2016;6(3):194–200.

64. Gortzak Y, et al. Prediction of pathologic fracture risk of the femur after combined modality treatment of soft tissue sarcoma of the thigh. *Cancer* 2010;116(6):1553–1559.

65. Helmstedter CS, et al. Pathologic fractures after surgery and radiation for soft tissue tumors. *Clin Orthop Relat Res* 2001;(389):165–172.

66. Cianni R, et al. Selective internal radiation therapy with SIR-spheres for the treatment of unresectable colorectal hepatic metastases. *Cardiovasc Intervent Radiol* 2009;32(6):1179–1186.

CHAPTER 42

BRAIN TUMORS IN CHILDREN

ANATOMY AND DEVELOPMENT

- There are no significant anatomic differences between the central nervous system (CNS) of a child and the CNS of an adult.
- The CNS in children reaches morphologic maturation during the first 2 years of life.
- The brain's neuronal complement and organization are essentially complete at birth; however, the myelin sheaths that cover the long nerve processes forming the connecting tracks or white matter of the brain and spinal cord are lacking. Myelinization occurs in a progressive anatomic sequence early in life, beginning with the corpus callosum centrally, and ending with the white matter of the cerebral hemispheres peripherally at 12 to 24 months of age.
- As functional maturation continues, the brain develops motor and sensory coordination during the first several years of childhood and progressive intellectual capacities throughout childhood and adolescence.
- The type and degree of neurologic and neurocognitive alterations associated with brain irradiation correlate with age-related developmental status.

MEDULLOBLASTOMA

- Medulloblastoma is an undifferentiated tumor believed to arise from the primitive multipotential medulloblast, embryologically located in the external granular layer of the cerebellum. It is classically identified as a primitive neuroectodermal tumor (PNET) presenting in the posterior fossa.
- After much debate, the World Health Organization preserved the term medulloblastoma and identified the supratentorial PNET as a specific undifferentiated embryonal neoplasm separate from classic embryonal tumors, with clear lines of differentiation (Table 42-1).

Table 42-1

Histopathologic Typing of Central Nervous System Tumors: World Health Organization Classification

Tumors of Neuroepithelial Tissue

Astrocytic tumors (astrocytoma, anaplastic astrocytoma, glioblastoma, pilocytic astrocytoma, pleomorphic xanthoastrocytoma, subependymal giant cell astrocytoma)

Oligodendroglial tumors (oligodendroglioma, anaplastic oligodendroglioma)

Ependymal tumors (ependymoma, anaplastic ependymoma, myxopapillary ependymoma)

Mixed gliomas (oligoastrocytoma, others)

Choroid plexus tumors

Neuronal tumors (gangliocytoma, ganglioglioma, desmoplastic infantile neuroepithelioma, dysembryoplastic neuroepithelial tumor)

Pineal tumors (pineocytoma, **pineoblastoma**)

Embryonal Tumors

Medulloepithelioma

Neuroblastoma

Ependymoblastoma

Primitive neuroectodermal tumors, medulloblastoma (posterior fossa, cerebellar), cerebral or spinal primitive neuroectodermal tumors

Tumors of Meningothelial Cells

Meningioma

Malignant meningioma

Tumors of Uncertain Histogenesis

Hemangioblastoma

Germ Cell Tumors

Germinoma

Embryonal carcinoma

Endodermal sinus tumor

Choriocarcinoma

Teratoma

Mixed germ cell tumors

Tumors of the Sellar Region

Pituitary adenoma

Craniopharyngioma

Note: Bold identifies embryonal tumors generically identified as primitive neuroectodermal tumors or PNETs.
Source: Kleihues P, Burger PC, Scheithauer BW, eds. *Histological typing of tumours of the central nervous system.* Berlin, Germany: Springer-Verlag, 1994.

Table 42-2

Chang Staging System for Medulloblastoma

Primary Tumor (T)	
T1	Tumor <3 cm in diameter
T2	Tumor ≥3 cm in diameter
T3a	Tumor >3 cm in diameter with extension into the aqueduct of Sylvius or into the foramen of Luschka
T3b	Tumor >3 cm in diameter with unequivocal extension into the brainstem
T4	Tumor >3 cm in diameter with extension up past the aqueduct of Sylvius or down past the foramen magnum (i.e., beyond the posterior fossa)
Distant Metastasis (M)	
M0	No evidence of subarachnoid or hematogenous metastasis
M1	Tumor cells found in cerebrospinal fluid
M2	Intracranial tumor beyond primary site (e.g., subarachnoid space or in the third or lateral ventricles)
M3	Gross nodular seeding in spinal subarachnoid space
M4	Metastasis outside the cerebrospinal axis (especially bone marrow, bone)

Note: T3b is generally defined by intraoperative demonstration of tumor extension into the brainstem.
Source: A pre-CT era system described by Chang CH, Housepian EM, Herbert C Jr. An operative staging system and a megavoltage radiotherapeutic technic for cerebellar medulloblastomas. *Radiology* 1969;93:1351, as modified by J. Langston (personal communication, 1988).

- The "staging" system is based on operative observation of tumor extent, now modified by imaging, and neuraxis staging, as suggested by Chang in the pre–computed tomography (CT) era (Table 42-2).
- Current data indicate that M stage correlates significantly with outcome, but local tumor extent (T stage, including T3b or brainstem invasion) has little impact in series reporting aggressive surgical resection (1).
- Risk stratification is performed following workup and resection and divides patients with medulloblastoma into either standard-risk or high-risk disease categories (Table 42-3).
- Recent genomic studies using genetic drivers for classification have further reliably identified and categorized medulloblastoma based on four subtypes (WNT, SHH, group C, and group D), each with well-defined clinical presentation, genetic abnormalities, and clinical outcomes. Ongoing studies are designed to match specific therapies to medulloblastoma subtypes (2).

Management

- The initial approach is gross total resection (GTR); complete or subtotal resection (STR) is achieved in 70% to 90% of children and is associated with improved disease control (1).
- Radiation therapy (RT) is often curative and is central in the management of medulloblastoma.

Table 42-3
Medulloblastoma Risk Stratification

Standard (Average) Risk
>3 years old
<1.5 cm² residual disease after resection
M0 by craniospinal MRI and CSF

High Risk
<3 years old
Subtotal resection, >1.5 cm² residual tumor
M+; leptomeningeal seeding
Location outside of posterior fossa (PNET)

- Medulloblastoma is sensitive to chemotherapy; high response rates have been documented with alkylating agents (especially cyclophosphamide) and platinum compounds (1).
- The combination of aggressive chemotherapy with incomplete or inadequate craniospinal irradiation (CSI) is associated with high rates of neuraxis recurrence (1).
- In patients receiving pre-CSI chemotherapy, the risk of neuraxis progression increases with the duration of chemotherapy (3).
- High-dose chemotherapy with autologous marrow rescue has occasionally been effective as a salvage regimen in recurrent disease (4).

Radiation Therapy

- Because the entire subarachnoid space is at risk, full neuraxis irradiation is mandatory.
- Adequate coverage at the subfrontal cribriform plate is particularly important; subfrontal recurrences are well documented and technically avoidable (5).
- CSI typically is performed with the patient in a prone position by means of an immobilizing cast or vacuum device.
- Lateral craniocervical fields adjoin a posterior spinal field (or two adjacent spinal fields in larger children).
- The junction between the lateral and posterior fields is critical and generally is achieved with correction for both superior divergence of the posterior spinal field (using a collimator angle for the lateral fields) and caudal divergence of the lateral fields (using a couch angle for the lateral fields). An "exact" three-dimensional (3D) junction is preferable, obviating the need for a "gap" yet requiring a shifting junction to minimize the potential for dosimetric inhomogeneity (6).
- A frequently used "moving junction" allows for the elimination (or marked decrease) of dose inhomogeneity at the craniospinal portal junction and minimizes failures or complications (7).
- Planning CSI delivery with proton pencil beam scanning can reduce dose inhomogeneity and matching pitfalls with gradient dose optimization (8).

- The staged intensity-modulated proton therapy (IMPT) technique has also been shown to improve setup error and sparing of critical structures compared to passive scatter, both of which can improve CSI plan quality and delivery (9).
- The posterior orbit is not included for central nervous system (CNS) tumors requiring CSI.
- The spinal subarachnoid space extends caudally to S2 or beyond based on magnetic resonance imaging (MRI) delineation.
- The lateral margins should dosimetrically include the width of the vertebral bodies and a 1- to 1.5-cm margin on the pedicles to ensure coverage of meninges and lateral nerve roots in the neural foramina.
- Use of electrons for spinal irradiation has been reported (10), but late results are unavailable. Electrons offer a potential advantage in limiting exit dose but require detailed attention to adequate coverage at depth and junctional homogeneity.
- Investigations of stereotactic radiosurgical technique in special are under evaluation (11).
- The usual sequence of therapy is CSI followed by posterior fossa boost. Therapy may need to be initiated with posterior fossa irradiation if neurologic or hematologic status initially precludes accurate CSI.
- Medulloblastoma is a relatively radiosensitive tumor. Local tumor control exceeds 80% with posterior fossa doses of 54 to 55 Gy in 1.6- to 1.8-Gy fractions (12).
- With postoperative irradiation alone, the standard neuraxis dose is 35 to 36 Gy (1.5 to 1.8 Gy per fraction) (13).
- A phase III trial of craniospinal radiation followed by chemotherapy demonstrated that average-risk patients may be treated safely with 23.4 Gy CSI (followed by a boost to posterior fossa to total 55.8 Gy) and concurrent vincristine followed by adjuvant chemotherapy (14).
- High-risk patients continue to require CSI doses of 36 Gy.
- COG ACNS0331 was a trial of standard-risk medulloblastoma in which conformal radiation boost volumes to the primary site were comparable to standard whole posterior fossa treatment volumes, but reduced CSI dose to 18 Gy compared to standard dose of 23.4 Gy had worse 5-year EFS and OS (15).
- A single-institution phase II trial has demonstrated among 59 patients with medulloblastoma treated with CSI proton therapy to a median dose of 23.4 Gy and boost of 54 Gy, only 9% of patients experienced grade III to IV ototoxicity. The 5-year PFS and OS were shown to be 80% (16).

EMBRYONAL TUMORS/PRIMITIVE NEUROECTODERMAL TUMORS AND MALIGNANT RHABDOID OR ATYPICAL TERATOID TUMORS

- The World Health Organization classification identifies the specific histotypes as medulloepithelioma, ependymoblastoma, or cerebral neuroblastoma; those without specific differentiation are classified as PNETs—medulloblastoma when located in the cerebellum and PNET when supratentorial (Table 42-1).
- Pineoblastomas are clinically grouped with the embryonal tumors.

Management

- Tumor extent and location often limit resectability of supratentorial PNETs, ependymoblastomas, pineoblastomas, and rhabdoid tumors.
- Cerebral neuroblastomas frequently are circumscribed lesions, with GTR reported in over 25% of cases (17).
- Postoperative neuraxis irradiation with local boost to the primary tumor site is standard in children older than 3 to 4 years of age.
- Guidelines for technique and dose are similar to those outlined for medulloblastoma: boost volumes for supratentorial or pineal region tumors are defined as wide local volumes with 2- to 3-cm margins, based on preoperative tumor extent and postsurgical anatomic changes.
- Limited data support local fields only for cerebral neuroblastoma; most series recommend CSI (18).
- Embryonal tumors in infants and young children generally are treated with initial chemotherapy (either lomustine [CCNU], vincristine sulfate, and prednisone or the "8-in-1" regimen) (17,19).

EPENDYMOMA

- Ependymomas are derived from the ependymal cells lining the ventricular system; they occur throughout the CNS.
- In children, 90% of ependymomas are intracranial neoplasms; 60% to 70% arise in the posterior fossa, primarily within the fourth ventricle.
- Supratentorial ependymomas occur predominantly in the parietal and frontal lobes, often contiguous with the ventricular system. They rarely occur as intraventricular tumors.
- Posterior fossa lesions classically arise along the floor of the fourth ventricle and frequently extend through the foramen of Luschka toward or into the cerebellopontine angle.
- In infants, tumors may originate in the cerebellopontine angle.
- Tumors grow through the foramen magnum in up to 50% of cases, usually as tongue-like projections extending to the C1 or C2 level; caudal extension may reach to C5 (20).

Prognostic Factors

- In a review of 37 children, univariate analysis showed that total surgical resection and median infratentorial location correlated with better outcome ($p < 0.002$). Loss of differentiating structures or a combination of necrosis, endothelial proliferation, and mitotic index higher than 5 were associated with poor prognosis. Adjuvant chemotherapy or RT significantly enhanced progression-free survival only in patients who had incomplete tumor resection (21).

Management

- Surgery and RT are standard treatment approaches for intracranial ependymomas (22).

- Maximal surgical resection is the optimal initial therapy (21), although it possibly should be delayed in infants in whom response to initial chemotherapy may permit more complete "secondary" resection.
- For supratentorial tumors, size and location may limit resectability.
- RT adds to disease control and survival. Two retrospective reviews indicate survival of 0% and 13% with surgery alone compared with 45% and 59% with irradiation ($p = 0.03$) (23).
- A St. Jude trial followed 153 children treated with aggressive surgery followed by immediate postoperative high-dose photon irradiation. The subgroup of patients treated without chemotherapy and without delayed irradiation (greater than 4.4 months after diagnosis) experienced a high 7-year PFS and OS of 77% and 85%, respectively. Predictors of PFS and OS include extent of resection, tumor grade, preirradiation chemotherapy, age, and race.
- Ependymomas are relatively sensitive to chemotherapy, especially alkylating agents and platinum compounds.
- Adjuvant chemotherapy has been the basis for multiple recent phase II and phase III trials, including the AIEOP and SIOP-EP-II studies.
- Based on the AIEOP trial, children with WHO grade II disease with NED after initial surgery were either given fractionated RT to 59.4 Gy or 6 cycles of chemotherapy (vincristine, etoposide, and cyclophosphamide) if younger than 3 years of age. Those with WHO grade III and NED received adjuvant postirradiation chemotherapy. Those with residual disease received second surgery, 4 cycles of chemotherapy, and radiation of 59.4 Gy followed by an 8 Gy boost. OS and PFS at 5 years were 65% and 81%, respectively.
- The SIOP-EP-II trial stratified patients to receive conventional chemotherapy with or without a histone deacetylase (HDAC) inhibitor. Results are pending.
- Recent research has identified potential epigenetic modifiers and targetable markers such as hypermethylated phenotypes in childhood ependymomas (24–26).

Radiation Therapy

- Debate continues regarding the appropriate irradiation volume for intracranial ependymomas.
- Some series indicate overt neuraxis dissemination at diagnosis in 3% to 16% of children; this is more often documented by cytology alone rather than by cranial and spinal imaging (23).
- Although historic data suggested a correlation between high-grade or anaplastic posterior fossa ependymomas and spinal seeding, subsequent data failed to substantiate a site- or histology-specific relationship (13,23,27).
- The incidence of neuraxis failure, either alone or in combination with local recurrence, is estimated to be 12% (28).
- In most series, neuraxis failure is associated with simultaneous local recurrence in at least 50% of cases.
- Disease control rates in contemporary series show no advantage to full cranial or craniospinal volumes compared with wide local fields, based on modern imaging (23).

- For tumors extending into the upper cervical spine, the inferior margin should be two vertebral levels below the preoperative tumor extent until field reduction at 45 Gy.
- For supratentorial ependymomas, local fields are defined by preoperative tumor extent, accounting for shifts in the normal brain postoperatively; margins of 2 to 3 cm are recommended (28).
- For documented intraventricular extension, full ventricular irradiation (45 Gy) is appropriate.
- Current guidelines call for 50 to 55 Gy to the primary tumor site, including field reduction at 45 Gy, to more narrowly encompass the tumor bed (20).
- Boost doses to 55 to 65 Gy have been recommended and are directed to small volumes of known residual disease, preferably using stereotactic radiosurgery or fractionated stereotactic irradiation (29).
- The COG trial ACNS0121 enrolled 378 patients based on (a) GTR followed by observation; (b) STR followed by chemotherapy, second surgery, and RT; (c) macroscopic GTR followed by conformal RT; and (d) microscopic GTR followed by conformal RT. Five-year EFS were 61%, 39%, 67%, and 70%, respectively. Primary failure was local, but a third of patients had a metastatic component of failure (30).

MALIGNANT BRAIN TUMORS IN INFANTS AND YOUNG CHILDREN

- Approximately 20% of pediatric brain tumors occur in infants and children younger than 3 years of age.
- Compared with tumors in older children, those occurring in this age group are more likely to be malignant by histology (embryonal tumors, malignant gliomas, choroid plexus carcinomas, and malignant rhabdoid tumors) and clinical behavior; supratentorial in location (especially during the first year of life); and associated with subarachnoid metastasis at diagnosis (23).
- Surgery is more difficult in the infant brain.
- The therapeutic index for RT is restrictive, with increased long-term neurologic and neurocognitive deficits leading to recommendations for dose reductions for children younger than 2 to 3 years of age (13).
- Results for medulloblastoma, ependymoma, and pineoblastoma show less favorable prognosis for children younger than 3 to 5 years of age (13,23).
- Supratentorial astrocytomas (especially optic chiasmatic/hypothalamic) are also common in young children; low-grade tumors are discussed elsewhere (28).

Management

- Data indicate successful treatment without irradiation in a small number of children with medulloblastoma and resected ependymoma.
- For children who progress during chemotherapy or have persistent disease at completion, aggressive CSI (30 to 35 Gy) has resulted in greater than 50% disease control at 5 years for medulloblastoma. Toxicities, although recognized, have been acceptable (31).

- The large Pediatric Oncology Group (POG) and Children's Cancer Group (CCG) "baby protocols," using 1 to 2 years of postoperative chemotherapy and systematic (POG) or selected (CCG) delayed irradiation, established progression-free survival rates of 37% at 2 years (all malignant cell types, POG) and 23% at 3 years (embryonal tumors and ependymomas, CCG) (32).
- Disease control has been moderately successful with malignant gliomas (3-year progression-free survival of 45%), medulloblastomas (38%), and ependymomas (45%), but poor with pineoblastomas (0%) (32).

LOW-GRADE GLIOMAS

- Almost 40% of pediatric brain tumors are low-grade gliomas (astrocytomas, oligodendrogliomas, mixed gliomas, and mixed neuroepithelial tumors).
- Astrocytomas present most often as supratentorial tumors; 60% occur in the diencephalon (hypothalamus, optic chiasm/optic pathways, and thalamus) and 40% in the cerebral hemispheres.
- Infratentorial astrocytomas involve the cerebellum or brainstem.
- Low-grade pediatric astrocytomas (WHO grade I to II) have excellent greater than 90% long-term PFS and OS and a much lower incidence of malignant transformation compared to similar than low-grade adult astrocytomas (33).
- Optic pathway tumors are low-grade gliomas (largely astrocytomas) in 90% of cases.
- Unique among childhood astrocytomas is the relative frequency of juvenile pilocytic astrocytoma (JPA), which is generally an indolent, circumscribed tumor.
- Oligodendroglioma is less common in children.
- Mixed gliomas most often include both oligodendroglial and astrocytic components.
- Although low-grade gliomas are classically localized, circumscribed tumors, they can show multifocal or disseminated disease; multiple tumor sites are seen in up to 20% of JPAs or ordinary astrocytomas, either at diagnosis or as a primary pattern of failure (34).
- Progression or transformation toward malignant glioma occurs in 10% to 15% of children with ordinary astrocytoma, especially if uncontrolled (35).
- Incomplete resection results in lower rates of 5-year PFS around 65%.

Low-Grade Diencephalic Gliomas (Optic Chiasmatic/Hypothalamic Gliomas, Low-Grade Thalamic Gliomas)

- It is difficult to differentiate tumors of the optic chiasm from those of the hypothalamus.
- By convention, suprasellar tumors that involve the visual pathways (optic nerve or tract) are termed optic chiasmatic tumors.
- Optic pathway gliomas are divided between anterior (40%, involving the optic nerve or chiasm) and posterior tumors (60%, involving the chiasm plus the hypothalamus, with or without extension into the optic tracts).
- Outcomes are based on location of the tumor with OS greater than 95% in patients with tumors confined to the optic nerve.
- Thalamic gliomas present throughout the pediatric age group, without specific association with neurofibromatosis type 1 (NF-1).

Management

- Tumors of the optic pathways may be relatively indolent (even asymptomatic), or, conversely, associated with significant vision loss or disabling diencephalic signs.
- Treatment is indicated for significant visual or neurologic deficits or for objective evidence of progression based on serial imaging or visual testing.
- Optic nerve glioma is managed by observation or resection, with the latter restricted to patients with disease anterior to the chiasm and little or no vision.
- Resection has been recommended for "exophytic" chiasmatic/hypothalamic tumors (36).
- RT was historically highly effective as a first-line treatment, but platinum-based chemotherapy is now favored (37).
- Radiation is reserved for progression after chemotherapy.
- Surgical intervention for thalamic glioma has been controversial (38). RT achieves durable disease control in approximately 50% of cases (13).
- Outcome is correlated with histology and is superior in JPA.
- Trials of chemotherapy have been prompted by radiation-related toxicities in very young children with optic chiasm/hypothalamic gliomas.

Radiation Therapy

- Local treatment volumes are used for optic pathway and hypothalamic tumors.
- Lesions confined to the chiasm and/or hypothalamus can be treated with conventional arcs or multiple coplanar configurations; early experience suggests excellent coverage with fractionated stereotactic irradiation or 3D conformal techniques (29,39).
- Optic pathway tumors that involve the optic nerves or optic tracts (sometimes extending posteriorly beyond the lateral geniculate bodies to the optic radiation) require opposed lateral high-energy fields, at least for a sizable component of the total irradiation dose.
- Children with NF-1 frequently exhibit "NF-1" lesions (characterized by the absence of enhancement and bright, focal signal on T2 sequences) that do not show neoplastic potential; such foci are common in the basal ganglia and brainstem and do not require radiation coverage.
- Dose levels of 50 Gy are recommended for children older than 3 years of age but are reduced to 45 Gy in infants.
- Thalamic gliomas usually require local treatment volumes; evidence of extension (into the midbrain or across the corpus callosum) calls for wider margins.
- Evolving experience with 3D planned therapies suggests efficacy for localized low-grade thalamic gliomas (29). A dose of 54 Gy is recommended (13).

Low-Grade Cerebral Hemispheric Gliomas

- Histologically, these tumors are predominately astrocytomas (JPA, ordinary astrocytomas); oligoastrocytomas are common (35).

Management

- Complete resection is the goal for most hemispheric gliomas (35).
- There is clearly no indication for adjuvant irradiation in completely resected low-grade astrocytomas. Similar recommendations are suggested for oligoastrocytoma and oligodendroglioma (35).
- For incompletely resected tumors, observation, radiation, or chemotherapy all have been proposed.
- Long-term disease control has been well documented after irradiation (13,40).
- Packer et al. has shown that younger age at diagnosis less than 5 years old is the most important factor in 3-year PFS (74% versus 39%).
- If planning to adjuvantly treat children less than 5 years old, chemotherapy should be initiated until child is 5 years old, at which time they should receive RT.
- Desmoplastic cerebral tumors (astrocytoma, infantile ganglioglioma, and desmoplastic neuroepithelial tumor) are often massive, superficial lesions that occur in infants and young children and are usually resectable despite their extent; adjuvant therapy is not indicated.

Radiation Therapy

- Local treatment volumes are indicated for low-grade gliomas.
- Use of 3D conformal techniques or fractionated stereotactic irradiation is of value in these circumscribed lesions (29).
- The recommended dose is 54 to 55 Gy; controlled studies of doses approximating 60 Gy with stereotactic techniques are ongoing (40).

Cerebellar Astrocytomas

- Cerebellar astrocytomas are benign, relatively common tumors occurring primarily in children 3 to 5 years of age.
- The tumors are classically cystic; approximately 85% are JPA histologically.

Management

- Complete resection, the treatment of choice, is achievable in 80% to 90% of cases (41).
- Recurrence after GTR is anecdotal (41).
- A clear indication for postoperative irradiation is unconfirmed in the literature.
- The availability of focal, fractionated radiation techniques raises the question of whether small areas of residual diffuse (i.e., not JPA) cerebellar astrocytomas might be best managed by judicious postoperative irradiation, thus avoiding the larger treatment volumes likely to be required with progressive tumors usually residual along the brainstem.

MALIGNANT GLIOMAS

- Malignant gliomas represent 7% to 10% of pediatric CNS tumors and approximately 15% of astrocytomas and common glial neoplasms.

- Histologically, 50% to 60% are anaplastic astrocytomas, 30% to 40% are glioblastomas, and 10% to 20% are anaplastic oligodendrogliomas and malignant mixed gliomas (42).
- The tumors are locally infiltrating; most series indicate a 5% to 10% rate of neuraxis dissemination at diagnosis.
- Peak incidence is at 9 years of age.
- Two third of malignant gliomas occur in cerebral hemispheres.
- Cells histologically display necrosis, high nuclear activity, cellular atypia, and microvascular proliferation.

Management

- Outcome is clearly superior after aggressive surgical resection for cerebral hemispheric malignant gliomas but can only be achieved around 75% of the time.
- It is rare to achieve more than biopsy or limited resection in thalamic tumors (17).
- Postoperative MRI is required within 24 to 48 hours of operation to evaluate extent of residual.
- RT is indicated postoperatively, except for children younger than 3 to 5 years of age who enter initial chemotherapy studies.
- The use of adjuvant chemoradiation therapy (CRT) by CCG-943, which tested postoperative irradiation versus combined irradiation and chemotherapy (vincristine sulfate, lomustine, and prednisone), has shown no difference in 5-year PFS (33%) or OS (36%) with the addition of chemotherapy. Fourteen percent, however, were not malignant gliomas but low-grade gliomas or ependymomas (43).
- ACNS0126 (Cohen et al.) has shown that childhood GBMs without O6-methylguanine-methyltransferase (MGMT) overexpression when treated with concurrent radiation with temozolomide (TMZ) and RT followed by adjuvant TMZ had no difference in EFS improvement. Although 2-year EFS rate was 17% among patients without MGMT overexpression and 5% among those with MGMT overexpression ($p = 0.045$), TMZ failed to improve outcome in children with high-grade astrocytomas (44).

Radiation Therapy

- Adjuvant RT in childhood malignant gliomas is similar to adjuvant RT in adult malignant gliomas.
- Adjuvant RT improves 5-year OS (10% to 30%) from surgery alone (0%).
- As in adults, current recommendations include wide local volumes for both thalamic and cerebral hemispheric tumors, based on preoperative tumor extent and reconfiguration of the brain after resection.
- CTV1 is defined as tumor bed (preoperative gross tumor volume [GTV] on T1 postcontrast MRI scans), residual disease, and edema on T2 scans with a 1.5- to 2.0-cm margin.
- PTV1 is defined as CTV1 with a 0.3- to 0.5-cm margin and is treated to 45 Gy.
- CTV2 boost is defined as a field reduction to residual disease on T1 postcontrast with an additional 1-cm margin.

- PTV2 is defined as CTV2 with a 0.3- to 0.5-cm margin and is treated to 54 to 59.4 Gy depending on location.
- There has been limited use of CSI in malignant gliomas.
- Although disseminated disease has been documented in up to 30% to 40% of children with supratentorial lesions, the incidence of isolated neuraxis failure remains at or below 10% (42).
- Limited data fail to indicate an advantage with "preventive" or therapeutic neuraxis irradiation. This is believed to be due to limited impact with tolerated doses of CSI (28).
- Use of stereotactic interstitial implants and radiosurgical boost therapy has been reported in pediatric malignant gliomas (29). Numbers are inadequate to draw conclusions, which must be based on the broader experience in young adults.

BRAINSTEM GLIOMAS

- Brainstem gliomas arise in the midbrain (or mesencephalon, including the tegmentum and tectal plate), pons, or medulla.
- Approximately 75% are pontine gliomas, presenting as diffusely infiltrating, expansile lesions that commonly extend longitudinally (to the medulla or midbrain) and into the cerebellopontine peduncles.
- Brainstem gliomas occur predominantly in children between 3 and 9 years of age.
- Brainstem tumors in children are classified as high or low grade. Fisher et al. (45) suggested that these tumors may be better biologically classified as (a) diffusely infiltrating, generally fibrillary astrocytomas, located in the ventral pons, and associated with a grim prognosis or as (b) focal, frequently pilocytic astrocytomas, arising outside the ventral pons, often with dorsal exophytic growth, and associated with excellent prognosis.
- Two-year overall survival is less than 10%.

Management

- The morbidity of biopsy within the pons and the lack of histology-specific therapeutic options virtually obviate indications for surgery for pontine gliomas (28).
- Dorsally exophytic brainstem gliomas require judicious surgical resection; a significant percentage will need ventriculoperitoneal (VP) shunt placement.
- Biopsy generally is indicated for tegmental midbrain tumors.
- Tectal plate tumors obstruct the aqueduct of Sylvius even when very small; VP shunt is indicated, followed by observation.
- Biopsy for typically indolent tectal plate tumors usually is deferred until documented growth requires therapeutic intervention (46).
- Intrinsic tumors at the cervicomedullary junction have been resected in some neurosurgical centers; further therapy is indicated only for the infrequent, high-grade neoplasms (28).

- RT is the primary treatment for brainstem gliomas arising in the pons (47). The radiation response and yet poor outcome have encouraged trials of hyperfractionated irradiation in this tumor system.
- Chemotherapy has little efficacy in pontine gliomas.

Radiation Therapy

- Infiltrating tumors of the pons require 2- to 3-cm anatomic margins in defining the target volume which may be reduced by anatomical barriers; T2 imaging is most accurate in outlining longitudinal (to the medulla and midbrain) and axial extension (to the cerebellopontine peduncles and into the cerebellum) as shown in a sample case (Fig. 42.1).
- Opposed lateral high-energy beam fields are used most often.
- The target volume for dorsally exophytic tumors is limited to the postoperative area of disease residual or progression along the posterior and/or lateral surface of the medulla or pons.

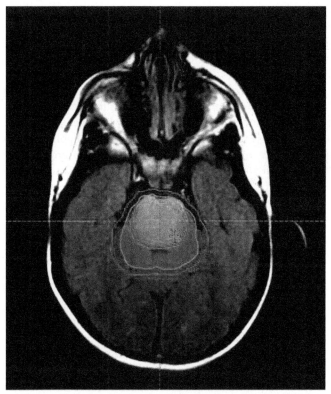

FIGURE 42-1. A 5-year-old girl with a diffuse intrinsic pontine glioma underwent definitive radiotherapy to 5,400 cGy. MRI scans including the T2 FLAIR were registered for treatment planning as the target was in the brainstem. The GTV (*light red*) contours the FLAIR enhancing tumor, the CTV (*orange*) contours the microscopic disease, and the PTV (*dark red*) contours a margin outside the CTV.

- Fractionated stereotactic irradiation or 3D conformal therapy may be ideal for these tumors.
- Focal tumors intrinsic to the pons or small lesions of the midbrain are ideally treated by standard coronal arc technique or the newer 3D modalities.
- The potential advantage of hyperfractionated irradiation in brainstem gliomas was reported using 72 Gy at 1 Gy twice daily (48).
- When disease control and toxicity data are combined, a "best" hyperfractionation regimen is suggested at 70.2 or 70.0 Gy, using 1.17- or 1.00-Gy fractions, respectively (47).
- A CCG trial of hyperfractionated irradiation in children with brainstem glioma suggested that altered fractionation could not be considered superior to conventional RT (49).
- Late toxicities with high-dose hyperfractionation, including neurocognitive deficits, hearing loss, leukoencephalopathy, diffuse microhemorrhages, and dystrophic calcifications on MRI, limit enthusiasm for routine use of hyperfractionated therapy for pontine gliomas or the more favorable brainstem presentations (39).
- For dorsally exophytic or focal brainstem tumors, "standard" irradiation regimens have used 50 to 55 Gy at fraction sizes approximating 1.8 Gy.
- Trials are under development in the cooperative groups to incorporate conventionally fractionated irradiation to the 55.8-Gy level.
- Use of conventionally fractionated dose schedules delivered by 3D techniques offers the most beneficial risk-benefit ratio based on available data.

CRANIOPHARYNGIOMA

- Craniopharyngioma is a benign tumor, arising from squamous cell rests derived from Rathke's pouch during embryogenesis, in the region of the pituitary stalk (classically from the tuber cinereum).
- Craniopharyngioma presents as a suprasellar tumor, frequently partially calcified and usually including an intrasellar component.
- Cystic or solid tumor extension may occur laterally into the middle cranial fossa or posteriorly into the posterior fossa.
- Endocrine deficits are apparent in 50% to 90% of children at diagnosis, most often related to growth hormone, thyroid-stimulating hormone, and adrenocorticotropic hormone; diabetes insipidus is present in 10% to 15% (50).

Management

- Treatment for craniopharyngioma is controversial.
- Total resection as the primary approach is attempted in most cases (51,52).
- Recurrence is relatively infrequent after imaging-confirmed resection; recent series indicate failure in 10% to 30% of cases (51,52).
- Postoperative imaging shows residual calcifications or frank tumor in up to 15% to 25% of cases coded at surgery as completely resected (52).

- Tumor control using limited surgery and irradiation results in durable disease control in 80% of children who are followed for 20 years after therapy (53).
- Numerous series document excellent progression-free survival rates at 10 to 20 years (28).
- Results of primary irradiation are superior to those with delayed therapy.
- For incompletely resected tumors, it is generally preferable to administer postoperative irradiation rather than await tumor progression (28).
- The cystic nature of craniopharyngioma has led to trials of intracystic applications of beta-emitting radionuclides such as yttrium-90 or phosphorus-32 (54).
- Use of stereotactic radiosurgery has been reported in selected cases of minimal residual or recurrent disease; most promising are early reports of fractionated stereotactic irradiation (54).
- There are no data regarding systemic chemotherapy for craniopharyngioma and only limited reports of intracystic bleomycin sulfate.

Radiation Therapy

- The target volume for craniopharyngioma is narrowly confined to the tumor volume, including the solid component and cyst(s).
- In cases with cyst aspiration or limited resection, it is important to cover the cyst wall.
- It is appropriate to limit the target volume to postoperative residual tumor if large cystic components are removed surgically.
- High-energy photons are used with two or three stationary fields or the classic coronal arc configuration.
- There is considerable enthusiasm for stereotactic irradiation or 3D conformal therapy, limiting the high-dose volume to the well-circumscribed neoplasm (7).
- Improved disease control has been reported with doses of 50 to 60 Gy using conventional fractionation (1.8 Gy once daily) (13).
- Toxicity (including optic neuropathy and brain necrosis) is associated with doses higher than 60 Gy (13).

PINEAL REGION TUMORS AND INTRACRANIAL GERM CELL TUMORS

- Pineal region tumors include a variety of histotypes arising in the posterior third ventricular region.
- Germ cell tumors (60% to 70%) and pineal parenchymal tumors (pineoblastoma or pineocytoma, 10% to 20%) are most common (55,56).
- As diagnostic imaging becomes more specific regarding pineal versus broader third ventricular origin, the proportion of cases represented by astrocytomas, ependymomas, other glial tumors, and arachnoid cysts has diminished.
- Intracranial germ cell tumors present as midline third ventricular tumors, occurring in the pineal region (50% to 60%) or the suprasellar region (30% to 35%); occasionally, they arise in the basal ganglia/thalamic region.

- All malignant and benign germ cell phenotypes occur as primary intracranial lesions: 60% to 70% are germinomas, 15% to 20% are "marker-secreting" types (embryonal carcinoma, endodermal sinus or yolk sac tumor, choriocarcinoma), and 15% to 20% are teratomas (benign, immature, or malignant) (28).
- Biochemical markers are noted in both serum and cerebral spinal fluid (CSF), with elevation of β-human chorionic gonadotropin (β-hCG) (typically measured in thousands) associated with choriocarcinoma and α-fetoprotein (AFP) elevation with endodermal sinus tumor or embryonal carcinoma. Levels up to 50 to 75 IU do not appear to negatively affect outcome after irradiation; levels greater than 50 are associated with unfavorable prognosis when "primary" chemotherapy is used (28).
- Germinomas may show mild elevation of serum or CSF β-hCG.

Management

- Biopsy is standard practice for suprasellar tumors and is preferable for pineal region tumors (56,57).
- VP shunt often is required (55).
- Histologic diagnosis may be obviated when elevated AFP levels are documented (diagnostic of an aggressive or "malignant" germ cell type) or, with less confidence, when multiple midline third ventricular tumors are noted in teenage boys (diagnostic of germinoma) (55).
- Histologic confirmation permits selection of treatment regarding irradiation parameters and adjuvant chemotherapy (18,55).
- Resection has no apparent role in germinoma; a potential gain in other types of germ cell tumors remains to be proven (57).
- An association between surgery and the risk of neuraxis or systemic dissemination has not been identified (55–57).
- RT is the standard treatment for intracranial germinomas, with levels of disease control often exceeding 90% (56,57), although there is considerable debate regarding appropriate dose and volume for primary irradiation.
- The radioresponsiveness of germinomas has encouraged a trial of local irradiation (20 to 25 Gy) for nonbiopsied pineal region tumors; documented early response was considered evidence of germinoma, and subsequent primary irradiation was administered. A lack of early responsiveness was considered evidence of an unfavorable germ cell tumor or, more likely, other tumor type; subsequent local irradiation or surgery was pursued (13,56).
- The current availability of relatively safe biopsy information renders the "radiodiagnostic" approach largely outdated (56).
- For other germ cell histotypes, irradiation is part of multimodality therapy, potentially including stereotactic RT.
- Data suggest that irradiation may be indicated for pineocytomas in children, although these tumors are benign in adults (58).
- Intracranial germ cell tumors are highly chemosensitive, with high rates of objective response to alkylating agents, platinum compounds, and traditional extraneural germ cell tumor regimens (57).

Radiation Therapy

- The variably reported incidence of subependymal and neuraxis seeding in intracranial germ cell tumors has focused debate on the appropriate irradiation volume.
- Earlier data from Columbia University indicated an actuarial rate of subarachnoid seeding approaching 37%, with the rate of spinal failure higher in suprasellar germinomas (43% at 5 years) than in the largely clinically diagnosed pineal region tumors (10%) (28).
- The rate of concurrent pineal and suprasellar lesions (multiple midline germinomas) ranges from 10% to more than 50% (18,56).
- Positive CSF cytology is reported in more than 60% of Japanese cases; the frequency in North American reports is approximately 15% (59).
- Several major series reporting disease control rates of over 90% are based on low-dose neuraxis irradiation followed by reduced-field boost (56,57), suggesting a role for CSI. Other series indicate a risk of spinal failure no higher than 10% after only local or cranial irradiation for histologically verified germinomas (56,59).
- Although each series consists of a small number of biopsy-proven germinomas, control rates of 90% are reported after local or wide-field cranial irradiation only (absent full CSI).
- Kun (28) favors CSI for all intracranial germinomas in children older than 10 to 12 years of age; for younger children, neuraxis irradiation (typically to dose levels of 25 Gy, in the absence of overt disease) may be obviated in favor of local irradiation (with recognition of a potentially higher risk of disease recurrence) including whole ventricular radiation (Fig. 42.2) or consideration of protocol-based therapy combining local irradiation (often at reduced dose) with chemotherapy (57).
- For other germ cell histotypes, CSI has been standard, but overall results with surgery and irradiation have been poor.
- Combined CRT is favored; some reports suggest that local irradiation may be adequate in conjunction with effective chemotherapy (57).
- Despite the recognized radiosensitivity of gonadal seminomas and the radioresponsiveness of histologically identical intracranial germinomas, most RT data for the latter tumor support a primary dose level approximating 50 Gy.
- The limited series reporting combined chemotherapy and irradiation suggest that a dose level of 35 to 40 Gy to the primary site may be adequate (57).
- Neuraxis dose levels for M0 disease may be limited to 25 Gy; with overt disease, a neuraxis dose of 30 Gy may be combined with third ventricular or local boost dose levels of 45 Gy, as appropriate (60).
- For malignant germ cell tumors, dose levels should approach tolerance, with 54 to 55 Gy to the primary tumor and neuraxis levels approximating 35 or 40 Gy, the latter with overt subarachnoid disease.
- Data regarding reduced dose levels in conjunction with chemotherapy are not available.

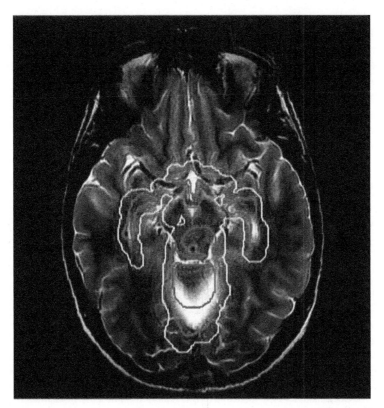

FIGURE 42-2. A 15-year-old male developed a nongerminomatous germ cell tumor with serum and cerebrospinal fluid markers showing elevated human chorionic gonadotropin. The patient underwent chemotherapy as well as radiotherapy. Using MRI scans including T2 FLAIR sequence, a whole-ventricle irradiation target delineation was created. The CTV (*blue*) contours the entire ventricle and PTV (*yellow*) contours provides a margin of the CTV.

SEQUELAE OF TREATMENT

- Acute and late irradiation side effects are related to the specific anatomic site treated.
- Growth disturbances are common in children. The majority of long-term survivors irradiated for brain tumors have been shown to develop growth hormone deficiency, and the adverse effects may be directly related to the biologically effective dose (48).
- Another radiation-related toxicity is the gradual onset of endocrine deficits, earliest and most commonly in growth hormone; subsequent treatment-related deficits in thyroid-stimulating hormone, adrenocorticotropic hormone, and gonadotropins are noted (50,61,62).
- Serious neurotoxicities are recorded in less than 10% of cases but are identifiable as late optic neuropathy or brain necrosis; the incidence is related to doses greater than 60 Gy (51,63).
- Secondary malignant neoplasms have been reported (anecdotally) after irradiation (51).

- Hyperfractionated regimens are associated with moderate acute epithelial toxicity (otitis, radioepidermitis) and dose-related subacute toxicity (prolonged steroid requirement and intralesional necrosis) (47,49,64,65).
- Late toxicities with high-dose hyperfractionation, including neurocognitive deficits and hearing loss clinically and leukoencephalopathy, diffuse microhemorrhages, and dystrophic calcifications on MRI, limit enthusiasm for routine use of hyperfractionated therapy for pontine gliomas or brainstem tumors (39).
- Decreased morbidity has been described in preliminary reports in children treated with proton beams (66,67).

References

1. Bailey CC, Gnekow A, Wellek S, et al. Prospective randomised trial of chemotherapy given before radiotherapy in childhood medulloblastoma. International Society of Paediatric Oncology (SIOP) and the (German) Society of Paediatric Oncology (GPO): SIOP II. *Med Pediatr Oncol* 1995;25(3):166–178.
2. Northcott PA, Korshunov A, Witt H, et al. Medulloblastoma comprises four distinct molecular variants. *J Clin Oncol* 2011;29(11):1408–1414.
3. Hartsell WF, Gajjar A, Heideman RL, et al. Patterns of failure in children with medulloblastoma: effects of preirradiation chemotherapy. *Int J Radiat Oncol Biol Phys* 1997;39(1):15–24.
4. Mahoney DH Jr, Strother D, Camitta B, et al. High-dose melphalan and cyclophosphamide with autologous bone marrow rescue for recurrent/progressive malignant brain tumors in children: a pilot pediatric oncology group study. *J Clin Oncol* 1996;14(2):382–388.
5. Halberg FE, Wara WM, Fippin LF, et al. Low-dose craniospinal radiation therapy for medulloblastoma. *Int J Radiat Oncol Biol Phys* 1991;20(4):651–654.
6. Tatcher M, Glicksman AS. Field matching considerations in craniospinal irradiation. *Int J Radiat Oncol Biol Phys* 1989;17(4):865–869.
7. Kiltie AE, Povall JM, Taylor RE. The need for the moving junction in craniospinal irradiation. *Br J Radiol* 2000;73(870):650–654.
8. Lin H, Ding X, Kirk M, et al. Supine craniospinal irradiation using a proton pencil beam scanning technique without match line changes for field junctions. *Int J Radiat Oncol Biol Phys* 2014;90(1):71–78.
9. Stoker JB, Grant J, Zhu XR, et al. Intensity modulated proton therapy for craniospinal irradiation: organ-at-risk exposure and a low-gradient junctioning technique. *Int J Radiat Oncol Biol Phys* 2014;90(3):637–644.
10. Maor MH, Fields RS, Hogstrom KR, et al. Improving the therapeutic ratio of craniospinal irradiation in medulloblastoma. *Int J Radiat Oncol Biol Phys* 1985;11(4):687–697.
11. Patrice SJ, Tarbell NJ, Goumnerova LC, et al. Results of radiosurgery in the management of recurrent and residual medulloblastoma. *Pediatr Neurosurg* 1995;22(4):197–203.
12. Hughes EN, Shillito J, Sallan SE, et al. Medulloblastoma at the joint center for radiation therapy between 1968 and 1984. The influence of radiation dose on the patterns of failure and survival. *Cancer* 1988;61(10):1992–1998.
13. Bloom HJ, Glees J, Bell J, et al. The treatment and long-term prognosis of children with intracranial tumors: a study of 610 cases, 1950–1981. *Int J Radiat Oncol Biol Phys* 1990;18(4):723–745.
14. Packer RJ, Gajjar A, Vezina G, et al. Phase III study of craniospinal radiation therapy followed by adjuvant chemotherapy for newly diagnosed average-risk medulloblastoma. *J Clin Oncol* 2006;24(25):4202–4208.

15. Michalski JM, Janss A, Vezina G, et al. Results of COG ACNS0331: A Phase III Trial of Involved-Field Radiotherapy (IFRT) and Low Dose Craniospinal Irradiation (LD-CSI) with Chemotherapy in Average-Risk Medulloblastoma: A Report from the Children's Oncology Group. *Int J Radiat Oncol Biol Phys* 2016;96(5):937–938.

16. Yock TI, Yeap BY, Ebb DH, et al. Long-term toxic effects of proton radiotherapy for paediatric medulloblastoma: a phase 2 single-arm study. *Lancet Oncol* 2016;17(3):287–298.

17. Jakacki RI, Zeltzer PM, Boyett JM, et al. Survival and prognostic factors following radiation and/or chemotherapy for primitive neuroectodermal tumors of the pineal region in infants and children: a report of the Childrens Cancer Group. *J Clin Oncol* 1995;13(6):1377–1383.

18. Linggood RM, Chapman PH. Pineal tumors. *J Neurooncol* 1992;12(1):85–91.

19. Reddy AT, Janss AJ, Phillips PC, et al. Outcome for children with supratentorial primitive neuroectodermal tumors treated with surgery, radiation, and chemotherapy. *Cancer* 2000;88(9): 2189–2193.

20. Goldwein JW, Leahy JM, Packer RJ, et al. Intracranial ependymomas in children. *Int J Radiat Oncol Biol Phys* 1990;19(6):1497–1502.

21. Figarella-Branger D, Civatte M, Bouvier-Labit C, et al. Prognostic factors in intracranial ependymomas in children. *J Neurosurg* 2000;93(4):605–613.

22. Merchant TE. Current clinical challenges in childhood ependymoma: a focused review. *J Clin Oncol* 2017;35(21):2364–2369.

23. Pollack IF, Gerszten PC, Martinez AJ, et al. Intracranial ependymomas of childhood: long-term outcome and prognostic factors. *Neurosurgery* 1995;37(4):655–666; discussion 66–67.

24. Rogers HA, Kilday JP, Mayne C, et al. Supratentorial and spinal pediatric ependymomas display a hypermethylated phenotype which includes the loss of tumor suppressor genes involved in the control of cell growth and death. *Acta Neuropathol* 2012;123(5):711–725.

25. Mack SC, Witt H, Piro RM, et al. Epigenomic alterations define lethal CIMP-positive ependymomas of infancy. *Nature* 2014;506(7489):445–450.

26. Witt H, Mack SC, Ryzhova M, et al. Delineation of two clinically and molecularly distinct subgroups of posterior fossa ependymoma. *Cancer Cell* 2011;20(2):143–157.

27. Kovalic JJ, Flaris N, Grigsby PW, et al. Intracranial ependymoma long term outcome, patterns of failure. *J Neurooncol* 1993;15(2):125–131.

28. Kun L. Brain tumors in children. In: Perez CA, Brady LW, eds. *Principles and practice of radiation oncology*, 3rd ed. Philadelphia, PA: Lippincott-Raven, 1998:2073–2105.

29. Grabb PA, Lunsford LD, Albright AL, et al. Stereotactic radiosurgery for glial neoplasms of childhood. *Neurosurgery* 1996;38(4):696–701; discussion 701–702.

30. Merchant TE, Bendel AE, Sabin N, et al. A phase II trial of conformal radiation therapy for pediatric patients with localized ependymoma, chemotherapy prior to second surgery for incompletely resected ependymoma and observation for completely resected, differentiated, supratentorial ependymoma. *Int J Radiat Oncol Biol Phys* 2015;93(3):S1.

31. Gajjar A, Mulhern RK, Heideman RL, et al. Medulloblastoma in very young children: outcome of definitive craniospinal irradiation following incomplete response to chemotherapy. *J Clin Oncol* 1994;12(6):1212–1216.

32. Duffner PK, Horowitz ME, Krischer JP, et al. Postoperative chemotherapy and delayed radiation in children less than three years of age with malignant brain tumors. *N Engl J Med* 1993;328(24):1725–1731.

33. Bandopadhayay P, Bergthold G, London WB, et al. Long-term outcome of 4,040 children diagnosed with pediatric low-grade gliomas: an analysis of the Surveillance Epidemiology and End Results (SEER) database. *Pediatr Blood Cancer* 2014;61(7):1173–1179.

34. Mamelak AN, Prados MD, Obana WG, et al. Treatment options and prognosis for multicentric juvenile pilocytic astrocytoma. *J Neurosurg* 1994;81(1):24–30.

35. Pollack IF, Claassen D, al-Shboul Q, et al. Low-grade gliomas of the cerebral hemispheres in children: an analysis of 71 cases. *J Neurosurg* 1995;82(4):536–547.

36. Wisoff JH, Abbott R, Epstein F. Surgical management of exophytic chiasmatic-hypothalamic tumors of childhood. *J Neurosurg* 1990;73(5):661–667.

37. Rodriguez LA, Edwards MS, Levin VA. Management of hypothalamic gliomas in children: an analysis of 33 cases. *Neurosurgery* 1990;26(2):242–246; discussion 246–247.

38. Bernstein M, Hoffman HJ, Halliday WC, et al. Thalamic tumors in children. Long-term follow-up and treatment guidelines. *J Neurosurg* 1984;61(4):649–656.

39. Freeman CR, Bourgouin PM, Sanford RA, et al. Long term survivors of childhood brain stem gliomas treated with hyperfractionated radiotherapy. Clinical characteristics and treatment related toxicities. The Pediatric Oncology Group. *Cancer* 1996;77(3):555–562.

40. Shaw EG, Daumas-Duport C, Scheithauer BW, et al. Radiation therapy in the management of low-grade supratentorial astrocytomas. *J Neurosurg* 1989;70(6):853–861.

41. Ilgren EB, Stiller CA. Cerebellar astrocytomas: therapeutic management. *Acta Neurochir (Wien)* 1986;81(1–2):11–26.

42. Marchese MJ, Chang CH. Malignant astrocytic gliomas in children. *Cancer* 1990;65(12):2771–2778.

43. Sposto R, Ertel IJ, Jenkin RD, et al. The effectiveness of chemotherapy for treatment of high grade astrocytoma in children: results of a randomized trial. A report from the Childrens Cancer Study Group. *J Neurooncol* 1989;7(2):165–177.

44. Cohen KJ, Pollack IF, Zhou T, et al. Temozolomide in the treatment of high-grade gliomas in children: a report from the Children's Oncology Group. *Neuro Oncol* 2011;13(3):317–323.

45. Fisher PG, Breiter SN, Carson BS, et al. A clinicopathologic reappraisal of brain stem tumor classification. Identification of pilocystic astrocytoma and fibrillary astrocytoma as distinct entities. *Cancer* 2000;89(7):1569–1576.

46. Robertson PL, Muraszko KM, Brunberg JA, et al. Pediatric midbrain tumors: a benign subgroup of brainstem gliomas. *Pediatr Neurosurg* 1995;22(2):65–73.

47. Packer RJ, Boyett JM, Zimmerman RA, et al. Outcome of children with brain stem gliomas after treatment with 7800 cGy of hyperfractionated radiotherapy. A Childrens Cancer Group Phase I/II Trial. *Cancer* 1994;74(6):1827–1834.

48. Schmiegelow M, Lassen S, Poulsen HS, et al. Cranial radiotherapy of childhood brain tumours: growth hormone deficiency and its relation to the biological effective dose of irradiation in a large population based study. *Clin Endocrinol (Oxf)* 2000;53(2):191–197.

49. Packer RJ, Boyett JM, Zimmerman RA, et al. Hyperfractionated radiation therapy (72 Gy) for children with brain stem gliomas. A Childrens Cancer Group Phase I/II Trial. *Cancer* 1993;72(4):1414–1421.

50. Sklar CA. Craniopharyngioma: endocrine abnormalities at presentation. *Pediatr Neurosurg* 1994;21(Suppl 1):18–20.

51. Sanford RA. Craniopharyngioma: results of survey of the American Society of Pediatric Neurosurgery. *Pediatr Neurosurg* 1994;21(Suppl 1):39–43.

52. De Vile CJ, Grant DB, Kendall BE, et al. Management of childhood craniopharyngioma: can the morbidity of radical surgery be predicted? *J Neurosurg* 1996;85(1):73–81.

53. Danoff BF, Cowchock FS, Kramer S. Childhood craniopharyngioma: survival, local control, endocrine and neurologic function following radiotherapy. *Int J Radiat Oncol Biol Phys* 1983;9(2):171–175.

54. Lunsford LD, Pollock BE, Kondziolka DS, et al. Stereotactic options in the management of craniopharyngioma. *Pediatr Neurosurg* 1994;21(Suppl 1):90–97.

55. Edwards MS, Hudgins RJ, Wilson CB, et al. Pineal region tumors in children. *J Neurosurg* 1988;68(5):689–697.

56. Jenkin D, Berry M, Chan H, et al. Pineal region germinomas in childhood treatment considerations. *Int J Radiat Oncol Biol Phys* 1990;18(3):541–545.
57. Calaminus G, Bamberg M, Baranzelli MC, et al. Intracranial germ cell tumors: a comprehensive update of the European data. *Neuropediatrics* 1994;25(1):26–32.
58. Schild SE, Scheithauer BW, Schomberg PJ, et al. Pineal parenchymal tumors. Clinical, pathologic, and therapeutic aspects. *Cancer* 1993;72(3):870–880.
59. Shibamoto Y, Oda Y, Yamashita J, et al. The role of cerebrospinal fluid cytology in radiotherapy planning for intracranial germinoma. *Int J Radiat Oncol Biol Phys* 1994;29(5):1089–1094.
60. Hardenbergh PH, Golden J, Billet A, et al. Intracranial germinoma: the case for lower dose radiation therapy. *Int J Radiat Oncol Biol Phys* 1997;39(2):419–426.
61. Fischer EG, Welch K, Shillito J Jr, et al. Craniopharyngiomas in children. Long-term effects of conservative surgical procedures combined with radiation therapy. *J Neurosurg* 1990;73(4):534–540.
62. Hetelekidis S, Barnes PD, Tao ML, et al. 20-Year experience in childhood craniopharyngioma. *Int J Radiat Oncol Biol Phys* 1993;27(2):189–195.
63. Flickinger JC, Lunsford LD, Singer J, et al. Megavoltage external beam irradiation of craniopharyngiomas: analysis of tumor control and morbidity. *Int J Radiat Oncol Biol Phys* 1990;19(1):117–122.
64. Freeman CR, Krischer JP, Sanford RA, et al. Final results of a study of escalating doses of hyperfractionated radiotherapy in brain stem tumors in children: a Pediatric Oncology Group study. *Int J Radiat Oncol Biol Phys* 1993;27(2):197–206.
65. Packer RJ, Zimmerman RA, Kaplan A, et al. Early cystic/necrotic changes after hyperfractionated radiation therapy in children with brain stem gliomas. Data from the Childrens Cancer Group. *Cancer* 1993;71(8):2666–2674.
66. Habrand JL, Mammar H, Ferrand R, et al. Proton beam therapy (PT) in the management of CNS tumors in childhood. *Strahlenther Onkol* 1999;175(Suppl 2):91–94.
67. Miralbell R, Lomax A, Bortfeld T, et al. Potential role of proton therapy in the treatment of pediatric medulloblastoma/primitive neuroectodermal tumors: reduction of the supratentorial target volume. *Int J Radiat Oncol Biol Phys* 1997;38(3):477–484.

CHAPTER 43

WILMS' TUMOR

NATURAL HISTORY

- Wilms' tumor is often localized at diagnosis. It is curable in most children.
- Spread throughout the peritoneal cavity may occur, especially if there has been preoperative rupture or the disease has been spilled at surgery. However, the results of the second National Wilms' Tumor Study (NWTS-2) demonstrated that tumor spillage at surgery, when localized to the flank, is less important prognostically than previously believed (1,2). Nevertheless, radiotherapy (RT) to the abdomen does reduce recurrences and improves survival, including in patients with peritoneal implants (3,4).
- The lungs are the most common metastatic site, followed by the liver. In NWTS-2, 57 patients (11.4%) had metastases at diagnosis; 47 of these had pulmonary metastases only (1).
- Genomic investigations suggest that mutations in the transcriptional repressor gene REST may confer increased likelihood to develop Wilms' tumor (5).
- TP53 mutations may predispose to development of anaplastic tumors (6).
- WT1 is a tumor suppressor gene, localizes at 11p13, encodes a transcription factor critical to normal kidney and gonadal development, and is associated with WAGR and Denys-Drash syndromes.
- WT2 is a protooncogene, located at 11p15, associated with IGF2 and Beckwith-Wiedemann syndrome.

PROGNOSTIC FACTORS

- Poor prognosis is seen in patients with extensive tumors, diploid tumors, unfavorable (anaplastic) histology, and chromosomal loss in 1p and 16q (7–9).
- Among favorable histology (FH), blastemal type has been identified as more aggressive as compared to epithelial predominant and the stromal predominant subtypes and is associated with a high risk in relapse. The benefit of more intensive chemotherapy to improve overall survival was only observed in stage I blastemal type (10).
- In various subsets of FH patients, microscopic residual disease, nodal involvement, and gain of 1q predict poorer prognosis (11–14).

- It has been suggested that loss of heterozygosity (LOH) of 11p15 as well as WT1 mutations are associated with higher relapse rates in very-low-risk disease (15), which could be why some data suggest that some very-low-risk tumors could be treated with surgery alone (16,17).
- NWTS-2 showed the importance of lymph node involvement as a prognostic factor.
- Liver involvement at diagnosis may not independently affect prognosis (18).

CLINICAL PRESENTATION

- The classic presentation for Wilms' tumor is that of a healthy child in whom abdominal swelling is discovered by the child's mother, pediatrician, or family practitioner during a routine physical examination.
- A palpable, smooth, firm, nontender mass (83%) on one side of the abdomen, abdominal pain (37%), fever (23%), or gross hematuria (21%) are common presentations (19).
- The child may be hypertensive or have nonspecific symptoms, such as malaise or fever.
- Only rarely does a patient present with symptomatic metastases.

DIAGNOSTIC WORKUP

- Plain films of the abdomen may demonstrate calcifications, which occur in 60% to 70% of neuroblastomas and 15% of Wilms' tumors.
- An excretory urogram (intravenous pyelogram) can differentiate renal tumors from other conditions. Cysts often appear as radiolucent areas. It now has largely been replaced by ultrasonography and computed tomography (CT) imaging.
- Ultrasonography may be helpful and is cost-effective. Duplex and color Doppler may be used to assess vessels for flow and tumor thrombus.
- Abdominal CT delineates the intrarenal tumor and demonstrates gross extrarenal spread, lymph node involvement, liver metastases, and the status of the opposite kidney.
- A direct comparison of CT with ultrasonography suggests that CT is a better diagnostic tool overall. Magnetic resonance imaging (MRI) is useful in identifying renal origin, vascular extension of the tumor, and nephrogenic rests.
- Clinical and imaging studies no not obviate the need for inspection at laparotomy.
- Plain chest radiography is essential. Chest CT may reveal some early lesions not visible on routine radiography, but it adds little when the chest radiographs are clearly positive.
- A complete blood count and urinalysis should be performed. Serum blood urea nitrogen and creatinine levels and liver function tests are routine.
- If neuroblastoma is not ruled out, a test for urinary catecholamines should be performed.
- Table 43-1 outlines the pretreatment investigations.

Table 43-1	
Pretreatment Workup	
History	Record preexisting conditions, family history of cancer, or congenital defects
Physical examination	Blood pressure, weight, height, presence of abdominal masses, congenital anomalies, particularly genitourinary, hemihypertrophy, and aniridia
Laboratory	Hemoglobin, white cell and differential counts, platelets, urinalysis, serum blood urea nitrogen, creatinine, protein, alanine and aspartate aminotransferases, alkaline phosphatase, and bilirubin
Radiology	CT or MRI scan of the abdomen and pelvis, abdominal ultrasonography, chest CT, chest x-ray, bone scan, and MRI of the brain for patients with clear cell sarcoma, rhabdoid tumor of the kidney, and renal cell carcinoma

Reprinted with permission from Kalapurakal JA, Thomas PRM. Wilms' tumor. In: Halperin EC, Wazer, DE, Perez CA, Brady LW, eds. *Principles and practice of radiation oncology*, 6th ed. Philadelphia, PA: Lippincott Williams & Wilkins, 2013. © Wolters Kluwer.

STAGING

- Tumor staging is performed by carefully examining the radiologic, operative, and histopathologic findings.
- The most current Children's Oncology Group (COG) staging system is given in Table 43-2; the most notable change from prior editions is that children with tumor spillage are upstaged from stage II to stage III (3).

PATHOLOGIC CLASSIFICATION

- Prognosis is affected by the particular variant of Wilms' tumor (20).
- Although histopathologists had attempted to relate appearance to prognosis, no generally acceptable classification was available until the report of Beckwith and Palmer (21) from the NWTS-1.
- The NWTS classifies all tumors as having FH or unfavorable histology (UH) for purposes of treatment. Of 1,465 randomized patients on NWTS-3, 163 (11.1%) had UH (22). Anaplasia (UH) may be focal or diffuse. The 4-year survival rates for stage II, III, and IV focal and diffuse anaplasia were 90% and 55%, 100% and 45%, and 100% and 4%, respectively (23).
- Renal cell carcinomas and congenital neuroblastic nephromas are not considered Wilms' tumor.
- Two monoplastic sarcomatous varieties are no longer considered true Wilms' tumors but have been included in NWTS protocols (24).
- Clear cell sarcoma infiltrates the parenchyma rather than forming a pseudocapsule and has the propensity to metastasize to bone (25). A skeletal survey and bone scan should thus be part of the workup.

Table 43-2

National Wilms' Tumor Study Staging System

Stage	Description
I	Tumor limited to the kidney, completely resected. The renal capsule is intact. The tumor was not ruptured or biopsied prior to removal. The vessels of the renal sinus are not involved. There is no evidence of tumor at or beyond the margins of resection. Note: For a tumor to qualify for certain therapeutic protocols as stage I, regional lymph nodes must be examined microscopically.
II	The tumor is completely resected, and there is no evidence of tumor at or beyond the margins of resection. The tumor extends beyond the kidney, as is evidenced by any one of the following criteria:
A	There is regional extension of the tumor (i.e., penetration of the renal capsule, or extensive invasion of the soft tissue of the renal sinus, as discussed below).
B	Blood vessels within the nephrectomy specimen outside the renal parenchyma, including those of the renal sinus, contain tumor. Note: Rupture of spillage confined to the flank, including biopsy of the tumor, is no longer included in stage II and is now included in stage III.
III	Residual nonhematogenous tumor present following surgery and confined to the abdomen. Any of the following may occur:
A	Lymph nodes within the abdomen or pelvis are involved by tumor. (Lymph node involvement in the thorax or other extra-abdominal sites is a criterion for stage IV.)
B	The tumor has penetrated through the peritoneal surface.
C	Tumor implants are found on the peritoneal surface.
D	Gross or microscopic tumor remains postoperatively (e.g., tumor cells are found at the margin of surgical resection on microscopic examination).
E	The tumor is not completely resectable because of local infiltration into vital structures.
F	Tumor spillage occurring either before or during surgery.
G	The tumor is treated with preoperative chemotherapy (with or without a biopsy regardless of type—Tru-cut, open or fine needle aspiration) before removal.
H	Tumor is removed in greater than one piece (e.g., tumor cells are found in a separately excised adrenal gland; a tumor thrombus within the renal vein is removed separately from the nephrectomy specimen). Extension of the primary tumor within vena cava into thoracic vena cava and heart is considered stage III, rather than stage IV even though outside the abdomen.
IV	Hematogenous metastases (lung, liver, bone, brain, etc.) or lymph node metastases outside the abdominopelvic region are present. (The presence of tumor within the adrenal gland is not interpreted as metastasis and staging depends on all other staging parameters present.)
V	Bilateral renal involvement by tumor is present at diagnosis. An attempt should be made to stage each side according to the above criteria on the basis of the extent of disease.

Reprinted with permission from the Children's Oncology Group protocol AREN0532.

- Malignant rhabdoid tumors of the kidney are the most lethal renal neoplasms in children. There is no conclusive evidence of skeletal muscle origin for this tumor, but a neuroepithelial derivative has been postulated.

GENERAL MANAGEMENT

- The diagnosis of Wilms' tumor is usually made preoperatively and confirmed at surgery; an incorrect diagnosis was made in only 30 of 606 patients (5%) registered in NWTS-1 (26).
- Preoperative therapy is not commonly practiced in the United States, although it has been examined in clinical trials. Emerging data evaluating response to preoperative chemotherapy have suggested omitting potentially deleterious doxorubicin as part of postoperative chemotherapy in treatment of stage II to III intermediate-risk Wilms' tumor when the histologic response to preoperative chemotherapy is incorporated into the risk stratification (27).
- Meticulous surgical techniques for exploring the abdomen through a transperitoneal incision are essential. The surgeon must excise all tumors, without spillage, if possible.
- Thorough assessment and sampling of lymph nodes from paraaortic, celiac, and iliac areas should be performed (19,28). It is no longer recommended to routinely explore the contralateral kidney owing to improved imaging capacity such as with CT and MRI scans.
- Most FH tumors are responsive to irradiation and chemotherapy (29). However, NWTS-3 showed that patients with stage II tumors do not require irradiation, and in stage III, 10 Gy to the tumor bed is sufficient (30).
- UH tumors are less responsive to either modality and generally are treated with aggressive multimodality regimens.

RADIATION THERAPY TECHNIQUES

- Anesthesia or sedation is often required for daily treatment of these children (31,32).
- Patients in whom irradiation was delayed for 10 days or more from surgery had a significantly higher chance of abdominal relapse, particularly those with UH tumors. Because the pathologist cannot always rule out UH quickly, all patients with Wilms' tumors should be scheduled to start irradiation within 10 days after surgery (33). For COG protocols, RT is recommended to start no later than day 14 after surgery.
- In NWTS-1 and NWTS-2, radiation doses to the operative bed were given according to the age of the patient; no significant dose response was detected (33).
- In NWTS-3, there was a randomization for patients with FH tumors, which resulted in elimination of irradiation for stage II FH and lung irradiation doses of 10 Gy for stage III FH and 12 Gy for stage IV FH (22,31). There are conflicting data regarding omission of pulmonary RT, especially regarding individual risk stratification (34,35).
- Data from NWTS-3 and NWTS-4 protocols showed few intra-abdominal relapses in patients with clear cell sarcoma and no dose response. There were more intra-abdominal relapses in patients with anaplastic tumors, but still no dose response (36). It was elected to treat all abdominal disease with 10 Gy.

- Parallel-opposed fields using 4- or 6-MV photons are preferred.
- Patients with disease confined to the operative site need only flank irradiation, even if there has been local spillage of tumor (for which careful intraoperative assessment by the surgeon is critical). The clinical target volume (CTV) should encompass the tumor bed, including outline of the excised kidney and associated tumor on the CT or MRI scans performed at diagnosis prior to chemotherapy. The entire width of the vertebrae should be included in CTV to minimize growth disturbances. Planning target volume is 1 cm beyond CTV.
- An example of a portal used for flank irradiation is presented in Figure 43-1 (33).
- When whole abdominal irradiation is administered, shaped portals must be used, and the femoral heads and acetabulum must be shielded (Fig. 43-2).
- In COG protocol AREN0533, whole-lung radiation is recommended for patients with lung metastases except those with favorite histology who achieve a complete response at week 6 (Fig. 43-2).
- Dosages for FH bilateral Wilms' tumor should be limited to 10 Gy to the second kidney.
- Radiation dose and volume recommendations from COG AREN0532, AREN0533, and AREN0321 are summarized in Table 43-3.

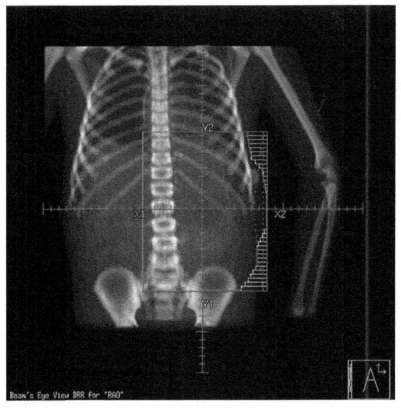

FIGURE 43-1. Anteroposterior portal of flank showing inclusion of entire width of vertebral body in irradiated volume.

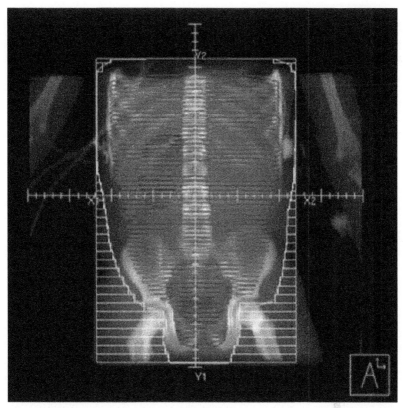

FIGURE 43-2. Anteroposterior portal for whole-abdomen irradiation in a patient with stage III Wilms' tumor. The upper margin of the abdominal field must include the diaphragm. The acetabulum and femoral head should be excluded from the irradiated volume to decrease the probability of slipped femoral epiphysis. PTV = CTV + 1 cm.

LATE EFFECTS OF TREATMENT

- Heaston et al. (37) reported that the skeletal effects of megavoltage irradiation were as frequent, but not as severe, as those of orthovoltage irradiation. Decreased irradiation doses and, more recently, three-dimensional conformal techniques, continue to decrease treatment morbidity (38) (Fig. 43-3).
- A series from Washington University confirmed a high incidence of scoliosis (14 of 26 patients) with a median dose of 30 Gy but suggested that functional disability was minimal (39). In another report, the incidence of scoliosis after 10 to 12 Gy, 12.1 to 23.9 Gy, and 24 to 40 Gy was 8%, 46%, and 63%, respectively (40).
- The cumulative frequency of congestive heart failure among patients on NWTS-1 through NWTS-4 at 20 years was 4.4% for patients treated with doxorubicin initially and 17.4% for patients treated with doxorubicin at first and subsequent relapse. Relative risk of congestive heart failure was increased in females, in patients given whole lung radiation, and in patients given left hemiabdominal radiation (41).

Table 43-3

Recommended Radiation Therapy Doses According to COG AREN0532, AREN0533, and AREN0321

Abdominal Stage and Histology	RT Dose/Field
Stage I and II FH	No radiation therapy
Stage III with tumor rupture or peritoneal metastases	10.5 Gy (in 7 fractions) to whole abdomen (a) Residual tumor will receive supplemental RT with 10.8 or 10.5 Gy (b) ≤12 months with stage III DA or RTK; RT dose is limited to 10.5 Gy (c) >12 months with stage III DA or RTK, whole abdomen to 10.5 Gy followed by supplemental flank boost 9 Gy
Stage III with diffuse unresectable peritoneal implants	21 Gy (in 14 fractions) to whole abdomen ≤12 months with stage III DA or RTK; RT dose is limited to 10.5 Gy
Stage III FH; age < 16 y: stage I–III FA, stage I–II DA, stage II–III CCSK; age ≤ 12 mo: stage I–III RTK	10.8 Gy (in 6 fractions) to flank And supplemental RT with 10.8 Gy to residual for those without rupture or peritoneal metastases
Stage III DA; age ≥ 16 y: stage I–III FA, stage I–II DA, stage I–III CCSK; age > 12 mo: stage I–III RTK	19.8 Gy (in 11 fractions) to flank for those without rupture or peritoneal metastases
Lung metastases	10.5 Gy (in 7 fractions) to whole lung if age < 12 mo 12 Gy (in 8 fractions) to whole lung if age > 12 mo
Brain metastases	21.6 Gy (in 12 fractions) followed by local boost of 10.8 Gy if age < 16 y 30.6 Gy (in 17 fractions) if age > 16 y
Liver metastases	19.8 Gy (in 11 fractions) to whole liver (a) Residual tumor will receive supplemental RT with 5.4–10.8 Gy (b) ≤12 mo: 10.8 Gy, no boost allowed
Bone metastases	25.2 Gy (in 14 fractions) to bone lesion + 3 cm if age < 16 y 30.6 Gy (in 17 fractions) to bone lesion + 3 cm if age > 16 y
Unresected lymph node metastases	19.8 Gy (in 11 fractions) FA/DA/CCSK/RTK: 30.6 Gy if age ≥ 16 y

CCSK, clear cell sarcoma of the kidney; DA, diffuse anaplasia; FA, focal anaplasia; FH, favorable histology; RT, radiation therapy; RTK, rhabdoid tumor of the kidney.
Adapted from the Children's Oncology Group AREN0321, AREN 0532, and AREN0533 protocols.

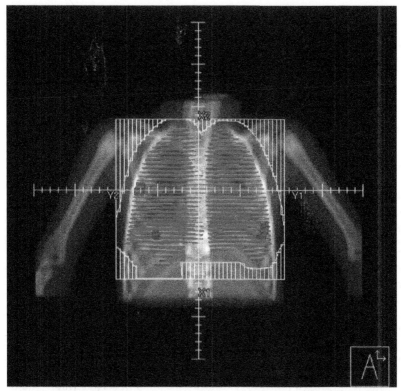

FIGURE 43-3. Anteroposterior portal for whole lung irradiation in a patient with stage IV Wilms' tumor. The lower margin of the lung field must include the diaphragm to ascertain inclusion of the anterior and posterior costophrenic angles. PTV = CTV + 1 to 1.5 cm (consider motion).

- Forty-three second malignant neoplasms were observed, whereas only 5.1 were expected with a cumulative incidence at 15 years of 1.6%. Abdominal irradiation increased the likelihood, and the risk was even greater if it was given to a dose of 35 Gy with doxorubicin (8 observed, 0.22 expected) (42).
- A recent investigation from the United Kingdom suggests that 75% of excess deaths in these patients occur from secondary malignancy and cardiac pathologies (43).
- Intestinal obstruction has been reported in 5% to 6% of patients; risk was greater when irradiation was initiated within 10 days of surgery (41).
- A few patients develop arterial hypertension or renal insufficiency (41).
- A retrospective study including 3,468 children cancer survivors with an average 30-year follow-up revealed a cumulative incidence of diabetes of 16% for pancreatic tail dose ≥10 Gy (44).
- Rates and causes of mortality in patients with Wilms' tumor were assessed in a study. Specific causes of death in the first 5 years were found to be original disease (94%), secondary cancer (1.3%), cardiac disease (0.7%), and end-stage renal failure (0.6%). The risk of death from treatment-related late effects in 5-year survivors increased to

17% for secondary cancer, 8.8% for cardiac disease, and 8.2% for end-stage renal failure and the original disease, the main cause of death decreased to 40% (45).

- Long-term survivors should be carefully monitored for late toxicity, including neuro-psychological sequelae and second malignant tumors. Some have postulated omitting routine pelvic CT scanning, but this likely does not apply to all patients (46).
- A summary of the late effects, by organ system, has been published (47).

References

1. D'Angio GJ, Evans A, Breslow N, et al. The treatment of Wilms' tumor: results of the Second National Wilms' Tumor Study. *Cancer* 1981;47(9):2302–2311.
2. Farewell VT, D'Angio GJ, Breslow N, et al. Retrospective validation of a new staging system for Wilms' tumor. *Cancer Clin Trials* 1981;4(2):167–171.
3. Kalapurakal JA, Li SM, Breslow NE, et al. Intraoperative spillage of favorable histology wilms tumor cells: influence of irradiation and chemotherapy regimens on abdominal recurrence. A report from the National Wilms Tumor Study Group. *Int J Radiat Oncol Biol Phys* 2010;76(1):201–206.
4. Kalapurakal JA, Green DM, Haase G, et al. Outcomes of children with favorable histology Wilms tumor and peritoneal implants treated in National Wilms Tumor Studies-4 and -5. *Int J Radiat Oncol Biol Phys* 2010;77(2):554–558.
5. Mahamdallie SS, Hanks S, Karlin KL, et al. Mutations in the transcriptional repressor REST predispose to Wilms tumor. *Nat Genet* 2015;47(12):1471–1474.
6. Ooms AH, Gadd S, Gerhard DS, et al. Significance of TP53 Mutation in Wilms Tumors with Diffuse Anaplasia: A Report from the Children's Oncology Group. *Clin Cancer Res* 2016;22(22):5582–5591; doi: 10.1158/1078-0432.CCR-16-0985.
7. Grosfeld JL. Risk-based management: current concepts of treating malignant solid tumors of childhood. *J Am Coll Surg* 1999;189(4):407–425.
8. Messahet B, Williams R, Ridolfi A, et al. Allele loss at 16q defines poorer prognosis Wilms tumour irrespective of treatment approach in the UKW1-3 clinical trials: a Children's Cancer and Leukaemia Group (CCLG) Study. *Eur J Cancer* 2009;45(5):819–826.
9. Graf N, van Tinteren H, Bergeron C, et al. Characteristics and outcome of stage II and III non-anaplastic Wilms' tumour treated according to the SIOP trial and study 93-01. *Eur J Cancer* 2012;48(17):3240–3248.
10. Van den Heuvel-Eibrink MM, van Tinteren H, Bergeron C, et al. Outcome of localised blastemal-type Wilms tumour patients treated according to intensified treatment in the SIOP WT 2001 protocol, a report of the SIOP Renal Tumour Study Group (SIOP-RTSG). *Eur J Cancer* 2015;51(4):498–506.
11. Ehrlich PF, Anderson JR, Ritchey ML, et al. Clinicopathologic findings predictive of relapse in children with stage III favorable-histology Wilms tumor. *J Clin Oncol* 2013;31(9):1196–1201.
12. Gratias EJ, Jennings LJ, Anderson JR, et al. Gain of 1q is associated with inferior event-free and overall survival in patients with favorable histology Wilms tumor: a report from the Children's Oncology Group. *Cancer* 2013;119(21):3887–3894.
13. Gratias EJ, Dome JS, Jennings LJ, et al. Association of Chromosome 1q Gain With Inferior Survival in Favorable-Histology Wilms Tumor: A Report From the Children's Oncology Group. *J Clin Oncol* 2016;34(26):3189–3194.
14. Chagtai T, Zill C, Dainese L, et al. Gain of 1q As a Prognostic Biomarker in Wilms Tumors (WTs) Treated With Preoperative Chemotherapy in the International Society of Paediatric Oncology (SIOP) WT 2001 Trial: A SIOP Renal Tumours Biology Consortium Study. *J Clin Oncol* 2016;34(26):3195–3203.

15. Perlman EJ, Grundy PE, Anderson JR, et al. WT1 mutation and 11P15 loss of heterozygosity predict relapse in very low-risk Wilms tumors treated with surgery alone: a children's oncology group study. *J Clin Oncol* 2011;29(6):698–703.

16. Shamberger RC, Anderson JR, Breslow NE, et al. Long-term outcomes for infants with very low risk Wilms tumor treated with surgery alone in National Wilms Tumor Study-5. *Ann Surg* 2010;251(3):555–558.

17. Fernandez CV, Perlman EJ, Mullen EA, et al. Clinical Outcome and Biological Predictors of Relapse After Nephrectomy Only for Very Low-risk Wilms Tumor: A Report From Children's Oncology Group AREN0532. *Ann Surg* 2017;265(4):835–840; doi: 10.1097/SLA.0000000000001716.

18. Ehrlich PF, Ferrer FA, Ritchey ML, et al. Hepatic metastasis at diagnosis in patients with Wilms tumor is not an independent adverse prognostic factor for stage IV Wilms tumor: a report from the Children's Oncology Group/National Wilms Tumor Study Group. *Ann Surg* 2009;250(4):642–648.

19. Kalapurakal J, Thomas P. Wilms' tumor. In: Halperin E, Perez C, Brady L, eds. *Principles and practice of radiation oncology*. Philadelphia, PA: Lippincott Williams & Wilkins, 2008:1850–1858.

20. Perez CA, Kaiman HA, Keith J, et al. Treatment of Wilms' tumor and factors affecting prognosis. *Cancer* 1973;32(3):609–617.

21. Beckwith JB, Palmer NF. Histopathology and prognosis of Wilms tumors: results from the First National Wilms' Tumor Study. *Cancer* 1978;41(5):1937–1948.

22. D'Angio GJ, Breslow N, Beckwith JB, et al. Treatment of Wilms' tumor. Results of the Third National Wilms' Tumor Study. *Cancer* 1989;64(2):349–360.

23. Faria P, Beckwith JB, Mishra K, et al. Focal versus diffuse anaplasia in Wilms tumor—new definitions with prognostic significance: a report from the National Wilms Tumor Study Group. *Am J Surg Pathol* 1996;20(8):909–920.

24. Beckwith JB. Wilms' tumor and other renal tumors of childhood: a selective review from the National Wilms' Tumor Study Pathology Center. *Hum Pathol* 1983;14(6):481–492.

25. Sandstedt BE, Delemarre JF, Harms D, et al. Sarcomatous Wilms' tumour with clear cells and hyalinization. A study of 38 tumours in children from the SIOP nephroblastoma file. *Histopathology* 1987;11(3):273–285.

26. D'Angio GJ, Evans AE, Breslow N, et al. The treatment of Wilms' tumor: results of the national Wilms' tumor study. *Cancer* 1976;38(2):633–646.

27. Pritchard-Jones K, Bergeron C, de Camargo B, et al. Omission of doxorubicin from the treatment of stage II-III, intermediate-risk Wilms' tumour (SIOP WT 2001): an open-label, non-inferiority, randomised controlled trial. *Lancet* 2015;386(9999):1156–1164.

28. Thomas P. Wilms' tumor. In: Perez C, Brady L, eds. *Principles and practice of radiation oncology*, 3rd ed. Philadelphia, PA: Lippincott-Raven, 1998:2107–2116.

29. Meisel JA, Guthrie KA, Breslow NE, et al. Significance and management of computed tomography detected pulmonary nodules: a report from the National Wilms Tumor Study Group. *Int J Radiat Oncol Biol Phys* 1999;44(3):579–585.

30. Thomas PR. Wilms' tumor: changing role of radiation therapy. *Semin Radiat Oncol* 1997; 7(3):204–211.

31. Thomas PR, Tefft M, Compaan PJ, et al. Results of two radiation therapy randomizations in the third National Wilms' Tumor Study. *Cancer* 1991;68(8):1703–1707.

32. Verma V, Beethe AB, LeRiger M, et al. Anesthesia complications of pediatric radiation therapy. *Pract Radiat Oncol.* 2016;6(3):143–154.

33. D'Angio GJ, Tefft M, Breslow N, et al. Radiation therapy of Wilms' tumor: results according to dose, field, post-operative timing and histology. *Int J Radiat Oncol Biol Phys* 1978;4(9–10):769–780.

34. Nicolin G, Taylor R, Baughan C, et al. Outcome after pulmonary radiotherapy in Wilms' tumor patients with pulmonary metastases at diagnosis: a UK Children's Cancer Study Group, Wilms' Tumour Working Group Study. *Int J Radiat Oncol Biol Phys* 2008;70(1):175–180.

35. Verschuur A, Van Tinteren H, Graf N, et al. Treatment of pulmonary metastases in children with stage IV nephroblastoma with risk-based use of pulmonary radiotherapy. *J Clin Oncol* 2012;30(28):3533–3539.

36. Green DM, Beckwith JB, Breslow NE, et al. Treatment of children with stages II to IV anaplastic Wilms' tumor: a report from the National Wilms' Tumor Study Group. *J Clin Oncol* 1994;12(10):2126–2131.

37. Heaston DK, Libshitz HI, Chan RC. Skeletal effects of megavoltage irradiation in survivors of Wilms' tumor. *AJR Am J Roentgenol* 1979;133(3):389–395.

38. Ludin A, Macklis RM. Radiotherapy for pediatric genitourinary tumors. Its role and long-term consequences. *Urol Clin North Am* 2000;27(3):553–562, x.

39. Thomas PR, Griffith KD, Fineberg BB, et al. Late effects of treatment for Wilms' tumor. *Int J Radiat Oncol Biol Phys* 1983;9(5):651–657.

40. Paulino AC, Wen BC, Brown CK, et al. Late effects in children treated with radiation therapy for Wilms' tumor. *Int J Radiat Oncol Biol Phys* 2000;46(5):1239–1246.

41. Green DM, Grigoriev YA, Nan B, et al. Congestive heart failure after treatment for Wilms' tumor: a report From the National Wilms' Tumor Study group. *J Clin Oncol* 2001;19(7):1926–1934.

42. Breslow NE, Takashima JR, Whitton JA, et al. Second malignant neoplasms following treatment for Wilm's tumor: a report from the National Wilms' Tumor Study Group. *J Clin Oncol* 1995;13(8):1851–1859.

43. Wong KF, Reulen RC, Winter DL, et al. Risk of Adverse Health and Social Outcomes Up to 50 Years After Wilms Tumor: The British Childhood Cancer Survivor Study. *J Clin Oncol* 2016;34(15):1772–1779.

44. De Vathaire F, El-Fayech C, Ben Ayed FF, et al. Radiation dose to the pancreas and risk of diabetes mellitus in childhood cancer survivors: a retrospective cohort study. *Lancet Oncol* 2012;13(10):1002–1010.

45. Cotton CA, Peterson S, Norkool PA, et al. Early and late mortality after diagnosis of Wilms tumor. *J Clin Oncol* 2009;27(8):1304–1309.

46. Kaste SC, Brady SL, Yee B, et al. Is routine pelvic surveillance imaging necessary in patients with Wilms tumor? *Cancer* 2013;119(1):182–188.

47. Green DM, Donckerwolcke R, Evans AE, et al. Late effects of treatment for Wilms tumor. *Hematol Oncol Clin North Am* 1995;9(6):1317–1327.

CHAPTER 44

NEUROBLASTOMA

- Neuroblastoma is the most common, extracranial pediatric solid tumor.
- Its clinical course is distinctly heterogenous with spontaneous regression or maturation to a benign ganglioneuroma in some cases or rapidly progressive, fatal progression in others.

NATURAL HISTORY

- Neuroblastoma, along with ganglioneuroma and ganglioneuroblastoma, may arise initially from any site along the sympathetic nervous system.
- The most common site of origin is the adrenal medulla (30% to 40%) or the paraspinal ganglia in the abdomen or pelvis (25%).
- Thoracic (15%) and head-and-neck primary tumors (5%) are slightly more common in infants than in older children.
- More than 70% of patients with neuroblastoma have metastatic disease at presentation; the most frequent sites are the lymph nodes, bone, bone marrow, skin (or subcutaneous tissues), and liver. The lung and central nervous system are rarely sites of metastatic involvement (1).
- Patients who present with metastatic disease have a less than 40% long-term survival rate (2).

CLINICAL PRESENTATION

- Pain is the most common presenting symptom, frequently due to bone, liver, or bone marrow metastases or local visceral invasion by the primary tumor.
- Other symptoms may include weight loss, anorexia, malaise, and fever.
- Respiratory distress as a result of massive hepatomegaly from liver metastases may be seen, especially in infants with stage 4S disease. This is known as "Pepper's syndrome."
- Horner's syndrome can accompany a primary tumor originating in the neck.

- Spinal cord compression with paralysis of the lower extremities can accompany the so-called dumbbell-shaped tumor that extends from its origin along the sympathetic ganglia through the adjacent neural foramina.
- Orbital metastases may cause proptosis and ecchymosis, known as "raccoon eyes."

DIAGNOSTIC WORKUP

- The diagnosis of neuroblastoma must be established by pathologic evaluation.
- It is important to attempt to determine if the tumor is more likely to be neuroblastoma as opposed to Wilms' tumor before biopsy, as a biopsy in the latter automatically upstages the patient to stage 3 requiring flank RT.
- Tumor tissue may be obtained from the suspected primary tumor site or involved lymph nodes, by excision (if the tumor is resectable) or incisional biopsy.
- Bone marrow aspirate and biopsy frequently show metastatic tumor deposits that can establish the diagnosis.
- Pathologic evaluation of bone marrow is a requirement for staging. Neuroblastoma in bone marrow appears in clumps and pseudorosettes, but the absence of pseudorosettes does not eliminate the possibility of neuroblastoma (1).
- Laboratory studies include measurement of urinary catecholamines and their metabolites; either homovanillic acid or vanillylmandelic acid (metabolites of dopa/norepinephrine and epinephrine, respectively) is elevated in more than 90% of patients with stage 4 neuroblastoma. A vanillylmandelic acid/homovanillic acid ratio exceeding 1.5 is associated with a favorable prognosis in patients with metastatic neuroblastoma.
- Anemia secondary to bone marrow involvement can be evaluated with a complete blood count.
- Serum ferritin, lactate dehydrogenase, and other liver functions should be assayed routinely.
- Imaging studies assist in staging and planning an approach to therapy. The specific imaging workup depends on the location of the primary tumor.
- Neck and chest tumors can be easily evaluated by computed tomography (CT). Abdominal or pelvic masses are often initially evaluated by abdominal ultrasound or CT.
- Unlike Wilms' tumor, which originates from the kidney and causes calyceal distortion, neuroblastoma often displaces a normal kidney inferiorly and laterally. X-ray studies show intrinsic speckled calcifications in 85% of neuroblastomas.
- Magnetic resonance imaging (MRI) scans are replacing the routine use of CT in evaluation of suspicious thoracic or abdominal masses. Although MRI cannot demonstrate intratumoral calcifications, it allows better evaluation of blood vessel encasement, intraspinal extension (dumbbell tumors), diffuse hepatic replacement, and bone marrow involvement (1). Each of these findings improves staging accuracy and facilitates the decision-making process regarding appropriate surgical interventions (3).
- Radionuclide bone scans are helpful in determining the extent of metastatic disease because neuroblastoma has a predilection for bony metastases.

- Metaiodobenzylguanidine (MIBG) is concentrated by neurosecretory granules of both normal and neoplastic tissues of neural crest origin. MIBG labeled with either ^{131}I or ^{123}I has a sensitivity of 85% to 90% and specificity of nearly 95% in the detection of metastatic neuroblastoma (4).
- The long-acting somatostatin analog octreotide, labeled with ^{123}I, has been used to image neuroblastoma, with a sensitivity comparable to that of ^{131}I MIBG (5). The expression of somatostatin receptors by neuroblastoma tissues is a favorable prognostic factor.

STAGING

- The most commonly used staging system is the International Neuroblastoma Staging System (INSS), initially published in 1988. It is based on clinical, radiographic, and surgical findings (6).
- The INSS system relies heavily on surgical resectability and thus is not well suited for pretreatment risk stratification.
- The International Neuroblastoma Risk Group (INRG) recently proposed a set of image-defined risk factors (IDRFs) based on the primary tumor site, in addition to the presence or absence of locoregional or metastatic disease for staging (Table 44-1) (7).
- The INRG staging system is increasingly being used and differs slightly from the INSS (Table 44-2).

PATHOLOGIC CLASSIFICATION

- Neuroblastomas are derived from primitive neural crest cells arising from within sympathetic ganglia.
- Three types of tumors are recognized, representing different degrees of differentiation.
- Ganglioneuroma consists of mature ganglion cells, Schwann's cells, and nerve bundles and is benign in appearance and nature. It is frequently calcified and may represent a matured neuroblastoma.
- Ganglioneuroblastoma is the intermediate form between ganglioneuroma and neuroblastoma; both mature ganglion cells and undifferentiated neuroblasts are evident.
- Neuroblastoma, a "small round blue cell" tumor composed of dense nests of hyperchromatic cells, is at the undifferentiated end of the spectrum of these neural crest tumors.
- Homer-Wright rosettes with a central fibrillary core can be present; necrosis, hemorrhage, and calcium are frequently seen.
- Immunohistochemical stains characteristically stain positive for neurofilaments, neuron-specific enolase, synaptophysin, and chromogranin A, and negative for muscle and leukocyte common antigens.
- Electron microscopy demonstrates neurosecretory granules, but it rarely is required to establish the diagnosis.
- The significance of the grading system for neuroblastoma proposed by Shimada et al. (8) has been confirmed by the Children's Cancer Group (9).

Table 44-1

International Neuroblastoma Risk Group Image-Defined Risk Factors

Ipsilateral tumor extension within two body compartments	Neck-chest Chest-abdomen Abdomen-pelvis
Neck	Tumor encasing carotid and/or vertebral artery and/or internal jugular vein Tumor extending to base of skull Tumor compressing the trachea
Cervicothoracic junction	Tumor encasing brachial plexus roots Tumor encasing subclavian vessels and/or vertebral and/or carotid artery Tumor compressing the trachea
Thorax	Tumor encasing the aorta and/or major branches Tumor compressing the trachea and/or principal bronchi Lower mediastinal tumor, infiltrating the costovertebral junction between T9 and T12
Thoracoabdominal	Tumor encasing the aorta and/or vena cava
Abdomen-pelvis	Tumor infiltrating the porta hepatis and/or the hepatoduodenal ligament Tumor encasing branches of the superior mesenteric artery at the mesenteric root Tumor encasing the origin of the celiac axis, and/or of the superior mesenteric artery Tumor invading one or both renal pedicles Tumor encasing the aorta and/or vena cava Tumor encasing the iliac vessels Pelvic tumor crossing the sciatic notch
Intraspinal tumor extension whatever the location provided that	More than one third of the spinal canal in the axial plane is invaded and/or the perimedullary leptomeningeal spaces are not visible and/or the spinal cord signal is abnormal
Infiltration of adjacent organs/structures	Pericardium, diaphragm, kidney, liver, duodenopancreatic block, and mesentery
Conditions to be recorded, but not considered IDRFs	Multifocal primary tumors Pleural effusion, with or without malignant cells Ascites, with or without malignant cells

Table 44-2

Neuroblastoma Staging Systems

International Staging System	International Neuroblastoma Risk Group Staging System
Stage 1	**Stage L1**
Localized tumor with complete gross excision, without microscopic residual disease; representative ipsilateral lymph nodes negative for tumor microscopically (nodes attached to and removed with the primary tumor may be positive).	Localized tumor not involving vital structures as defined by the list of image-defined risk factors and confined to one body compartment
Stage 2A	**Stage L2**
Localized tumor with incomplete gross excision; representative ipsilateral nonadherent lymph nodes negative for tumor microscopically.	Locoregional tumor with presence of one or more image-defined risk factors
Stage 2B	
Localized tumor with or without complete gross excision, with ipsilateral nonadherent lymph nodes positive for tumor. Enlarged contralateral lymph nodes must be negative microscopically.	
Stage 3	
Unresectable unilateral tumor infiltrating across the midline,[a] with or without regional lymph node involvement; or localized unilateral tumor with contralateral regional lymph node involvement; or midline tumor with bilateral extension by infiltration (unresectable) or by lymph node involvement.	
Stage 4	**Stage M**
Any primary tumor with dissemination to distant lymph nodes, bone, bone marrow, liver, skin, and/or other organs (except as defined for stage 4S).	Distant metastatic disease (except stage MS)
Stage 4S	**Stage MS**
Localized primary tumor as defined for stages 1, 2A, or 2B with dissemination limited to skin, liver, and/or bone marrow[b] (limited to infants <1 year of age).	Metastatic disease in children younger than 18 months with metastases confined to skin, liver, and/or bone marrow

Note: Multifocal primary tumors (e.g., bilateral adrenal primary tumors) should be staged according to the greatest extent of disease, as defined in the table, followed by a subscript letter M (e.g., 3M).
[a]The midline is defined as the vertebral column. Tumors originating on one side and crossing the midline must infiltrate to or beyond the opposite side of the vertebral column.
[b]Marrow involvement in stage 4S should be minimal—that is, less than 10% of total nucleated cells identified as malignant on bone marrow biopsy or on marrow aspirate. More extensive marrow involvement would be considered to be stage 4. The MIBG scan (if performed) should be negative in the marrow.

PROGNOSTIC FACTORS

- In general, more than 75% of infants and children less than 2 years old will survive, as well as 90% to 100% of children with INSS stages 1 or 2 (10,11).
- Infants less than 12 months old with metastatic disease confined to the liver, bone marrow (not bone), or skin (stage 4S) have a good prognosis; more than 75% survive with little or no treatment (10).
- Patients with more differentiated tumors, such as ganglioneuroma or ganglioneuroblastoma, fare better than do children with poorly differentiated or undifferentiated neuroblastomas.
- *MYCN* (N-*myc*) is a protooncogene that resides on the short arm of chromosome 2. An increased number of *MYCN* gene copies are associated with an extremely poor prognosis (less than 5% survival) (12). *MYCN* amplification has been associated with the multidrug-resistance *MDR* gene and may account for this tumor's resistance to therapy.
- Neuroblastoma is associated with loss of heterozygosity on chromosome 1p36 and, occasionally, deletions on 14q and 17q. Patients with advanced disease often have amplification of the N-*myc* oncogene, 1p36 deletions, unfavorable histology, and diploid tumors (13).
- A tumor with a deoxyribonucleic acid index of 1 (diploid or near diploid) gives a worse prognosis than do tumors that are aneuploid (14).
- 11q chromosomal aberration was found to be the most significant factor in determining prognosis among patients with MYCN-nonamplified stage 2, 3 tumors over 18 months and among MYCN-nonamplified stage 4S patients under 18 months old.
- The INRG recently proposed a new risk stratification system incorporating the INRG stage, age, histologic category, tumor grade, MYC-N amplification status, presence or absence of 11q aberration, and DNA ploidy (15).
- Radiation is typically only used in the definitive treatment for high-risk neuroblastoma. According to the INRG classification, this includes stages L1, L2, and MS with myc-n amplification or any stage M regardless of myc-n status.

GENERAL MANAGEMENT

- Because of the biologic heterogeneity of neuroblastomas, the following treatment recommendations should be considered as guidelines.
- Low-risk patients have an excellent prognosis after complete gross surgical excision. Adjuvant chemotherapy or irradiation has not improved the outcome in children with completely resected tumors with favorable biologic features (16,17). In such patients, positive surgical margins or microscopic residual disease does not always require more aggressive therapy.
- Unresectable tumors that are of otherwise low stage may require preoperative chemotherapy to convert them to resectable lesions. Complete resection can be achieved in

nearly two thirds of previously unresectable stage 3 to 4 primary tumors. Second-look surgery may be necessary.

- Infants less than 1 year of age should undergo complete resection of the primary tumor and receive adjuvant chemotherapy (18).
- Radiation therapy plays a key role in the management of patients with high-risk disease.
- In general, high-risk patients receive five to six cycles of induction chemotherapy including cisplatin, cyclophosphamide, doxorubicin, etoposide, topotecan, and vincristine followed by surgical resection of the primary tumor. This is followed by myeloablative chemotherapy and tandem autologous hematopoietic stem-cell rescue and then radiation therapy.
- Postconsolidation treatment with immunotherapy with antiganglioside 2 chimeric 13.18 antibody and interleukin (IL)-2 cytokines plus isotretinoin was shown to improve overall and event-free survival in patients after the above regimen and represents the current standard of care for high-risk patients (19).
- On current Children's Oncology Group (COG) protocols, radiation for high-risk disease is given to the primary tumor and any sites of metastatic disease that remained MIBG active after induction chemotherapy.
- Intraspinal extension of neuroblastoma poses a unique problem. These patients were historically treated with laminectomy and surgical debulking, with or without irradiation and chemotherapy (20). Because the morbidity of this approach is significant, a number of investigators have used primary chemotherapy.
- Systemic radionuclide therapy with ^{131}I MIBG has been tested in several centers in Europe and the United States with early, encouraging results (21,22).

RADIATION THERAPY TECHNIQUES

- Treatment of children with cancer must minimize the risk of late effects without compromising the chance for tumor control and cure.
- Radiation guidelines from recent COG protocols recommend targeting the postinduction presurgical primary tumor volume (GTV1) followed by a boost to any residual tumor (GTV2).
- For metastatic sites, only the postinduction volume is targeted.
- A margin of 1.5 to 2 cm to each GTV is recommended for the clinical target volume (CTV).
- When the vertebral body is included in the CTV, the entire vertebral body should be included to prevent future growth deformities.
- The dose to the primary site GTV1 and any metastatic sites is 21.6 Gy. The boost dose for residual primary tumor is 9 Gy.
- Either three-dimensional conformal radiotherapy or intensity-modulated radiation therapy may be appropriate based on the tumor location and relationship to the organs at risk.

SEQUELAE OF TREATMENT

Early Complications

- Acute side effects of therapy, expected for any patient receiving irradiation, depend on tumor site and fields of treatment.
- Skin reactions and mucositis may be enhanced if concurrent chemotherapy is used.

Late Effects

- Long-term effects from radiation therapy and chemotherapy depend on the site irradiated and the total dose of both irradiation and chemotherapy agents used.
- Age at the time of treatment may influence the risk and severity of skeletal anomalies (23), which may include limb shortening or spinal deformities such as kyphosis and scoliosis.
- Generally, younger children are more prone to late radiation injury than are older children.
- Chemotherapy may increase the risk of irradiation sequelae, and the expected tolerance may be reduced (24).

References

1. Mansur DB, Michalski JM. Neuroblastoma. In: Halperin EC, Perez CA, Brady LW, eds. *Principles and practice of radiation oncology*, 5th ed. Philadelphia, PA: Lippincott Williams & Wilkins, 2008:1859–1871.
2. Matthay KK, Villablanca JG, Seeger RC, et al. Treatment of high-risk neuroblastoma with intensive chemotherapy, radiotherapy, autologous bone marrow transplantation, and 13-cisretinoic acid. Children's Cancer Group. *N Engl J Med* 1999;341:1165–1173.
3. Siegel MJ, Jamroz GA, Glazer HS, et al. MR imaging of intraspinal extension of neuroblastoma. *J Comput Assist Tomogr* 1986;10(4):593–595.
4. Shapiro B. Imaging of catecholamine-secreting tumours: uses of MIBG in diagnosis and treatment. *Baillieres Clin Endocrinol Metab* 1993;7(2):491–507.
5. Nitschke R, Smith EI, Shochat S, et al. Localized neuroblastoma treated by surgery: a Pediatric Oncology Group Study. *J Clin Oncol* 1988;6(8):1271–1279.
6. Brodeur GM, Seeger RC, Barrett A, et al. International criteria for diagnosis, staging, and response to treatment in patients with neuroblastoma. *J Clin Oncol* 1988;6(12):1874–1881.
7. Monclair T, Brodeur GM, Ambros PF, et al. The International Neuroblastoma Risk Group (INRG) staging system: an INRG Task Force report. *J Clin Oncol* 2009;27:298–303.
8. Shimada H, Chatten J, Newton WA Jr, et al. Histopathologic prognostic factors in neuroblastic tumors: definition of subtypes of ganglioneuroblastoma and an age-linked classification of neuroblastomas. *J Natl Cancer Inst* 1984;73(2):405–416.
9. Chatten J, Shimada H, Sather HN, et al. Prognostic value of histopathology in advanced neuroblastoma: a report from the Childrens Cancer Study Group. *Hum Pathol* 1988;19(10):1187–1198.
10. Evans AE, Baum E, Chard R. Do infants with stage IV-S neuroblastoma need treatment? *Arch Dis Child* 1981;56(4):271–274.
11. Evans AE, D'Angio GJ, Propert K, et al. Prognostic factor in neuroblastoma. *Cancer* 1987;59(11):1853–1859.

12. Seeger RC, Brodeur GM, Sather H, et al. Association of multiple copies of the N-myc oncogene with rapid progression of neuroblastomas. *N Engl J Med* 1985;313(18):1111–1116.

13. Grosfeld JL. Risk-based management: current concepts of treating malignant solid tumors of childhood. *J Am Coll Surg* 1999;189(4):407–425.

14. Look AT, Hayes FA, Shuster JJ, et al. Clinical relevance of tumor cell ploidy and N-myc gene amplification in childhood neuroblastoma: a Pediatric Oncology Group study. *J Clin Oncol* 1991;9(4):581–591.

15. Cohn SL, Pearson AD, London WB, et al. The International Neuroblastoma Risk Group (INRG) classification system: an INRG Task Force report. *J Clin Oncol* 2009;27:289–297.

16. Ninane J, Wese FX. Treatment of localized neuroblastoma. *Am J Pediatr Hematol Oncol* 1986;8(3):248–252.

17. Nitschke R, Smith EI, Altshuler G, et al. Postoperative treatment of nonmetastatic visible residual neuroblastoma: a Pediatric Oncology Group study. *J Clin Oncol* 1991;9(7):1181–1188.

18. Shorter NA, Davidoff AM, Evans AE, et al. The role of surgery in the management of stage IV neuroblastoma: a single institution study. *Med Pediatr Oncol* 1995;24(5):287–291.

19. Pearson AD, Pinkerton CR, Lewis IJ, et al. High-dose rapid and standard induction chemotherapy for patients aged over 1 year with stage 4 neuroblastoma: a randomised trial. *Lancet Oncol* 2008;9:247–256.

20. Plantaz D, Rubie H, Michon J, et al. The treatment of neuroblastoma with intraspinal extension with chemotherapy followed by surgical removal of residual disease. A prospective study of 42 patients—results of the NBL 90 Study of the French Society of Pediatric Oncology. *Cancer* 1996;78(2):311–319.

21. Lashford LS, Lewis IJ, Fielding SL, et al. Phase I/II study of iodine 131 metaiodobenzylguanidine in chemoresistant neuroblastoma: a United Kingdom Children's Cancer Study Group investigation. *J Clin Oncol* 1992;10(12):1889–1896.

22. Meller S. Targeted radiotherapy for neuroblastoma. *Arch Dis Child* 1997;77(5):389–391.

23. Wallace WH, Shalet SM. Chemotherapy with actinomycin D influences the growth of the spine following abdominal irradiation. *Med Pediatr Oncol* 1992;20(2):177.

24. Wallace WH, Shalet SM, Morris-Jones PH, et al. Effect of abdominal irradiation on growth in boys treated for a Wilms' tumor. *Med Pediatr Oncol* 1990;18(6):441–446.

CHAPTER 45

RHABDOMYOSARCOMA

ANATOMY

- Rhabdomyosarcoma is a highly malignant soft tissue sarcoma that arises from unsegmented, undifferentiated mesoderm or myotome-derived skeletal muscle.
- It may occur in any site in the body. The most frequently involved sites are the orbit (9%); head and neck (excluding parameningeal tumors) (10%); parameningeal (16%); genitourinary (24%); extremity (19%); and other miscellaneous sites (22%) (1).

NATURAL HISTORY AND PATTERNS OF SPREAD

- Rhabdomyosarcoma is heterogeneous and arises in multiple sites (2).
- Tumors of the head and neck area occur throughout childhood and are commonly embryonal.
- Tumors arising in the trunk and extremity occur in adolescents and are usually alveolar or undifferentiated.
- Tumors arising in the urinary bladder and vagina occur primarily in infants and often are embryonal or botryoid. This locally invasive tumor spreads along fascial or muscle planes and by lymphatic extension, and may have hematogenous dissemination.
- Lymph node metastases are rare in orbital tumors but occur in approximately 7% of tumors at other head and neck sites, 20% to 30% of paratesticular tumors, 3% of truncal tumors (3), and 20% to 40% of extremity (4).
- Hematogenous metastases are detected at the time of presentation in approximately 16% of patients (5–7). The common sites of hematogenous dissemination are lungs (47%), bone marrow (38%), bone (34%), and distant nodes (26%) (8).

PROGNOSTIC FACTORS

- In 439 patients with rhabdomyosarcoma treated with complete resection and chemotherapy (with or without irradiation), poor prognostic factors included tumor larger than 5 cm, alveolar or undifferentiated histology, primary tumor site, and treatment modalities (9).
- Distant metastasis at the time of diagnosis is a poor prognostic factor (10,11).
- Following diagnostic standardization and histologic re-review of rhabdomyosarcoma (RMS) cases enrolled during this era, analysis of low-risk (D9602) and intermediate-risk (D9803) RMS studies showed that fusion status rather than histology best predicts prognosis for patients with RMS.
- A recent analysis of high-risk COG studies D9802 and ARST0431 revealed that fusion-negative RMS had a superior EFS to fusion-positive RMS; however, poorer outcome for metastatic RMS was most related to clinical risk factors including age, primary site, and number of metastatic sites (12).

CLINICAL PRESENTATION

- Rhabdomyosarcoma usually presents as an asymptomatic mass. When symptoms are present, they relate to mass effect on associated organs (13).
- Tumors of the orbit may cause proptosis and ophthalmoplegia.
- Parameningeal tumors often present with cranial nerve palsy, headache, and nasal, aural, or sinus obstruction.
- Genitourinary tumors may cause hematuria, urinary obstruction, or constipation.

DIAGNOSTIC WORKUP

- The extent of the primary tumor is best determined with a multidisciplinary, expeditious workup by a radiation oncologist, pediatric oncologist, and appropriate subspecialty surgeon.
- Recommended baseline evaluations are shown in Table 45-1 (14).

STAGING

- The clinical grouping classification used extensively by the Intergroup Rhabdomyosarcoma Study (IRS) is somewhat of a misnomer because it actually requires surgical-pathologic evaluation (Table 45-2).
- Pretreatment staging uses a tumor-node-metastasis system, which emphasizes characteristics of the primary tumor site, size and invasiveness, nodal status, and systemic spread (Table 45-3) (15).

Table 45-1	
Recommended Workup for Tumors at Various Sites	
All Patients	**Optional**
History	
Physical examination by several observers	Examination under anesthesia for infants and youngsters
Laboratory studies	
Complete blood cell count	
Liver function tests	
Renal function tests	
Urinalysis	
Imaging studies	
PET/CT (may replace chest/abdomen/pelvis CT and bone scan)	Plain films of bones abnormal on scan Abdomen-pelvis CT, MRI, or ultrasound
MRI or CT of primary tumor	
Bone marrow biopsy and aspirate	
Head and neck	
MRI or CT of primary tumor (with contrast)	Plain films of area Dental evaluation and x-rays Paranasal sinus and skull films
Lumbar puncture with cytologic examination of fluid in parameningeal primary tumors	MRI of spine if cerebrospinal fluid is positive or patient is symptomatic
Genitourinary	
CT or MRI of abdomen-pelvis (with contrast)	Ultrasound of pelvis
Pelvic examination under anesthesia	Cystoscopy
Extremity and truncal lesions	
MRI or CT of primary lesion (with contrast)	Plain films of primary site Ultrasound Barium gastrointestinal contrast studies

Reprinted with permission from Breneman JC, Donaldson SS. Rhabdomyosarcoma. In: Halperin EC, Perez CA, Brady LW, eds. *Principles and practice of radiation oncology*, 6th ed. Philadelphia, PA: Lippincott Williams & Wilkins, 2013:1677. © Wolters Kluwer.

PATHOLOGIC CLASSIFICATION

- The classic classification of rhabdomyosarcoma, used by the IRS investigators, consists of four histologic subtypes: embryonal, botryoid subtype of embryonal, alveolar, and pleomorphic.
- More recently, investigators have observed a subset of patients with a "solid" alveolar pattern, considered a subtype of alveolar rhabdomyosarcoma (16).
- A lack of agreement among pediatric pathologists has led to the new International Classification of Rhabdomyosarcoma, based on a review of IRS-II data, which divides subgroups into distinct prognostic groups (Table 45-4).

Table 45-2

Intergroup Rhabdomyosarcoma Study Clinical Grouping Classification

Group I	Localized disease, completely resected
A	Confined to organ or muscle of origin
B	Infiltration outside organ or muscle of origin; regional nodes not involved
Group II	Compromised or regional resection
A	Grossly resected tumor with microscopic residual disease
B	Regional disease, completely resected, in which nodes may be involved or extension of tumor into adjacent organ may exist
C	Regional disease with involved nodes, grossly resected, but with evidence of microscopic residual disease
Group III	Incomplete resection or biopsy with gross residual disease
Group IV	Distant metastases at diagnosis

Reprinted with permission from Mauer HM. The Intergroup Rhabdomyosarcoma Study: objectives and clinical staging classification. *J Pediatr Surg* 1980;15:371–372.

Table 45-3

IRSG Presurgical Staging Classification

Stage	Sites	Tumor (T)	Node (N)	Metastases (M)
I	Favorable sites	Any T	Any N	M0
II	Unfavorable sites	T1a or T2a	N0 or Nx	M0
III	Unfavorable sites	T1a or T2a T1b or T2b	N1 Any N	M0
IV	All	Any T	Any N	M1

Favorable sites: orbit, head and neck (excluding parameningeal), genitourinary (nonbladder/nonprostate), and biliary track.
Unfavorable sites: bladder/prostate, extremity, cranial, parameningeal, and other (includes trunk, retroperitoneum, and so on).
Tumor (T): T1a, confined to anatomic site of origin and ≤5 cm; T1b, confined to anatomic site of origin and >5 cm; T2a, extension and/or fixative to surrounding tissue and ≤5 cm; T2b, extension and/or fixative to surrounding tissue and > 5 cm.
Node (N): N0, regional nodes not clinically involved; N1, regional nodes clinically involved by neoplasm; Nx, clinical status of regional nodes unknown;
Metastasis (M): M0, no distant metastasis; M1, metastasis present.
Data from Crist WM, Anderson JR, Meza JL, et al. Intergroup rhabdomyosarcoma study-IV: results for patients with nonmetastatic disease. *J Clin Oncol* 2001;19(12):3091–3102.

Table 45-4

International Classification of Rhabdomyosarcoma

I. Superior prognosis
   a. Botryoid rhabdomyosarcoma
   b. Spindle cell rhabdomyosarcoma
II. Intermediate prognosis
   a. Embryonal rhabdomyosarcoma
III. Poor prognosis
   a. Alveolar rhabdomyosarcoma
   b. Undifferentiated sarcoma
   c. Anaplastic rhabdomyosarcoma
IV. Subtypes whose prognosis is not presently evaluable
   a. Rhabdomyosarcoma with rhabdoid features

Reprinted with permission from Breneman JC, Donaldson SS. Rhabdomyosarcoma. In: Halperin EC, Perez CA, Brady LW, eds. *Principles and practice of radiation oncology*, 6th ed. Philadelphia, PA: Lippincott Williams & Wilkins, 2013:1677. © Wolters Kluwer.

- The botryoid subtype, a polypoid variant of embryonal rhabdomyosarcoma, has a grape-like appearance; it is usually noninvasive and localized and presents in mucosal-lined organs such as the vagina, urinary bladder, middle ear, biliary tree, and nasopharynx.
- The spindle cell subtype of embryonal rhabdomyosarcoma has a spindled appearance and is frequently found in paratesticular sites.
- Patients with embryonal rhabdomyosarcoma have intermediate outcome; the mesenchymal cells tend to differentiate into cross-striated muscle cells. Immunohistochemistry may demonstrate actin- or desmin-positive reactions. Ultrastructural studies exhibit evidence of myogenesis. The presence of cross-striations confirms the diagnosis.
- Embryonal histology occurs in 60% of cases and is found most commonly in the orbit, head and neck, and genitourinary sites.
- The poor-prognosis group includes alveolar, undifferentiated sarcomas and anaplastic rhabdomyosarcoma.
- Approximately 20% of rhabdomyosarcomas are the alveolar subtype, most commonly found in adolescents with truncal, retroperitoneal, and extremity tumors. The projected outcome for this group is 54% at 5 years (17).
- The pleomorphic type is extremely rare; many cases formerly classified as pleomorphic are currently considered to be malignant fibrous histiocytoma.
- Cases previously classified as extraosseous Ewing's sarcoma are now more appropriately included in the Ewing's family of tumors and are managed as such.
- Molecular profiling: Alveolar characterized by translocation between (2:13) (q35:q14) (70%) or (1;13) (p36;q14) (20%); Embryonal has loss of heterozygosity (LOH) at 11p15.

GENERAL MANAGEMENT

- A multidisciplinary approach using surgery, irradiation, and chemotherapy is critical in the management of rhabdomyosarcoma; the optimal sequence and specific application of each modality are under investigation. Early local progression during

Table 45-5
Prognostic Subgroups from ARST Protocols

I.   Low risk
    a. Embryonal histology
    b. Subset 1: stage 1 or 2 group I or II, stage 1 group III (orbit only)
    c. Subset 2: stage 1 group III nonorbit, stage 3 group I or II N0
II. Intermediate risk
    a. Alveolar: stage 1–3 group I–III
    b. Embryonal/botryoid/spindle cell: stage 2–3 group III
III. High risk
    a. Metastases (stage 4, group IV)

Data from Children's Oncology Group protocol ARST0331, ARST0531, and ARST0431. National Cancer Institute, www.cancer.gov.

induction chemotherapy in intermediate-risk rhabdomyosarcoma has been reported in a small proportion of patients (2.2%); therefore, earlier radiotherapy could potentially improve outcome by preventing early local progression (18).

- General management depends on risk stratification (Table 45-5):
  - For low-risk subset 1 (per ARST0331): VAC × 4 → RT week 13 (if needed) with VA → VA × 4.
  - For low-risk subset 2 (per ARST0331): VAC × 4 → RT week 13 (if needed) with VA → VA × 12.
  - For intermediate risk (per ARST0531): VAC (standard arm) versus VAC alt with V/I, VI will be concurrent with RT; RT starts at week 4 except parameningeal sites with intracranial extension (RT starts at week 0).
  - For high risk (per ARST0431): V/I × 6 weeks → V/D/C alt with IE at q 2-week intervals, concurrent with RT; RT starts at week 20 except parameningeal sites with intracranial extension (RT starts at week 0).

Orbit

- Historically, orbital exenteration was used. However, this procedure should be reserved for salvage treatment and enucleation for the management of posttreatment ocular complications.
- High-dose irradiation provides local tumor control of 90%, and when combined with systemic chemotherapy, results in cure rates of more than 90% (1,19).
- Traditionally, when irradiation alone was used, the entire orbit was included in the tumor volume; with a combined-modality approach, the site of tumor involvement with a margin is treated using doses of 45 to 50 Gy with systemic chemotherapy, without irradiating the entire orbit.
- Chemotherapy alone (i.e., without irradiation) results in local relapse, poor event-free survival, and loss of functional vision.

Head and Neck: Parameningeal Sites

- Nonorbital rhabdomyosarcomas of the head and neck sites are grouped into parameningeal sites (mastoid, middle ear, nasopharynx, nasal cavity, pterygopalatine fossa, infratemporal fossa, paranasal sinuses, and parapharyngeal space) or nonparameningeal sites, based on differences in natural history, treatment, and prognosis (1,20). Tumors in the parameningeal sites tend to invade into the base of the skull, resulting in cranial nerve palsy and direct extension into the central nervous system.
- It was previously thought that as many as 35% of children with tumors arising in a parameningeal site later developed meningeal extension. However, the prognosis of these patients is markedly improved with appropriate imaging, multiagent chemotherapy, and adequate irradiation of the primary tumor and adjacent meninges (14).
- Former irradiation regimens for these tumors used whole-brain irradiation as part of central nervous system prophylaxis; more recent studies show that this approach is unnecessary, and that adequate local tumor control can be achieved with local-field irradiation plus a margin, even with direct intracranial tumor extension (21).
- Patients with known meningeal dissemination throughout the neuraxis should receive craniospinal irradiation.

Head and Neck: Nonparameningeal Sites

- Nonparameningeal head and neck tumors may be more amenable to complete gross surgical excision than parameningeal tumors.
- Children with tumors in nonparameningeal head and neck sites tend to have a better outcome than those with parameningeal tumors (1).
- Nonparameningeal head and neck sites include the scalp, parotid, oral cavity, larynx, oropharynx, and cheek.
- Approximately 15% of these patients present with regional lymph node metastasis (14).
- Radiotherapeutic management is based on the amount of residual tumor after surgery.
- Draining regional lymph nodes are not routinely irradiated unless they contain metastatic tumor.

Pelvis

- Pelvic tumors are usually divided into anatomic subgroups, as the natural history, treatment, and prognosis are different for each site.

Bladder and Prostate

- Bladder and prostate primary tumors account for approximately one half of all pelvic rhabdomyosarcomas (20); more than 90% of these tumors are of the embryonal histologic subtype, with approximately one third having a botryoid morphology.
- In males, it is often difficult to differentiate a tumor of prostatic origin from one of bladder origin, as disease usually involves both structures. However, patients with prostate tumors have significantly inferior survival than do those with localized tumor confined to the bladder (22).

- Anterior pelvic exenteration, when combined with multiagent chemotherapy and irradiation for microscopic or gross residual disease, is associated with a survival rate of approximately 70% (23,24).
- A partial cystectomy may be acceptable for a small tumor arising from the dome of the bladder, where the entire tumor can be grossly excised (25,26).
- IRS-III intensified the therapy with the systematic use of planned irradiation 6 weeks after the start of treatment, and added cisplatin and doxorubicin chemotherapy (25).
- The goals of IRS studies are to preserve bladder function without compromising survival. The results of IRS-III showed a bladder retention rate of 60% and a overall survival rate of 90% for patients presenting with local or regional disease at 4 years. The results of IRS-IV showed a bladder preservation rate of close to 70% and a overall survival rate of 82% at a mean follow-up of 6 years.

Paratesticular

- Paratesticular tumors may arise anywhere along the spermatic cord, from the inter-scrotal area through the inguinal canal. They usually present as painless scrotal or inguinal masses that do not transilluminate.
- Most boys with paratesticular rhabdomyosarcoma present with early-stage disease, which is amenable to complete resection and is associated with cure rates approaching 90%.
- Retroperitoneal node metastases can occur along the external iliac and spermatic vessels, aorta, and vena cava. In early reports, the clinical incidence of periaortic and renal hilar lymph node involvement was as high as 40% (4); more recently, imaging studies and selected lymph node sampling show a lower incidence. In IRS-III patients, 81% of paratesticular patients had clinically uninvolved retroperitoneal lymph nodes on imaging studies (27).
- The incidence of retroperitoneal lymph node involvement varies with the age of the patient and method of staging. In the IRS-III study, retroperitoneal lymph node sampling was done in most patients, showing a 14% incidence of node involvement for children younger than 10 years of age and a 47% incidence for those aged 10 years or older. In IRS-IV, thin-cut CT without surgical sampling was used for staging, and the incidence of detected nodes dropped to 4% and 13% for the two age groups, respectively (28).
- For COG ARST protocol, staging ipsilateral retroperitoneal lymph node dissection is required for all patients 10 years of age or older with paratesticular tumors given that this group of children has a high risk of nodal and for patients younger than 10 years with clinically or radiographically involved lymph nodes (except when extensive lymph node involvement, defined as two or more lymph nodes greater than 2 cm in dimension, is identified by imaging studies). However, a recent study results from the "Cooperative Weichteilsarkom Studiengruppe" Trials CWS-86, -91, -96, and -2002P concluded that primary lymph node sampling seemed to have no impact on the EFS and should not be recommended. However, patients with positive lymph nodes had a poor prognosis and require additional local therapy (29).
- The recommended surgical procedure is inguinal orchiectomy.

- Regional lymph node irradiation to the periaortic and ipsilateral iliac nodes is recommended for nodal spread (4).
- Surgical violation of the scrotum or tumor extension to this structure is an indication for scrotal irradiation.

Gynecologic Tumors

- Tumors arising in the vulva, vagina, cervix, and uterus are approximately one third as common as bladder and prostate primary tumors, with the vagina being the most common site (30). Botryoid morphology is common.
- Initial surgery is primarily used for diagnosis, although gross tumor resection is occasionally possible without cosmetic or functional deformity.
- These tumors are often quite sensitive to chemotherapy, and unlike with bladder and prostate tumors, some of these children may not require irradiation for local tumor control (12–30).
- Preservation of bladder and sexual function is often possible with vaginal tumors, although vulvar and uterine tumors may not be as amenable to organ-preserving therapy, when surgery is used for primary therapy (30).
- Radiation therapy is usually reserved for patients with residual disease after resection, or as part of a preoperative regimen to help limit the extent of surgery.
- Intracavitary and interstitial brachytherapy are useful in these sites, compared with external beam irradiation, to provide sparing of normal tissues (31).

Other Pelvic Sites

- These tumors include perianal, perirectal, and perineal primary sites. Regional lymph node involvement may be high.
- If excision demands exenteration with urinary and fecal diversion procedures, combined chemotherapy and irradiation is recommended instead of primary surgical procedures.

Extremity

- Tumors arising in the extremity are often alveolar or undifferentiated subtypes. They tend to be large and deeply invasive at diagnosis and are associated with a high probability of lymphatic and hematogenous metastasis (32).
- Complete surgical resection usually requires extensive dissection, and alone is associated with a high risk of residual disease.
- Because irradiation and multiagent chemotherapy provide excellent local control, it is advisable to avoid disfiguring and mutilating surgical procedures; limb-salvage procedures are recommended instead.
- Regional lymph node sampling or sentinel lymph node procedure is required for histologic evaluation in patients with extremity tumors (ARST0531). Patients with lymph node involvement have a particularly poor prognosis (32).

- Radiation therapy for extremity primary tumors requires careful immobilization techniques, sparing of nonirradiated skin for lymphatic drainage, and use of shrinking fields.
- Physical therapy during and after radiation therapy is important for optimal functional results.

Chemotherapy

- Several drugs have demonstrated single-agent activity against rhabdomyosarcoma; reported response rates are as follows: vincristine sulfate, 59%; dactinomycin (actinomycin D), 24%; cyclophosphamide, 54%; doxorubicin (Adriamycin), 31%; dacarbazine, 11%; mitomycin-C, 36%; cisplatin, 15% to 21%; etoposide, 15% to 21%; ifosfamide, 86%; irinotecan, 23%; and topotecan, 46% (14).
- The most extensive experience in combination chemotherapy is with a vincristine sulfate, dactinomycin, and cyclophosphamide regimen (VAC) or VAC plus doxorubicin (VACA).
- For intermediate-risk rhabdomyosarcoma, VAC alternating with vincristine, topotecan, and cyclophosphamide does not significantly improve failure-free survival compared with VAC (33).
- For high-risk rhabdomyosarcoma, the combination of vincristine and irinotecan is highly active (33).

RADIATION THERAPY TECHNIQUES

- Adequate irradiation requires careful attention to volume and dose.
- Careful examination by the radiation oncologist at the time of initial diagnosis, even before neoadjuvant chemotherapy, is essential for treatment planning.
- It is important to evaluate the soft tissue extent of the primary lesion by computed tomography or magnetic resonance imaging; rhabdomyosarcoma tends to infiltrate tissue planes, and tumors often extend beyond a fascial compartment and obvious visible or palpable margins.
- Per ARST protocols, GTV is defined as the visible and/or palpable disease defined by physical examination, CT, MRI, or PET scan prior to any surgical debulking or chemotherapy. For patients who undergo initial surgery, operative notes and pathology reports may be helpful. For patients with initial tumors that extend into body cavities (i.e., thorax, abdomen), the GTV may require modification. If the tumor has been resected or responded to chemotherapy and the normal tissues have returned to their normal positions, the GTV excludes the volume which extends into the cavity.
- CTV: If there are no sites that warrant irradiation for potential occult tumor, then the CTV is defined as GTV + 1 cm (but not extending outside of the patient). It also includes regional lymph node chains for clinically or pathologically involved nodes. For tumors with no evidence of nodal involvement (N0), the draining regional lymph nodes are not irradiated. For some sites, the definition of CTV is modified to account for specific anatomic barriers to tumor spread. When lymph nodes

are clinically or pathologically involved with tumor, the entire lymph node drainage chain should be included in the CTV.

- PTV = CTV + 5 mm.
- In ARST protocol, volume reduction is permitted for patients whose total dose will be 5,040 cGy. In cases where there is a rapid, substantial decrease in tumor size, a cone down may be performed after 3,600 cGy. The GTV cone down is defined as residual visible or palpable tumor as assessed by CT, MRI, PET scan, or physical exam following induction chemotherapy.
- Compared to IRS III and IV results, reduced-dose radiotherapy on COG D9602 did not compromise local control for low risk patients with microscopic tumor after surgical resection (36 Gy for microscopic residual and uninvolved nodes and 41.4 Gy for involved nodes) or with orbital primary tumors (45 Gy) when cyclophosphamide was added to the treatment program (34).
- In patients with tumors at parameningeal sites (middle ear, paranasal sinuses, nasopharynx, nasal cavity, infratemporal fossa, and parapharyngeal area), irradiation portals should cover the adjacent meninges to prevent meningeal relapse (1,20).
- For orbital tumor, technique is very important for minimizing corneal and lacrimal gland dose and preserving useful vision in the treated eye. Photon irradiation with the eyelid open minimizes corneal dose when an anterior field is used and may be associated with improved long-term functional outcome (35). Proton has been used for treating orbital tumor (36).
- Three-dimensional conformal therapy (coplanar or noncoplanar) or IMRT is required to minimize dose to normal tissue. IMRT improves target dose coverage compared with 3DCRT (37). Proton therapy is associated with reduced late toxicity (38,39) without an increased risk of marginal failure (40).
- Radiation doses according to histology, clinical group, and site are listed in Table 45-6.
- Dose to the brain or spinal cord axis is 30 Gy in 1.5- to 2.0-Gy fractions (41).
- IRS-IV investigators studied the efficacy of a higher hyperfractionated irradiation dose (59.4 Gy in 1.1-Gy fractions, twice daily, at 6-hour intervals) for children with gross

Table 45-6

Radiation Doses per ARST Protocols

Clinical Group	Total Dose (cGy)
I, embryonal/botryoid/spindle cell	0
I, alveolar/undifferentiated/anaplastic	3,600
II, node negative	3,600
II, node positive	4,140
III, orbit only	4,500
III, all others	5,040

Data from Children's Oncology Group protocol ARST0331, ARST0531, and ARST0431. National Cancer Institute, www.cancer.gov.

residual disease (42). Results were comparable to conventionally fractionated RT (15). Prognostic subgroups were established in this trial and are listed in Table 45-5.

- Immobilization techniques that ensure reproducible portals are essential.
- Sedation or anesthesia may be necessary to ensure adequate implementation of the treatment plan.
- These complex programs are best conducted in regional centers by an experienced team.
- Interstitial irradiation, including high dose rate brachytherapy, may play an important role as primary treatment or as a boost after external beam therapy for selected sites (43,44).
- Although radiation therapy is often delayed for several weeks to allow administration of neoadjuvant chemotherapy, some data suggest that earlier irradiation, particularly in high-risk patients, may provide better local tumor control and survival (1,20,45).
- Interaction between irradiation and some commonly used chemotherapeutic drugs can produce undesirable early and late effects, particularly with dactinomycin and doxorubicin. Radiation therapy given concurrently with these agents should be avoided; both drugs accentuate a "recall" of radiation injury if given during or immediately after radiation therapy. Systemic treatment with drugs such as vincristine sulfate and cyclophosphamide can often be continued concurrently with irradiation.
- Brachytherapy has been used in the treatment of pediatric soft tissue sarcomas, both alone and in combination with external beam irradiation. Local tumor control is excellent, and morbidity is acceptable (46).

SEQUELAE OF THERAPY

- Newer protocols using more aggressive therapy, including cisplatin, dacarbazine, etoposide, and other agents, carry acute side effects (e.g., renal and electrolyte imbalance) that demand close monitoring.
- Radiation toxicity is related to the regions irradiated and the dose administered.
- Prompt attention to skin care with moisturizers and steroid creams is important.
- After orbital irradiation, an acute inflammatory reaction of the cornea and conjunctiva occurs, resulting in pain and photophobia. Steroids should be administered under the direction of an ophthalmologist.
- Cataracts developed in 65 of 79 irradiated patients (82%), and 43 (66%) underwent surgery (47). Twenty-four patients had a dry eye, and 22 had chronic keratitis. In 48 of 82 patients, there was orbital hypoplasia; ptosis and enophthalmos occurred in 22 patients.
- Of 469 children with nonorbital soft tissue sarcomas of the head and neck who were treated with multiagent chemotherapy and radiation therapy (except in three cases), 213 survived relapse-free for 5 years or longer (27). Hypoplasia or tissue asymmetry was seen in 74, poor dentition or malformed teeth in 61, impaired vision in 37, and decreased learning in 36 patients. Thirty-six patients (19%) required growth hormone injections.
- Acute otitis externa or media with hyperemia and swelling of the membranes of the eustachian tube is common during or soon after treatment of head and neck areas.

- Erythematous mucositis occurs after head and neck irradiation and after drug therapy—and almost universally if the two are used simultaneously. Mouth washes such as salt and soda, 1% hydrogen peroxide, or combinations of diphenhydramine elixir, hydrocortisone, and antibiotics partially alleviate the reaction.
- Bacterial or fungal superimposed infection requires specific drug management.
- Pretreatment evaluation by a dentist is very important to correct preexisting problems and to provide fluoride applications.
- Acute gastrointestinal sequelae, such as vomiting and diarrhea, are usually managed by supportive care and appropriate medication. Nutritional support with hyperalimentation may be necessary.
- Late radiation effects are related to the irradiated site, the irradiation dose, and the age of the child at the time of treatment. Effects include bone and soft tissue growth disturbances, cataract, hypopituitarism, gonadal dysfunction, induction of second malignant tumors (particularly bone sarcomas), and chronic organ dysfunction (48–50). Combined-modality treatment programs are significantly implicated in many of these complications.

References

1. Arndt CA, Crist WM. Common musculoskeletal tumors of childhood and adolescence. *N Engl J Med* 1999;341(5):342–352.
2. Breneman JC, Wiener ES. Issues in the local control of rhabdomyosarcoma. *Med Pediatr Oncol* 2000;35(2):104–109.
3. Lawrence W, Hays DM, Heyn R, et al. Lymphatic metastases with childhood rhabdomyosarcoma. A report from the Intergroup Rhabdomyosarcoma Study. *Cancer* 1987;60:910–915.
4. LaQuaglia MP, Ghavimi F, Penenberg D, et al. Factors predictive of mortality in pediatric extremity rhabdomyosarcoma. *J Pediatr Surg* 1990;25(2):238–244.
5. Crist W, Gehan EA, Ragab AH, et al. The Third Intergroup Rhabdomyosarcoma Study. *J Clin Oncol* 1995;13:610–630.
6. Maurer HM, Beltangady M, Gehan EA, et al. The intergroup rhabdomyosarcoma study-I. *Cancer* 1988;61:209–220.
7. Maurer HM, Gehan EA, Beltangady M, et al. The intergroup rhabdomyosarcoma study-II. *Cancer* 1993;71:1904–1922.
8. Oberlin O, Rey A, Lyden E, et al. Prognostic factors in metastatic rhabdomyosarcomas: results of a pooled analysis from United States and European cooperative groups. *J Clin Oncol* 2008;26:2384–2389.
9. Wolden SL, Anderson JR, Crist WM, et al. Indications for radiotherapy and chemotherapy after complete resection in rhabdomyosarcoma: a report from the Intergroup Rhabdomyosarcoma Studies I to III. *J Clin Oncol* 1999;17(11):3468–3475.
10. McDowell HP, Foot AB, Ellershaw C, et al. Outcomes in pediatric metastatic rhabdomyosarcoma: results of the international society of pediatric oncology (SIOP) study MMT-98. *Eur J Cancer* 2010;46:1588–1595.
11. Oberlin O, Rey A, Lyden E, et al. Prognostic factors in metastatic rhabdomyosarcomas: results of pooled analysis from United States and European cooperative groups. *J Clin Oncol* 2008;26:2384–2389.
12. Rudzinski ER, Anderson JR, Chi YY, et al. Histology, fusion status, and outcome in metastatic rhabdomyosarcoma: a report from the Children's Oncology Group. *Pediatr Blood Cancer* 2017;64(12). doi: 10.1002/pbc.26645.

13. Constine LS, Tarbell NJ, Halperin EC, eds. Chapter 11. Rhabdomyosarcoma. In: *Pediatric radiation oncology*, 6th ed. Philadelphia, PA: Wolters Kluwer, 2016.

14. Halpern, EC, Wazer, DE, Perez CA, et al., eds. Chapter 87. Rhabdomyosarcoma. In: *Principles and practice of radiation oncology*, 6th ed. Philadelphia, PA: Lippincott Williams & Wilkins, 2013.

15. Crist WM, Anderson JR, Meza JL, et al. Intergroup rhabdomyosarcoma study-IV: results for patients with nonmetastatic disease. *J Clin Oncol* 2001;19(12):3091–3102.

16. Tsokos M, Webber BL, Parham DM, et al. Rhabdomyosarcoma. A new classification scheme related to prognosis. *Arch Pathol Lab Med* 1992;116(8):847–855.

17. Newton WA Jr, Gehan EA, Webber BL, et al. Classification of rhabdomyosarcomas and related sarcomas. Pathologic aspects and proposal for a new classification—an Intergroup Rhabdomyosarcoma Study. *Cancer* 1995;76(6):1073–1085.

18. Minn AY, Lyden ER, Anderson JR, et al. Early treatment failure in intermediate-risk rhabdomyosarcoma: results from IRS-IV and D9803—a report from the Children's Oncology Group. *J Clin Oncol* 2010;28:4228–4232.

19. Crist WM, Garnsey L, Beltangady MS, et al. Prognosis in children with rhabdomyosarcoma: a report of the intergroup rhabdomyosarcoma studies I and II. Intergroup Rhabdomyosarcoma Committee. *J Clin Oncol* 1990;8(3):443–452.

20. Maurer HM, Gehan EA, Beltangady M, et al. The Intergroup Rhabdomyosarcoma Study-II. *Cancer* 1993;71(5):1904–1922.

21. Gasparini M, Lombardi F, Gianni MC, et al. Questionable role of CNS radioprophylaxis in the therapeutic management of childhood rhabdomyosarcoma with meningeal extension. *J Clin Oncol* 1990;8(11):1854–1857.

22. LaQuaglia MP, Ghavimi F, Penenberg D, et al. Factors predictive of mortality in pediatric extremity rhabdomyosarcoma. *J Pediatr Surg* 1990;25(2):238–243; discussion 243–244.

23. Maurer HM, Beltangady M, Gehan EA, et al. The intergroup rhabdomyosarcoma study-I. A final report. *Cancer* 1988;61(2):209–220.

24. Rodary C, Gehan EA, Flamant F, et al. Prognostic factors in 951 nonmetastatic rhabdomyosarcoma in children: a report from the International Rhabdomyosarcoma Workshop. *Med Pediatr Oncol* 1991;19(2):89–95.

25. Hays DM. Bladder/prostate rhabdomyosarcoma: results of the multi-institutional trials of the Intergroup Rhabdomyosarcoma Study. *Semin Surg Oncol* 1993;9(6):520–523.

26. Hays DM, Raney RB, Wharam MD, et al. Children with vesical rhabdomyosarcoma (RMS) treated by partial cystectomy with neoadjuvant or adjuvant chemotherapy, with or without radiotherapy. A report from the Intergroup Rhabdomyosarcoma Study (IRS) Committee. *J Pediatr Hematol Oncol* 1995;17(1):46–52.

27. Raney RB, Asmar L, Vassilopoulou-Sellin R, et al. Late complications of therapy in 213 children with localized, nonorbital soft-tissue sarcoma of the head and neck: a descriptive report from the Intergroup Rhabdomyosarcoma Studies (IRS)-II and -III. IRS Group of the Children's Cancer Group and the Pediatric Oncology Group. *Med Pediatr Oncol* 1999;33(4):362–371.

28. Wiener ES, Anderson JR, Ojimba JI, et al. Controversies in the management of paratesticular rhabdomyosarcoma: is staging retroperitoneal lymph node dissection necessary for adolescents with resected paratesticular rhabdomyosarcoma? *Semin Pediatr Surg* 2001;10:146–152.

29. Seitz G, Fuchs J, Martus P, et al. Outcome, treatment, and treatment failures in patients suffering localized embryonal paratesticular rhabdomyosarcoma: results from the "Cooperative Weichteilsarkom Studiengruppe" trials CWS-86, -91, -96, and -2002P. *Ann Surg* 2016;264(6):1148–1155.

30. Hays DM, Shimada H, Raney RB Jr, et al. Clinical staging and treatment results in rhabdomyosarcoma of the female genital tract among children and adolescents. *Cancer* 1988;61(9):1893–1903.

31. Gerbaulet A, Panis X, Flamant F, et al. Iridium afterloading curietherapy in the treatment of pediatric malignancies. The Institut Gustave Roussy experience. *Cancer* 1985;56(6):1274–1279.

32. Mandell L, Ghavimi F, LaQuaglia M, et al. Prognostic significance of regional lymph node involvement in childhood extremity rhabdomyosarcoma. *Med Pediatr Oncol* 1990;18(6):466–471.

33. Arndt CAS, Stoner JA, Hawkins, DS, et al. Vincristine, actinomycin, and cyclophosphamide compared with vincristine, actinomycin, and cyclophosphamide alternating with vincristine, topotecan, and cyclophosphamide for intermediate-risk rhabdomyosarcoma: Children's Oncology Group Study D9803. *Clin Oncol* 2009;27:5182–5188.

34. Breneman J, Meza J, Donaldson SS, et al. Local control with reduced-dose radiotherapy for low-risk rhabdomyosarcoma: a report from the Children's Oncology Group D9602 Study. *Int J Radiat Oncol Biol Phys* 2012;83(2):721–726.

35. Sagerman RH. Orbital rhabdomyosarcoma: a paradigm for irradiation. *Radiology* 1993;187(3): 605–607.

36. Yock T, Schneider R, Friedmann A, et al. Proton radiotherapy for orbital rhabdomyosarcoma: clinical outcome and a dosimetric comparison with photons. *Int J Radiat Oncol Biol Phys* 2005;63:1161–1168.

37. Lin C, Donaldson SS, Meza JL, et al. Effect of radiotherapy techniques (IMRT vs. 3D-CRT) on outcome in patients with intermediate-risk rhabdomyosarcoma enrolled in COG D9803—a report from the Children's Oncology Group. *Int J Radiat Oncol Biol Phys* 2012;82(5):1764–1770.

38. Weber DC, Ares C, Albertini F, et al. Pencil beam scanning proton therapy for pediatric parameningeal rhabdomyosarcomas: clinical outcome of patients treated at the Paul Scherrer Institute. *Pediatr Blood Cancer* 2016;63(10):1731–1736.

39. Childs SK, Kozak KR, Friedmann AM, et al. Proton radiotherapy for parameningeal rhabdomyosarcoma: clinical outcomes and late effects. *Int J Radiat Oncol Biol Phys* 2012;82(2):635–642. doi: 10.1016/j.ijrobp.2010.11.048.

40. Vern Gross TZ, et al. Patterns of failure in pediatric rhabdomyosarcoma after proton therapy. *Int J Radiat Oncol Biol Phys* 2016;96(5):1070–1077.

41. Paulino AC, Simon JH, Zhen W, et al. Long-term effects in children treated with radiotherapy for head and neck rhabdomyosarcoma. *Int J Radiat Oncol Biol Phys* 2000;48(5):1489–1495.

42. Donaldson SS, Asmar L, Breneman J, et al. Hyperfractionated radiation in children with rhabdomyosarcoma—results of an Intergroup Rhabdomyosarcoma Pilot Study. *Int J Radiat Oncol Biol Phys* 1995;32(4):903–911.

43. Healey EA, Shamberger RC, Grier HE, et al. A 10-year experience of pediatric brachytherapy. *Int J Radiat Oncol Biol Phys* 1995;32(2):451–455.

44. Nag S, Grecula J, Ruymann FB. Aggressive chemotherapy, organ-preserving surgery, and high-dose-rate remote brachytherapy in the treatment of rhabdomyosarcoma in infants and young children. *Cancer* 1993;72(9):2769–2776.

45. Koscielniak E, Jurgens H, Winkler K, et al. Treatment of soft tissue sarcoma in childhood and adolescence. A report of the German Cooperative Soft Tissue Sarcoma Study. *Cancer* 1992;70(10):2557–2567.

46. Merchant TE, Parsh N, del Valle PL, et al. Brachytherapy for pediatric soft-tissue sarcoma. *Int J Radiat Oncol Biol Phys* 2000;46(2):427–432.

47. Raney RB, Anderson JR, Kollath J, et al. Late effects of therapy in 94 patients with localized rhabdomyosarcoma of the orbit: report from the Intergroup Rhabdomyosarcoma Study (IRS)-III, 1984–1991. *Med Pediatr Oncol* 2000;34(6):413–420.

48. Abramson DH, Notis CM. Visual acuity after radiation for orbital rhabdomyosarcoma. *Am J Ophthalmol* 1994;118(6):808–809.

49. Kaste SC, Hopkins KP, Bowman LC. Dental abnormalities in long-term survivors of head and neck rhabdomyosarcoma. *Med Pediatr Oncol* 1995;25(2):96–101.

50. Raney B Jr, Heyn R, Hays DM, et al. Sequelae of treatment in 109 patients followed for 5 to 15 years after diagnosis of sarcoma of the bladder and prostate. A report from the Intergroup Rhabdomyosarcoma Study Committee. *Cancer* 1993;71(7):2387–2394.

CHAPTER 46

LYMPHOMAS IN CHILDREN

- Lymphomas constitute the third most common childhood cancer.
- Pediatric Hodgkin's lymphoma (HL) is more common than non-Hodgkin's lymphoma.

HODGKIN'S LYMPHOMA

- There is a bimodal age distribution. The childhood form occurs in patients age 14 years or younger and is rare in children less than 4 years of age. The young adult form affects people aged 15 to 34 years of age.
- There is a strong association between HL and the Epstein-Barr virus (EBV). EBV-positive tumor genomes are more frequent in children younger than 10 years of age and who live in developing countries (1).

Pathologic Classification

- The World Health Organization's (WHO) classification system classifies HL into two main groups. They are classical type (positive for CD 15 and CD 30) and nodular lymphocyte predominant type (positive for CD 20 and lacking CD 15 and CD 30). The classical type have four subtypes: nodular sclerosing, mixed cellularity, lymphocyte rich, and lymphocyte depleted.
- Nodular sclerosing HL is the most common subtype in all age groups; it is more frequent in adolescents (77%) and adults (72%) than in younger children (44%) (2).
- In an analysis of 2,238 patients, lymphocyte-predominant HL was relatively more common (13%) in younger children (age less than 10 years), whereas lymphocyte-depleted HL was exceedingly rare (2).
- Mixed cellularity HL is more common in younger children (33%) than in adolescents or adults (11% to 17%) (2).

Clinical Presentation

- Most children (80%) present with cervical lymphadenopathy.
- Mediastinal involvement is present in approximately 75% of adolescents, but in only 33% of children 1 to 10 years old.
- One third of patients have one or more "B" symptoms at diagnosis (unexplained fever greater than 38°C and recurrent during the previous month, drenching night sweats during the previous month, or weight loss of greater than 10% in the 6 months preceding diagnosis) (3).

Diagnostic Workup

- The diagnosis of HL is made by lymph node biopsy and confirmed pathologically by the presence of Reed-Sternberg cells and the mononuclear variants.
- Recommended procedures for pretreatment evaluation in the child with HL are similar to those for the adult.

Staging

- As with adults, children with HL are staged according to the system devised at the Ann Arbor Staging Conference in 1970.
- The distribution of stages observed in children is different than in adults. Among 2,238 patients treated consecutively at Stanford University, stage I or stage II disease was present in 60%. Stage I was slightly more common in younger children (18%) than in adolescents (8%); stage II disease was seen in 40% to 50% of all age groups; stage IV disease was observed in younger children (3%) less often than in adolescents (15%) (2).

Prognostic Factors

- Several factors influence the choice and success of therapy; stage, bulk, and biologic aggressiveness are frequently codependent.
- Stage of disease is the most significant prognosticator of treatment outcome.
- Bulk of disease is reflected in the disease stage. Large mediastinal adenopathy (LMA) (more than one third of the maximum transthoracic diameter) and multiple sites of involvement (most often defined as more than three) with extensive splenic disease (more than four nodules) are associated with increased risk of recurrence after irradiation alone (4).
- Stage IV disease has exceptionally poor prognosis when managed with conventional therapeutic techniques.
- Systemic symptoms (B disease) correlate with an increased risk of relapse (3).
- Adverse prognostic factors include stage IIB, IIIB, IV; B symptoms; bulky disease; male gender; WBC count greater than 11,500 per mm^3; and hemoglobin less than or equal to 11 g per dL.

- Lymphocyte-depleted histology confers a worse outcome than do the other subtypes (4).
- Mixed cellularity disease is associated with an increased risk of subdiaphragmatic relapse in pathologically staged patients who have disease apparently confined to supradiaphragmatic areas.
- Children 10 years of age or younger fare better than do older patients (2).
- In relapsed cases, response to initial salvage chemotherapy predicts for survival (5).

General Management

- Although the biology and natural history of HL in children are similar to those in adults, treatment regimens used in adults can produce substantial treatment-related late toxicities when they were administered to children.
- To decrease the morbidity from radiation therapy, investigators at Stanford pioneered the use of multiagent chemotherapy in combination with lower doses of irradiation for young children with both early- and advanced-stage disease. This combined modality approach has resulted in excellent local control rates (6).
- Low-dose (15 to 25.5 Gy) involved-field radiation remains a critical component of combined modality treatment.
- Involved-field radiation therapy (IFRT) guidelines are outlined generally in Table 46-1.
- Recently, guidelines for implementation of involved-site radiation therapy (ISRT) have been published (7). In doing so, precise information regarding pre- and post-therapy structural (contrast-enhanced CT) and functional (PET) imaging is required. Though several clinical protocols still use IFRT, ISRT is rapidly becoming the standard of care in terms of radiotherapeutic management of HL.

Radiation Therapy Alone

- The use of radiation therapy to extended fields to a dose of 30 to 40 Gy produced the first cures in patients with HL. However, radiation therapy doses used in adults and the extended fields can produce significant late effects in pediatric patients.
- Radiation therapy alone has been largely abandoned as a treatment strategy in children.

Chemotherapy Alone

- Since the initial use of mechlorethamine hydrochloride, vincristine sulfate (Oncovin), procarbazine hydrochloride, and prednisone (MOPP) in the 1960s, marked improvement in cure rates has been achieved in the management of pediatric HL.
- Subsequent therapies have built upon the MOPP backbone. Doxorubicin (Adriamycin), bleomycin sulfate, vinblastine sulfate, and dacarbazine (ABVD) were developed as an alternative effective regimen in an attempt to improve survival and decrease long-term effects of treatment such as sterility and second malignancy (8,9).

Table 46-1

Involved-Field Radiation Guidelines

Involved Node(s)	RT Field
Unilateral neck	Unilateral neck + ipsilateral supraclavicular The superior border should extend from the midpoint of the chin through the midtragus. This should provide a minimum of 2 cm margin at the tip of the mastoid. The inferior border must be 1.5 cm below the clavicle. The lateral field border should be determined by the most lateral extent of disease on the CT study of the neck.
Supraclavicular	Supraclavicular + mid/low neck + infraclavicular
Axilla	Axilla +/− infraclavicular/supraclavicular
Mediastinum +/− hila	Mediastinum + hila + infraclavicular/supraclavicular The superior field border should encompass the initial superior extent of disease plus a 2-cm margin. The lower border should be placed 2 cm or at least one full vertebral body below the lowest initial extent of disease. The inferior border does not need to extend as low as the diaphragm if disease was never present in this region. The lateral field borders will be treated based on the width of the disease and the mediastinum after chemotherapy, not the width of the original mass. A 1.5-cm margin should be given on any residual mass and the normal mediastinal contour. The lateral margins of the mediastinal portals should cover the bilateral hila.
Spleen	Spleen +/− adjacent paraaortics If initially involved, the entire spleen should be treated with a 1.5–2-cm margin to account for respiratory movement. The postchemotherapy spleen volume should be used, as defined by CT scan. If the paraaortic lymph nodes were not involved, then they do not need to be specifically included. The splenic field should extend medially to 1.5 cm beyond the contra-lateral edge of the vertebral bodies to prevent asymmetric radiation of the spine. Only those vertebral bodies adjacent to the spleen should be included. This will result in treatment of the superior paraaortic lymph nodes even when they were not involved.
Paraaortics	Paraaortics +/− spleen The superior edge of the field is generally placed at the insertion of the diaphragm, with the inferior border at the level of the aortic bifurcation. Laterally, the fields should cover the initial extent of disease with a 1.5-cm margin or should be at least 2 cm lateral to the vertebral bodies on each side. The spleen or splenic pedicle should be included with this field.

Table 46-1	
Involved-Field Radiation Guidelines *(continued)*	
Involved Node(s)	RT Field
Iliac	Iliacs + inguinal/femoral Generally, the iliac and inguinofemoral chains are targeted with CT-based planning. If superficial inguinal and/or femoral lymph nodes are involved in the absence of iliac disease, then treatment may be limited to this region. The depth of the lymph nodes should be carefully measured on a CT scan. If adequate superficial and deep coverage of these nodes can be obtained using only an anterior field with photons or an electron beam of appropriate energy, this is encouraged. The upper border is typically 2 to 3 cm above and parallel to the inguinal fold. Inferiorly, the lower border should parallel the upper border. The medial border should be the medial border of the obturator canal; the lateral border should be the lateral border of the acetabulum.

In the treatment of children, the medial field border nearly always must cross the midline and include all of the vertebral body in order to have the appropriate margin for treatment.

Source: AHOD0431 (low risk), AHOD0031 (intermediate risk), and AHOD0831 (high risk) protocols.

- Different combinations of MOPP and ABVD were also developed.
- Currently, treatment with chemotherapy alone is preferred by investigators desiring to avoid long-term sequelae of radiation, including musculoskeletal growth impairment, cardiovascular dysfunction, and radiation-induced solid cancer. However, single-modality chemotherapy treatment usually involves more cycles of chemotherapy with higher cumulative doses of chemotherapy agents, which is associated with potential significant long-term adverse outcomes including gonadal toxicity, cardiac toxicity, and secondary leukemia. Combined-modality therapies prescribe low-dose, involved-field radiation in lieu of several chemotherapy cycles.
- Chemotherapy alone offers the advantage of eliminating the potential toxicities of irradiation; disadvantages include the toxicities associated with intensive drug therapy and the increased likelihood of disease recurrence in sites of bulky disease without use of radiotherapy (9,10).
- Earlier randomized pediatric trials prospectively comparing outcomes in patients treated with chemotherapy alone to those treated with combined-modality therapy have not definitively established the superiority of one treatment approach over the other (9,11).
- The subset analysis of COG5942 shows that patients with lymphocyte-predominant HL who had a complete response to 4 and 6 monthly cycles of cyclophosphamide, vincristine, prednisone, procarbazine, doxorubicin, bleomycin, and vinblastine (COPP/ABV) had an excellent EFS and OS without the addition of radiotherapy (12).

Combined Chemotherapy and Radiation Therapy

* In a randomized study of children with stage III to IV HL, the Children's Cancer Group reported a 4-year disease-free survival rate of 87% in 57 patients treated with ABVD and low-dose extended-field irradiation versus 77% in 54 patients treated with MOPP/ABVD (9).
* Despite excellent tumor control with ABVD, bleomycin sulfate and doxorubicin cause pulmonary and cardiovascular damage (respectively), the intensity of which may be exacerbated by the addition of mediastinal or mantle irradiation (13,14). In an attempt to decrease alkylator therapy and potential cardiotoxicity, the Pediatric Oncology Group (POG) developed a series of studies built upon the ABVD backbone, substituting dacarbazine with etoposide.
* In efforts to eliminate alkylating agents, the VAMP (vinblastine, doxorubicin, methotrexate, prednisone) regimen has been shown efficacious and safe in select low-risk HL cases (15). Moreover, a nonrandomized trial of favorable-risk HL patients demonstrated an acceptably high event-free survival when omitting RT if achieving a complete response to 2 cycles of VAMP (16). This was recapitulated in a randomized study using ABVD with or without dexrazoxane (17), along with another randomized subset of early-stage HL who were complete responders to 2 cycles of vincristine, prednisone, procarbazine, and doxorubicin (OPPA) or vincristine, prednisone, etoposide, and doxorubicin (OEPA) (18).
* The German cooperative groups have built upon COPP chemotherapy in both pediatric and adult Hodgkin's disease. The DAL-HD-90 study uses OEPA/COPP for males and OPPA/COPP for females, both followed by IFRT (19).
* Children's Cancer Group investigators compared COPP/ABV hybrid chemotherapy and low-dose, involved-field radiation to treatment with COPP/ABV chemotherapy alone. Significantly higher 3-year event-free survival was seen in patients randomized to receive combined-modality therapy. Early follow-up did not demonstrate a significant difference in overall survival among the groups because of the successful salvaging of relapsed patients (20).

Risk-Adapted Therapy

* An emerging focus of major ongoing investigation for both HL and non-Hodgkin's lymphomas (per below) centers on risk stratification and potential changes in management based on rapidity and quality of response to initial chemotherapy (21–23).
* The Children's Oncology Group (COG) closed a phase III study for the treatment of children and adolescents with newly diagnosed low-risk (stage IA, IIA without bulky disease) Hodgkin's disease (AHOD0431) and concluded that 3 cycles of AVPC is not adequate therapy for low-risk HL of nodular sclerosis histology. PET response after 1 cycle of AVPC is highly predictive of outcome.
* The intermediate-risk HL protocol (COG AHOD0031) treats patients with stage IA/IIA bulky, IB, IIB, IIIA, or IVA disease with 2 cycles of ABVE-PC prior to response evaluation. Those with a rapid early response to 2 cycles of chemotherapy

(greater than 60% reduction in tumor dimension) who then go on to achieve a complete response after an additional 2 cycles of the same chemotherapy are randomized to 21 Gy IFRT or no additional treatment. Patients with slow early response to 2 cycles of chemotherapy are randomized to either standard therapy (an additional 2 cycles of ABVE-PC + 21 Gy IFRT) or intensified therapy (2 cycles of ABVE-PC, 2 cycles of DECA [dexamethasone, etoposide, cisplatin, cytarabine] + 21 Gy IFRT). (COG AHOD0031: A Phase III Study of Dose-Intensive, Response-Based Chemotherapy and Radiation Therapy for Children and Adolescents with Newly Diagnosed Intermediate-Risk Hodgkin Disease.) Early results show no survival improvement with radiation therapy in the rapid early responders ($p = 0.07$). However, the 3-year event-free survival for rapid early responders (87%) was significantly higher than the slow early responders (78%) ($p = 0.0001$).

- The high-risk HL protocol (AHOD0831) is also completed. The results show that among pediatric patients with very high-risk HL (IIIB, IVB), a response-directed approach utilizing limited chemotherapy (4 cycles of ABVE-PC for RER; 4 cycles of ABVE-PC and 2 cycles of ifosfamide/vinorelbine for SER) and risk-directed radiation therapy did not reach the ambitiously high prespecified target for 4-year second EFS (greater than or equal to 95%). However, 4-year EFS (82%) and OS rates (93%) are comparable with results of recent trials for this population (POG 9425: IIIB/IVB) (24).

Radiation Therapy Techniques

- Because most radiation is delivered as part of a combined modality regimen, the dose ranges from 15 to 25 Gy. The dose depends on the protocol on which the child is enrolled.
- For COG protocols (AHOD0031, AHOD0431, and AHOD0831), IFRT was used to deliver 21 Gy in 14 fractions of 1.5 Gy per day. For IFRT, the gross tumor volume (GTV) includes any lymph node measuring greater than 1.5 cm in a single axis as defined on computed tomography. The clinical target volume (CTV) is the anatomical compartment. The planning target volume (PTV) is a 1.0-cm margin around the CTV to account for patient motion and setup variability. This can be modified at the discretion of the treating radiation oncologist if there are concerns of extended treatment of normal tissue. Anatomical compartments that are contiguous to involved compartments will also need to be treated if they contain lymph nodes greater than 1.0 cm in size as seen on CT scan. Treatment fields must be designed to include the original extent of disease.
- For the new generation COG protocols, ISRT is used to deliver 21 Gy in 14 fractions of 1.5 Gy per day. For ISRT, targets at noncontiguous sites need to be separately identified. The prechemotherapy GTV includes nodal and nonnodal tissues that were involved with lymphoma prior to any treatment. Postchemotherapy GTV including GTVPET positive: an area of imaging abnormality demonstrating the lymph node(s) that remain PET avid (Deauville score greater than 2), uptake greater than mediastinal blood pool and GTVPET negative: an area of imaging abnormality on

CT demonstrating the lymph node(s) as no longer PET avid (Deauville score 1 to 2). Delineation of the CTV requires consideration of the expected routes of disease spread and the quality of pretreatment imaging. The CTV should include the lymph nodes/tissues originally involved with lymphoma (i.e., the prechemotherapy GTV), but must take into account the reduction in axial diameter that has occurred with chemotherapy. As a guideline, CTV = GTV + 1.5 cm. The internal target volume (ITV) encompasses the CTV with an added margin to account for variation in shape and motion within the patient. PTV = ITV + 5 mm.

- Involved-nodal radiotherapy (INRT) was introduced in Europe for HL and markedly reduced the irradiated volume. INRT design requires accurate prechemo or prebiopsy information obtained in the treatment position. This technique is not used in pediatric Hodgkin's in the United States at this time.

NON-HODGKIN'S LYMPHOMA

- Childhood non-Hodgkin's lymphomas (NHLs) are generally diffuse, high grade, and poorly differentiated; extranodal involvement is common, and dissemination occurs early and often. This differs from adult NHL, in which low- and intermediate-grade nodal disease predominate.
- In younger children, NHL is more frequent than HL; the converse is true for adolescents.

Pathologic Classification

- Pediatric NHLs are grouped into four major histopathologic subtypes: (a) small, non-cleaved cell (SNCC) lymphoma (Burkitt's and non-Burkitt's subtypes), (b) lymphoblastic lymphoma, (c) diffuse large B-cell lymphoma, and (d) anaplastic large cell lymphoma.
- The histologic categories for the commonly used classification systems of NHL for the pediatric age group are presented in Table 46-2 (25).

Prognostic Factors

- Prognostic factors in pediatric NHL are stage of disease (which takes into account other known prognostic variables such as tumor burden, site, and extent of involvement) (26), serum lactate dehydrogenase (27), and soluble interleukin-2 receptor levels (which may reflect either disease burden or biologic aggressiveness).
- Most cases of pediatric NHL are of the high-grade and diffuse aggressive subtypes; this may obscure the prognostic value of histology.
- The clinical relevance of genetic abnormalities, such as the translocation t(2;5) (p23;q35) nonrandomly expressed in Ki-1–positive anaplastic large cell lymphomas, c-myc rearrangements in diffuse large B cell and small noncleaved B-cell lymphomas, and the translocation t(8;14) characteristic of Burkitt's cells, has only recently been elucidated in childhood lymphomas (28).

Biologic Characteristics of the Four Major Subtypes of Childhood Non-Hodgkin's Lymphoma as Defined by Histology and Immunophenotype

Histology	Immunology	Cytogenetics	Molecular Genetics
Burkitt lymphoma	B cell (sIg+)	t(8;14)(q24;q32) t(2;8)(p11;q24) t(8;22)(q24;q11)	IgH/c-myc Igκ/c-myc Igλ/c-myc
Lymphoblastic lymphoma	Immature T cell (80%)	T(1;14)(p32;q11) T(11;14)(p13;q11) T(11;14)(p15;q11) T(10;14)(q24;q11) T(7;19)(q35;p13) And others	TCRad/TAL1 TCRad/RHOM B2 TCRad/RHOM B1 TCRad/HOX11 TCRb/LYL1 Ig gene
	Precursor B cell (20%)	Hyperdiploid	rearrangement
Diffuse large B-cell lymphoma (mediastinal large B cell)	B cell (of germinal center or postgerminal center) (B cells of medullary thymus)		Ig gene rearrangement
Anaplastic large cell lymphoma	T cell (mostly), null cell, or natural killer cell	T(2;5)(p23;q25)	NPM/ALK

Not all tumors in each category contain one of the translations or molecular lesions described.
Reprinted with permission from Monika L, et al. Lymphomas in children. In: Halperin EC, Wazer DE, Perez CA, et al., eds. *Principles and practice of radiation oncology*, 6th ed. Philadelphia, PA: Lippincott Williams & Wilkins, 2013. © Wolters Kluwer.

Clinical Presentation

- Clinical presentation depends on the site(s) of involvement.
- Children with NHL usually present with extranodal disease, most frequently in the abdomen (approximately 30% of cases). Most gastrointestinal (GI) lymphomas are of the small noncleaved cell type, and most often present with abdominal pain, a palpable mass, and an increase in abdominal girth.
- The second most frequently involved single site is the mediastinum (25% of patients). Most of these cases are of lymphoblastic histology and present with dyspnea as the most common complaint.
- Thirty percent of cases involve the head and neck region (including Waldeyer's ring or cervical lymph nodes), with the remaining cases represented by peripheral lymph nodes outside the neck (7%), as well as other extranodal involvement inclusive of the bone, skin, and thyroid (27).
- Central nervous system (CNS) involvement at diagnosis was detected in 36 of 445 children with NHL (lymphoma cells in cerebrospinal fluid in 23, cranial nerve palsy in 9, and both features in 4) (29).

- Systemic symptoms are relatively rare in childhood NHL, except in anaplastic large cell lymphoma.
- Bone marrow involvement is a relatively common feature of childhood NHL.

Diagnostic Workup

- The diagnostic workup of pediatric NHL is similar to that of the adult.
- Tissue diagnosis and extent of disease workup should be performed expeditiously because of the extremely rapid growth rate of many pediatric NHLs.
- Bone marrow biopsy should be performed; omitting this procedure may result in understaging.
- To evaluate the abdomen in very young children, ultrasound studies may be more helpful than CT scanning because of children's relative lack of retroperitoneal fat.
- With abdominal or head and neck presentations (in which concomitant GI involvement, although rare in childhood cases, is a possibility), contrast studies of the GI tract are recommended (30).

Staging Systems

- The Ann Arbor staging system (commonly used in adult NHL) is limited in scope in pediatric NHL because of a preponderance for extranodal presentation, a tendency to evolve into leukemia and involve the CNS at relapse, and the aggressiveness with which cases with mediastinal involvement evolve.
- The clinical staging system proposed at the St. Jude Children's Research Hospital has been widely accepted. This system relies on noninvasive procedures that can be carried out quickly; primary site and extent of disease are considered in assigning a clinical stage (26).
- A recent revision to the staging system has now been recently reported (31).

General Management

- With the development of effective multiagent chemotherapy regimens, radiation therapy for local control of primary disease (exclusive of bone) or for CNS prophylaxis has virtually been eliminated.
- Irradiation is reserved for the following circumstances: emergency treatment of mediastinal disease or spinal cord compression; treatment for patients who fail to obtain a complete remission after induction chemotherapy; palliation of pain or mass effect; consolidation before bone marrow transplantation in patients with recurrent disease; overt CNS lymphoma at diagnosis or relapse; and leukemic transformation at diagnosis.
- Use of the international pediatric NHL response criteria in children and adolescents receiving therapy for NHL incorporates data obtained from new and more sensitive technologies that are now being widely used for disease evaluation, providing a standardized means for reporting treatment response (32).

Radiation Therapy

- Primary site/involved-field irradiation (exclusive of bone primary lesions).
- Radiation therapy to the primary site was incorporated into early chemotherapy trials; doses of 30 to 40 Gy were used (26). With growing concern for the significant toxicities observed, protocols reduced the local-field dose to 20 Gy and the volume of tumor margin from 5 cm to 2 to 3 cm (30).
- Results of these limited radiation therapy trials showed similar local control and survival rates as those achieved with more aggressive local-field therapy in early-stage NHL (23).
- Most investigators have abandoned the use of involved-field irradiation in localized, early-stage pediatric NHL.
- Local residual disease, after induction chemotherapy or at relapse after complete remission, is most often managed with local-field irradiation, with doses ranging from approximately 30 Gy for the small cell lymphocyte/blast to approximately 45 Gy for the large cell histiocytic subtypes.
- For palliation, irradiation at total doses as low as 10 Gy (given as conventional fractionation) often results in rapid relief of symptoms associated with superior vena cava syndrome, acute respiratory distress, spinal cord compression, or orbital proptosis.
- Palliation of cranial nerve deficits requires higher total doses of local-field irradiation (20 to 30 Gy) (33).

Primary Non-Hodgkin's Lymphoma of Bone

- The role of involved-field irradiation in primary NHL of bone (PBL) has not been studied in a randomized trial.
- Patients have been treated with 37.5 Gy to the involved bone, in addition to chemotherapy (23).
- Although some reports support the practice of eliminating radiation therapy in the treatment of children with PBL, its role in the management of pediatric PBL remains to be clarified.

Central Nervous System Prophylaxis and Overt Central Nervous System Disease

- CNS relapse is observed in 30% to 35% of children (10).
- CNS prophylactic cranial radiotherapy was incorporated into the treatment of childhood NHL with excellent results. This has been replaced by intrathecal chemotherapy because of the concern for increased neurotoxicity with cranial irradiation.
- Cranial irradiation currently is limited to patients with overt CNS lymphoma at diagnosis or relapse and those with leukemic transformation at diagnosis; patients with cranial nerve palsies should receive irradiation to the skull base or whole cranium.

Testicular Lymphoma

- Testicular involvement at diagnosis is uncommon (5% to 10% of children with disseminated small noncleaved cell NHL).

- Most of these patients undergo orchiectomy, although the efficacy of scrotal irradiation is unclear. However, the poor prognosis of patients with testicular involvement and relapses in the testes argue in favor of local therapy with orchiectomy or irradiation (25 Gy) as a component of therapy (34).

Sequelae of Radiation Therapy

Acute Effects

- Acute side effects most often associated with mantle irradiation include temporary loss or change in taste, xerostomia, sore throat, esophagitis, low posterior scalp epilation, skin erythema, and occasionally dyspepsia and nausea/vomiting.
- Acute effects of paraaortic irradiation include early-onset nausea and vomiting, which usually abates after the second or third treatment without antiemetic therapy.

Long-Term Effects

- Second malignant neoplasms are the most clinically significant complication of treatment for HL. The 15-year actuarial risk ranges from 8% to 15% (13). The risk of leukemia, which plateaus after 10 to 15 years, is associated primarily with the use of alkylating agents (13). Women surviving pediatric HL were found to have a 37-fold increase in the risk of breast cancer (35); it is the most common solid second malignant neoplasm, particularly with doses greater than 20 Gy. Twenty-year follow-up with lower dose RT (as low as 15 Gy) produces a second neoplasm rate of roughly 17% (36).
- Relating to potential secondary neoplasms caused by other forms of irradiation, a study posits that surveillance CT scans need not occur after the first year in certain subsets of HL (37).
- Long-term sequelae specific to irradiation include impairment of muscle and bone development and injury to the lung, heart, thyroid gland, and reproductive organs (10).
- Height reduction is most severe in prepubertal children treated with full-dose irradiation (38).
- Slipped capital femoral epiphysis occurs in up to 50% of young children whose femoral heads have been irradiated. A threshold dose of 25 Gy for such slippage was reported (39). Shielding the femoral heads essentially prevents development of this complication. Higher irradiation doses (30 to 40 Gy) and steroid administration increase the risk of avascular necrosis, with rates as high as 15%.
- Radiation doses of 20 to 40 Gy to the mandible may result in dental abnormalities (40).
- Cardiac sequelae, including pericarditis, valvular thickening, and coronary artery disease, are observed with irradiation to the heart and are related to dose (41). Doses of less than 30 Gy, adequate cardiac shielding, and the avoidance of an anterior weighting of the treatment fields appear to reduce the risk of cardiac complications.
- Pulmonary complications, most typically pneumonitis, occur in up to 5% of patients treated with standard-dose irradiation. With doses of 25 Gy or less, the incidence is low except when used in combination with pulmonary toxic chemotherapeutic agents (e.g., bleomycin sulfate).

- Thyroid dysfunction, which may result from neck, mediastinal, or mantle field irradiation, is most often manifested by an elevated serum concentration of thyroid-stimulating hormone and is dose related (10,42).
- Infertility and impaired secretion of sex hormones are potential complications of pelvic irradiation. Oophoropexy in females may allow preservation of ovarian function (43).
- Normal pregnancies, without increased risk of fetal wastage, spontaneous abortion, or birth defects, have been reported after pelvic irradiation (43).
- In males irradiated to the pelvis, oligospermia is common but may be reversible (usually within 18 to 24 months) if the irradiation dose scattered to the shielded testes is small. However, permanent oligospermia may occur after full-dose pelvic irradiation (43).
- In 20 children treated with MOPP, MOPP/ABVD, or COMP (5 received inverted-Y irradiation, 15.5 to 40.0 Gy), azoospermia was noted in 8 patients and oligospermia in 8 (44).
- Small bowel obstruction may be observed in patients who receive paraaortic irradiation, particularly after surgical exploration. Obstruction requiring surgical intervention is related to the total irradiation dose given (1% for less than 35 Gy and 3% for doses greater than 35 Gy) (10).

References

1. Ambinder RF, Browning PJ, Lorenzana I, et al. Epstein-Barr virus and childhood Hodgkin's disease in Honduras and the United States. *Blood* 1993;81(2):462–467.
2. Cleary SF, Link MP, Donaldson SS. Hodgkin's disease in the very young. *Int J Radiat Oncol Biol Phys* 1994;28(1):77–83.
3. Crnkovich MJ, Leopold K, Hoppe RT, et al. Stage I to IIB Hodgkin's disease: the combined experience at Stanford University and the Joint Center for Radiation Therapy. *J Clin Oncol* 1987;5(7):1041–1049.
4. Specht L, Nordentoft AM, Cold S, et al. Tumor burden as the most important prognostic factor in early stage Hodgkin's disease. Relations to other prognostic factors and implications for choice of treatment. *Cancer* 1988;61(8):1719–1727.
5. Metzger ML, Hudson MM, Krasin MJ, et al. Initial response to salvage therapy determines prognosis in relapsed pediatric Hodgkin lymphoma patients. *Cancer* 2010;116(18):4376–4384.
6. Donaldson SS, Link MP. Combined modality treatment with low-dose radiation and MOPP chemotherapy for children with Hodgkin's disease. *J Clin Oncol* 1987;5(5):742–749.
7. Hodgson DC, Dieckmann K, Terezakis S, et al.; International Lymphoma Radiation Oncology Group. Implementation of contemporary radiation therapy planning concepts for pediatric Hodgkin lymphoma: guidelines from the International Lymphoma Radiation Oncology Group. *Pract Radiat Oncol* 2015;5(2):85–92.
8. Fryer CJ, Hutchinson RJ, Krailo M, et al. Efficacy and toxicity of 12 courses of ABVD chemotherapy followed by low-dose regional radiation in advanced Hodgkin's disease in children: a report from the Children's Cancer Study Group. *J Clin Oncol* 1990;8(12):1971–1980.
9. Hutchinson RJ, Fryer CJ, Davis PC, et al. MOPP or radiation in addition to ABVD in the treatment of pathologically staged advanced Hodgkin's disease in children: results of the Children's Cancer Group Phase III Trial. *J Clin Oncol* 1998;16(3):897–906.
10. Constine L, Mandell L. Lymphomas in children. In: Perez C, Brady L, eds. *Principles and practice of radiation oncology*, 3rd ed. Philadelphia, PA: Lippincott–Raven, 1998:2145–2165.

11. Weiner MA, Leventhal B, Brecher ML, et al. Randomized study of intensive MOPP-ABVD with or without low-dose total-nodal radiation therapy in the treatment of stages IIB, IIIA2, IIIB, and IV Hodgkin's disease in pediatric patients: a Pediatric Oncology Group study. *J Clin Oncol* 1997;15(8):2769–2779.

12. Appel BE, Chen L, Buxton A, et al. Impact of low-dose involved-field radiation therapy on pediatric patients with lymphocyte-predominant Hodgkin lymphoma treated with chemotherapy: a report from the Children's Oncology Group. *Pediatr Blood Cancer* 2012;59(7):1284–1289.

13. Landman-Parker J, Pacquement H, Leblanc T, et al. Localized childhood Hodgkin's disease: response-adapted chemotherapy with etoposide, bleomycin, vinblastine, and prednisone before low-dose radiation therapy-results of the French Society of Pediatric Oncology Study MDH90. *J Clin Oncol* 2000;18(7):1500–1507.

14. Tucker MA, Meadows AT, Boice JD Jr, et al. Leukemia after therapy with alkylating agents for childhood cancer. *J Natl Cancer Inst* 1987;78(3):459–464.

15. Donaldson SS, Link MP, Weinstein HJ, et al. Final results of a prospective clinical trial with VAMP and low-dose involved-field radiation for children with low-risk Hodgkin's disease. *J Clin Oncol* 2007;25(3):332–337.

16. Metzger ML, Weinstein HJ, Hudson MM, et al. Association between radiotherapy vs no radiotherapy based on early response to VAMP chemotherapy and survival among children with favorable-risk Hodgkin lymphoma. *JAMA* 2012;307(24):2609–2616.

17. Tebbi CK, Mendenhall NP, London WB, et al. Response-dependent and reduced treatment in lower risk Hodgkin lymphoma in children and adolescents, results of P9426: a report from the Children's Oncology Group. *Pediatr Blood Cancer* 2012;59(7):1259–1265.

18. Dorffel W, Ruhl U, Luders H, et al. Treatment of children and adolescents with Hodgkin lymphoma without radiotherapy for patients in complete remission after chemotherapy: final results of the multinational trial GPOH-HD95. *J Clin Oncol* 2013;31(12):1562–1568.

19. Schellong G, Potter R, Bramswig J, et al. High cure rates and reduced long-term toxicity in pediatric Hodgkin's disease: the German-Austrian multicenter trial DAL-HD-90. The German-Austrian Pediatric Hodgkin's Disease Study Group. *J Clin Oncol* 1999;17(12):3736–3744.

20. Nachman JB, Sposto R, Herzog P, et al. Randomized comparison of low-dose involved-field radiotherapy and no radiotherapy for children with Hodgkin's disease who achieve a complete response to chemotherapy. *J Clin Oncol* 2002;20(18):3765–3771.

21. Friedman DL, Chen L, Wolden S, et al. Treatment of children and adolescents with Hodgkin lymphoma without radiotherapy for patients in complete remission after chemotherapy: final results of the multinational trial GPOH-HD95. *J Clin Oncol* 2014;32(32):3651–3658.

22. Charpentier AM, Friedman DL, Wolden S, et al. Predictive Factor Analysis of Response-Adapted Radiation Therapy for Chemotherapy-Sensitive Pediatric Hodgkin Lymphoma: Analysis of the Children's Oncology Group AHOD 0031 Trial. *Int J Radiat Oncol Biol Phys* 2016;96:943–950.

23. Link MP, Donaldson SS, Berard CW, et al. Results of treatment of childhood localized non-Hodgkin's lymphoma with combination chemotherapy with or without radiotherapy. *N Engl J Med* 1990;322(17):1169–1174.

24. Kelly KM, Cole PD, Chen L, et al. Phase III Study of Response Adapted Therapy for the Treatment of Children with Newly Diagnosed Very High Risk Hodgkin Lymphoma (Stages IIIB/IVB) (AHOD0831): A Report from the Children's Oncology Group. *Blood* 2015;126(23):3927.

25. Committee Nn-HsCPW. Classification of non-Hodgkin's lymphomas. Reproducibility of major classification systems. NCI non-Hodgkin's Classification Project Writing Committee. *Cancer* 1985;55(1):91–95.

26. Wollner N, Burchenal JH, Lieberman PH, et al. Non-Hodgkin's lymphoma in children. A comparative study of two modalities of therapy. *Cancer* 1976;37(1):123–134.

27. Murphy SB, Fairclough DL, Hutchison RE, et al. Non-Hodgkin's lymphomas of childhood: an analysis of the histology, staging, and response to treatment of 338 cases at a single institution. *J Clin Oncol* 1989;7(2):186–193.

28. Heerema NA, Bernheim A, Lim MS, et al. State of the Art and Future Needs in Cytogenetic/Molecular Genetics/Arrays in childhood lymphoma: summary report of workshop at the First International Symposium on childhood and adolescent non-Hodgkin lymphoma, April 9, 2003, New York City, NY. *Pediatr Blood Cancer* 2005;45(5):616–622.

29. Sandlund JT, Murphy SB, Santana VM, et al. CNS involvement in children with newly diagnosed non-Hodgkin's lymphoma. *J Clin Oncol* 2000;18(16):3018–3024.

30. Wollner N, Mandell L, Filippa D, et al. Primary nasal-paranasal oropharyngeal lymphoma in the pediatric age group. *Cancer* 1990;65(6):1438–1444.

31. Rosolen A, Perkins SL, Pinkerton CR, et al. Revised International Pediatric Non-Hodgkin Lymphoma Staging System. *J Clin Oncol* 2015;33(18):2112–2118.

32. Sandlund JT, Guillerman RP, Perkins SL, et al. International Pediatric Non-Hodgkin Lymphoma Response Criteria. *J Clin Oncol* 2015;33(18):2106–2111.

33. Ingram LC, Fairclough DL, Furman WL, et al. Cranial nerve palsy in childhood acute lymphoblastic leukemia and non-Hodgkin's lymphoma. *Cancer* 1991;67(9):2262–2268.

34. Kellie SJ, Pui CH, Murphy SB. Childhood non-Hodgkin's lymphoma involving the testis: clinical features and treatment outcome. *J Clin Oncol* 1989;7(8):1066–1070.

35. Basu SK, Schwartz C, Fisher SG, et al. Unilateral and bilateral breast cancer in women surviving pediatric Hodgkin's disease. *Int J Radiat Oncol Biol Phys* 2008;72(1):34–40.

36. O'Brien MM, Donaldson SS, Balise RR, et al. Second malignant neoplasms in survivors of pediatric Hodgkin's lymphoma treated with low-dose radiation and chemotherapy. *J Clin Oncol* 2010;28:1232–1239.

37. Voss SD, Chen L, Constine LS, et al. Surveillance computed tomography imaging and detection of relapse in intermediate- and advanced-stage pediatric Hodgkin's lymphoma: a report from the Children's Oncology Group. *J Clin Oncol* 2012;30(21):2635–2640.

38. Willman KY, Cox RS, Donaldson SS. Radiation induced height impairment in pediatric Hodgkin's disease. *Int J Radiat Oncol Biol Phys* 1994;28(1):85–92.

39. Silverman CL, Thomas PR, McAlister WH, et al. Slipped femoral capital epiphyses in irradiated children: dose, volume and age relationships. *Int J Radiat Oncol Biol Phys* 1981;7(10):1357–1363.

40. Maguire A, Craft AW, Evans RG, et al. The long-term effects of treatment on the dental condition of children surviving malignant disease. *Cancer* 1987;60(10):2570–2575.

41. Hancock SL, Donaldson SS, Hoppe RT. Cardiac disease following treatment of Hodgkin's disease in children and adolescents. *J Clin Oncol* 1993;11(7):1208–1215.

42. Sklar C, Whitton J, Mertens A, et al. Abnormalities of the thyroid in survivors of Hodgkin's disease: data from the Childhood Cancer Survivor Study. *J Clin Endocrinol Metab* 2000;85(9):3227–3232.

43. Ortin TT, Shostak CA, Donaldson SS. Gonadal status and reproductive function following treatment for Hodgkin's disease in childhood: the Stanford experience. *Int J Radiat Oncol Biol Phys* 1990;19(4):873–880.

44. Ben Arush MW, Solt I, Lightman A, et al. Male gonadal function in survivors of childhood Hodgkin and non-Hodgkin lymphoma. *Pediatr Hematol Oncol* 2000;17(3):239–245.

CHAPTER 47

RADIATION TREATMENT OF BENIGN DISEASE

- Though radiation oncologists are primarily involved in the care of malignant tumors, radiation therapy also plays a role in many benign diseases. The inherent risks of late skin injury, carcinogenesis, leukemogenesis, and genetic damage must be carefully considered before treating any patient with ionizing radiation. However, radiation oncologists are ideally suited to treat even those patients with benign disease, as they have great proficiency in utilizing all clinical and technical aspects of ionizing radiation. A survey by Order and Donaldson assessed almost 100 indications of radiation therapy for benign diseases and found that only 10 indications are actually treated by greater than 90% of American radiation oncologists. Furthermore, only 30 radiation oncologists of those surveyed treated 30 or greater indications (1).

TECHNICAL CONSIDERATIONS

The report of the Committee on Radiation Treatment of Benign Disease of the Bureau of Radiological Health recommends the following:
- Before institution of therapy, the quality of the radiation, total dose, overall treatment time, underlying organs at risk, and shielding factors should be considered.
- Infants and children should be treated with ionizing radiation only in very exceptional cases and only after careful evaluation of the potential risks compared with the expected benefit.
- Direct irradiation of regions overlying organs, which are particularly prone to late effects such as the thyroid, eye, gonads, bone marrow, and breast, should be avoided.
- Meticulous radiation protection techniques, including cones and lead shields, should be employed in all instances.
- The depth of penetration of the x-ray beam should be chosen in accordance with the depth of the pathologic process.
- Kopicky and Order (2) analyzed the current use of radiation therapy for benign disease by radiation oncologists. On the basis of replies from those surveyed, 70 diseases mentioned in the questionnaire were divided into the categories of "acceptable for treatment" and "unacceptable for treatment" (at most centers).

RADIATION THERAPY TECHNIQUES

- There are wide differences of opinion among radiation oncologists about the optimal dose and fractionation for treatment of most diseases.
- The choice of beam energy depends on the depth of the target volume, and every effort should be made to spare underlying normal tissue in superficial lesions.
- The appropriate energy depends on the type of modality used: electrons, low-energy x-rays, high-energy photons, or protons.
- Special consideration should be made for the usage of lead shields when appropriate.

EYE

Thyroid Ophthalmopathy

- Thyroid ophthalmopathy occurs in 25% to 50% of patients diagnosed with Graves' disease (3). The pathogenesis is believed to be an autoimmune reaction directed toward orbital fibroblasts in which activated T lymphocytes invade the orbit. This stimulates glycosaminoglycan production by fibroblasts, resulting in a hyperosmotic shift causing tissue edema and marked enlargement of the extraocular muscles.
- Signs and symptoms of Graves' ophthalmopathy include bilateral exophthalmos, extraocular muscle dysfunction, diplopia, blurred vision, eyelid and periorbital edema, chemosis, lid lag, and compressive optic neuropathy. The clinical signs are grouped according to the NOSPECS system, which classifies six disease categories and three degrees of severity; the sum of the parameters constitutes the ophthalmopathy index.
- Historically, corticosteroids have been used as the first line of therapy for patients with Graves' ophthalmopathy, whereas surgical decompression has typically been reserved for patients with advanced disease or those who failed first-line therapy. There is a meta-analysis that shows that corticosteroid therapy improves symptoms in 65% of patients. However, proptosis often persists and many patients relapse following corticosteroid taper, eventually requiring surgical intervention or orbital radiation therapy (4).
- As lymphocytes and fibroblasts are quite sensitive to radiation, retrobulbar irradiation is a logical method of treatment. Radiation is most effective for soft tissue symptoms such as redness, edema, and chemosis.
- In 311 patients treated with orbital irradiation, 80% showed improvement or complete resolution of soft tissue symptoms (5). A significant response was demonstrated in more than 75% of the patients with corneal manifestations such as stippling and ulceration. Extraocular dysfunction and proptosis were improved in 61% and 52% of patients, respectively. Defects in visual acuity responded in 41% to 71% of patients. After irradiation, corticosteroid therapy was successfully discontinued in 76% of patients. Corrective or cosmetic eye surgery was necessary in only 29% after radiation therapy, and in most instances, it was done to correct diplopia.
- Marquez et al. (6) have recorded 453 patients receiving retrobulbar radiation therapy for Graves' ophthalmopathy. One hundred ninety-seven had more than 1 year

of follow-up. There was an improvement or resolution in the size of soft tissue findings in 89% of patients. Additionally, patients had improvements in proptosis (70%), extraocular muscle dysfunction (85%), corneal abnormalities (96%), and vision (67%).

- Prummel et al. (7) conducted a randomized study comparing prednisone and retrobulbar radiation, which showed equal outcomes, approximately 50%, for both treatments. However, there was a much higher rate of minor, moderate, and major complications with prednisone.
- In another randomized trial, the addition of radiation showed no significant symptomatic benefit for thyroid ophthalmopathy categories I through III, but substantial benefit for advanced thyroid ophthalmopathy, categories IV and V. The authors concluded that radiation is best utilized for thyroid categories IV through VI, orbitopathy index of greater than 4, and in those patients with nonrecurrent symptoms of grades 2 and 3 (8).
- Megavoltage external-beam irradiation using precise planning with high-resolution computed tomography (CT), along with complete patient immobilization, is required for optimization of the dose distribution and to avoid unwanted irradiation of sensitive structures, such as the lens and pituitary gland.
- Small opposed bilateral fields are used to encompass both retrobulbar volumes with customized blocks to shield periorbital structures.
- A split-beam technique or gantry of bilateral opposing beam so that the anterior beam edges are matched posteriorly to the lens to limit lens dose are reasonable.
- A total dose of 20 Gy to the midplane given in 10 fractions over a 2-week period is recommended; doses greater than 20 Gy do not improve the outcome.
- Photons in the range of 6 to 10 MV are used.
- Special care should be exercised in the selection of beams and calculation of doses to avoid excessive dose to the optic nerve and other sensitive ocular structures.
- Special attention should be paid to the total dose administered to the midline structures when concurrent opposing lateral portals are used; the dose contribution from each portal should be taken into account.
- Radiation therapy produces an effective and safe treatment for progressive Graves' ophthalmopathy, with a 96% overall response rate, 98% patient satisfaction rate, and no irreparable long-term sequelae with follow-ups extending 20 years or more. The most common late effect observed is the development of cataracts, which occurs more frequently in older patients and is reversible with extraction. Overall, if appropriately indicated and precisely administered, radiation therapy for advanced thyroid ophthalmopathy offers a favorable risk-benefit ratio.

Orbital Pseudotumor

- Lymphoid diseases of the orbit represent a spectrum of diseases and are classified into three groups: pseudolymphoma (which includes orbital pseudotumor and reactive hyperplasia), atypical lymphoid hyperplasia, and malignant lymphoma.
- Orbital pseudotumor is a benign, idiopathic orbital inflammation that can simulate Graves' exophthalmos or tumor. Though the etiology is unclear, three possible

causative mechanisms have been postulated: an infectious process, an autoimmune process (circulating antibodies against extraocular muscle proteins), or a fibroproliferative process.

- Typically, unilateral orbital involvement with acute onset of retrobulbar pain, exophthalmos, and impaired eye motility are seen, though bilateral involvement can be present in up to 50% of patients.
- There may be a palpable mass or proptosis with progressive loss of vision.
- CT or magnetic resonance imaging (MRI) is helpful in differentiating pseudotumor from Graves' disease, if the retro-orbital muscles are primarily involved, but biopsy is usually required to define the disease process.
- Corticosteroids are the primary therapy, but up to 50% of patients have an insufficient response or have to discontinue steroids secondary to untoward effects. If the disease is not appropriately treated, it can lead to progression with subsequent permanent deterioration of visual acuity.
- A 4- to 6-MV photon beam is used with unilateral or bilateral temporal fields posterior to the lens, or with a split-beam technique for better lens protection.
- The most commonly utilized dose is 20 Gy in 10 fractions over a 2-week period.
- Local tumor control ranges from 73% to 100% (9,10).
- Responses include expected 45% complete tapering of steroids, 5% complete resolution of symptoms with decreased steroid dose, and 35% improvement in symptoms without increase in steroid dose (11).
- Patients with bilateral tumors seemed to have higher response rates, because of either treatment setup (opposed lateral fields in bilateral tumors versus conformal fields in unilateral tumors which can lead to more marginal misses) or a more aggressive tumor biology (12).
- Patients should be monitored closely because subsequent progression to systemic lymphoma has been reported in up to 29% of patients (9).

Pterygium

- Pterygium consists of fibrovascular proliferative tissue, which most commonly originates from the medial bulbar conjunctiva and extends onto the cornea.
- Symptoms include tearing, foreign body sensation, and visual impairment.
- Treatment is indicated if there is encroachment of the pupil or if the patient is symptomatic.
- The treatment of choice for pterygium is surgery; however, the recurrence rate is 20% to 30% with this modality alone (13).
- Radiation is typically indicated after relapse or adjunctly after local resection of a pterygium, though a few centers have used primary or preoperative radiation therapy.
- Van den Brenk (14) reported a recurrence rate of only 1.4% in 1,300 pterygia in 1,064 patients treated with prophylactic postoperative beta-ray therapy with a ^{90}Sr applicator. Treatment consisted of 8 to 10 Gy given for each of three applications on days 0, 7, and 14 after the operation. Comparable results with similar radiation doses have been reported by others (15–17).

- In a randomized controlled trial of 25 Gy in 1 fraction of beta radiation versus sham radiation, there was a significantly lower relapse rate with postoperative radiation, 93% versus 33%. Furthermore, at a mean follow-up of 18 months, there were no major treatment complications observed (18).
- A prospective study showed that beta-irradiation was more effective when given at the time of surgery rather than 4 days later (19). Similar data were reported by others (17,20).

Age-Related Macular Degeneration

- Age-related macular degeneration is the leading cause of severe blindness in the United States today.
- The incidence increases with age, with the disease afflicting 11% of patients between 65 and 74 years of age and 28% of patients older than 75 years of age (21).
- The neovascular (wet) type occurs in 10% of patients and is due to choroidal vessels penetrating Bruch's membrane and proliferating beneath the retinal pigment epithelium, leading to choroidal neovascularization, subretinal hemorrhage, and serous retinal detachment.
- When the choroidal neovascular membrane is subfoveal, the visual prognosis is poor, with severe vision loss in more than 75% of patients at 2 years (22).
- Antivascular endothelial growth factor receptor agents such as ranibizumab, given as intraocular injections into the vitreous cavity, have revolutionized the management of this disease entity. These agents are the mainstay of current therapy for choroidal neovascularization, regardless of the location in the macula (23,24). However, patients require frequent treatment to fully benefit.
- In one randomized trial, visual acuity improved by 15 or more letters in 33.8% of the patients receiving 0.5-mg intravitreal injections of ranibizumab, as compared with 5.0% of the sham-injection group (24).
- Brachytherapy, photons, and protons have all been utilized for treatment; however, no comparative studies have been performed.
- Hypofractionated doses seemed to have better responses in early studies. However, stereotactic radiation therapy seemed to have limited benefit in visual acuity and membrane size. UC Davis group published their experience of incremental doses from 20 to 40 Gy and found moderate delayed radiation retinopathy after 10 years (25).
- Proton therapy appears to have greater radiation retinopathy risk, but is minimized when treated over 12 fractions or greater (26).
- The rationale for using local irradiation for choroidal neovascular membrane is based on the radiosensitivity of proliferating endothelial cells, reduction in the inflammatory response, and possible occlusion of aberrant vessels.
- Chakravarthy et al. (27) reported results in 19 patients with subfoveal neovascular membranes because of age-related macular degeneration treated with 10 Gy at 2 Gy per fraction or 15 Gy at 3 Gy per fraction. Using patients who declined treatments as controls, the data indicated that at 12 months, visual acuity was maintained or improved in 63% of patients and significant neovascular regression was recorded in 77% of treated patients. Visual acuity deteriorated in six of seven controls, and all showed progressive enlargement of membranes. There was no significant difference in outcome between the two dose regimens.

- In an update from the same institution, significant improvement in visual acuity and reduced subretinal scarring were reported in 35 treated eyes, compared with the untreated eyes in the same patients (28).
- Bergink et al. (29) reported their findings of comparing four different dose regimens. The best results were seen with 12 Gy in 2 fractions, 18 Gy in 3 fractions, or 24 Gy in 4 fractions. Stable visual acuity was reported in 21 of 30 patients treated.
- Freire et al. (30) reported on 41 patients treated with 14.4 Gy in 8 fractions of 1.8 Gy each. CT-simulation treatment planning was performed using a unilateral oblique 6-MV photon field, half-beam blocked anteriorly to spare the ipsilateral lens and contralateral globe. Preliminary results at 2 to 3 months after treatment showed subjective visual acuity to be stable in 66%, improved in 27%, and worse in 7%.
- Alberti et al. (31) published the results of various investigations into the treatment of wet macular degeneration. There was a significant positive impact seen in a large number of patients.

CENTRAL NERVOUS SYSTEM

Arteriovenous Malformations

- Congenital disorder of abnormal vasculature forms a shunt between the high pressure arterial system and low pressure venous system, bypassing the capillary bed. Arteriovenous malformations (AVMs) are usually fragile and therefore are predisposed to bleeding, carrying with it significant morbidity and mortality.
- Speltzer-Martin Grading System is a widely used grading system to assess outcomes after microsurgical management. It is calculated by size, eloquent versus noneloquent hemisphere involvement, and superficial versus deep vein involvement. High grade AVMs are generally inoperable.
- Surgery, utilizing microsurgical techniques, is often the first-line treatment for AVMs as obliteration of the lesion from radiation can take up to 3 years. However, AVMs in deep or eloquent regions of the brain are often treated with stereotactic radiosurgery.
- AVMs of the brain are treated with stereotactic radiosurgery using a single fraction of high-dose radiation to a stereotactically defined small volume to sclerose the AVM and prevent hemorrhage.
- Minimum doses of 15 to 30 Gy are prescribed in the periphery of the target; complete obliteration of the AVM is seen in 71% to 89% of patients within 2 years (32).
- In a series by Maruyama, 500 patients were treated with stereotactic radiosurgery with mean dose of 21 Gy. The cumulative obliteration rate was 81% and 91% at 4 and 5 years, respectively. The hemorrhage risk was reduced by 54% during the latency period, and by 88% once there was complete obliteration (33).
- Effective obliteration of the AVM after stereotactic radiosurgery correlates with the minimum dose delivered, but not with the maximum dose or volume treated (34).
- Stereotactic radiosurgery is more effective when the AVM is less than 2 cm and when all feeder vessels are irradiated.
- Stereotactic radiotherapy with 2 to 3 sessions of 8 to 10 Gy is equally effective.

- Results of conventional fractionated radiation therapy appear inferior to those of stereotactic radiosurgery. Doses of 40 to 55 Gy in 1.8- to 3.5-Gy fractions yielded complete responses in 20% of patients (10).
- For extracerebral cavernous hemangioma of the middle fossa, a preoperative dose of 30 Gy has been reported to increase resectability and decrease intraoperative hemorrhage.

SKIN

Keloids

- Reaction to skin trauma with excessive production of fibrous tissue that extends beyond the wound, becomes hyalinized, and does not regress spontaneously is known as keloids, which frequently cause itching and pain.
- They may occur in susceptible individuals after infection or burns, but most commonly occur after traumatic or surgical wounds, with most common locations being the face and trunk.
- The preferred treatment is excision, followed by a procedure tailored to prevent fibroblast proliferation (which could lead to recurrence).
- Although good results have been reported with local injections of triamcinolone, postoperative irradiation is effective and more comfortable for patients. Typically, radiation is indicated for repeated recurrences postoperatively or high-risk situations such as an unfavorable location, marginal resection, and more extensive lesions.
- Other common treatments prior to definitive surgery and radiation include intralesional 5-fluorouracil (5-FU) (in combination with triamcinolone), silicone gel sheets, pressure therapy, and cryotherapy.
- Radiation therapy is usually started within 24 hours after excision. Typically, 100- to 140-kV x-rays with a 1- to 7-mm aluminum half-value layer (HVL) or low-energy electrons (6 MeV) with appropriate bolus are used.
- The irradiation field should be custom-designed to fit the area to be treated with a 0.5-cm margin around the suture lines.
- When treating earlobes, they should be taped away from the face, and a direct anteroposterior field (with a small cone) should be used.
- Total dose is 10 to 15 Gy in 2 to 5 fractions.
- Excellent cosmetic results are found in 92% of sites treated (35).
- Ten-year overall control rate was 73% (36), with negative prognostic factors being size greater than 2 cm, prior treatment, and male gender. High-dose-rate brachytherapy using Ir-192 in the perioperative setting, commonly administered in 3 to 4 fractions of 5 to 6 Gy to 0.5 cm depth. One study of recurrent keloids treated in 3 fractions of 6 Gy to 0.5 cm depth found of 32 keloids treated, 2 recurred and 2 were mildly hypertrophied after 30-month follow-up (37).
- Treatment of primary keloids with irradiation alone is not as successful, but may be attempted in the case of inoperability. It can have acceptable results if radiation is initiated within about 6 months of the initial trauma. Conversely, there is a poor

response to radiation if the keloid has fully matured. Good results with 4 Gy given once a month for one to five treatments with energies of 60 to 90 kV have been reported (38,39).

Plantar Warts

- Plantar warts can be extremely painful and disabling.
- Surgical treatment, including desiccation and curettage, leads to incapacity during the long period of healing and may leave painful scars.
- Salicylic ointment has been used with success rates of approximately 65% (10).
- Liquid nitrogen cryosurgery produces cure rates of 90% (10).
- Carbon dioxide laser surgery has an overall success rate of 75% (10).
- Intralesional injections of bleomycin sulfate control 77% of extremity warts (10).
- Radiation treatment for plantar warts can be simple, safe, and effective. A single treatment of 10 Gy with 100 kV and a HVL of 4.3 mm of aluminum, using closed lead shielding to define the treated field, is recommended.
- Preliminary paring is not necessary, and the wart usually separates and falls off in 3 to 4 weeks without sequelae.

Keratoacanthoma

- Keratoacanthoma is a rapidly growing benign tumor that may be locally invasive.
- It occurs most commonly in sun-exposed areas of the skin in middle-aged or elderly light-skinned men.
- It tends to regress spontaneously and may be difficult to differentiate histologically from squamous cell carcinoma.
- Aggressive treatment is recommended, that is, complete excision with adequate margins.
- Radiation therapy is recommended for recurrences after surgery or when surgery would result in poor cosmesis.
- Use of 40 Gy in 4-Gy fractions twice weekly with orthovoltage techniques, given approximately 1 month after treatment, gives rise to complete regression with satisfactory cosmesis in all patients.
- In another study, 18 patients with 29 lesions received doses from 35 Gy in 15 fractions to 56 Gy in 28 fractions. They reported complete regression and good cosmetic results for all lesions (40).

HEMANGIOMAS

Cutaneous Hemangiomas

- The treatment of cavernous hemangiomas of the skin in infants, by repeated doses of radium in surface applicators, was commonplace many years ago. However, the use of radiation therapy has largely been abandoned in recent years because of the potential for late effects in the pediatric patient population and because the treatment is usually unnecessary.

- After an initial growth phase, most of these lesions regress spontaneously and disappear by the patient's 5th year. One must consider the risk of radiation-induced malignancies when treating benign disease, particularly in children.
- Furst et al. (41) reported a dose-response relationship for thyroid cancer, neoplasms of bone and soft tissues, and breast hyperplasia in children irradiated for skin hemangiomas at the Radiumhemmet.
- Port wine stain or capillary hemangioma is somewhat resistant to radiation therapy.
- Furst et al. (42) reported results of radiation therapy in 20,012 patients with hemangiomas. Most patients (99%) were younger than 2 years of age when treated. All lesions improved; 72% had excellent cosmetic results, and the remainder had some blemishes, although the results were acceptable.
- For minor superficial hemangiomas, contact radiation therapy, with a HVL of 0.2 to 2.5 mm of aluminum, is most suitable.
- The dose to the skin is 5 to 10 Gy per treatment given in 1 to 3 sessions at weekly intervals.
- For thicker lesions, orthovoltage irradiation is recommended with doses of 1 to 4 Gy per treatment. The treatment regimen may be repeated once or twice if there is continued growth or poor regression.
- Megavoltage photons or electrons can be used, depending on the clinical situation. Doses of 2 to 18 Gy have been used to treat hemangiomas in single or multiple fractions, with complete responses expected in 35% to 40% of patients and partial responses in 45% to 50% (10).

Ocular Angiomas

- Orbital hemangiomas can become symptomatic, causing hemorrhage and a loss of vision.
- They are effectively managed with radiation therapy using doses of 12 Gy in 8 fractions of 1.5 Gy each. This regimen results in complete reabsorption of the subretinal fluid without reaccumulation.
- Gamma knife radiosurgery may also be an option. One study treated 23 patients with orbital cavernous hemangioma to a median tumor margin dose of 15 Gy (range 12 to 20 Gy), with no tumor progression after 12 months, and orbital pain in 3 patients and chemosis in 2 patients (43).

Cavernous Hemangioma of the Liver

- Cavernous hemangioma of the liver is a congenital anomaly that is most often asymptomatic, unless the lesion bleeds. It is a benign vascular tumor found at autopsy in 2% to 3% of asymptomatic patients. The incidence of clinically significant lesions is substantially lower.
- Fever or anemia occurs in 6% of patients (10).
- Clinically evident hepatomegaly occurs in 50% of patients. Although rare, simultaneous hemorrhage, thrombocytopenia, and hypofibrinogenemia have been described.

- Radiation therapy has been used for symptomatic and surgically unresectable (multiple, diffuse, or massive) hemangiomas of the liver, as well as in pediatric patients with hyperconsumptive coagulopathy (44).
- Doses of 10 to 30 Gy (in 1 to 3 weeks) result in symptomatic improvement in all patients and tumor regression in a significant number of patients.
- Recommended doses are 10 Gy or less for children and 20 to 30 Gy (in 3 to 4 weeks) for adults.
- If no response is observed in 4 to 6 months, an additional 10 to 15 Gy (in 1 to 2 weeks) may be given.
- Common complications include radiation hepatitis, veno-occlusive disease, and hepatoma.

SOFT TISSUE

Bursitis and Tendinitis

- Repeated strain or trauma to the tendons in various regions of the body can lead to an acute or chronic inflammation of the tendon or bursa.
- Bursitis and tendinitis are ailments that most commonly affect the shoulder, elbow (tennis/golfers elbow), or ankle joint (plantar fasciitis).
- Patients often have associated pain, tenderness, or decreased range of motion.
- Management includes immobilization and protection of the joint during the acute phase. These conservative measures frequently lead to complete resolution of symptoms within a few weeks. Other commonly used adjunct therapies include local application of cold and heat, analgesics, corticosteroids, and physical therapy. Occasionally, shock wave therapy, electrotherapy, and acupuncture have been used with some success, though the level of evidence for these modalities is limited.
- Radiation therapy is indicated when conservative measures have been ineffective, prior to the use of surgery. There is often a period of intensification of pain before the onset of relief with radiation.
- Typically, limited opposed fields are used to encompass only the joint. Occasionally, a single anterior field is utilized.
- Total doses of 6 to 10 Gy, in 1.5- to 2.0-Gy fractions, are given in 3 to 5 successive days (10).
- One or two additional treatments may be added after 1 to 2 weeks in chronic cases where the initial results are unsatisfactory.

Desmoid Tumor

- Desmoid tumor, also known as aggressive fibromatosis, is a low-grade, locally invasive, and nonmetastasizing tumor of connective tissue. Its origin is probably related to other fibromatoses such as keloids, Peyronie's disease, plantar and palmar fibromatosis, fibromatosis coli, and progressive myositis fibrosa.

- These tumors are deeply infiltrating and nonencapsulated. They merge imperceptibly into the surrounding muscle, resulting in a high frequency of positive margins after resection.
- Most common presentations include extremities, abdominal wall, and abdominal cavity (45).
- MRI has significant utility in detailing the size and extent of infiltration of the lesion.
- Surgical resection is the primary treatment modality, but local recurrences range from 10% to 100%, depending on the extent of the surgical resection.
- For R0 resections, no further treatment is warranted. However, for R1 and R2 resections as well as inoperable cases, radiation is indicated. With total radiation doses of greater than 50 Gy, the recurrence rate is decreased from 60% to 80% to 10% to 30%. The local control rate for primary radiation does not differ significantly from that of adjuvant radiation.
- The recommended postoperative dose is 50 to 55 Gy at 1.8 to 2.0 Gy per fraction. For inoperable or recurrent desmoids, the usual dose is 60 to 65 Gy.
- The irradiation fields are generous and encompass the entire aponeurotic compartment, with 5-cm margins around the tumor volume.
- McCollough et al. (46) reported 5 failures in 30 irradiated cases, and Leibel et al. (47) reported 6 failures in 19 cases.
- In most studies, tumor size had no prognostic influence on local control.
- Some institutions practice observation in patients undergoing gross total resection with involved surgical margins. The group at Massachusetts General Hospital reported that local control was achieved in 17 of 21 patients with effective salvage therapy (18). However, they advocated this approach only in patients committed to regular follow-up and did not recommend observation for those patients who had recurrent disease.

Peyronie's Disease

- Painful angulation of the erect penis was described by Peyronie in 1743.
- It is caused by inflammatory lesions of the corpora cavernosa that progress to hard plaques, nodules, or bands that may be localized or extensive.
- The plaque is usually on the dorsum of the penis, with curvature or angulation in the direction of the plaque, which may precede the development of pain.
- The cause is unknown, but there is an association with connective tissue disorders such as Dupuytren's contracture. Other risk factors include diabetes mellitus, vascular disease, and a genetic predisposition.
- Peyronie's disease may resolve spontaneously over a period of months to years.
- Many believe that radiation therapy is effective and hastens the regression of symptoms. Pain is particularly well treated with radiation, as it is relieved in more than 75% of patients.
- Other therapies that are effective in relieving symptoms to varying degrees are local corticosteroid injections, systemic corticosteroids, procarbazine hydrochloride, and surgery.
- During radiation therapy, careful lead shielding of the gonads, pubic hair, and glans (if not involved) is required.

- The penis can be drawn through a hole in a lead sheet, and a single dorsal field may be used.
- Effective doses range from 5 Gy in 1 fraction, which may be repeated in 1 month, to 3 Gy daily for 6 or 7 fractions (10).

Prevention of Vascular Restenosis

- Percutaneous transluminal coronary angioplasty is a common technique used to treat coronary stenotic lesions in many patients with atherosclerotic coronary artery disease.
- The most important long-term limitation of balloon angioplasty is restenosis. It is defined as a greater than 50% decrease in vessel diameter at follow-up angiography. The incidence of restenosis is 30% to 50%, with most restenosis occurring during the first 4 months after balloon angioplasty.
- Vascular brachytherapy (VBT) for in-stent restenosis has been rigorously investigated, and its efficacy has been shown in several multi-institutional randomized trials. All the trials testing the various isotope systems were positive with a decrease of in-stent restenosis from about 40% to 10% (48–51).
- Only one randomized trial of VBT for *de novo* lesions in native coronary vessels has been conducted, and it was a negative trial (52).
- Three isotopes (^{192}Ir, ^{90}Sr/Y, and ^{32}P) have been used in over 95% of the clinical trials involving catheter-based VBT systems. However, the Betacath system is the only system currently manufactured for in-stent restenosis. It uses ^{90}Sr, which is a pure β emitter with a 28.5-year half-life and 546-keV maximum β energy. The daughter isotope, ^{90}Y, is the one primarily used for therapy because the majority of the ^{90}Sr β particles are absorbed by the stainless steel encapsulation and the surrounding catheter. ^{90}Y is also a pure β emitter with a 64-hour half-life and 2.27-MeV maximum β energy.
- There are four main components to the Betacath system: the source train, transfer device, delivery catheter, and accessories. The sources are stored in a small transfer device and are advanced and retracted by a closed-loop hydraulic system using sterile water. The advantages of the Betacath system are minimal exposure to staff and short treatment times (3 to 5 minutes). Because of its long half-life, the isotope need only be exchanged once every 6 months, and treatment times need not change during the 6-month period. The potential disadvantages of the system are attenuation by calcifications or the stent, an inferior depth-dose gradient compared with a γ source, and the lack of utility in larger vessels (53).
- The recommended dose is 18.4 Gy for vessels with a reference diameter of 2.7 to 3.3 mm, and 23 Gy for a reference diameter between 3.4 and 4.0 mm. The dose is prescribed at a 2-mm radius from the center of the source axis (54,55).
- In terms of treatment planning, the gross tumor volume (GTV) is the stenotic area, the clinical target volume (CTV) is the dilated portion of the vessel, and the planning target volume (PTV) is 5 to 10 mm proximal and distal to the CTV. Restenosis after VBT is found at the treatment edge in up to 50% of cases, and the most likely etiology of the edge failure is inadequate radiation dose to the lesion margins. Therefore, a wide treatment margin on either side of the injured vessel is utilized to optimize outcomes (56–58).

- With the advent of the drug-eluting stent (DES), the role of VBT has significantly diminished. The RAVEL (sirolimus-eluting stent) and TAXUS I to IV (palitxel-eluting stent) trials have shown a substantial reduction in the occurrence of restenosis with the use of DESs over bare metal stents for *de novo* lesions (59–63).
- There are also now two major randomized trials, which have been completed, comparing VBT with DESs for in-stent restenosis. The TAXUS V trial utilized a paclitaxel-eluting stent, and showed that at 9 months the rate of major adverse coronary events was reduced by 43% in the DES arm compared to the VBT arm. The SIRS trial used a sirolimus-eluting stent, and it showed superior clinical and angiographic outcomes with the use of DESs versus VBT (64,65).
- Though VBT has become limited in its role, it still has some utility in the following circumstances: small diameter vessels, bifurcation regions, and recurrent multi-DES resistant lesions.

Arrhythmias

- Sustained monomorphic ventricular tachycardia (SMVT) is a cardiac arrhythmia with poor prognosis. Patients who are hemodynamically stable on presentation may become unstable rapidly and without warning.
- Initial treatments include pharmacologic or electrical cardioversion. Recurrent or refractory patients are next investigated for an underlying cause (myocardial infarction [MI], electrolyte abnormality, drug toxicity) and considered for an implantable cardioverter defibrillator (ICD).
- Radiofrequency catheter ablation (RFA) and catheter ablation are suggested for patients with ICDs and antiarrhythmic agent with recurrent SMVTs. RFA alter or eliminate reentry circuits or foci, commonly present because of cardiac rearrangement after infarcts.
- Recent efforts are examining the potential use for stereotactic body radiation therapy (SBRT) as an alternative to RFA, treating electrogenic foci with external radiation.
- A Washington University study included five patients who were treated with SBRT with 25 Gy in a single fraction, treating to foci mapped by electrocardiographic imaging maps. During a 6-week follow-up, there were 4 episodes of ventricular tachycardia over 46 patient-months, a reduction from baseline of 99.9% (66).
- Although highly promising, this is considered experimental at this time and should only be performed as part of clinical trial, despite positive findings in a feasibility study.

BONE

Aneurysmal Bone Cyst

- An aneurysmal bone cyst is a benign vascular-cystic lesion that usually appears as an expansive and eccentric cavity in the metaphyseal ends of bones. It typically does not involve the epiphysis, and it often protrudes into the surrounding soft tissues.

- Treatment is primarily surgical curettage or resection, but the recurrence rate after curettage is 30% to 60%.
- Radiation therapy is reserved for those lesions that are inoperable, repeatedly recur, or are difficult to curette properly because of size and location.
- A radiation dose of approximately 40 to 45 Gy in 4 to 5 weeks generally produces excellent results.

Vertebral Hemangioma

- Vertebral hemangiomas are not uncommon. About 10% of the population has asymptomatic lesions, which are found at autopsy.
- Lesions are generally diagnosed by the typical radiographic appearance of rarefaction with vertical dense trabeculations of a honeycomb pattern. The lesions often extend into the lacunae, pedicles, or transverse or spinous processes.
- Vertebral expansion, tumor extension into the extradural space, hemorrhage, or compression fracture (rarely) may lead to cord compression.
- Surgical decompression may be required after preliminary arteriography, but it may be difficult to perform because of the risk of hemorrhage.
- Usually, only limited removal of the tumor is possible; therefore, postoperative irradiation is typically recommended (30 to 40 Gy in 3 to 4 weeks) with excellent results.
- Outcomes include no impact of radiotherapy on reossification, as well as increase in pain relief and decrease in analgesic need at higher doses (67).

Heterotopic Bone Formation

- Heterotopic bone formation (heterotopic ossification) occurs in 30% of patients undergoing hip arthroplasty.
- The incidence is greater than 80% in patients who have a history of ipsilateral or contralateral heterotopic ossification, and more than 60% in patients with other high-risk factors such as hypertrophic osteoarthritis, ankylosing spondylitis, and diffuse idiopathic skeletal hyperostosis.
- Treatment traditionally is given in the immediate postoperative period, with radiation doses ranging from 7 or 8 Gy in a single fraction to 10 Gy in 4 to 5 fractions (68). Comparable results have been described with 7 Gy in a single dose given preoperatively (69).
- There is no difference between single or multiple fractions and treatment given preoperatively or postoperatively.

GLANDULAR TISSUE

Gynecomastia

- Gynecomastia occurs in as many as 90% of patients receiving estrogens or flutamide, compared with only 8% of patients undergoing orchiectomy. Patients on gonadotropin-releasing hormone agonists have a 3% to 15% incidence of gyneco-mastia, whereas the incidence is 19% in those patients receiving a combination of flutamide and gonadotropin-releasing hormone agonists (70).

- Prophylactic breast irradiation prior to the initiation of treatment can be effective in preventing gynecomastia, particularly in patients being given estrogens. Radiation is less effective if given after estrogens have been started.
- Treatment modalities include orthovoltage irradiation, 9- to 12-MeV electrons, ^{60}Co, or 4-MV photons using tangential fields.
- A single dose of 9 Gy or 4 to 5 Gy daily for three treatments is effective in controlling gynecomastia (10).
- In patients treated after estrogen therapy, 20 Gy in 5 fractions is recommended.
- Response typically includes 33% reduction in patients with existing gynecomastia, and 39% improvement or resolution in pain (71).

Parotitis

- Acute postoperative parotitis is rare; typically, it occurs 4 to 6 days after surgery in debilitated and profoundly dehydrated patients. It is associated with decreased sali-vary secretions and a dry mouth.
- Treatment consists of correction of dehydration, mouth care, broad-spectrum antibi-otic therapy, and surgical drainage if necessary.
- Radiation therapy combined with the above measures is effective and may avoid the necessity for incision and drainage.
- The response to irradiation is often rapid and dramatic, with improvement in pain, induration, and swelling within 12 to 14 hours after the onset of treatment. Typically, all evidence of disease is gone in 3 to 6 days.
- Recommended doses are 7.5 to 10.0 Gy in 3 to 5 fractions using orthovoltage x-rays, ^{60}Co, or 9- to 12-MeV electrons. Treatment is directed through a laterally placed portal encompassing the parotid gland, with 2-cm margins around the volume being treated.

Sialorrhea

- Excessive drooling, or sialorrhea, is commonly found in neurologic diseases, includ-ing 80% of Parkinson's disease as well as ALS and strokes.
- Often associated with poor oral and facial muscle control leading to swallowing difficulties.
- Mild symptoms are treated with conservative management, including observation, oromotor control and dental malocclusion, postural changes, and biofeedback.
- Anticholinergics are first-line medications used, with glycopyrrolate being the most drying properties. Botulinum toxin injections have shown some benefit in the long-term for severe symptoms.
- Recommended dose for radiation therapy 12 Gy over 2 fractions. Studies have shown no superiority of electron therapy versus photon therapy.

- Field set up is parallel opposed fields, targeting the inferior two-thirds of the bilateral parotid glands, bilateral submandibular glands, and a portion of the oral cavity and oropharynx.
- The response to radiation was 81% in one systematic review (72). Symptom relief is first felt within 2 months of treatment, though duration varied from 3 months to 5 years.
- Short-term toxicity (72–74) is estimated at 24% to 40%, including xerostomia, mucositis, dysgeusia, and skin reaction. Long-term toxicity is estimated at 12%.

CONCLUSION

- Practice guidelines are systematically developed statements to assist the radiation oncologist and the patient in decisions regarding care for a specific clinical circumstance. These guidelines should include validity, reliability, reproducibility, clinical applicability, multidisciplinary process, review of evidence, and documentation.
- Utilization of these guidelines will lead to improved patient outcome and will minimize the wide variation in daily practice.
- Few clinical studies are available to explain the underlying radiobiologic mechanisms in the use of radiation therapy in the treatment of benign disease. However, the basic biologic data are known to substantiate such use. The potential hazards for tumor induction or somatic changes following radiation exposure for benign disease are well known, but the risk is very small. Furthermore, the overall contribution to anyone's general lifetime risk remains unclear.
- Therefore, patients older than 30 to 40 years of age are reasonable candidates for treatment with radiation therapy. However, in younger patients where there is a higher risk of carcinogenesis, one should carefully weigh the risks versus the benefits of treatment. Modern prospective clinical trials are needed to determine the appropriate criteria for treatment with radiation therapy for benign disease.
- Currently, very few clinical trials are being carried out involving patients with benign disease.

References

1. Order SE, Donaldson SS. *Radiation therapy of benign diseases: a clinical guide, 2nd rev ed. Medical radiology: radiation oncology series.* Berlin, Heidelberg, Germany: Springer-Verlag, 1998.
2. Kopicky J, Order SE. Survey and analysis of radiation therapy of benign disease. In: Council NR, ed. *A review of the use of ionizing radiation for the treatment of benign disease,* vol. II. Rockville, MD: US Department of Health, Education and Welfare, Bureau of Radiological Health, 1977:13.
3. Marius NS, James AG, Rebecca SB. The evaluation and treatment of graves ophthalmopathy. *Med Clin North Am* 2012;96(2):311–328. doi: 10.1016/j.mcna.2012.01.014
4. Prummel MF, Wiersinga WM. Immunomodulatory treatment of Graves' ophthalmopathy. *Thyroid* 1998;8(6):545–548.
5. Petersen IA, Kriss JP, McDougall IR, et al. Prognostic factors in the radiotherapy of Graves' ophthalmopathy. *Int J Radiat Oncol Biol Phys* 1990;19(2):259–264.
6. Marquez SD, Lum BL, McDougall IR, et al. Long-term results of irradiation for patients with progressive Graves' ophthalmopathy. *Int J Radiat Oncol Biol Phys* 2001;51(3):766–774.

7. Prummel MF, Mourits MP, Blank L, et al. Randomized double-blind trial of prednisone versus radiotherapy in Graves' ophthalmopathy. *Lancet* 1993;342(8877):949–954.

8. Mourits MP, van Kempen-Harteveld ML, Garcia MB, et al. Radiotherapy for Graves' orbitopathy: randomised placebo-controlled study. *Lancet* 2000;355(9214):1505–1509.

9. Austin-Seymour MM, Donaldson SS, Egbert PR, et al. Radiotherapy of lymphoid diseases of the orbit. *Int J Radiat Oncol Biol Phys* 1985;11(2):371–379.

10. Serber W, Dzeda MF, Hoppe RT. Radiation treatment of benign disease. In: Perez CA, Brady LW, eds. *Principles and practice of radiation oncology*, 3rd ed. Philadelphia, PA: Lippincott–Raven, 1998:2167–2185.

11. Prabhu RS, Kandula S, Liebman L, Wojno TH, et al. Association of clinical response and long-term outcome among patients with biopsied orbital pseudotumor receiving modern radiation therapy. *Int J Radiat Oncol Biol Phys* 2013;85(3):643–649.

12. Marks LB. Association of clinical response and long-term outcome among patients with biopsied orbital pseudotumor receiving modern radiation therapy: in regard to Prabhu et al. *Int J Radiat Oncol Biol Phys* 2013;86(5):808.

13. Camerol ME. *Pterygium throughout the world*. Springfield, IL: Charles C Thomas Publisher, 1965.

14. Van den Brenk H. Results of prophylactic postoperative irradiation in 1300 cases of pterygium. *Am J Roentgenol* 1968;103:723.

15. Brenner DJ, Merriam GR Jr. Postoperative irradiation for pterygium: guidelines for optimal treatment. *Int J Radiat Oncol Biol Phys* 1994;30(3):721–725.

16. Paryani SB, Scott WP, Wells JW Jr, et al. Management of pterygium with surgery and radiation therapy. The North Florida Pterygium Study Group. *Int J Radiat Oncol Biol Phys* 1994;28(1):101–103.

17. Wilder RB, Buatti JM, Kittelson JM, et al. Pterygium treated with excision and postoperative beta irradiation. *Int J Radiat Oncol Biol Phys* 1992;23(3):533–537.

18. Jurgenliemk-Schulz IM, Hartman LJ, Roesink JM, et al. Prevention of pterygium recurrence by postoperative single-dose beta-irradiation: a prospective randomized clinical double-blind trial. *Int J Radiat Oncol Biol Phys* 2004;59(4):1138–1147.

19. Aswad MI, Baum J. Optimal time for postoperative irradiation of pterygia. *Ophthalmology* 1987;94(11):1450–1451.

20. Campbell OR, Amendola BE, Brady LW. Recurrent pterygia: results of postoperative treatment with Sr-90 applicators. *Radiology* 1990;174(2):565–566.

21. Bressler NM, Bressler SB, Fine SL. Age-related macular degeneration. *Surv Ophthalmol* 1988;32(6):375–413.

22. Guyer DR, Fine SL, Maguire MG, et al. Subfoveal choroidal neovascular membranes in age-related macular degeneration. Visual prognosis in eyes with relatively good initial visual acuity. *Arch Ophthalmol* 1986;104(5):702–705.

23. Brown DM, Kaiser PK, Michels M, et al. Ranibizumab versus verteporfin for neovascular age-related macular degeneration. *N Engl J Med* 2006;355(14):1432–1444.

24. Rosenfeld PJ, Brown DM, Heier JS, et al. Ranibizumab for neovascular age-related macular degeneration. *N Engl J Med* 2006;355(14):1419–1431.

25. Trikha R,Morse LS, Zawadzki RJ, Werner JS, Park SS. Ten-year follow-up of eyes treated with stereotactic fractionated external beam radiation for neovascular age-related macular degeneration. *Retina.* 2011;31(7):1303–1315. doi:10.1097/IAE.0b013e318203ee46.

26. Kishan AU, Modjtahedi BS, Morse LS, Lee P. Radiation therapy for neovascular age-related macular degeneration. *Int J Radiat Oncol Biol Phys* 2013;85(3):583–597. doi:10.1016/j.ijrobp.2012.07.2352.

27. Chakravarthy U, Houston RF, Archer DB. Treatment of age-related subfoveal neovascular membranes by teletherapy: a pilot study. *Br J Ophthalmol* 1993;77(5):265–273.

28. Hart PM, Archer DB, Chakravarthy U. Asymmetry of disciform scarring in bilateral disease when one eye is treated with radiotherapy. *Br J Ophthalmol* 1995;79(6):562–568.

29. Bergink GJ, Deutman AF, van den Broek JF, et al. Radiation therapy for subfoveal choroidal neovascular membranes in age-related macular degeneration. A pilot study. *Graefes Arch Clin Exp Ophthalmol* 1994;232(10):591–598.

30. Freire J, Longton WA, Miyamoto CT, et al. External radiotherapy in macular degeneration: technique and preliminary subjective response. *Int J Radiat Oncol Biol Phys* 1996;36(4):857–860.

31. Alberti WE, Richard G, Sagerman RH. *Age-related macular degeneration: current treatment concepts.* Berlin, Heidelberg, Germany: Springer-Verlag, 2001.

32. Steiner L, Lindquist C, Adler JR, eds. Clinical outcome of radiosurgery for cerebral arteriovenous malformations. *J Neurosurg* 1992;77(1):1–8.

33. Maruyama K, Kawahara N, Shin M, et al. The risk of hemorrhage after radiosurgery for cerebral arteriovenous malformations. *N Engl J Med* 2005;352(2):146–153.

34. Flickinger JC, Pollock BE, Kondziolka D, et al. A dose-response analysis of arteriovenous malformation obliteration after radiosurgery. *Int J Radiat Oncol Biol Phys* 1996;36(4):873–879.

35. Borok TL, Bray M, Sinclair I, et al. Role of ionizing irradiation for 393 keloids. *Int J Radiat Oncol Biol Phys* 1988;15(4):865–870.

36. Kovalic JJ, Perez CA. Radiation therapy following keloidectomy: a 20-year experience. *Int J Radiat Oncol Biol Phys* 1989;17(1):77–80.

37. Jiang P, Baumann R, Dunst J, et al. Perioperative interstitial high-dose-rate brachytherapy for the treatment of recurrent keloids: feasibility and early results. *Int J Radiat Oncol Biol Phys* 2016;94(3):532–536. doi:10.1016/j.ijrobp.2015.11.008.

38. Doornbos JF, Stoffel TJ, Hass AC, et al. The role of kilovoltage irradiation in the treatment of keloids. *Int J Radiat Oncol Biol Phys* 1990;18(4):833–839.

39. Inalsingh CH. An experience in treating five hundred and one patients with keloids. *Johns Hopkins Med J* 1974;134(5):284–290.

40. Donahue B, Cooper JS, Rush S. Treatment of aggressive keratoacanthomas by radiotherapy. *J Am Acad Dermatol* 1990;23(3 Pt 1):489–493.

41. Furst CJ, Lundell M, Holm LE. Tumors after radiotherapy for skin hemangioma in childhood. A case-control study. *Acta Oncol* 1990;29(5):557–562.

42. Furst CJ, Lundell M, Holm LE. Radiation therapy of hemangiomas, 1909–1959. A cohort based on 50 years of clinical practice at Radiumhemmet, Stockholm. *Acta Oncol* 1987;26(1):33–36.

43. Liu X, Xu D, Zhang Y, Liu D, Song G. Gamma Knife surgery in patients harboring orbital cavernous hemangiomas that were diagnosed on the basis of imaging findings. *J Neurosurg* 2010;113(suppl):39–43.

44. Toro A, Mahfouz AE, Ardiri A, et al. What is changing in indications and treatment of hepatic hemangiomas. A review. *Ann Hepatol* 2014;13(4):327–339.

45. Peng PD, Hyder O, Mavros MN, et al. Management and recurrence patterns of desmoids tumors: a multi-institutional analysis of 211 patients. *Ann Surg Oncol* 2012;19(13):4036–4042. doi:10.1245/s10434-012-2634-6.

46. McCollough WM, Parsons JT, van der Griend R, et al. Radiation therapy for aggressive fibromatosis. The Experience at the University of Florida. *J Bone Joint Surg Am* 1991;73(5):717–725.

47. Leibel SA, Wara WM, Hill DR, et al. Desmoid tumors: local control and patterns of relapse following radiation therapy. *Int J Radiat Oncol Biol Phys* 1983;9(8):1167–1171.

48. Betriu A, Masotti M, Serra A, et al. Randomized comparison of coronary stent implantation and balloon angioplasty in the treatment of de novo coronary artery lesions (START): a four-year follow-up. *J Am Coll Cardiol* 1999;34(5):1498–1506.

49. Leon MB, Teirstein PS, Moses JW, et al. Localized intracoronary gamma-radiation therapy to inhibit the recurrence of restenosis after stenting. *N Engl J Med* 2001;344(4):250–256.

50. Teirstein PS, Massullo V, Jani S, et al. Catheter-based radiotherapy to inhibit restenosis after coronary stenting. *N Engl J Med* 1997;336(24):1697–1703.
51. Waksman R, Raizner AE, Yeung AC, et al. Use of localised intracoronary beta radiation in treatment of in-stent restenosis: the INHIBIT randomised controlled trial. *Lancet* 2002;359(9306): 551–557.
52. Kuntz RE, Speiser B, Joyal M, et al. Acute and midterm clinical outcomes after use of 90Sr/90Y beta radiation for the treatment of native coronary artery obstructions: acute results from the Novoste Beta-Cath System Trial. *American College of Cardiology, 49th Annual Scientific Session.* Anaheim, CA; March 2000.
53. Azeem T, Adlam D, Gershlick A. Evolution of vascular brachytherapy over time: data from the RENO-registry analysis. *Int J Cardiol* 2005;100(2):225–228.
54. Giap H, Massullo V, Teirstein P, et al. Theoretical assessment of late cardiac complication from endovascular brachytherapy for restenosis prevention. *Cardiovasc Radiat Med* 1999;1(3): 233–238.
55. Giap H, Tripuraneni P, Teirstein P, et al. Theoretical assessment of dose-rate effect in endovascular brachytherapy. *Cardiovasc Radiat Med* 1999;1(3):227–232.
56. Kim HS, Waksman R, Kollum M, et al. Edge stenosis after intracoronary radiotherapy: angiographic, intravascular, and histological findings. *Circulation* 2001;103(17):2219–2220.
57. Tripuraneni P, Parikh S, Giap H, et al. How long is enough? Defining the treatment length in endovascular brachytherapy. *Catheter Cardiovasc Interv* 2000;51(2):147–153.
58. Urban P, Serruys P, Baumgart D, et al. A multicentre European registry of intraluminal coronary beta brachytherapy. *Eur Heart J* 2003;24(7):604–612.
59. Colombo A, Drzewiecki J, Banning A, et al. Randomized study to assess the effectiveness of slow-and moderate-release polymer-based paclitaxel-eluting stents for coronary artery lesions. *Circulation* 2003;108(7):788–794.
60. Grube E, Silber S, Hauptmann KE, et al. TAXUS I: six- and twelve-month results from a randomized, double-blind trial on a slow-release paclitaxel-eluting stent for de novo coronary lesions. *Circulation* 2003;107(1):38–42.
61. Morice MC, Serruys PW, Sousa JE, et al. A randomized comparison of a sirolimus-eluting stent with a standard stent for coronary revascularization. *N Engl J Med* 2002;346(23):1773–1780.
62. Stone GW, Ellis SG, Cox DA, et al. A polymer-based, paclitaxel-eluting stent in patients with coronary artery disease. *N Engl J Med* 2004;350(3):221–231.
63. Tanabe K, Serruys PW, Grube E, et al. TAXUS III Trial: in-stent restenosis treated with stent-based delivery of paclitaxel incorporated in a slow-release polymer formulation. *Circulation* 2003;107(4):559–564.
64. Neumann FJ, Desmet W, Grube E, et al. Effectiveness and safety of sirolimus-eluting stents in the treatment of restenosis after coronary stent placement. *Circulation* 2005;111(16): 2107–2111.
65. Stone GW, Ellis SG, O'Shaughnessy CD, et al. Paclitaxel-eluting stents vs vascular brachytherapy for in-stent restenosis within bare-metal stents: the TAXUS V ISR randomized trial. *JAMA* 2006;295(11):1253–1263.
66. Cuculich PS, Schill MR, Kashani R, et al. Noninvasive cardiac radiation for ablation of ventricular tachycardia. *N Engl J Med* 2017;377(24):2325–2336. doi: 10.1056/NEJMoa1613773.
67. Miszczyk L, Tukiendorf A. Radiotherapy of painful vertebral hemangiomas: the single center retrospective analysis of 137 cases. *Int J Radiat Oncol Biol Phys* 2012;82(2):e173–e180. doi: 10.1016/j.ijrobp.2011.04.028.
68. Kolbl O, Knelles D, Barthel T, et al. Randomized trial comparing early postoperative irradiation vs. the use of nonsteroidal antiinflammatory drugs for prevention of heterotopic ossification following prosthetic total hip replacement. *Int J Radiat Oncol Biol Phys* 1997;39(5):961–966.

69. Seegenschmiedt MH, Keilholz L, Martus P, et al. Prevention of heterotopic ossification about the hip: final results of two randomized trials in 410 patients using either preoperative or postoperative radiation therapy. *Int J Radiat Oncol Biol Phys* 1997;39(1):161–171.

70. Kirschenbaum A. Management of hormonal treatment effects. *Cancer* 1995;75:1983–1986.

71. Widmark A, Fossa SD, Lundmo P, et al. Does prophylactic breast irradiation prevent antiandrogen-induced gynecomastia? Evaluation of 253 patients in the randomized Scandinavian trial SPCG-7/SFUO-3. *Urology.* 2003;61(1):145–151.

72. Hawkey NM, Zaorsky NG, Galloway TJ. The role of radiation therapy in the management of sialorrhea: a systematic review. *Laryngoscope* 2016;126(1):80–85. doi: 10.1002/lary.25444.

73. Assouline A, Levy A, Abdelnour-Mallet M, et al. Radiation therapy for hypersalivation: a prospective study in 50 amyotrophic lateral sclerosis patients. *Int J Radiat Oncol Biol Phys* 2014;88(3):589–595. doi: 10.1016/j.ijrobp.2013.11.230.

74. Borg M, Hirst F. The role of radiation therapy in the management of sialorrhea. *Int J Radiat Oncol Biol Phys* 1998;41(5):1113–1119.

CHAPTER 48

PALLIATION: BRAIN, SPINAL CORD, BONE, AND VISCERAL METASTASES

BRAIN METASTASES

Epidemiology and Natural History

- Population-based studies show an incidence of brain metastases (BM) ranging from 7 to 14 per 100,000 population per year. However, because of significant inaccuracies with population and pathologic studies, this is likely an underestimation (1).
- Headache and impaired cognition are the most common presenting symptoms.
- The incidence of BM is increasing due to the availability of improved diagnostic imaging techniques such as magnetic resonance imaging (MRI) and an increase in long-term survival of patients treated with systemic agents that do not cross the blood-brain barrier.
- The most common sources of BM are tumors of the lung, breast, and melanoma (1,2). Melanoma has a high predilection for metastasizing to the brain with up to 37% of patients with stage IV melanoma developing clinical BM, a number which can reach 75% on autopsy series (2,3).
- BM from melanoma and renal cell carcinoma are most likely to be hemorrhagic (1,4,5).

Prognostic Factors

- The Disease-Specific Graded Prognostic Assessment (DS-GPA) is a multi-institutional, multinational collaboration that studied the prognosis of patients with BM treated between 1985 and 2007 (6).
- Prognostic factors include KPS, age, presence of extracerebral metastases, and number of metastases, but not all factors are prognostic in all cancer types. Age is strongly prognostic in NSCLC but not prognostic in melanoma, renal cell carcinoma, or GI cancer.
- Median survival ranges from 4.9 months (small cell lung cancer) to 13.8 months (breast cancer) and could be as high as 25 months in breast cancer patients with a DS-GPA of 3.5 to 4.0

- The recursive partitioning analysis (RPA) study, although a more approximate estimation of prognosis, is easy to remember and still in use clinically. Three RPA classes are described: RPA class I (Karnofsky performance score [KPS] ≥ 70, controlled primary, age less than 65 years, brain metastasis only), II (not meeting requirements of classes I or III), and III (KPS less than 70) (7).

Diagnostic Workup

- Contrast-enhanced MRI is a more sensitive test than computed tomography (CT) to detect BM, especially those less than 5 mm in size.
- Surgical excision for histologic confirmation should be performed in the absence of a primary site.

General Management

- Corticosteroids are recommended to improve neurologic symptoms or to prevent them when treating patients with significant peritumoral edema. In asymptomatic patients with little edema or mass effect, corticosteroids may be reserved until the first sign of symptoms.
- A reasonable corticosteroid regimen is a 10-mg intravenous bolus of dexamethasone followed by 16 mg PO divided QID or BID. The dose is then tapered over 2 to 4 weeks.
- Large metastases in the cerebral hemispheres or the posterior fossa can be managed with initial surgical excision for rapid relief of mass effect, edema, impending herniation, and hydrocephalus.
- Postoperative WBRT improves local control, rate of neurologic death, and distant brain control, without improving overall survival (8,9). A recent study of postoperative SRS versus WBRT to the surgical cavity in patients with a limited number of BMs found improved neurocognition and QOL with SRS and equivalent OS. This suggests postoperative SRS may be preferable to WBRT (10).
- Radiosurgery is becoming the standard treatment for patients with a limited number of intact metastases to avoid the detrimental effects of WBRT on cognition and quality of life.
- The maximum number of metastases that can be treated with SRS is currently a matter of debate. A cutoff of 5 to 10 metastases is often used, but certain centers, in the right patient, will treat more.
- There is limited evidence that SRS improves overall survival in young patients with good KPS and a single metastasis (11,12).
- If a patient has received upfront whole-brain radiotherapy (WBRT) for a limited number of metastases, a boost with SRS should be considered to improve local control.
- WBRT is used to salvage patients after radiosurgery, or upfront, where the number or size of metastases is too great. WBRT is also used to palliate metastases from SCLC and when there is leptomeningeal spread.
- The recent QUARTZ randomized trial evaluated the benefit of WBRT in patients with BM from NSCLC unsuitable for SRS or surgery and found that WBRT was equivalent to corticosteroids and best supportive care in a population of patients with poor KPS (38% had KPS ≤ 60).

- Patients with multiple small metastases from EGFR + NSCLC treated with EGFR inhibitors crossing the blood-brain barrier may be effectively controlled without upfront radiation. Other targeted agents in lung, melanoma, and other cancers are under investigation.
- Patients with SCLC and 1 to 2 small BM, and patients with germ cell tumors, may be initially controlled with upfront cytotoxic chemotherapy, although frequent imaging should be obtained and radiation administered if there are any signs of intracranial disease progression.
- Cancer of the breast is the most common primary site to metastasize to the orbit or choroid, causing proptosis and diplopia. A dose of 20 Gy in 5 fractions is well tolerated and achieves tumor stability or regression in the majority of patients (13).

Radiation Therapy Techniques

Radiosurgery

- Stereotactic radiosurgery (SRS) can be delivered with Gamma Knife (GK) or linear accelerator–based systems.
- Single-fraction SRS doses vary according to target size and location to keep rates of radionecrosis less than 10% as detailed in RTOG 90-05 (14):
  - Less than 20 mm—24 Gy
  - 21 to 30 mm—18 Gy
  - 31 to 40 mm—15 Gy
- BM in or near the brain stem and those in eloquent areas such as the motor and sensory cortex can receive 15 to 18 Gy (15–17).
- In GK SRS, doses are often prescribed to the 50% isodose line. With LINAC-based SRS, the dose is typically prescribed approximately to the 80% isodose line.
- GK SRS systems with an invasive stereotactic frame need no CTV nor PTV for intact lesions. A 2-mm CTV is recommended for cavity treatments.
- Frameless GK SRS has recently come into use employing a thermoplastic mask for immobilization and an infrared camera for intrafraction motion assessment. It allows for multifraction SRS, usually in 3 to 5 fractions, which is an attractive option for lesions too large to be treated safely and effectively with single-fraction SRS dose constraints.

Whole-Brain Radiotherapy

- WBRT doses of 20 Gy in 5 fractions, 30 Gy in 10 fractions, or 37.5 Gy in 15 fractions are commonly used.
- If WBRT reirradiation is attempted, a dose of 20 to 25 Gy in 10 fractions can be used.
- WBRT is often delivered with opposed lateral fields (Fig. 48-1). Recommended field borders are:
  - Superior and posterior: flash the skin of the cranium by 2 cm.
  - Inferior: at C1-2, or C2-3 in cases of leptomeningeal spread to ensure full coverage of the fourth ventricle and foramen magnum.
  - Anterior: shielded with MLCs to cover the lens and approximately 1 cm away from the base of skull ensuring coverage of the cribriform plate and middle cranial fossa.

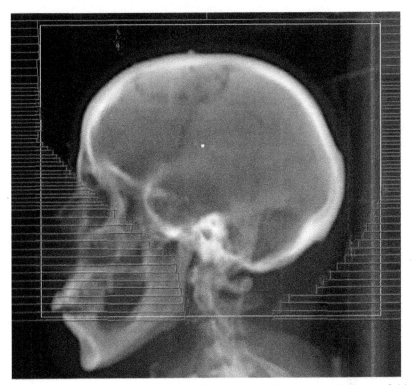

FIGURE 48-1. Lateral digitally reconstructed radiograph of a whole-brain radiotherapy field. Note the inferior border at C2-3 because of leptomeningeal involvement.

- The isocenter can be placed at the level of the orbit to minimize exit dose through the lenses. Segments can be used, usually inferiorly, to improve coverage or homogeneity.
- WBRT with hippocampal avoidance and the use of memantine (a drug used in Alzheimer's disease) are strategies under investigation to decrease toxicity from WBRT.

SPINAL CORD COMPRESSION

Natural History

- Approximately 5% to 10% of cancer patients are estimated to develop metastatic epidural spinal cord compression (MESCC) during the course of their disease (18,19).
- If left untreated, the natural history of MESCC leads to increasing pain, paralysis, sensory loss, and sphincter dysfunction. Avoiding such debilitating complications at the end of life is the purpose of local control in MESCC.

Prognostic Factors

- According to a large retrospective review of 1,852 patients with MESCC, factors associated with improved OS include ambulatory status at presentation, greater than

15-month interval between diagnosis and MESCC, greater than 2 weeks to develop motor deficits, histology (breast, prostate, myeloma, lymphoma), and absence of visceral metastases (20).
- Factors associated with improved LC include long-course RT and absence of visceral metastases.

Clinical Presentation

- At presentation, 90% of patients suffer of pain and about 50% of patients are either unable to walk or have bladder and bowel dysfunction (18).

Diagnostic Workup

- MESCC is defined by both clinical and radiographic criteria. There should be clinical symptoms with at least indentation of the thecal sac by an extradural tumor at that level. Subclinical MESCC is defined as the presence of radiographic features of cord compression without neurologic symptoms.

General Management

- Corticosteroids are indicated for patients with neurologic deficits and suspected or confirmed MESCC. A reasonable regimen is dexamethasone 10-mg IV bolus followed by 16 mg PO divided BID or QID.
- The trial by Patchell et al. randomized 101 patients with MESCC (excluding cauda equina) to surgical decompression and adjuvant RT to 30 Gy/10 or RT alone. Patients in the surgery + RT group were more likely to maintain ambulation (84% versus 57%) and had better urinary continence, functional status, and improved overall survival (126 days versus 100 days). The trial was criticized for its small sample size and long accrual (10 years) (21).
- A retrospective matched control study by Rades et al. found no difference between RT alone or combined with surgery (22).
- Surgical decompression is generally recommended in operable patients with good performance status and an expected survival of at least 3 months, in cases of spinal instability/fracture, or if a histologic diagnosis is needed. A surgical consultation should be sought within 24 hours of a diagnosis of MESCC.
- Postoperative RT should start after wound healing is complete, usually 1 to 4 weeks after surgery.
- Primary RT should be considered on an urgent basis for patients who are not candidates for surgical intervention. Because of the time required to plan stereotactic body radiotherapy (SBRT) treatments to the spine, it is not commonly used in symptomatic MESCC.
- Patients with recurrent MESCC should be considered for surgical decompression if operative candidates. Reirradiation with conventional fractionation or SBRT can be considered in patients with adequate prognosis on an individual basis or best supportive care if prognosis and performance status are poor.

Radiation Therapy Techniques

- Common fractionations include 20 Gy/5, 30 Gy/10, and 37.5 Gy/5. Patients with poor performance status and limited prognosis can be treated with a single fraction of 8 Gy.
- Reirradiation doses should be limited to a total biologic equivalent dose (BED) of 135 Gy using a cord α/β of 2, when the treatment interval is ≥ 6 months (23). Conventional reirradiation doses include 8 Gy/1, 20 Gy/8, and 25 Gy/10.
- Radiation fields are commonly 8 to 9 cm wide and extended superiorly/inferiorly to the interspace of one vertebral body above and below to allow for a margin and facilitated future treatments.
- Simple PA or AP/PA beams are commonly used in the thoracic and lumbar spine.
- Lateral opposed beams with a thermoplastic mask can be used in the cervical spine to spare the oropharynx and esophagus.
- Three-field techniques with laterals and a PA beam can be used in the low lumbar and sacral spine.
- Antiemetics can prevent RT-induced nausea when a significant volume of bowel is in field.

BONE METASTASES

Natural History

- Bone metastases can lead to severe complications such as debilitating pain, pathologic fracture, hypercalcemia, and spinal cord compression.
- Bone metastases are the second most common cause of pathologic fractures after osteoporosis.
- A predictive model for survival in patients with metastatic cancer was developed to include three risk factors: primary cancer site, site of metastases (bone versus other than the bone), and KPS (24).
- Patients with bone-only metastases from breast or prostate cancer can have median survivals in the range of 21 to 51 months (25,26).
- The most common cancers to metastasize to bones are breast, prostate, thyroid, kidney, lung, and multiple myeloma. Multiple myeloma and renal cell carcinoma metastases are most often osteolytic, whereas breast and prostate cancers are most often osteosclerotic (27,28).

Diagnostic Workup

- Plain radiographs are useful as first-line imaging to assess patients with bone pain.
- Bone scans are very sensitive in the detection of bone metastases but may miss purely osteolytic metastases such as in multiple myeloma.
- CT scans are useful to assess fractures or fracture risk and to confirm abnormal radionuclide uptake on bone scan.
- MRI of the entire spine is useful to assess areas of cord compression or impending compression and the number of vertebral metastases.
- FDG-PET-CT is sensitive and specific for the detection of bone metastases and has improved detection of osteolytic lesions over bone scan (29).

- Bone biopsy can be performed for diagnostic purposes, such as in patients presenting with no identifiable primary, or in equivocal cases where confirming metastatic disease would alter the overall management. Although the diagnostic yield of core bone biopsies for lytic lesions can approach 90%, biopsies of sclerotic lesions have a yield of only 50% to 60% (30,31).

General Management

Surgery

- Patients with mechanical instability in the vertebral column should be evaluated for surgical intervention. The Spinal Instability Neoplastic Score (SINS) predicts tumor-related instability in the vertebral column based on location, pain, nature of the lesion, spinal alignment, vertebral collapse, and involvement of posterolateral elements (32). Patients with SINS score ≥7 require surgical consultation. The Tokuhashi score estimates survival of patients with spinal metastases (33).
- Patients with impending fractures in long bones can benefit from surgical fixation. The Mirels criteria quantify the risk of pathologic fracture in long bones using site, nature, size, and symptoms from a metastatic deposit (34). Lesions with scores of ≥8 may benefit from prophylactic internal fixation.
- Postoperative RT with 30 Gy/10 or 20 Gy/5 is commonly started after a healing period of 2 to 4 weeks (35,36).

Radiation

- Single-fraction and multifraction RT regimens lead to equivalent pain response rates of 40% to 70%. Multifraction regimens decrease the need of retreatment from 20% to 8% (24,37–40).
- Common fractionations include 8 Gy/1, 20 Gy/5, and 30 Gy/10.
- Reirradiation can achieve a complete pain response in 20% of patients and partial response in 50%, including in initial nonresponders (41).
- Reirradiation with 8 Gy/1 or 20 Gy/5 showed similar rates of response in bone metastases (42). Reirradiation for vertebral metastases should take into account a careful assessment of previous spinal cord dose, overlap, and interval between treatments (see Spinal Cord Compression—Radiation Therapy Techniques).
- Pathologic fracture rates are estimated at 3% after a first course of RT and 5% to 7% after reirradiation (38,39,42).
- Dexamethasone 8 mg PO daily × 5 days has been shown in a double-blind RCT to decrease the incidence of pain flare after palliative RT, from 35% to 26% (37).
- Bone marrow suppression can occur in patients treated with large radiation fields and high doses of RT, elderly patients, and those receiving chemotherapy.
- Patients with a limited number of bone metastases may benefit from aggressive treatment such as SBRT. In a phase II RCT by Gomez et al., patients with stage IV NSCLC and ≤3 metastases (including 10 with bone metastases) who were treated with high-dose RT had improved PFS compared to usual care (43).
- Prolonged DFS is achieved in about 20% of patients with oligometastatic disease treated with SBRT (44).

Spine Stereotactic Body Radiotherapy

- Spine SBRT delivers high-dose, highly conformal treatments to the vertebral bodies using near-rigid patient immobilization and image guidance.
- The Neurologic-Oncologic-Mechanical-Systemic (NOMS) decision framework outlines an approach to patients with spinal metastatic disease, including the need to assess spinal stability (45).
- The Bilsky grade describes the degree of spinal compression on T2-weighed MR images (46).
- SBRT is indicated in clinical scenarios where local control is particularly important such as oligometastases, oligoprogression, radioresistant histology, recurrence after conventional RT, and extraosseous disease.
- SBRT for pain control achieves a complete response in 50% to 60% of patients and overall improvement in 80% (47,48). A randomized study on spine SBRT versus conventional RT for pain control is currently underway (Canadian Cancer Trials Group SC24).
- SBRT is generally contraindicated in patients with mechanically unstable spine, disease in greater than 3 contiguous levels, high-grade cord compression (Bilsky 3), patients less than 5 months from prior conventional RT, patients unable to undergo spine MRI (or CT myelogram), and those with poor performance status or limited survival.
- The role for SBRT in moderate (Bilsky 2) radiologic epidural disease without clinical cord compression is controversial. Approaches include separation surgery + SBRT, SBRT alone, or conventional RT.
- One-year local control after SBRT is generally 80% to 90%.
- Compression fractures after SBRT occur in approximately 12% of patients. Pain flare has been reported in 23% to 65% of patients (49,50). Radiation myelopathy is a feared complication, but with strict cord dose constraints, the risk is estimated between 0% and 3% (48).

Other Therapies

- Osteoclast inhibitors such as bisphosphonates and denosumab reduce skeletal related events (pathologic fractures, need for RT/surgery, spinal cord compression, hypercalcemia) by an absolute 10% to 20%, decrease pain, and improve quality of life.
- Side effects include hypocalcemia and osteonecrosis of the jaw. Patients should be monitored with blood work for renal function, calcium, and electrolytes, and regular assessments of oral health.
- Bone-targeted radioisotopes (e.g., strontium-89, samarium-153, radium-223) localize to areas of osteosclerotic bone metastases.
- Radium-223 is an alpha-particle–emitting agent, which was shown in a double-blind RCT to improve OS by 4 months in patients with bone metastases from castration-resistant prostate cancer. There was also a reduction in skeletal related events, pain, and spinal cord compression (51,52).
- The recommended dose for radium-223 is 50 kBq/kg every 4 weeks for 6 doses. Patients should be monitored with blood work for anemia and thrombocytopenia

and assessed for any signs of active infection before the administration of the following dose.

- Strontium-89 and samarium-153 are beta-particle–emitting radioisotopes that can provide pain relief in 40% to 95% of patients. The most common toxicity is myelosuppression (53).
- Vertebroplasty and kyphoplasty are percutaneous injection techniques that may provide pain relief in patients with malignant vertebral compression fractures, but data on this are modest. Contraindications include spinal compression and retropulsion of bone fragments.

Radiation Therapy Techniques

- On long bones, an anatomical CTV margin of 2 cm is recommended.
- Conventional RT for vertebral metastases: see section on spinal cord compression.

Spine Stereotactic Body Radiotherapy

- SBRT to the spine can be delivered in a single fraction or in 2 to 5 fractions. Postoperative spine SBRT is most often fractionated.
- Thin-slice MRI with T1- and T2-weighed images is useful for delineating the spinal cord or thecal sac and any paraspinal extension. A CT myelogram can be used in patients unable to undergo an MRI or where postoperative hardware obscures visualization of the spinal cord.
- Consensus guidelines exist regarding volume definition in the definitive or postoperative setting. Generally, the entire vertebral body is included unless there is limited disease in the lamina, spinous process, or pedicle (54,55).
- Patient setup includes a near-rigid immobilization system, a treatment delivery system capable of couch corrections in 6 degrees of freedom, and daily cone-beam CT. Strict tolerance levels should be maintained for translational and rotational variation (less than 1 to 2 mm and less than 1 to 2 degrees).
- With careful positioning and quality assurance, PTV can be reduced to 2 mm and spinal cord PRV to 1.5 to 2 mm (56,57).

SUPERIOR VENA CAVA OBSTRUCTION

- Superior vena cava obstruction (SVCO) requires prompt intervention to re-establish venous return to the right atrium and decrease SVC venous pressure.
- SVCO is caused by external compression or invasion by tumor in 60% to 90% of cases. NSCLC, SCLC, and non-Hodgkin lymphoma account for the vast majority of responsible malignancies (58). Other causes include aortic aneurysms, SVC thrombus from intravascular catheters or pacemakers, and fibrosing mediastinitis.
- Classical symptoms are facial swelling and flushing, venous redistribution in the chest, shortness of breath, cough, stridor, dysphagia, and hoarseness. Cerebral edema is a dangerous complication that can lead to ischemia, herniation, and neurologic damage.

- Most symptoms improve over time because of the development of collateral venous circulation; therefore, SVCO is in most cases not immediately life-threatening. However, patients with stridor from airway obstruction, severe laryngeal edema, and neurologic symptoms represent oncologic emergencies requiring urgent treatment.

Diagnosis

- Most patients with SVCO have an abnormal mediastinal widening on chest radiograph.
- Contrast-enhanced CT scan is a useful initial imaging modality that can confirm SVCO and identify its underlying cause.
- Histologic diagnosis should be obtained before initiating therapy in most clinically stable patients. If lymphoma is suspected, steroids should be held until an adequate biopsy has been obtained.

Treatment

- Elevating the bed above the level of the heart and supplemental oxygen are measure that can improve symptoms.
- The treatment of SVCO depends on the clinical scenario. Steroids, SVC stent placement, RT, and chemotherapy can all be used alone or in combination.
- SVC stents provide rapid relief of symptoms in 95% of patients while the histologic diagnosis is being investigated (59).
- RT is widely used in SVCO with palliative doses (e.g., 20 Gy/5 or 30 Gy/10) providing symptom relief in the majority of patients. RT can obscure subsequent histologic diagnosis and should be preceded by tissue confirmation whenever possible.
- Chemotherapy is an appropriate initial therapy for chemosensitive malignancies such as SCLC, lymphoma, and germ cell tumors.

Thoracic Symptoms

- RT is most effective for hemoptysis, chest pain, dyspnea, postobstructive pneumonia, dysphagia from esophageal compression, and SVCO. RT is less effective for malignant pleural effusion (60).
- There are limited data that longer courses of RT achieve better palliation, although higher doses such as 30 Gy/10 can cause more toxicity (mainly esophagitis).
- A Canadian RCT compared 20 Gy/5 to 10 Gy/1 for the palliation of thoracic symptoms from lung cancer not suitable for curative treatment. It found improved symptom palliation and QOL without increased toxicity in the 20 Gy/5 arm. There was a small yet significant 2-month increase in OS for patients with good performance status and no metastases (61).
- Trials from the Medical Research Council in the United Kingdom have reported similar palliation with short or long courses of RT (39 Gy/13 versus 17 Gy/2; 30 Gy/10 versus 17 Gy/2; 17 Gy/2 versus 10 Gy/1), although it was noted that 3 patients treated with 17 Gy/2 and 2 patients treated with 39 Gy/13 developed radiation myelopathy (62).

- Endobronchial HDR brachytherapy can be used for patient with endobronchial disease causing obstructive symptoms or for hemoptysis uncontrolled by external beam RT. A wide variety in schedules exists, usually 10 to 16 Gy in 1 to 3 weekly sessions delivered at 1 cm depth with a 1- to 1.5-cm proximal/distal PTV.
- Endobronchial brachytherapy provides no immediate relief and may cause transient swelling. High-grade airway obstruction with airway compromise should be considered for more immediate interventions such as laser or argon plasma coagulation, electrocautery, or stent insertion. Other relative contraindications include lesions causing bronchial fistulae or those involving (or in close proximity with) large vessels because of the risk of fistula formation and fatal hemorrhage.

Liver Metastases

- Selected patients with a limited number of liver metastases from colorectal cancer—and others—have prolonged survival with surgical resection or local ablation. Nonsurgical options include systemic and regional chemotherapy, RT (SBRT, conformal RT, or whole-liver RT) radiopharmaceuticals, radiofrequency ablation, intratumoral instillations, or cryotherapy.
- Liver SBRT is effective where local control of liver metastases is clinically important, such as patients with good performance status, controlled extrahepatic disease, oligometastases, or oligoprogression.
- SBRT doses ranging from 30 to 60 Gy and schedules of 3 to 6 fractions have been used, according to the volume of metastases and the ensuing dose to normal liver (63,64).
- Local control at 1 year is 60% to 90%. Median OS after SBRT ranges from 10 to 34 months (65,66).
- Ideal candidates for liver SBRT include patients with no active extrahepatic disease, ≤5 metastases, less than 6 cm in size, greater than 5 mm from luminal GI structures, greater than 700 cc of uninvolved liver, and life expectancy greater than 3 months.
- Liver SBRT requires careful consideration of patient positioning. Simulation should include assessment of tumor motion (e.g., 4D CT scan or breath-hold technique) and daily cone-beam CT scans. MRI images can be fused to aid in contouring. Careful attention should be paid to OARs including the stomach, bowel, biliary structures, and kidneys.
- Whole-liver RT can achieve improvement in pain in 50% to 80% of patients, but doses should be limited to avoid RT-induced liver disease (65). Whole-liver RT below 27 to 30 Gy in 2 Gy fractions is unlikely to cause RT-induced liver disease. 8 Gy/1 was well tolerated in patients premedicated with granisetron and 2 mg dexamethasone 1 hour before RT (67).

Hemorrhage

- Treatment of malignant hemorrhage should be individualized in the context of disease burden, life expectancy, intent of treatment, and goals of care.
- Some patients may be controlled with packing, hemostatic agents, and pressure dressings alone. Systemic agents such as tranexamic acid for gynecologic bleeding and

octreotide for gastric bleeding can be used in combination with interventions, RT, or on their own.

- Interventions such as cauterization, arterial embolization, and laser coagulation can be considered in patients with reasonable performance status and life expectancy.
- RT is very effective for the palliation of bleeding from nearly all tumors including gynecologic, thoracic, gastric, rectal, head and neck, and urinary malignancies. Bleeding can be controlled in greater than 70% of patients (68–70).
- Single fractions of 8 to 10 Gy are effective, as are longer palliative regiments (71,72). High-dose palliation with 40 Gy/15 or 50 Gy/20 can provide additional local control. A convenient schedule of 8 Gy × 3 on days 0, 7, and 21 can achieve rapid hemostasis with additional local control on subsequent visits depending on the patient's performance status (73).

References

1. Nayak L, Lee EQ, Wen PY. Epidemiology of brain metastases. *Curr Oncol Rep* 2012;14(1):48–54.
2. Fox BD, et al. Epidemiology of metastatic brain tumors. *Neurosurg Clin N Am* 2011;22(1):1–6, v.
3. Amer MH, et al. Malignant melanoma and central nervous system metastases: incidence, diagnosis, treatment and survival. *Cancer* 1978;42(2):660–668.
4. Wronski M, Arbit E. Surgical treatment of brain metastases from melanoma: a retrospective study of 91 patients. *J Neurosurg* 2000;93(1):9–18.
5. Wronski M, et al. Surgical resection of brain metastases from renal cell carcinoma in 50 patients. *Urology* 1996;47(2):187–193.
6. Sperduto PW, et al. Summary report on the graded prognostic assessment: an accurate and facile diagnosis-specific tool to estimate survival for patients with brain metastases. *J Clin Oncol* 2012;30(4):419–425.
7. Gaspar L, et al. Recursive partitioning analysis (RPA) of prognostic factors in three Radiation Therapy Oncology Group (RTOG) brain metastases trials. *Int J Radiat Oncol Biol Phys* 1997;37(4):745–751.
8. Kocher M, et al. Adjuvant whole-brain radiotherapy versus observation after radiosurgery or surgical resection of one to three cerebral metastases: results of the EORTC 22952-26001 study. *J Clin Oncol* 2011;29(2):134–141.
9. Patchell RA, et al. Postoperative radiotherapy in the treatment of single metastases to the brain: a randomized trial. *JAMA* 1998;280(17):1485–1489.
10. Brown PD, et al. Postoperative stereotactic radiosurgery compared with whole brain radiotherapy for resected metastatic brain disease (NCCTG N107C/CEC.3): a multicentre, randomised, controlled, phase 3 trial. *Lancet Oncol* 2017;18(8):1049–1060.
11. Andrews DW, et al. Whole brain radiation therapy with or without stereotactic radiosurgery boost for patients with one to three brain metastases: phase III results of the RTOG 9508 randomised trial. *Lancet* 2004;363(9422):1665–1672.
12. Tsao M, Xu W, Sahgal A. A meta-analysis evaluating stereotactic radiosurgery, whole-brain radiotherapy, or both for patients presenting with a limited number of brain metastases. *Cancer* 2012;118(9):2486–2493.
13. Hahn E, et al. Clinical outcomes of hypofractionated radiation therapy for choroidal metastases: symptom palliation, tumor control, and survival. *Pract Radiat Oncol* 2017;7(6):388–395.
14. Shaw E, et al. Single dose radiosurgical treatment of recurrent previously irradiated primary brain tumors and brain metastases: final report of RTOG protocol 90-05. *Int J Radiat Oncol Biol Phys* 2000;47(2):291–298.

15. Dea N, et al. Safety and efficacy of Gamma Knife surgery for brain metastases in eloquent locations. *J Neurosurg* 2010;113(Suppl):79–83.

16. Koyfman SA, et al. Stereotactic radiosurgery for single brainstem metastases: the cleveland clinic experience. *Int J Radiat Oncol Biol Phys* 2010;78(2):409–414.

17. Luther N, et al. Motor function after stereotactic radiosurgery for brain metastases in the region of the motor cortex. *J Neurosurg* 2013;119(3):683–688.

18. Loblaw DA, et al. A 2011 updated systematic review and clinical practice guideline for the management of malignant extradural spinal cord compression. *Int J Radiat Oncol Biol Phys* 2012;84(2):312–317.

19. Loblaw DA, et al. Systematic review of the diagnosis and management of malignant extradural spinal cord compression: the Cancer Care Ontario Practice Guidelines Initiative's Neuro-Oncology Disease Site Group. *J Clin Oncol* 2005;23(9):2028–2037.

20. Rades D, et al. Prognostic factors for local control and survival after radiotherapy of metastatic spinal cord compression. *J Clin Oncol* 2006;24(21):3388–3393.

21. Patchell RA, et al. Direct decompressive surgical resection in the treatment of spinal cord compression caused by metastatic cancer: a randomised trial. *Lancet* 2005;366(9486):643–648.

22. Rades D, et al. Matched pair analysis comparing surgery followed by radiotherapy and radiotherapy alone for metastatic spinal cord compression. *J Clin Oncol* 2010;28(22):3597–3604.

23. Nieder C, et al., Update of human spinal cord reirradiation tolerance based on additional data from 38 patients. *Int J Radiat Oncol Biol Phys* 2006;66(5):1446–1449.

24. Chow E, et al. Predictive model for survival in patients with advanced cancer. *J Clin Oncol* 2008;26(36):5863–5869.

25. Halabi S, et al. Meta-analysis evaluating the impact of site of metastasis on overall survival in men with castration-resistant prostate cancer. *J Clin Oncol* 2016;34(14):1652–1659.

26. Niikura N, et al. Treatment outcome and prognostic factors for patients with bone-only metastases of breast cancer: a single-institution retrospective analysis. *Oncologist* 2011;16(2):155–164.

27. Coleman RE. Metastatic bone disease: clinical features, pathophysiology and treatment strategies. *Cancer Treat Rev* 2001;27(3):165–176.

28. Coleman RE. Clinical features of metastatic bone disease and risk of skeletal morbidity. *Clin Cancer Res* 2006;12(20 Pt 2):6243s–6249s.

29. Costelloe CM, et al. Imaging bone metastases in breast cancer: techniques and recommendations for diagnosis. *Lancet Oncol* 2009;10(6):606–614.

30. Li Y, et al. Factors influencing diagnostic yield of CT-guided percutaneous core needle biopsy for bone lesions. *Clin Radiol* 2014;69(1):e43–e47.

31. Wu JS, et al. Bone and soft-tissue lesions: what factors affect diagnostic yield of image-guided core-needle biopsy? *Radiology* 2008;248(3):962–970.

32. Fisher CG, et al. A novel classification system for spinal instability in neoplastic disease: an evidence-based approach and expert consensus from the Spine Oncology Study Group. *Spine (Phila Pa 1976)* 2010;35(22):E1221–E1229.

33. Tokuhashi Y, et al. A revised scoring system for preoperative evaluation of metastatic spine tumor prognosis. *Spine (Phila Pa 1976)* 2005;30(19):2186–2191.

34. Mirels H. Metastatic disease in long bones: a proposed scoring system for diagnosing impending pathologic fractures. 1989. *Clin Orthop Relat Res* 2003;(415 Suppl):S4–S13.

35. Drost L, et al. Efficacy of postoperative radiation treatment for bone metastases in the extremities. *Radiother Oncol* 2017;124(1):45–48.

36. Willeumier JJ, van der Linden YM, Dijkstra PD. Lack of clinical evidence for postoperative radiotherapy after surgical fixation of impending or actual pathologic fractures in the long bones in patients with cancer; a systematic review. *Radiother Oncol* 2016;121(1):138–142.

37. Chow E, et al. Dexamethasone in the prophylaxis of radiation-induced pain flare after palliative radiotherapy for bone metastases: a double-blind, randomised placebo-controlled, phase 3 trial. *Lancet Oncol* 2015;16(15):1463–1472.

38. Chow R, et al. Efficacy of multiple fraction conventional radiation therapy for painful uncomplicated bone metastases: a systematic review. *Radiother Oncol* 2017;122(3):323–331.

39. Lutz S, et al. Palliative radiation therapy for bone metastases: update of an ASTRO Evidence-Based Guideline. *Pract Radiat Oncol* 2017;7(1):4–12.

40. McDonald R, et al. Effect of radiotherapy on painful bone metastases: a secondary analysis of the NCIC Clinical Trials Group Symptom Control Trial SC 23. *JAMA Oncol* 2017;3(7):953–959.

41. Wong E, et al. Re-irradiation for painful bone metastases—a systematic review. *Radiother Oncol* 2014;110(1):61–70.

42. Chow E, et al. Single versus multiple fractions of repeat radiation for painful bone metastases: a randomised, controlled, non-inferiority trial. *Lancet Oncol* 2014;15(2):164–171.

43. Gomez DR, et al. Local consolidative therapy versus maintenance therapy or observation for patients with oligometastatic non-small-cell lung cancer without progression after first-line systemic therapy: a multicentre, randomised, controlled, phase 2 study. *Lancet Oncol* 2016;17(12):1672–1682.

44. Tree AC, et al. Stereotactic body radiotherapy for oligometastases. *Lancet Oncol* 2013;14(1):e28–e37.

45. Laufer I, et al. The NOMS framework: approach to the treatment of spinal metastatic tumors. *Oncologist* 2013;18(6):744–751.

46. Bilsky MH, et al. Reliability analysis of the epidural spinal cord compression scale. *J Neurosurg Spine* 2010;13(3):324–328.

47. Guckenberger M, et al. Safety and efficacy of stereotactic body radiotherapy as primary treatment for vertebral metastases: a multi-institutional analysis. *Radiat Oncol* 2014;9:226.

48. Huo M, et al. Stereotactic spine radiosurgery: review of safety and efficacy with respect to dose and fractionation. *Surg Neurol Int* 2017;8:30.

49. Chiang A, et al. Pain flare is a common adverse event in steroid-naive patients after spine stereotactic body radiation therapy: a prospective clinical trial. *Int J Radiat Oncol Biol Phys* 2013;86(4):638–642.

50. McDonald R, et al. Incidence of pain flare in radiation treatment of bone metastases: a literature review. *J Bone Oncol* 2014;3(3–4):84–89.

51. Parker C, et al. Alpha emitter radium-223 and survival in metastatic prostate cancer. *N Engl J Med* 2013;369(3):213–223.

52. Sartor O, et al. Effect of radium-223 dichloride on symptomatic skeletal events in patients with castration-resistant prostate cancer and bone metastases: results from a phase 3, double-blind, randomised trial. *Lancet Oncol* 2014;15(7):738–746.

53. Finlay IG, Mason MD, Shelley M. Radioisotopes for the palliation of metastatic bone cancer: a systematic review. *Lancet Oncol* 2005;6(6):392–400.

54. Cox BW, et al. International Spine Radiosurgery Consortium consensus guidelines for target volume definition in spinal stereotactic radiosurgery. *Int J Radiat Oncol Biol Phys* 2012;83(5):e597–e605.

55. Redmond KJ, et al. Consensus contouring guidelines for postoperative stereotactic body radiation therapy for metastatic solid tumor malignancies to the spine. *Int J Radiat Oncol Biol Phys* 2017;97(1):64–74.

56. Li W, et al. Impact of immobilization on intrafraction motion for spine stereotactic body radiotherapy using cone beam computed tomography. *Int J Radiat Oncol Biol Phys* 2012;84(2):520–526.

57. Tseng CL, et al. Magnetic resonance imaging assessment of spinal cord and cauda equina motion in supine patients with spinal metastases planned for spine stereotactic body radiation therapy. *Int J Radiat Oncol Biol Phys* 2015;91(5):995–1002.

58. Rice TW, Rodriguez RM, Light RW. The superior vena cava syndrome: clinical characteristics and evolving etiology. *Medicine (Baltimore)* 2006;85(1):37–42.

59. Rowell NP, Gleeson FV. Steroids, radiotherapy, chemotherapy and stents for superior vena caval obstruction in carcinoma of the bronchus: a systematic review. *Clin Oncol* 2002;14(5):338–351.

60. Rodrigues G, et al. Palliative thoracic radiotherapy in lung cancer: an American Society for Radiation Oncology evidence-based clinical practice guideline. *Pract Radiat Oncol* 2011;1(2):60–71.

61. Bezjak A, et al. Randomized phase III trial of single versus fractionated thoracic radiation in the palliation of patients with lung cancer (NCIC CTG SC.15). *Int J Radiat Oncol Biol Phys* 2002;54(3):719–728.

62. Macbeth FR, et al. Radiation myelopathy: estimates of risk in 1048 patients in three randomized trials of palliative radiotherapy for non-small cell lung cancer. The Medical Research Council Lung Cancer Working Party. *Clin Oncol (R Coll Radiol)* 1996;8(3):176–181.

63. Hong TS, et al. Phase II study of proton-based stereotactic body radiation therapy for liver metastases: importance of tumor genotype. *J Natl Cancer Inst* 2017;109(9).

64. Lee MT, et al. Phase I study of individualized stereotactic body radiotherapy of liver metastases. *J Clin Oncol* 2009;27(10):1585–1591.

65. Hoyer M, et al. Radiotherapy for liver metastases: a review of evidence. *Int J Radiat Oncol Biol Phys* 2012;82(3):1047–1057.

66. Kavanagh BD, et al. Interim analysis of a prospective phase I/II trial of SBRT for liver metastases. *Acta Oncol* 2006;45(7):848–855.

67. Soliman H, et al. Phase II trial of palliative radiotherapy for hepatocellular carcinoma and liver metastases. *J Clin Oncol* 2013;31(31):3980–3986.

68. Inoperable non-small-cell lung cancer (NSCLC): a Medical Research Council randomised trial of palliative radiotherapy with two fractions or ten fractions. Report to the Medical Research Council by its Lung Cancer Working Party. *Br J Cancer* 1991;63(2):265–270.

69. A Medical Research Council (MRC) randomised trial of palliative radiotherapy with two fractions or a single fraction in patients with inoperable non-small-cell lung cancer (NSCLC) and poor performance status. Medical Research Council Lung Cancer Working Party. *Br J Cancer* 1992;65(6):934–941.

70. Pereira J, Phan T. Management of bleeding in patients with advanced cancer. *Oncologist* 2004;9(5):561–570.

71. Cameron MG, et al. Palliative pelvic radiotherapy for symptomatic incurable prostate cancer—a prospective multicenter study. *Radiother Oncol* 2015;115(3):314–320.

72. van Lonkhuijzen L, Thomas G. Palliative radiotherapy for cervical carcinoma, a systematic review. *Radiother Oncol* 2011;98(3):287–291.

73. Yan, J., et al. A hypofractionated radiotherapy regimen (0-7-21) for advanced gynaecological cancer patients. *Clin Oncol (R Coll Radiol)* 2011;23(7):476–481.

CHAPTER 49

PAIN MANAGEMENT IN RADIATION ONCOLOGY

INTRODUCTION

- Managing pain in cancer patients is a fundamental component of comprehensive oncologic care. Poorly controlled or uncontrolled pain can lead to significant psychologic and spiritual distress (1,2).
- Pain is common in patients with cancer. Initial prevalence studies found that approximately 30% to 50% of cancer patients undergoing treatment for their disease and up to 90% of patients with advanced cancer have pain severe enough to warrant opioid therapy (3,4).
- Pain can be classified, taxonomically, as nociceptive (somatic or visceral), neuropathic, idiopathic, or psychogenic.
- Pain in cancer patients is most often a result of direct effects of the tumor (e.g., bony metastases or plexopathy); less commonly, it is due to complications of cancer therapy (e.g., radiation-induced mucositis or chemotherapy-induced neuropathy) or unrelated to the cancer or its treatment (e.g., chronic, nonmalignant musculoskeletal back pain).
- Optimal pain management requires ongoing clinical assessments, knowledge of basic opioid pharmacology, management of opioid-related side effects, and use of adjuvant analgesics, as appropriate.
- There are a number of nonpharmacologic and integrative approaches (e.g., meditation, cognitive behavioral therapy, yoga, etc.) that can be offered in conjunction with pharmacotherapy, though with various levels of evidence supporting their use in the treatment of cancer-related pain.
- Interventional procedures, for example, spinal drug delivery and neurolytic blocks, are supported by controlled trials and should be considered in select patients, but are beyond the scope of this chapter.

ASSESSMENT

- A comprehensive assessment of the patient's pain includes a thorough history of the pain complaint (Table 49-1); physical exam, including a detailed neurologic exam; and a review of the relevant laboratory and radiologic studies performed.

Table 49-1	
Pain History	
Location	Where is the pain?
Onset	When did the pain start?
Quality	Can you describe the pain? (Try not to give leading descriptors; allow the patient to answer)
Radiation	Does it move anywhere? (If yes, where?)
Severity	"On a scale of 0 to 10, with 0 being no pain and 10 being the worst pain you could imagine, how would you rate your pain currently?" "How would you rate the pain at its worst in the last 24 hours?"
Timing	"Is it constant or intermittent?"
Alleviating Factors	"What makes the pain better?"
Aggravating Factors	"What makes the pain worse?"
Impact	"How has the pain impacted your life?" "What has it prevented you from accomplishing?"

- *Nociceptive somatic pain (e.g., bony metastases)* is sustained predominantly by tissue injury or inflammation. It is often described as "sharp," "aching," "stabbing," "throbbing," or "pressure."
- *Nociceptive visceral pain* is often poorly localized; it is described as "crampy" pain (e.g., obstruction of hollow viscus) or as "aching" and "stabbing" (e.g., pain secondary to splenomegaly).
- *Neuropathic pain* is sustained by abnormal somatosensory processing in the PNS (peripheral nervous system) or CNS (central nervous system). It is typically described as "burning," "shocklike," and "electrical," but may also be "sharp" or "stabbing." It often occurs in a paroxysmal fashion. On physical examination, patients may have allodynia (pain induced by nonpainful stimuli) and hyperalgesia (increased perception of painful stimuli).
- *Psychogenic pain* refers to pain that is believed to be sustained predominantly by psychologic factors. It is rarely seen in the cancer population.
- In the absence of evidence sufficient to label pain as either nociceptive or neuropathic, we may use the term *idiopathic*. In patients with cancer, so-called *idiopathic pain* should lead to additional workup and a search for an underlying etiology and pathophysiology.
- The clinician should evaluate the impact that the pain has on the patient's functioning, social roles, psychologic coping, and spiritual well-being.
- The degree of pain perceived by each patient will be influenced by comorbid psychiatric disorders (including anxiety, depression), perceived lack of benefit of analgesics based on past experiences, existential or spiritual distress, acuity of illness, and personal or family history of previous drug use (whether illicit drugs or opioids). A thorough exploration of this history is essential.
- Past pharmacotherapy and use of other therapeutics should be reviewed. Both their analgesic affect and side effects should be assessed.

Mitigating Risk

- The opioid crisis in the United States, with high rates of overdoses, has been the subject of a national debate and has led to public health strategies seeking to reduce the use of opioids in chronic nonmalignant pain.
- Although cancer pain management is generally not included in these public health guidelines to mitigate risk and overprescribing, for example, the CDC Guideline for Prescribing Opioids for Chronic Pain (5), the need to assess patients with cancer-related pain for risks of opioid misuse remains. Clinicians should employ simple tools (e.g., Opioid Risk Tool) to identify patients who may be at higher risk, for example, younger patients and patients with a personal or family history of substance abuse or alcoholism or comorbid psychologic conditions.
- Identification of aberrant drug-taking behaviors is an important aspect of the assessment. These behaviors include asking for or demanding more medication or specific medications, hoarding, selling medications, seeing multiple prescribers to obtain pain medications, etc. Some behaviors (e.g., selling medications) may be more likely to be associated with medication abuse or addiction than others (e.g., asking for a specific dose of hydromorphone), which may be associated with inadequate analgesia, or so-called pseudoaddiction. Patients with significant psychopathology may also demonstrate these behaviors. Comanagement with experts in pain, palliative care, and addiction is sometimes necessary, especially when initial management strategies are not successful at mitigating the behaviors, or the patient is at high risk for misuse per screening tool.
- For patients already on opioid therapy, evaluation of the "4As" (analgesia, adverse effects, aberrant drug-taking behaviors, and activities of daily living), developed by Passik and Portnoy, can be a helpful heuristic to use for ongoing assessment and documentation of a patient with chronic pain (6).

PHARMACOLOGIC TREATMENT OF CANCER PAIN

- When formulating a cancer pain treatment plan, it is important to consider the underlying pathophysiology—nociceptive somatic, nociceptive visceral, or neuropathic—as this will provide the clinician with a rationale for choosing particular therapies (Table 49-2).
- The main classes of medications used to treat cancer-related pain are nonopioid analgesics (e.g., acetaminophen), nonsteroidal anti-inflammatory drugs (NSAIDs), opioids, anticonvulsants, antidepressants, bisphosphonates, and steroids.
- The WHO (World Health Organization) has developed a stepwise approach that has served as a basic guide for the management of cancer-related pain. Recent modification of this "analgesic ladder" now incorporates interventional approaches (nerve blocks, epidurals) and neurosurgical procedures. In short, the approach moves in a stepwise approach—up or down the ladder—depending on the acute or chronic nature of the pain. For acute pain or the management of a pain crisis, an epidural or

Table 49-2

Etiology of Cancer-Related Pain and Suggested Pharmacotherapy and Other Treatments

Etiology of Pain	Treatment Options	Indications	Contraindications/Cautions	Notable Adverse Effects
Nociceptive somatic (e.g., constant, localized, changing with movement) For example, bone metastases, wounds, soft tissue tumors, arthritis	**NSAIDs** *Naproxen 500 mg PO Q8H (max 1,500 mg QD) Ibuprofen 400–800 mg PO Q6–8 H (max 3,200 mg QD)*	Mild to moderate pain	Renal/hepatic impairment, history of gastrointestinal (GI) bleed	Gastrointestinal (gastritis, bleed), renal insufficiency, cardiac
	Acetaminophen *Acetaminophen 325–650 mg PO Q4–6H (max 4 g QD)*	Mild to moderate pain	Excessive dosing may lead to liver toxicity	Liver toxicity
	Bisphosphonates *Pamidronate 60–90 mg IV infused over 90–120 min Zoledronate 4 mg IV over 15 min*	Bone metastases	Avoid zoledronate, as higher dosages are associated with increased creatinine	Nausea, fever, renal dysfunction, hypocalcemia, and rarely osteonecrosis of the jaw
	Corticosteroids *Dexamethasone 1–4 mg PO/SC/IV BID-TID (max 16 mg QD)*	Metastases	Consider time-limited trial, given multiple adverse effects with long-term use; also be mindful of potential for adrenal insufficiency in the context of rapid withdrawal or tapering	Short-term: impaired glucose control, thrush, dyspepsia, insomnia, delirium, anxiety, HTN, immunosuppression Long-term: Cushingoid habitus, proximal myopathy, osteoporosis, and aseptic necrosis
	Opioids	Moderate to severe pain	Caution in opioid-naïve patients, or patients with renal or hepatic insufficiency	Sedation, nausea, constipation, rarely respiratory arrest

	Intervention	Indication	Side effects / comments
	Nerve Blocks		
	Peripheral nerve or plexus block	Somatic pain in discrete dermatomes	Rash, pruritus, injection site soreness, bleeding, infection
	Ganglion impar block	Pain originating from anorectal area or lower part of the vagina	Less common but more severe: nerve injury, local anesthetic systemic toxicity (LAST) ranging from mild systemic symptoms to central nervous system and cardiovascular events
	Radiopharmaceuticals		
	Strontium-89, samarium-153	Multiple, painful osteoblastic lesions	
	Surgery		
	Orthopedic procedures (decompressive surgery)	Spinal cord metastases, hip fracture repair, and fracture fixation	
Nociceptive visceral (e.g., deep, aching, cramping, poorly localized) For example, bowel obstruction, bulky liver metastases	**Anticholinergics**		
	Scopolamine 1 patch	Caution in elderly patients	Delirium, lethargy, constipation, urinary retention
	Hyoscyamine 0.125–0.25 mg PO/SC/IV Q4H (max 12 tabs QD)		Same as above, but often better tolerated
	Glycopyrrolate 0.2–0.4 mg IV/SC Q4H PRN		Same as above, but often better tolerated. Glycopyrrolate does not cross the blood-brain barrier

continued

Table 49-2

Etiology of Cancer-Related Pain and Suggested Pharmacotherapy and Other Treatments *(continued)*

Etiology of Pain	Treatment Options	Indications	Contraindications/Cautions	Notable Adverse Effects
	Opioids			
	See section on opioid dosing	Moderate to severe pain	Caution in opioid-naïve patients, or patients with renal or hepatic insufficiency	Sedation, nausea, constipation, rarely respiratory arrest
	Nerve Blocks			
	Celiac plexus	Pain from upper abdominal viscera: pancreas, gallbladder, liver, mesentery, GI tract from the stomach to transverse colon, and adrenal glands		
	Hypogastric plexus	Pain from pelvic viscera: descending and sigmoid colon, rectum, bladder, testes, uterus, and ovaries		
	External Beam Radiation Therapy			
		Solitary, localized lesions; painful bony, visceral, or cutaneous disease; spinal cord compression; brain metastases		Myelosuppression, upper field—alopecia, radiation pneumonitis, lower field—nausea, vomiting, diarrhea
	Surgery			
	Vascular procedures (stenting, amputation)	Peripheral arterial disease		

Neuropathic (e.g., burning, shooting, tingling, shocklike) For example, postherpetic neuralgia, diabetic neuropathy, compression radiculopathies	**Tricyclic Antidepressants (TCAs)**		
	Nortriptyline or desipramine, start at 10–25 mg QHS (nortriptyline max 150 mg QD, desipramine 300 mg QD); increase every 3–7 days as tolerated	Can be helpful adjunctive medication in patients with comorbid depression	Sedation, anticholinergic effects, cardiac arrhythmias
		Avoid if patient is too sedated at baseline, as it can be very sedating. Monitor QT interval with initiation of therapy and with dosage changes. Be mindful of potential drug-drug interactions	
	Selective Serotonin and Norepinephrine Reuptake Inhibitors (SNRIs)		
	Venlafaxine 37.5 mg QD; increase by 37.5–75 mg Q week as tolerated (max 225 mg QD)	Caution in patients with hepatic impairment, decrease dosage in patients with renal impairment and avoid duloxetine if CrCl < 30 mL/min	Nausea
	Duloxetine start at 30 mg QD; titrate to 60 mg after a week if tolerated	Decrease dosage in patients with renal impairment, as 90%–100% is excreted through urine	Sedation, peripheral edema, dizziness
	Anticonvulsants		
	Gabapentin 100–300 mg QHS; increase as tolerated (max 3,600 mg QD) Pregabalin 25–50 mg TID (max 600 mg QD in divided doses)		
	Opioids		
	See section on opioid dosing	Moderate to severe pain, adjunctive therapy	Caution in opioid-naive patients, or patients with renal or hepatic insufficiency	Sedation, nausea, constipation, rarely respiratory arrest

continued

Table 49-2

Etiology of Cancer-Related Pain and Suggested Pharmacotherapy and Other Treatments (*continued*)

Etiology of Pain	Treatment Options	Indications	Contraindications/Cautions	Notable Adverse Effects
	Topical Analgesics			
	Lidocaine patch TD 5%, 1–3 patches up to 12 h/day		Caution for lidocaine in advanced liver failure secondary to decreased clearance	Rash, local erythema (lidocaine), burning sensation (capsaicin)
	Capsaicin cream			
	Spinal Infusions			
	Epidural opioid +/– bupivacaine +/– clonidine	Chest wall pain over several dermatomes, abdominal pain, lumbosacral pain, perineal pain, and lower extremity pain		Ambulation can be compromised for patients for lumbosacral and lower extremity involvement
	Intrathecal opioid +/– bupivacaine +/– clonidine	Same indications as epidural infusions		Associated with more numbness and weakness
	Surgery			
	Neurosurgical ablative procedures (cordotomy, trigeminal tractotomy)			

Adapted from Quill T, Bower K, Holloway RG, et al, eds. *Primer for palliative care*, 6th ed. Chicago, IL: American Academy of Hospice and Palliative Medicine, 2014:36–40.

patient-controlled analgesia (PCA) may be considered first, with subsequent addition of nonopioid analgesics and adjuvants to supplement (Fig. 49-1).

- Indeed, acute cancer-related pain in the setting of progression of disease (e.g., new pleuritic pain from pleural metastases) or complication (e.g., pathologic fracture) should be managed with IV opioids.
- Frequent bolus doses with rapid adjustments to reach a satisfactory degree of analgesia are recommended. The National Comprehensive Cancer Network (NCCN) has proposed a rational consensus guideline (7) for assessment and management of acute cancer pain that can be applied as a standard practice. See http://www.jnccn.org/content/11/8/992.full.pdf+html.
- The use of patient-controlled analgesic devices, by those trained to use them, may offer another effective way to quickly and safely mitigate the severity of pain while optimizing patient control.
- The general prescribing principles for cancer-related pain include selecting the proper drug, dosing to optimize effects, treating opioid-related side effects, and managing the poorly responsive patient.
- Drug selection should include patient preference and experience, availability of appropriate dosing forms and routes of administration (e.g., fentanyl TD may not be well absorbed in very thin patients because of lack of adipose tissue), drug pharmacokinetics (e.g., avoiding morphine in patients with renal failure), and cost.
- In an opioid-naïve patient, a short-acting opioid, for example, oral oxycodone 5 to 10 mg, or morphine 15 mg, can be prescribed *as needed* every 1 to 4 hours for moderate to severe cancer-related pain. A long-acting opioid formulation can then be initiated equal to

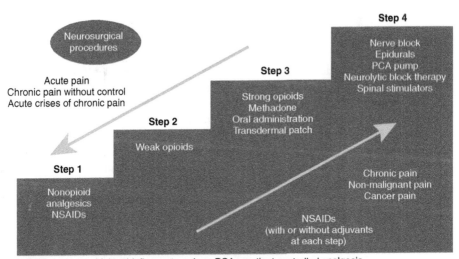

NSAID – nonsteroidal anti-inflammatory drug, PCA – patient-controlled analgesia

FIGURE 49-1. The World Health Organization analgesic ladder for treating cancer pain. (Reprinted with permission from Vargas-Schaffer G. Is the WHO analgesic ladder still valid? *Can Fam Physician* 2010;56(6):514–517; originally adapted from World Health Organization. *Traitement de la douleur cancéreuse.* Geneva, Switzerland: World Health Organization, 1987.)

75% to 100% of the 24-hour dose of short-acting opioid used to achieve acceptable analgesia. Continuation of a short-acting opioid equal to 10% to 25% of the 24-hour dose of the background, i.e., long-acting opioid therapy, is often suggested. For example, a patient using oxycodone 5 mg four to five times per day with good analgesic effect can be started on OxyContin 10 mg BID with oxycodone 5 mg as needed every 1 to 4 hours for "rescue doses" for episodic worsening of pain, or breakthrough pain.

- Transdermal fentanyl is generally used for stable, chronic pain in patients that have been tolerant to at least 30 mg of oral morphine equivalent daily dose. The patient should be counseled that it takes up to 12 to 24 hours for onset and discontinuation of action. Heat (e.g., fevers, hot temperatures), hydration, and nutritional status may affect absorption.
- Transmucosal Immediate Release Fentanyl (TIRF) products (e.g., Actiq, Fentora, Onsolis, Abstral, Lazanda, and Subsys) are FDA indicated, and have the most evidence for use in the opioid-tolerant cancer patient with breakthrough pain (8). These medications are individually dosed for the patient. The medications are generally applied to the mucosa of either the buccal or nasal cavity for rapid absorption given fentanyl's lipophilic nature. They have a short onset and duration of action and may be particularly helpful in patients in whom nausea, esophagitis, or gastritis from radiation treatment may affect oral dosing.
- Several strategies exist to manage the poorly opioid-responsive patient: better management of adverse effects, adoption of pharmacologic strategies to lower the opioid requirement (e.g., spinal route of administration or addition of a nonopioid or adjuvant analgesic), consideration of rotation to another opioid, or implementation of a nonpharmacologic strategy (e.g., biofeedback) to lower the opioid requirement.

MANAGEMENT OF NEUROPATHIC PAIN

- Neuropathic pain is defined by the 2008 International Association for the Study of Pain (IASP) as "pain caused by a lesion or disease of the somatosensory system." (9) It can be especially challenging to address as the targets of current treatments are directed toward nerves with pathologic responses to noxious and nonnoxious stimuli.
- Current evidence recommends a multimodal approach, utilizing four main classes of medications: antidepressants, anticonvulsants, opioids, and topical agents. Table 49-2 outlines these agents with modes of action and duration of treatment. Although there is no consensus on which combinations are most effective, studies have shown that the addition of oxycodone to gabapentin (10), morphine to gabapentin (11), nortriptyline to gabapentin (12), and topical lidocaine to pregabalin (13) is more effective at lower combined doses than as single agents.
- Among antidepressants, tricyclic antidepressants (TCAs) and serotonin and norepinephrine reuptake inhibitors (SNRIs) have been most effective in patients with neuropathic pain and comorbid depression, particularly in the setting of diabetic neuropathy, nerve injury, postherpetic neuralgia, and central poststroke pain. Selective serotonin reuptake inhibitors, on the other hand, have not been shown to be effective in the treatment of neuropathic pain (14).

- A significant degree of variation exists among patients, as does their responsiveness to different analgesics and combinations thereof. As such, it is not uncommon to give trials of the aforementioned medications and to periodically assess for the degree of analgesia and uptitrate medications as indicated, as well as to monitor for adverse effects.
- Typically, trials with TCAs are conducted over 6 to 8 weeks, with at least 2 weeks at the maximum tolerated dose, whereas trials with SNRIs are conducted over 4 to 5 weeks. Anticonvulsants and opioids can be trialed for up to 4 weeks, whereas topical agents can be trialed for up to 2 weeks.

MANAGEMENT OF BONE PAIN

- Opioid therapy is the mainstay for managing pain because of bony metastases, but is often used in combination with adjuvant analgesics.
- Adjuvant analgesics for bone pain include NSAIDs, corticosteroids, bisphosphonates (15,16), and the radiopharmaceuticals, strontium chloride (^{89}Sr) (17) and samarium lexidronam (^{153}Sm) (18).
- Multiple studies have demonstrated the efficacy of bisphosphonates in reducing skeletal complications and pain from bone metastases. Pamidronate and zoledronate are recommended in patients with multiple myeloma and other malignancies with painful bone lesions. It should be noted that the long-term use of bisphosphonates is associated with a small, but meaningful, risk of osteonecrosis of the jaw.
- The limitations of radiopharmaceuticals include their cost and the potential for development of cytopenias. As such, their use is typically limited to patients with refractory multifocal bone pain whose blood counts are adequate and are not expected to require myelosuppressive chemotherapy in the near future.

Management of Opioid-Related Side Effects

- There are certain predictable side effects of opioid use, which can be anticipated and managed accordingly.
- The most common side effects include constipation, nausea, pruritus, and sedation, with the development of tolerance to all opioid side effects while on a stable opioid dose, except for constipation.
- Tolerance to sedation typically occurs within 36 to 72 hours, whereas tolerance to nausea and pruritus usually occurs within 7 to 10 days (19).

Constipation

- As patients with cancer often have a multifactorial etiology of constipation, and the incidence of opioid-induced constipation is high, the current recommendation is to initiate a bowel regimen in any patient on opioids.
- Although extensive detail regarding the various pharmacologic agents to treat constipation is beyond the scope of this chapter, it can be helpful to keep a few principles in mind:
  - The goal of laxative therapy is to achieve comfortable defecation every 1 to 2 days.
  - An escalation of laxatives is recommended every 2 days, if constipation is refractory to initial treatment.

- The major categories of laxative therapies that are recommended are stool soften-ers (*docusate sodium*), osmotic or surfactant laxatives (*lactulose, sorbitol, magnesium citrate, polyethylene glycol*), stimulant laxatives (*senna, bisacodyl*), rectal laxatives (*suppositories and enemas for refractory constipation*), and peripherally acting mu-opioid receptor antagonists (PAMORAs) methylnaltrexone, naloxegol, and nadlemedine.
- Though evidence is lacking, a standard bowel regimen in use is docusate sodium 100 mg orally three times daily with senna 1 or 2 tabs every night. Addition of an osmotic or surfactant laxative to senna and docusate sodium is often suggested when constipa-tion persists.
- PAMORAs should be considered in patients who are refractory to standard laxa-tive therapy, e.g., methylnaltrexone 8-12mg (dosing is weight based) subcutaneously every other day.

Nausea

- Nausea is a common, but fortunately often time-limited, adverse effect of opioid therapy. As such, it is important to both manage and to educate patients about it, in order to reduce the likelihood of refusal or early termination of a given opioid.
- Opioid-induced nausea is believed to be caused by stimulation of dopaminergic and serotonergic activation in the chemoreceptor trigger zone (CTZ) within the area pos-trema of the brain. Activation of receptors in the area postrema leads to stimulation of the vomiting center, resulting in nausea and emesis.
- Applying a systematic approach based on the most likely underlying etiology of nausea, the most commonly agents used to treat CTZ-induced nausea are ondanse-tron or other 5-HT3 receptor antagonists and haloperidol (which acts on dopamine receptors).

Pruritus

- Although not typical, some patients may experience pruritus. Although the effect often self-resolves, patients can be treated with diphenhydramine or other antihista-mines as needed.
- Morphine tends to be more pruritogenic than other opioids by inducing the release of histamine from mast cells.

Sedation

- Sedation can be concerning for some patients (e.g., those with tenuous respiratory status) and not as concerning for others (e.g., those who have insomnia secondary to chronic pain). The depressant effects of opioids on the central nervous system have been well-studied, and although this effect is likely to resolve over time, it requires vigilant monitoring and management.
- Experienced providers recognize opioid-induced sedation prior to the development of respiratory arrest, which allows for dose titration.
- Once a patient is sedated, opioid dosages can be decreased by 25% to 50%, or the dosage intervals can be increased (e.g., from every 4 hours to every 8 hours).

Neurotoxicity

- Myoclonus, hyperalgesia, seizures, and delirium are examples of opioid-induced neurotoxicity and upon occurrence should lead to discontinuation of the opioid, administration of intravenous fluids, and rotation to an equianalgesic dose of another opioid.

Respiratory Depression

- Although rare in cancer patients being titrated rationally with opioids, opioid-induced respiratory depression may occur.
- Patients at higher risk are those with comorbid pulmonary disease, for example, chronic obstructive pulmonary disease (COPD) or idiopathic pulmonary fibrosis (IPF), or patients using other sedatives, for example, benzodiazepines. Patients on methadone may have higher risk as well.
- Respiratory depression or opioid overdose is defined by inability to be aroused to verbal or tactile stimuli *or* O_2 saturation less than 90% *OR* greater than 5% drop from baseline (if less than 90% normally) *AND* a respiratory rate less than 8/minute.
- When treating respiratory depression, the goal is to reverse sedation and the respiratory depressant effects of the opioids without reversing analgesia.
- In hospital settings, the provider can dilute 1 ampule of naloxone (0.04 mg/mL) with 9 cc of sterile saline and push 1 to 2 cc (0.04 to 0.08 mg) every 1 to 2 minutes until the patient wakes up. Naloxone only lasts 45 to 60 minutes, so an infusion may be needed if the patient is on a long-acting opioid.
- A prescription for naloxone nasal spray be warranted in patients on high doses of opioids or those with higher risk of overdose because of comorbid diseases or polypharmacy.

Opioid Rotation

- For the patient who is having a poor response to the initial opioid despite appropriate titration, intolerable adverse effects, or renal and/or hepatic dysfunction, rotation to another opioid may be appropriate, as there is a large intraindividual variation in response to different opioids.
- The respective potency of one opioid to another can be approximated by using an equianalgesic table (Table 49-3).
- Given that patients may have incomplete cross-tolerance (i.e., the new drug may be more effective because of differences in potency or drug bioavailability), when converting to a different opioid, the equianalgesic dose should be reduced by 25% to 50%.
- For example, a patient receiving hydromorphone 4 mg by mouth every 6 hours, but develops significant sedation, can be rotated to morphine in the following way: hydromorphone 4 mg × 4 doses/24 hours = hydromorphone 16 mg/24 hours, which is roughly equivalent to 64 mg of oral morphine. When reducing for incomplete cross-tolerance by 25%, the resulting dose is 48 mg of morphine. Thus, the patient may be started on morphine ER 15 mg PO TID.

Table 49-3

Relative Potencies (Equianalgesic Doses) and Duration of Action of Opioid Analgesics

Opioid Agonist	Parenteral Dose (IV/SC/IM)	Oral/Rectal Dose	PO:IV Ratio	Duration of Action (hours)
Morphine	10 mg	30 mg	3:1	3–4
Morphine, long-acting (MS Contin, Avinza, Kadian)	—	30 mg	—	8–12
Hydrocodone	—	30–45 mg	—	3–5
Oxycodone	—	20 mg	—	3–5
Oxycodone, long-acting (OxyContin)	—	20 mg	—	12
Oxymorphone (Opana)	1 mg	10 mg	10:1	3–6
Oxymorphone, long-acting (Opana ER)	—	10 mg	—	12
Hydromorphone (Dilaudid)	1.5 mg	7.5 mg	5:1	2–3
Codeine	130 mg	200 mg	1.5:1	4
Fentanyl[a]	0.1 mg (100 µg)	—	—	1–2
Methadone[b]	—	—	—	—

[a]When rotating from a continuous fentanyl infusion, use an equianalgesic ratio of 100 µg/h of fentanyl to 4 mg/h of morphine intravenously. Fentanyl can also be administered as a transdermal patch; when rotating from morphine to transdermal fentanyl, divide the oral morphine equivalent daily dose in milligrams by 2 for the equianalgesic dose of transdermal fentanyl in micrograms per hour. The duration of action of transdermal fentanyl is 48 to 72 hours.

[b]Methadone has a complicated pharmacodynamic and pharmacokinetic profile that makes equianalgesic dosing difficult. Consult with an experienced clinician before initiating or adjusting doses of methadone.

Strategies for Refractory Pain

- More invasive options of achieving analgesia exist, including ketamine, lidocaine, and epidural infusions, intrathecal pumps, peripheral nerve blocks, neurolytic sympathetic blocks, and neurosurgical procedures (e.g., myelotomy).
- For refractory pain at the end of life, palliative sedation may be considered.
- These options are beyond the scope of this chapter, but referral to a pain or palliative care specialist would be warranted in cases of refractory pain.

References

1. Massie MJ, Holland JC. The cancer patient with pain: psychiatric complications and their management. *Med Clin North Am* 1987;71:243–258.
2. Cleeland CS. The impact of pain on the patient with cancer. *Cancer* 1984;54:2635–2641.
3. Kanner RM. The scope of the problem. In: Portenoy RK, Kanner RM, eds. *Pain management: theory and practice.* Philadelphia, PA: FA Davis, 1996:40.

4. Vainio A, Auvinen A. Prevalence of symptoms among patients with advanced cancer: an international collaborative study. *J Pain Symptom Manage* 1996;12:3–10; World Health Organization. *Cancer pain relief with a guide to opioid availability*, 2nd ed. Geneva, Switzerland: World Health Organization, 1996.

5. https://www.cdc.gov/mmwr/volumes/65/rr/rr6501e1.htm

6. Passik SD, Weinreb HJ. Managing chronic nonmalignant pain: overcoming obstacles to the use of opioids. *Adv Ther* 2000;17:70–80.

7. https://www.nccn.org/

8. Brant JM, et al. Breakthrough cancer pain: a systematic review of pharmacologic management. *Clin J Oncol Nurs* 2017;21(3):71–80.

9. Jensen TS, Baron R, Haanpaa M, et al. A new definition of neuropathic pain. *Pain* 2011;152:2204–2205.

10. Hanna M, O'Brien C, Wilson MC. Prolonged-release oxycodone enhances the effects of existing gabapentin therapy in painful diabetic neuropathy patients. *Eur J Pain* 2008;12:804–813.

11. Gilron I, Bailey JM, Tu D, et al. Morphine, gabapentin, or their combination for neuropathic pain. *N Engl J Med* 2005;352:1324–1334.

12. Gilron I, Bailey JM, Tu D, et al. Nortriptyline and gabapentin, alone and in combination for neuropathic pain: a double-blind, randomised controlled crossover trial. *Lancet* 2009;374(9697):1252–1261.

13. Baron R, Mayoral V, Leijon G, et al. Efficacy and safety of combination therapy with 5% lidocaine medicated plaster and pregabalin in post-herpetic neuralgia and diabetic polyneuropathy. *Curr Med Res Opin* 2009;25:1677–1687.

14. Hwang U, Wattana M, Todd KH. *Evidence-based practice of palliative medicine*, 1st ed. Philadelphia, PA: Elsevier Saunders, 2013:55–56.

15. Cascinu S, Graziano F, Alessandroni P et al. Different doses of pamidronate in patients with painful osteolytic bone metastases. *Support Care Cancer* 1998;6:139–143.

16. Finley RS. Bisphosphonates in the treatment of bone metastases. *Semin Oncol* 2002;129(Suppl 4):132.

17. Robinson RG, Preston DF, Baxter KG et al. Clinical experience with strontium-89 in prostatic and breast cancer patients. *Semin Oncol* 1993;20(Suppl 2):44.

18. Serafini AN, Houston SJ, Resche I et al. Palliation of pain associated with metastatic bone cancer using samarium-153 lexidronam: a double-blind placebo-controlled trial. *J Clin Oncol* 1998;16:1574–1581.

19. Goldberg GR, Smith CB. *Evidence-based practice of palliative medicine*, 1st ed. Philadelphia, PA: Elsevier Saunders, 2013:5.

COMMONLY PRESCRIBED DRUGS

Antibiotics

Name	Usual Dose	Comments
Amoxicillin	• 250–500 mg t.i.d. • Tablet 125, 250 mg • Liquid 125, 250 mg/5 mL	Commonly used for ear, nose, and throat or skin infections from *Streptococcus pneumoniae, Staphylococcus* spp., or *Haemophilus influenzae*
Amoxicillin/clavulanate potassium (Augmentin)	• 250–500 mg t.i.d., 875 mg b.i.d • Tablet 250, 500, and 875 mg • Liquid 125, 200, 250, 400 mg/5 mL	Commonly used for acute sinusitis, skin and UTI infected with beta-lacta-mase–producing strains of *S. aureus, Escherichia coli,* and *Klebsiella* spp.
Amoxicillin/clavulanate (Augmentin)	• Tablet 1,000 mg b.i.d.	
Azithromycin (Z-pak)	As directed	Commonly used for acute bacterial sinusitis, pelvic inflammatory disease, community-acquired pneumonia, uncomplicated skin infections
Bacitracin	Topical, OTC apply b.i.d., t.i.d.	
Sulfamethoxazole/trimethoprim (Bactrim DS)	800 mg/160 mg 1–2 b.i.d.	UTI uncomplicated: 3–5 d Pyelonephritis: 14 d Skin: 10 d
Cephalexin (Keflex)	• 500 mg b.i.d., max 4 g daily • Tablet 250, 500, 750 mg • Liquid 125, 250 mg/5 mL	Cystitis uncomplicated: 7–14 d
Ciprofloxacin (Cipro)	• Tablet 250–750 mg b.i.d. • ER tablet 500, 1,000 mg q.d. • IR tablet 250, 500, 750 mg	Prostatitis: 500 mg b.i.d. 6 wk UTI uncomplicated: • IR 250 mg b.i.d. 3 d • ER 500 q.d. 3 d UTI complicated: • IR 250 mg b.i.d. 7 d • ER 1,000 q.d. 7 d

continued

Antibiotics *(continued)*

Name	Usual Dose	Comments
Clarithromycin (Biaxin)	• 250, 500 mg b.i.d. • 1,000 mg q.d. • Tablet 250, 500 mg	Bronchitis: 250 mg b.i.d. 7–14 d 1,000 mg q.d. 7 d Pharyngitis: 250 mg b.i.d. 10 d Skin: 250 mg b.i.d. 7–14 d
Clindamycin (Cleocin)	• 150–450 mg q.i.d. • Capsule 75, 150, 300 mg	Skin MSSA, nonaerobic coverage 300–450 mg q6h 7–14 d
Levofloxacin (Levaquin)	• 500–750 mg q.d. • Tablet 250, 500, 750 mg • Liquid 25 mg/mL	Prostatitis chronic: 500 mg q.d. 4 wk Skin uncomplicated: 500 mg q.d. 10 d Skin complicated: 750 mg q.d. 14 d UTI uncomplicated: 250 mg q.d. 3 d UTI complicated: 250 mg q.d. 10 d 750 q.d. 7 d
Mupirocin (Bactroban)	Topical, apply b.i.d., t.i.d.	
Neosporin	Topical, apply b.i.d./t.i.d.	
Polysporin	Topical, apply b.i.d./t.i.d.	
Silvadene cream 1%	Topical, apply b.i.d./t.i.d.	

Antivirals

Name	Usual Dose	Comments
Acyclovir (Zovirax)	• Tablet 400, 800 mg	H. simplex: 400 mg 5× daily 7 d H. zoster: 800 mg 5× daily 7–10 d
Famciclovir (Famvir)	• 250–1,500 mg • Tablet 125, 250, 500 mg	H. simplex: 500 mg b.i.d. 7 d H. zoster: 500 mg t.i.d 7 d Suppressive therapy: 250 mg q.d.
Valacyclovir (Valtrex)	• Capsule 500, 1,000 mg	H. simplex: 1,000 mg b.i.d. 10 d H. zoster: 1,000 mg t.i.d. 7–10 d
Antifungals		
Clotrimazole (Lotrimin)	Topical, apply b.i.d.	
Clotrimazole (oral)	Oral 10 mg dissolved	10 mg dissolved 5× daily 14 d
Fluconazole (Diflucan)	• Tablet 50, 100, 150, 200 mg	200 mg day 1, then 100 mg q.d.
Ketoconazole	• Tablet 200, 400 mg q.d.	200 mg q.d. 14 d, if no response increase to 400 mg q.d.
Terbinafine (Lamisil)	Topical, apply b.i.d.	

Skin Reactions

Dry desquamation can be treated with Aquaphor or hydrocortisone cream. Noninfected moist desquamation and impending moist desquamation can be treated with saline soaks and Aquaphor after drying the open area.

Name	Usual Dose	Comments
Dry Desquamation		
Aquaphor/Hydrophor/ Calendula	Topical, apply b.i.d.–t.i.d.	
Benzocaine (Dermoplast)	Topical, apply t.i.d.	Topical anesthetic spray or lotion
Desoximetasone (Topicort)	Topical, apply b.i.d. • cream 0.05, 0.25% • gel 0.05% • spray 0.25%	
Hydrocortisone 1%, 2.5%	Topical, apply b.i.d–q.i.d.	Nonaerosol spray, ointment, cream
Lidocaine	Topical • cream 3% • gel 2, 4%	Apply topically for local analgesia
Miaderm	Topical b.i.d.–t.i.d.	Calendula, hyaluronate, aqueous cream, and aloe vera
Miaderm-L	Topical b.i.d.–t.i.d.	Calendula, hyaluronate, aqueous cream, aloe vera, 4% lidocaine
Neomycin sulfate/dexameth-asone sodium phosphate (Neo-Decadron Cream)	Topical, apply t.i.d.	
Pure lanolin cream (TheraCare)	Topical, apply p.r.n.	
Moist Desquamation		
Aluminum acetate (Domeboro)	Dissolve 1 tab/packet in water, apply moist soak for 20 min t.i.d.	
Aquaphor/Hydrophor/ Calendula	Topical, apply b.i.d.	
Aquaphor/Xylocaine 5% Aquaphor/lidocaine 1%	Topical, apply t.i.d.	
Desoximetasone (Topicort)	Topical, apply b.i.d. • Cream 0.05, 0.25% • Gel 0.05% • Spray 0.25%	

continued

Skin Reactions *(continued)*

Name	Usual Dose	Comments
Hydrogel wound dressings (Vigilon, Geliperm)	Topical, apply p.r.n.	
EMLA cream	Lidocaine 2.5%, prilocaine 2.5%, apply p.r.n.	
Ketoconazole (Nizoral 2% cream)	Topical, apply q.d.	Cutaneous candidiasis: 2 wk
Lidocaine 2.5% L.M.X.4 (4%) L.M.X. 5 (5%) Miaderm (4%)	Topical, apply p.r.n.	
Lidoderm patch (5%)	Topical, apply for 12 h q.d.	3 patches at a time for wound coverage
Polymyxin B sulfate/bacitracin zinc/neomycin sulfate (Neosporin)	Topical, apply q.d.–t.i.d.	
Silver sulfadiazine (Silvadene)	Topical, apply t.i.d. • cream 1%	For moist desquamation
Nonstick adhesive pads (Telfa)	Cover wound or ulceration p.r.n.	
Saline soaks	Saline soaks 15 min b.i.d.	Facilitate healing and removal of necrotic skin tissue
Zinc	8 mg p.o. q.d.	

Ulceration: Slow Healing

Antibiotics and Wound Infections

Name	Usual Dose	Comments
Acetic acid 0.05%	Topical, apply q.d. or q.o.d. to open wound	For superficial *Pseudomonas* infection, avoid 0.1% acetic acid as it delays granulation tissue
Acyclovir (Zovirax)	See "Antivirals"	
Cephalexin (Keflex)	See "Antibiotics"	
Ciprofloxacin (Cipro)	See "Antibiotics"	
Clindamycin (Cleocin)	See "Antibiotics"	
Fluconazole (Diflucan)	200 mg p.o. day 1, then 100 mg p.o. q.d., for 14 d • Tablet 50, 100, 150, 200 mg	Prescribe for frank thrush or esophagitis symptoms early (first 2 wk) in thoracic RT course
Hydrocolloid (DuoDERM)	Replace dressing q3 days	

Skin Reactions *(continued)*

Name	Usual Dose	Comments
Ketoconazole (Nizoral)	200 mg p.o. q.d.; 400 mg q.d. if insufficient initial response	Decreased effectiveness with H2 blockers Tablet (200 mg)
Metronidazole (Flagyl)	500 mg p.o. q6h; maximum 4,000 mg/d	For anaerobic infections Tablet (250 and 500 mg)
Polymyxin B sulfate/ bacitracin zinc/neomycin sulfate (Neosporin)	Topical, apply q.d.–t.i.d.	
Generalized Pruritus		
Diphenhydramine hydrochloride (Benadryl)	25–50 mg p.o. q4–8h	
Hydroxyzine (Vistaril)	25 mg p.o. t.i.d.–q.i.d. • Capsule 25, 50, 200 mg	Sedating
Methylprednisolone (Medrol Dosepak)	6-d prescription as directed	
Promethazine hydrochloride (Phenergan)	25.0 mg p.o. q.d. (or p.r.) 12.5 mg b.i.d. • Tablet 12.5, 25, 50 mg • Suppository 12.5, 25, 50 mg	Strong H1 blockers; may potentiate CNS depressants; has antiemetic properties
Silicone foam dressing (Mepilex)	Replace dressing q2 days	
Vasolex (trypsin, Balsam Peru, castor oil)	Topical, apply b.i.d.	
Vitamin E	1,000 IU p.o. q.d.	

Head and Neck

Name	Usual Dose	Comments
Eye		
Artificial tears	Topical, apply q.h.s.	
Cortisporin Ophthalmic	Topical, apply ointment or 4 gtts of suspension q3–4h up to 10 d	Combination steroid and antimicrobial Contraindicated for viral infections or ulcerative keratitis and after foreign body removal
Cyclosporine emulsion (0.05%) (Restasis)	1 gtt b.i.d.	Increased tear production

continued

Head and Neck *(continued)*

Name	Usual Dose	Comments
Lacrisert sterile ophthalmic insert	Insert as directed q.d.	Consider for severe dryness
Neosporin Ophthalmic	Topical, apply ointment or 1–2 gtts of suspension q4h	
Proparacaine hydrochloride 5%	Per manufacturer's instructions	Topical anesthetic for procedures to conjunctiva

Ear and Sinuses

Name	Usual Dose	Comments
Amoxicillin	See "Antibiotics"	
Amoxicillin/clavulanate (Augmentin)	See "Antibiotics"	
Antipyrine-benzocaine (Auralgan)	q1–2h p.r.n. pain	For acute otitis
Chlorpheniramine and phenylephrine (e.g., Actifed)	4–6 mg p.o. q4–6h	Avoid if patient is on MAO inhibitor or has hypertension, DM, asthma, glaucoma, or urinary retention
Benzocaine	4 to 5 gtts; repeat q1–2h if necessary	Topical anesthetic ear drops for otitis externa
Ciprofloxacin and dexamethasone (Ciprodex)	4 gtts b.i.d. 7 d	
Ciprofloxacin and prednisone (Cipro HC Otic)	3 gtts b.i.d. 7 d	
Cortisporin Otic	4 gtts t.i.d.–q.i.d ≥ 10 d.	
Diphenhydramine hydrochloride (Benadryl)	25–50 mg p.o. q4–8h	
Fexofenadine (Allegra)	60 mg b.i.d. XR: 180 mg q.d.	
Guaifenesin (Mucinex)	IR: 200–400 mg q4h ER: 600–1,200 mg b.i.d. Liquid 200–400 mg q4h	
Loratadine (Claritin)	10 mg QD, 5 mg b.i.d.	
Methylprednisolone (Medrol Dosepak)	6-day prescription as directed	
Pseudoephedrine hydrochloride (decongestant, e.g., Sudafed)	60 mg q4–6h ER: 120 mg p.o. b.i.d.	Avoid if patient is on MAO inhibitor or has hypertension, DM, asthma, glaucoma, or urinary retention
Trimethoprim/sulfamethoxazole (Bactrim, Bactrim DS)	See "Antibiotics"	

Head and Neck *(continued)*

Name	Usual Dose	Comments
Mucositis, Dysphagia		
Acetaminophen	500–1,000 mg q.i.d. p.r.n.	Do not exceed 4 g daily
Acetaminophen with codeine	15–60 mg codeine/acetaminophen 300–100 mg • Tablet 15 mg codeine-300 mg acetaminophen (#2); 30 mg codeine-300 mg acetaminophen (#3); 60 mg codeine-300 mg acetaminophen (#4) • Solution 12 mg codeine-120 mg acetaminophen/5 mL	Maximum daily dose codeine 360 mg/d maximum, maximum daily dose acetaminophen 4 g/d • Discontinuation titration, decrease dose by 25%–50% every 2–4 d
Baking soda mouthwash	Mix 1 tbs baking soda and 1 tbs salt in 1 quart water Gargle and spit b.i.d.	Reduces inflammation and restores oral pH
Benzydamine (topical NSAID)	Gargle and spit 15 mL q3h for pharyngitis	Not available in United States
Chlorhexidine gluconate (Peridex)	½ oz, swish 30 sec and spit b.i.d.	Used as a prophylactic oral antibiotic or for mucositis
Clotrimazole (Mycelex)	Dissolve one 10 mg lozenge in mouth, up to five times a day, for 14 consecutive days	For oropharyngeal candidiasis
Lidocaine (Xylocaine 2% jelly, 2% Xylocaine Viscous)	Xylocaine oral spray 10 mg per dose Xylocaine Viscous 2%—2 tsp swish and swallow	For pain
Mucositis mouthwash	Mix 4 oz Maalox, 4 oz Benadryl elixir, 100 mL viscous Xylocaine, and 1 oz Mycostatin suspension 1 tsp 20 min before meals; swish and swallow	
Polyvinylpyrrolidone-sodium hyaluronate (Gelclair)		Barrier protection
Oral infection, Mucositis, and Candidiasis		
Amoxicillin/clavulanate (Augmentin)	See "Antibiotics"	
Chlorhexidine gluconate (Peridex)	½ oz, swish 30 sec and spit b.i.d.	Used as a prophylactic oral antibiotic or for mucositis 1 pint dispenser

continued

Head and Neck *(continued)*

Name	Usual Dose	Comments
Clindamycin (Cleocin)	See "Antibiotics"	
Fluconazole (Diflucan)	See "Antifungal"	
Hydrogen peroxide gargle	Mix 1:1 water:hydrogen peroxide 1–3 tsp gargle p.r.n.	
Ketoconazole (Nizoral)	See "Antifungal"	
Nystatin suspension, generic	5 mL swish 2 min and swallow q.i.d.	Continue through 2 d after resolution of symptoms
Miracle mouthwash	Mix 60 mL tetracycline oral suspension (125 mg/5 mL), 30 mL Mycostatin oral suspension (100,000 u/mL), 30 mL hydrocortisone oral suspension (10 mg/5 mL), and 240 mL Benadryl syrup (12.5 mg/5 mL) 2 tsp p.o., swish and swallow/swish and spit q.i.d.	For mucositis, stomatitis, esophagitis
Sucralfate (Carafate) suspension	2 tsp, swish and swallow q.i.d. Suspension: 1 g/10 mL (smoother texture vs. slurry) Slurry alternative: dissolve 1-g tablet in 2 tbs water, swish and swallow q.i.d.	For oral/esophageal mucositis
Triple mix (FIRST Magic Mouthwash BLM)	Mix 1:1:1 Benadryl elixir:Maalox:viscous Xylocaine 2% 2 tsp p.o. 10 min q.a.c. and q.h.s.	

Xerostomia		
Artificial saliva	Apply to oral mucosa p.r.n. Carbonated beverages; diet	Biotene 15 mL t.i.d. Salivart: 25- and 75-g containers Xero-Lube: 180-mL pump spray bottle Moi-Stir: 120-mL spray bottle SalivaSure 1 lozenge/hour Saliva substitute: 120-mL squirt bottle
Baking soda mouthwash	Mix 1 tbs baking soda and 1 tbs salt in 1 quart water Gargle and spit b.i.d.	Reduces inflammation and restores oral pH
Biotene dry mouth toothpaste (OTC)	b.i.d.	

Head and Neck *(continued)*

Name	Usual Dose	Comments
Biotene Dental Gum (OTC)	1–2 pieces daily p.r.n.	
Fluoride carriers	Via dental consultation	
Glycerine	Mix 1/4 tsp in 8 oz water Use p.r.n.	
Guaifenesin (Mucinex, OTC)	IR: 200–400 mg q4h ER: 600–1,200 mg b.i.d Liquid 200–400 mg q4h	
Pilocarpine hydrochloride (Salagen)	• Tablet 5, 7.5 mg t.i.d.	For xerostomia; caution if cardiovascular disease, COPD, retinal disease Tablet (5 mg)
PreviDent (fluoride toothpaste)	Use in lieu of regular tooth-paste as needed	
Salt/baking soda mouthwash	Use p.r.n. swish, gargle, and spit	Mix 1 tsp salt and 1 tbs bak-ing soda in 1 qt warm water

Thorax

Name	Usual Dose	Comments
	Dyspnea	
Alprazolam (Xanax)	0.25–0.5 mg t.i.d. • Tablet 0.25, 0.5, 2 mg	Maximum daily dose 4 mg Titrate dose every 3–4 d
Alprazolam ER	0.5–1.0 mg q.d. • Tablet 0.5, 1, 2, 3 mg	Maximum daily dose 6 mg
Codeine	30 mg p.o. q4–6h • Tablet 15, 30, 60 mg • Liquid 15 mg/5 mL	
Diazepam (Valium)	2–10 mg p.o. b.i.d.–t.i.d. • Tablet 2, 5, 10 mg IM, IV 2–10 mg q3–4h prn	
Lorazepam (Ativan)	0.5–2 mg p.o. b.i.d.–q.i.d. • Tablet 0.5, 1, 2 mg	Maximum daily dose 10 mg
Morphine sulfate	10–30 mg p.o. q4h • Tablet 10, 15, 30 mg • Liquid 10, 20 mg/5 mL • *IV* 2.5–5 mg q3–4h • *IM/SubQ* 5–15 mg q4h	Doses for opioid naive
	Bronchial Dilators and Antispasmodics	

Albuterol or metaproterenol (same mechanism) may be alternated q2h with Atrovent (different mechanism).

continued

Thorax *(continued)*

Name	Usual Dose	Comments
Albuterol sulfate (Proventil, Proventil Repetabs, Ventolin)[a]	Aerosol: 2 puff q4–6h Regular release: 2–4 mg t.i.d.–q.i.d. ER: 8 mg q12h • Tablet 2, 4 mg • Tablet ER 4, 8 mg • Liquid 2 mg/5 mL	Regular release maximum daily dose 32 mg ER maximum daily dose 32 mg
Beclomethasone dipropionate (Beclovent)	40–80 mcg b.i.d.	Maximum daily dose 320 mcg b.i.d.
Flunisolide, steroid (Aerobid)	160 mcg b.i.d.	Maximum daily dose 320 mcg b.i.d.
Ipratropium bromide (Atrovent)[a]	2 inhalation q6h	Maximum daily dose 12 inhalations (408 mcg)
Metaproterenol sulfate	Oral: 20 mg t.i.d.–q.i.d. • Tablet 10 mg, 20 mg • Syrup 10 mg/5 mL	
Triamcinolone (Azmacort)	2 puffs t.i.d.–q.i.d.	240 dose oral inhaler

Cough		
Acetaminophen with codeine phosphate (Tylenol with Codeine)	15–60 mg codeine/acetaminophen 300–100 mg • Tablet 15 mg codeine-300 mg acetaminophen (#2); 30 mg codeine-300 mg acetaminophen (#3); 60 mg codeine-300 mg acetaminophen (#4) • Solution 12 mg codeine-120 mg acetaminophen/5 mL	Maximum daily dose codeine 360 mg/d maximum, maximum daily dose acetaminophen 4 g/d • Discontinuation titration, decrease dose by 25%–50% every 2–4 d
Diphenhydramine (Benadryl)	25 mg p.o. q4h • Tablet 25, 50 mg	Avoid if COPD, asthma, glaucoma, urinary retention Maximum daily dose 150 mg
Chlorpheniramine and phenylephrine (Actifed)	• Liquid 1 mg chlorpheniramine-2.5 mg phenylephrine per 1 mL; 4 mL q4h • Liquid 4 mg chlorpheniramine-10 mg per 4 mL; 5 mL q4–6h • Tablet 4 mg chlorpheniramine-10 mg phenylephrine; 1 tablet q4–6h • Tablet 4 mg chlorpheniramine-20 mg phenylephrine; 1–2 tablets q12h	Maximum daily dose 24 mL Maximum daily dose 30 mL Maximum daily dose 6 tabs Maximum daily dose 4 tabs

Thorax *(continued)*

Name	Usual Dose	Comments
Cetirizine (Zyrtec)	10 mg q.d. • Tablet 10 mg	
Benzonatate (Tessalon Perles)	100–200 mg p.o. t.i.d	Maximum daily dose 600 mg
Codeine	30 mg p.o. q4–6h • Tablet 15, 30, 60 mg • Liquid 15 mg/5 mL	
Dextromethorphan hydro-bromide and guaifenesin (Mucinex DM)	Available in liquid and tablet forms. General dosing guidelines: Guaifenesin 200–400 mg q4h Dextromethorphan 10–20 mg q4h	Maximum daily dose guaifen-esin 2,400 mg, dextrometho-rphan 120 mg
Hydromorphone hydro-chloride/guaifenesin, class II (Dilaudid cough syrup)	1–2 tsp p.o. q3–4h • liquid guaifenesin 100 mg	Hydromorphone hydro-chloride (1 mg/guaifenesin 100 mg/5 mL syrup)
Guaifenesin (e.g., Robitussin)	Liquid 200–400 mg q4h Tablet IR 200–400 mg q4h Tablet ER 600–1,200 mg q12h • Liquid 100 mg/5 mL • Tablet IR 200, 400 mg • Tablet ER 400 mg	Mucolytic
Guaifenesin with codeine phosphate (e.g., Robitussin AC)	• Liquid: guaifenesin 100 mg—codeine 6.33 mg per 5 mL; 15 mL q4–6h • Liquid: guaifenesin 100–200 mg—codeine 8–10 mg per 5 mL; 10 mL q4–6h • Liquid: guaifenesin 225 mg—codeine 7.5 mg per 5 mL; 7.5 mL q4–6h	Maximum daily dose 90 mL Maximum daily dose 60 mL Maximum daily dose 45 mL
Humibid LA and DM	1–2 tablets p.o. q12h • Tablet LA 600 mg • Tablet DM-ER 600 mg	LA: 600 mg guaifenesin DM-ER: 600 mg guaifene-sin/30 mg dextromethorphan hydrobromide
Hydrocodone bitartrate (Hycodan)	5 mg p.o. q4h • Tablet 5 mg • Syrup 5 mg/5 mL	Tablet (5 mg) or alcohol-free syrup (5 mg/5 mL)
Hydrocodone and chlor-pheniramine (Tussionex) extended-release suspension	Capsule: hydrocodone 10 mg-chlorpheniramine 8 mg; 1 capsule b.i.d Liquid: hydrocodone 10 mg-chlorpheniramine 8 mg per 5 mL; 5 mL q4–6h	

continued

Thorax *(continued)*

Name	Usual Dose	Comments
Infectious Processes		
Amantadine hydrochloride (Symmetrel)	100 mg p.o. b.i.d. • Tablet 100 mg • Capsule 100 mg • Syrup 50 mg/5 mL	Antiviral for influenza A, prophylaxis or treatment. Start within 24–48 h of symptoms
Amoxicillin/clavulanate potassium (Augmentin)	See "Antibiotics"	
Azithromycin dihydrate (Zithromax)	See "Antibiotics"	
Ciprofloxacin (Cipro)	See "Antibiotics"	
Clindamycin (Cleocin)	See "Antibiotics"	
Erythromycin	See "Antibiotics"	
Rimantadine hydrochloride (Flumadine)	Prophylaxis: 100 mg p.o. b.i.d. Treatment: 100 mg b.i.d for 5–7 d	For prophylaxis, 7 d after last known exposure; for treatment, start within 48 h of symptom onset
Trimethoprim/sulfamethoxazole (Bactrim, Bactrim DS)	See "Antibiotics"	
Radiation Pneumonitis		

Basic treatment is steroidal and nonsteroidal anti-inflammatories. The inhalable steroids can be used as supplements to lower systemic therapy and when weaning. Be cautious regarding a possible infectious etiology.

Name	Usual Dose	Comments
Beclomethasone dipropionate (Beclovent)	40–80 mcg b.i.d. • 40 mcg/actuation • 80 mcg/actuation	Maximum daily dose 320 mcg
Flunisolide (Aerobid)	160 mcg b.i.d. • 80 mcg/actuation	Maximum daily dose 320 mcg
NSAIDs		
Ibuprofen (IBU)	400 mg p.o. q6h • Tablet 200, 400, 600, 800 mg	
Indomethacin (Indocin)	25 mg b.i.d.–t.i.d. • Capsule 25, 50 mg • Capsule ER 75 mg • Liquid 25 mg/5 mL	
Naproxen (Naprosyn)	500 mg b.i.d. • Liquid 125 mg/5 mL • Tablet 250, 375, 500 mg maximum, 200 mg per d	Maximum daily dose 1,000 mg

Thorax *(continued)*

Name	Usual Dose	Comments
Prednisone	20 mg p.o. q8h (or 60 mg p.o. q.d.) • Tablet 2.5, 5, 10, 20, 50 mg	2–4 wk with a gradual taper over 3–12 wk Consider *Pneumocystis* pneumonia prophylaxis
Triamcinolone (Azmacort)	2 puffs t.i.d.–q.i.d.	Oral inhaler: 240 dose unit

*a*Usual requirement is six cans q.d.

Breast

Name	Usual Dose	Comments
	Hormonal Therapy	
Anastrozole (Arimidex)	1 mg p.o. q.d. • Tablet 1 mg	
Clonidine (Catapres)	0.1 mg p.o. b.i.d. • Tablet 0.1 mg • Transdermal patch weekly	Hot flashes, off-label Maximum daily dose 0.6 mg p.o.
Gabapentin	Initially 300 mg p.o. q.d. Increase to 600–1,200 mg b.i.d.–t.i.d. over 3–12 d • Tablet 100, 300, 400 mg	Hot flashes, off-label
Medroxyprogesterone (Depo Provera)	150 mg IM q3 mo	Hot flashes, persistent, off-label
Megestrol acetate (Megace)	20 mg p.o. b.i.d. • Tablet 20, 40 mg	Hot flashes
Methyldopa (Aldomet)	250 mg p.o. b.i.d. • Tablet 125, 250, 500 mg • Liquid 250 mg/5 mL	Hot flashes, off-label
Paroxetine (Paxil)	12.5 mg p.o. daily • Tablet 12.5, 25, 37.5 mg	Hot flashes Maximum daily dose 60 mg
Raloxifene hydrochloride (Evista)	60 mg p.o. q.d. • Tablet 60 mg	
Tamoxifen citrate (Nolvadex)	20 mg p.o. q.d. • Tablet 10, 20 mg	
Venlafaxine (Effexor)	Initially 37.5 mg p.o. q.d. Increase by 37.5 mg/wk • Tablet/capsule 37.5, 75, 150 mg	Hot flashes, off-label Maximum daily dose 150 mg

Gastrointestinal

Name	Usual Dose	Comments
Antacids and Antiflatulents		
Aluminum, magnesium, and simethicone (combination)	Tablet: aluminum 200 mg/ magnesium 200 mg/simethicone 25 mg; 1–4 tab q.i.d. Liquid: aluminum 200 mg/ magnesium 200 mg/simethicone 20 mg per 5 mL; 10–20 mL between meals and at bedtime Liquid: aluminum 400 mg/ magnesium 400 mg/simethicone 40 mg per 5 mL	Maximum daily dose 12–16 tabs or 80–120 mL (40–60 mL double strength)
Cimetidine (Tagamet)	Prophylaxis: 200 mg p.o. 30 min prior to eating/drinking trigger foods Treatment: 200 mg p.o. q.d. • Tablet 200, 300, 400, 800 mg • Solution: 300 mg/5 mL	Maximum daily dose 400 mg
Famotidine (Pepcid)	10–20 mg p.o. b.i.d. • Liquid 40 mg/5 mL • Tablet 10, 20, 40 mg	Maximum daily dose 40 mg
Omeprazole (Prilosec)	20 mg p.o. q.d. for 4–8 wk • Tablet 10, 20, 40 mg • Liquid 2 mg/mL	
Ranitidine hydrochloride (Zantac)	Prophylaxis: 75–150 mg 30–60 min prior to eating/ drinking trigger Treatment: 75–150 mg p.o. q.d.–b.i.d. • Tablet 75, 150, 300 mg • Liquid 15 mg/mL, 75 mg/5 mL, 150 mg/10 mL	
Simethicone	40–125 mg q.i.d. as needed or 160–500 mg qd • Tablet 125, 180 mg • Chewable: 80, 125 mg • Liquid 20 mg/0.3 mL	Maximum daily dose 500 mg
Antidiarrhea		
Initiate a low-residue, low-fat, nonspicy diet. If further intervention is required, use Imodium.		
Bismuth subsalicylate (Pepto-Bismol)	524 mg q30–60 min • Liquid 262 mg/15 mL • Tablet 262 mg	

Gastrointestinal *(continued)*

Name	Usual Dose	Comments
Cholestyramine (Questran)	4 g q.d.	Maximum daily dose 36 mg Increase by 4 g at weekly intervals
Difenoxin hydrochloride/ atropine sulfate(Motofen)	2 tablets initially, 1 after each loose stool • Tablet 1–0.025 mg	Maximum daily dose 8 tablets
Diphenoxylate hydro- chloride/atropine sulfate (Lomotil)	5 mg q.i.d. • Tablet 2.5–0.025 mg • Liquid 2.5–0.025 mg/5 mL	Reduce dose to as low as 25% once control achieved
Loperamide hydrochloride (Imodium AD)	Initial 4 mg p.o., 2 mg p.o after each loose stool • Tablet 2 mg • Liquid 1 mg/5 mL, 1 mg/7.5 mL	

Appetite Stimulants

Cyproheptadine hydrochloride (Periactin)	Initial 4 mg t.i.d. Maintenance 4 mg q.i.d. • Tablet 4 mg • 2 mg/5 mL	Maximum daily dose 0.5 mg/kg
Dronabinol (Marinol)	2.5 mg p.o. b.i.d. or 5.0 mg p.o. q.h.s. • Capsule 2.5, 5, 10 mg • Liquid 5 mg/mL	
Megestrol acetate (Megace)	160–800 mg p.o. q.d. Liquid, start 625 mg q.d. • Tablet 20, 40 mg • Liquid 40 mg/mL • Liquid 625 mg/5 mL	Doses ranging from 160 to 800 mg have been effective (off label); titrate as needed
Prednisone	10–40 mg q.d. • Tablet 1, 2.5, 5, 10, 20, 50 mg	

Esophagitis

If early esophagitis develops, especially in the setting of steroid use, suspect *Candida* infection and treat with antifungal. For radiation esophagitis, topical anesthetics may provide some relief to assist with oral intake; consider systemic pain medications as needed.

Fluconazole (Diflucan)	See "Antifungal"
Famotidine (Pepcid)	See "Antacids and antiflatulents"
Hurricane mixture	Mix 1:1 20% benzocaine: Maalox 1–2 tsp p.o. q4h

continued

Gastrointestinal *(continued)*

Name	Usual Dose	Comments
Ketoconazole (Nizoral)	See "Antifungal"	Tablet (200 mg)
Miracle mouthwash	Mix 60 mL tetracycline oral suspension (125 mg/5 mL), 30 mL mycostatin oral suspension (100,000 u/mL), 30 mL hydrocortisone oral suspension (10 mg/5 mL), and 240 mL Benadryl syrup (12.5 mg/5 mL) 2 tsp p.o. swish and swallow/ swish and spit q.i.d.	
Sucralfate (Carafate suspension)	2 tsp swish and swallow q.i.d. Liquid 1 g/10 mL Tablet 1 g	For oral/esophageal mucositis Tablet can be dissolved in 2 tbs water, swish and swallow
Triple mix	Mix 1:1:1 Benadryl elixir: Maalox: viscous Xylocaine 2% 2 tsp p.o. 10 min q.a.c. and q.h.s.	

Hiccups

Name	Usual Dose	Comments
Baclofen	5–10 mg t.i.d. • Tablet 10, 20 mg 25 mg p.o. t.i.d—50 mg p.o. q.i.d.	Maximum daily dose 75 mg
Chlorpromazine (Thorazine)	• Tablet 10, 25, 50, 100, 200 mg • Liquid 10 mg/5 mL	Drug of choice for refractory hiccups
Metoclopramide (Reglan)	10 mg p.o. t.i.d. • Tablet 5 mg, 10 mg • Liquid 5 mg/5 mL	Maximum daily dose 40 mg

Motility Factors and Ulcer Medications

Carafate protects the stomach with a coating action and may have some prophylactic benefit. The H2 blockers (Tagamet Pepcid, Prilosec, and Zantac) are especially used for prophylaxis during steroidal and nonsteroidal anti-inflammatory therapy.

Name	Usual Dose	Comments
Cimetidine (Tagamet)	300 mg p.o. ti.d. 400 mg p.o. b.i.d 800 mg p.o. q.h.s. • Tablet 200, 300, 400, 800 mg • Liquid 300 mg/5 mL	
Dicyclomine hydrochloride (Bentyl)	20 mg p.o. q.i.d., increase to 40 mg p.o. q.i.d. if tolerated • Tablet 10, 20 mg • Solution 10 mg/mL, 10 mg/5 mL	Maximum daily dose 80 mg

Gastrointestinal *(continued)*

Name	Usual Dose	Comments
Donnatal (antispasmodic)	1–2 tablets or tsp p.o. t.i.d.–q.i.d. 5–10 mL p.o. t.i.d–q.i.d • Tablet hyoscyamine sulfate 0.1037 mg, atropine sulfate 0.0194 mg, scopolamine hydrobromide 0.0065 mg, phenobarbital 16.2 mg Liquid hyoscyamine sulfate 0.1037 mg, atropine sulfate 0.0194 mg, scopolamine hydrobromide 0.0065 mg, phenobarbital 16.2 mg per 5 mL; 120 mL, 480 mL	
Famotidine (Pepcid)	40 mg p.o. q.h.s, maintenance 20 mg p.o. q.h.s. • Liquid 40 mg/5 mL • Tablet 10, 20, 40 mg	
Hyoscyamine Levsin	0.125–0.25 mg q.i.d. • Tablet 0.125 mg • Liquid 0.125 mg/5 mL	Maximum daily dose 1.5 mg
Metoclopramide (Reglan)	10 mg p.o. t.i.d • Tablet 5 mg, 10 mg • Liquid 5 mg/5 mL	Maximum daily dose 40 mg
Omeprazole (Prilosec)	See "Antacids and antiflatulents"	
Ranitidine hydrochloride (Zantac)	See "Antacids and antiflatulents"	
Sucralfate (Carafate)	Active ulcer 1 g q.i.d. for 4–8 wk Maintenance 1 g b.i.d. • Tablet 1 g • Liquid 1 g/10 mL	Avoid taking within 30 min of antacids

Nausea and Vomiting

Name	Usual Dose	Comments
Chlorpromazine (Thorazine)	10–25 mg p.o. q4–6h 25–50 mg i.m. q3–4h until vomiting stops • Tablet 10, 25, 50, 100, 200 mg • Liquid 25 mg/mL, 50 mg/mL	
Dronabinol (class II) (Marinol)	2.5–10 mg p.o. t.i.d—q.i.d • Tablet 2.5, 5, 10 mg • solution 5 mg/mL	
Lorazepam (Ativan)	0.5–2 mg q6h	Off-label

continued

Gastrointestinal *(continued)*

Name	Usual Dose	Comments
Ondansetron (Zofran)	8 mg p.o. q8h • Tablet 4, 8, 24 mg • Liquid 4 mg/5 mL	For prevention of radiation therapy–induced nausea, administer 1–2 h prior to RT
Prochlorperazine (Compazine)	5–10 mg p.o. up to q.i.d. • Tablet 5, 10 mg • Suppository 25 mg (b.i.d.)	Maximum daily dose 40 mg
Promethazine (Phenergan)	12.5–25 mg up to q4h • Tablet 12.5, 25, 50 mg • Liquid 6.25 mg/5 mL • Suppository 12.5, 25 mg	Sedating, may potentiate CNS depressants

Laxatives

Name	Usual Dose	Comments
Bisacodyl (Dulcolax, laxative)	5–15 mg p.o. q.d. 10 mg rectal q.d. • Tablet 5 mg • Suppository 10 mg	
Docusate sodium (Colace, stool softener)	50–360 mg p.o. q.d.—divided 283/5 mL rectal q.d.—t.i.d • Tablet 50, 100, 250 mg • Enema 283/5 mL	
Docusate and senna (Senokot-S)	Up to 4 tabs daily • Tablet 8.6 mg/50 mg	
Lactulose (e.g., Cephulac)	10–40 g p.o. daily Packet 10 g Liquid 10 g/15 mL	For significant constipation, as with high-dose morphine sulfate
Magnesium citrate	1 bottle p.o. p.r.n. 195–300 mL	
Mineral oil	15–45 mL p.o. (liquid) q.d.–t.i.d. 30–90 mL p.o. (suspension) q.d.–t.i.d. 118 mL p.r. (enema) q.d. • Oil 30, 472, 273, 500, 1,000, 4,000 mL • Enema 135 mL	Maximum daily dose liquid 45 mL, suspension 90 mL
Psyllium metamucil	1–3 tsp in juice daily with meals	Bulking agent
Sodium phosphate (Fleet Enema)	1–2 as directed p.r. p.r.n. • Enema 15 mL	Maximum daily dose 3 enemas
Texas cocktail	30 mL mineral oil in 8 oz juice; follow in 1 h with 10 oz magnesium citrate	

Gastrointestinal *(continued)*

Name	Usual Dose	Comments
	Proctitis and Tenesmus	
Anusol HC-1 (1% hydrocortisone)	• Topical, q.i.d.	
Anusol HC 2.5% (2.5% hydrocortisone)	• Topical, q.i.d.	
Anusol HC 25-mg suppositories	p.r.n b.i.d.–t.i.d.	Package of 12 or 24
Dibucaine (Nupercainal) Hemorrhoidal and anesthetic ointment	Apply to rectum up to q.i.d. after each bowel movement • Topical 1% cream	
Hydrocortisone retention enema (Cortenema)	1 p.r.n. q.h.s.; retain for 1 h	Supplied as single-dose units
Mesalamine	• Retention enema 4 g nightly, retained overnight • Rectal suppository (Canasa) 1,000 mg retained 1–3 h nightly	
Preparation H	Topical 0.25% q.i.d. Suppository 1 p.r.n. up to q.i.d.	
Proctofoam HC, 2.5% Cortifoam	Topical p.r.n. up to q.i.d. • Aerosol	
	Oral and Enteral Nutritional Supplements	
Usual requirement is six cans per day		
Boost		240 cal/8 oz, 10 g protein Prefilled container, protein powder
Ensure		250 cal/8 oz, 11 g protein 8-oz container, 1-qt can, 14-oz can powder
Ensure Plus		355 cal/8 oz, 13 g protein 8-oz container, 1-qt can, 1-L prefilled container
Osmolite		250 cal/8 oz, 8.8 protein 8-oz containers, 1-qt can, 1-L prefilled container
Osmolite HN		355 cal/8 oz, 10.5 g dietary protein 8-oz containers, 1-qt can, 1-L prefilled containers
Sustacal		240 cal/8 oz, 14.4 g protein 8-, 12-, and 32-oz can
Sustacal HC		360 cal/8 oz, 14.4 g protein 8-oz cans

Genitourinary

Name	Usual Dose	Comments
Analgesics and Antispasmodics		
Belladonna/opium	1 suppository p.r. q.d.–b.i.d. • Suppository belladonna extract 16.2 mg/opium 30 mg	Maximum daily dose 4/d Controlled substance C-II; for moderate-to-severe pain associated with ureteral spasms not responsive to nonopioids
Flavoxate hydrochloride (Urispas)	100–200 mg p.o. t.i.d.–q.i.d. • Tablet 100 mg	
Oxybutynin chloride (Ditropan)	IR 5 mg p.o. b.i.d.–t.i.d. ER 5–10 mg p.o. q.d.	Maximum daily dose (IR) 5 mg q.i.d., (ER) 30 mg q.d.
Pentosan polysulfate sodium (Elmiron)	100 mg p.o. t.i.d. • Tablet 100 mg	For interstitial cystitis
Phenazopyridine hydrochloride (Pyridium)	200 mg p.o. t.i.d. • Tablet 100, 200 mg	For interstitial cystitis; with or after meals; turns urine orange
Tolterodine tartrate (Detrol)	IR 2 mg p.o. b.i.d. ER 4 mg p.o. q.d. • Tablet (IR) 1, 2 mg • Tablet (ER) 2, 4 mg	For overactive bladder
Bladder Outlet Obstruction		
Tamsulosin hydrochloride (Flomax)	0.4–0.8 mg p.o. q.d. • Tablet 0.4 mg	
Terazosin hydrochloride (Hytrin)	1 mg p.o. q.h.s (initial dose); increase stepwise to 2, 5, or 10 mg daily • Tablet 1, 2, 5, 10 mg	Maximum daily dose 20 mg/d Warning: Can cause postural hypotension
Antibiotics		
Ciprofloxacin (Cipro)	See "Antibiotics (General Information)"	
Doxycycline (Vibramycin)	200 mg p.o. q.d. day 1, then 100 mg p.o. q.d. • Tablet 50, 75, 100 mg • Liquid 25 mg/5 mL	
Nitrofurantoin (Macrobid)	Macrodantin: 50–100 mg p.o. q6h for 7 d • Tablet 25, 50, 100 mg Macrobid: 100 mg p.o. b.i.d. For 7 d • Tablet 100 mg	

Genitourinary *(continued)*

Name	Usual Dose	Comments
Trimethoprim/ sulfamethoxazole (Bactrim, Septra)	See "Antibiotics (General Information)"	
Preimplant prophylaxis	Cefazolin 1 g IV Levofloxacin 500 mg IV	
Preimplant prophylaxis for risk of bacterial endocarditis	Ampicillin 2 g or vancomycin 1 g, and gentamicin 1.5 mg/kg 30 min before implant. Give ampicillin 1 g at 6 h post implant	

Nervous System

Name	Usual Dose	Comments
Edema		
Dexamethasone (e.g., Decadron)	Radiation-induced symptomatic edema: 2–6 mg p.o. q8h	If insomnia develops, daily dose should be taken by late morning or early afternoon
	Tumor-induced edema: 16–25 mg i.v. initially, then 4–10 mg i.v./p.o. q6h Severe sudden symptoms/ impending herniation: 100 mg i.v. initially, then 25 mg q6h • Tablet 0.5, 0.75, 1, 1.5, 2, 4, and 6 mg) • Solution 0.5 mg/5 mL	If given with lung irradiation, steroids should be tapered over 6–8 wk
Seizures		
Carbamazepine (Tegretol)	*Seizure prophylaxis*: 200 mg p.o. t.i.d.–q.i.d. • Tablet 200 mg • Liquid 100 mg/5 mL *Trigeminal neuralgia*: 200 mg p.o., titrating up to 800 mg daily Maintenance 400–800 mg daily • Tablet 200 mg • Liquid 100 mg/5 mL	Maximum daily dose 1,600 mg Maximum daily dose 1,200 mg

continued

Nervous System *(continued)*

Name	Usual Dose	Comments
Levetiracetam (Keppra)	Initial 500 mg p.o. b.i.d., titrate up by 500 mg b.i.d. every 2 wk • Tablet 250, 500, 750, 1,000 mg • Liquid 500, 1,000, 1,500 mg/100 mL	Maximum daily dose 1,500 mg b.i.d.
Phenobarbital	*Seizure prophylaxis:* Maintenance 60–200 mg q.d. or 50–100 mg up to t.i.d. • Tablet 15, 16.2, 30, 32.4, 60, 64.8, 97.2, 100 mg	
Phenytoin (Dilantin) for seizure prophylaxis	Initial 100 mg t.i.d., maintenance 300–600 mg q.d. (tablet) Initial 125 mg t.i.d., maintenance up to 625 mg q.d. (liquid) Therapeutic range: 10–20 μg/mL • Tablet IR 30, 50 mg • Tablet ER 100, 200, 300 mg • Liquid 125 mg/5 mL	
Pregabalin (Lyrica)	Initial 75 mg p.o. b.i.d., titration schedule variable • Tablet 25, 50, 75, 100, 150, 200, 225, 300 mg • Liquid 20 mg/mL	Maximum daily dose 600 mg q.d.
Topiramate (Topamax) for seizure prophylaxis	Initial 25 mg p.o. b.i.d., titrate up by 50 mg per dose • Tablet 25, 50, 100, 200 mg	Maximum daily dose 200 mg b.i.d.
Valproate (Depakote)	Initial 15 mg/kg/d, titrate up by 5–10 mg/kg/d each week • Tablet IR 250 mg • Tablet ER 250, 500 mg • Liquid 250 mg/5 mL	Maximum daily dose 60 mg/kg/d

Vertigo

Name	Usual Dose	Comments
Meclizine hydrochloride (Antivert)	12.5–50.0 mg p.o. b.i.d. • Tablet 12.5, 25, 50 mg	
Scopolamine patch (Transderm Scop)	Apply patch to dry skin behind the ear q3day	Each patch contains 1.5 mg of scopolamine and is programmed to deliver 1.0 mg over 3 d

Pain Management

Name	Initial Dose	Comments
Nonopioid Analgesics		
Acetaminophen (Tylenol)	IR 650 mg p.o. q4–6h ER 1,000 mg p.o. q6h Extended release 1,300 mg q8h • Tablet 325, 500, 650 mg • Liquid 500 mg/5 mL	Maximum daily dose < 4 g/d
Aspirin	325–650 mg p.o. q4h 500–1,000 mg p.o. q4–6h 300–600 p.r. q4h • Tablet 235, 500 mg • Suppository 300, 600 mg	Maximum daily dose < 4 g/d
Celecoxib (Celebrex)	Initial dose 400 mg, followed by 200 mg b.i.d. • Tablet 50, 100, 200, 400 mg	Reduce dose by 50% for patients with CYP2C9 mutations
Ibuprofen	200–400 mg p.o. q4–6h • Tablet 200 mg	Maximum daily dose 3,200 mg/d
Ketorolac (Toradol)	Injectable: 60 mg i.m. initially, then 30 mg q6h • Solution 60 mg/2 mL	Maximum daily dose 120 mg/d IM
	Oral: 20 mg p.o. initially, 10 mg q4–6h • Tablet 10 mg	Maximum daily dose 40 mg/d
Naproxen (Naprosyn)	IR 500–750 mg initially, then 250–500 mg q6–12h ER 750–1,000 mg q.d. • Tablet 250, 375, 500 mg • Tablet (ER) 375, 500 mg	(IR) Maximum daily dose 1,500 mg/d < 6 mo (ER) Maximum daily dose 1,500 mg/d
Tramadol (Ultram)	Immediate release 50–100 mg q4–6h Extended release 100 mg q.d.	(IR) Maximum daily dose 400 mg/d (ER) Maximum daily dose 300 mg/d
Opioid Analgesics for Mild to Moderate Pain		
Codeine	15–60 mg q4h • Tablet 15, 30, 60 mg	Maximum daily dose 360 mg/d maximum • Discontinuation titration, decrease dose by 25%–50% every 2–4 days

continued

Pain Management *(continued)*

Name	Initial Dose	Comments
Codeine/acetaminophen (Tylenol with codeine #2, #3, #4)	15–60 mg codeine/acetaminophen 300–100 mg • Tablet 15 mg codeine-300 mg acetaminophen (#2); 30 mg codeine-300 mg acetaminophen (#3); 60 mg codeine-300 mg acetaminophen (#4) • Solution 12 mg codeine-120 mg acetaminophen/5 mL	Maximum daily dose codeine 360 mg/d maximum, maximum daily dose acetaminophen 4 g/d • Discontinuation titration, decrease dose by 25%–50% every 2–4 d
Codeine/guaifenesin (Robitussin A-C)	*Cough:* 10 mL p.o. q4h • Syrup 10 mg codeine-100 mg guaifenesin/5 mL	Maximum daily dose 60 mL/24 h
Hydrocodone (Hysingla, Zohydro)	Hysingla ER 20 mg q.d., increase by 10–20 mg every 3–5 d until adequate analgesia achieved Zohydro ER 20 mg b.i.d, increase by 10 mg b.i.d every 3–7 d until adequate analgesia achieved • Hysingla ER 20, 30, 40, 60, 8, 100, 120 mg • Zohydro ER 10, 15, 20, 30, 40, 50 mg	
		Tablet (5 mg) or syrup (5 mg/5 mL), nonalcoholic
Hydrocodone/acetaminophen	Hydrocodone 2.5–10 mg q4–6h • Tablet codeine 2.5–10 mg—acetaminophen 300–750 mg • Liquid hydrocodone 7.5 mg—acetaminophen 325 mg per 15 mL; • Liquid hydrocodone 7.5 mg—acetaminophen 500 mg per 15 mL	Maximum daily acetaminophen dose 4 g/d
Hydrocodone/guaifenesin (Vicodin TUSS)	Liquid hydrocodone 5 mg—guaifenesin 400 mg; 10 mL q4–6h	Maximum daily dose hydrocodone 30 mg, guaifenesin 2,400 mg/24 hours

Pain Management *(continued)*

Name	Initial Dose	Comments
Opioid Analgesics for Severe Pain (Class II Narcotics)		
Fentanyl	i.v. i.m. initial 25–35 mcg or 0.35–0.5 mcg/kg qh Infusion: 50–700 mcg or 0.7–10 mcg/kg/h p.o. lozenge initial 200 mcg, followed by 200 mcg in 15 min if pain unresolved. Next dose in 4 h Sublingual spray initial 100 mcg, followed by 100 mcg in 30 min if pain unresolved. Next dose in 4 h, 2 sprays per dose • Sublingual spray 100, 200, 400, 600, 800, 1,200, 1,600 mcg • p.o. lozenge 200, 400, 600, 800, 1,200, 1,600 mcg	Maximum daily dose 4 lozenges
Fentanyl transdermal system (Duragesic)	25 µg/h +, q 3-d patch • Patch 12, 25, 37.5, 50, 62.5, 75, 87.5, 100 mcg/h	See *Physicians' Desk Reference* tables for conversion factors
Hydromorphone hydrochloride (Dilaudid)	p.o. IR initial tablet 2–4 mg q4–6 h p.o. IR initial liquid 2.5–10 mg q3–6h i.v. 0.2–1 mg q2–3h • Tablet 2, 4, 8 mg • Liquid 1 mg/mL • i.v. 10 mg/mL	i.v./i.m. to p.o. conversion factor: 5
Meperidine hydrochloride (Demerol)	i.m. sub-Q 50–150 mg q3–4h • Tablet 50, 100 mg • Liquid 50 mg/5 mL • i.v. 10–25 mg/mL	Oral form available; i.v./i.m. to p.o. conversion factor: 4 For discontinuation, reduce dose by 25% q2–4 d as tolerated
Methadone hydrochloride	p.o. i.m. i.v. sub-Q initial 2.5 mg q8–12h Titrate up by 2.5 mg per dose each week • Tablet 5, 10 mg • Liquid 5 mg/mL • i.v. 10 mg/mL	Please use manufacturer-provided tables when converting opioid to methadone

continued

Pain Management *(continued)*

Name	Initial Dose	Comments
Morphine sulfate	p.o. initial dose 10–30 mg q4h i.v. initial dose 2.5–5 mg q4h, titrate end point for pain relief or until sedation, oxygen saturation <95% • Tablet 15, 30 mg • Liquid 10, 20, 100 mg/5 mL or 20 mg/mL	Adhere to institutional protocol
Oxycodone	IR initial 5–15 mg q4–6h ER initial 10 mg q12h • Tablet IR 5 mg • Tablet ER 9 mg • Liquid 5 mg/5 mL, 100 mg/5 mL • Roxicodone (IR) tablet 5, 15, 30 mg • Oxycontin (ER) tablet 10, 15, 20, 30, 40, 60, 80 mg	
Oxycodone/acetaminophen (Paracetamol, Percocet, Roxicet) IR	IR 2.5–10 mg oxycodone q6h • Tablet 2.5, 5, 7.5, 10–325 mg • Liquid 5–325/5 mL	Daily dose limited by acetaminophen content 4 g daily
Oxycodone/aspirin (Percodan)	Initial one 4.835–325 mg q6h • Tablet 4.835–325 mg	Maximum daily dose 12 tabs (oxycodone 58.02 mg and aspirin 3,900 mg)
Narcotic Antagonist		
Naloxone hydrochloride (Narcan)	IV or IM: initially 0.01 mg/kg or 0.4–2 mg since dose, repeat at 0.1 mg/kg every 2–3 min • Syringe/ampule 0.4 and 1 mg/mL Intranasal spray 4 mg, repeat every 2–3 min • Nasal spray 4 mg/0.1 mL • IV 0.4 mg/mL, 4 mg/10 mL	

Psychotropic Medications

Name	Initial Dose	Comments
Antianxiety		
Alprazolam (Xanax)	0.25–0.5 mg p.o. t.i.d. • IR tablet 0.25, 0.5, 1, 2 mg • ER tablet 0.5, 1, 2, 3 mg	Maximum daily dose 4 mg/d Titrate every 3–4 d for desired effect
Chlordiazepoxide (Librium)	Mild-moderate anxiety: 5–10 mg p.o. t.i.d.–q.i.d. Severe anxiety: 20–25 mg p.o. t.i.d.–q.i.d. • Tablet 5, 10, 25 mg	
Diazepam (Valium)	Oral 10 mg p.o. t.i.d–q.i.d. first 24 hours, then 5 mg p.o. t.i.d–q.i.d I.M. 10 mg i.m. initially, 5–10 mg 3–4 hours later • Tablet 2, 5, 10 mg • Injection 10 mg/2 mL	
Lorazepam (Ativan)	*Anxiety:* 1 mg p.o. b.i.d—t.i.d initially, then 2–6 mg daily in divided doses (range 1–10 mg daily) *Antinausea:* 0.5–2 mg p.o. q6h • Tablet 0.5, 1, 2 mg • Liquid 2 mg/mL	
Benzodiazepine receptor antagonist		
Flumazenil (Romazicon)	i.v. initial 0.2 mg i.v. over 15 sec, q 1 min • i.v. 0.5 mg/5 mL	Maximum episodic dose 1 mg, maximum hourly dose 3 mg
Antidepressants		
Amitriptyline (Elavil)	Initial therapy: 25–50 mg p.o. q.h.s. • Tablet 10, 25, 50, 75, 100, 150 mg	Maximum daily dose 300 mg daily
Fluoxetine (Prozac)	20 mg p.o. q.am • Tablet 10, 20, 60 mg	After several weeks, may increase by 20 mg daily Maximum daily dose 80 mg/d
Nortriptyline (Pamelor)	25 mg p.o. t.i.d.–q.i.d. • Tablet 10, 25, 50, 75 mg • 10 mg/5 mL	Maximum daily dose 150 mg/d

continued

Psychotropic Medications *(continued)*

Name	Initial Dose	Comments
Paroxetine (Paxil)	20 mg p.o. q a.m.; increase by 10 mg/d at weekly intervals • IR tablet 10, 20, 30, 40 mg • IR liquid 10 mg/5 mL • ER tablet 12.5, 25. 37.5 mg	Maximum daily dose 50 mg/d
Sertraline (Zoloft)	50 mg p.o. q.d.; increase by 25–50 mg weekly • Tablet 25, 50, 100 mg • Liquid 20/mL	Maximum daily dose 200 mg/d

Antipsychotics

Name	Initial Dose	Comments
Chlorpromazine hydrochloride (Thorazine)	10–50 mg p.o. t.i.d. • Tablet 10, 25, 50, 100, and 200 mg • Syrup 10 mg/5 mL	
Fluphenazine hydrochloride (Prolixin)	1 mg p.o. t.i.d.–2.5 mg p.o. q.i.d. Maintenance: 1–5 mg p.o. q.d. Debilitated: 1.0–2.5 mg p.o. Q.d. • Tablet 1, 2.5, 5, and 10 mg • Elixir 2.5 mg/5 mL	
Haloperidol (Haldol)	Moderate: 0.5–2.0 mg p.o. t.i.d. Severe: 3.0–5.0 mg p.o. t.i.d. • Tablet 0.5, 1, 2, 5, 10, and 20 mg • Liquid 2 mg/mL	
Thioridazine (Mellaril)	25 mg p.o. t.i.d.–50 mg p.o. q.i.d. Severe psychoses: 100 mg p.o. t.i.d.–200 mg p.o. q.i.d. • Tablet 10, 15, 25, 50, 100, 150, and 200 mg • Liquid 30 and 100 mg/mL	

Hypnotics and Sleep Aids

Name	Initial Dose	Comments
Diphenhydramine hydrochloride (Benadryl)	50 mg p.o. q.h.s. • Tablet 25, 50 mg • Liquid 12.5 mg/5 mL	
Estazolam (Prosom)	Initial 1 mg p.o. q.h.s. • Tablet 1, 2 mg	
Flurazepam hydrochloride (Dalmane)	Initial 15 mg elderly, 15 mg female, 15–30 mg male q.h.s • Tablet 15, 30 mg	

Psychotropic Medications *(continued)*

Name	Initial Dose	Comments
Temazepam (Restoril)	7.5–30.0 mg p.o. q.h.s. • Tablet 7.5, 15, 22.5, 30 mg	
Triazolam (Halcion)	0.25 mg p.o. q.h.s. Elderly patients: 0.125–0.25 mg p.o. q.h.s. • Tablet 0.125, 0.25 mg	
Zolpidem tartrate (Ambien)	IR 5 mg (female) 5–10 mg (male) ER 6.25 mg (female) 6.25–12.5 mg (male) • IR tablet 5, 10 mg • ER tablet 6.25, 12.5 mg	
Promethazine (Phenergan)	For nausea, p.o. i.m. i.v. rectal 12.5–25 mg q4–6h • Tablet 12.5, 25, 50 mg • Liquid 6.25 mg/5 mL • i.v. 25, 50 mg/mL • Rectal 12.5, 25, 50 mg	

Gynecologic

Name	Initial Dose	Comments
Aci-Jel therapeutic vaginal jelly	1 applicator full administered intravaginally every morning and evening	
Clonidine patch	0.1 mg/24 h patch • Patch 0.1, 0.2, 0.3 mg/24 h	
Estradiol vaginal cream 0.01% (Estrace)	*Cream*: 2–4 g daily for 1–2 wk; maintenance: 1 g 1–3 times/wk *Vaginal ring*: 2 mg p.v. 90 d *Tablet* 1 tab p.v. q.d. 2 wk, maintenance 1 tab p.v. twice weekly • Cream 1 mg/g • Ring 2 mg/ea • Tablet 10 µg	Hormone replacement; see risk warnings
Estrogen (Premarin)	0.3 mg p.o. q.d. 0.5 g p.v. q.d., 3 wk on, 1 wk off • Tablet 0.3 mg • Cream 0.625 mg/g	For vaginal atrophy, fibrosis Hormone replacement, see risk warnings

continued

Gynecologic *(continued)*

Name	Initial Dose	Comments
Megestrol acetate (Megace)	20 mg p.o. b.i.d. initially, maintenance 10 mg p.o. q.d. or q.o.d. • Tablet 20, 40 mg • Solution 40 mg/mL	
Paroxetine (Paxil, Brisdelle)	Brisdelle 7.5 mg p.o. q.h.s Paxil CR 12.5–25 mg p.o. Q.d. • Tablet 7.5, 10, 20, 30 mg	
Venlafaxine (Effexor)	37.5–150 mg p.o. q.d. • IR tablet 25, 37.5, 50, 75, 100 mg • ER tablet 37.5, 75, 150, 225 mg	

Muscle Relaxants

Name	Initial Dose	Comments
Carisoprodol (Soma)	p.o. 250, 250 mg q.i.d. • Tablet 250, 350 mg	Maximum duration 2–3 wk
Carisoprodol/aspirin (Soma Compound)	1–2 tablets p.o. q.i.d. • Tablet 200 mg carisoprodol—325 mg aspirin	Maximum daily dose 8 tablets (carisoprodol 1,600 mg, aspirin 2,600 mg) Maximum duration 2–3 wk
Carisoprodol/aspirin/codeine phosphate (Soma Compound with Codeine)	1–2 tablets p.o. q.i.d. • Tablet carisoprodol 200 mg—aspirin 325 mg—codeine 16 mg	Maximum daily dose 8 tablets (carisoprodol 1,600 mg, aspirin 2,600 mg, codeine 128 mg) Maximum duration 2–3 wk
Cyclobenzaprine hydrochloride (Flexeril)	p.o. IR 5 mg t.i.d. p.o. ER 15 mg daily May increase to 30 mg daily • Tablet IR 5, 7.5, 10 mg • Tablet ER 15, 30 mg • Liquid 1 mg/mL	Therapy should be limited to 3 wk maximum Tablet (10 mg)
Diazepam (Valium)	p.o. 2–10 mg b.i.d.–q.i.d. i.m. i.v. 2–10 mg • Tablet 2, 5, 10 mg • Liquid 1 mg/mL • i.v. 5 mg/mL	See "Anxiety" for nonmuscle relaxant application

Muscle Relaxants *(continued)*

Name	Initial Dose	Comments
Methocarbamol (Robaxin)	p.o. 1.5 g q.i.d. × 2–3 d i.m. i.v. 1 g q8h × 2–3 d • Tablet 500, 750 mg • i.v. 1,000 mg/10 mL	Maximum daily dose 3 g for 3 d; may repeat course after 48 h drug-free interval
Orphenadrine citrate (Norflex)	p.o. 100 mg b.i.d. i.m. i.v. 60 mg b.i.d. • Tablet 100 mg • i.v. 30 mg/mL	

Erectile Dysfunction

Name	Initial Dose	Comments
	Alprostadil	
Caverject	Intracavernosal injection: 2.5–60.0 mcg Initial dose 2.5 mcg, first titration upward in health care provider setting by 2.5 mg, then by 5–10 mcg increments until response achieved and not lasting more than 1 h. No more than two doses during initial titration to be within 24-h period • Vial 6–40 µg	
Muse	Urethral suppository: 125–1,000 mcg • Suppository 125, 250, 500, 1,000 mcg	Cartons containing 6 systems
Sildenafil citrate (Viagra)	50 mg (maximum recommended dose, 100 mg) • Tablet 25, 50, and 100 mg	

Cancer Therapy Hyperuricemia

Name	Initial Dose	Comments
Allopurinol (Zyloprim)	300–400 mg p.o. b.i.d. × 2–3 d, then 300 mg p.o. b.i.d. • Tablet 100, 300 mg	

CNS, central nervous system; ER, extended release; IR, immediate release; IV, intravenous; MSSA, methicillin-sensitive *Staphylococcus aureus*; OTC, over the counter; RT, radiation therapy; sub-Q, subcutaneous; UTI, urinary tract infection.
Information adapted from *Commonly prescribed medications in radiation oncology*, 10th ed. Austin, TX: Texas Oncology, Austin Midtown Radiation Oncology, 2012, with permission.

Note: Page numbers followed by f indicate figures, and page numbers followed by t indicate tables.